EXPLORING THE DIMENSIONS OF

Human Sexuality

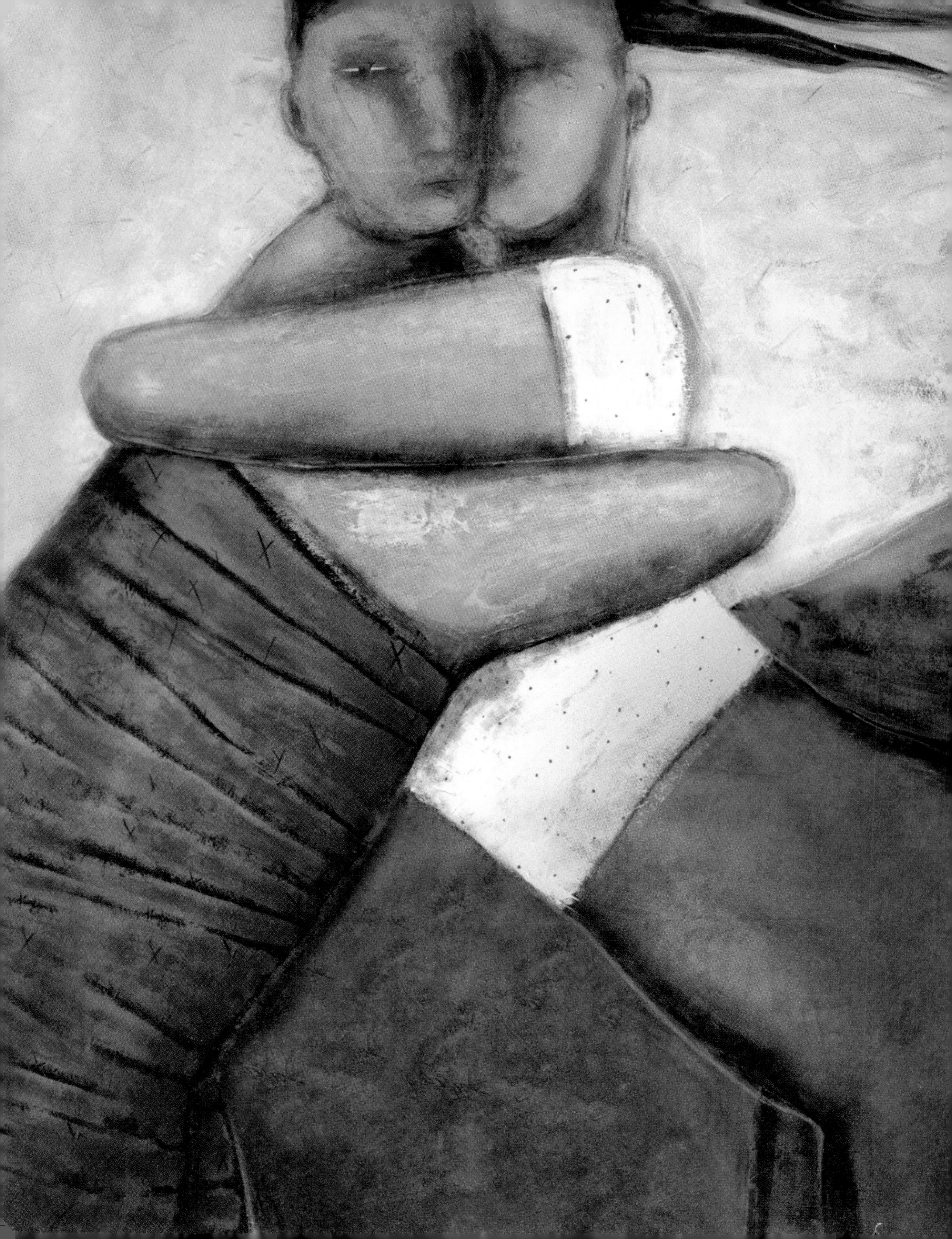

EXPLORING THE DIMENSIONS OF

Human Sexuality

SECOND EDITION

Jerrold S. Greenberg
University of Maryland

Clint E. Bruess
Birmingham-Southern College

Debra W. Haffner
Religious Institute on Sexual Morality, Justice, and Healing

JONES AND BARTLETT PUBLISHERS
Sudbury, Massachusetts
BOSTON TORONTO LONDON SINGAPORE

World Headquarters

Jones and Bartlett Publishers
40 Tall Pine Drive
Sudbury, MA 01776
978-443-5000
info@jbpub.com
www.jbpub.com

Jones and Bartlett Publishers
Canada
2406 Nikanna Road
Mississauga, ON L5C 2W6
CANADA

Jones and Bartlett Publishers
International
Barb House, Barb Mews
London W6 7PA
UK

Production Credits
Chief Executive Officer: Clayton Jones
Chief Operating Officer: Don Jones, Jr.
Executive V.P. and Publisher: Robert W. Holland
V.P., Design and Production: Anne Spencer
V.P., Manufacturing and Inventory: Therese Bräuer
V.P., Sales and Marketing: William J. Kane, Jr.
Acquisitions Editor: Jacqueline Ann Mark
Senior Production Editor: Julie C. Bolduc
Editorial Assistant: Nicole Quinn
Marketing Manager: Ed McKenna
Manufacturing Buyer: Amy Bacus
Interior Design: Anne Spencer
Illustration: Imagineering Scientific and Technical Artworks, Vincent Perez
Composition: Graphic World, Inc.
Cover Design: Kristin E. Ohlin
Cover Image: © John Nelson, Veer
Printing and Binding: Courier Kendallville
Cover Printing: Lehigh Press

Chapter 12 is adapted from Debra Haffner, *Beyond the Big Talk,* Newmarket Press, 2001, with permission from the author.

Library of Congress Cataloging-in-Publication Data

Greenberg, Jerrold S.
Exploring the dimensions of human sexuality / Jerrold S. Greenberg, Clint E. Bruess, Debra W. Haffner. — 2nd ed.
p. cm.
Includes bibliographical references and index.
ISBN 0-7637-0735-X
1. Sex. 2. Sex (Psychology) 3. Hygiene, Sexual. 4. Interpersonal relations. 5. Sexual Ethics. I. Bruess, Clint E. II. Haffner, Debra. III. Title.
HQ21.G67118 2004
306.7—dc22 2003016536

Printed in the United States of America
08 07 06 05 04 10 9 8 7 6 5 4 3 2 1

Brief Contents

Contents

Features

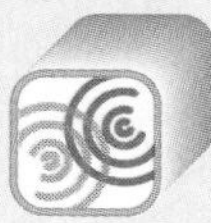

Communication Dimensions

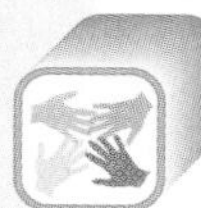

Multicultural Dimensions

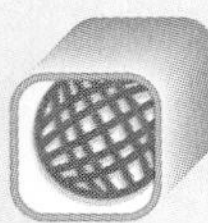

Global Dimensions

Gender Dimensions

Features

Ethical Dimensions

Preface

The authors of this book feel strongly about the importance of understanding human sexuality as part of a healthy personality. In addition, we have seen numerous positive and negative examples of what can happen when people do or do not understand how human sexuality can be related to human well-being. We have had examples of this with our own children.

Let us start with a positive example. When one of our daughters was 11 years old, she and her parent had watched a TV program about an unmarried girl who became pregnant and decided to have an abortion. The next day her parent asked her how she felt about the program — fully expecting to hear something about the daughter's views on abortion. Instead, the young girl said, "I thought it was stupid." Surprised by this response, the parent said, "Why did you think it was stupid?" The girl said, "If the girl didn't want to be pregnant, why did she get pregnant in the first place?" That is pretty good insight for an 11-year-old. The parent was pleased that the daughter seemed to have her priorities straight when it came to decisions related to causing pregnancy. There did not seem to be much reason to think that young girl would be pregnant before she made a conscious decision to do so.

When the son of one of the authors was entering fifth grade, school personnel organized a committee of parents to review instructional materials for the sexuality education course. As luck would have it, one of the authors was selected to serve on this committee. At the first committee meeting, the author was surprised to learn that the program focused exclusively on reproductive anatomy and physiology. The author asked, with an inquiring tone, "How will you help your students process their feelings regarding sexuality?" The answer was that the reproductive system would be taught just as any other body system would, rather than highlighted by including discussion of feelings associated with it. At that point the author volunteered to resign from the parent review committee and asked to join the "Digestive System Parent Review Committee." Of course, there was none. That allowed the author to point out that there really is a distinction between education regarding sexuality and education pertaining to health in general. And that this distinction needs to be addressed with students. We do that in this book by exploring the varied dimensions of human sexuality.

In many regards, human sexuality today does not differ from that of our ancestors' times. In a biological sense, human reproduction occurs the same way. Religion and culture have long played a role in our sexuality; so has public policy. However, we have noted that a greater awareness now exists of the many dimensions that shape our sexuality.

As longtime sexuality educators, we saw clearly that no one aspect of sexuality can be separated from the others, and no one aspect is more important. We have written a text that presents all aspects of sexuality as interconnected and significant. Throughout this text you will find an emphasis on health and well-being based on the assumption that we are all sexual beings and that sexuality should be viewed in its totality — with biological, spiritual, psychological, and sociocultural dimensions.

Because we realize that learning best occurs when students are actively involved, we have created a text that goes beyond merely presenting factual knowledge about the varied dimensions of human sexuality. We want students to explore the varied dimensions and see how each affects their personal sexuality.

ABOUT THE AUTHORS

Jerrold S. Greenberg, EdD, is a professor in the Department of Public and Community Health at the University of Maryland. He has authored over forty books and is the founder–manager of the Service–Learning in Health Education Interest Group and listserv. He has received many awards from professional associations including the Scholar Award from the American Association for Health Education.

Clint E. Bruess is Dean Emeritus of the School of Education and Professor Emeritus of Health Education at the University of Alabama at Birmingham. He is currently Chair of the Division of Education at Birmingham-Southern College. He has coauthored more than 15 textbooks in the areas of human sexuality, sexuality education, personal health, and school health programs. In addition, he has published numerous articles in professional journals and served in elected and appointed positions for the American School Health Association (also a Fellow), American Association for Health Education (also a Fellow), and Society of Public Health Educators.

Debra Haffner, MPH, M Div, is the Director of the Religious Institute for Sexual Morality, Justice, and Healing. She served as the President and CEO of the Sexuality Information and Education Council of the United States from 1988 to 2000. She is the author of two award-winning books for parents on educating their children about sexuality issues, and has published more than 70 articles on sexuality and sexuality education. The Reverend Haffner is an ordained Unitarian Universalist minister.

At the same time, however, this exploration is facilitated by having accurate and up-to-date knowledge. To help ensure this, the content in this text has been updated twice. It was revised for the 2002 update and again for this 2004 edition. Therefore, there is an abundance of 21st century references used throughout the text.

The dimensions discussed in the book can be broken down into biological, psychological, and sociocultural categories. Here are some examples:

Biological Dimensions

Physiology The basis of understanding sexuality is knowledge about the physiology of how our bodies work. Factual information lays the foundation of critical thinking — without the facts, you cannot begin to think critically about your sexuality. The greater your knowledge, the more likely you are to take responsibility for your sexual health.

Gender The physiological differences between genders create the foundation for the development of psychological and social wellness and strongly influence our perceptions of sexual wellness. Gender Dimensions receive a full chapter and boxed treatment in every chapter.

Psychological Dimensions

Psychology Developing a positive image of self and sexuality is critical to developing sexual wellness. For example, a positive body image lends itself to your overall wellness; a negative self-image can lead to drug abuse (steroids or diet pills) or psychological disorders (anorexia, bulimia, binge eating disorder, or muscle dysmorphia). Body image is so important that we devote a minichapter to the topic — the most comprehensive coverage in the market!

Spiritual Religious and spiritual beliefs influence feelings about sexual behavior, premarital sexual activity, adultery, divorce, contraception, abortion — even masturbation. Spiritual issues are discussed in Multicultural Dimensions boxes and in the opening chapter.

Sociocultural Dimensions

Multicultural Cultures within the United States and around the world differ in their views of sexuality. From seminude beaches in the south of France to Middle Eastern Muslim communities where women are covered from head to hand to foot, ours is a world of diversity. Sometimes these diverse behaviors are a part of the culture, and other times they are forced. We saw a vivid example of this when behaviors changed quickly in 2001 and 2002 in Afghanistan when abrupt changes occurred in who was running the country. Your ability to respect your sexual partner's cultural beliefs and feelings will result in a higher level of satisfaction for both of you. To help students better understand sexual diversity, each chapter contains one boxed example of a culture within the United States and one from elsewhere in the world.

Ethics Ethical decision making takes on legal and moral implications in the area of sexuality. The law and courts become involved in such far-flung areas as access to abortion clinics, workplace sexual harassment, and ownership of frozen embryos. Moral implications include sexual coercion and underscore the importance of taking responsibility for your sexual wellness. Ethical Dimensions boxes appear in every chapter, as well as in Chapter 18, Sexual Ethics, Morality, and the Law.

Public Policy Even public policy affects our sexual behavior! The Healthy People 2010 project attempts to use health promotion to establish acquired immune deficiency syndrome (AIDS) and sexually transmitted infection (STI) awareness, decrease unwanted teenage pregnancies, and increase the number of women who receive prenatal care. Public policy on free speech continues to allow the uncontrolled distribution of pornographic material on the Internet. Furthermore, access to proper health care, birth control, and positive sexual role models is often lacking for the poor.

Integration

Integrated Theme With so many factors influencing our sexual behavior, we have created a striking full-page feature: Exploring the Dimensions of Human Sexuality, an integrated approach that ties all these strands together. This feature helps students understand how many different aspects affect their sexual health and influence their sexual behavior. Our intent is to help students envision the convergence of the many aspects of sexuality and help them choose sexual practices that lead to a lifetime of sexual health and wellness.

Integrated Web Site Exploring the Dimensions of Human Sexuality also links to our web site (**sexuality.jbpub.com**), where each dimension is presented in greater depth. Students will be able to click on a particular dimension and find self-assessments, exercises, research links, and information that allows them to explore further their own dimensions of human sexuality. Integrating the book and web site actively engages the students in the learning process.

See the Visual Walkthrough on page xx for an example of this feature.

Pedagogy

Throughout, numerous ways of organizing content are presented to enhance student learning.

In Focus Minichapter on Body Image We offer a comprehensive look at the concept of body image in a minichapter, the first of its kind in a human sexuality text. Together in one place we discuss how body image affects self-esteem and sexuality; how the quest for a perfect body creates problems ranging from eating disorders to cosmetic surgery and steroid abuse; and how body image affects both genders. There are also three other In Focus chapters: Unexpected Pregnancy Outcomes, HIV and AIDS, and Atypical Sexual Behaviors.

The Dimensions of Human Sexuality Boxed Feature Program A carefully designed boxed feature program reinforces the dimensions theme of the textbook with five distinct boxes in each chapter: Multicultural Dimensions, Global Dimensions, Gender Dimensions, Communication Dimensions, and Ethical Dimensions. *Please refer to page xx of the Visual Walkthrough for detailed descriptions of these features.*

Critical Thinking Exploring the dimensions of human sexuality requires students to think critically about how the multifaceted dimensions relate to them. To that end, we have embedded the text with critical thinking questions to help students reflect on the subject matter and understand its implications for their sexual health. Critical thinking questions are found in boxes, in photo captions, and in the end-of-chapter section — including application questions related to the chapter-opening story, critical thinking questions about material, and a critical thinking minicase. Critical thinking questions help students recall information and synthesize new material with existing knowledge and stimulate students to make informed judgments about the information provided.

Myth vs. Fact and Did You Know . . . Boxes Students' sexual health and wellness are also influenced by sexual myths and folklore. Many of our brief sidebars are designed to set students straight on such myths. Did You Know . . . boxes add whimsical and high-interest information to engage the student further.

Chapter-Opening Story Each chapter opens with an engaging real-life story that explores the concepts to be discussed in the chapter. Students are drawn into the chapter material with a high-interest case and introduced to the topics that will be discussed. At the end of the chapter, students are asked to relate the chapter's information to application questions about the opening story.

Reviewing the Dimensions of Human Sexuality Each chapter ends with an interactive feature designed to help students take responsibility for their sexual health and wellness. Reviewing the Dimensions of Human Sexuality includes an interactive self-assessment designed to help students understand and clarify their own feelings about sexuality issues presented in that chapter. It also includes discussion questions, application questions pertaining to the opening story, critical thinking questions, a critical thinking minicase, and a self-assessment.

Changes in the New Edition Throughout this new edition, extensive updates have been made to focus on information and statistics of recent developments. This includes an in-depth discussion of new contraceptive methods such as the contraceptive patch, NuvaRing, male contraceptive implants, Implanon, Jadelle, Lea's shield, and Essure. There is an expanded section on hepatitis B, a presentation on sexual abuse and the church, and a discussion of sexual orientation in the context of sports and other social institutions. Also covered is the latest research pertaining to hormone replacement therapy and the issues related to HRT, as well as an in-depth discussion of sexual disabilities.

An Introduction to Service–Learning Appendix We recognize the responsibility our readers have for the sexual health of the communities in which they live and study. Although we are all rightfully concerned with our own sexual health and well-being, we must also recognize our responsibility to take action to contribute to the sexual health of the communities in which we reside. One way in which we encourage this action is by including the Introduction to Service–Learning appendix at the conclusion of the text. The activities suggested here employ a service–learning methodology: That is, readers provide service while learning chapter content. This feature represents a unique approach to sexual responsibility and does not appear in other sexuality texts.

Writing this book has, itself, been a service–learning activity for us. We did abundant and thorough research to identify state-of-the-art knowledge and attitudes pertaining to sexuality and learned a great deal in doing so. That was the learning part of the service–learning equation. The service part relates to our interest in helping to enhance the sexual health and wellness of our readers. As such, we hope you find the information we included, the issues we raised and discussed, and the myths we debunked useful as you live and express your sexuality. If that is the case, the time, effort, and energy we have devoted to writing this text will have been well worth that investment.

Acknowledgments

First of all, we would like to thank the many reviewers who guided us throughout the many stages of this project. Their voice, criticism, and support have truly made this a better text.

We would also like to thank members of the Jones and Bartlett Health team for their work on the text and its supplements, as well as Dr. Sue Tendy, Ed.D. of the United States Military Academy at West Point for revising the material on Sexual Harassment in the Military; Stephanie Chisolm of James Madison University for updating the Instructor's Manual, PowerPoints, and web material; and Michael Maina of Valdosta State University for updating the Test Bank.

I would like to thank my family; Karen, Todd, Keri, and my mother, Bess Greenberg, for their encouragement and support.

Jerrold Greenberg
Department of Public and Community Health
University of Maryland

To Susan J. Laing with appreciation for her part in a wonderful relationship.

Clint Bruess
Division of Education
Birmingham-Southern College

I would like to thank my family; Ralph Tartaglione, Alyssa Haffner Tartaglione, and Gregory Haffner Tartaglione, for their support, as well as the parents, children, and teenagers who have shared their stories with me.

Debra W. Haffner
Religious Institute on Sexual Morality, Justice, and Healing

REVIEWERS

Veanne N. Anderson
Indiana State University
Betsy Bergen
Kansas State University
Charles Chase
West Texas A&M University
Susan Clark
Ball State University
Judy Drolet
Southern Illinois University, Carbondale
Lyndall Ellingson
California State University, Chico
Nora Few
University of Illinois at Urbana-Champaign
Patricia Goodson
University of Texas at San Antonio
Anthony Parrillo
East Carolina University
Miguel Perez
University of North Texas
Catherine Sherwood-Puzzello
Indiana University
Stanley Snegroff
Adelphi University
Susan Sprecher
Illinois State University
Richard Stacy
University of Nebraska at Omaha
Susan Tendy
United States Military Academy, West Point
Maria Theresa Wessel
James Madison University
Susan Woods
Eastern Illinois University
Donna Videto
SUNY College at Cortland
Emilia Patricia Zarco
University of the Philippines

Features of Exploring the DIMENSIONS of Human Sexuality, Second Edition

A Visual Walkthrough

Exploring the Dimensions of Human Sexuality, Second Edition is designed around the central theme that our feelings, attitudes, and beliefs regarding sexuality are continually influenced by our internal and external environments. All aspects of sexuality—biological, spiritual, psychological, and sociocultural—are interconnected and significant. The boxed feature program, additional pedagogy, and ancillaries of this new textbook have been designed around these core concepts.

BOXED FEATURES

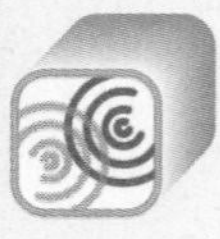

Communication Dimensions

These boxes discuss communication issues that arise around sexuality between the genders, partners from different ethnic groups, and others.

Multicultural Dimensions

To better appreciate how various people view sexuality we offer a multicultural boxed feature. These boxes deal exclusively with diversity issues within the United States.

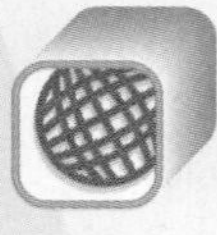

Global Dimensions

Sexuality is viewed very differently outside of the United States. Issues such as divorce in China and international differences in discussing sexuality are discussed in the Global Dimensions boxes.

Gender Dimensions

Issues arising from gender are integrated throughout the text, discussed in detail in the Gender Dimensions chapter, and featured in the Gender Dimensions boxes found in each chapter. Topics covered in these boxes include communication breakdown between genders, responsibility for contraception, and many others.

Ethical Dimensions

The importance of ethics in sexuality is underscored in the Ethical Dimensions box features. This is where topics such as abstinence-only education and the ethics surrounding technological advances are discussed.

Pedagogical Design

Chapter-Opening Pedagogy Each chapter-opening spread gives the reader a glimpse of what is to come with chapter objectives, a list of the Dimensions of Human Sexuality boxed features that will follow, and a list of topics also explored on the companion web site. In addition, a high-interest and engaging real-life story draws students into the chapter material and introduces them to the topics that will be discussed. This opening story is revisited at the end of the chapter in the application questions.

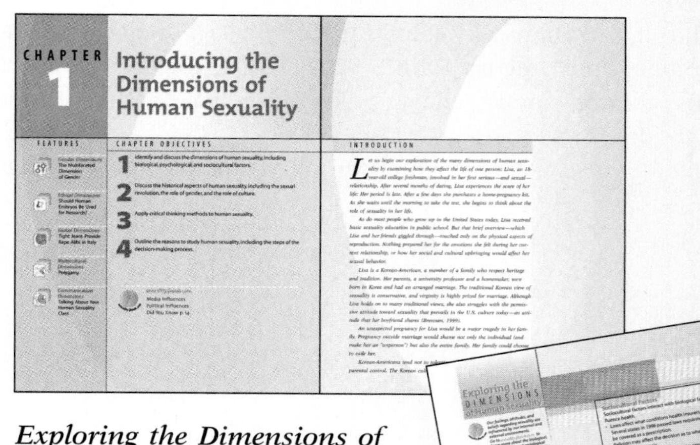

CHAPTER 1

Introducing the Dimensions of Human Sexuality

FEATURES

CHAPTER OBJECTIVES

INTRODUCTION

Exploring the Dimensions of Human Sexuality This feature organizes the multifaceted issues in each chapter into biological, psychological, and sociocultural factors. This visual element is integrated with the companion web site where instructors and students can further explore these dimensions.

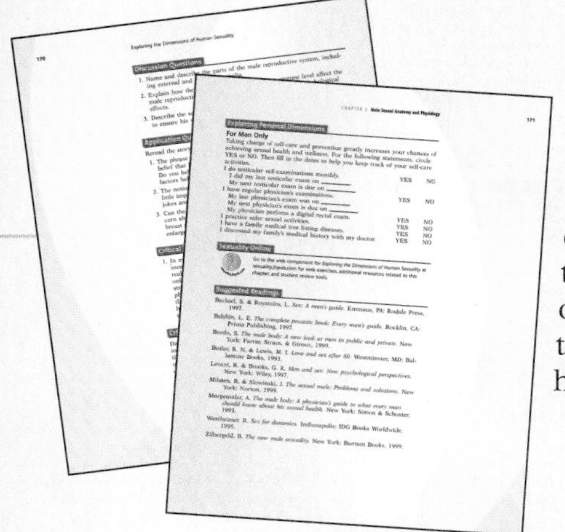

Reviewing the Dimensions of Human Sexuality This end-of-chapter activity gives students the opportunity to review and apply key chapter concepts. Items in this section include discussion questions, critical thinking questions, and application questions that relate to the chapter-opening story. The Exploring Personal Dimensions section directs students to focus on personal choices and take responsibility for their sexual health and well-being.

Teaching and Learning Aids

Exploring the Dimensions of Human Sexuality Online The companion web site is integrated with the Exploring the Dimensions of Human Sexuality feature found in each main chapter of the text and offers four central components:

- Content links to give the instructor the ability to integrate the web into the curriculum.
- Student activities such as web exercises and self-assessments involve students in the dimensions of human sexuality in a structured online environment.
- Online student study tools offer students the opportunity to review chapter concepts and prepare for anatomical review, practice, quizzes, flashcards, and crossword puzzles.
- Reference links offer lists of references related to chapter content.

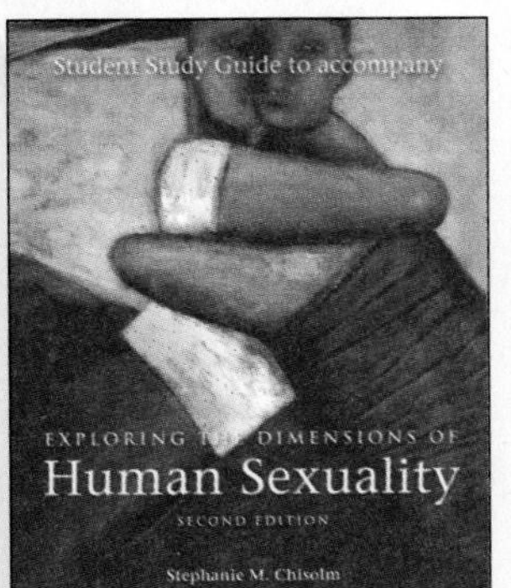

This workbook and note-taking guide is the perfect learning companion for students.

Visit sexuality.jbpub.com

Instructor's ToolKit CD-ROM offers the instructor maximum flexibility in preparing for class, designing and presenting lectures, and generating tests. The ToolKit features an instructor's manual, PowerPoint lecture presentations, an image bank, a table bank, and a computerized test bank. Content can be implemented into many of the common distance learning programs. (Available for both PC and Macintosh.)

SPECIAL FEATURES

Myth vs. Fact Students' sexual health and wellness are influenced by sexual myths and folklore. Myth vs. Fact features common myths associated with the material presented in each chapter along with the fact to dispel each myth.

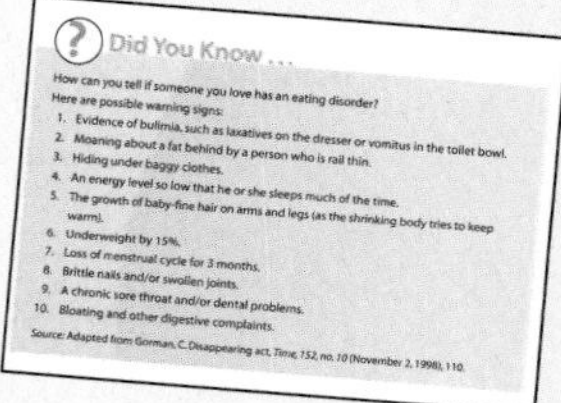
Myth vs Fact

Myth: Being assertive means standing up for your basic rights at the expense of someone else's rights.
Fact: Being aggressive is standing up for your basic rights at the expense of someone else's. Being assertive means standing up for your

Brief **Did You Know. . .** sidebars add whimsical and high-interest information to further engage the student.

In Focus Minichapters The authors have included focused minichapters which delve into topics that affect student's lives. These take a fully comprehensive look at subjects such as body image, unexpected pregnancy, HIV & AIDS, and atypical sexual behaviors. The concentrated chapters offer today's students a deeper understanding of issues about which they should be informed.

Service–Learning Appendix Although we are all rightfully concerned with our own sexual health and well-being, the authors encourage readers to also recognize the responsibility to contribute to the sexual health of the communities in which they reside. An Introduction to Service–Learning appendix at the end of the text gives an overview of the concept of service–learning and suggests specific activities through which the reader can contribute to their community's sexual health. These activities employ a service–learning methodology; that is, students provide service while learning chapter content at the same time.

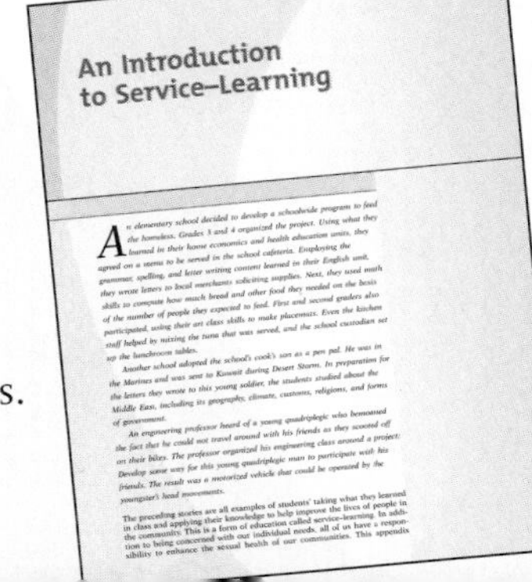
An Introduction to Service–Learning

CHAPTER 1

Introducing the Dimensions of Human Sexuality

FEATURES

Gender Dimensions
The Multifaceted Dimension of Gender

Ethical Dimensions
Should Human Embryos Be Used for Research?

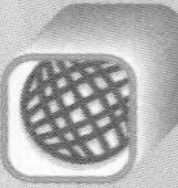

Global Dimensions
Tight Jeans Provide Rape Alibi in Italy

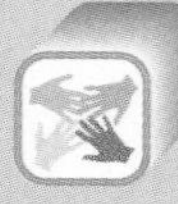

Multicultural Dimensions
Polygamy

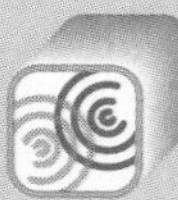

Communication Dimensions
Talking About Your Human Sexuality Class

CHAPTER OBJECTIVES

1. Identify and discuss the dimensions of human sexuality, including biological, psychological, and sociocultural factors.
2. Discuss the historical aspects of human sexuality, including the sexual revolution, the role of gender, and the role of culture.
3. Apply critical thinking methods to human sexuality.
4. Outline the reasons to study human sexuality, including the steps of the decision-making process.

sexuality.jbpub.com
Media Influences
Political Influences
Did You Know

INTRODUCTION

Let us begin our exploration of the many dimensions of human sexuality by examining how they affect the life of one person: Lisa, an 18-year-old college freshman, involved in her first serious—and sexual—relationship. After several months of dating, Lisa experiences the scare of her life: Her period is late. After a few days she purchases a home-pregnancy kit. As she waits until the morning to take the test, she begins to think about the role of sexuality in her life.

As do most people who grow up in the United States today, Lisa received basic sexuality education in public school. But that brief overview—which Lisa and her friends giggled through—touched only on the physical aspects of reproduction. Nothing prepared her for the emotions she felt during her current relationship, or how her social and cultural upbringing would affect her sexual behavior.

Lisa is a Korean-American, a member of a family who respect heritage and tradition. Her parents, a university professor and a homemaker, were born in Korea and had an arranged marriage. The traditional Korean view of sexuality is conservative, and virginity is highly prized for marriage. Although Lisa holds on to many traditional views, she also struggles with the permissive attitude toward sexuality that prevails in the U.S. culture today—an attitude that her boyfriend shares (Brennan, 1999).

An unexpected pregnancy for Lisa would be a major tragedy in her family. Pregnancy outside marriage would shame not only the individual (and make her an "unperson") but also the entire family. Her family could choose to exile her.

Korean-Americans tend not to tolerate secrecy by children and exert strict parental control. The Korean culture discourages open discussion of feelings and seeking out of psychological counseling. Thus, Lisa is in a crisis because she feels she cannot tell her parents, but she also cannot tell anyone else (who may in turn tell her parents). In fact, Lisa has yet to tell her boyfriend what is upsetting her.

Religion plays a major role in many people's sexuality. For Lisa's parents, whose cultural traditions in Korea can be traced to Confucianism, abortion may be a possibility (as a means of saving face for the family). But many Korean-American immigrants are members of fundamentalist Christian groups, who often prohibit abortion. Lisa wonders what she will do if, in fact, she is really pregnant.

Lisa is lucky: She is not pregnant. But Lisa has realized that she has to start taking greater responsibility for her sexual behavior. How can she incorporate the many dimensions affecting her sexuality into her personal sexuality?

This chapter begins our exploration of the many dimensions of sexuality and how they affect our lives.

The Dimensions of Human Sexuality

human sexuality
A part of your total personality. It involves the interrelationship of biological, psychological, and sociocultural dimensions.

essentialism
Belief that once the cultural and historical aspects are taken away, the essence of sexuality is biological.

When you think about human sexuality, what do you think of? Some form of physical contact? Human reproduction? Feelings when you see an attractive person? Human sexuality is all that and more. **Human sexuality** is a part of your total personality. It involves the interrelationship of biological, psychological, and sociocultural dimensions.

The Sexuality Information and Education Council of the United States (SIECUS) defines *human sexuality* as encompassing the sexual knowledge, beliefs, attitudes, values, and behaviors of individuals. Its various dimensions include the anatomy, physiology, and biochemistry of the sexual response system; identity, orientation, roles, and personality; and thoughts, feelings, and relationships. The expression of sexuality is influenced by ethical, spiritual, cultural, and moral concerns (SIECUS, 1995).

The Alberta Society for the Promotion of Sexual Health (ASPSH) indicates that sexuality means many things: feelings about ourselves, roles we play in society, and reproduction. It is not limited to how we behave sexually. It is the total of our physical, emotional, and spiritual responses, thoughts, and feelings. Sexuality is more about who we are than about what we do (ASPSH, 2003).

Sexuality is a natural part of life. The concepts of human sexuality are learned. From our viewpoint, human sexuality involves at least three dimensions—biological, psychological, and sociocultural. Each dimension has many subdimensions. The interactive relationship of these dimensions describes an individual's total sexuality.

The Interactive Nature of Sexual Dimensions

A complex set of biological, psychological, and sociocultural variables plays a role in all our sexual interactions. The decision to be sexually active is a result of many factors. Sexual arousal is a physiological function. Psychologically, our body image and feelings of self-worth may inhibit getting involved ("I'm not good enough for her"; "I'm not attractive enough for him"). A lack of self-worth may also inhibit arousal. Our culture helps us develop a sense of what is attractive—height, weight, hair style, skin tone. In addition, religious beliefs affect our sexual undertakings, as do legal and ethical considerations. Role models set by family and friends influence us as well.

All these dimensions constantly interact and influence our sexuality. Although we discuss them separately for clarity, remember that almost all decisions related to sexuality we make are influenced by more than one dimension.

Biological Dimension

The basis of understanding sexuality is physiological knowledge about how our bodies work. Factual information lays the foundation of decision making—without the facts, you cannot begin to think critically about your sexuality. The greater your knowledge, the more likely you are to take responsibility for your sexual health.

Until relatively recently, most of the research into human sexuality focused on physiology. For example, a model of the human sexual response cycle, published by the well-known researchers Masters and Johnson in 1966, focused mainly on physiology.

Fisher (1992) emphasizes the genetic aspects of behavior. In her view, humans have a common nature, a set of unconscious tendencies that are encoded in our genes. She believes that although we are not aware of these predispositions, they still motivate our actions. Although she recognizes that culture plays a role in one's sexuality, she also seems to support **essentialism,** the belief that the essence of sexuality is biological.

Gender DIMENSIONS

The Multifaceted Dimension of Gender

The first words our parents heard after we emerged from the womb declared our biological gender: "It's a boy!" or "It's a girl!" Our parents bought crib sheets and clothes that were pink or blue to match our gender. As children, we heard Mr. Rogers sing to us, "Boys are special on the outside, / Girls are special on the inside."

We soon learned the sociocultural meanings of gender: Boys and girls are socialized to play in different styles and usually learn to prefer different sets of toys. Our moms and/or dads tended to do gender-specific chores. Teenage boys are somehow allowed to be sexually active, whereas girls are discouraged from such activities (a concept known as the "double standard").

Psychologically, girls are encouraged to show their emotions, whereas boys learn to suppress emotions. This leads to differing communication styles as well: Females are generally more expressive verbally than males. (Of course, there are many expressive men and inexpressive females. Remember that Lisa in our opening story has been culturally socialized to suppress open discussion of feelings.)

Socially, there are many gender inequalities that will be covered in detail throughout this text. In the workplace, a woman earns 83 cents for every dollar a man earns (a concept known as the "wage gap") and faces a tougher time getting promoted into upper management (a concept known as the "glass ceiling"). After a woman goes home from work, she does more household chores (known as the "second shift") than her spouse.

Why are such topics covered in a human sexuality course? Because our gender—who we are as men and women and how we experience ourselves as male and female—is an essential component of our sexuality.

Research into sexual dysfunction has relied, until relatively recently, on psychological therapy. Erectile disorder (the inability to achieve erection), for example, was long believed to be mostly psychological in nature. However, it is now clear that 70–80% of cases are biological (physiological) in nature (Crenshaw, 1984; Nidus Information Service, 1998; Stipp, 1987), and wonder drugs such as sildenafil citrate (Viagra) are able to help men overcome erectile disorder.

Our physiological state affects sexuality; thus, a person who has a spinal-cord injury may experience sexual pleasure in a manner different from that experienced by many other people. Also, as we age, physical, hormonal, neural, and vascular changes can affect sexual functioning and behavior (Sanders, 1999).

The physiological differences between the sexes help to lay the groundwork for the development of psychological and social wellness, and our gender strongly influences our perceptions of sexual wellness. For example, the sexual double standard, in which men are expected to be promiscuous and women are not, is a belief held by many people in the United States. In our human sexuality classes we always ask students to complete the sentences "A man who carries a condom in his wallet is ______" and "A woman who carries a condom in her purse is ______." The man is routinely described as "responsible," the woman as "a slut."

Psychological Dimensions

Although sexual activity is definitely physical, it also involves psychology—our sense of being. The noted sexual therapist Dr. Ruth Westheimer has a favorite saying, that sexual behavior "is all between the ears."

A major psychological factor that affects our sexual wellness is body image. A positive body image lends itself to a feeling of overall wellness; a negative self-image can lead to drug abuse (use of steroids or diet pills) or psychological disorders (anorexia, bulimia, binge eating disorder, or muscle dysmorphia). Body image is so important that we have devoted a minichapter to the topic (In Focus: Body Image).

The introduction of the drug Viagra caused more than physiological changes for some of the 30 million U.S. men who suffer from erectile disorder. For instance, men with erectile disorder are often depressed; however, Viagra may restore their interest in sexual activity because it causes the fear of failure to evaporate. The renewed confidence may enhance the frequency of sexual relations (Renshaw, 1999).

Men are not alone in benefiting from Viagra: Women who have tried it have reported enhanced sexual feelings. Some people believe this enhancement to be a placebo effect but also point out that it indicates that women wish they had a similar pill (Renshaw, 1999). Older women, however, may not be happy about their husband's sudden and frequent requests for intercourse. Of course, they may also feel relieved to know that their partner's disorder was physiological and not the result of their inability to arouse him (Sanders, 1999).

Sociocultural Dimensions

social constructionism
The belief that sexual identities are acquired from and influenced and modified by an ever-changing social environment.

The biological and psychological components of sexuality are affected by society and culture. The sociocultural dimension of sexuality is the sum of the cultural and social influences that affect our thoughts and actions.

In contrast to a perception of sexuality's being controlled mainly by biological or genetic characteristics, Tiefer (1995) promotes the idea of **social constructionism,** which proposes that sexual identities and experiences are acquired from and influenced and modified by an ever-changing social environment. According to social constructionists, people acquire and assemble meanings, skills, and values from the people around them. From birth onward, we receive signals from all around us telling us how to think and act. For instance, we may learn how people of our gender should behave, that some words are "wrong" or "dirty," that certain parts of our bodies are untouchable and unmentionable (at least in certain circumstances), and that we should hide our feelings if we think they are unacceptable to others.

Indeed, we are surrounded by social influences on our sexuality. Among the sources of influence are religion, multiculturalism, socioeconomic status, ethics, the media, and politics. We will look at each influence here briefly and will revisit them throughout the text.

Myth vs Fact

Myth: Human sexuality relates mainly to biological functioning.
Fact: Human sexuality includes a biological dimension but also includes psychological and sociocultural dimensions.

Myth: Most people are well informed about human sexuality.
Fact: Unfortunately, most people still have relatively poor knowledge of sexuality. Therefore, many myths about human sexuality still exist.

Myth: Sexual "normality" is similar among various cultures.
Fact: Sexual attitudes and behaviors differ greatly among cultural groups. There is no set standard for "normality."

Religious Influences

Religious and spiritual beliefs influence feelings about morality, sexual behavior, premarital sexual behavior, adultery, divorce, contraception, abortion, and masturbation.

A comprehensive survey of college freshmen—taken annually since 1966 by the UCLA Higher Education Research Institute—finds that young adults are looking for a return to religious or more traditional moral values after the legacy left by the 1980s and the baby boomers.

In 1999 only 40% of freshmen agreed that it is OK for two people who like each other to have sexual intercourse, even if they have known each other for only a short time. In 2001, this number increased only slightly, to 41.8%, and in 2002 it was 42.2%. This represents lower support than previously for casual sexual behavior among the entering class—down from an all-time high of 52% in 1987. Interestingly, in 2002 this idea was supported by 55.2% of males and only 31.7% of females. Only half of 1999's freshman class backed efforts to keep abortion legal. This was after a record low figure after 6 years of decline, but in 2001 the proportion increased to 53.9%, and in 2002 it was 55%. In 2002 the number supporting this attitude was about equal for males and females. Support for laws protecting abortion peaked in 1990 at 65% (Characteristics of freshmen, 2001; The nation: Attitudes and characteristics of freshmen; Srinivasan, 1999, 2002).

In 2003 the percentage of freshmen supporting the legal right of gay couples to marry grew to 59.3%, up from 57.9% the year before. A record low percentage of students—24.8%—said they supported laws prohibiting gay relationships. The percentage who believed married women should confine their activities to the home and family remained at the 2002 15-year low of 21.5% (Rooney, 2003).

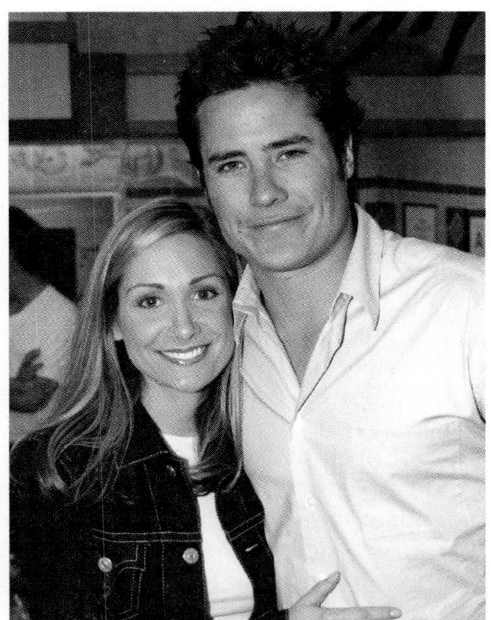

Romance reality shows have been successful with television viewers. With so many people looking for love, networks have no shortage of candidates, but it remains to be seen whether real romance can blossom in front of the camera. Do you watch romance reality shows? Why do you think society has embraced them? Do you think it's healthy to make a game out of love?

Religion plays a major role in many people's sexuality, including Lisa from the opening story. For Lisa's parents, whose cultural traditions in Korea can be traced to Confucianism, abortion might have been a possibility (as a means of saving face for the family).

Religion can also play a role in use or nonuse of medical services related to sexuality. For example, in 2001 the nation's Roman Catholic bishops voted 209–7 to prohibit

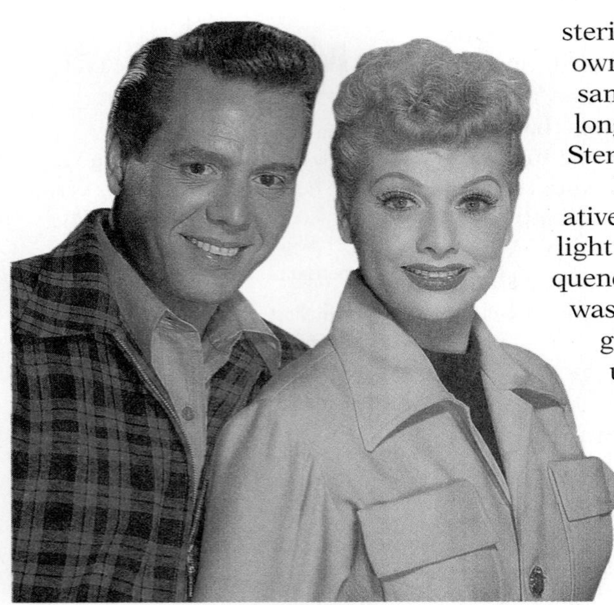
In its infancy, television was reluctant to show a biracial couple. When Lucille Ball and Desi Arnaz proposed the *I Love Lucy* show in the early 1950s, television executives wanted a white actor to play opposite Lucy, fearing problems of showing a white-and-Latino couple. Lucy and Desi were forced to put up $5,000 of their own money to create a pilot, which was, of course, a success.

sterilizations at Catholic hospitals or at non-Catholic hospitals owned by the Catholic church. This policy put sterilization on the same footing with abortion and euthanasia, both of which have long been condemned by the Catholic church (Catholic bishops: Sterilization evil, 2001).

Religiosity (an intense religious belief) has been found to be negatively correlated with number of sexual partners, the frequency of light and heavy petting, extensiveness of sexual experiences, frequency of thinking about sexuality, and ideal frequency of coitus. It was positively correlated with age at first intercourse. Highly religious males had a tendency to reverse the usual sequence of sexual behaviors—they often had oral sexual experience before intercourse. This was probably because of a strong emphasis on the male's obtaining sexual experience but also a prohibition of intercourse outside marriage (Mahoney, 1980).

Religiosity, measured by church attendance, has also been negatively related to premarital sexual permissiveness standards for both men and women. Men and women who had strong religious interest and attended church frequently were less sexually active. People with relatively conservative sexual standards were also likely to have close friends with similar standards (Sack, Keller, & Hinkle, 1984).

Religious beliefs have been shown to influence sexual attitudes and behavior in other ways as well. For example, couples who attend religious services regularly report high rates of marital satisfaction (Wilson & Filsinger, 1986). We do not know, however, whether attending religious services stabilizes marriages or whether people who attend religious services regularly are more stable and committed to marriage in the first place.

Laumann and associates (1994) found additional relationships between religiosity and sexual behavior. They found that conservative religious beliefs may restrain sexual experience. Those who reported no religion or more liberal religious beliefs reported a higher number of sexual partners than those who reported more conservative religious beliefs. Also, they found that religion seems to restrain oral sexual activity. About 34% of the men and 36% of the women in the study who said they had no religion reported having engaged in oral sexual activity at some time in their lives, but for Christians the percentages varied from the midteens to the lower 20s for females and from the lower to upper 20s for males.

Multicultural Influences

Cultures within the United States differ in their views of sexuality. Your ability to respect your sexual partner's cultural beliefs and feelings will result in a higher level of satisfaction for both of you.

First we must distinguish between ethnic background and ethnicity. A person's ethnic background is usually determined by birth and is related to country of origin, native language, race, and religion. **Ethnicity** refers to the degree of identification an individual feels with a particular ethnic group (Harrell & Frazier, 1999).

ethnicity
The degree of identification an individual feels with a particular ethnic group.

Our opening story underscores this concept. Had Lisa been pregnant, she would have found herself torn between her parents' strong ethnicity and the individual cultural beliefs and practices that she learned in school and college. Such excruciating cultural conflicts would place some people in Lisa's position at high risk for depression, even suicide (Brennan, 1999).

Cultural influences from citizens of other countries also play a dramatic role in U.S. culture. This is especially important for college students in the United States, since 1 in 10 students is from another country. These students' local cultural understandings of the body, health, and morality shape their use of contraceptive methods and abortion. For example, in the United States, abortion is not viewed as a method of contraception. In contrast, Russians tend to view abortion as a primary means of birth control; many Russian women have four or five abortions (Caron, 1998).

In Greece, where policies of both church and state frown on most medical contraceptive alternatives, abortion is estimated to have been responsible for almost half of the sharp postwar decline in the Greek birth rate—despite its illegality until 1980. Even after the legalization of abortion, female contraceptive methods continue to be rejected by the great majority of Greek women. Abortion and male barrier methods continue to be the primary means of fertility control (Georges, 1996).

In Ireland, however, abortion is still illegal unless the mother's life is at risk. It is estimated that about 4,500 Irish women travel to other countries for abortions each year (Caron, 1998).

Another example of a cultural influence are the governmental policies of the People's Republic of China to limit reproduction. The government has aggressive birth-control programs and emphasizes the necessity of the one-child family. People who limit their family to one child receive incentives, such as a monthly subsidy and free education for their child. There are even reports that the government forces some women to have abortions or become sterilized. In addition, those who do not follow these policies may lose their jobs and be publicly ostracized (Beck, Rohter, & Friday, 1984; Chen & Kols, 1982; Personal correspondence, 1998).

In 2001, Turkey's health minister announced that high school girls training to be nurses must be virgins. He also said that the virginity test he was authorizing would protect the nation's youth from prostitution and underage sexual intercourse. The regulations allow principals in state schools that train nurses, midwives, and other health workers to expel girls who have had sexual intercourse. Virginity is highly valued in mainly Muslim Turkey. Forced virginity tests were common until the practice was banned in 1999 after five girls took rat poison rather than submit to the test. However, in 2001 the health minister again authorized use of virginity tests (Turkey says only virgins can be nurses, 2001).

A look at cultural influences on sexuality would not be complete without consideration of Sweden. Nearly everyone has heard something about Sweden when it comes to sexuality. Like the United States, Sweden is highly industrialized and modern. Sexual behaviors in Sweden are much like ours, but meanings might be quite different. A certain degree of permissiveness in thinking about sexuality seems to be prevalent. In Sweden teenagers are more likely to know about sexuality, including contraception. Abortion is available and subsidized by the government for the first 18 weeks of pregnancy. Families, schools, and medical networks are supportive when it comes to sexuality, and parents are likely to know

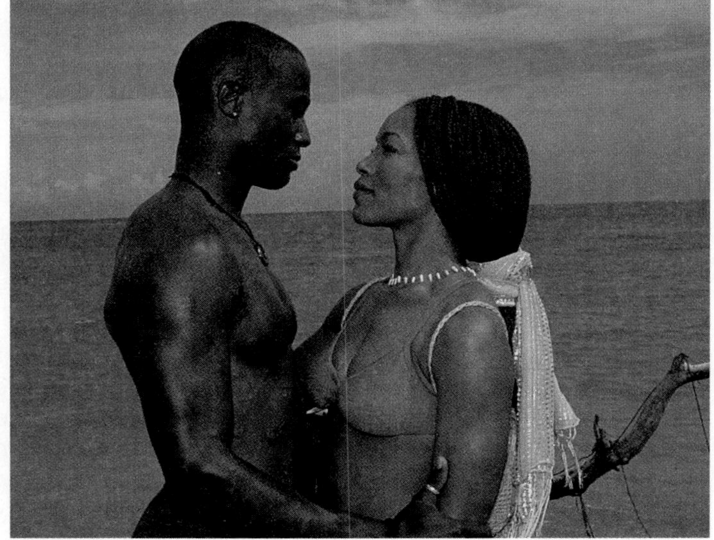

The movie *How Stella Got Her Groove Back* received flack over one line about the prevalence of AIDS in Jamaica. The offending line was deleted when the movie was released on home video in 1999. Such sensitivity to diversity is becoming more commonplace in almost all media.

about their children's sexual activities. Interestingly, these attitudes and practices consistently result in lower rates of teen pregnancy and overall rates of sexually transmitted infections (STIs), including human immunodeficiency virus/acquired immunodeficiency syndrome (HIV/AIDS), than commonly found in the United States (Caron, 1998).

Socioeconomic Influences

Socioeconomic status and education also influence sexual attitudes and behaviors, at least within the same ethnic group. Low-income individuals often think and act differently than middle-class individuals. People with low socioeconomic status may be more likely to engage in sexual intercourse at an earlier age and to have children outside marriage. In this case, it is possible that sexual activity may be a means of obtaining status and not necessarily a means of showing intimacy (Michael, et al., 1994).

Educational levels are also indicators of sexual behavior. For whatever reason, people with more education masturbate more than do less-educated persons (Michael, et al., 1994). Further, education may be a liberalizing influence. People with at least some college education tend to have more sexual partners than those who did not attend college.

Socioeconomic status influences more than just sexual activities. The poor have less access to proper health care, birth control, care during pregnancy, day care for children, and positive sexual role models.

Lisa, from our opening story, is affected by her family's high socioeconomic status. The prevailing indicator of success among second-generation Korean-Americans is high academic achievement at prestigious universities, followed by pursuit of professional careers. Lisa's academic performance to this point has reflected this cultural value. An unexpected and unwanted pregnancy creates a major obstacle to achieving the expected success and thus creates an added intergenerational cultural conflict (Brennan, 1999).

Ethical Influences

The ethics of sexuality involves questioning the way we treat ourselves and other people. Examples of sexually oriented ethical dilemmas include the following:

- Should I or should I not participate in a certain sexual behavior?
- Is it ethical to use a prostitute?
- Is it ethical not to disclose my full sexual history to a new partner?
- Is it ethical to engage in sexual behaviors with a person who is underage?
- Is it ethical to use a position of power to obtain sexual partners?

Ethical issues are not necessarily the same as legal concerns. For example, prostitution is illegal in the United States except in a few counties in Nevada. However, the ethical question of prostitution would look at the morality of hiring a prostitute—who may be selling her body as a last resort to survive. Also, the age of maturity in your state (the age at which you are deemed legally of age to engage in sexual activity) is probably 16 or 17 years old. Thus, it would be illegal to have a sexual partner below that age. However, in Tokyo, Japan, the legal age for girls is 12 years. Is it ethical for you to have a sexual partner who is of age in the country you are visiting, even if she is very young?

How we consider such questions and ultimately decide what is right and wrong profoundly shapes our sexuality. Ethical decision making underscores

Ethical DIMENSIONS

Should Human Embryos Be Used for Research?

In May 1999, the National Bioethics Advisory Commission released a draft report suggesting that Congress should lift a part of its ban on federal spending for embryonic research. The commission, which was President Clinton's top advisory panel on medical ethics, said the research showed such promise for the betterment of mankind that it merited the recommendations.

The commission specifically recommended allowing controlled experiments to obtain so-called stem cells from embryos left over from "procedures" (namely, abortions) at fertility clinics. Stem cells have been shown in recent years to be building blocks for almost all human tissue. Scientists believe the cells' capability to grow into virtually any tissue raises the possibility of growing spare body parts or correcting disorders such as Parkinson's disease or diabetes.

But not everyone agrees. The proposal of government-funded embryonic research raised outrage among prolife groups. Because embryos are destroyed in the process of harvesting stem cells, such research raised an emotional debate in Congress and elsewhere—between people on both sides of the abortion question. At least 75 members of Congress said all stem cell research violates the federal research ban, which has been extended annually since its enactment in 1994.

Janet Parshall, the chief spokeswoman for the Family Research Council, criticized the recommendation. "I think it's the worst kind of utilitarianism . . . to say we will destroy these so those can live," she said. "One would only hope that common sense and compassion would rule the day rather than scientific advancement."

Committee members agreed that women should not be allowed to terminate a pregnancy to donate the fetal material for research. In discussing a possible abortion, the possibility of research on the aborted material should not be mentioned by the physician unless asked. A fetus would only be used with the consent of the parents.

This ethical issue was taken a step further in August 2001, when President Bush decided to allow stem cell research to proceed, but very carefully. By allowing federal funding for research only on stem cells that had already been harvested, he could argue that he upheld his campaign promise not to promote research that requires destroying embryos and at the same time allowed funding for some research (Gibbs & Duffy, 2001).

Sources: Sanders, A. L. Presidential panel set to ok embryo research, *Time online,* May 24, 1999; Associated Press, Bioethics panel urges embryo study, *AP Wire Service Online,* May 24, 1999; Mann, W. C. Top advisors see medical applications for embryos, *ABCNews.com,* May 24, 1999.

the importance of taking responsibility for your sexual wellness. Chapter 18 explores ethical, moral, and legal issues relating to sexuality in detail.

Media Influences

It has long been recognized that the media help shape public attitudes on many topics (Folkerts, Lacy, & Davenport, 1998)—especially sexuality, gender roles, and sexual behaviors. The depictions of sexuality we encounter in the media are there mainly to entertain and sell products. Consequently, the media do not provide us with realistic depictions.

Television shows are filled with portrayals of sexual activity and "double-meaning" comments. The number of programs containing sexual content increased from 56% to 68% from the 1997/98 season to the 2000/01 season (Sex on TV, 2001). The music industry has countless sexual images. Listen to the words of many currently popular songs and you will hear the sexual content. Magazines, tabloids, and books contribute to the many sexual themes that bombard us. Next time you are in the checkout line at the supermarket, take a look

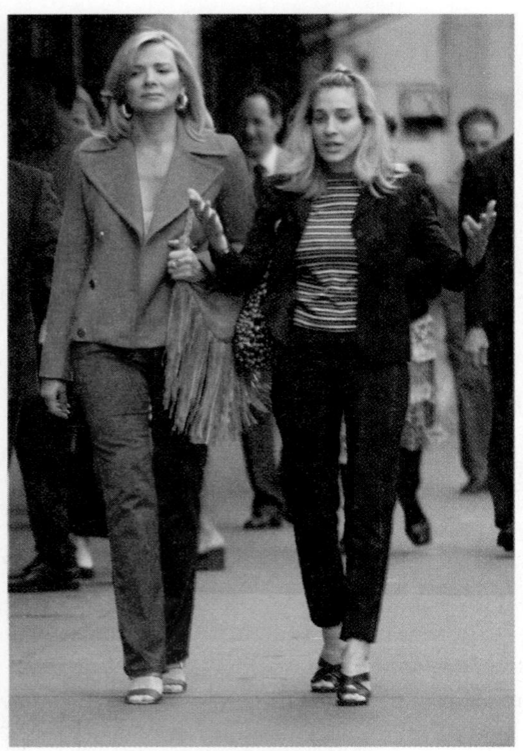

On the surface, *Sex and The City* seems to present four successful, single women living, loving, and having it all in New York City. Beneath the shoes, clothes, and beautiful faces in beautiful places, some see the show as an insightful commentary on loss, loneliness, and the failure of sexual liberation.

at the number of magazine covers that relate to sexuality. Numerous advertisements also use sexual themes to sell products. We are told that if we buy the right soap, toothpaste, clothes, or cars we will look sexier and be more attractive.

If they would so choose, the media could enhance sexual health by communicating accurate information and portraying realistic situations. The National Coalition to Support Sexuality Education encourages writers, producers, filmmakers, programming executives, performers, program hosts, reporters, advertising professionals, Internet access providers, and others to do the following when possible (Sexuality education in the schools: Issues and answers, 1998).

- Include the portrayal of effective communication about sexuality and personal relationships.
- Show typical sexual interactions between people as verbally and physically respectful.
- Suggest intimate behaviors other than intercourse to inform the public about the possibility of alternative, pleasurable, consensual, and responsible sexual activity.
- Recognize and show that healthy sexual encounters are anticipated events, not spur-of-the-moment responses to the heat of passion. Model the communications about upcoming sexual encounters, including expressions of partners' wishes and boundaries.
- When describing, alluding to, or portraying sexual intercourse, include steps that should be taken for prevention, such as using contraceptives and condoms to prevent unwanted pregnancy and getting information about the full spectrum of sexually transmitted infections.

Representatives of the media can do a lot to influence thinking about sexuality if they so choose. Images we are exposed to every day are an important form of sexuality education.

For many years several types of media have influenced dancing styles. For example, in the 1960s and 1970s the way Elvis Presley moved his hips was condemned by some people. Dances such as the twist, the bump, and the dog raised questions about so-called sexual movements among several generations.

Some feel that some recent teen dancing strains the limits of what adults consider decent (DeJesus & McCarron, 2002). The "freak" is characterized by overt sexual gestures to the beat of pulsating music. Boys grind their pelvises against girls' backsides while hands grope freely. The dance can involve two or three teens, usually a girl sandwiched between two boys. Girls sometimes straddle their dance partners on the floor; boys sometimes pin the girls against the wall to play out erotic moves. The "freak" is considered by many parents and teachers to be too suggestive. Many teens do not see reasons for concern. They say, "This is just the way we dance." In response, some school chaperones are equipped with flashlights to patrol dance floors and pry apart entangled bodies. Others have banned straddling, fondling, or lying down while dancing.

Political Influences

Even public policy affects our sexual behavior. For example, the U.S. government's Healthy People 2000 and 2010 projects attempt to use health promotion to establish AIDS and STI awareness, decrease unwanted teenage

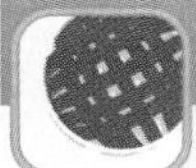

Global DIMENSIONS

Tight Jeans Provide Rape Alibi in Italy Can a woman wearing jeans be raped? Not according to the Italian Supreme Court in a February 1999 ruling. Stemming from a 1992 rape case, Italy's highest court ruled that "it is common knowledge . . . that jeans cannot even be partly removed without the effective help of the person wearing them . . . and it is impossible if the victim is struggling with all her might."

The case, which sparked a furor in Italy, also illustrates the gender dimension: Males continue to play a dominant role in many countries. Italy's Supreme Court, for example, has 410 male judges and only 10 female judges. The insensitivity of the "jeans alibi," as well as further "evidence" cited later, shows a lack of compassion and understanding of gender differences.

The case also illustrates the legal dimension of sexuality: Until 1996, rape in Italy was viewed as a "crime of honor" against the victim's family. A defendant could avoid punishment by merely agreeing to marry his victim! New laws passed in 1996 reclassified sexual assault from a moral offense to a criminal felony.

The "jeans alibi" case began in 1992 in the quaint Italian village of Muro Lucano, 60 miles from Naples. During the course of a driving lesson, the male 45-year-old instructor drove his 18-year-old female student to an isolated spot and, in the student's words, raped her. The instructor maintained that the sexual activity was consensual. He was convicted in his first trial of the lesser charge of indecent exposure. On appeal, he was convicted of rape and sentenced to 34 months in prison.

The Supreme Court of Appeals in Rome then overturned that decision, citing lack of evidence. In addition to the jeans alibi, the court cited the fact that the woman had gone home after the rape but waited several hours before telling her parents.

The gender insensitivity of the jeans alibi was explained by the court: "It should be noted that it is instinctive, especially for a young woman, to oppose with all her strength the person who wants to rape her. It is illogical to say that a young woman would passively submit to a rape, which is a grave violence, for fear of undergoing other hypothetical and no more serious offenses to her physical safety."

Alessandra Mussolini (granddaughter of Italy's former fascist leader Benito Mussolini and one of the drafters of the new rape laws) said, "The judges obviously have no sensitivity to the psychology of rape—no understanding of how victims think or how real life works."

Sources: Burke, G. Judged by her jeans, *Time*, vol. 153, no. 8, March 1, 1999; Judge in rape case sparks imbroglio, *ABCNews.com*, February 12, 1999; and Stanley, A. Ruling on tight jeans and rape sets off anger in Italy, *The New York Times online*, February 16, 1999.

pregnancies, and increase the number of women who receive prenatal care. And, the U.S. constitutional right to free speech allows the uncontrolled distribution of some pornographic material on the Internet.

Even political elections—including choosing elected officials and voting on ballot initiatives—can have a profound effect on policies and on thinking about human sexuality. Consider the political ramifications of the 1998 elections:

1. Representative Tammy Baldwin (D-WI) made history in 1998 by becoming the first lesbian member of Congress and the first member of Congress to be open about her or his sexuality before being elected. With the reelections of Jim Kolbe (R-AZ) and Barney Frank (D-MA) in 1998, the number of openly gay and lesbian members of the House of Representatives was three. As of 2003, there were no openly gay or lesbian senators.

2. Many senators who support sexual health (access to information and services, funding for sexual issues, and so on) were able to hold on to their seats despite strong opposition.
3. In some states, prochoice governors who were elected were able to capitalize on their opponents' antichoice positions.
4. Abortion rights advocates defeated two ballot initiatives (in Washington and Colorado) that would have made partial birth abortions a felony unless the mother's life was in danger.
5. Voters in Colorado approved 55% to 45% a measure that required parental consent for abortions for minors. It required notification of *both* parents for teens seeking an abortion in the state and a 48-hour waiting period. It did not provide for a judicial bypass, and reproductive rights supporters have occasionally mounted a legal challenge to this kind of legislation.
6. Hawaii and Alaska had ballot initiatives stemming from the issue of same-sex marriage. In Hawaii 58% voted for the initiative; thus the Hawaii legislature amended the state constitution to define marriage as between a man and a woman. The Alaska measure (with 60% support) directly amended the constitution to define marriage as between a man and a woman.

As a result of the 2002 elections, for the first time in decades the same political party (in this case, the Republicans) that occupied the White House also controlled the U.S. House and the Senate. This provided an opportunity for that political party to influence various policy issues, including those related to sexuality, strongly. The Republican Party has openly supported limiting the right of women to get abortions. It also has clearly desired to emphasize abstinence from sexual activity as the major way to control pregnancies and sexually transmitted infections among young people. It has gone so far as to provide federal funding for certain types of educational programs only if they emphasize abstinence. It will be interesting to see how far this political party can go in its efforts to implement its policies related to sexuality.

We saw a different kind of political influence when Miss America 2003 wanted to promote abstinence from sexual activity before marriage as part of her platform. Miss America Pageant officials directed her not to do this. They said she should promote youth violence prevention instead of abstinence and attempted to prevent reporters from asking questions about her abstinence views. Miss America said she would "not be bullied" into avoiding the topic of teen abstinence (Pageant officials advise Miss America 2003 to stop promoting teen abstinence, 2002). Various political means can be used to try to influence sexuality.

Historical–Cultural Influences on Sexuality

Just as many sociocultural influences have affected human sexuality, so have some interesting historical–cultural influences. Because we cannot consider all of them, and because most of these topics are covered in greater depth elsewhere in this text, we briefly focus on some from a historical standpoint—namely, the sexual revolution, control of sexual behavior, conception, contraception, and gender roles. As you read about these historical–cultural influences, think about how you and people you know may have been affected by them.

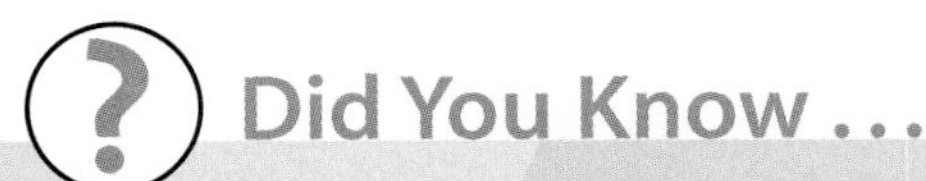

It appears that rates of premarital sexual intercourse may have recently decreased, in contrast to a rather steady increase during the first six to seven decades of the 1900s. For example, the proportion of 15- to 19-year-old females participating in premarital sexual intercourse increased from 28.6% in 1970 to 53% in 1988 and 55% in 1990. In 1997 50% reported having premarital intercourse (Department of Health and Human Services, 1998).

The number of teens who have ever had sexual intercourse increases dramatically with grade level: from 16% among 7th and 8th graders to 60% among 11th and 12th graders. Additionally, teenagers who are black or members of low-income or single-parent families are more likely to have had sexual intercourse than their peers (Dailard, 2001).

In 1998 it was reported that 7.2% of all students had their first sexual intercourse before age 13 (4% of whites, 21.7% of African-Americans, and 7.7% of Hispanics). In addition, 48.4% of all students in grades 9–12 had had sexual intercourse (Kann, et al., 1998).

The Sexual Revolution

No doubt you have heard references to the sexual revolution. The meaning of this term varies according to the speaker; however, it is clear that many changes related to sexuality have occurred in the past 80 to 100 years. Whether or not there has been an actual revolution—or perhaps an evolution—is for you to decide after considering some facts and observations.

Many people talk about a sexual revolution in reference to rates of sexual intercourse before marriage. Many of our history books would lead us to believe that in the past, Americans were sexually chaste before marriage. If we read between the lines, however, we find that this is not necessarily true. Reiss (1973) informs us that in the late 1700s in Massachusetts, one of three women in a particular church confessed fornication to her minister (the actual number was probably higher yet). The U.S. western frontier society relied heavily on prostitution. The women's liberation movement of the 1870s revealed numerous sexual affairs. And the first vulcanized rubber condom was displayed at the Philadelphia World's Fair in 1876. These are not isolated events, and they should make us question what we think about the sexual purity and innocence of our forebears (Bruess & Greenberg, 1994).

Even out-of-wedlock childbearing may not be more prevalent now than several generations ago. For example, rates of white out-of-wedlock births in 1970 did not differ greatly from those in 1850. However, in 1985 about 25% of U.S. births were to unmarried women, up from about 5% in 1960 (Newcomer, 1990). In 1994 the proportion of children born to unmarried women was 26%, and in 2000 it was 31% (Fertility of American women: June 2000, 2001).

Studies done between 1920 and 1945 do seem to indicate that the greatest increases in rates of premarital sexual intercourse occurred in the early 1900s (Bell, 1966). This means that the so-called sexual revolution began early in the 20th century and not in more recent years. Many older people who seem so concerned about changes in sexual behavior were in the middle of the sexual revolution themselves. Our best research tells us that approximately 35% to 45% of females and 55% to 65% of males participated in sexual intercourse before marriage during most of the first six to seven decades of the 20th century (Bruess & Greenberg, 1994).

Myth vs Fact

Myth: Rates of premarital intercourse increased rapidly in the first 60–70 years of the 20th century.
Fact: There was a rather steady rate of premarital sexual intercourse during the first six to seven decades of the 20th century.

Myth: We have long known that early childhood experiences are important to sexual development.
Fact: It was not until at least the middle of the 20th century that it was recognized that early childhood experiences are important to a child's healthy development.

Did You Know . . .

During the Middle Ages, some people believed in witches, whom they accused of having sexual relations with the devil. Because that was not generally acceptable behavior, something had to be done about it. Some women who were sexually "loose" were simply ignored, but others were labeled as witches, and witch-hunts were common. Women were put on trial, and, if they were found guilty of witchcraft, attempts were made to free them from the devil. This was done by a "laying on of hands" by an appropriate religious leader. If these attempts failed, it was sometimes thought better to kill the witch than to let her live.

It is certain that many changes that influence our thinking about sexuality occurred during this time. For example, as traditional moral viewpoints were questioned, people began to wonder whether any one standard of morality could apply universally. Social scientists talked about people's defining their own morality, while religious leaders often saw morality as determined by an order higher than that of mere humans.

By the dawn of the 20th century, sexuality was still not a topic for daily conversation, although it was no longer considered evil or dirty. Several events occurred that contributed to a trend toward more receptivity to the subject. For example, wars exposed many people to other cultures, and the uncertainty of survival contributed to a philosophy of "Live tonight, for tomorrow we may die." The result was a change in the concept of sexual morality.

The rise in the status of women also had a significant effect on our receptivity to the subject of sexuality. Women became better educated, were a more significant part of the work force, were more aggressive, and became more active partners in sexual activity. The "new" woman wanted freedom similar to that of males (Murstein, 1974, 419).

Rapid improvements in communication and transportation also had a tremendous effect. First the telephone became a convenient way to promote interpersonal relationships, and today the Internet provides a means for people to meet, send quick love letters, and stay in touch. Magazines and films spread the word about flirting, dating, sexual feelings, and a variety of sexual behaviors. Dancing became more prominent as a social activity to develop intimate relationships. The car became a "bedroom on wheels," providing an opportunity for having private sexual activity or a means for getting somewhere privacy would be guaranteed.

It is now accepted that early childhood experiences are important to sexuality. This idea is in direct contrast to earlier thinking that children should be treated as asexual beings, and it has ramifications for sexuality education programs for children of all ages.

Alfred Kinsey's research on human sexual behavior in males and females in the 1940s and 1950s provided statistics and information about people and their sexual behaviors. Research findings such as Kinsey's continue to influence us today.

Many of today's adults were influenced by significant events during the 1950s and 1960s. Although innocuous by today's standards, the first nationwide television appearance of Elvis Presley in 1956 was considered obscene by many. Also, the introduction of the bikini swimsuit in 1959 had an effect on thinking about sexuality. During this time, the lyrics of popular songs rapidly became more sexually suggestive as well. Record smashing (and later tape smashing) by opponents of these songs occurred in an attempt to censor the music.

The 1960s work of William Masters and Virginia Johnson on human sexual response also greatly contributed to our knowledge of how we function sexually and how and why we sometimes do not function. In addition to basic information about sexual functioning, their research provided the foundation for sexual counseling and methods for dealing with human sexual inadequacy.

Increasingly reliable contraceptives, especially the pill (introduced in the United States in 1960), were developed and accepted by large numbers of people. Today many reliable and relatively safe contraceptive methods are available, and the vast majority of married couples use contraception.

In the late 20th century and early 21st century, books, classes, and radio and television programs about sexuality, as well as numerous web sites related to sexuality, became common. The press reports the findings of virtually every new study, and discussions about sexuality in American society are out of the closet and into public forums.

Myth vs Fact

Myth: Contraceptive methods were not available until the 20th century.
Fact: Methods used to prevent pregnancy are as old as recorded history.

Control of Sexual Behavior

Throughout the history of Western culture there have been many attempts to control sexual behavior. Most of these are found in moral and legal codes of the time. For example, early Christian moralists taught that since sexual activity outside marriage had a purpose other than **procreation,** it was a sin. Even within marriage, sexual union was lawful only if it was performed for the purpose of begetting children. Almost all medieval theologians emphasized that it was a mortal sin to embrace one's spouse solely for pleasure (Aries & Bejin, 1985, 115).

procreation
Sexual intercourse for the purpose of reproduction.

Early Christians also thought that marital sexual behavior was to be stable and rational. Intercourse was objectionable on all fast or feast days, during the days a female was menstruating, for 40 days after childbirth, during pregnancy, and during breastfeeding. In addition, intercourse between husband and wife was supposed to take place in the "natural" position, that is, with the woman stretched out on her back with the man on top. All other positions were considered scandalous or "unnatural" (Aries & Begin, 1985, 120).

Furthermore, according to the church, it was only the lowest type of demon who engaged in oral–genital sexual activity or anal intercourse. Homosexuality was considered an abomination punishable by death. Some people interpreted the church's prohibitions literally. To prove their loyalty to God, they wore uncomfortable shirts made of hair, donned heavy iron girdles, slept on hard wooden boards, and made a point of never completely satisfying their hunger and thirst. Thousands of people practiced these forms of self-torture until the mid-1300s, when the pope declared such behavior to be heretical. During this time many people were guided more by biological drives than by the church. They mouthed adherence to the principle of sexual restraint but ignored it in practice.

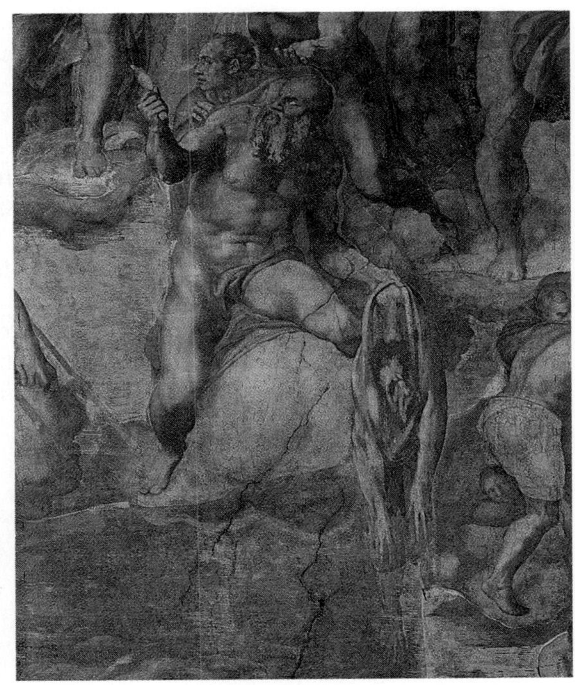

Michelangelo's amazing fresco for the Sistine Chapel altar, "The Last Judgment," created quite a stir in its day because of its depiction of nudity. Pope Paul IV told Michelangelo in 1555 to "make it suitable"; Michelangelo replied, "Let him make the world a suitable place and painting will soon follow suit." The Council of Trent resolved the matter by decreeing that the nudity be concealed.

A belief in witchcraft was another means of controlling sexual behavior. Strong feelings, especially lust and passion, were believed to arise from evil spirits, and since women (and not men) inspired lust, some religious leaders saw women as witches or agents of the devil. Witches were tortured, ostensibly to drive the devil out of them, or killed. Bewitchment was said to account for the mysterious and overwhelming emotional effects that women had on men, sometimes driving them to irrational acts. Witch trials were held throughout the Middle Ages, particularly during the 15th century (Sadock, Kaplan, & Freedman, 1976).

In 17th-century England, the Puritan influence was responsible for legislation to prevent amusements such as dancing, singing, and the theater. Women were treated as prostitutes if they wore long hair or makeup. On Sundays any activities not related to worship were banned.

By the end of the 18th century, sexual behavior was subdued and spontaneity inhibited. People conducted their lives very discreetly. Harsh negative attitudes toward same-gender sexual behavior were common during this time, and many people who practiced that behavior were reportedly put to death. So strong were fears and feelings during the period that people who asked for leniency for those convicted of sodomy (which includes almost any sexual behavior one wishes to prohibit) were themselves in danger of persecution. Eighteenth-century studies of sexuality emphasized physiology and generally concluded that excessive sexual activity—specifically, expelling of semen to excess—had debilitating physical consequences.

In the 19th century, during Victorian times, sexual drives were generally repressed. Though it was believed that men had natural and spontaneous sexual desires, women supposedly had dormant sex drives unless subjected to undue excitation. Children, it was believed, had no sexual feelings.

Much was done to protect the people of Victorian times from sexual arousal. Sexual references in literature and general conversation were suppressed, as were most sexual feelings. Masturbation, a particularly repudiated activity, was called the "secret sin," "self-pollution," and the "solitary vice." Devices were even developed to place around the male's penis at night to prevent **spermatorrhea** (more commonly called **nocturnal emissions** or **wet dreams**) (Figure 1.1).

spermatorrhea (wet dreams, or nocturnal emissions)
Emission of semen during sleep.

ovist
Adherent to the 17th-century belief that the preformed baby was contained within the female body and that the male's sperm simply activated its development.

In the early 20th century, as conservative morality about sexuality diminished and people argued that sexual expression was natural and normal, some secular attempts were made to legislate sexual morality. This resulted in censorship, prohibition, and the revival of old statutes against certain sexual behaviors, such as homosexuality, oral–genital relations, and sodomy.

Theoretically, in the United States there is a separation of church and state, but legal debates about such subjects as abortion, access to sexual

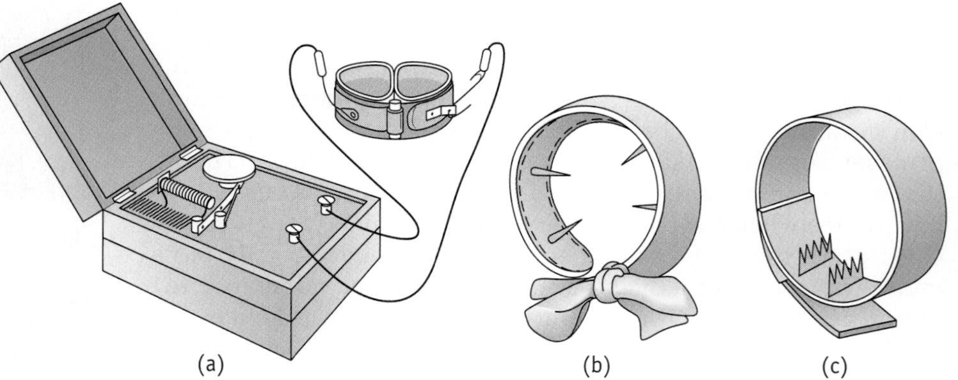

FIGURE 1.1 Devices designed to prevent wet dreams. One device caused a bell to ring when erection occurred (a). For some devices, no bell was needed (b and c).

information and services, homosexuality, and other sexual behaviors have prompted some people to wonder about that separation.

Conception

Much of our information about prehistoric peoples is obtained by analyzing the remains of their art. In addition, we can make inferences from the art of primitive cultures that exist today. Prehistoric cave paintings indicate that more than 30,000 years ago sexuality was an important part of culture. Some of these stone engravings suggest human intercourse, and some show women and men with exaggerated body parts.

Despite the attention to sexuality in their art and perhaps their religion, prehistoric peoples apparently did not understand its role in reproduction. Consequently, theorists believe that a number of explanations for childbirth existed. One notion may have been that children were sent by ancestral deities; sexual intercourse was reserved solely for pleasure. Or a woman became pregnant by sitting over a fire on which she had roasted a fish received from the prospective father. An Australian tribe believed that a woman conceived by eating human flesh. Some cultures thought it was possible for a man to become pregnant (Tannahill, 1980). Some of these theories might seem humorous, but they are really no more peculiar, or at least no more wrong, than such modern superstitions as "You can't get pregnant if you do it only once." By the time of the first written records, however, it appears that humans were aware that they played some part in reproduction, even if they did not know how.

Throughout recorded history, many theories and myths about conception existed. For example, Aristotle theorized that the human fetus resulted from the mixture of menstrual blood and seminal fluid. One hundred years before Aristotle, the Greek poet Aeschylus believed that a child was conceived by a male alone (Where do babies come from? 1982).

The Ashanti of Ghana also believed that conception occurred by mixing the woman's menstrual blood and the man's ejaculate. They felt the mother's blood became the blood of the child and the father's semen became the child's spirit and life force. Many Australian cultures believed that pregnancy occurred when the spirit of a child entered the womb, where it was nurtured until birth. Supposedly, the man's psychic powers caused the fetal spirit to enter the female's body. Similarly, inhabitants of the Trobriand Islands believed that a spirit invaded the body through the head of a sexually mature woman. The spirit was nurtured by the woman's blood; for that reason menstrual periods ceased during pregnancy (Davenport, 1976).

The microscope allowed scientists to see sperm for the first time. In 1677, the Dutch naturalist Anton van Leeuwenhoek described the human sperm discovered by one of his students. Many scientists, however, refused to accept that sperm could be responsible for creating human life. Other scientists claimed they had seen tiny humans inside sperm. This thinking led to the belief that a tiny, fully formed person would not grow until he or she reached the female "nest." At the same time other scientists, known as **ovists,** claimed

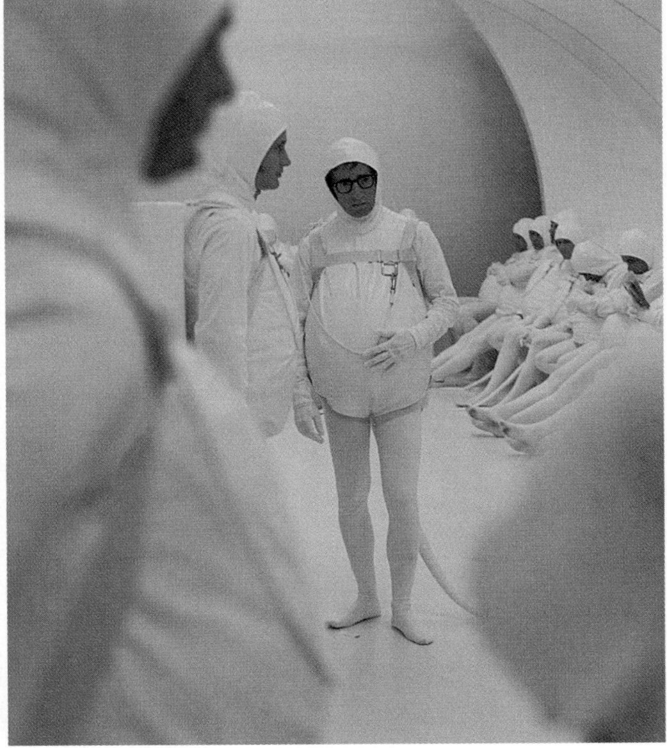

Woody Allen's farcical treatment of sperm cells in *Everything You Always Wanted to Know about Sex*... reflects what was once thought true. When sperm cells were discovered by a magnifying glass in 1677, scientists believed that they saw tiny men (called *animalcules*) inside sperm cells. Other scientists even claimed to see microscopic horses in horse sperm!

that the preformed baby was contained in the female and the sperm served only to activate its development. It was not until 1875 that it was demonstrated that the sperm penetrates and combines with the egg (Where do babies come from? 1982).

It is impossible to know the overall effect of the accurate understanding of conception; however, it would seem that such knowledge was useful to both males and females. The understanding that sexual intercourse could result in conception must have influenced sexual behavior and made it possible to have at least some control over whether or not to procreate. The control of reproduction is possible today; throughout most of history it was not.

Contraception

contraception
Means of preventing pregnancy in spite of sexual intercourse.

Although the process of reproduction was not understood until relatively recently, **contraception**—methods employed to prevent pregnancy—is as old as recorded history. More than 4,000 years ago Egyptian women used medicated tampons as contraceptives. Lint, moistened in a mixture of acacia tips ground with honey, was placed into the vagina. Many other practices, some of them dangerous, were used in the centuries that followed (The ecology of birth control, 1971). Among these were inserting spongy or absorbent fabrics into the vagina or mixing crocodile dung with a paste and inserting the mixture into the vagina. It is said that Persian women placed lemon-soaked sponges in the vagina to prevent pregnancy. It is interesting to note that these methods have some merit. Most of them attempted to form a barrier or alter the acid–base relationship within the vagina. In fact, many of today's contraceptive methods are based on these same principles.

The first modern contraceptive device, which was eventually called the condom, appeared in the mid-16th century. It was designed to protect the wearer against the plague of syphilis then spreading throughout Europe. The condom was first made of fine linen, then of animal intestine, and finally of rubber. Even though its original use was for protection from disease, its potential as a contraceptive was quickly noticed (The ecology of birth control, 1971).

In the middle of the 19th century the German physician Mensinga perfected the rubber diaphragm. He believed that women should have equal rights with men and that their lives would be improved by controlling the number of children they conceived. In the United States, the diaphragm was generally unknown until after World War I. Although condoms were not as effective as diaphragms, and although they depended on the male's willingness to use them, they were manufactured in great quantities at the end of the 19th century and thus became cheaper and more available (Bullough, 1976a, 651). Today, 5.5 billion condoms are manufactured in the United States each year.

The idea of the intrauterine device (IUD) was borrowed from an ancient practice of camel drivers, who put a round stone (or an apricot pit, according to some accounts) into the uterus of a female camel to prevent pregnancy on long trips. During the 1920s, a German gynecologist modernized the idea by substituting a ring of surgical silk or silver (The ecology of birth control, 1971). It was not until experiments with IUDs were performed in Israel and Japan in 1959, however, that their use became widespread.

A number of effective spermicides appeared on the market at the end of the 19th century. The early ones, marketed in a suppository form, probably worked by blocking the cervix with an oily film. Numerous other chemicals soon appeared on the market (Bullough, 1976a, 651). Foams and jellies were introduced in the early 20th century. The most effective method of preventing pregnancy is the oral contraceptive; research on an oral contraceptive was widespread in the 1950s, but it was not until 1960 that the first oral contraceptive was approved for public use. It can probably be said that this event marked the beginning of the modern era of contraception.

It was 30 years later, in 1990, that the U.S. Food and Drug Administration approved levonorgestrel (Norplant). This hormonal contraceptive implant system consists of six capsules 34 mm long, inserted beneath the skin of a woman's upper arm. Its release marked the first time long-term (in this case, up to 5 years) hormonal control of conception was available in the United States (FDA OKs hormonal implant, 1990).

Not necessarily considered a form of contraception, abortion is a means of controlling births. Abortion early in pregnancy was legal in ancient China and Europe. In the 13th century the Roman Catholic church indicated that the soul developed 40 days after conception in males and 90 days after conception in females, and abortion was allowed within those intervals. In the late 1860s the Catholic church declared that life begins at conception; that doctrine led to its abortion ban (O'Keefe, 1995).

Early American law allowed abortion until the woman felt fetal movement, but during the 1860s abortion became illegal in the United States except to save the woman's life. In addition to the religious beliefs of some people, reasons for this included health problems related to crude abortion procedures, the belief that population growth was needed for economic reasons, and maybe a male-dominated political system's response to more women's seeking independence and equality (Sheeran, 1987). It was not until 1973 that the U.S. Supreme Court in its famous *Roe* v. *Wade* decision legalized a woman's right to decide to terminate her pregnancy before the fetus could survive independently of the woman's body. Debates about this issue continue.

Gender Roles

"The paramount destiny and mission of women are to fulfill the noble and benign offices of wife and mother. This is the law of the Creator." Words of a time long past? Not quite. This is actually an excerpt from a Supreme Court opinion rendered in the first case tried under the Fourteenth Amendment in 1873. The court's decision upheld the denial of the right of women to practice law (Bardes, Shelley, & Schmidt, 1998).

Historically, the role of the woman as a sexual partner has been to satisfy male needs. In India, for example, women were viewed as nothing without men. In the West, women who enjoyed sexual activity dared not speak of it publicly because of the severe penalties for doing so. Throughout the ages women were viewed as property of men (Spielvogel, 1997). In most societies, if a woman committed adultery, was raped, or lost her virginity, she was considered damaged property. A woman's father or husband could expect to gain compensation for this damage, or, in the case of adultery, he might even kill her and her partner if they were caught (Bullough, 1976b, 677–679).

In many societies men enjoyed a status vastly superior to that of women. This status can probably be accounted for by (1) men's greater physical strength, (2) women's repeated pregnancies in the absence of reliable contraceptive methods, and (3) the ideology that disparity in male and female roles was divinely ordained. Men used their greater physical strength to trap animals and handle livestock, to defend themselves, and to intimidate women. Since women were often pregnant and spent much of their time caring for children, little time was left to alter their inferior status. Those who felt male and female roles had a divine origin saw any attempts to change these roles as antireligious (Murstein, 1974, 566).

Myth vs Fact

Myth: Open discussion about sexuality will have negative results—people will be more likely to be sexually permissive.
Fact: Healthy communication about sexuality will help people develop into sexually healthy adults—open discussions do not have negative results.

Myth: The relatively open attitudes in thinking about sexuality in Sweden have resulted in higher rates of teen pregnancy and sexually transmitted infections.
Fact: Swedish attitudes and practices related to sexuality have resulted in lower rates of teen pregnancy and sexually transmitted infections.

Myth: Abortion has been illegal throughout most of the history of the United States.
Fact: Early American law allowed abortion until a woman felt fetal movement. In the 1860s abortion became illegal in the United States, but in 1973 the Supreme Court legalized a woman's right to terminate her pregnancy.

Myth: What is sexually arousing to people is very much the same regardless of the culture.
Fact: In different cultures the idea of what is sexually arousing varies a great deal.

The ancient Greeks believed that men were primarily mental and spiritual in their makeup and that women were primarily physical and earthy. Because the Greeks believed the mind and body were separate entities, this meant men had a higher nature and deserved greater privileges. Several centuries later, however, Jesus insisted on the basic equality of the sexes. He opposed Jewish divorce law, which allowed women to be disposed of as property (Nelson, 1978).

Throughout medieval times, women were thought to be inferior to men. Their motives were suspect, they were thought to be sinful, and their female functions were belittled. Some still believed Aristotle's earlier claim that the female was little more than an incomplete male. Both religious and scientific thinking seemed to support these ideas (Bullough, 1976b).

In the early 1800s there were more male children than female children in the western states and territories of the United States. Some researchers have thought this was because nutrition and health of young females were neglected, since their labor was not as economically valued. Others have indicated that this imbalance simply occurred because more boys were born in, survived childhood in, or moved to western regions (Courtwright, 1990). This presents another example in which it is difficult to determine the real reasons for the situation.

However, the mid- to late 1800s and the early 1900s witnessed many advances in the status of women in the United States. After the first major organized meeting on the rights of women in 1848, there was a sort of legal emancipation, an opening of work opportunities, and an ideological acceptance of the equality of the sexes. Actual changes in behavior, however, did not keep pace with this verbal acceptance. The average woman was probably more interested in receiving greater respect and consideration, and in receiving the right to vote, than in having equal professional rights. Most articles advocating the causes important to women today were written by highly educated men and women, and probably the majority of Americans were not even aware of these new ideas (Murstein, 1974, 379). Nonetheless, the seeds of the women's rights movement were planted.

The women's suffrage movement began in the late 19th century with the goal of obtaining for women the right to vote. The passage in 1920 of the Nineteenth Amendment to the U.S. Constitution guaranteed women the right to vote. World War II created an environment for increased gender equality. As men were required to leave home for military duty, thousands of women left their traditional roles in the home and took paying jobs for the first time. It was not until the 1960s, however, after many postwar marriages, the baby boom, and continued disappointment about women's roles, that a new movement for gender equality became evident.

Some people had thought that the ratification of the Nineteenth Amendment would end the struggle for women's rights, but this had not happened. In 1963 the Equal Pay Act, which stated that women must receive pay equal to that of men if they perform the same work, was enacted. In 1964 women were included in the protections of the Civil Rights Act. This made it clear that equality of opportunity for women was endorsed by the federal government (Degler, 1980, 442). Still, by the late 1990s women earned an average 83 cents for every dollar men earned.

In 1963 Betty Friedan published *The Feminine Mystique,* which helped create a widespread movement for women's rights. She urged women to make a life for themselves in addition to their homes and families. The case for women's equality was also championed in a number of other books. In 1966 Friedan organized the National Organization for Women

Multicultural DIMENSIONS

Polygamy When speaking of culture, sociologists generally refer to the "learned values, beliefs, norms, behaviors, and even material objects that are passed from one generation to the next." Within the culture of the United States, however, are many subcultures—groups of people with shared values within the overall culture. Each subculture has a distinctive way of looking at life that sets it off from the prevalent culture. In the United States, these groups may be defined by ethnicity, age, religion, sexuality, geographical location, and national origin. The Multicultural Dimensions boxes look at varied subcultures within the United States.

The first subculture we explore is defined by the sexual practice of polygamy, or having multiple wives. Although polygamy is practiced around the world—it is the preferred arrangement in some parts of Africa, the Middle East, and Asia—it is illegal in the United States. Still, anywhere between 20,000 and 60,000 Americans are living in families in which one man is "married" to multiple wives. Most of these families live in Utah or surrounding states and practice the Mormon religion.

The practice of polygamy caused the Mormons to be driven out of several states before they finally settled in the 1800s in Utah, which was then a wilderness. Even there the federal government would not let them practice polygamy, and Utah's statehood was made conditional on its acceptance of monogamy. Utah outlawed polygamy in 1896, and the Mormon church officially has denounced it.

Yet the practice never ended. Some fundamentalist Mormons believe that polygamy is part of their religious heritage. Others believe that the Mormon church merely denounced polygamy for political reasons. One reason the practice continues is that the state is reluctant to prosecute polygamy cases, in light of the disastrous results of one such prosecution in 1953: A major raid on a polygamist compound was covered by *Life* magazine. Instead of receiving support for upholding the moral law, the state was ridiculed for breaking apart a "family."

But the reality of modern Mormon polygamy appears to have a darker side than previously known: Some women have stepped forward, and, instead of portraying a happy "village" sharing responsibilities for housework and children, they allege a world of repression and sexual crimes. Allegations include forcing teenage girls to marry relatives.

In one 1999 trial a 16-year-old girl alleged that her father forced her to become the 15th wife of her uncle. During her attempt to flee, her father whipped her. The girl's uncle, David O. Kingston, was charged with three counts of incest and one count of unlawful sexual conduct. Her father, John Kingston, was charged with child abuse. Yet no charges of polygamy were filed.

In a 2001 legal test for polygamy, Tom Green was taken to court on bigamy charges. At the time he had 26 children, 5 wives, and 3 more children on the way. Green's case divided Utah, where polygamy is still widely practiced. His critics accused him of exploiting his wives. He said his wives, all of whom were from polygamous families, were just following the original tradition of Mormonism. In an attempt to persuade the jury that he had a loving family, he took his entire clan into court. He was convicted anyway (McCarthy/Partoun, 2001).

Sources: Egan, T. The persistence of polygamy, *The New York Times Magazine* (February 28, 1999), 50–55; Henslin, J. M. *Essentials of sociology: A down-to-earth approach,* 2e. Needham, MA: Allyn & Bacon, 1998; and Tavris, C. *The mismeasure of women.* New York: Touchstone, 1992.

(NOW), which has consistently advocated women's rights. By 1970 a number of other organizations that pushed for women's equality were formed, including the Women's Equity Action League and the Women's Political Caucus. So successful was the women's movement that it has been considered "possibly the most lasting legacy of the . . . period of protests" (Degler, 1980, 446).

In recent years many issues related to women's roles have been raised. Women now work in a variety of jobs previously thought to be only for males, and there are more women in positions of authority. Discrimination against pregnant women in the workplace has lessened, many women delay having children to pursue other interests, and there is an increased acceptance of child care while women work. Varied opinions about women's roles continue. For example, in 1984 it was a shock to some and a victory to others when Geraldine Ferraro was selected as a vice-presidential candidate. Studies about gender and leadership style, gender differences in work, family conflict, gender and the influence of achievement evaluations, gender in the college classroom, among others, continue to provide reams of information about women and their roles and status. But whether we have achieved equality between the sexes is still a matter of debate.

Thinking Critically About Human Sexuality

You have probably observed that, when it comes to many topics related to health and sexuality, there are "experts" everywhere. The concept of critical thinking is important to being able to judge the accuracy of what these people say as well as lots of other information you hear related to sexuality. In this case, the word *critical* does not mean being negative or criticizing people or things. It means being careful and somewhat analytical.

In essence, then, **critical thinking** is thinking that prevents blindly accepting conclusions or arguments (or headlines) and instead closely examines all assumptions. This includes carefully evaluating existing evidence and cautiously assessing all conclusions (Baron, 1998).

Critical thinking is like scientific methods you may have used in other classes. In practice, it involves guidelines such as these (Baron, 1998):

1. Never jump to conclusions; gather as much information as you can before making up your mind about any issue.
2. Keep an open mind; do not let your existing views blind you to information or new conclusions.
3. Always ask "How?" as in "How was this evidence gathered?"
4. Be skeptical; always wonder about *why* someone is making an argument, offering a conclusion, or trying to persuade you.
5. Never be stampeded into accepting some view or position by your own emotions—or by arguments and appeals designed to play on your emotions.

Not every guideline will apply in every situation, but the important goal is to develop a style of thinking using as many of the guidelines as seem appropriate in a given situation.

critical thinking
Thinking that avoids blind acceptance of conclusions or arguments and closely examines all assumptions.

correlation
A relationship between two events.

causation
A relationship in which one event causes another event to occur.

Correlation Versus Causation

A research study found that for people 60 years and older, the 62% who drank coffee still enjoyed active sex lives, compared with only 37% of those who were not coffee drinkers (Plotnik, 1993). Does coffee lead to a better sex life for seniors? Or are the two events just coincidental? The study shows a **correlation,** a relationship between two events. But it does not necessarily show a **causation,** a relationship in which one event causes the other.

It is easy to show that a correlation exists. But correlations do not necessarily show cause and effect. There is a high correlation between the winning conference of the Super Bowl and the stock market: When the NFC wins, the stock market goes up in most years; when the AFC wins, the market goes down in most years. In fact, from 1972 to 1985 there was a perfect correlation. However, no scientific study is needed to understand that the Super Bowl does not cause the stock market to go up or down.

Returning to the coffee example, perhaps people more than 60 years old who are in good health enjoy both coffee and sexual activity. However, there does not appear to be a causal link between caffeine use and sexual activity. In contrast, a study showing a correlation between the drug Viagra and an active sex life would appear to have a causal link. So, correlations can sometimes help predict behavior and point to possible causes of behavior. Further studies can help validate the causation.

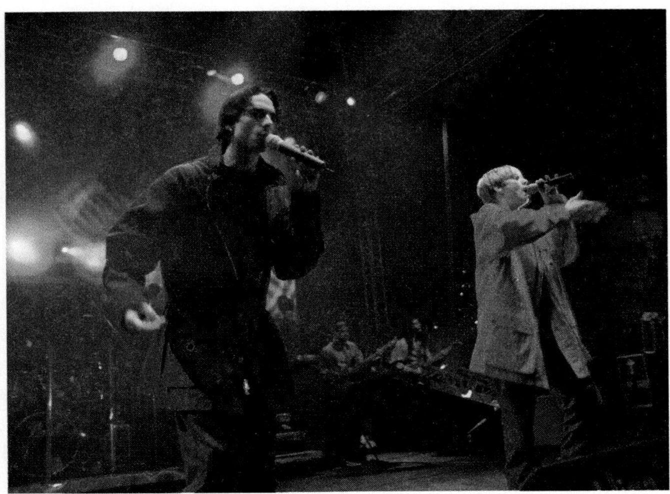

The Backstreet Boys made a hit with lyrics such as "Don't care what is hidden in your history,/As long as you're here with me./Don't care who you are,/Where you're from,/What you did,/As long as you love me." However, such thoughts show a lack of responsibility. You should care where your lover is from, because sociocultural dimensions matter. You should care what your lover has done in the past, because you could be at risk for an STI or HIV. Accepting sexual responsibility is paramount in achieving sexual health and wellness.

Being a Good Consumer of Sexual Information

We are bombarded with information—and misinformation—about sexuality issues. In fact, most best-selling newsstand periodicals lure readers with information about "new" sexual techniques or sex surveys. It is important to keep the principles of the scientific method in mind when reading popular literature.

Consider a study that garnered a great deal of media attention: In 1996, the medical anthropologists Sidney Ross Singer and Soma Grismaijer surveyed 4,700 women and concluded that their odds of having breast cancer increased the longer women wore bras. Their hypothesis was that the cinching effect of a bra suppresses the lymphatic system below a woman's armpit, blocking an internal network of vessels that are intended to flush toxic wastes from the body. Over time, these toxins accumulate in the breast tissue and create an environment in which cells can turn cancerous.

The results of the survey appear to confirm their hypothesis: Of women who wore bras 24 hours a day, in three of four breast cancer developed; of women who wore bras less than 12 hours a day, in one in seven breast cancer developed; of women who rarely wore bras, in only 1 in 168 did breast cancer develop (Joseph, 1998).

The study appears to have found a *correlation* between length of bra-wearing time and breast cancer. However, few medical scientists would agree that a *causation* exists; many would even question the correlation. First, consider the design of the survey on which the conclusion was based: Participants were not randomly selected, following accepted statistical guidelines. For example, women who have had breast cancer might be more willing to participate in a breast-cancer study. Nor were participants questioned about preexisting breast-cancer risks. In addition, participants answered only 12 questions regarding their bra-wearing habits.

A scientific approach to the correlation of bra use and breast cancer would be to find a large, randomly selected sample of women who wear bras for specific lengths of time each day. The women would need to be prescreened for breast-cancer risk and would need to undergo medical exams before participating. Family history of cancer, age, race, body mass, weight, diet, exercise, alcohol or drug consumption, and other factors would have to be controlled in some manner. A matching control group (not selected by bra-wearing time) would add further validity. The study could follow the women across a long period, perhaps 15 to 25 years.

Thus, a critical review of the study quickly calls into doubt the causal factor between bra use and breast cancer. Even the correlation appears to be contrived. However, it does open the door for further studies.

A final point about the scientific method should be made here: When this study first appeared in popular print media, the information provided varied by the source. News media presented the story as provocative and quirky but with powerful opposition voiced by medical doctors and cancer specialists. But one popular "health" magazine reported the study in a way that suggested a causal link—and placed an ad on the opposite page for a "health drug" claiming to lower risk of breast cancer. Always remember to think about why someone is publishing the study. In this case, it was clearly done to help sell a product.

Why Study Sexuality?

There are many reasons for studying human sexuality, including obtaining accurate sexual knowledge, clarifying personal values, improving sexual decision making, learning the relationship between human sexuality and personal well-being, and exploring how the varied dimensions of human sexuality influence one's sexuality.

Sexual Knowledge

A major reason for studying human sexuality is to acquire a sound foundation of sexual knowledge. Only knowledge can dispel sexual myths, superstitions, and misinformation that block understanding, inhibit communication, and create confusion. Correct information lays the groundwork for sexual decision making. The greater your knowledge, the more likely you are to take responsibility for your sexual health. Studies have found that college students want specific factual information (probably pertaining to a sexual encounter), as well as the answer to the age-old question "Am I normal?" (Caron & Bertran, 1988).

The issue of sexual and physical normality underscores the psychological dimensions of human sexuality. It is normal to wonder whether your appearance and/or sexual desires are normal. Many men worry about the size and shape of their penis, and women often worry about the size and shape of their breasts. Learning about the wide variety in appearances, as you will in the anatomy and physiology chapters (Chapters 4 and 5), may help you feel better about yourself. Learning more about sexuality can often increase your sense of personal worth, or **self-esteem.**

self-esteem Sense of personal worth.

values Those beliefs to which we attach the most worth.

Factual knowledge can also help you interpret sociocultural traditions or myths. History is filled with examples of myths about the biological nature of sexuality. Aristotle, for example, thought that menstrual fluid was the substance from which the embryo was formed, a belief held for centuries. Leonardo da Vinci's anatomical drawings show a tube running from the uterus to the breasts of a woman, depicting the common belief that the menstrual fluid that did not flow during pregnancy was diverted to the breasts to make milk—this in spite of the fact that he had dissected female cadavers and certainly never saw such a tube! The U.S. culture is by no means free of sexual myths, as you will discover throughout this text.

A major issue relating to sexual knowledge involves how to engage in "safer sex." What activities can lead to the transmission of STIs and HIV? Is your partner, for example, in a high-risk group? What can be done to lower the risk of transmitting STIs and HIV? (These questions will be answered in later chapters.) Does your partner share your knowledge—and concern—about such issues? If not, should you be willing to engage in sexual activity with that person?

Personal Values

A second reason for studying sexuality is to clarify personal sexual **values,** those beliefs to which we attach the most worth. By exploring your own dimensions of human sexuality, you may come to understand the origins and nature of your sexual values, as well as the values of others.

Remember Lisa from our opening story. She began to understand how sexuality fit into her personal values, especially those involving her family. The values that her family and culture held were very important to Lisa, and she fretted over the prospect of becoming an "unmember" of her family, were she to become pregnant outside marriage.

Responsible Sexual Decision Making

A third reason for studying sexuality is to improve your sexual decision-making skills. Most people have had some sexual experience. Among college students, somewhere between 50% and 80% have had sexual intercourse, and almost all have participated in some form of sexual activity (Porter, 1998; Selingo, 1997). But experience alone does not necessarily provide wisdom or skill in sexual decision making. The study of sexuality provides a sound foundation of sexual information, promotes an understanding of sexual attitudes, and examines a broad range of sexual issues.

For example, assume you were dating Lisa in the opening story. Without an understanding of the many social and cultural factors that influence her sexuality, you would find it hard to understand her feelings. Her communication style is restricted by her cultural background, which discourages openly discussing feelings and seeking psychological counseling. Lack of understanding of why Lisa holds in her feelings could lead to a deterioration of your relationship.

Dr. Drew, the dry-witted host of *Loveline,* a radio and TV talk show that answers viewers' sexuality questions, often suggested that listeners think about their actions before they get involved in sexual situations. A frequently occurring situation on the show was that of having sexual activity with a roommate's lover, which callers often claimed "just happened." Dr. Drew responded that, in most cases, it does not just happen—the two parties consciously flirt, possibly dress enticingly, and in the end must find a time and place to be alone. Dr. Drew suggested that had the parties stopped to think about the actions they were taking, they could have made the sexually responsible decision not to engage in sexual activity.

A Decision-Making Model

A simple but formal model of the decision-making process consists of the following steps (Bruess & Richardson, 1995).

1. *Recognition.* Only with the recognition of an issue can a decision be made. For example, a couple who consider engaging in sexual

intercourse need to recognize the risk of pregnancy, transmission of STIs or HIV, and overstepping of a partner's personal dimensions.

The best decision making requires defining the issue as precisely as possible: For example, what forms of contraception are acceptable? What forms are unacceptable? What can be done to promote safer sexual activity? How does my partner feel about this? What physiological or cultural dimensions might influence my partner's decisions?

2. *Evaluation.* Having recognized a need to make decisions, it is time to gather relevant information, analyze the possible choices, and decide on the best alternative. For example, the latex condom might be a choice for contraception and lowering of the possibility of STI transmission. But the condom also has a lower rate of contraception effectiveness than some other methods. Another choice might be using a contraceptive method with a higher effectiveness rate—such as the pill—combined with a latex condom for STI protection. Further consideration might be necessary if one person is unwilling to use contraceptives because of religious beliefs. Or perhaps one partner has an allergy to latex condoms (in which case polyurethane condoms could be substituted). The decision to remain abstinent could also be discussed.
3. *Implementation.* When a decision has been reached, the plan needs to be put into action. A decision to combine the pill with latex condoms is not effective unless you can delay intercourse until the woman has received a prescription for the pill and taken it for about a month and the man has purchased latex condoms (and learned how to use them).
4. *Review.* After putting the decision into practice, there should be a periodic review. Are the desired results being achieved, or should another alternative be tried? Perhaps after making the decision, something new is learned about the issues that raises questions about the choice. For example, Lisa's pregnancy scare would likely make her seek out a more effective contraceptive method. If so, the decision-making process can be started again. In fact, you will find yourself renewing the decision-making process throughout your life, according to how your circumstances change. The opening story of the contraception chapter (Chapter 8) illustrates the changes in one woman's contraceptive use throughout her life.

Sexual Health and Wellness

Finally, sexual education can contribute to safer sexual behavior. Given that some sexual behaviors can result in pregnancies and/or the spread of sexually transmitted infections (including HIV), it is important for people of all ages to understand which practices can result in safer sexual behavior and to incorporate such practices into personal relationships.

Note that, although we use the term *safer sex,* no sexual activity can be deemed *perfectly* safe. Although knowing a partner's sexual history, using latex condoms consistently, and avoiding certain sexual behaviors can *reduce* your risk of STIs and HIV, they do not *eliminate* the risk. Condoms can break or be improperly used. Your partner may not wish to disclose a complete sexual history (especially embarrassing or abusive situations). Alcohol can also get in the way of judgment.

Communication DIMENSIONS

Talking About Your Human Sexuality Class Expect to find a great deal of interest when you tell people you are taking a class in human sexuality. Inevitably, many of your friends, colleagues, neighbors, and family members will ask, "What are you learning?" How you answer that question says a great deal about your tactfulness, how people perceive your knowledge, and how interestingly and humorously you can present delicate information. We have dealt with this question for years, and here are some suggestions:

- Be careful talking about sexual information at work. One *Seinfeld* episode revolved around Jerry's being unable to remember a new girlfriend's name—except that it rhymed with a female body part. Eventually, he remembers her name is Dolores—which rhymes (sort of) with clitoris. One man embarrassed a sexually inhibited female colleague by describing the episode at work. The woman, who did not know the term *clitoris,* was further embarrassed when the man showed her the definition in a dictionary (in front of several colleagues). She complained to human resources, and he was fired. He sued the company and won a settlement, which is currently in the appeals process. Do not give people sexual information they do not want to hear! As illustrated in the *Seinfeld* case, it is best to change subjects—or even apologize—if someone is uncomfortable with what you are saying. Watch for nonverbal cues as well. Pressing a point may cost you friends.
- Do not go into detail. Use the KISS method (Keep It Simple and Sincere). If you find the human sexual response cycle (Chapter 7) interesting, discuss it in general terms: "I was surprised to learn that males and females have the same physiological response to sexual activity." If asked further questions, simply arrange for the person to borrow your book.
- Do not gross people out. In general, people do not want to hear sordid stories relating to sexuality. Information on atypical sexual behaviors (In Focus: Atypical Sexual Behaviors), female genital mutilation (Chapter 4), or sexual slavery (Chapter 17) is not usually dinnertime conversation. Recognize diversity. In fact, many people will be highly offended by hearing such information.
- Do not be afraid to say something in a straightforward manner. Show comfort with the subject matter by using sexual terminology in a polite, accurate manner. No one will be offended by the use of the word *penis* or *vagina* if used in context—especially if you are answering someone's question.
- Do not lecture. No matter how hard you try (or how sincere you are), you simply will not change friends' sexual behavior by telling them what they are doing wrong.

Practicing safer sexual behaviors does not end with youth. The Centers for Disease Control and Prevention (CDC) report that more than 10% of the total AIDS cases in the United States occur in people aged 50 years and older, and that HIV rates are increasing among people in their 60s and 70s (Broom, 1999).

Practicing safer sexual behavior can promote sexual health and wellness, as well as improve self-esteem. The failure to practice safer sexual behavior can result in physiological, psychological, and social trauma. Although many STIs are "curable," some (such as genital herpes) can only be controlled. Knowing that you have herpes or genital warts may lead to lower self-esteem and a reluctance to seek out partners. Contracting HIV would mean a lifetime of treatment to prevent contracting AIDS. An unwanted pregnancy can have devastating results for both the parents and the child. For Lisa, pregnancy outside marriage could have resulted in losing her family.

Throughout this text, we emphasize safer sexual behaviors. We discuss the aspects of safer sexual behavior with each form of contraception in Chapter 8 and with each atypical behavior discussed in a minichapter.

Service–Learning Projects in Your Community

service–learning
Educational method by which students learn through active participation in organized service experiences.

One of the best ways to learn about the social and cultural environment in your community is through direct involvement. **Service–learning** is an educational method by which students learn through active participation in organized service experiences. Service–learning has equal focuses on the benefits of the service to the recipient and the benefits of learning to the student (Greenberg, 1997).

Service–learning requires that you be directly engaged with other people—both those providing services and those being served. These engagements can bring about significant learning experiences by

- having people work together in a group to plan and carry out service activities
- adjusting these activities to fit the tastes and needs of people who are often very different from one another (perhaps in age, cultural background, or viewpoints about sexual issues)
- providing opportunity for reflection on the meaning of the service–learning activities in your life and the lives of those for whom you provide services
- giving a chance to develop effective habits of performance in joint endeavors and to assume growing responsibilities in such relationships
- putting emphasis on helping others in ways that develop "habits of the heart," which cannot be measured with standard tests (Howe, 1997)

Examples of service–learning activities, which can be found in the Appendix, range from advocating ratings on CDs containing sexually explicit content to volunteering at a rape crisis center.

Exploring the DIMENSIONS of Human Sexuality

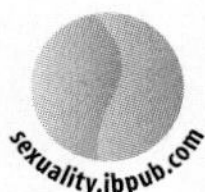

Our feelings, attitudes, and beliefs regarding sexuality are influenced by our internal and external environments. Go to sexuality.jbpub.com to learn more about the biological, psychological, and sociological factors that affect your sexuality.

Sociocultural Factors

- Socioeconomic status
- Laws
- Religion
- Culture
- Ethnic heritage
- Media and ad information
- Family, neighbors, and friends
- Ethics

Biological Factors

- Gender
- Genetics
- Reproduction
- Fertility control
- Sexual arousal and response
- Physiological cycles and changes
- Physical appearance
- Growth and development

Psychological Factors

- Emotions
- Experience
- Self-concept
- Motivation
- Expressiveness
- Learned attitudes and behaviors
- Body image

CASE STUDY

Many factors influence our sexuality. Throughout the text we will help you explore the many dimensions of human sexuality. Each chapter will explore how these dimensions interact in a specific instance. For example, consider your physical appearance. At first glance, it appears to be a biological factor, set by genetics. But your body image, or self-concept of your appearance, is psychological. Sociocultural factors also come into play—your perception is influenced by the culture in which you live and conveyed by the media that surround you.

Discussion Questions

1. List the three main dimensions of sexuality and their subdivisions and give examples of each.
2. Trace the historical aspects of human sexuality, including the sexual revolution and the changing roles of gender and culture.
3. Explain a method for critical thinking and differentiate between correlation and causation. Give examples to back up your answer.
4. Explain the main reasons for studying human sexuality.

Application Questions

Reread the chapter-opening story and answer the following questions.

1. If Lisa were pregnant, what advice would you give her? Consider Lisa's sexual dimensions, including reaction of family, religion, and communication style.
2. If you were Lisa's lover, how might you respond to the situation? To answer this, you need to reconcile your sexual dimensions with Lisa's.
3. Do all Korean-Americans have the same set of sexual dimensions? How might such dimensions differ, depending on age? length of time in the United States? geographic location? socioeconomic status?

Critical Thinking Questions

1. Consider your own sexuality. Write about how each of the three dimensions affects you. Which has the greatest effect on you? the least? Explain your answers.
2. Use the decision-making model to decide whether or not to engage in a sexual activity that you have not yet done. Having thought it through, would you proceed? What precautions might you take to promote safer sexual behavior?

Critical Thinking Case

Should an Artificial Womb Be Used?

People often need to focus on ethical questions related to conception. For example, an article in the *New York Times Magazine* by Perri Klass (September 29, 1996, 117–119) reports that Japanese researchers developed a technique called *extrauterine fetal incubation* (EUFI). They took goat fetuses, supplied them with oxygenated blood, and suspended them in incubators that contained artificial amniotic fluid (the fluid that surrounds a fetus in a pregnant woman's uterus) heated to body temperature. So far, the researchers have been able to keep goat fetuses alive for 3 weeks, but they are confident they can extend the length of time and ultimately be able to apply this technique to humans. When they do, we will have an artificial womb. This will allow us to have more control over conception and birth than ever before.

If it were ever possible, should an artificial womb be used for human pregnancies? What circumstances would warrant the use of an artificial womb for human births? Consider the case in which a woman had fertile eggs but had had her uterus removed as a result of cancer. Should she be able to use EUFI to have a baby? What about the female executive who wants a family but worries that a pregnancy (and postpartum leave) will sideline her career? What about the couple who would otherwise use a human surrogate womb?

Consider further social consequences: Should insurance companies pay for the cost of using the artificial womb? Should the government allot Medicaid money for the socioeconomically deprived who wish to use such a service? Or should such a service be available only to the wealthy?

Exploring Personal Dimensions

Sexuality and Human Relations

A number of internal and external forces in your life influence the decisions you make regarding sexual behavior. What you do may be in harmony with some of these forces and in conflict with others.

Directions

Give a value to the following forces in your life as they pertain to your sexual behavior (i.e., what makes you be sexually active or what makes you refrain from sexual activity). If you are married, apply this tool to a specific sexual behavior such as your degree of fidelity to your spouse or your degree of sexual activity with your spouse.

a = a major force influencing my sexual behavior
b = a moderate force influencing my sexual behavior
c = an insignificant force influencing my sexual behavior

1. Religious influence	a	b	c
2. Family influence	a	b	c
3. How it feels when we kiss and hug	a	b	c
4. My own self-image (how I think I look to others)	a	b	c
5. My sense of right or wrong	a	b	c
6. Radio, television, or movies	a	b	c
7. How it feels to touch someone	a	b	c
8. How I learned to act	a	b	c
9. The way I feel inside	a	b	c
10. Literature (books, magazines) or music	a	b	c
11. Pleasure	a	b	c
12. My judgment	a	b	c
13. My sense of what I should and should not do	a	b	c
14. Friends' influence	a	b	c
15. Physical stimulation	a	b	c
16. Introversion or extroversion (how outgoing I am)	a	b	c
17. My morals or values	a	b	c
18. The expectations/relationship I have with boyfriend/girlfriend (for marrieds, consider friends other than spouse)	a	b	c
19. Fear of, or anticipation of, pregnancy	a	b	c
20. Desire to feel good about myself	a	b	c

Scoring

a = 3 b = 2 c = 1

Total values as follows from top to bottom of the four columns

	Column A	*Column B*	*Column C*	*Column D*
	1. ____	2. ____	3. ____	4. ____
	5. ____	6. ____	7. ____	8. ____
	9. ____	10. ____	11. ____	12. ____
	13. ____	14. ____	15. ____	16. ____
	17. ____	18. ____	19. ____	20. ____
Totals	____	____	____	____

Interpretation

Column A represents the degree to which your morals and values or beliefs influence your sexual behavior and decisions.

Column B represents the degree to which social forces influence your sexual behavior.

Column C represents the degree to which biological factors influence your sexual behavior and decisions.

Column D represents the degree to which psychological forces influence your sexual behavior and decisions.

The relative influences can be compared directly with each other to see which area is the strongest or whether they are equal. You may interpret the results as follows:

11–15 major influence
6–10 moderate influence
1–5 insignificant influence

Sexuality Online

Go to the web component for *Exploring the Dimensions of Human Sexuality* at sexuality.jbpub.com for web exercises, additional resources related to this chapter, and student review tools.

Suggested Readings

Bruess, C. E. & Greenberg, J. S. *Sexuality education: Theory and practice,* 2nd ed. Sudbury, MA: Jones and Bartlett, 2004.

Caron, S. L. *Cross-cultural perspectives on human sexuality.* Needham Heights, MA: Allyn & Bacon, 1998.

Haffner, D. W. Moving toward a health paradigm of teen development: Helping young people develop into sexually healthy adults, *SIECUS Report, 18, no. 4* (April/May 1990), 12–14.

Henshaw, S. K. Unintended pregnancy in the United States, *Family Planning Perspectives, 30, no. 1* (Jan./Feb. 1998), 26.

Hutcherson, Hilda. *What your mother never told you about sex.* New York: Penguin Putnam Publishers, 2002.

Laumann, E. O., Gagnon, J. H., Michael, R. T., & Michaels, S. *The social organization of sexuality.* Chicago: University of Chicago Press, 1994.

Levine, J. Promoting pleasure: What's the problem? *SIECUS Report 30, no. 4* (April/May 2002), 19–22.

Shannon, D. & Dwyer, C. Sexuality education and the Internet: The next frontier, *SIECUS Report, 25* (1996), 3–6.

Suggs, R. & Miracle, A., eds. *Culture and human sexuality.* Pacific Grove, CA: Brooks/Cole, 1993.

CHAPTER 2

Sexuality Research

FEATURES

Multicultural Dimensions
The Wyatt Surveys on African American and White Women in Los Angeles

Ethical Dimensions
Permission to Do Research on Sexual Behavior

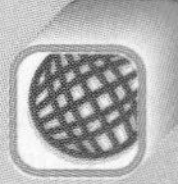

Global Dimensions
The Liu Report: Sexual Behavior in Modern China

Gender Dimensions
Differences in Research Results

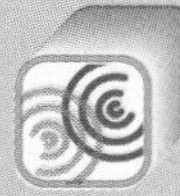

Communication Dimensions
Talking About Sexuality Research Results

CHAPTER OBJECTIVES

1. Describe the various methods used in sexuality research, including the steps in the scientific process.
2. Identify the ethical issues involved in sexuality research.
3. Describe the work of early sexuality researchers and how they set the stage for modern research.
4. Summarize the contributions of major modern sexuality researchers.

sexuality.jbpub.com

Ethical Dimensions: Permission to Do Research on Sexual Behavior
Alfred Kinsey
William Masters and Virginia Johnson
Youth Risk Behavior Surveillance System

INTRODUCTION

You have probably heard the joke "My mind is made up; don't confuse me with the facts." Unfortunately, when it comes to sexuality research, this attitude too often prevails. For example, a few years ago one of our students mentioned that one of his parents had asked him how his courses were going that term. When he mentioned he was learning about research on human sexuality, there were a few seconds of silence.

He explained that he had been raised in a home where sexuality was not discussed. He asked his parent about the silence, and the answer came back that it was a little difficult to think about research on such a topic. What did the researchers do? How did they do it? Why would they even want to do research on sexuality?

Our student explained that for a few minutes he felt he was the parent while he tried to answer these questions. Fortunately, he had already read the early chapters of his text, so he thought he did a pretty good job.

This is not an isolated instance of lack of understanding, or even of repression, when it comes to sexuality research. For instance, in many places in this text you will find references to the National Health and Social Life Survey (NHSLS). In 1988, a team of researchers at the University of Chicago won a federal government grant competition to conduct an extensive research study on sexual behavior. In 1989, however, conservative members of Congress attacked its research for a number of reasons (Laumann, et al., 1994). They said it was a plot by homosexuals to legitimate the normality of gay and lesbian lifestyles; it was an unwarranted intrusion by the government in private matters; it was not needed; it should not be supported with taxpayers' money; and the project staff had an antifamily agenda.

During a federal governmental review, facts about the research were widely misrepresented. It was also claimed that the researchers had published statements that they had not, and statements were taken out of context in an attempt to show that the researchers should not be doing the research. As a result, the previously approved government grant was cancelled. The research was then completed with private funding. Since the study of human sexuality still prompts anxiety and even fear in some people, as well as a hesitancy to talk about the subject with other people, sexuality research can be difficult.

In this chapter we present some of the major 20th- and 21st-century research on sexuality to show you how knowledge about human sexuality is obtained and to discuss some of the findings that researchers believe can aid individuals in accepting and understanding the sexual parts of their personalities. We turn to the findings after identifying some of the methodology used in sexuality research.

Research Methods

Research is undertaken to expand our knowledge about specific factors in our environment. Our current knowledge of human sexuality is based on relatively few studies. Perhaps by reading about issues and techniques related to research in general, you will better understand and evaluate the studies we discuss, as well as ask yourself how valid the findings are.

The first task of any researcher, regardless of the subject, is to ask an explicit question. The next is to design a way of gathering the relevant information. In sexuality research the most common methods used are surveys, case studies, and experimental research. Less common is the method of direct observation, a method used more in sexual research clinics but also used extensively in the research of Masters and Johnson (discussed shortly). Each method of research has its advantages and disadvantages, some of which are discussed here.

A good researcher chooses a method according to the particular problem and population being studied. For example, a survey would be used when a large number of responses are desired, as in a study of adolescent behavior. Observation might be desirable when a small number of subjects are involved, as in measuring responses of people who are engaging in a sexual behavior while being electrically monitored.

The Scientific Method

Sexology is the study of sexuality. To study sexuality appropriately, it is necessary to use the **scientific method**—that is, research conducted in an atmosphere free from bias—because it is the most objective way to establish new knowledge in any field. Scientists must always approach research studies without preconceived ideas of what their studies will show. In addition, they cannot have preconceived agendas to show what sexual behavior *should* be. Researchers do not set out to "prove" something but instead conduct research scientifically to discover what *is*—not necessarily just what they want it to be. Researchers follow proper procedures and discover information through research that can then be generalized to the real world outside the study.

sexology
The study of sexuality.

scientific method
Research conducted in an atmosphere free from bias.

hypothesis
A tentative proposal or an educated guess about the results of a research study.

variable
A measurable event that varies or is subject to change.

volunteer bias
Characteristics of volunteers that are likely to influence research results.

As we will explain, the scientific method involves the following steps:

1. *Identifying a research question* (which could be based on personal interest or experience, on social concerns, or on the interests of those funding the research, such as government agencies or private industry)
2. *Reviewing the literature*
3. *Formulating a hypothesis (or two or more hypotheses)*
4. *Operationalizing variables*
5. *Collecting data*
6. *Analyzing the data to test the hypotheses*

The scientific method first involves identifying a research question. Not all questions about sexuality lend themselves to scientific research, because many involve subjective values, morals, and philosophical questions. (However, scientific research can provide information that can help us address even these types of questions.)

Second, to inform themselves adequately, researchers must review literature related to the research question. Thus the researchers learn what is already known about the topic, think of ways to conduct the desired research, and possibly even come up with new research questions.

Third, a hypothesis is formulated. A **hypothesis** is a tentative proposal or an educated guess about the results of a research study. It often deals with the relationship between two variables. A **variable** is a measurable event that varies or is subject to change (such as frequency of sexual behavior, use of contraceptives, or amount of alcohol ingested).

Fourth, operationalizing the variables means specifying how they are going to be measured. For example, some variables, such as gender or income level, are easy to measure. Others, such as sexual desire or satisfaction in a relationship, are not. There are many ways to measure these variables, and the research has to state clearly how this will be done.

Fifth, collecting the data involves using methods such as survey research, case studies, experimental research, and direct observation. Each of these is explained in greater detail shortly.

Sixth, the data are analyzed to test the hypotheses. Data can be analyzed to describe situations, to show a relationship between variables, or to show that one situation causes another. Each of these methods of analysis demands the use of appropriate statistical methods.

Various forms of bias can be problematic. For example, in addition to possible bias of researchers, there could be bias of research subjects. If all subjects are college educated, they will probably be biased. Or, if some subjects are really not willing to participate or to be honest even if they agree to participate, they will also be biased. This type of bias is referred to as **volunteer bias**—characteristics of volunteers that are likely to influence research results.

One of the goals of the scientific method is to find information that can be generalized to the real world outside the study. Obviously, when researchers are trying to learn more about human sexuality, they cannot

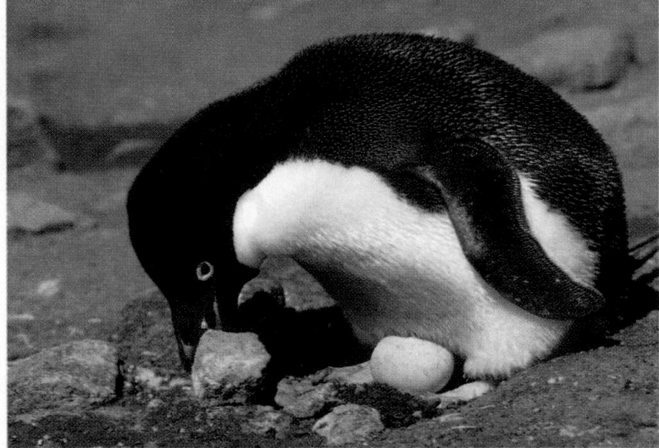

Researchers on Antarctica's Ross Island have noted that female penguins, desperate for stones for their real nest, were willing to engage in "courtship" with an unpaired male penguin in exchange for stones. The penguin expert Eric Bennett decided to try an experiment at the Baltimore Zoo: He dressed up as a penguin and surrounded himself with lots of rocks. Within minutes, female penguins began presenting themselves for courtship. Does Bennett's experiment reflect the scientific method?

get information from *all* human beings. Therefore, they must study a relatively small group of people from which the results may be generalized to a larger population. **Generalization,** the ability to conclude that the same results would be obtained outside the study, can occur only if all aspects of the scientific method are properly planned, carried out, and controlled as much as possible.

The **population** is the group being studied in a research project. Usually only a **sample** (a segment of the larger population) participates, because the total population would be too large and unwieldy. A **random sample** represents the larger population and is chosen in a way that eliminates bias. If the sample is selected properly, the researcher can generalize findings to the larger population.

generalization
The ability to conclude that the same results would be obtained outside the study.

population
The group being studied in a research project.

sample
A segment of the larger population.

random sample
A sample that represents the larger population and that is chosen without bias, so that every member of the larger population had an equal chance to be selected.

survey
Research in which people complete questionnaires or are personally interviewed.

interview
Oral research method designed to gather information.

questionnaire
Written instrument designed to gather information.

self-report data
The respondents' descriptions of something.

frequency
How often something occurs or has occurred.

duration
How long something occurs or has occurred.

case study
In-depth study of individual(s) or small groups.

experiment
Observation of behavior (or effects) under controlled conditions.

experimental group
In an experiment, the group subjected to a particular event or condition.

control group
In an experiment, the group not subjected to a particular event or condition.

observation
Watching subjects in a particular setting.

Survey Research

Much information about human sexuality has been obtained by **surveys** asking people about sexual attitudes and experiences. It can be obtained orally (face-to-face interviews) or in written form (pencil-and-paper questionnaires). Researchers use surveys when information from a large number of people is desired. For example, they might use a survey to find out how people feel about condom advertisements on television.

The **interview** allows the interviewer to explain the purpose and value of the survey, to clarify and explain the questions, and to report answers clearly. However, some individuals may not report their sexual experiences and views honestly because they may be embarrassed to admit particular behaviors and thoughts to a stranger. Also, the subjects being interviewed may be equally embarrassed to admit they do not participate in certain sexual activities.

Questionnaires are less expensive than interviews, which require many people to conduct the interviews. A questionnaire that the subject can fill out at his or her convenience makes many people feel more relaxed and reinforces anonymity; the privacy may also ensure more honest answering. In addition, the questionnaire eliminates the subject's being influenced by the interviewer's facial or bodily gestures.

The major concern with any **self-report data** is that subjects may include inaccuracies. Accuracy is obviously necessary to reliable research. For instance, people often have difficulty recalling past events, and events can become highly embellished or minimized the longer the time between experience and reporting. Recall involves estimating **frequency** and/or **duration** of behaviors, and many people have problems remembering numbers.

Case Studies

Case studies are in-depth studies of individuals or small, select groups of individuals. Those under study are generally followed over a period of months or years. Case studies provide a chance to look at specific behaviors or characteristics in great depth. Also, because case studies generally cover a relatively long period, the researcher is able to explore cause-and-effect relationships in detail. For example, much information about sex offenders and people with sexual-response difficulties has been obtained through case studies.

With case studies, however, there is no way to use proper sampling techniques, making it difficult to generalize case-study results to the rest of the population. For instance, how do we know that sex offenders or those receiving treatment for sexual-response problems are like the rest of the population?

Ethical DIMENSIONS

Permission to Do Research on Sexual Behavior

A faculty member at Mercer University in Macon, Georgia, was told by the president of the university that he could not conduct research in the form of a survey of sexual behavior of undergraduate students at Mercer (Wilson, 2002). The president said the project simply was not appropriate at a Baptist institution.

The president was concerned that the survey's explicit questions might offend students and their parents. Even though a 13-member campus review board unanimously approved the survey, top university administrators said that the survey was also subject to their approval. This was a procedural step that had never before been invoked. One of the vice presidents said that such a survey could have negative impacts on admissions and parents' attitudes about the school.

On the other hand, the researchers involved in the study said that better safe-sex programs were needed for Mercer undergraduates, and that a well-done survey about sexual behavior would be a good place to start. The faculty and students working together on the project hoped to publish the results in a scholarly journal. They indicated that preventing them from conducting the survey denied them academic freedom. They were upset that the result was an apparently arbitrary decision of senior administrators.

What do you think? Was it ethical for the researchers to conduct the survey? Was it ethical for the president to tell them they could not conduct the survey? Should the senior administrators have allowed the survey to be conducted even if they did not like the idea of the survey's being done on their campus?

Source: Wilson, Robin. "An Ill-Fated Sex Survey." *The Chronicle of Higher Education,* 48, no. 47, Aug. 2, 2002, A10–A12.

Experimental Research

In an **experiment,** behavior can be studied under controlled conditions. A common experimental design is one in which two groups are matched and compared. The groups are identical but for one important difference—the **experimental group** is subjected to a particular event or condition, whereas the **control group** is not. Both groups are observed, and the results are compared to determine whether the experimental condition had an effect. For example, a researcher could compare the responses of different groups of people (perhaps grouped by sex or age) to erotic materials.

Experimental research allows control over variables thought to influence responses or behavior. At the same time, the somewhat artificial setting may influence behavior or response. Merely knowing you are in a study or being in a laboratory might alter your reaction.

Direct Observation

Observation is a method in which subjects are watched in a laboratory, a class, a natural setting, or the workplace. It can be an accurate way to collect sexual information—particularly if the researcher controls the setting. A prime example of observational research has been the human sexual-response research of Masters and Johnson.

The major drawback of direct observation is the required expenditure of time and money. In addition, people are likely to be reluctant to perform sexual activity in a laboratory where they are being observed. In addition, some people question the ethics of participating in observational research either as the researcher or as the subject. When people do feel relatively

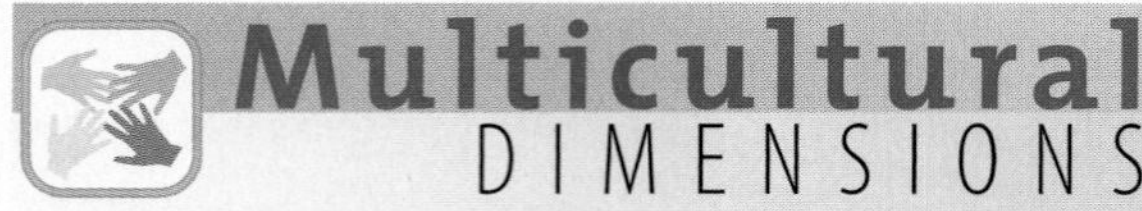

The Wyatt Surveys on African American and White Women in Los Angeles

In several places in this book you will see research findings indicating differences in sexual behaviors and attitudes between people of different races. Care is needed when interpreting such findings, because it is often hard to differentiate between what may be a result of racial culture, what may be a result of socioeconomic differences, and what may be random or coincidental. A good example of this is provided by the Wyatt surveys.

Wyatt and her colleagues used Kinsey-style face-to-face interviews to examine the sexual behavior of 122 white and 126 African American 18- to 36-year-old women in Los Angeles. The two samples were balanced in relation to demographic characteristics such as age, education, number of children, and marital status.

Wyatt reported that by age 20, 98% of the people in her study (both white and African American) had experienced premarital sexual intercourse. When social class differences were considered, the ages of first intercourse for African American and white women were similar.

To control for demographic differences between white and African American women, Wyatt limited the subjects to demographically similar (age, education, social class) women. Her sample of African American women then matched the demographic characteristics of the larger African American Los Angeles population. However, because of Wyatt's efforts to use demographically similar groups, the white sample did not match the demographic characteristics of the larger white Los Angeles population because it contained a greater proportion of white women from lower-income families. This is an example of a trade-off in research. Wyatt wanted to be sure her two groups were demographically similar but in doing so ended up with one group that was not demographically similar to its larger population. This is not necessarily bad; however, it illustrates that we must understand what the researchers have done to interpret the results accurately.

Sources: Wyatt, G. E. The sexual abuse of Afro-American and white American women in childhood, *Child Abuse and Neglect, 9*(1985), 5, 7, 19; Wyatt, G. E. Reexamining factors predicting Afro-American and white American women's age at first coitus, *Archives of Sexual Behavior, 18*(1989), 271–298; Wyatt, G. E., Peters, S. D., & Guthrie, D. Kinsey revisited, Part I: Comparisons of the sexual socialization and sexual behavior of white women over 33 years, *Archives of Sexual Behavior, 17*(3, 1988a), 201–209; Wyatt, G. E., Peters, S. C., & Guthrie, D. Kinsey revisited, Part II: Comparisons of the sexual socialization and sexual behavior of black women over 33 years, *Archives of Sexual Behavior, 17*(4, 1988b), 289–332.

comfortable and volunteer for observational research related to sexuality, one must always ask whether their sexual responses in such a setting replicate those obtained in the privacy of their normal environment. Another important question is whether people who are comfortable doing this are similar to the majority of people who aren't—put another way, can the findings be generalized?

Issues in Sexuality Research

Despite the care and planning that go into implementing a research project, the success of a project depends on the cooperation of the subjects. The most difficult task in studying humans is finding a large group who will stay with the project to completion. When mail questionnaires are used, for example, the response rate is generally less than 40% of the total number distributed—and often close to 20%. Interviews are expensive, but the response rate can be high, depending on the interviewer's expertise and awareness. The interviewer must establish rapport with the subjects so that they are not embarrassed, intimidated, or totally unresponsive.

When asked to be surveyed about sexual behavior, many people will refuse, but others will participate. Therefore, those who do participate may be more or less sexually experienced and liberated than those who choose not to take part. This volunteer bias may allow us to draw conclusions from the study results about how some people view sexual matters, but it does not allow us to conclude that people in general behave or believe that way. When people answer surveys or consent to be interviewed, there are always problems of reporting accuracy, ability to recall past experiences as they really occurred, and willingness to be truthful, particularly about sexual matters, when facing an interviewer. Consider, for example, that reporting and evaluating how we feel now are easier than reporting how we felt sometime in the past. In recalling how and where we learned about sexuality or what sexual activities we were involved in as children, we are easily influenced by events that took place in intervening years, by changes in behavior socially defined as normal (or at least permissible), and by our own maturity. Even if subjects want and intend to give honest responses, they may feel reluctant to share the intimate details of their activities with a stranger, worry about the researcher's attitude toward their sexual behavior—particularly in an interview—or be afraid that their responses are not genuinely confidential.

Research on sexuality faces some additional problems. Many conditions affect our sexuality, including broad cultural and social definitions of sexuality roles and proper sexual behavior, as well as characteristics such as ethnic origin, religion, personal experience, and education. Such conditions and their effects may be too complex to measure or control. Also, cooperative subjects may be hard to find, because in our culture people feel anxiety, self-consciousness, and a reluctance to share private thoughts, experiences, and memories about sexuality. For example, many people would not want to talk about their experiences with forcible sexual behavior. Even talking about whether or not one masturbates and, if so, how frequently, is not something most people are eager to do.

Adding to the difficulty of gathering accurate information is the influence of the researcher's own values and biases. The researcher may have very strong opinions about issues in the study and may—perhaps unintentionally—phrase questions in favor of his or her views, emphasize certain words in a face-to-face interview, and/or have certain racial, ethnic, or cultural views that affect rapport with the subjects in the study. Interviewers and writers of questionnaires may have perceptions about the group they are surveying, which can also influence how questions are asked or phrased. When the information is collected and interpreted, the researcher must consciously prevent personal feelings and attitudes from affecting analysis and reporting. For example, a researcher who might be either strongly for or strongly against abortion would need to be very careful when asking questions about abortion and recording the answers of a research subject. It would be wise to have several researchers with different views work together to check questionnaires and procedures to be sure there is as much **objectivity** as possible: that is, be sure the results are the same no matter who asks the questions or records the answers.

objectivity
Being sure the results are the same no matter who asks the questions or records the answers.

Ethical Issues in Sexuality Research

Recently there has been increased attention to the need to protect the people participating in any form of human research. Because of the intimate

informed consent
Document required to participate in a research study after the purposes, risks, and benefits of the study have been explained.

vaginal plethysmography
Insertion of a probe into a woman's vagina to measure changes in blood volume.

penile strain gauge
A wire or cuff placed around the penis to measure physiological changes over time.

plethysmograph
A laboratory measuring device that charts physiological changes over time.

nature of sexual research, the ethical issues involved in this field are particularly important.

An ethical issue of particular concern is obtaining the **informed consent** of participants; subjects of research studies must agree in writing to participate *after* the purposes, risks, and benefits of the study have been explained to them. Consent is obtained to ensure that subjects both understand what the project entails and agree to undergo the experience as described. This requirement protects subjects against physical and psychological abuse by irresponsible researchers and protects researchers against claims that subjects were taken advantage of. Investigators are now required by law to obtain an individual's consent to be subjected to the project as described; those testing minors must also obtain parental or guardian permission.

Researchers do not have the right to coerce people to participate in a study, and they must be honest when presenting information about the research. They also have a responsibility to protect the confidentiality of their participants. They must be sure that personal facts can never be connected to a given individual. It is obvious that participants must also be protected from physical and psychological harm. Many methods must be used to guarantee the anonymity of participants and to be sure confidential information is never released.

Human-research review committees commonly exist in government agencies and in universities. These committees must review and approve any research designs and procedures that will use human subjects. Such committees consider the value of the research and compare it to any potential risks to the participants. It can be difficult for committees to decide whether to allow a researcher to carry out a particular study—especially if children are involved. This is one reason why we do not have better information about the sexual thoughts and experiences of young people.

Additional ethical questions arise in studies of the sexual behaviors and attitudes of various racial groups. Some people argue that such research is important to better understanding of diverse feelings and practices. In contrast, others feel that describing sexual behaviors and attitudes according to racial groups contributes to stereotypical thinking.

Another interesting ethical issue arises from the ways that have been developed to measure physiological changes in the vagina or the penis due to sexual stimulation. **Vaginal plethysmography** involves inserting a probe into a woman's vagina to measure increased blood volume, an indication of sexual arousal. Changes in blood volume over time can be charted with this device. Similarly, a **penile strain gauge** can be used. This is a wire or cuff placed around the penis that is attached to a **plethysmograph,** a laboratory measuring device that charts physiological changes over time and records changes in the girth of the penis as it responds to sexual arousal or loss of arousal.

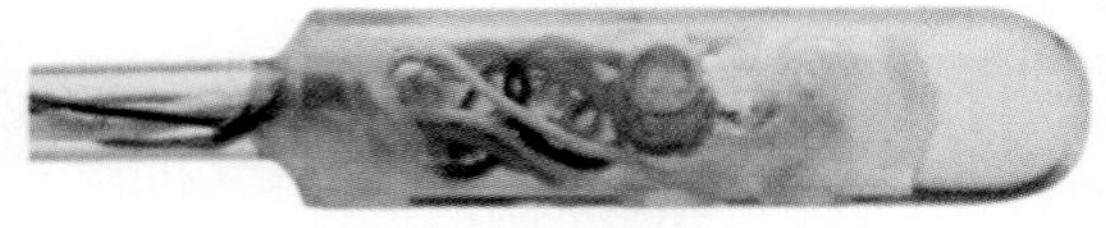

The vaginal plethysmograph is used to measure sexual response by detecting changes in the amount of blood in the vaginal walls. The device is used in sexuality research.

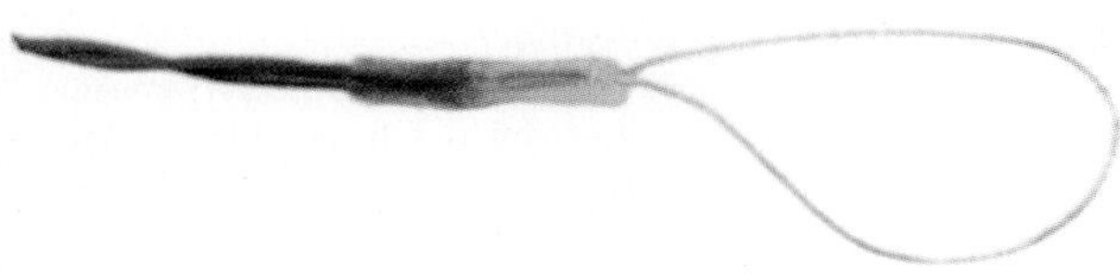

The penile strain gauge is used to measure erectile response by detecting changes in the circumference of the penis. The device is used in sexuality research.

Plethysmography has been used to see whether a person has certain sorts of sexual interests, such as a sexual interest in children. For example, if it were suspected that a person were sexually attracted to children, the device might provide additional information that could lead to a referral for possible treatment. Following treatment, the device could be used again to see whether the degree of sexual interest in children has decreased. However, because people can sometimes learn to control their physiological responses, this is not a foolproof test. Also, it would be a mistake to base too many assumptions about a person's future sexual behaviors on one measure of physiological response. Use of penile and vaginal plethysmography is likely to be debated for years to come.

Finally, it is crucial to be sure a test has **validity:** that is, that it tests what it is supposed to test. For example, a sexual-knowledge test must be a good representation of overall sexual knowledge. This might be shown by a comparison to a known good test or by expert ratings.

validity, validation
Demonstration that tests measure what they are designed to measure.

Most research on sexual feelings, attitudes, responses, and behavior depends on participants' reporting about themselves. Some people believe that sexuality research is useless and meaningless because subjects can lie about their sexual behavior, exaggerate their experiences, or feel too embarrassed to discuss personal sexual matters openly and honestly. Others believe that we need information about sexual matters and must encourage research, even while acknowledging its limitations. Although it is difficult to validate information that people include on a questionnaire or divulge in an interview, validation is frequently done by asking for the same information in another part of the survey or in conversation and cross-checking whether the information given is the same in both instances.

Given the variety of attitudes toward sexuality in our society, the many different opinions concerning moral and ethical issues related to sexuality, and even the disagreement as to whether sexuality should be researched at all, researchers have a difficult job. They must design a scientifically sound study, create confidence in that study, and guarantee their subjects' privacy.

Early Sexuality Researchers

As discussed in Chapter 1, we have some information about sexual practices throughout human history. Although not all of the information was gathered in a systematic way, in Western civilization attempts to study human sexual behavior systematically date back at least to the ancient Greeks. Physicians, such as Hippocrates, and philosophers, such as Plato and Aristotle, are the forefathers of sexuality research. They made extensive observations and offered the first elaborate theories regarding sexual responses and dysfunctions, reproduction and contraception, abortion, legislation related to sexuality, and sexual ethics (The Kinsey Institute, 1998).

In Rome, Greek physicians such as Soranus and Galen further advanced sexual knowledge. Their work prompted later Islamic scholars to spend much time on sexual questions. These studies, together with the Greek and Roman manuscripts, became standard texts at medical schools and stimulated a rebirth of anatomical research in the 16th, 17th, and 18th centuries. In the 19th century, new concerns about overpopulation and sexual psychology intensified efforts to study the topic of sexuality. Finally, at the turn of the 20th century, the investigation of sexuality became a legitimate endeavor in its own right (The Kinsey Institute, 1998).

Richard von Krafft-Ebing

Richard von Krafft-Ebing (1840–1902) wrote during a period when Victorian standards strongly suppressed thinking about human sexuality. Because he was a product of this period, and because he was a physician who worked primarily with sexually disturbed people, von Krafft-Ebing's writings (1902) indicated that sexual activity is something to fear.

He supported what we now know as the double standard, whereby men have sexual freedoms that women do not. He may have supported this because of his apparent discomfort with the sexuality of women.

von Krafft-Ebing's writings had a tremendous influence on many physicians as well as the public. Even though he seemed to be biased and made some false assumptions, his writings convinced some physicians and researchers that the study of sexuality was legitimate. This helped prepare the way for Ellis and Freud.

Henry Havelock Ellis

Henry Havelock Ellis (1859–1939), an English psychologist and physician who studied human sexuality, grew up in fear of what he had been told about the danger of nocturnal emissions. He was also concerned about his general ignorance of human sexuality. Between 1896 and 1910 Ellis published a six-volume series entitled *Studies in the Psychology of Sex,* which included the following beliefs:

1. Masturbation is common for both sexes.
2. Orgasm in males and females is very much the same.
3. Homosexuality and heterosexuality are a matter of degree.
4. Women do have sexual desire, contrary to Victorian thought.
5. There is no one norm for human sexuality. Thoughts and acts vary among individuals and cultures.
6. There should be sexuality education for both sexes starting at early ages.
7. There should not be laws against contraception or private sexual behavior.

Ellis wrote about sexual behavior from anthropological, cultural, psychological, and medical viewpoints. Most of his findings were from case studies and life histories.

Ellis approached sexual phenomena from experience or experiment and even used his personal experiences in sexual matters for research purposes. He discussed nocturnal emission, masturbation, and other sexual behaviors and concluded that there is wide variation in normal sexual behavior. Two aspects in particular made Ellis's writings significant: the fact that he provided accurate information from a somewhat scientific viewpoint and his ability to divorce himself from the repressive Victorian climate of his time. Victorian society defined sexuality in negative terms, labeling many behaviors as diseases and deviations. Thus this early researcher, who viewed sexual behavior in a normative framework, influenced many of the attitudes about sexuality that are held in our society today.

It is clear that Ellis's ideas were controversial and ahead of their time, particularly his support of sexuality education. In fact, some people today still have difficulty accepting his beliefs. Ellis's work influenced the later pursuits of many sexuality researchers and writers.

Sigmund Freud

Sigmund Freud (1856–1939), a psychological researcher, developed theories about human development, personality, and psychopathology that have influenced our thinking. To develop into a well-adjusted person, according to Freud, one had to progress successfully through a number of psychosexual stages.

Freud viewed sexuality and sexual pleasure as a central part of human life and felt that people naturally sought to have as much pleasure and as little pain as possible. He indicated that sexual activity was natural and that procreation was secondary to pleasure, and he cautioned against severe restrictions on sexual instincts. People, he maintained, could become neurotic if denied natural expression of their sexual instincts.

One of Freud's important contributions was his suggestion that early childhood experiences had strong consequences for adult functioning. Largely because of Freud's work, sexual thoughts and behaviors are still considered to be major influences on contemporary life in general.

20th-Century Sexuality Researchers

The 19th-century model of sexuality and sexual behavior was a medical one. Individuals who differed from the accepted norms were considered ill or, in scientific terms, deviant or pathological; however, little was known about sexual attitudes, behaviors, and activities. There was a dearth of knowledge about human sexuality from the psychological, psychosocial, and physiological perspectives. Research into sexual attitudes and behaviors lacked respectability, and many institutions would not fund or support it. In the 1930s changes in public attitudes in the United States, desire for contraception (both for child spacing and for population control), and a more open interest in the scope of sexual behavior led to greater acceptance of human sexuality as a legitimate field for research.

What follows is an overview of the more prominent research in human sexual behavior during the past 60 or 70 years. Although some of this work was done in the late 1930s, you will find that many of the issues are not very different from those you are concerned with and possibly are experiencing now.

Our overview covers two categories—scientific literature and popular literature. In most instances it is obvious which category applies, but admittedly in a few cases the point is arguable. We hope that a review of these studies will not only add to your sum of information but also help you to expand and develop your sexuality and interpersonal relationships.

Scientific Literature

Alfred C. Kinsey: Establishing Scientific Sex Research

Alfred Kinsey, a biologist and zoologist, joined the faculty of Indiana University in 1920. He gained academic recognition early in his career through his writings in biology. In 1937 Kinsey became the teacher of a newly introduced course in marriage and sexuality education. As his interest in the subject grew, he began to amass information concerning sexual activities and beliefs about sexuality. Dr. Kinsey's scientific background led him to gather facts and statistical data, and by 1939 he had collected 733 sex histories. Realizing the need to standardize his data-collecting methods, he then developed a detailed list of 521 interview questions. By means of this list, Kinsey gathered the largest amount of information on human sexuality ever collected.

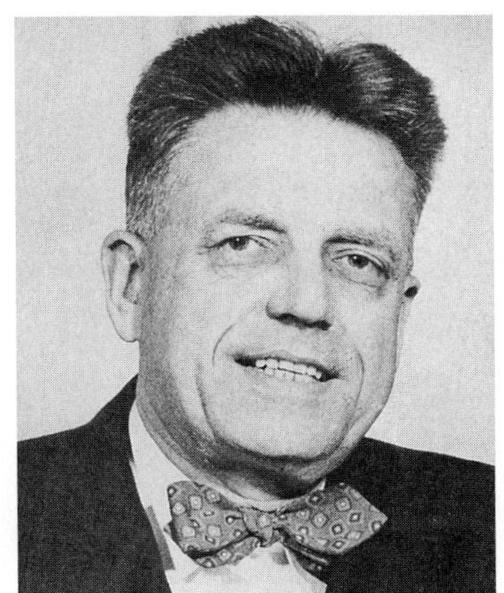

Alfred Kinsey and his colleagues were at the forefront of using scientific methodology to study human sexuality. His research, begun in 1938, was revolutionary in that it covered a wide range of sexual activities and applied statistical methods to sexuality research.

The interviews covered six ways in which males and females achieve orgasm in our culture: masturbation, nocturnal sex dreams and emissions, heterosexual petting, heterosexual premarital intercourse, homosexual intercourse, and sexual contact with animals. The questions focused on nine major areas: social and economic data, marital history, sexuality education, physical and physiological data, nocturnal sex dreams, masturbation, heterosexual history, homosexual history, and animal contacts. Using these highly specific interviews, Kinsey and his associates collected data from only white males and females. They represented rural and urban areas in each state and a range of ages, marital statuses, educational levels, occupations, and religions. The sample contained a disproportionately high number of better-educated people living in cities. All subjects were volunteers. Kinsey's studies may be the best-known example of survey research related to sexuality, but his sample cannot be viewed as representative of the U.S. population.

Sexual Behavior in the Human Male (1948) is based on interviews with 5,300 males, *Sexual Behavior in the Human Female* (1953) on interviews with 5,900 females. Kinsey was not the first researcher in America to conduct a sexual survey by questionnaire or interview. Rather, his contribution to sexuality research was revolutionary in that he covered a wide variety of sexual activities and applied quantitative statistical research methods to sexuality.

Americans had little knowledge about sexual behavior in this culture until Kinsey presented his findings. His conclusions generated a great deal of public reaction. Kinsey concluded that there was a relationship between sexual behaviors and attitudes on the one hand and education and socioeconomic characteristics on the other. In males, the lower the educational level, the higher the premarital activity. For women, the findings were the opposite—the higher the educational level, the more likely the premarital activity. He found that those women who had experienced premarital orgasm were more likely to experience marital orgasm. Most of the married females reported orgasm response through coital and noncoital sexual behavior. Only about 2% of women reported a complete lack of sexual arousal. A great many of Kinsey's subjects reported childhood sexual experiences, which reinforced Freud's belief that sexual expression is experienced in childhood. Kinsey concluded from all the data that people are sexual from early childhood through adulthood.

Since Kinsey's sample comprised a disproportionately large number of educated, urban, Protestant young people, with underrepresentation of less educated, rural, and older persons, his findings were not representative of the population in general. Kinsey defended his work by explaining that the nature of sexual behavior made it hard to get answers from large numbers of people; too many refused. He did ask clubs, groups, and associations for interviews, and he interviewed all willing members.

Despite its limitations, Kinsey's work was hailed as the first large-scale study of sexual behavior. The books had a significant effect on subsequent sexual research and on our society in general by opening the subject of sexuality for discussion and academic study. Despite the criticism it evoked—some of it justified—Kinsey's work was generally acknowledged at the time for its objectivity, scholarly approach, and scope.

Some of Kinsey's major findings are described in the following paragraphs. Keep in mind when reading Kinsey's findings that he had ventured into an area that was taboo in American society—frank and open discussion of sexual matters. His findings influenced a whole generation—that of your parents or, for many of you, your grandparents—by increasing their awareness about what sexual activities were actually being engaged in by Americans. In addition, they prodded people to rethink their own attitudes about these behaviors.

Masturbation Close to 92% of males in Kinsey's sample stated that they had masturbated at some point in their lives, with the highest incidence reported between 16 and 20 years of age; about 62% of all females reported that they had masturbated. The higher the educational level, the greater the incidence of masturbation in both men and women. In both males and females the stronger the religious adherence, the lower the incidence of masturbation.

Nocturnal Dreams About Sex Dreams about sex were experienced by both sexes. From the data Kinsey concluded that 70% of females had dreams about sex. About 90% of the females who reported sex dreams had heterosexual dreams with sexual partners they could not identify. About 37% of 45-year-old women had experienced dreams that led to orgasm. The highest incidence of nocturnal emissions was reported by 71% of single males aged 21 to 25 years.

Heterosexual Petting Kinsey defined *heterosexual petting* as "a deliberate attempt to effect erotic arousal through any physical contact that does not involve intercourse." His study found that 88% of all males had engaged in petting or would engage in some mode of petting before marriage. More than 25% of the males had experienced orgasm through petting before marriage. The highest incidence of heterosexual petting in males occurred between 16 and 20 years of age, with tremendous variation in frequency. Petting in males occurred primarily among those in high school and college, with 92% of males in this group actively involved before marriage.

Kinsey found that 40% of the females in his study had experienced heterosexual petting by 15 years of age, and between 69% and 95% had such an experience by age 18. Petting to the point of orgasm during their late teens was reported by 23% of females. The average frequencies of petting among single females between the ages of 15 and 25 ranged from once a week to once a month, with an average of once in 2 weeks for the typical female. In the total range, 90% of females had some petting experience before marriage.

Premarital Intercourse With regard to heterosexual premarital intercourse, Kinsey found that 22% of all adolescent males had experienced intercourse. Among college males 67% had experienced premarital intercourse. Males of lower social class reported greater frequency of premarital intercourse than those of higher social class. Nearly 50% of the females reported premarital intercourse. About two-thirds of the married females reported sexual orgasm before marriage through any one of five techniques: masturbation, nocturnal dreams, heterosexual petting, heterosexual coitus, and homosexual contacts. At all social levels, males and females who were devoutly religious reported much less premarital intercourse than nondevout subjects. Kinsey also found that people who married earlier had experienced premarital intercourse at a younger age, and those who married later had begun premarital intercourse at a later age.

Homosexual Activity Kinsey found homosexual incidence highest in high school males. About 37% of all males had some homosexual experience between adolescence and old age. Twenty-five percent of females aged 30 years and over had been erotically aroused by other females, and 17% had experienced sexual contact with other females. Female homosexual contact was greatest in the college and graduate school groups.

The Kinsey Institute is still operating. It is called the Kinsey Institute for Research in Sex, Gender, and Reproduction and is located at Indiana University.

William Masters and Virginia Johnson: The Physiology of Sexual Response The research efforts and studies of Masters and Johnson are probably the most widely known and cited of all sex-related data. These researchers were the first to observe people's sexual behaviors in a laboratory setting and to identify physiological changes during sexual arousal. William Masters was a gynecologist and Virginia Johnson a psychologist. Together they were the directors of what was the Reproductive Biology Research Foundation in

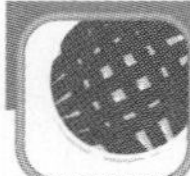

Global DIMENSIONS

The Liu Report: Sexual Behavior in Modern China Dalin Liu and associates (1997) interviewed 23,000 Chinese people over a period of 18 months. The nationwide survey about sexual attitudes and behavior, a Chinese "Kinsey Report," was the first conducted in China. Liu reported the following:

1. For high school students, the mean age of first ejaculation was 14.4 years.
2. College students were highest in their masturbation rates (59% for males and 17% for females) as compared to high school students (13% for males and 5% for females), city married subjects (33% for males and 12% for females), and village married subjects (9% for males and 11% for females).
3. Thirteen percent of the college student males and 6% of the college student females had experienced premarital sexual activity. This compared with 22% of the city married men and 16% of the city married women, and 35% of the village married men and 15% of the village married women.
4. Among all groups, college students had the highest proportion of those who had homosexual behavior (8%) as compared to less than 1% of city married subjects and just over 2% of village married subjects.
5. Sexual satisfaction was reported by 55% of married males and 67% of married females.
6. Ninety-five percent of the college students and 67% of the married subjects felt positively about the female's initiating sexual activity. Four percent of the college students and 11% of the married subjects felt negatively about this idea.
7. Fifty-six percent of college students, as compared to 10% of married subjects, approved of extramarital sexual activity. Thirty-nine percent of the college students and 79% of the married subjects felt very negative about extramarital sexual activity.
8. Most Chinese couples engage in little or no foreplay before initiating intercourse. Many wives report some discomfort during intercourse as a result of insufficient vaginal lubrication.
9. Women are more likely than men to initiate divorce proceedings (three of five divorces are requested by women).

Source: Liu, Dalin, Man Lun Ng, Li Ping Zhou, & Haeberle, E. J. *Sexual behavior in modern China.* New York: Continuum, 1997.

Saint Louis and is now the Masters and Johnson Institute. In 1966 they published their data in *Human Sexual Response,* and in 1970 they published *Human Sexual Inadequacy.*

William Masters began his research in 1954 by talking to prostitutes about female sexual functioning. One of the prostitutes was a woman with a Ph.D. in sociology working as a call girl to supplement her income. This woman told Masters that he would never understand women without an "interpreter." In response to this suggestion, he launched a search for a female research partner, a quest that led him to Virginia Johnson and the establishment of their research team.

Once the two started their research, they realized that prostitutes were not the best subjects for a study of normal sexual response. They then informed university contacts and professionals that they were in search of volunteer study subjects. Of the 1,273 volunteers who initially applied, Masters and Johnson selected 694—276 married couples, 106 unmarried women, and 36 unmarried men. Ninety-eight of the single people had been married previously.

The investigators obtained social and sexual histories for all their subjects, gave them information to explain the studies, and introduced them to the laboratory setting. For experiments involving sexual intercourse, married couples were used as subjects; in studies other than intercourse (such as masturbation and controlled vaginal tests with an artificial phallus), unmarried subjects participated.

Through direct observation, filming, and monitoring with instruments, Masters and Johnson recorded a variety of changes in the physiology of the body in general and in the genitals and reproductive organs in particular. Most of their findings related to physiological responses to sexual arousal that had never before been measured or documented. Their major finding, generally accepted as true since the results were published, was the existence of a cycle of physiological events in response to sexual stimulation. The whole cycle, known as the *human sexual response,* occurs in both sexes in four phases, always in order: excitement, plateau, orgasm, and resolution. (The human sexual response cycle is discussed in detail in Chapter 7.) This research showed that males and females have many similar responses, as well as responses specific to the physiology of each sex. The research of Masters and Johnson now serves as the basis for modern therapy, education, and counseling; cross-disciplinary research; and general information about sexual functioning. Both professionals and nonprofessionals can discuss sexual behavior and sexuality more knowledgeably since the publication of *Human Sexual Response.*

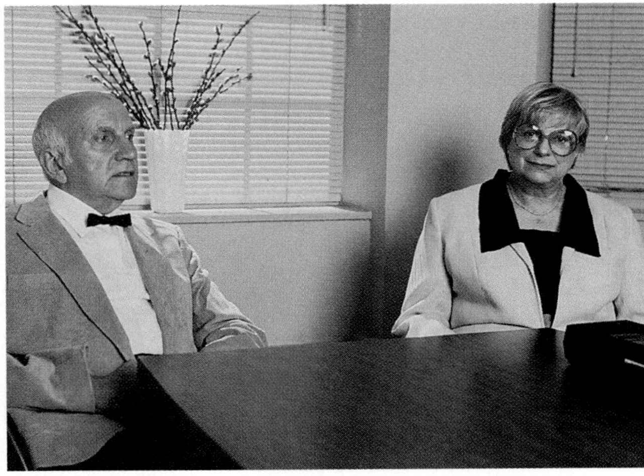

William Masters and Virginia Johnson were the first sexuality researchers to observe people's sexual behaviors in a laboratory setting. Among their many contributions to sexuality research is the human sexual response cycle (Chapter 7).

The second major Masters and Johnson study, *Human Sexual Inadequacy,* was published in 1970. This study of sexual dysfunction (a topic discussed in Chapter 15) put the relationship of the physiology and the psychology of sexual response in sharper focus. Causes of sexual dysfunction, the relationship of the partners who experienced dysfunction, and sexual interaction in general were the concerns of this book. Masters and Johnson defined *sexual dysfunction* as an inability to respond emotionally and physically to sexual arousal. They were able to give a range of dysfunctions, defining six basic types—three for women and three for men. The dysfunctions were also defined in terms of the phases of the sexual response cycle. The physiological, psychological, and emotional (or situational) causes were suggested and defined, with treatment developed to deal with the causes and symptoms presented. Their research has provided a great deal of knowledge of physiological changes that occur in the body during sexual activities.

In doing the research that was published as *Human Sexual Response,* Masters and Johnson studied a group that was not representative of the overall American population. They were volunteers who were better educated than average, had all been sexually active, and were mainly white. But because these researchers were concerned primarily with observing and measuring physiological responses, a true representation of the population may not be as crucial as it could be in other studies.

In 1980 two psychologists, Bernie Zilbergeld and Michael Evans, wrote a critical review of the research of Masters and Johnson. They had examined their research methods in order to replicate their research using a different population group. (**Replication** plays an important role in research. When one does research the methodology should be described clearly and specifically so other researchers can replicate it and verify findings.) Zilbergeld and Evans questioned Masters and Johnson's conclusions about the efficacy of their treatments for sexual dysfunctions, the criteria they used to define the low relapse rates in patients, and the small number of patients who were followed up.

replication
Repetition of a research study done in the same way as the previous study.

In 1979 Masters and Johnson published *Homosexuality in Perspective.* This study of the sexual response of homosexuals added much information to the human sexuality literature. The data were gathered by studying the sexual response cycles of 38 lesbian couples and 42 male homosexual couples between 1957 and 1970. The researchers reported that there was little difference between homosexuals and heterosexuals in sexual functioning and response to sexual stimulation. However, homosexuals appeared to communicate with partners more effectively during sexual activity than heterosexuals. The broadest conclusion reported in this publication was that homosexuality is not a disease and that homosexuals, like heterosexuals, are individuals who have sexual concerns.

Homosexuals who had problems concerning their homosexuality were studied as well. Some of these individuals expressed a desire to learn to function within the lifestyle more effectively, and some professed a desire to change to a heterosexual lifestyle.

Masters and Johnson and You The work of Masters and Johnson affects your sexual life in many ways. Both you and your partner can now better understand your bodies' responses to sexual stimulation. Knowing that you proceed through several identifiable phases during your sexual response cycle (see Chapter 7) will make you and/or any sexual partner more willing to proceed at a sexual pace in synchrony with your physiology. The results will be greater sexual satisfaction and, as we shall see in Chapter 15, less sexual dysfunction. Because of the work of Masters and Johnson and that of others motivated by Masters and Johnson's studies, a person experiencing problems with sexual functioning has access to a whole warehouse of effective sexual therapy modalities. As with the work of Kinsey, the studies of Masters and Johnson not only broke ground for sexual research as a profession, but also produced some very useful information for the general public.

Robert Sorenson: Adolescent Sexuality in the 1970s

In 1973 Robert Sorenson published *Adolescent Sexuality in Contemporary America*, in which he reported the data gathered from approximately 400 adolescents, 13 to 19 years of age. Parental permission was required for participation, because many of the potential subjects were minors. Forty percent of adults refused permission for their teenagers to participate, and some teenagers themselves refused participation, a situation that highlights the difficulty of conducting sexuality research. Sorenson's was the first nationwide study of adolescent sexual behavior since Kinsey's study. His findings showed a dramatic increase in premarital coitus among adolescents in America: 45% of girls and 60% of boys in the study had participated by age 19. He reported that 70% of the total U.S. population in their late teens were involved in premarital intercourse. Sorenson also found that teenagers were concerned with values, communication, and emotional aspects of sexual activity. As a whole teens seek love, are tolerant or acceptant of the sexual behavior of their peers, and, although not ready for commitment, have feelings for a partner.

Sorenson used good sampling procedures. However, because of parental and adolescent refusal to participate, a question is raised concerning the possible differences between teenagers who did and did not participate. Did restrictive parents affect the attitudes of the children who did not participate? Are, then, the responses of those who did participate really representative of teenagers in America? Furthermore, Sorenson's questionnaire was 38 pages long, and its length may have influenced the accuracy of responses, particularly to the later items in the instrument.

Melvin Zelnik and John Kantner: Sexual Behavior of Young Women

In 1971, 1976, and 1979, Melvin Zelnik and John Kantner studied the sexual behavior of white and black American females aged 15 to 19 years. They gath-

Myth vs Fact

Myth: Most women prefer a sexual partner who has a large penis.
Fact: Surveys indicate this is not true. Plus, we know that a female's vagina can adjust to different size penises and that there is far less difference in the sizes of erect penises than of soft penises.

Myth: Sexual activity usually ends soon after age 60.
Fact: Most people older than 60 years in relatively good health continue to participate in many forms of sexual activity.

Myth: Masturbation is physically harmful.
Fact: Masturbation does not harm the body in any way.

Myth: Anal intercourse between uninfected people can transmit human immunodeficiency virus (HIV).
Fact: If there is no infection, there will be no HIV transmission. To contract acquired immunodeficiency syndrome (AIDS) a person must first be infected with HIV.

Myth: Most husbands have extramarital affairs.
Fact: The rates may vary in different studies, but the National Health and Social Life Survey reported that 25% of men and 15% of women had extramarital affairs.

Myth: Few women masturbate.
Fact: Most men and women, married and unmarried, occasionally masturbate. About 50–68% of females masturbate at least once a month.

Myth: Most normal women have orgasms from penile thrusting alone.
Fact: Different women prefer different kinds of stimulation. Many do not reach orgasm from penile thrusting alone.

Myth: A man cannot have an orgasm without an erection.
Fact: He can have an orgasm even if he does not have an erection.

ered from several hundred women data on sexual activity, contraceptive use, premarital pregnancy, and abortion, using probability sampling techniques. It was found that in 1976 1 in 5 American women had experienced sexual intercourse by age 16 and two-thirds by age 19. The numbers for each age group were higher than in the 1971 group. Also in 1976, 1 in 10 young women reported at least one pregnancy by age 17, and 1 in 4 by age 19. Black teenage women were more likely to become pregnant than white teenage women, although the numbers of whites who became pregnant were growing because of increasing sexual activity. White women, however, made greater use of abortion services, which resulted in a decline in births to whites between 1971 and 1976. The use of contraception also increased between 1971 and 1976. Zelnik and Kantner further found that the older a woman was at first intercourse, the more likely it was that she used contraception.

In 1980 Zelnik and Kantner published the combined results of their three studies. The incidence of premarital intercourse for women was above 30% in 1971, 43% in 1976, and 50% in 1979. The proportion of coital-experienced whites increased from 26% in 1971 to 38% in 1976 and to 47% in 1979. The proportion of coital-experienced blacks increased from 54% in 1971 to 66% in both 1976 and 1979. Blacks were more likely to initiate coitus 1 year earlier than whites; the average age of the men at first intercourse was 15.5 years for blacks and 16.4 years for whites. The premarital pregnancy rate among teenagers was 9% in 1971, 13% in 1976, and 16% in 1979.

Contraceptive methods used in 1976 and 1979 differed as well. Use of the pill and intrauterine device (IUD) declined by 41% in the 3 years, whereas use of withdrawal and the rhythm method rose by 86%. In 1976 the first methods used by teenagers who ever practiced contraception were, in order of frequency, condom, pill, and withdrawal; in 1979 they were withdrawal, condom, and pill. Although less effective methods were being used in 1979, it was evident that more teenagers were using some method of contraception than in 1976. Yet pregnancy rates continued to climb. This may be due to earlier exposure to intercourse, less use of the most effective contraceptive method (the pill), and factors (behavioral and otherwise) that are still not known.

Zelnik and Kantner revealed much information about the sexual experiences of and the contraceptive use by teenage women in the 1970s, showing a consistent increase in coital activity and, despite greater use of contraception in 1979, an increase in the pregnancy rate.

Alan Bell and Martin Weinberg: Homosexuality

Alan Bell and Martin Weinberg studied the sexual lives of homosexual men and women in the San Francisco area and published their findings in 1978 under the title *Homosexualities: A Study of Diversities Among Men and Women.* The 979 men and women who made up the sample were from divergent social, economic, and occupational strata. A matched sample of 477 homosexuals was not random, because subjects were recruited from gay organizations and bars and thus did not represent homosexuals in general. Still this broad study of the lifestyles of homosexuals has contributed much to our knowledge.

Bell and Weinberg concluded that the term *homosexual* should really be *homosexualities,* because they found that distinct types of relationships exist among homosexuals. They developed the following categories of homosexual relationships: (1) closed couples—those living together in committed, stable relationships; (2) open couples—those living together with less emotional involvement and dependency and having intercourse outside the relationship; (3) functionals—sexually active people uncommitted to any partner; (4) dysfunctionals—sexually active people with sexual problems who were unhappy about being homosexual; and (5) asexuals—those who were not happy about being homosexual and who were less active sexually.

Myth vs Fact

Myth: Erectile dysfunction (sometimes referred to as "impotence" by the layperson) usually cannot be treated successfully.

Fact: With counseling, medical treatments, surgical treatments, and better sexual knowledge alone or in combination, most instances of erectile dysfunction can be treated.

June Reinisch and Ruth Beasley found these nine myths to be commonly believed. More information about these myths can be found in later chapters in this book and in their book *The Kinsey Institute new report on sex* (1991). New York: St. Martin's.

Bell and Weinberg found that homosexual and heterosexual men were much alike, though homosexuals tended to be lonelier and have less self-esteem. Lesbians were also like heterosexual women, though they too differed with respect to self-esteem. The investigators found that male homosexuals tended to be more promiscuous than heterosexual men but that lesbians differed from male homosexuals in that they tended to have more stable relationships and fewer partners.

This is one of the most comprehensive studies of homosexual lifestyles. One of Bell and Weinberg's important conclusions is that homosexuals who are adjusted to their lifestyle "are no more distressed psychologically than are heterosexual men and women" (Bell & Weinberg, 1978).

Bell and Weinberg collaborated with S. K. Hammersmith and published their results in 1981 in *Sexual Preference: Its Development in Men and Women.* They report that sexual preference is not greatly influenced by parenting practices or other psychosocial influences. Although they are not specific about causal factors, they suggest there is a biological reason for sexual orientation. The topic of homosexuality is covered in detail in Chapter 11.

Philip Blumstein and Pepper Schwartz: Relationships Among Couples

In 1983 Philip Blumstein and Pepper Schwartz published *American Couples,* which contained information about trends in couples, married and cohabiting, heterosexual and homosexual. They distributed questionnaires to 11,000 couples recruited from television, radio, and newspaper advertisements. Their 55% response rate resulted in a sample of 4,314 heterosexual couples and 1,757 homosexual couples (969 gay males and 788 lesbians). Their well-designed questionnaire, high response rate, and large national sample are obvious strengths. As with almost any survey about sexuality, results are criticized for underrepresentation of some population groups.

Both heterosexual and homosexual cohabiting couples seemed to have fewer difficulties in their relationships than married heterosexual couples. It was hypothesized that this occurred because cohabitation is based more on equal participation by both partners. Blumstein and Schwartz also found that it was very rare to find serious problems in relationships in which sexual activity was quite regular. It would be interesting to know whether the regular sexual activity contributed to the positive relationship, or vice versa. What do you think?

The National Health and Social Life Survey

A University of Chicago research team conducted the first comprehensive survey of adult sexual behavior since Kinsey's research (Laumann, et al., 1994). The National Health and Social Life Survey (NHSLS) was designed to assess the incidence and prevalence of a broad range of sexual practices and attitudes within the U.S. population.

When the AIDS epidemic began in the 1980s, experts were not well informed about contemporary sexual practices. Believing that such data might help prevent the spread of HIV, in 1987 an agency within the U.S. Department of Health and Human Services asked for proposals to study adult sexual attitudes and practices. The research team from the University of Chicago was awarded a grant in 1988 to support a survey of 20,000 people.

As mentioned earlier, after 2 years of planning, federal funds for the project were withdrawn. In 1991, because conservative members of Congress were offended by the idea of using government funds for research on sexual behavior, legislation was passed to eliminate federal funding for such studies.

The research team then obtained funding from several private foundations. They were able to proceed, but with a much smaller sample. After sampling techniques were used to select a representative sample of 4,369 18- to 59-year-old Americans, 79% of the sample agreed to participate. This gave them a sample size of 3,432.

Although they did have a high participation rate, they had been forced to limit their sample size. This resulted in a population that was representative of white Americans, black Americans, and Hispanic Americans; however, there were too few representatives of other groups to provide useful information about them.

The research team trained 220 professional interviewers, and all 3,432 subjects were interviewed face-to-face. The interviewers made sure the respondents understood all questions. The questionnaire also had internal checks to measure consistency of answers and to validate the responses.

You will see references to NHSLS data in other parts of this book, and here are a few examples of findings: (1) Of married persons 93.7% had had only one sexual partner in the last year as compared with 38% of those never married and not cohabitating; (2) married people were much more likely than singles to report being extremely or very happy; (3) 9.1% of men and 4.3% of women reported engaging in any same-sex activity since puberty (for nearly half of these men the behavior occurred only before the age of 18 years). About 1.4% of the women and 2.8% of the men reported a homosexual identity.

Popular Literature

Nancy Friday: What Do Women and Men Fantasize About?

Nancy Friday, rather than asking people about their behavior, asked about their imaginations and fantasies. She wrote two books, *My Secret Garden* (1973) and *Forbidden Flowers* (1975), in which she compiled the many sexual fantasies shared by women. Friday found that women wanted to share their experiences and to hear the experiences of others. Society permitted men to discuss sexuality with other men; women believed they had not been given this privilege. She asserted that "women needed and were waiting for some kind of yardstick against which to measure ourselves" (Friday, 1973). These women wrote to Friday and discussed fantasies about intimacy, intercourse, sexual techniques, masturbation, and their feelings about fantasizing.

On the last page of *Forbidden Flowers,* Friday asked male readers to send her descriptions of their sexual fantasies. She received letters from more than 3,000 men describing fantasies related to masturbation, sexual techniques, sharing, voyeurism, and exhibitionism, and she published a selection of them in the book *Men in Love* (1980). Men's fantasies revealed lust, rage, anger, compassion, eroticism, loving and caring feelings, and a variety of attitudes about women and other men.

Because Friday's research was anecdotal, no statistical inference could be made. Women and men saw themselves involved in the whole spectrum of sexual activity and expressed a variety of feelings about interpersonal relations. Both genders were imaginative, and their fantasies defied stereotyping.

Morton Hunt: Urban Adult Sexual Behavior

Early in the 1970s the Playboy Foundation funded a study of contemporary sexual behavior. Morton Hunt conducted this study and reported his findings in the book *Sexual Behavior in the 1970s* (1974). In this study 24 cities were selected as representative of urban America, and subjects were randomly chosen from telephone directories in each city. The 2,026 subjects (1,044 females and 982 males) met in small groups to discuss sexual behaviors. After participating in the discussion, they were asked to complete a

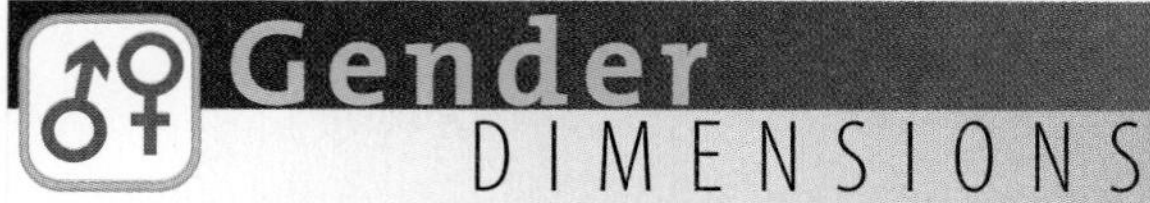

Gender DIMENSIONS

Differences in Research Results

When reviewing research results, researchers have historically commonly found relatively large differences between genders in the amount of heterosexual sexual behavior. Even when comparing the amounts for males and females of the same age, it is common to see much higher rates for males than females. The reasons for this are not known, but this situation makes for interesting discussion because one must wonder who the males are having heterosexual behavior with if the numbers are much smaller for females.

Gender differences also often exist when it comes to reasons for first sexual intercourse (Laumann, et al., 1994). For example, among those females who wanted their first vaginal intercourse to happen when it did, just over half the males were motivated by a curiosity about sexual behavior, but a little less than one-quarter of the females were. However, about one-quarter of the males had intercourse because of affection for their partner, whereas 47.5% of the females did it for this reason. Only about 3% of the females said that physical pleasure was their main reason, compared to about four times as many men (12%) who said this.

Watch for these kinds of comparisons as you consider research on sexuality behavior and think about reasons why gender differences might exist.

questionnaire. Four separate questionnaire forms were used, each related to the subjects' marital status: unmarried women, married women, unmarried men, married men. There were 1,000 to 1,200 items to be answered, depending on the individual's status.

Hunt was criticized for not informing participants in advance of the length of the questionnaire. Another limitation of this study was the possibility that the discussions in which subjects participated before filling out the questionnaire could have influenced their responses. In addition, because sampling from the telephone directory eliminated individuals with unlisted numbers, those who could not afford telephone service, and those who lived in institutions (such as colleges), the resulting group was considered unrepresentative of the total population. Because 80% of the people contacted refused to participate, generalizing of this survey was further limited. Nevertheless Hunt's study did gather some new data on adult sexual practices. It found a wider variety of coital positions, longer foreplay and coital duration, more common occurrence of premarital sexual encounters, a greater acceptance of oral–genital sexual behavior, and more frequent marital sexual intercourse than previous studies had reported.

Carol Tavris and Susan Sadd: The Redbook *Report on Women*

"The *Redbook* Report on Female Sexuality," which focused on the sexual practices of women, was written from data gathered from a 60-item multiple-choice questionnaire that appeared in the October 1974 issue of *Redbook*. More than 100,000 female readers responded, and results were published in the September and October 1975 issues. Although again the sample consisted of volunteers, raising the question of how representative it was of the general population, the size of the sample alone made it noteworthy. The major findings of the report were that the women who responded were active sexually, that they frequently initiated sexual activity, that almost all respondents had experienced oral–genital sexual behavior, that a third had been involved in extramarital sexual behavior, and that religion influenced their participation in sexual activities (the more deeply religious reported less sexual activity). A most interesting point in this study was an apparent relationship between premarital intercourse and extramarital intercourse. The younger a respondent had been at the time of her initial premarital sexual involvement, the more probable was her involvement in extramarital intercourse. Most of the women involved in extramarital intercourse reported that such affairs were casual, did not affect the marriage, and were rarely continued.

***Shere Hite: Women's Sexuality, Men's Sexuality, and* Women and Love** Between 1972 and 1976, when the findings were published in *The Hite Report,* Shere Hite mailed more than 100,000 60-item essay-type questionnaires to such women's groups as the National Organization for Women, university women's organizations, and women's newsletters. She also placed notices in *The Village Voice, Mademoiselle, Brides, Ms.,* and *Oui* magazines asking women to send for questionnaires. Hite received completed questionnaires from 3,109 women, who expressed their personal feelings about masturbation, orgasm, intercourse, clitoral stimulation, lesbianism, sexual slavery (satisfying males' needs during sexual activity and ignoring their own needs), and the sexual revolution. Many women reported that they experienced orgasm more frequently from clitoral stimulation than from coitus and that they achieved deep orgasm from masturbation. Furthermore, they described a history of orgasm in general. Of the sample, 8% preferred sexual activity with other women, 53% said that they preferred sexual activity with themselves, and 17% preferred no sexual activity at all. Although the question was not directly asked, many women offered the information that they were curious about and might be interested in a sexual encounter with another woman. The majority of older women said that sexual pleasure increased with age, but many respondents older than 45 years reported difficulty in finding new sexual partners.

The findings published in *The Hite Report* were of great interest, for despite the fact that only a relatively small portion of the total female population was reached, no study had previously afforded such large numbers of women the opportunity to express their preferences and desires in matters of sexuality. However, remember that Hite recruited her subjects by inserting a notice in magazines such as *Oui, The Village Voice, Ms.,* and *Mademoiselle.* Rather than being representative of all women, this small, select group of women is considered to be what is called a biased sample. Hite did not statistically analyze her data; rather, she used what are described as anecdotal reports—essays written by individuals describing their sexual activities and the feelings they experienced.

In 1981 Hite published *The Hite Report on Male Sexuality* using the same anecdotal analysis, this time presenting the views of 7,200 men. Men preferred intercourse to masturbation or oral–genital sexual activity. They were generally unaware that women could achieve orgasm by means other than intercourse. They expressed ignorance of when a female orgasm occurs and expressed anxious feelings about not knowing. Some of the males expressed anger over always being the initiators of sexual activity yet volunteered that sexually aggressive women were difficult for them to deal with. Many men stated that they grew up not being allowed to express themselves emotionally, for the culture demanded that men be strong and showing emotion was not defined as indicating strength. Again, because the Hite study of males was anecdotal, it is not considered to be of statistical note.

In 1987 Hite published *Women and Love: A Cultural Revolution in Progress.* After spending 7 years analyzing surveys from 4,500 women, she concluded that women are fed up with men. Despite women's liberation and the sexual revolution, Hite reported that women remain oppressed, and even abused, by men. Four of five women in her study said they still had to fight

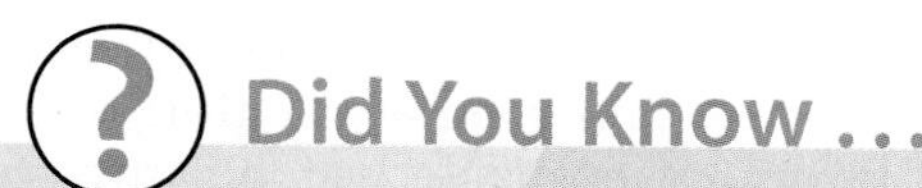

Remember that the main purpose of sexual themes in newspapers, magazines, and on radio and TV may be to sell newspapers and magazines and raise ratings of the programs. Also, there is a motivation to entertain people. It may be possible to get some sound information about sexuality through these sources; however, caution is needed if you are going to be a wise consumer. It is probably healthy to be skeptical until you have a chance to verify the information in accepted professional journals.

for their rights within relationships, 87% said that men became more emotionally dependent than women, 92% complained that men communicate with women in language that indicates "condescending, judgmental attitudes," 95% reported forms of "emotional and psychological harassment," 79% said they seriously question whether they should put so much energy into love relationships, 98% wished for more verbal closeness with male partners, 70% of the women married 5 years or more said they had extramarital affairs more often for emotional closeness than for sexual activity, and 87% of the married women said they have their deepest emotional relationship with a woman friend.

Many respectable researchers, both male and female, questioned Hite's findings. Criticisms pointed to a highly self-selected sample—only a 4.5% return from more than 100,000 questionnaires distributed to a variety of women's groups in 43 states—and a likely disproportion of unhappy people, because unhappy people were probably more willing to answer the questions than were happy people. Hite indicated a desire for men to see what women feel works in relationships, but others feared that Hite's book encouraged women to take the easy way out and blame everything on men.

Lorna Sarrel and Philip Sarrel: The Redbook *Report on Sexual Relationships*

In 1980 *Redbook* magazine published a sexuality questionnaire to which approximately 20,000 women and 6,000 men responded. The questionnaire was primarily concerned with the quality of relationships and the interpersonal communication of couples. More than half of the men (60%) and less than half of the women said that sharing feelings was very important to their relationships. Seventy-five percent of those who answered the questionnaire rated their current sexual relationships as being good or excellent. Fifteen percent reported sexual dysfunction, and these people said that they spoke about sexuality with their partner very little. Of particular interest is the fact that 40% of men and women who were parents said that lack of privacy interfered in some way with their enjoyment of sexual activity. Many individuals accepted sexual activity to satisfy a partner even if they did not want to make love at the time, and half of those who did said they "end up enjoying it."

This study is not indicative of sexual relationships of the population in general, because the readership of *Redbook* in 1980 tended to be youthful, married, better educated, and financially more secure than the general population. However, these people do represent a very large group of our population and they certainly do show an interest in sexual matters, are comfortable with the subject, and possess a willingness to discuss sexuality and interpersonal relationships. It is fair to believe that they did represent many couples in the society (Sarrel & Sarrel, 1980).

June Reinisch and Ruth Beasley: The Kinsey Institute New Report on Sex

The inclusion of a 1991 book within our popular literature section may be debatable, but it is indeed written for the general public. In fact, one of its authors said, "It's a great book to have in the bathroom, when you have time to read bits and pieces. It is designed to be a 'friendly encyclopedia,' telling readers in question-and-answer format almost everything they wanted to know about sexuality" (Dolan, 1990).

Research from the Kinsey Institute and the results of a Roper poll of 2,000 adults show that knowledge about sexuality is still at a very low level. For example, half of the adults tested did not know that a lubricant such as Vaseline or baby oil can cause microscopic holes in a condom or a diaphragm in as little as 60 seconds. This lack of understanding hardly contributes to safer sex practices.

Of women aged 30 to 44 years, only 55% received a passing grade on the test, and 52% of men in the same age group did. Men answered correctly more often on matters of sexual practices, and women knew more about their own sexual health. People living in the Midwest had the highest scores, and those in the South and the Northeast had the lowest.

Seventeen *Magazine and The Kaiser Family Foundation: SexSmarts Survey on Teen Sexual Behavior*

The latest in a series of surveys of teens aged 15–17 years found that only 1 in 10 teens who have had sexual intercourse discussed his or her sexual plans with parents ahead of time, and more than a third did not tell their parents about their sexual history at all. Forty-eight percent of all survey respondents and 56% of sexually active respondents never talked with a parent about "how to know when you are ready to have sex." Eighty percent of respondents said teens do not discuss sexual issues with their parents because they worry that their parents will disapprove or will assume that they are already participating in sexual behavior if they discuss the subject with them (Kaiser Family Foundation and *Seventeen* magazine release latest SexSmarts Survey on teen sexual behavior, 2002).

Eighty-four percent of all respondents said they had never talked with a health care provider about how to know when one is prepared for sexual behavior. More than two-thirds had not discussed contraception, HIV and AIDS, condoms, or STIs with a health care provider. Nearly two-thirds had spoken with a sexual partner about "what they are comfortable doing sexually." Fifty-eight percent had never discussed STIs with a partner, 56% had never discussed HIV and AIDS with a partner, and 53% of all respondents and 28% of sexually active teens had never discussed contraception with a partner. Most cited lack of knowledge about sexual issues, fear of what a partner might think, and embarrassment as reasons they do not discuss sexual issues with partners.

Other Examples of Recent Research

It is almost impossible to count the many research studies related to human sexuality done in recent years. And until these studies stand the test of time, it is difficult to tell which, if any, might become classics. The following is a summary of selected, more recent, research studies.

Studies on Premarital Sexual Attitudes and Behavior

Using data collected from undergraduate students at a small southern university between 1970 and 1981, Earle and Perricone (1986) found significant increases in rates of premarital intercourse, significant decreases in average age at first experience, and significant increases in average number of part-

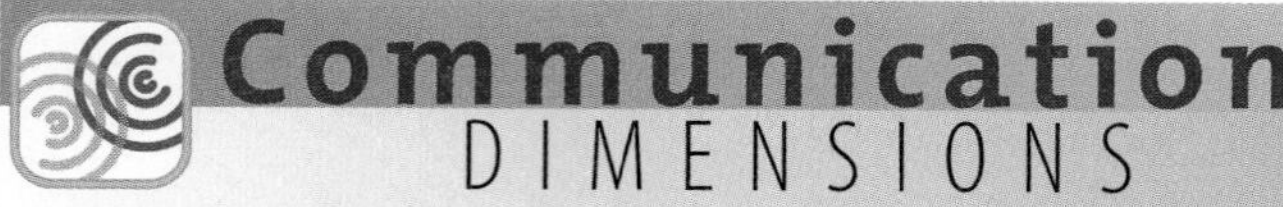

Talking About Sexuality Research Results

It is not easy to analyze findings of sexual research, and it is common to hear others talking about some "new findings" they just heard about. What if someone tells you about some sexual "research" and some interesting findings? What can you suggest to help the person (and you) analyze whether or not the research seems sound? Here are some possibilities for questions and conversational points.

- Was the scientific method used? This method does not rely just on testimonials or someone's opinion. It requires proper sampling techniques, accurate measurement and observation, and appropriate statistical analysis of the findings to reach valid conclusions.
- Is the study replicable? One study, taken alone, seldom proves anything. To be valid, one researcher's findings must be repeatable by others.
- Have the research findings been properly used? For example, conclusions based on data from one population may not apply to another population, and the results from animal studies cannot be applied with certainty to humans.
- Were the proper statistics used and were they used correctly? Many people tend to accept statistical data without question, although statistical errors do occur.
- What is the competency of the author or researcher? Does the person have a record of excellent previous research? What kinds of expertise does the author or researcher have?
- Has the research been reviewed by peers? Peer review is the process in which the work of a scientist is reviewed by others who have equal or superior knowledge. It may be done while the study is being developed or afterward, as when results of the study are being considered for publication in a scientific journal.

Even these questions will not guarantee appropriate judgments about the accuracy of sexual research, but it can be very helpful to see whether there are good answers to them. They may also inspire some very interesting conversation.

ners. Although differences between males and females still existed, the differences were much more evident in attitudes than in behavior.

Also looking at trends over time, Sherwin and Corbett (1985) examined changes in sexual norms at the same university in 1963, 1971, and 1978. Campus sexual norms did become more liberal, but they did not change from "nothing" to "anything goes." Increased expectations of sexual intimacy were more noticeable in male–female relationships that involved affection and commitment rather than in casual relationships. Female behaviors changed more during the 15-year period from 1963 to 1978 than did those of males. Hofferth, Kahn, and Baldwin (1987) reported that, during that period, levels of sexual experience had increased among both black and white teenage women. Although the rate has increased over this period, a leveling off has since occurred.

Newcomer and Udry (1987) reported that females living in a mother-only home were more likely to participate in premarital intercourse, but the same was not true for boys. Fisher (1986) found no significant differences in sexual attitudes, knowledge, or contraceptive choices of young people who communicated well with their parents about sexuality as compared to those who did not communicate well with parents. Moore, Peterson, and Furstenberg (1986) found that females in a traditional two-parent home who communicated well with their parents about sexuality were less likely to have intercourse.

Roche (1986) investigated what people think is proper premarital sexual behavior, what they do, and what they think others do at various stages of dating. The persons questioned were most restrictive in what they believed was proper conduct, more permissive in their reported behavior, and most permissive in their perception of what others were doing. In the early stages of dating, males' and females' attitudes differed greatly about what was considered proper behavior.

Wyatt, Peters, and Guthrie (1988a & 1988b) compared their data with Kinsey's data, which were approximately 40 years older. They found that their female subjects began intercourse earlier, were less likely to report that their first partner was a fiancé or husband, reported a higher number of sexual partners, and participated in a broader range of sexual behaviors. Women in this study were also more likely to report instances of child sexual abuse. These findings were the same for both white and black females.

DeBuono and colleagues (1990) concluded that the sexual behavior of college women changed very little from 1975 to 1989. They found no significant changes in the proportion of women who were sexually experienced, in the sexually active women's average number of male partners, or in the proportion of women engaging in high-risk sexual practices. However, the proportion of sexually experienced women who regularly used condoms rose from 6% in 1975 to 25% in 1989. And although this percentage indicates increased attention to safer sexual behavior, 25% is still very low.

Forrest and Singh (1990) compared 1988 data from the National Survey of Family Growth with 1982 data and concluded that the proportion of U.S. women aged 15 to 44 years who had sexual intercourse rose slightly, from 86% to 89%. The proportion of sexually active teenagers rose from 47% to 53%. Thirty-four percent of women 18 to 19 years and half of all males the same age had had multiple partners in a 1-year period.

Data from the U.S. Department of Health and Human Services (Premarital sexual experience among adolescent women—United States, 1970–1988, 1991) indicated that the proportion of adolescent women (15 to 19 years old) who reported having premarital intercourse increased steadily from 28.6% in 1970 to 51.5% in 1988. The largest relative increase occurred among those 15 years of age (from 4.6% in 1970 to 25.6% in 1988). It was also found that the initiation of sexual intercourse early in life is associated with an increased number of sexual partners and a greater risk for sexually transmitted infections.

Sroka (1991) summarized other research studies and provided valuable insights. For example, the average age for first-time sexual intercourse in this country is 16 years for females and 15.5 for males. Every 30 seconds a teenage girl becomes pregnant, and every 13 seconds a teenager contracts a sexually transmitted infection. There are an estimated 1 million teenage pregnancies a year, and 3 million teenagers—one of six—contract a sexually transmitted infection each year. AIDS is the leading cause of death for those aged 15 to 24 years.

Rubinson and DeRubertis (1991) studied trends in sexual attitudes and behaviors of a college population over a 15-year period. Eighty-nine percent of the males and 70% of the females reported having engaged in premarital intercourse. The most frequent age at first intercourse was 17 years. Study results indicated that both males and females tended to have fairly liberal attitudes about premarital sexual intercourse, and these remained steady over time. One changing trend was that actual intercourse behavior, unlike 15 years earlier, began to reflect attitudes and become more liberal.

In 1994 the Sexuality Information and Education Council of the United States (SIECUS) reported the findings from a national telephone survey of 503 high school students in grades 9–12. More than three-quarters had engaged in "deep kissing," more than half in "petting," and more than one-third in sexual intercourse. However, only 57% always used a condom. Among sexually active teens, the average age at the time of first intercourse was just below 15 years. In fact, 40% of all sexually active teens experienced sexual intercourse at the age of 14 years or younger. The average number of sexual partners among all sexually active teens was 2.7, and 21% had had four or more partners.

In 1995 de Gaston, Jensen, and Weed reported the results of a survey of 1,228 parochial school students in the eastern United States. Most of the students were Roman Catholic, and 75% attended church at least once weekly. About 75% of the students had not yet participated in sexual intercourse. Of those who were sexually active, nearly half reported first sexual intercourse before age 14 years. Contrary to the authors' expectations, only 3.5% reported forced sexual intercourse, and 13.3% reported pressured sexual activity at the time of their first intercourse. Most activity (81.1%) was voluntary and desired by both partners. Females were twice as likely as males to wish they had waited.

In 1996 Sprecher and Hatfield reported on the sexual attitudes of 1,043 U.S. college students. They found that men were more tolerant of their own sexual behavior than that of other men, but women were less permissive when judging their own behavior than when judging that of other women. Men tended to endorse a traditional double standard of sexual behavior for early relationship stages; however, women were not willing to accept this gender-based standard.

Sprecher and Hatfield (1996) also compared U.S. sexual standards with those in Russia (401 subjects) and Japan (223 subjects). It was evident that people's sexual standards were influenced by culture and gender. American students were the most tolerant of premarital sexual intercourse; the Japanese were the least tolerant. In the United States and Russia, men were far more permissive than were women; in Japan, men and women did not differ in their sexual permissiveness. Russian students were most likely to endorse a double standard; American students were least likely to advocate such a dual standard. Whereas in the United States men were far more willing than were women to accept a traditional double standard, in Russia and Japan men and women were equally likely to accept or reject the double standard.

As part of the Youth Risk Behavior Surveillance System (YRBS), in 1995 the Centers for Disease Control and Prevention surveyed 10,094 students in grades 9–12 (Centers for Disease Control and Prevention, 1996). Fifty-three percent of the students had had sexual intercourse. Black students (73.4%) were significantly more likely than white (48.9%) and Hispanic students (57.6%) to have had sexual intercourse. Nine percent of the students had initiated sexual intercourse before age 13 years. Thirty-eight percent of the students had had sexual intercourse during the 3 months preceding the survey.

In 1997 the Centers for Disease Control updated the YRBS and surveyed 16,262 students in grades 9–12 (Centers for Disease Control and Prevention, 1998). This time 48.4% of the students had had sexual intercourse. Black students (72.7%) were significantly more likely than white (43.6%) and Hispanic students (52.2%) to have had sexual intercourse. Just above 7% of the students had initiated sexual intercourse before age 13 years. Thirty-four percent of the students had had sexual intercourse during the 3 months preceding the survey. In each instance, you will note that the numbers are slightly smaller than the 1996 YRBS numbers. It would be too soon to conclude that rates of sexual intercourse are going down for U.S. students in grades 9–12; however, it is through repeated studies like this that we can eventually see trends.

In 1997, 218 students aged 13–18 years were asked their reasons for initiating or postponing the onset of sexual intercourse (Alexander & Hickner,

1997). Reasons for engaging in first intercourse reflected both active choices and loss of control. Reasons stated for refraining included fear of pregnancy and sexually transmitted infections, lack of developmental readiness and opportunity, and social sanctions. Morality was cited infrequently as a reason for postponing sexual behavior.

In 1998 the Office of Population Affairs of the U.S. Department of Health and Human Services provided information about adolescent sexual activity (U.S. Department of Health and Human Services, 1998b). In regard to trends, the office reported that the number of females aged 15–19 years who had experienced sexual intercourse in 1970 was 29%, and in 1980 it was 42%. Data for the first half of the 1980s seemed to level off (44%), but another increase was shown for 1988 (52%). Data for 1995 showed another leveling off. For 17- to 19-year-old males, data showed an increase in the proportion of those who had ever had sexual intercourse from 66% in 1979, to 76% in 1988, to 82% in 1990.

In 1997 Secretary of Health and Human Services Donna E. Shalala announced that the percentage of teenagers who had had sexual intercourse had declined for the first time after increasing steadily for more than two decades (U.S. Department of Health and Human Services, 1998a). As part of the National Survey of Family Growth (NSFG), which has been conducted periodically since 1970, almost 9,000 women 15–19 years of age participated in personal interviews about their sexual behavior. In 1997, 50% of the women reported participating in sexual intercourse. Previous survey results had shown a steady increase—29% in 1970, 36% in 1975, 47% in 1982, 53% in 1988, and 55% in 1990.

Dailard (2001) reported on the findings of the National Longitudinal Study of Adolescent Health (more commonly called the "Add Health Survey"). She indicated that teens' reports of ever having had sexual intercourse increase dramatically with grade level, from 16% among 7th and 8th graders to 60% among 11th graders. Teenagers who are black or in low-income or single-parent families are more likely to have had sexual intercourse than their peers. In addition, the Add Health Survey strongly indicates that whether or not a teenager has ever had sexual intercourse is largely explained by that individual's own sexual history and his or her perceptions about the costs and benefits of having sexual intercourse. In sharp contrast, the data indicate other major risk behaviors—such as cigarette smoking, drug and alcohol use, weapons-related violence, and suicidal thoughts and attempts—are shaped more by factors such as problems with school or work or the number of friends who regularly smoke or drink.

In 2001 a correlation between the level of adolescent–parent communication and abstinence from initiation of sexual intercourse was reported (Karofsky, 2001). High levels of communication with the mother was most closely associated with abstinence from sexual intercourse.

In 2002 the Kaiser Family Foundation reported the results of a national survey of 1,200 adolescents and young adults 13–24 years old (Substance use and risky sexual behavior, 2002). It concluded that for many teens and young adults alcohol use and drug use are closely linked to sexual decision making and risk taking. Nearly 90% say their peers use alcohol or drugs before having sexual intercourse at least some of the time, and many young people report that condoms are often not used when people are drinking or using drugs. More than a third of sexually active young people report that alcohol or drugs have influenced their decisions about sex. Almost as many have "done more" sexually than they had planned while under their influence. As a result, they report they worry about STIs and pregnancy.

It is interesting that most sexually active teenagers had sexual intercourse for the first time in their parents' homes, late at night (Most sexually active teens first had sex at home, 2002). On the basis of a national survey that had tracked 8,000 children aged 12–16 years since 1997, the study found that 56% of those who had been sexually active said they first had sexual intercourse at their family's home or at the family home of a partner, 12% said at a friend's house, 4% said in a vehicle, 3% said at an outdoor location, 3% said at a hotel or motel, and 10% said at another location. In addition, 42% said they first had sexual intercourse between 10 P.M. and 7 A.M. and 28% said between 6 P.M. and 10 P.M. Only 15% of respondents said they had intercourse for the first time between 3 P.M. and 6 P.M. This study dispels the myth that teens most often have sexual intercourse after school, when parents are at work.

Changes in sexual risk behavior among U.S. high school students (grades 9–12) over a 10-year period were reported in 2002 (Trends in sexual risk behaviors among high school students, 2002). The percentage who reported ever having had sexual intercourse decreased by 16%. In 1991 56% had participated, but in 2001 only 46% had done so. Also, the overall proportion who had had four or more partners dropped by 24%—from 19% in 1991 to 14% in 2001.

The overall prevalence of "current sexual activity"—defined as having intercourse at any point during the 3 months preceding the survey—did not change between 1991 and 2001. It was reported by about one-third of the respondents. Condom use rose between 1991 and 1999 but had "leveled off" since then. In 2001 about 58% of sexually active teens used condoms, compared to about 46% in 1991. The percentage of sexually active students who had used drugs or alcohol before their most recent intercourse increased 18% between 1991 and 2002.

Studies on Ethnic Differences in Sexual Attitudes and Behavior

Only relatively recently have researchers looked at the influence of ethnic differences in sexual attitudes and behavior. Examples of such studies are given in the following discussion.

Data indicating some ethnic differences in the proportion of women 15–19 years of age who have ever had sexual intercourse were reported in the National Survey of Family Growth (Abma, et al., 1997). For example, 55% of the Hispanics, 49.5% of the whites, and 59.5% of the blacks reported having participated in sexual intercourse.

Gender and ethnic differences in the timing of first sexual intercourse were reported in 1998 (Upchurch, et al., 1998). In an ethnically diverse sample of 877 Los Angeles County youths, there was an overall median age of first sexual intercourse of 16.9 years. Black males had the lowest median (15.0), and Asian-American males the highest (18.1) age. White and Hispanic males, and white and black females, reported similar ages (about 16.5 years). Hispanic and Asian-American females had rates of first sexual intercourse about half that of white females. Even after controlling for background characteristics, black males had rates of first sexual intercourse that were about three to five times the rates of the other groups.

Quadagno and associates (1998) indicated that previous investigators had reported ethnic differences in the expression of sexual decision making and sexual behaviors in women. They examined the influence of ethnicity on who makes decisions on the timing and type of sexual activity. Their results showed that ethnicity had little direct effect on most variables. The main exception was that ethnicity influenced joint decision making regarding the timing and type of sexual activities for Hispanic but not for African-American women. They concluded that ethnicity contributes to differences in sexual behaviors but that other variables are equally important.

Did You Know . . .

Many studies of sexual behavior have examined only whether a person reports ever having had sexual intercourse. When investigating the safety of sexual behavior, it is also helpful to know how often people have participated in sexual intercourse in a recent time, with whom, and what types of sexual practices have been used. For example, we know that teenagers and nonwhite women are at greater risk of contracting HIV than are older women, but teenagers are less consistently sexually active than are older women (Klitsch, 1990). Similarly, nonwhite women are statistically more likely to contract sexually transmitted infections than white women; however, they are less consistently sexually active than white women. Again, researchers need to consider the type of behavior or practice, not just the amount, to determine the degree to which safe sexual behavior is practiced.

Ford and coworkers (2001) reported that the sexual partners of white and black adolescents are likely to be similar to them. In contrast, the sexual partners of Latino adolescents and of adolescents of "other" race or ethnicity are more likely to be of a different racial or ethnic group. As adolescents get older, their partners become more heterogeneous.

Studies on the Use of Contraception

Countless factors have been considered as influencing contraceptive use. Studer and Thornton (1987) found that adolescents with a deep religious commitment were less likely to participate in sexual intercourse, but when they did participate, they were also less likely to use reliable contraception. Yarber (1986) found that overall health habits were not related to whether young females sought prescription contraception.

Sack, Billingham, and Howard (1985) found that, to predict contraceptive use, seven independent variables could be used: the age an individual started engaging in intercourse, frequency of intercourse, frequency of dating, length of time partners knew each other, number of partners, anticipation or nonanticipation of intercourse, and the number of close friends who were thought to use birth control. Schwartz and Darabi (1986) found that a feared pregnancy, advice from significant others, and situational factors were the greatest motivators for adolescents to make a first visit to a family planning clinic.

Silverman, Torres, and Forrest (1987) found that a negative attitude toward contraceptives was an important reason for not using them and for relying on nonprescription methods. Individuals used more reliable contraceptive methods if a more positive attitude toward contraceptive methods was encouraged and if improved access to and knowledge of inexpensive, personalized family planning services were provided.

Nearly all 20- to 29-year-old women who had ever had sexual intercourse used a contraceptive method at some time, but a high proportion did not start using contraception until an average of 8 months after their first experience. Catholic women were no less likely to have had sexual intercourse, to be currently sexually active, or to use contraceptives (Tanfer & Horn, 1985).

Kegeles, Adler, and Irvin (1989) found that convenience and social considerations had a greater effect on teenagers' intentions to use condoms than did knowledge of the health benefits of condom use. The factors most strongly related to intention to use condoms during the next year were the beliefs that condoms are easy to use, that they permit one to engage in sexual intercourse spontaneously, and that they are popular with adolescents' peers. In addition, both males and females who intended to use condoms believed it important for the male to share the responsibility for contraceptive use.

Hingson (1990) also examined which teenagers will use condoms. Interestingly, those with the most sexual partners in the preceding year were the least likely to have used condoms. Those who thought condoms protect well against HIV and those who did not believe that condoms reduce sexual pleasure were more than three times as likely to have been consistent condom users. Those who carried condoms with them, those who were not embarrassed if asked to use a condom, and those who did not drink were also significantly more likely to use condoms at every act of intercourse. If you worked in a community agency and were interested in promoting the use of condoms among sexually active young people, how would these two studies influence your strategy?

Mosher (1990) found that the use of oral contraceptives by married women declined markedly between 1973 and 1982 but then remained steady. Reliance on female sterilization continued to increase, however, and it was still the leading method among currently and formerly married women. IUD use dropped by two-thirds (from 2.2 million to 0.7 million women) between 1982 and 1988. Condom use increased most sharply among teenagers and rose among never-married white and black women, but the pill was still the leading method by far in these groups. Overall, about 60% of U.S. women 15 to 44 years of age were using contraception in 1988: 24% relied on either male or female sterilization, whereas 37% used reversible methods.

It is always interesting to consider why pregnant adolescents say they did not use contraception. Stevens-Simon and associates (1996) surveyed 200 poor and pregnant 13- to 18-year-olds in an adolescent-oriented maternity program. The most frequently cited reasons for not using contraceptives before conception were "I don't mind getting pregnant" (17.5%), followed by "I was using birth control but it didn't work (broke)" (12%), "I thought there was something wrong with me and I couldn't get pregnant" (9%), and "I just didn't get around to it" (9%).

Changes in the initiation of adolescent sexual and contraceptive behavior in the United States between 1978 and 1988 were reported by Cooksey, Rindfuss, and Guilkey (1996). They found that the overall patterns of earlier initiation of sexual intercourse and increased use of condoms were not found in all population segments. Overall, patterns through the decade suggested that pressures from parents, religious groups, and others led to a later age at first intercourse or use of contraceptives, but not both. A notable exception is that increased maternal education leads to both a later age at first intercourse and a higher likelihood of using contraception at first intercourse.

In 1996 Peipert and colleagues surveyed the frequency of condom use of 147 women at a private university in New England and compared their results to those of similar surveys done in 1975, 1986, and 1989. In 1995 74% of the sexually active women said their partners "always or almost always" used condoms during sexual intercourse, compared with 11% in 1975, 21% in 1986, and 41% in 1989.

In a nationally representative sample of sexually experienced youths aged 14–22 years, 37% of females and 52% of males said the condom was the primary method used to prevent pregnancy at last intercourse. An additional 8% and 7%, respectively, used a condom for noncontraceptive purposes. Condom use was reported at last intercourse by 25% of males whose partner was using the pill (Santelli, et al., 1997).

Although the proportion of adolescent females who have experienced sexual intercourse has increased over time, their likelihood of pregnancy has decreased. Increases in contraceptive use by adolescent females contribute to this change. For example, adolescent females who used a contraceptive at first intercourse increased from 48% in 1982 to 65% in 1983–1988 (U.S. Department of Health and Human Services, 1998b).

Related closely to contraceptive use is the fact that in 1998 it was reported that births among unmarried black girls were plunging (National Center for Health Statistics, 1998b). The birthrate of 74.4 per 1,000 women represented a 40-year low. The sharpest drop was among 15- to 17-year-olds, whose birthrate had declined 20% since 1990. Although they were not sure exactly what caused the change, experts thought reasons included a fear of AIDS, girls' increased insistence on condom use, desire to prevent "kids holding me down," and attachment of an old stigma to unwed motherhood. This last factor is particularly interesting because it could mean the renewal of shame. In other words, those who have recently become pregnant may be cast out by their friends.

The National Survey of Family Growth (Abma, et al., 1997) included a number of interesting statistics related to the use of contraception. For example, the leading method of contraception remains female sterilization (10.7 million women), followed by the oral contraceptive pill (10.4 million), the male condom (7.9 million), and male sterilization (4.2 million). Condom use at first intercourse increased from 18% in the 1970s to 36% in the late 1980s and 54% in the 1990s. Also, at first intercourse, some method of contraception was used by 36.2% of Hispanic women, 50.1% of black women, and 64.8% of white women.

Ford and colleagues (2001) reported that the less similar adolescents and their sexual partners are to one another—whether because of a difference in age, grade, or school—the less likely they are to use condoms and other contraceptive methods. The likelihood of having sexual relations with adolescents with different characteristics increases as adolescents get older.

Oncale and King (2001) reported that many college students either have tried to talk their sexual partners out of using a condom or have had a partner try to dissuade them from condom use. Nearly 14% of women and nearly 17% of men who had engaged in sexual intercourse admitted to having actively tried to dissuade a partner from the couple's using condoms. Thirty percent of men and 41% of women said that a sexual partner had tried to dissuade them. The most frequent reasons cited were (1) that sexual intercourse feels better without a condom, (2) that the woman will not get pregnant, and (3) that the person will not get a sexually transmitted infection.

Related to control of births, in 2002 it was reported that the overall U.S. abortion rate declined throughout the 1990s, but "rose sharply" for low-income women. The abortion rate among U.S. women of childbearing age fell from 24 per 1,000 women in 1994 to 21 per 1,000 women in 2000—an 11% decrease. However, the rate among women earning less than the federal poverty level rose by 25% during this period, and the rate for women earning less than two times the poverty level—or $34,000 for a family of four—rose by 34%. The rate among teens 15–17 years old fell by 40% from 24 per 1,000 girls in 1994 to 15 per 1,000 girls in 2000. The majority (56%)

of women who have abortions are in their 20s. Two-thirds have never been married, and 61% have one or more children. More than three-quarters reported having a religious affiliation—43% Protestant, 27% Catholic, and 8% other religions (U.S. abortion declines overall but increases among low-income women, report says, 2002).

Other Representative Studies

Studies have also been done on a variety of other topics. For example, Weisman and associates (1986) found newly trained female obstetrician–gynecologists to have more favorable attitudes toward abortion than similarly trained males. Abortion attitudes were a strong indicator of whether or not physicians provided abortions. On a different note, Tanfer (1987) found that heterosexual cohabitation was a common occurrence among 20- to 29-year-old women. This did not seem to be a permanent replacement for marriage but rather a new dimension of the courtship process.

Continuing with the theme of living styles, Saluter (1990) reported that more than five times as many couples were cohabiting in 1989 as in 1970 (2.8 million versus 523,000), and almost 60% of the cohabiting people had never been married. Also, in 1989 13.4 million 18- to 24-year-olds and nearly 5 million 25- to 34-year-olds were living with their parents. The median age at first marriage for both men and women had reached the highest level since such data were first recorded in 1890—26.2 years for men and 23.8 years for women.

Family structure also seems to have an effect on risky behavior. Flewelling and Bauman (1990) found that children from single-parent or stepparent households were substantially more likely than children from intact families to smoke cigarettes, use drugs, and have sexual intercourse. In a similar vein, Shrier and associates (1997) studied the association of sexual risk behaviors and problem drug behaviors in high school students. They found that increased frequency of drug use behaviors and more years of sexual intercourse were associated with an increased number of sexual partners and recent condom nonuse.

Pregnancy and other risk behaviors among adolescent girls has also been studied (Rome, Rybikci, & Durant, 1998). The purpose of the study was to determine whether teenage girls who had been pregnant were more likely to engage in other risk or problem behaviors than girls who had had sexual intercourse without becoming pregnant. Results indicated that girls who had been pregnant also had engaged in other risk behaviors, including recent weapon carrying and cocaine use. A history of previous sexually transmitted infections plus increasing numbers of partners added to the risk of pregnancy.

Information related to adolescent pregnancy risks and outcomes is also interesting (Sexuality Information and Education Council of the United States, 1988). For example, 94% of teens believe that if they were involved in a pregnancy they would stay in school; in actuality, only 70% eventually complete high school. Fifty-one percent of teens believe that if they were involved in a pregnancy they would marry the mother or father; in actuality 81% of teenage births are to unmarried teens. Thirty-two percent of teens say they would consider an abortion; in actuality, 50% of pregnancies of unmarried teens end in abortion.

Moore (2001) reported that nationally the teen birth rate dropped 22% between 1991 and 2000. Southern and southeastern states had the highest teen birth rates; northeastern and some northern states had much lower birth rates. Interestingly, teens overestimated the number of their peers who had engaged in sexual intercourse. Teens estimated that 38% of their peers had engaged in sexual intercourse by age 15 years, whereas only 25% of girls and 27% of boys had done so.

A report from the U.S. Centers for Disease Control (Births: preliminary data for 2000, 2001) indicated that several factors have contributed to the decline in the teen birth rate. Sexual activity has leveled off, reversing the steady increases over the preceding two decades. Many initiatives have focused on the prevention of pregnancy through abstinence and many teens have heard the message. Finally, more sexually active teens are using contraception including the more effective newer forms.

Kirby (2001) pointed out that despite declining rates of teen pregnancy, more than 4 in 10 girls become pregnant at least once before age 20, a proportion that translates into nearly 900,000 teen pregnancies per year. When teens give birth, they become less likely to complete school and more likely to be single parents. Their children have less supportive and stimulating home environments, poorer health, lower cognitive development, worse educational outcomes, more behavior problems, and greater likelihood of becoming teen parents themselves. Many teens do not use contraceptives correctly and consistently every time they have sexual intercourse.

The issue of equality in sex roles has been studied frequently. For example, Thornton (1989) reported that contemporary adults and teenagers advocated more equality in sex roles and felt less bound by social imperatives to marry, stay married, have children, and remain faithful to their spouses as compared with their counterparts 25 years before.

For years it has been accepted that men have a higher incidence of sexual activity than women. Phillis and Gromko (1985) pointed out that this might be because there are more females than males in society. So, the actual numbers of persons of both sexes involved in heterosexual activity might be similar even though the proportions might be different.

More and more studies examine the issue of AIDS. A majority of Americans reported that they have not changed their attitudes toward homosexuals as a result of the AIDS epidemic. Also, little change was noted since 1982 in the public's views about homosexual relations between consenting adults (Gallup poll finds majority opinion of gays unchanged by AIDS, 1986).

As part of an anti-AIDS program, the practice of making condoms available to young people in schools and agencies has been attacked by some people. However, a study of the effects of a condom distribution program at a Los Angeles County high school showed: (1) The percentage of sexually active males who reported using a condom every time they had vaginal intercourse increased from 37% to 50% after the condom program started; (2) the percentage of boys at the school who reported using a condom the first time they engaged in intercourse increased from 65% to 80%; (3) the percentage of boys engaging in vaginal intercourse did not increase (Condoms from schools encourage safe sex, not more sex, 1998).

The U.S. surgeon general reported (2001) that almost 775,000 AIDS cases had been reported in the United States since 1981 and that about 900,000 persons were living with HIV. About one-third were aware of their status and were in treatment, one-third were aware and not in treatment, and one-third had not been tested and were not aware. About 40,000 new HIV infections occur each year.

Sternberg (2001) reported that from about 1995 to 1998 new AIDS cases and AIDS deaths dropped because of potent new AIDS drugs. In 1998 they leveled off, and 1998 to 2001 they increased. Reasons for this increase seem to be related to the fact that some people delay getting tested for HIV, AIDS drugs do not work against some strains of HIV, and in some groups there is an increase in risky sexual behavior.

In 2002 it was reported that the age at which girls begin menstruating had declined since the 1970s. For African-American girls it decreased markedly, dropping by 9.5 months. For white girls it decreased by 2 months. Overall,

African-American girls on average began menstruating about 3 months earlier than white girls (12.3 years versus 12.6 years) and were 40% more likely than white girls to begin menstruation before age 11 years. The reasons for early menstruation are not well understood (Age at first menstruation continues to decline, especially among African Americans, study says, 2002).

The number of married U.S. teenagers increased by 50% during the 1990s. In 2000 4.5% of teens were married compared to 3.4% in 1990. The exact reasons for this are not known; however, some people attribute the change to abstinence education and others attribute it to the increased number of immigrants from countries in which teenage marriage is more common (Number of married U.S. teens increased by 50% in 1990s, 2002).

Interestingly, high school– and college-aged Americans indicated stronger support than their parents' generation for some traditionally "conservative" stances, including opposition to abortion. Forty-four percent of survey respondents between 15 and 22 years old said they supported government-imposed restrictions on abortion rights in the United States, whereas 34% aged 26 years and older supported such restrictions (Young Americans more likely than their parents' generation to oppose abortion, 2002).

Finally, in 2003 the Henry J. Kaiser Family Foundation released a comprehensive survey of young people about the factors that shape and inform their knowledge and decision making (National Survey of Adolescents and Young Adults, 2003). The study involved a nationally representative survey of 1,800 young people aged 13–24 years. The main findings reflected interviews with 1,552 young people between 15–24 years. More young people reported that sexual health issues are "big concerns" for people their age, more than any other issue. A summary of key findings include the following:

1. Young people report great pressure to participate in sexual activity.
2. One-third of adolescents have participated in oral sexual activity; 1 in 5 are unaware that this behavior can transmit STIs.
3. Pregnancy remains a serious concern for young people, and many have faced pregnancy scares or have been pregnant themselves.
4. Many young people remain reluctant to discuss sexual health issues with partners, family, and health providers.
5. Young people report that alcohol and drugs often play a dangerous role in their sex lives.
6. A surprisingly high number of young people are misinformed about safer sexual activity.
7. While most young people agree that sexual activity without a condom is risky, many young people see sexual activity without condoms occasionally as "not a big deal."
8. When it comes to sex and relationships, young people say they get their information from a variety of places, including their parents, sexuality education, friends, and the media.
9. Young people express a strong desire for more information about sexuality and sexual health.

The study's authors pointed out that in the past decade there has been an increase in the use of condoms among sexually active young people, and a small but significant decline in teen birth rates. However, 10 percent of the girls between age 15–19 years have become pregnant, nearly two-thirds of the high school seniors have had sexual intercourse, and an alarming percentage of sexually active adolescents and young adults engaged in unsafe sexual behaviors. Nearly 1 in 4 sexually active young people contracted an STI every year, and one-half of all new HIV infections in this country occurred among people under the age of 25 years.

Research on Sexuality Education

Research has been done to evaluate the effect of sexuality education programs (see Chapter 1). For example, Eisen, Zellman, and McAlister (1990) found that good sexuality education programs help delay the onset of sexual intercourse for teenagers. Those students who were already sexually active and had participated in good sexuality education programs were more likely to have used an effective contraceptive at most recent intercourse. Also, the programs increased the consistent use of effective methods. Along with positive effects on sexual knowledge, good sexuality education programs can have important behavioral effects.

The positive influence of sexuality education on behavior has been verified in many studies. For example, Kirby and Coyle (1994) reported that education programs do not hasten the onset of sexual intercourse and may increase the use of contraception in general and/or condoms in particular. They indicate that specific programs have delayed the onset of intercourse, increased the use of protection against pregnancy or STIs and HIV, and/or reduced the number of sexual partners. Using appropriate behavior-change theories has enhanced the potential for altering students' risk-taking behaviors.

Kirby (2001) reported that some sexuality and HIV education programs can delay the onset of intercourse, reduce the number of partners, reduce the frequency of sexual intercourse, increase condom or contraceptive use, and thereby decrease sexual risk taking. Also, some programs that have addressed nonsexual risk or protective factors (such as attachment to family, parental monitoring, and attachment to school) have reduced sexual risk taking. Characteristics of effective programs include the following: (1) They focus on reducing one or more behaviors that lead to unintended pregnancy or STIs; (2) they provide basic, accurate information about the risks of teen sexual activity and about ways to avoid intercourse or use methods of protection against pregnancy and STIs; (3) they provide examples of practice with communication, negotiation, and refusal skills; (4) they continue for a sufficient length of time; and (5) they employ teaching methods designed to involve the participants and induce them to personalize the information.

Eighty-nine percent of teenagers take a sexuality education class by the time they finish high school. Unfortunately, 46% of them have said such classes fail to teach them how to discuss contraception and STI with their partners and do not address emotional consequences of sexual activity. Almost half of the students said they did not receive enough information in the classes. Many teachers want to do more but are prevented by their school districts from expanding the curricula (Teens unsatisfied with sex ed classes, 2001).

Unfortunately, evaluations of comprehensive sexuality education have tended to focus mainly on whether the programs have helped young people delay sexual activity and prevent unwanted pregnancy and disease (Haffner & Goldfarb, 1998). Other goals, such as helping young people develop an appreciation of their bodies or communicate effectively with peers and partners, are often overlooked. Evaluations of sexuality education need to be improved so they reflect broad program goals. In the meantime, many evaluations have found that high-quality sexuality education programs increase knowledge, clarify values, increase parent–child communication, help young people delay the initiation of sexual intercourse, increase the use of contraception and condoms, do not encourage young people to begin intercourse, and do not increase the frequency of sexual intercourse.

The Future of Sexuality Research

More sexuality research is definitely needed. Not only do we need to have more information on sexual behavior itself; we also need to explore how we make decisions to engage in sexual activity, how the quality of relationships can be improved, and what factors will be important in helping people achieve sexual satisfaction throughout the life cycle. A variety of cultural and societal factors (age, religion, education) have always affected sexual decision making, but recently a change in societal attitudes toward marriage, divorce, childbearing, and sexual relationships has become evident. The stresses these new attitudes bring to bear on personal relationships need to be explored in the near future.

There are real challenges related to sexuality research. Tiefer (1994), in her presidential address to the International Academy of Sex Research, emphasized three crises facing sexology. First, the media are inundating the public with sexual topics. Second, many people in academic circles still hesitate to accept sexuality research as being as legitimate as other forms of research. Finally, there is a tendency for sexuality research to focus only on medical topics and not on the comprehensive nature of people and society. We have learned a great deal through sexuality research; however, even better research methods are needed to fit together the psychological, the biological, and the sociological aspects of sexuality research.

In closing, Tables 2.1 and 2.2 summarize the sexuality research of selected researchers.

TABLE 2.1 Selected Sexuality Researchers and Their Studies (Grouped by Type of Method)

Author(s)	Date	Title
Interview survey		
Scientific literature		
Kinsey, Pomeroy, & Martin	1948	*Sexual behavior in the human male*
	1953	*Sexual behavior in the human female*
Bell & Weinberg	1978	*Homosexualities: A study of diversity among men and women*
Bell, Weinberg, & Hammersmith	1981	*Sexual preference: Its development in men and women*
Mosher	1990	*Contraceptive practice in the United States, 1982–1988*
U.S. Centers for Disease Control	1991	*Premarital sexual experience among adolescent women—United States, 1970–1988*
U.S. Centers for Disease Control	1998	*National survey of family growth*
Carolina Population Center	2001	National longitudinal study of adolescent health (The "Add Health Survey")
Popular literature		
Hunt	1974	*Sexual behavior in the 1970s*
Reinisch & Beasley	1991	*The Kinsey Institute new report on sex*
Kaiser Family Foundation and *Seventeen* magazine	2002	SexSmarts survey on teen sexual behavior

TABLE 2.1 Selected Sexuality Researchers and Their Studies (Grouped by Type of Method) ***(continued)***

Author(s)	Date	Title
Questionnaire survey		
Scientific literature		
Sorenson	1973	*Adolescent sexuality in contemporary America*
Zelnik & Kantner	1977	Sexual and contraceptive experience of young unmarried women in the United States, 1976 and 1971
	1978	First pregnancies to women aged 15–19: 1976 and 1971
	1980	Sexual activity, contraceptive use, and pregnancy among metropolitan-area teenagers: 1971–1979
Blumstein & Schwartz	1983	*American couples*
Kegeles, Adler, & Irvin	1989	Adolescents and condoms: Associations of beliefs and intentions to use
DeBuono, et al.	1990	Sexual behavior of college women in 1975, 1986, and 1989
Flewelling & Bauman	1990	Family structure as a predictor of initial substance abuse and sexual intercourse in early adolescence
Hingson, et al.	1990	Beliefs about AIDS, use of alcohol and drugs, and unprotected sex among Massachusetts adolescents
Rubinson & De Rubertis	1991	Trends in sexual attitudes and behaviors of a college population over a 16-year period
Laumann, Gagnon, Michael, & Michaels	1994	*The social organization of sexuality*
deGaston, Jensen, & Weed	1995	Closer look at adolescent sexual activity
Peipert, et al.	1996	College women and condom use
Sprecher & Hatfield	1996	Premarital sexual standards among U.S. college students: Comparison with Russian and Japanese students
Stevens-Simon, et al.	1996	Why pregnant adolescents say they do not use contraceptives prior to conception
U.S. Centers for Disease Control	1996	Youth risk behavior surveillance system
Alexander & Hickner	1997	First coitus for adolescents: Understanding why and when
Shrier, et al.	1997	The association of sexual risk behaviors and problem drug behaviors in high school students
Rome, et al.	1998	Pregnancy and other risk behaviors among adolescent girls in Ohio
U.S. Centers for Disease Control	1998	Youth risk behavior surveillance system
	2000	Youth risk behavior surveillance system
Karofsky	2001	Parent–teen communication and the initiations of sexual intercourse
Popular literature		
Tavris & Sadd	1975	The *Redbook* report on female sexuality
Hite	1976	*The Hite report*
	1981	*The Hite report on male sexuality*
	1987	*Women and love: A cultural revolution in progress*
Sarrel & Sarrel	1980	The *Redbook* report on sexual relationships
Direct observation		
Scientific literature		
Masters & Johnson	1966	*Human sexual response*
	1970	*Human sexual inadequacy*
	1979	*Homosexuality in perspective*

TABLE 2.2 Examples of Additional Research

Author(s)	Date	Title
Phillis & Gromko	1985	Sex differences in sexual activity: Reality or illusion?
Sack, Billingham, & Howard	1985	Premarital contraceptive use: A discriminant analysis approach
Sherwin & Corbett	1985	Campus sexual norms and dating relationships: A trend analysis
Tanfer & Horn	1985b	Contraceptive use, pregnancy, and fertility patterns among single American women in their 20s
Earle & Perricone	1986	Premarital sexuality: A ten year study of attitudes and behavior on a small university campus
Fisher	1986	Parent–child communication about sex and young adolescents' sexual knowledge and attitudes
Gallup Poll	1986	Gallup Poll finds majority opinion of gays unchanged by AIDS
Moore, Peterson, & Furstenberg	1986	Parental attitudes and the occurrence of early sexual activity
Roche	1986	Premarital sex: Attitudes and behavior by dating stage
Schwartz & Darabi	1986	Motivations for adolescents' first visit to a family planning clinic
Weisman, et al.	1986	Abortion attitudes and performance among male and female obstetrician–gynecologists
Yarber	1986	Delay in seeking prescription contraception and the health lifestyle and health locus of control of young women
Hofferth, Kahn, & Baldwin	1987	Premarital sexual activity among U.S. teenage women over the past three decades
Newcomer & Udry	1987	Parental marital status effects on adolescent sexual behavior
Silverman, Torres, & Forrest	1987	Barriers to contraceptive services
Studer & Thornton	1987	Adolescent religiosity and contraceptive usage
Tanfer	1987	Patterns of premarital cohabitation among never-married women in the United States
Wyatt, Peters, & Guthrie	1988a	Kinsey revisited, part I: Comparisons of the sexual socialization and sexual behavior of white women over 33 years
	1988b	Kinsey revisited, part II: Comparisons of the sexual socialization and sexual behavior of black women over 33 years
Thornton	1989	Changing attitudes toward family issues in the United States
Eisen, Zellman, & McAlister	1990	Evaluating the impact of a theory-based sexuality and contraceptive education program
Forrest & Singh	1990	The sexual and reproductive behavior of American women, 1982–1988
Klitsch	1990	Subgroups of U.S. women differ widely in exposure to sexual intercourse
Saluter	1990	Marital status and living arrangements: March 1989
Sroka	1991	Common sense on condom education
Sexuality Information and Education Council of the United States	1994	Teens talk about sex
Cooksey, Rindfuss, & Guilkey	1996	The initiation of adolescent sexual and contraceptive behavior during changing times
Santelli, et al.	1997	The use of condoms with other contraceptive methods among young men and women
National Center for Health Statistics	1998	The opposite of sex

TABLE 2.2 **Examples of Additional Research** *(continued)*

Author(s)	Date	Title
U.S. Dept. of Health and Human Services, Office of Population Affairs	1998b	Trends in adolescent pregnancy and childbearing
Upchurch, et al.	1998	Gender and ethnic differences in the timing of first sexual intercourse
Quadagno, et al.	1998	Ethnic differences in sexual decisions and sexual behavior
Oncale & King	2001	Comparison of men's and women's attempts to dissuade sexual partners from the couple using condoms
Kirby	2001	Emerging answers: Research findings on programs to reduce sexual risk-taking and teen pregnancy
Office of the Surgeon General	2001	The surgeon general's call to action to promote sexual health and responsible sexual behavior
Ford, et al.	2001	Characteristics of adolescents' sexual partners and their association with use of condoms and other contraceptive methods
Kaiser Family Foundation	2002	Substance use and risky sexual behavior: Attitudes and practices among adolescents and young adults
Child Trends	2002	National longitudinal survey of youth (Most sexually active teens first had sex at home, late at night, survey shows)
Youth Risk Behavior Surveillance System	2002	Trends in sexual risk behaviors among high school students
Alan Guttmacher Institute	2002	U.S. abortion rate declines overall but increases among low-income women
Centers for Disease Control Study	2002	Age at first menstruation continues to decline
U.S. Bureau of the Census	2002	Number of married U.S. teens increased by 50% in 1990s
University of California-Berkeley	2002	Young Americans more likely than their parents' generation to oppose abortion
Kaiser Family Foundation	2003	National survey of adolescents and young adults: Sexual health knowledge, attitudes, and experiences

Exploring the DIMENSIONS of Human Sexuality

sexuality.jbpub.com

Our feelings, attitudes, and beliefs regarding sexuality are influenced by our internal and external environments. Go to sexuality.jbpub.com to learn more about the biological, psychological, and sociological factors that affect your sexuality.

Biological Factors

- The medical model was the focus of sexuality research in the 19th century.
- The sexual response cycle was discovered by the researchers Masters and Johnson.
- Physiological changes in the vagina or penis can be monitored by the vaginal plethysmograph and penile strain gauge, respectively.

Sociocultural Factors

- The gender "double standard" research goes back to the 19th century, when discomfort with women's sexuality prompted such beliefs.
- Education leads to both a later age of first intercourse and a higher likelihood of using contraception at first intercourse.
- Religious adolescents are less likely to participate in sexual intercourse; when they do, they are less likely to use reliable contraceptives.
- Ethical considerations abound in sexuality research.

Psychological Factors

- The NHSLS data found that married people were much more likely than single people to report being extremely or very happy.
- Behaviors and practices, as well as frequency of sexual activity, need to be accounted for in sexuality research.
- Motivation to respond to a sexual research survey may create a bias in the sample.
- Learned attitudes and behaviors may influence answers given on sexuality surveys.

CASE STUDY

It's amazing how many factors are involved in even basic research on sexuality. Political forces have banned the use of government money for research dealing with sexuality, so monies must be provided by private foundations or companies, which may have a political or financial agenda of their own.

Learned behaviors prompt many people to answer questions as they think they should be answered, instead of with the truth, and that tendency can create survey bias. And the limited number of people willing to respond to a sexuality survey, especially in lower socioeconomic classes, also hinders researchers.

Finally, cultural, ethnic, and religious biases may hinder researchers from getting the data needed. For example, a survey of sexual behavior based on religious affiliation would do poorly, because many Muslim (the number-two religion in the United States) women would not allow interviews or would do so only with their husband present.

Discussion Questions

1. Compare and contrast the varied methods of sexuality research.
2. Describe the ethical issues involved in sexuality research, citing examples of each.
3. Who were the early sexuality researchers, and what did they figure out? Is their research still considered valid?
4. List the major modern sexuality researchers and describe their contributions. How has their research changed sexuality?

Application Questions

Reread the story that opens the chapter and answer the following questions.

1. Imagine your parents asked you to explain what sexuality researchers do—and why. Prepare a brief response to their query.
2. Explain which dimensions of human sexuality would influence congressional funding for a study on sexuality. Would representatives from some states be more willing to support sexuality research? Explain your answer.
3. For over a year, allegations of sexual relations between President Clinton and the former White House intern Monica Lewinsky rocked the news. Evaluate why, in light of a sexual scandal, the president's approval ratings continued to climb.

Critical Thinking Questions

1. What motivates a person to take the time and effort to respond to a human sexuality research questionnaire? Could that motivation lead to a sample bias?
2. As you will learn in the chapter on sexual arousal and response, Masters and Johnson were not the only team to discover a human sexual response cycle. How is it possible that different research groups obtained different results regarding a physiological response?
3. In 1991, the U.S. federal government pulled support from the NHSLS research project and passed legislation prohibiting the spending of federal funds on sexuality research. Although this was clearly a political move, it raises the question, Why should the government support such research? Put another way, how does sexuality research help the American people?
4. Imagine that you and/or your lover read a popular magazine sex survey that showed that a large percentage of people were doing a sexual activity that you had never tried. Would that motivate you to try something new? Would you encourage your lover to try it? How would you feel if your lover asked you to try it?

Critical Thinking Case

During the 1970s, it was widely reported that Russian track and field athletes were encouraged to have sexual relations the night before a major meet. In fact, reports claimed that those who did so performed better (closer to their potential). Imagine that the coach of your college's track team has just learned this information. He has asked you to design a sexuality research project, using scientific methodology, to prove or disprove the hypothesis that sexual activity leads to improved athletic performance.

Which method(s) of research would give you the best results? Explain why. Is it possible to prove the validity of such a hypothesis? What other factors might be involved? What ethical issues might you encounter? How could those issues be overcome?

Exploring Personal Dimensions

Sexuality Research

Mark each of the following statements "true" or "false."

_____ 1. All research completed as part of the National Health and Social Life Survey was financially supported by the U.S. federal government.

_____ 2. The first step in the scientific method is identifying a research question.

_____ 3. A hypothesis is a statement based upon research results.

_____ 4. Kinsey's research is an example of survey research.

_____ 5. The research of Masters and Johnson is an example of experimental research.

_____ 6. A plethysmograph is used in the laboratory to measure and chart physiological changes over time.

_____ 7. Most normal women have orgasms from penile thrusting alone.

_____ 8. Blumstein and Schwartz reported that both heterosexual and homosexual cohabiting couples seemed to have fewer difficulties in their relationships than married heterosexual couples.

_____ 9. The Liu Report can be correctly referred to as a Chinese National Health and Social Life Survey.

_____10. Over half the U.S. students in grades 9–12 have participated in sexual intercourse.

_____11. Both the proportion of adolescent females in the United States who have experienced sexual intercourse and their likelihood of pregnancy have increased in recent years.

_____12. Good sexuality education programs do not hasten the onset of sexual intercourse and may increase the use of contraception—particularly condoms.

Interpretation

All of the even-numbered statements are true and all of the odd-numbered statements are false. If you were correct on at least 10 statements, you did well. If you were not correct on at least 10 statements, find the correct answers in the chapter. All of the correct answers are in this chapter on sexuality research.

Sexuality Online

Go to the web component for *Exploring the Dimensions of Human Sexuality* at sexuality.jbpub.com for web exercises, additional resources related to this chapter, and student review tools.

Suggested Readings

The "Add Health" Survey. National Longitudinal Study of Adolescent Health. Carolina Population Center, University of North Carolina-Chapel Hill, 2001. [Online]. Available: www.cpc.unc.edu/projects/addhealth/

Bogaert, A. F. Volunteer bias in human sexuality research: Evidence for both sexuality and personality differences in males, *Archives of Sexual Behavior, 25, no. 2* (April 1996), 125–140.

Brecher, E. *The sex researchers.* New York: Signet Books, 1969.

Cassell, C. Let it shine: Promoting school success, life aspirations to prevent school-age parenthood, *SIECUS Report 30, no. 3* (February–March 2002), 7–12.

Kirby, D. *Emerging answers: Research findings on programs to reduce sexual risk-taking and teen pregnancy.* Washington, DC: The National Campaign to Prevent Teen Pregnancy, 2001.

Michael, R. T., Gagnon, J. H., Laumann, E. O., & Kolata, G. *Sex in America.* Boston: Little, Brown, 1994.

Parker, R. & Gagnon, J., eds. *Conceiving sexuality: Approaches to sex research in a postmodern world.* New York: Routledge, 1995.

Pomeroy, W. *Dr. Kinsey and the Institute for Sex Research.* New York: Harper & Row, 1972.

Santelli, J. S., Warren, C. W., Lowry, R., Sogolow, E., Collins, J., Kann, L., Kaufmann, R. B., & Celentano, D. D. The use of condoms and other contraceptive methods among young men and women, *Family Planning Perspectives, 29, no. 6* (Nov.–Dec., 1997), 280–283.

The surgeon general's call to action to promote sexual health and responsible sexual behavior. Rockville, MD.: Office of the Surgeon General, 2001.

Upchurch, D. M., Lillard, L. A., Aneshensel, C. S., & Li, N. F. Inconsistencies in reporting the occurrence and timing of first intercourse, *Journal of Sex Research 39, no. 3* (August 2002), 196–206.

CHAPTER 3 Sexual Communication

FEATURES

Multicultural Dimensions
Female and Male Subcultures?

Ethical Dimensions
Ethics, Communication, and Date Rape

Gender Dimensions
Sexual Behavior in Marriage

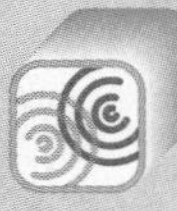

Communication Dimensions
Clarity in Sexual Communication

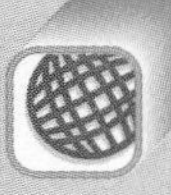

Global Dimensions
International Differences in Discussing Sexuality

CHAPTER OBJECTIVES

1. Describe the process of sexual communication, including nonverbal communication.
2. Identify barriers to sexual communication, including gender differences, attitudes about sexuality, and sexual language.
3. Discuss techniques for improving sexual communication.

sexuality.jbpub.com

Attitudes About Sexuality
Learning Assertiveness
Global Dimensions: International Differences in Discussing Sexuality

INTRODUCTION

Two for the Road (1967) *is a movie starring Audrey Hepburn as Joanna and Albert Finney as Mark. When they first meet on the road in Europe, Joanna is in a touring girls' choir and Mark is a struggling architect. The film follows their life together—through courtship and marriage, infidelity, and parenthood—all on the road in a variety of cars (hence the title), through a score of time-shifting vignettes.*

The film presents a lovely portrayal of a young couple growing in—and eventually out of—love. It not only shows the life cycle of a 12-year relationship, but also brilliantly portrays how communication changes during that life cycle.

As the couple meets and falls in love at a dizzying pace, conversation flows. It seems there is nothing that Joanna and Mark cannot talk about. They openly share their worlds together, delighting in the pleasure of each other. They communicate with touch, holding hands, kissing, making love (although in a 1967 family movie the lovemaking is only implied).

In one blissful scene, the young lovers are shown to their table in a French restaurant. Joanna and Mark hold hands, giggle, smile, make eye contact while walking across the restaurant. But they notice an older married couple who are eating their dinner. The couple is simply eating—no conversation, no touching, no eye contact. Mark turns to Joanna and suggests, "I guess married people don't talk."

But as their relationship and life change, so does their communication style. In time, Joanna and Mark have experienced life together, and they do not talk about it as much as they used to talk about their lives before they met. The mistakes they made as youths disappear into their sophisticated adulthood. There are no silly mistakes to giggle about anymore.

In time, they begin to know each other so well that each can anticipate what the other is going to say or wants to do. Verbal expression becomes infrequent, because it no longer seems very important.

And their lives change, too: They become parents, and Mark becomes a well-known architect. Children and work decrease the amount of time they have for each other. Again, life changes alter communication styles.

Eventually, Joanna and Mark are back in the same French restaurant, but this time as a married couple—no talk, no touch, no eye contact. A young couple, holding hands and giggling, looks at them; he whispers something in her ear. Joanna and Mark have come full circle—they are the married couple who do not talk!

Of course, one of the pleasures of being in a long-term relationship is that there is such a high level of comfort that sometimes you do not have to talk. Yet the very essence of a relationship is communication. Over time, if you rely on your assumptions about what the other person wants, needs, or thinks, the relationship begins to break down—and knowing what your partner wants all the time can become old hat. As people do in real life, Joanna and Mark fail to bridge the gap between not needing to talk constantly and not communicating.

Joanna and Mark's relationship deteriorates. They meet new people, have affairs—all in an effort to relive those days of carefree expression, of newness and excitement. Eventually the marriage ends; the full cycle of the relationship has been portrayed in less time than it may take you to read this chapter!

Many of you who have had long-term relationships can probably relate to the story of Joanna and Mark. When partners fail to communicate freely about sexuality or other topics, their relationship is bound to be limited—in scope and time. You have a great opportunity to enrich your relationships and sexual experiences when you can communicate with your partner about arousing mind and body experiences, your feelings about each other, and the other's preferences in life and in sexuality.

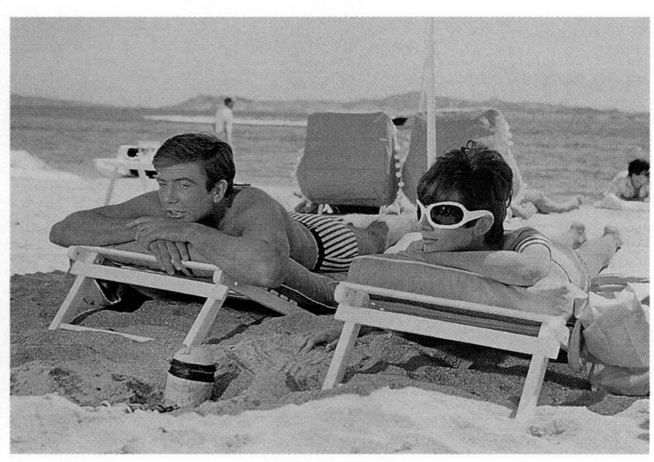

The movie *Two for the Road* (1967) explores the life cycle of a relationship, as well as the way communication changes through the cycle. From your own personal experience, does communication change in a relationship over the long term?

The Process of Communicating Sexually

Effective communication begins with an understanding of how communication works. The basic communication model (Figure 3.1) illustrates the five steps of the communication process. Let us consider how the basic commu-

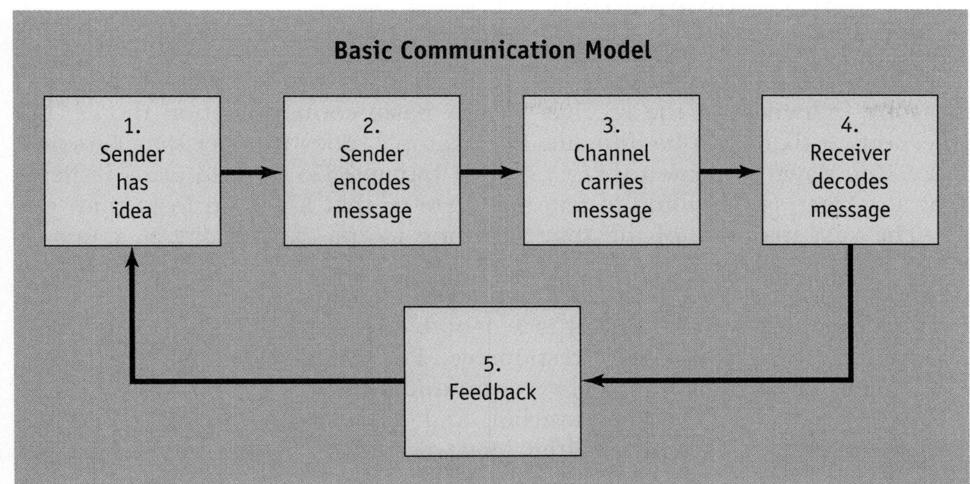

FIGURE 3.1 The basic communication model.

nication model might work in a relationship in which partners are participating in some sexual activity.

First, the sender has an idea. Partner A (the sender) does not want to have sexual intercourse. The nature of the idea is influenced by many factors, such as the context of the situation and the sender's mood, background, culture, and frame of reference. For example, Partner A may be too tired or upset, perhaps it is already too late at night, or perhaps Partner A does not know enough about Partner B. Whatever the reasons, Partner A does not want to participate.

Second, the sender encodes the idea in a message. **Encoding** means converting the idea into words or gestures to convey meaning. Partner A says, "I do not want to have sexual intercourse." A potential problem is that words have different meanings for different people. If misunderstandings result from missed meanings, that process is called **bypassing.** For example, Partner B may think all forms of sexual behavior except sexual intercourse are acceptable to Partner A. It may also be possible that Partner B thinks Partner A is just "saying" this and does not really mean it.

Third, the message travels over a channel. Channels include speech, telephones, fax machines, computers, and written correspondence. In this case, the channel contains speech and gestures. Partner A's voice tones, inflections, and gestures are part of the channel.

Fourth, the receiver (Partner B) decodes the message. **Decoding** means translating the message from its symbol form into meaning. Communication can be successful only when decoding is accurate. Various forms of "noise," however, can distort the message. In its simplest sense the noise of a crowded room makes hearing difficult. Noise can also be represented by misinterpretation of words, voice tones, or gestures; emotional reactions; or the use of alcohol or other drugs. In our example, after having several drinks, Partner B hears "Come and convince me."

Fifth, the receiver responds verbally or nonverbally—this is called **feedback.** Feedback helps the sender know whether or not the message was received and understood. In view of what Partner B heard, feedback is sent in the form of further sexual advances, because "noise" disturbed the transmission of Partner A's message.

Note that in Figure 3.1 the model provides for continual sending, receiving, and feedback. In our example, it is likely that the feedback provided by Partner B will result in additional communication from Partner A, and so the process continues.

encoding
Converting an idea into words or gestures to convey meaning.

bypassing
When misunderstandings result from missed meanings.

decoding
Translating the message from its symbol form into meaning.

feedback
When the receiver responds verbally or nonverbally.

Nonverbal Communication

Nonverbal communication includes all unwritten and unspoken messages. These may be sent intentionally or unintentionally. These silent signals exert a strong influence on the receiver in our basic communication model, but interpreting them can be difficult. For example, does the fact that Person A is looking down indicate modesty or just fatigue? Do crossed arms indicate that a person is unwilling to communicate or that a person feels cold?

The vast majority of message meaning (some experts say as much as 93%) (Guffey, 1999) is sent nonverbally. Messages can be difficult to decipher when verbal and nonverbal messages seem to contradict each other. For example, if Person A says it is acceptable to participate in sexual intercourse but then is not very responsive, Person B may have a problem knowing what Person A is really communicating.

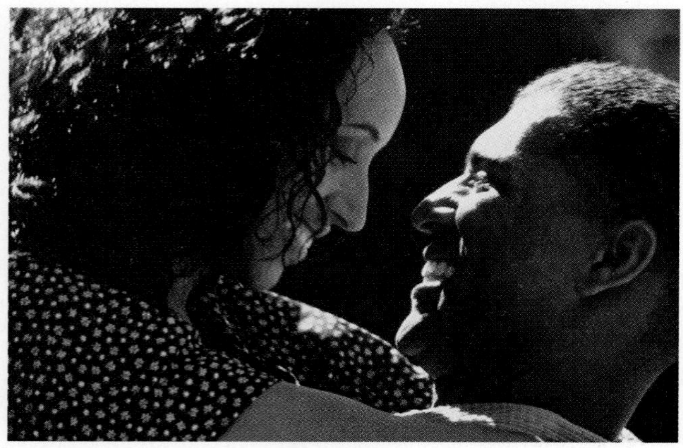

You can show interest in your partner with nonverbal communication. Gazing into each other's eyes, leaning in toward each other, smiling, and touching are all ways of conveying interest in one another.

When verbal and nonverbal messages conflict, receivers often have more faith in the nonverbal cues than what is said. It is important to recognize the significance of nonverbal communication, but it is unwise to attach a specific meaning to each gesture in every situation.

Note the body posture of your classmates. During an interesting class activity, most of them will probably be leaning or looking toward the lecturer or the center of the group, indicating that they are involved in what is happening. During a boring class, they will probably be leaning away from the lecturer or group. We call this physical behavior *body language*. Communicating by body posture often conveys as much as, or more than, the spoken word. When people feel uncomfortable about expressing their thoughts or feelings verbally, body language may be the only form of communication in which they participate.

We all recognize the importance of communicating nonverbally: We smile when we say hello, scratch our heads when perplexed, and hug a friend to show affection. (We also have an array of body terms to describe our nonverbal behavior: "Keep a stiff upper lip," "I can't stomach him," "She has no backbone," "I'm tongue-tied," "He caught her eye," "I have two left feet," "That was spine-tingling.") We show appreciation and affection, revulsion and indifference with expressions and gestures. We tell people we are interested in them by merely making eye contact and, as the male peacock displays his feathers, we display our sexuality by the ways we dress and walk and even by the way we stand.

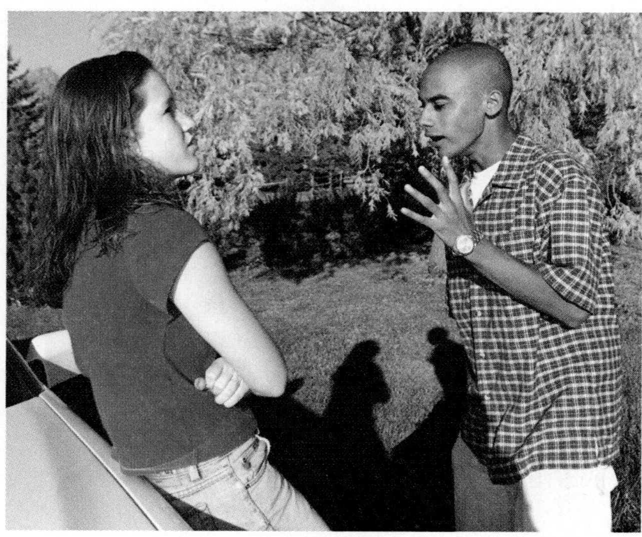

Misinterpretation of your partner's body language can often lead to conflict in a relationship.

Unfortunately, the nonverbal expression of feelings and thoughts is easy to misinterpret. For example, there is a tendency for people to view their own actions differently from the way their partners view those actions. In addition, people are more likely to notice negative than positive nonverbal behaviors (Manusov, 1997). There can also be differences in male and female nonverbal communication. Women tend to be more expressive and more skilled at sending and receiving nonverbal messages. Examples include smiling, gazing, having an expressive face, using the hands to communicate,

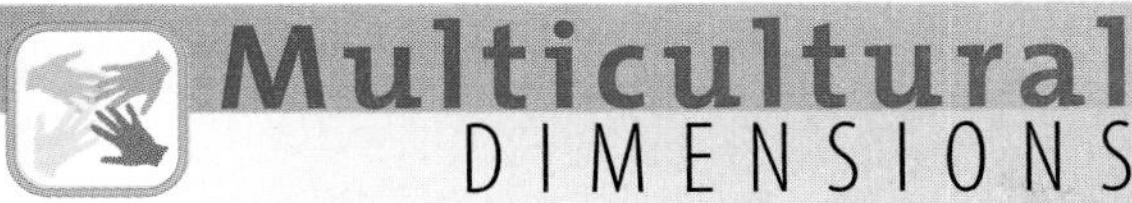

Multicultural DIMENSIONS

Female and Male Subcultures? Male–female communication is related to gender issues. In the business world males and females seem to be members of different subcultures: Even though meetings in the executive suite increasingly are coed gatherings, there are often real differences in the behavior of females and males.

It could be called the "bad-boy/good-girl" clash. Men seated around conference tables often start acting like adolescents—putting on a show of bravado while trading "witty" put-downs to protect themselves from the pain of criticism. As a prerequisite to success, their culture has taught them to be both self-effacing and self-promoting.

Women, by contrast, have learned from their culture to be earnest perfectionists, eager to show they have done all their homework by explaining every point; yet they are quick to admit mistakes. A woman executive reported seeing this at a meeting where a female colleague began her presentation with many apologies. She told the group that all the information she needed was not available, that she had been rushed, that her slides probably contained typos. She said she was sorry several times but then went on to give a flawless presentation with perfect slides. The man who followed her launched right into his presentation with no apologies whatsoever—and his slides were much less well put together.

Another time the woman executive said she felt frustrated listening to a man who used one incomprehensible acronym after another. Finally, she raised her hand and asked him what one acronym meant. After he explained, the guy sitting next to her leaned over and said, "I'm so glad you asked; I had no idea what he was talking about." She realized that men will not ask questions that make them look uninformed.

Men will, however, take up room at conference tables, spreading out papers, stretching or leaning back, and swiveling around in their chairs. Men are often observed standing up at meetings when they want to make a point or stretching in their seats. Some walk around the room when speaking, asserting their power position.

On average, men talk more at meetings than women, and so their ideas typically are adopted more often. Men also are more comfortable making up things, so if someone asks about a particular financial figure, for example, they may offer one. A woman is more likely to say, "I'm not sure about that." Women give the impression that they do not know what they are talking about, whereas many men seem confident whether they know a little or a lot.

However, it is probably possible to change behaviors and expectations in different cultures. For example, at Eddie Bauer & Co. in Seattle, where half of all managers are women, female executives report a "comfort level" about speaking freely at meetings that they did not feel working at other places. Style differences seem to relate more to job categories than to gender.

Of course, we cannot assume that all males or females will behave exactly as those described do. The point is that we need to be aware of possible subcultural differences in our personal relationships as well as in our business relationships. Understanding these possible differences can be helpful in improving communication in all relationships.

Source: Hymowitz, C. Men, women fall into kids' roles in meetings, *The Birmingham News* (December 20, 1998), D1–D2.

and having an expressive voice. Men tend to be louder and more likely to interrupt and to be more nervous and uneasy about the use of nonverbal messages. Examples include using speech stammers and false starts, interrupting others, having restless feet and legs, interspersing speech with "um" and "ah," speaking loudly, and touching themselves during interactions (Briton & Hall, 1995).

Consequently, to depend on nonverbal communication alone to express yourself sexually is to risk being misunderstood. Furthermore, if your partner is depending on nonverbal communication to express feelings to you, it is up to you to find out—verbally—whether you are getting the right message. Without such a reality check, your partner, although totally failing to connect, might assume that he or she is communicating effectively. For example, imagine that a man and woman on their first date begin hugging, kissing, and caressing each other after a movie. The woman's breathing speeds up, and the man, taking this as a sign of sexual arousal and interest, presses onward. When the woman suddenly pushes free and complains that the man is too impatient, he is confused. The problem here is one of interpretation rather than incompatibility: The rapid breathing that the man took as a sign of arousal was really a sign of nervousness. If these people had been more effective verbal communicators, they would have been able to clarify the situation in the beginning. Instead they reached a silent impasse, with him confused and her resentful. It can work the other way around, too; both people may want to touch each other but feel too awkward to show it and thus are disappointed.

Although there are many forms of nonverbal communication, probably three of the most important are proximity, eye contact, and touching. Another name for proximity is *nearness*. Even in our example of students' leaning in the direction of the speaker if they are interested, they are showing nearness. Most often, however, proximity refers to the face-to-face distances between people. Although there are differences, in most cultures moving closer indicates increased interest or intimacy, and moving farther away indicates the opposite.

Making eye contact with another person shows interest. This can be true when one is simply listening to another person; however, making eye contact with another person for a little longer than usual can also be a signal of interest in a relationship.

Touching can be very important in a relationship, and it can show interest, intimacy, and emotional closeness. It can range from a slight touch to show concern or connection to the intimate touching associated with sexual relationships. Touch must be used with caution. For example, if someone you do not know very well touches you, that action could be offensive to you. Also, in social and work situations it is important to be careful in using touch to prevent appearing overly intimate and to avoid giving any suggestion of sexual harassment.

Barriers to Effective Sexual Communication

The basic communication model is successful only when the receiver understands the message as intended by the sender. In real life, that is hard to accomplish. Consider all the times that you thought you had delivered a clear message, only to be misunderstood. Most messages reach their destination but are disrupted by communication barriers. The most common barriers to successful communication are bypassing, frame of reference, and lack of language and listening skills (Guffey, 1999). To this list we add mind-altering drugs (which include alcohol). Figure 3.2 summarizes ways that barriers play a part in sexual miscommunication.

- *Bypassing:* We all attach meanings to words, but individuals may attach different meanings. Consider the confusion that results if your partner does not want to engage in "sexual relations." You may back off all physical contact. Yet some people—including the former president Bill Clinton—consider sexual relations to refer only to penile–vaginal intercourse. So it is important to understand what meaning your partner attaches to a word.

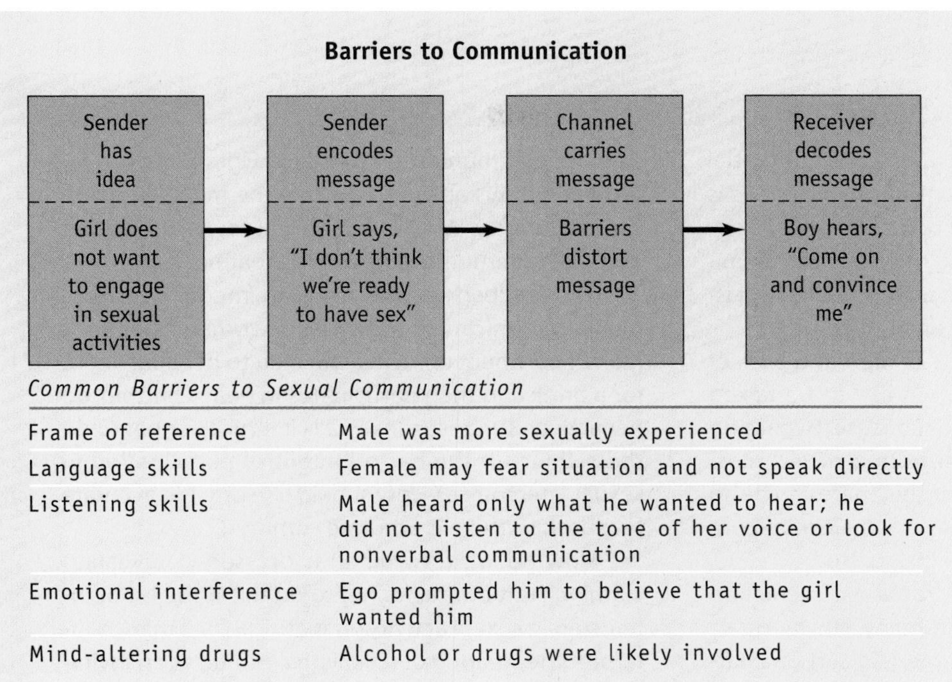

Common Barriers to Sexual Communication

Frame of reference	Male was more sexually experienced
Language skills	Female may fear situation and not speak directly
Listening skills	Male heard only what he wanted to hear; he did not listen to the tone of her voice or look for nonverbal communication
Emotional interference	Ego prompted him to believe that the girl wanted him
Mind-altering drugs	Alcohol or drugs were likely involved

FIGURE 3.2 Common barriers to communication.

- *Frame of reference:* Your frame of reference is your unique set of experiences. Your sociocultural upbringing strongly influences your style of communication. A belief in the sexual double standard, in which men pursue women and women "give in" to men, affects the male's frame of reference in our example. As you may remember from Chapter 1's opening story about Lisa, the Korean culture often discourages open discussion of feelings and seeking out of psychological counseling. Thus, Lisa was unable to tell her boyfriend of her pregnancy scare.
- *Lack of language skill:* In a new situation, you may not be prepared to communicate effectively. For example, one partner may fear the situation and not know how to communicate effectively that the other's sexual pursuit is unwelcome.
- *Lack of listening skills:* We often listen selectively and interpret messages to our advantage. In our example, the male heard only what he wanted to hear ("Come on and convince me"). He failed to listen to the tone of his partner's voice or look for nonverbal cues.
- *Mind-altering drugs:* Use of alcohol and drugs creates a powerful barrier to communication. More than half of all date rapes involve alcohol. As your inhibitions and ability to communicate clearly fade, so does your ability to control the situation.

Gender Communication Issues

In a popular magazine, Sheidlower (1997) indicated that communication difficulties between the sexes are related to a lack of vocabulary. Men and women are unable to reach a mutual understanding of certain concepts because they cannot describe them to each other. He compares the reality of situations with the words women use in their language ("she-speak"). Here

Ethical DIMENSIONS

Ethics, Communication, and Date Rape

One example of potential communication difficulties is sexual behavior on a date. Keeping our basic communication model in mind, let us consider some ethical issues related to communication and date rape.

It has been found that 69% of men and 54% of women believe that some women like to be talked into having sexual intercourse. Because bypassing (misunderstanding that results from a mixed message) can occur if a male believes this, there can be an ethical responsibility for the male or female to be sure certain messages are accurately interpreted.

There are cultural images of romantic interaction in sexual situations that lead to many ethical questions about date rape. For example, is it part of a dating ritual for a woman to resist a man's initial sexual advances? What is her ethical responsibility to be sure she is sending accurate—and not misleading—messages?

If a woman is drunk or has used other chemical substances that can influence judgment, what is the ethical responsibility of the male in regard to his actions? Should the female have considered the ethics of putting herself (and himself) in that situation in the first place? If she is under the influence of chemical substances, she may send (encode) a message in a way she does not intend.

If a male is drunk or has used other chemical substances that can influence his judgment, the "noise" (see the communication model in Figure 3.2) can interfere with his ability to decode the message being sent accurately. What is his ethical responsibility for accurate communication in this situation?

The feedback being sent is an important part of our communication model. If a woman goes to a man's apartment or invites the man to her apartment for a drink and then participates in heavy petting, do her actions suggest consent? Is it ethical for her to do these things if she has no intent of participating in sexual intercourse? How should she provide accurate feedback so there is accurate communication?

How about if a woman is dressed in revealing clothing? Is it ethical for her to do this if she is not interested in sexual activity? Is it ethical for a man to interpret the wearing of revealing clothing as an invitation for sexual activity?

Date rape may be a result of miscommunication. Following the steps of our basic communication model (sender's having an idea, sender's encoding the message, message's traveling over a channel, receiver's decoding the message, and feedback's traveling to the sender) and considering how bypassing can occur and how noise can interfere with accurate communication give us many ethical issues related to communication and date rape to consider. Clear communication is needed to help prevent date rape.

Source: Is there a date rape crisis in society? in Vail, A., ed. *Taking sides: Clashing views on controversial issues in family and personal relationships,* 4th ed. Guilford, CT: Dushkin/McGraw-Hill, 1999.

are two examples (***the authors recognize that these examples are quite sexist, but we include them because many people, unfortunately, believe in these stereotypes***):

- "He-speak": A new car has "331 horsepower, five-speed transmission, V-8, four valves per cylinder, dual overhead cam, and a twin turbocharger." "She-speak": "It's red."
- "He-speak": A new amplifier has "twin mono-blocks, low THD, only 40 watts per channel, but it's a small room, so the low-impedance speakers will still work; it'll be expensive if we blow any Gold Aero KT-88 output tubes." "She-speak": "That thing is not going in *my* living room."

Gender DIMENSIONS

Sexual Behavior in Marriage

Listen to this couple in their mid- to late 20s, married nine years:

Wife: I don't understand him. He's ready to go any time. It's always been a big problem with us right from the beginning. If we've hardly seen each other for two or three days and hardly talked to each other, I can't just jump into bed. If we have a fight, I can't just turn it off. He has a hard time understanding that. I feel like that's all he wants sometimes. I have to know I'm needed and wanted for more than just jumping into bed.

Husband: She complains that all I want from her is sex, and I try to make her understand that it's an expression of love. I'll want to make up with her by making love, but she's as cold as the inside of the fridge. I get mad when that happens. Why shouldn't I? Here I'm trying to make up and make love, and she's holding out for something—I don't know what.

Wife: He keeps saying he wants to make love, but it just doesn't feel like love to me. Sometimes I feel bad that I feel that way, but I just can't help it.

Husband: I don't understand. She says it doesn't feel like love. What does that mean, anyway? What does she think love is?

Wife: I want him to talk to me, to tell me what he's thinking. If we have a fight, I want to talk about it so we could maybe understand it. I don't want to jump in bed and just pretend it didn't happen.

Husband: Talk! Talk! What's there to talk about? I want to make love to her and she says she wants to talk. How's talking going to convince her I'm loving her?

In sexual behavior, as in other matters, the barriers to effective communication are high and the language people use only further confuses and mystifies them. He says he wants to make love, but she says, "It doesn't feel like love." Neither quite knows what the other is talking about; both feel vaguely guilty and uncomfortable, aware only that somehow they're not connecting. He believes that he has already given her a profound declaration of love: he married her and they share a home.

Yet she says, "Just once, I'd like him to love me without it ending up in sex. But when I tell him that, he thinks I'm crazy."

For him, perhaps, it does seem crazy. Sexual activity may be the one way in which he can allow himself the expression of deep feeling. His wife, however, finds it difficult to be comfortable with her feelings in the same area. She keeps asking for something that she can understand and is comfortable with—a demonstration of his feelings in nonsexual ways. He keeps giving her the one thing he can understand and is comfortable with—his feelings wrapped up in a blanket of sex. Thus some husbands and wives find themselves in an impossibly difficult bind, one that stems from the cultural context in which girls and boys grow to adulthood.

We are suggesting that the man's ever-present sexual readiness is not simply an expression of urgent sexual need but is also a complex response to a socialization process that restricts the development of the emotional side of his personality. Conversely, the woman's insistent plea for a nonsexual emotional statement is a response to a process that encourages the development of the emotional side of her personality.

Sheidlower's point is that if we want to have high-quality relationships, we have to make an effort. Whether or not there is a difference in vocabulary between the genders is for each of us to decide, but we can also do our part to reduce the possibility of a problem of miscommunication.

Gender roles can strongly shape our communication patterns. Because men have traditionally focused on their place in the hierarchy, they tend to be good at public speaking. Women, who have traditionally focused on nurturing relationships, tend to be better at speaking in private. On the emotional level, women tend to be good at verbalizing thoughts and feelings in close relationships. Men, in contrast, tend to be good at dismissing their feelings or keeping them to themselves. For men, expressing feelings does not help determine their status or help them compete in the outside world. It can be helpful to be aware of the context and the power of gender roles to influence what we hear, what we say, and what is the purpose of our communication (Worden & Worden, 1998).

Because emotions are involved in the use of language, remembering that gender differences may affect people's responses to emotion can be helpful. For example, men and women may have subtle differences in their responses to a number of emotions, including anger, sadness, and jealousy (Guerrero, 1998).

Do males and females naturally communicate differently, or are their communication behaviors learned just as other behaviors are? Some people believe that males are socialized to be more assertive and direct, in both verbal and nonverbal communication. Eye contact, body placement, and rough physical contact by males can communicate intention, superiority, and territoriality. Historically, women have generally been socialized to have a less pronounced presence. They tend, for example, to listen empathetically, communicate and elicit emotions, and process conflict. As a result, a familiar complaint of women in heterosexual relationships is that male partners "never want to talk about things," "aren't sensitive to their needs," and "just don't understand." Conversely, males often wonder how a seemingly innocuous comment could cause their female partner's sudden silence or desire to talk about where the relationship is going. People internalize the values attached to gendered communication to the point that men become used to living within conflict and women prefer the roles of peacemaker and relationship builder. Some people argue that looking at gender exclusively as the source of different communication styles is a mistake and that such elements as upbringing, socioeconomic status, culture, and ethnicity must be considered within this context (Do women and men communicate differently? 2003).

Attitudes About Sexuality

Some people are prevented from communicating openly by attitudes learned at home. Some parents "protect" young children from references to sexuality. When as teenagers these children are exposed to talk about sexuality—on the street or at school—they often feel guilty for participating in or eavesdropping on such forbidden conversations. When parents fail to acknowledge our sexuality as children, we should not be surprised if suppressed feelings permeate our adult sexual lives.

There is a debate over whether or not men and women have different talking styles (Do men and women speak different languages? 1999). Some people believe that men have a need for control in their social relationships. During conversations they try to capture the floor, state their issues with forthright clarity, and make decisions confidently. They do not like being interrupted and revel in giving information and advice. By contrast, the argument goes, women are predisposed to being inclusive and nurturing in their conversational style. They wait their turn for the floor and make cooperative decisions after hearing all sides. Women like to keep the conversation flowing, interrupt one another, fill silences, and ask questions. Expressing sympathy and sharing similar feelings are regular elements of women's conversations.

Those who believe that these patterns of communication exist say that the contrasting styles may lead to misunderstanding between men and women in close relationships. Further, to improve rational quality it is necessary to develop understanding and sympathy for differences in the ways men and women talk and to make sincere efforts to listen and appreciate the other's way of speaking. Opponents of this view believe that we must dig deeper than sex differences to understand people's communication problems. Communication may depend more on social status and power of the speaker than on gender.

Deborah Tannen, a professor of linguistics, has written extensively about male and female communication styles. She indicates that many women feel it is natural to consult their partners at every turn, whereas men automatically make more decisions without consulting their partners. This may show a real difference in conceptions of decision making. For example, women expect decisions to be discussed first and made by consensus; however, many men feel oppressed by lengthy discussions about what they see as minor decisions, and they feel hemmed in if they cannot act without talking first. Tannen further indicates that communication is a continual balancing act, juggling conflicting needs for intimacy and independence (Tannen, 1991).

Some writers suggest that men often do not communicate well with women because they have a "fear of intimacy" that is really a fear of rejection. One way to deal with this is for men to learn to talk about their lives more openly, as women have learned to do. Developing their own friendships with other men can help men acquire personal skills that will also improve their relationships with women (Dickson, 2000).

Parent–Teen Communication

An excellent example of the importance of good communication is that between parents and their children—especially their adolescent children. Karofsky (2001) reported a correlation between the level of adolescent–parent communication, as perceived by the teenager, and abstinence from initiation of sexual intercourse. High levels of communication with mothers were most closely associated with abstinence. The amount of parent–teen communication declined as the teen got older. The authors suggest two possibilities: (1) As communication declined at home, teenagers sought a replacement for intimacy with their parents and then participated in sexual intercourse; (2) as teenagers became sexually active, they were reluctant to discuss these and other personal issues with their parents, and therefore communication declined.

Dailard (2001) reported that teenagers who feel their parents are warm, caring, and supportive are more likely to delay sexual activity than their peers. Teens who feel highly satisfied with their relationship with their mother are more likely to use contraception and to delay sexual activity and are less likely to have an unplanned pregnancy.

When it comes to communicating with their children about sexuality, many parents consider the task a daunting one, for which they feel ill equipped. Parents often do not have meaningful conversations with sons and daughters because they do not know what to say or how to begin, fearing that talking to children about sexuality may either scare children or encourage them in sexual behaviors at a young age. Most parent–child discussions about sexuality are limited, indirect, and uncomfortable. Yet, parents' failure to provide adolescents with appropriate information and decision-making skills may place teens at risk for negative outcomes such as pregnancy or STI. Only about 15% of adolescents have had conversations about sexuality with their parents. Mothers are more likely than fathers to discuss birth control, adolescent pregnancy, and sexual morality with both sons and daughters (Filomeno, 2002).

Sexual Language

One of us was invited to speak with a group of elderly people about sexuality. Proceeding with undaunted courage, he began the session with exercises designed to neutralize the emotional impact of sexual words. He showed slides containing one or two words and instructed the participants to shout in unison the word appearing on the slide. The first slide was shown and the audience shouted *love* with much enthusiasm. Buoyed up by the group's cooperation and interest, he projected the next slide—*hug.* The audience again shook the room with their shouts. From that point on, however, it was all downhill. With each successive word, the decibel level of the voices lowered—no small wonder, considering the remaining words: *kiss, caress, pet, sexual intercourse, oral sex, penis,* and *vagina.* The point was made: People are uncomfortable with sexual language. How can sexual communication be effective if we cannot even speak the language?

When discussing sexual topics, people often find that the words themselves prevent rational, thoughtful, comfortable interaction. Some words

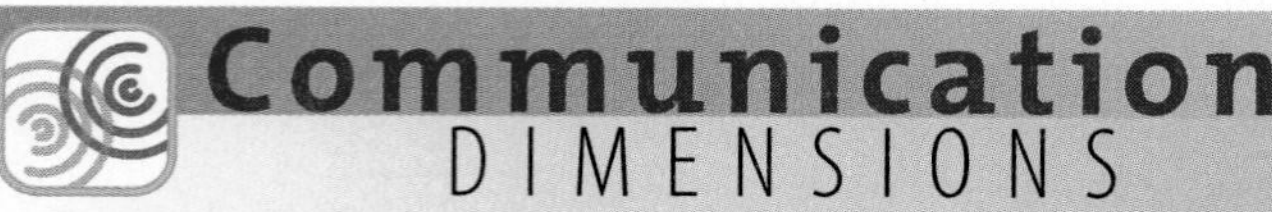

Clarity in Sexual Communication

In the communication process, the idea sent and the message actually received are ideally the same. But as you likely know from experience, it does not always work that way. Often, the words chosen, the tone of voice, the body language, or the context in which the message is delivered blurs the true intent of the sender. When you add the ambiguity of sexual language, communicating clearly becomes even more difficult.

Consider the President Bill Clinton and his now-infamous words in a press conference on January 26, 1998: "I did not have sexual relations with that woman—Miss Lewinsky." To President Clinton, "sexual relations" specifically referred to penile–vaginal intercourse, sexual activity in which he and Monica Lewinsky did not participate.

In his own parlance, Clinton was telling the truth. Yet few would agree with him. One reason was the context of the comment—a formal press conference in the White House. Also, the delivery of the comment—with strong body language and tersely delivered words—made it appear that there was no relationship at all between Clinton and Lewinsky.

Now consider how such language ambiguity might affect a newer relationship.

Let us say that you suggest beginning a more "serious relationship" with someone. Your partner responds that the relationship is not ready for "sexual relations." At this point, it is not clear what either party has said. A "serious relationship" could imply having sexual activity, but it could also imply seeing each other more often or not seeing other people. The "sexual relations" comment in the context of an intimate conversation could be construed to refer to any sexual activity.

Thus, it is important to be clear in communicating about sexuality with a partner. If you or your partner cannot talk about sexuality, that may be a sign that you are not ready to be involved in a sexual relationship.

A good way to start a conversation is to talk about sexual histories. By starting the conversation and opening it up for participation, you will make it more comfortable for your partner. Talk about sexual activities that you have enjoyed and would like to share with your partner.

Before entering into a sexual relationship, you should talk about any STIs that you or a partner may have had, and any STI and/or HIV testing you have had (and why you had it done). In addition, you should discuss using latex condoms to prevent STI transmission, as well as using a contraceptive method to prevent pregnancy.

evoke such strong emotions—embarrassment, guilt, shame, or anger—that they interfere with thoughtful discourse. Generally, the greater the emotion, the greater the interference.

For example, it may be that the term used influences what a partner hears: "Penis," "dick," and "cock" may all have different connotations for different people. Calling a vagina a "vagina" may sound very clinical to one person, whereas calling it a "pussy" or a "cunt" may sound sexy, dirty, or just fine to someone else. The sexual language used can promote communication and relationships, or it can inhibit them.

Techniques for Improving Sexual Communication

There are no magical methods for attaining free, open, and comfortable communication about sexual topics, but we do have some suggestions.

Planning

One common barrier to good sexual communication is the complete avoidance of the subject by both partners. We suggest that partners set aside time to discuss sexuality as they would any other topic of mutual interest and of significance to their relationship. In setting up a time for such a discussion, it is wise to make the following plans.

1. Make sure you have plenty of time for your discussion. Do not be cut short when one of you has to run off somewhere.
2. Do not allow others to interrupt your discussion by calling you or by barging in on you.
3. Accept all feelings and the right to express these feelings verbally. For example, it is just as appropriate to say, "I feel angry when . . . " as it is to say, "I feel terrific when. . . . "
4. Take a risk—really describe your thoughts and needs. Do not expect your partner to guess what they are.
5. Approach the discussion with both understanding that the goal is to improve your relationship rather than to see who can shock whom.
6. Expect changes but not miracles. Sexual communication requires continued dialogue. You might want to seek the help of other family members, friends, peer counselors, members of the clergy, psychologists, sexuality counselors, or others who can contribute to your ability to communicate sexually.

Working to improve your sexual communication will help you and your partner develop a deeper trust, a greater sense of intimacy, and a feeling of adventure about your relationship.

Flooding

A technique for learning to use and become comfortable with sexual language is called **flooding.** In one use of this technique, people stand in front of a mirror, look themselves in the eye, and repeat over and over again the words they feel uncomfortable using. We are not necessarily referring to profanity. We are talking about sexual language. Learning to feel comfortable with these words and being able to use them should be your goals.

flooding
Experiencing something so frequently that you no longer are aroused by it. This is a technique used to become more comfortable with sexual terminology.

Learning Assertiveness

Some people just have a tough time communicating—period. Inevitably they have trouble communicating sexually. When this is the case, working to improve only the sexual side of communication is a mistake. Therefore, we turn now to a topic that concerns one's ability to express oneself with confidence in all areas—the quality of assertiveness and the means to develop it.

assertiveness
Standing up for one's basic rights without violating anyone else's rights.

aggressiveness
Standing up for one's basic rights, but at the expense of someone else's basic rights.

nonassertiveness
Giving up your basic rights so others may achieve theirs.

The first step toward grasping what it means to be assertive is to distinguish assertive, aggressive, and nonassertive behaviors. **Assertiveness** means standing up for your basic rights *without violating* anyone else's. **Aggressiveness** means standing up for your basic rights (or more) *at the expense* of someone else's rights. **Nonassertiveness** means *giving up* your basic rights so that other people can achieve theirs.

For example, an assertive style of verbal sexual communication would be one in which you stand up for your own sexual rights and needs by expressing your wishes, while allowing your partner the same freedom.

Body language, too, can be aggressive, nonassertive, or assertive. Aggressive body language includes a pointing finger, leaning toward the other person, glaring, and using a loud, angry tone of voice. Nonassertive body language is characterized by slumped posture, a lack of eye contact, hand-wringing, hesitant speech, nervous whining or laughing, and not saying or doing what you want to. Assertive behavior, by contrast, entails sitting or standing tall, looking directly at the person you are talking to, speaking in explicit statements with a steady voice, and using the gestures or physical contact that is right for you.

As a first step toward learning to be assertive, consider this formula, developed by Bower and Bower (1976), for organizing assertive verbal responses. The formula, which they call DESC, involves

1. ***D***escribing the other person's behavior or the situation as objectively as possible (as in sentences taking the form "When you . . .")
2. ***E***xpressing your feelings about the other person's behavior or the situation that you just described (as in statements beginning with "I feel . . .")
3. **S**pecifying changes you would like to see made ("I would like . . ." or "My preference is . . .")
4. ***C***hoosing the consequences you are prepared to accept (a) if the situation changes to our satisfaction and (b) if it does not ("If you . . . , I will . . ." or "If you don't . . . , I will . . .")

Using the DESC form, then, let us look at an example of assertive sexual communication: "When you expect me to become sexually aroused in two minutes of foreplay (Describe), I feel as though I'm being used (Express). I would like us to spend more time touching, kissing, and hugging (Specify). If you agree to devote more time to foreplay, I will relax and pay special attention to your sexual needs. If you don't agree to devote more time to foreplay, I won't have intercourse with you (Choose)." Note that our imaginary speaker describes the situation from a personal point of view, expressing his or her own feelings and preferences, as well as the consequences of the listener's choice.

The form of the DESC message just described suggests the philosophical basis of the assertion theory: We are in control of ourselves alone; we have no right to tell others how to behave; we need not tolerate the other person's behavior when it is contrary to our own desires. The basis of assertive behavior is the combination of self-respect with respect for others. One could find no better formula for effective sexual communication.

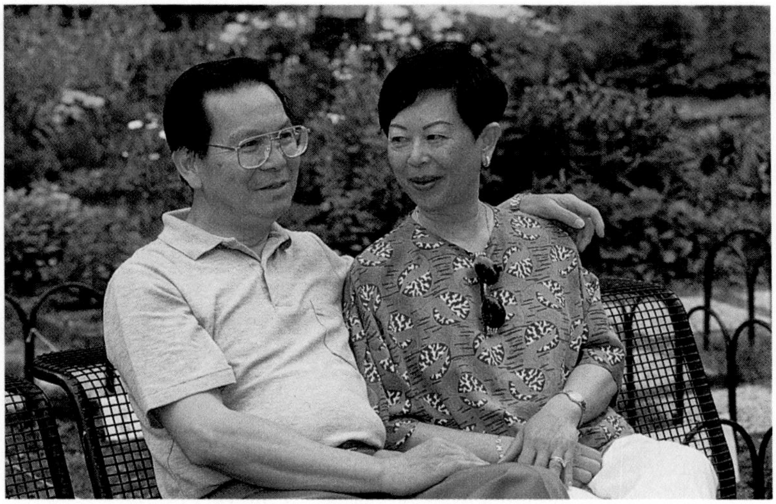

Sitting close together, touching, and smiling are all ways to show you care. Nonverbal communication is important; expressing feelings in words is also vital.

Expressing Yourself Nonverbally

Words are important, but they do not say it all. Do not be afraid to smile, wink, hug, touch, kiss, or in other ways communicate your affection for another. As we said earlier, in the way you walk, sit, gesture, and so on, you are "talking" to your partner, whether you intend to or not. But you can also consciously use those gestures to help get your message across.

Seeking Information (Listening)

Verify your interpretation of the other person's verbal, and especially nonverbal, communication. Listen actively, and ask whether your understanding of your partner's feelings and intentions is accurate. Listening is often hard and takes real skill. If you want to hear what others say effectively, make sure you are not a

- *Mind reader:* You hear little or nothing as you think, "What is this person really thinking or feeling?"
- *Rehearser:* Your mental tryouts for "Here's what I'll say next" tune out the speaker.
- *Filterer:* Some call this selective listening—hearing only what you want to hear.
- *Dreamer:* Drifting off during a face-to-face conversation can lead to an embarrassing "What did you say?" or "Could you repeat that?"
- *Identifier:* If you refer everything you hear to your experience, you probably did not hear what was said.
- *Comparer:* When you get side-tracked assessing the messenger, you are sure to miss the message.
- *Derailer:* Changing the subject too quickly tells others you are not interested in anything they have to say.
- *Sparrer:* You hear what is said but quickly belittle it or discount it. That puts you in the same class as the derailer.
- *Placater:* Agreeing with everything you hear just to be nice or to prevent conflict does not make you a good listener (Why don't we hear others? 1996).

The leadership expert Stephen Covey speaks of "attentive" and "empathetic" listening—not the fake or manipulative kind but rather "listening with the intent to understand." Covey speaks and writes about situations related to business; however, the basics of good listening skills apply to intimate relationships as well. Good listeners are rare; most of us have to squelch our natural inclination to talk.

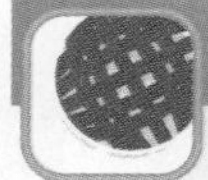

Global DIMENSIONS

International Differences in Discussing Sexuality In many chapters of this book, we have seen examples of international differences related to the topic of human sexuality. One way to gain understanding of these differences is to consider how sexuality education is viewed in some countries. Here are some examples.

1. In Mexico, it is the government's policy to stabilize growth. Family planning is supposed to be implemented by means of education and public services. At the same time, the conservative Catholic church opposes sexuality education.
2. In Chile, sexuality is not a subject that is talked about by family members or in schools.
3. In China, there is virtually no institutional sexuality education. People rely on folklore, sexually explicit materials, and approved marriage manuals for sexuality information.
4. In Denmark, sexuality and social-life education has been a compulsory subject in schools since 1970, and it was a tradition long before then.
5. In Egypt, discussion of sexuality is socially unacceptable. Egypt uses an approach that emphasizes repression rather than education.
6. In Greece, sexuality education does not exist in the school curriculum. Greece is one of the few European countries without sexuality education.
7. In India, sexuality education is not offered in schools because society believes it would "spoil the minds" of children.
8. In Iran, to get a marriage license, couples must take a segregated course in family planning.
9. In Japan, sexuality education in schools (typically focused on reproductive issues) is mandated, beginning at age 10 or 11 years. The Ministry of Education believes that teachers should teach HIV and AIDS prevention to students without mentioning sexual intercourse.
10. In Kenya, the government opposes sexuality education in schools. Young people turn to their peers for sexuality information.
11. In Romania, sexuality education was removed from the schools in the early 1980s. The major sources of contraception and sexuality information are friends, mass media, and health care providers.
12. In Singapore, women are highly ignorant about their bodies, including being unable to locate the vagina. Women complain also of pain during intercourse, because of lack of foreplay. Some women who believe they are barren actually turn out to be virgins.
13. In Sweden, sexuality education has been a compulsory subject in schools since 1955. It is well integrated into the school curriculum. In addition, Swedish children receive their first sexuality education at home, from their parents.
14. In Thailand, there are strong taboos surrounding the discussion of sexuality and disease. HIV/AIDS education has been stifled and many do not know how the disease is spread.
15. In the United Kingdom, sexuality education has been required in secondary schools since 1993. In Northern Ireland, it is not mandated, but it is encouraged in the teaching of health education. In Scotland, jurisdiction over the provision of sexuality education lies with the local education authority. In general, teens report that they believe their parents should be their main source of sexuality information; however, in practice they are more likely to turn to their friends for information.

Although it is difficult to draw definite conclusions from this information, it appears that there can be real differences in the ability of people from various countries to engage in effective communication about human sexuality. For example, think about the differences that are likely to exist between people from Sweden and those from Thailand or from Egypt. Of course, we cannot generalize about all people from any country, because many differences are possible within countries. But these differences can strongly influence communication about sexuality.

Source: Caron, S. L. *Cross-cultural perspectives on human sexuality.* Boston: Allyn & Bacon, 1998.

The characteristics of good listeners are as follows:

1. The most visible characteristic is body language—nodding encouragingly, perhaps leaning into the conversation, not glancing around the room or looking for something.
2. Good listeners demonstrate that they are mentally engaged in what you are saying by making brief comments from time to time and asking focused questions—patiently waiting for the answer before providing one.
3. They listen with the "third ear," seeking to understand those thoughts that are not expressed.
4. They try to understand, rather than first being understood. They try to see the topic of conversation from the speaker's standpoint first. Good listeners push back the urge to express personal opinions until they are asked or until the time is appropriate.
5. Good listeners have to be trusted. They never repeat confidences and personal problems without consent of the party involved (Listening to understand, 1998).

Hostile settings and other communication hindrances can defeat even the best listeners. Here are a few steps to avoid those pitfalls:

1. Choose the physical environment. Find a quiet, nonthreatening place to talk if you want to ensure true understanding.
2. Cut the butt-ins. It can be difficult to communicate if the phone rings or if a person pops in at the door.
3. Recognize differences. People communicate best in different ways. Some of us are primarily auditory, whereas others are visual or "hands-on."
4. Persist. Refuse to believe that you cannot understand another person's message.

Steps Toward Change

Counselors often work with couples to help them improve their communication skills. In summary, the counselor (1) encourages **active listening;** (2) elicits feedback from each partner by asking each to summarize what he or she just heard; (3) facilitates the expression of feelings and thoughts directly and succinctly; (4) requests the use of **"I" statements** (beginning each sentence with "I" to express personal feelings better and avoid blaming the other partner) instead of questions; and (5) prohibits interruptions and blaming (Worden & Worden, 1998). These techniques will help all of us communicate much more effectively.

active listening
Paraphrasing what someone has said to demonstrate interest and understanding.

"I" statement
Statement that begins with an "I" to express personal feelings.

Resolving Conflicts

In relationships—even the best of relationships—conflicts arise. Too often poor communication skills (such as improper listening), a combative or offensive stance geared toward winning rather than communicating, an inability to acknowledge another's point, or a refusal to consider alternative solutions interferes with the healthy resolution of these conflicts. As a result, conflicts threaten the continuation of the relationship and, at the least, tear little pieces from it, potentially leaving the relationship bankrupt. To gain a sense of how these poor communication skills impair effective conflict resolution, consider the following dialogue.

> Paul: *Well, Barbara, as you know, I really care for you, and I hope we can continue to develop our relationship. We can't go any further tonight, though, because I'd like you to be tested for HIV.*
> Barbara: *Now you ask—right in the middle of this romantic time! Why didn't you say something about this before?*
> Paul: *You've got some nerve. You should have realized this is something we need to consider.*
> Barbara: *I should have realized? How was I supposed to know you were concerned about HIV status? You never said anything about it.*
> Paul: *Why should I take the chance of getting HIV? You're pretty selfish, aren't you?*
> Barbara: *I've had it! Either we're going to trust each other and move ahead in our relationship or you can say good-bye right now.*
> Paul: *In that case, GOOD-BYE!*

In this example, both Paul and Barbara are trying to win: Paul wants Barbara to have an HIV test, and Barbara wants Paul to have faith and move ahead with their relationship. Neither Paul nor Barbara can possibly win this battle, although they are probably unaware of this. If they proceed with their relationship (including sexual intercourse and other intimate behaviors), Paul will be uneasy because of his concern about HIV. He will probably feel his concerns are not very important, will resent Barbara's lack of concern, and will have a difficult time participating freely in the relationship.

However, if Barbara agrees to the HIV test, she will feel that Paul did not trust her and "forced" her to take the test. She may also feel he waited to spring the idea on her and wonder why it did not arise earlier.

It becomes evident, then, that regardless of which way they go, one or the other will be resentful. This resentment will probably result in a weakening, or possibly a dissolution, of their relationship. So, no matter who wins, both really lose.

This situation is not totally hopeless, though. Consider the effect on resolving their conflict if Paul and Barbara had communicated as follows:

> Paul: *Well, Barbara, as you know, I really care for you, and I hope we can continue to develop our relationship. We can't go any further tonight, though, because I'd like you to be tested for HIV.*
> Barbara: *Now you ask—right in the middle of this romantic time! Why didn't you say something about this before?*
> Paul: *You feel we should have discussed this earlier?*
> Barbara: *Yes, and HIV status is something we both need to be concerned about.*
> Paul: *You have a concern about my HIV status, too?*
> Barbara: *You bet! And I think it is only fair that we treat ourselves and each other equally in this situation.*
> Paul: *You think that it would be a problem if you got the HIV test and I didn't?*
> Barbara: *Yes.*
> Paul: *Would you be embarrassed if other people knew you had taken the test?*
> Barbara: *Yes, I guess I would.*
> Paul: *It sounds like my request might have hurt you at least a little?*
> Barbara: *Yes, I guess it did.*
> Paul: *I'm glad that you also care about our relationship. But HIV is really a serious health problem today, and I am worried about it. And I'm bothered that you didn't understand my concern.*

Barbara: *I guess you do have a reason to be concerned. I'm sorry.*
Paul: *Well, let's see what alternatives we have.*
Barbara: *Maybe I should just go ahead and be tested.*
Paul: *Or perhaps we should both be tested.*
Barbara: *How about agreeing that we will honestly share the results with each other but also that the results are private and not anyone else's business?*
Paul: *That's fine with me. In fact, we don't even need to tell anyone else we took the tests. That is our private matter.*
Barbara: *Would it make sense to agree to take the tests as soon as possible so we both know the results as soon as we can?*
Paul: *That seems sensible, and since your schedule in the next couple of weeks is so busy, I'll be happy to work around your schedule.*
Barbara: *Okay. Remember, though, the next time either of us has concerns or suggestions we need to bring them up as early as possible.*

In this example, Paul took the initiative in resolving his interpersonal conflict with Barbara. He began by employing a technique known as *active listening,* or *reflective listening.* The key to this technique is that the listener paraphrases the words of the speaker to indicate that he or she comprehends the meaning of the speaker's message. The listener tries to pick up on hidden messages and feelings not actually verbalized and paraphrases those as well. For example, Paul understood that Barbara would be embarrassed if other people knew she had taken the test, even though she never explicitly stated that. When Paul was able to understand and listen so well to Barbara—well enough to identify feelings she had not verbalized—Barbara was convinced that Paul cared enough to understand her needs. *Then* Barbara was ready to hear about Paul's needs and became more receptive to his viewpoint. Paul next expressed his opinion and the reasons for his feelings. The point of reflective listening is to enable each participant to acknowledge the other's view and to be less insistent in arguing for his or her own.

The next step in this technique is to propose as many alternative solutions as possible through brainstorming. The result is a win–win, rather than a no-win, situation, reached through a mutual agreement that it is possible to agree. Paul agrees that they both will be tested and that they will treat the testing and the results confidentially. He also shows respect for Barbara's busy schedule and says he is willing to work around it.

In addition, Paul and Barbara have improved their relationship *because* of this conflict. The conflict instigates a discussion about their needs and, therefore, provides the opportunity for them to demonstrate their feelings for each other by organizing to satisfy those needs. Instead of threatening the relationship, the conflict has actually improved it.

To reiterate, the steps in this conflict resolution process are as follows:

1. *Active listening:* Reflecting to the other person his or her own words and feelings.

2. *Identifying your position:* Stating your own thoughts and feelings about the situation, and explaining why you feel this way.

3. *Proposing and exploring alternative solutions:* First brainstorming and then evaluating the possibilities.

Although you may feel awkward using this technique initially, and your conversations may seem stilted, with practice it will become a part of your style and will be very effective. The payoffs are huge; do not give up on it.

A similar way to resolve conflict involves four steps (Resolve conflict in 4 steps, 1995): (1) *Identify the interests* of each person. Ask each person,

Myth vs Fact

Myth: For most people, good communication comes naturally.
Fact: Although some people may seem to be naturally better than others at communication, good communication is a lot of work for almost everyone.

Myth: Because sexuality is such an open topic today, most people can discuss it rather easily.
Fact: Even though sexuality seems more open, many people still experience much difficulty in talking about sexual topics and personal relationships.

Myth: Communication skills are basically the same in all cultures.
Fact: Although most skills may be quite similar, communicating with people from another culture can be challenging. Even though the language may be the same, communication methods and meanings may greatly differ.

Myth: Because men and women now have the same rights and are equal, they communicate in the same ways.
Fact: Conditions can be slow to change. Even though men and women have equal rights, we still need to be sensitive to differences in learning and motivation related to communication.

Myth: The most important part of communication is the meaning of the words we use.
Fact: It has often been said that "actions speak louder than words." It is also true that nonverbal communication is often more important, and revealing, than words used.

Myth: It is a bad idea to take a risk when trying to communicate with another person. The technique may backfire.
Fact: There are risks in most things we do, and developing and using good communication skills can involve disclosing personal feelings and desires. In a trusting relationship, this should not be too risky.

Myth vs Fact

Myth: Being assertive means standing up for your basic rights at the expense of someone else's rights.
Fact: Being aggressive is standing up for your basic rights at the expense of someone else's. Being assertive means standing up for your basic rights without violating anyone else's.

Myth: Conflicts will always get in the way of good relationships.
Fact: It is true that conflicts are a part of life, but if we learn how to deal with them effectively they can help us grow and have better relationships.

"What do you want?" Then listen carefully to the answers. (2) *Identify higher levels of interest* by asking, "What does having that do for you?" It is important to understand what each of us really wants. (3) *Create an agreement frame* by asking, "If I could show you how to get X, would you do Y?" X is the person's real interest, and Y is what you want from the person. (4) *Brainstorm for solutions.* Do not just give a solution and expect the other person to accept it. Commitment results from being involved in finding a solution. The solutions must satisfy the interests of all parties.

Giving and Receiving Criticism

Imagine a "sex critic" to evaluate your sexual functioning as a movie critic critiques movies! All of us would probably feel threatened, and because of that, our abilities to function normally would most likely be compromised. Well, in a very real sense, our sexual partners are our sex critics. They evaluate what we do in terms of how pleasing it is for both them and us. It would be nice if we could receive our "sex critique" without feeling threatened by it, without feeling that it denigrated our self-esteem. It would also be nice if we were open enough both to give and to receive feedback about our sexual functioning in a way that enhanced our sexual lives and those of our partners. Well, we can learn both to receive and to give criticism in a way that is truly constructive. Here are a few hints:

1. Find a private, relaxing place to discuss thoughts and feelings about your sexual relationship. You do not want to feel uncomfortable in your environment while discussing such a sensitive topic. Feeling uncomfortable will not be conducive to either receiving or giving feedback on such a sensitive issue.
2. Devote sufficient time to such a discussion. It would be unfortunate if you were beginning to communicate well on significant matters just as one of you had to leave.
3. Limit distractions so that your attention is focused on the conversation. Rather than wondering who might overhear you or who might inadvertently hit you in the head with a Frisbee, find a quiet, private place for your discussion.
4. It is probably not wise to do these things just before or just after a sexual encounter. Plan a relaxed time for this discussion.

In addition to these general suggestions, when *giving criticism* try to remember to

1. Begin your comments on a positive note. "You know, when you kiss me I really feel great." Then move to the behavior you would like to change. "I enjoy your touches so much that it would be terrific if you could. . . ."
2. Be specific regarding the change you are recommending. Rather than announcing, "You don't hold me enough," suggest, "When we watch television, I'd really like it if you would put your arm around me."
3. Be aware of the limitations of your partner. Do not expect more than your partner is able to give. To critique something that cannot or will not be changed may harm the relationship. If your partner is slow to arouse, asking him or her to speed up is unrealistic and, we might add, unfair. It is criticism given for no useful purpose.

When *receiving criticism* try to remember to

1. Separate your partner's suggestions and recommendations from your self-worth. You are no less of a person because you might need to adjust some of your sexual behavior. In fact, if you were not open to suggestion, then you might suspect you have a problem.
2. Assume a nondefensive attitude. Rather than attempting to justify your present actions, ask questions to understand the criticism better. Then, if you disagree, you will know why you disagree.
3. If the criticism is too general, ask for specific suggestions to help you make the recommended change. In addition, inquire as to how your partner can help make this change more likely to occur. Ask your partner to participate in remedying the situation or action being criticized.
4. Whether or not you agree with the criticism, thank your partner for being honest enough to express the concern to you. Acknowledge that it is not easy to discuss such matters and you appreciate the opportunity to consider something you have been doing or not been doing that is causing a problem. Encourage future suggestions that have the potential to improve your relationship.

With these recommendations for giving and receiving criticism, your relationship should improve. That is because not only will the specific suggestions lead to actual changes, but the practice of opening up your relationship to discussions of problems will, in itself, help foster a style of communicating that will serve you well in all aspects of your relationship. It will then be easier to discuss matters that bother you, and it will be easier to express emotions such as love, caring, and wonderment. The relationship will improve with this style of communication.

Final Thoughts on Sexual Communication

In this chapter we have discussed the importance of word meanings, nonverbal communication, cultural and personal backgrounds, and attitudes toward sexuality to communication. We have also seen that there are many ways to improve our ability to communicate significantly but that doing so usually takes a great deal of effort.

At the same time, however, to be effective, communication must be truthful. In practice, this is often not the case. For example, lying is common in relationships involving college students (Saxe, 1991). The majority of these lies (41%) were about relations with other partners. In another study, respondents said they did not regard their lies as serious, did not plan them, and did not worry about getting caught. They averaged about two lies each day (DePaulo, et al., 1996).

Communication difficulties may even increase the level of risk—especially for females. Rickert and associates (2002) reported that about 20% of women believe they never have the right to stop foreplay, including at the point of intercourse; refuse to have sexual intercourse, even if they have had intercourse with that partner before; make their own decisions about contraception, regardless of their partner's wishes; ask their partner whether he has been examined for STIs; or tell their partner that they want to make love differently or that he is being too rough. Moreover, more than 40% of young women believe that they never have or only sometimes have the right to tell a relative they are not comfortable with being hugged or kissed in certain ways. These findings show that some young women may be unable to communicate their sexual beliefs and desires clearly and are therefore at risk for undesired outcomes.

Finally, it is interesting to note what a number of leading sexologists have said about communication. They were asked to relate the most important information they had learned about sexuality over the years. Here are some of the ideas they expressed about communication (Haffner & Schwartz, 1998):

1. It is hard to be honest about past sexual experiences with a new partner.
2. Some sexual secrets—unless they pose a health threat—are better left unshared.
3. Nonverbal communication often works better than words in bed.
4. Talking during sexual activity—sharing fantasies, using forbidden words—can be very sexy.
5. Couples who have nothing to say to each other in restaurants are usually married—and they may be in trouble.
6. Open, honest communication is the most important foundation for a relationship.
7. You cannot underestimate the value of humor.
8. After humor, consideration is the second most important ingredient in a sexual relationship. Most people appreciate a sensitive and thoughtful partner.
9. Most people are not comfortable talking about sexual issues.
10. Consent requires communication.
11. It is better to talk about sexual feelings, desires, and boundaries in relationships.
12. Talking about scenes in movies or books can sometimes be a good way to communicate what you like in sexual behavior and relationships.

Exploring the DIMENSIONS of Human Sexuality

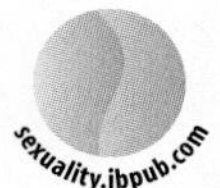

Our feelings, attitudes, and beliefs regarding sexuality are influenced by our internal and external environments. Go to sexuality.jbpub.com to learn more about the biological, psychological, and sociological factors that affect your sexuality.

Biological Factors

- Physiological reactions—such as blushing or erections—are nonverbal means of communicating sexual attraction.
- Alcohol or drugs can distort the communication process.
- Physical touching can indicate interest, intimacy, and emotional closeness.
- Hearing loss over time can inhibit communication and frustrate a partner.

Sociocultural Factors

- Media strongly influence sexual communication.
- Gender affects style of communication.
- Sexuality education may increase confidence.
- Cultures influence communication style.
- Religion may influence the sexual activities in which one participates.
- Family and peers set an example of sexuality.

Psychological Factors

- Emotions can overwhelm the ability to communicate.
- The role of the double standard in thinking may alter the communication process.
- Ego may get in the way of listening to a partner.
- Self-image and body image may distort communication.

CASE STUDY

Your ability to communicate sexually plays an important role in your sexual wellness and self-image. Your capacity to discuss sexual histories, contraceptives, and safer sexual activities can help prevent unwanted pregnancy and transmission of STIs and HIV.

From a psychological standpoint, a positive self-image as a communicator gives you confidence. A negative self-image may hinder your ability to ask for dates, to ask for sexual activities that you like, or to ask for safer sexual activities.

Sexual communication is influenced by virtually all social and cultural phenomena, including religion, ethnic heritage, language, family traditions, peers, geographical region, and even mass media.

Gender plays a pervasive role: Men and women communicate in different styles and express emotions differently.

Consider the confusion of sexual language: If your partner suggested that you were not close enough to engage in "sexual relations," you might back off any type of physical contact. It is important to talk with your partner to make sure each of you understands what the other wants.

Discussion Questions

1. Describe the steps of the communication process. Explain how they would work in discussing specific relationship or sexuality issues.
2. What are the barriers to effective sexual communication? How can they be overcome?
3. How can you improve your communication abilities? Which techniques would work best for you? Which would not work for you? Explain why.

Application Questions

Reread the chapter-opening story and answer the following questions.

1. If you were teaching this course, and Joanna and Mark were students, what information would you want them to leave with from your course?
2. The changes in communication style across the life cycle of the relationship can enhance or harm it. For example, anticipating what your partner wants can lead to a strengthened relationship, but it can also lead to deterioration of communication. What could Joanna and Mark have done to maintain interest in their relationship? (You may want to think about what successful couples you know do to stay happy.)

Critical Thinking Questions

1. Should sexual partners communicate all they think and feel so that they can better respond to each other's needs? Or should sexual partners be selective in relating their innermost thoughts and feelings? Explain why or why not. Would your opinion change from situation to situation?
2. You are excited about an upcoming first date when you overhear a conversation describing your date as someone who has had many sexual partners in the past. You have no idea whether the information is correct. Later, on your date, your partner implies a willingness to engage in sexual activity. Although you like the person and are sexually attracted, you are unable to forget what you overheard. How can you open the discussion of sexual histories without offending your date?
3. On the last episode of MTV's *Road Rules Latin America* (1999), all five of the campers (three males and two females) climb naked into a Jacuzzi™ as a final "gathering of friends." In real life, if you climbed naked into a Jacuzzi™ with some "close friends," what kind of sexual message might that be sending? What if you climbed into the Jacuzzi™ with just one other person whom you wanted to get to know better?

Critical Thinking Case

The following is a true date-rape case that occurred at Georgetown University in the mid-1990s. Kim and Mark (names changed) decided to go to the senior black-tie dance together. Both had agreed beforehand that it would not be a "real date." But during the long evening of drinking and dancing, their plans changed.

They met at 8:30 and went to two parties, the dance, and a bar before returning to Mark's apartment about 4:00 A.M. Kim had lost her key and had agreed to go back to his apartment. "I decided I wouldn't mind kissing him." They kissed, undressed, and climbed into his bed. Kim said later that she had frequently shared a bed with her previous boyfriend without having sexual intercourse and assumed she could do the same with Mark. When Mark asked whether he should get a condom, Kim said they did not know each other well enough to have sex. At that point, the stories diverge.

Kim said she told Mark, "I've never had sex before, and I don't want to have it on a whim." Then, "all of a sudden, he was on top of me, forcing himself into [me]. . . . I kept trying to push him off with my hands and squirming around, and I kept saying I didn't want to have sex."

Mark said in an affidavit that she was "kissing me and thrusting her pelvis against me. . . . At no time during our sexual activity did I use any kind of physical force against Kim. Nor did I threaten Kim verbally."

How could communication have gone so awry? Consider the dimensions of human sexuality as you explain what went wrong. Then describe what could have been done to prevent the incident.

Exploring Personal Dimensions

Measure Your Assertiveness

Indicate how characteristic or descriptive each of the following statements is of you by using the code given.

+3 very characteristic of me, extremely descriptive

+2 rather characteristic of me, quite descriptive

+1 somewhat characteristic of me, slightly descriptive

−1 somewhat uncharacteristic of me, slightly nondescriptive

−2 rather uncharacteristic of me, quite nondescriptive

−3 very uncharacteristic of me, extremely nondescriptive

_____ 1. Most people seem to be more aggressive and assertive than I am.

_____ 2. I have hesitated to make or accept dates because of "shyness."

_____ 3. When the food served at a restaurant is not done to my satisfaction, I complain about it to the waiter or waitress.

_____ 4. I am careful to avoid hurting other people's feelings, even when I feel that I have been injured.

_____ 5. If a salesperson has gone to considerable trouble to show me merchandise that is not quite suitable, I have a difficult time in saying no.

_____ 6. When I am asked to do something, I insist upon knowing why.

_____ 7. There are times when I look for a good, vigorous argument.

_____ 8. I strive to get ahead as well as most people do.

_____ 9. To be honest, people often take advantage of me.

_____ 10. I enjoy starting conversations with new acquaintances and strangers.

_____ 11. I often don't know what to say to attractive persons of the opposite sex.

_____ 12. I will hesitate to make phone calls to business establishments and institutions.

_____ 13. I would rather apply for a job or for admission to a college by writing letters than by going through personal interviews.

_____ 14. I find it embarrassing to return merchandise.

_____ 15. If a close and respected relative were annoying me, I would smother my feelings rather than express my annoyance.

_____ 16. I have avoided asking questions for fear of sounding stupid.

_____ 17. During an argument I am sometimes afraid that I will get so upset that I will shake all over.

_____ 18. If a famed and respected lecturer makes a statement that I think is incorrect, I will have the audience hear my point of view as well.

_____ 19. I avoid arguing over prices with clerks and salespeople.

_____ 20. When I have done something important or worthwhile, I manage to let others know about it.

_____ 21. I am open and frank about my feelings.

_____ 22. If someone has been spreading false and bad stories about me, I see him/her as soon as possible to "have a talk" about it.

_____ 23. I often have a hard time saying "no."

_____ 24. I tend to bottle up my emotions rather than make a scene.

_____ 25. I complain about poor service in a restaurant and elsewhere.

_____ 26. When I am given a compliment, I sometimes just don't know what to say.

_____ 27. If a couple near me in a theater or at a lecture were conversing rather loudly, I would ask them to be quiet or to take their conversation elsewhere.

_____ 28. Anyone attempting to push ahead of me in a line is in for a good battle.

_____ 29. I am quick to express an opinion.

_____ 30. There are times when I just can't say anything.

Scoring

To score this scale, first change the signs (+ or −) to the opposite for items 1, 2, 4, 5, 9, 11, 12, 13, 14, 15, 16, 17, 19, 23, 24, 26, and 30. Next, total the plus (+) items, then total the minus (−) items, and, last, subtract the minus total from the plus total to obtain your score. This score can range from −90 through zero to +90. The higher the score (closer to +90), the more assertively you usually behave. The lower the score (closer to −90), the more nonassertive is your typical behavior. This particular scale does not measure aggressiveness.

Source: Rathus, S. A. A 30-item schedule for assessing assertive behavior, *Behavior Therapy, 4* (1973), 398, 406. Copyright © 1973 Academic Press, Orlando, FL.

Sexuality Online

Go to the web component for *Exploring the Dimensions of Human Sexuality* at sexuality.jbpub.com for web exercises, additional resources related to this chapter, and student review tools.

Suggested Readings

Atkisson, A. What makes love last? *New Age Journal* (September/October 1994), 74–79.

Donahue, M. C. How active is your listening? *Current Health, 2, no. 23* (1996), 27–29.

Gossett, J. & Bellas, M. You can't put a rule around people's hearts. . . can you? Consensual Relationship Policies in Academia, *Sociological Focus, 35, no. 3* (August 2002), 267–284.

Hoyt, C. 22 minutes to a better marriage, *McCall's, 124* (1997), 124+.

Lewis, M. Love talk that can perk up your marriage, *New Choices, 37* (1997), 89.

Sprecher, S. Sexual satisfaction in premarital relationships: Associated with satisfaction, love, commitment, and stability, *Journal of Sex Research 39, no. 3* (August 2002), 190–196.

Tannen, D. *You just don't understand.* New York: Morrow, 1990 (also available in paperback from Ballantine, 1991).

Ting-Toomey, S. & Korzenny, F., eds., *Cross-cultural interpersonal communication.* Newbury Park, CA: Sage Publications, 1991.

Wipond, R. Do we actually want open discussion? *The Humanist, 56* (1996), 35–36.

CHAPTER

4

Female Sexual Anatomy and Physiology

FEATURES

Ethical Dimensions
Should PMS Be Used as an Excuse for Socially Unacceptable Behaviors?

Gender Dimensions
Breast Self-Examination

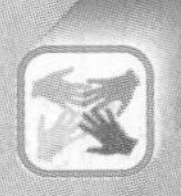

Multicultural Dimensions
Breast Cancer More Deadly in African Americans

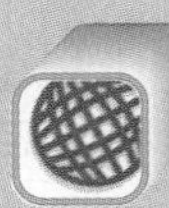

Global Dimensions
Female Genital Mutilation in Various Parts of the World

CHAPTER OBJECTIVES

1. Name and describe the parts of the female reproductive system, to include external and internal genitalia.
2. Discuss the role of breasts in sexual arousal and response, as well as in the reproductive function of lactation.
3. Explain the role of hormones as they pertain to sexuality.
4. Describe what occurs during menstruation, to include menarche, the menstrual cycle, perimenopause, and problems associated with each.
5. Cite various diseases that can affect the female reproductive system and the self-care procedures, as well as medical treatments, associated with these diseases.

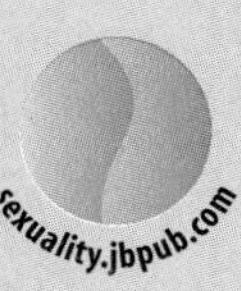

sexuality.jbpub.com

Global Dimensions: Female Genital Mutilation
Amenorrhea
Symptoms of Perimenopause and Menopause
Treatment for Menopause
Breast Cancer

INTRODUCTION

One of the authors of this text was sitting at his desk preparing for an upcoming class. On the desk were diagrams of the female and male reproductive systems, colored pictures with various parts differentiated from others by different pastel colors and shading. Before long, a colleague walked into the office. The visitor was a professor of educational administration and the proud recipient of a baccalaureate degree in mathematics, a master's degree in counseling, and a doctorate in educational administration. In short, this was an educated man, one on whom students and family relied and whose opinions were accorded the respect someone of his stature deserves. As he entered the office, he glanced at the desk and was fascinated with the reproductive system diagrams. When he inquired as to their purpose, he was told that they were to be used in a sexuality education class to help students learn about their sexual organs. It was then that he sheepishly admitted his own ignorance about the structure and function of the reproductive system. For the next 20 minutes, he and his colleague proceeded to discuss the reproductive systems of females and males, referring to the diagrams on the desk.

The only surprising aspect of this incident was the openness with which this educated man admitted his ignorance. In general, people know less about themselves, both physically and psychologically, than they know about cars or ecology or sports or politics or contemporary musicians or any of the hundreds of topics people care about or find fascinating. The less we know about our bodies, the less well equipped we are to keep them healthy. The more we know, the more choices we have and the better decisions we can make. Appropriate health maintenance should be valued similarly by males and females, and both genders need to adopt certain behaviors, such as periodic medical screenings, to maintain their health. However, men's and women's reproductive health issues are not the same.

The purpose of this chapter and the next is to describe the anatomy of the female and male reproductive systems as a step toward creating a comprehensive picture of human sexuality.

The Female Reproductive System

vulva
The female external genitalia.

mons pubis (mons veneris, mount of Venus)
The rounded, soft area above the vaginal opening that becomes covered with hair at puberty.

labia majora
Two large folds of skin whose main function is to protect the external genitalia and the opening of the vestibule (defined later).

labia minora
Two folds of skin lying inside the labia majora, which contain numerous blood vessels and nerve receptors.

Bartholin's glands
Small glands located within the labia minora that secrete a few drops of fluid during sexual arousal.

clitoris
The structure located at the upper part of the labia minora that is homologous to the penis and is very sensitive to stimulation.

corpora cavernosa
A cavernous structure located within the clitoris and the penis that fills with blood during sexual excitement, causing erection.

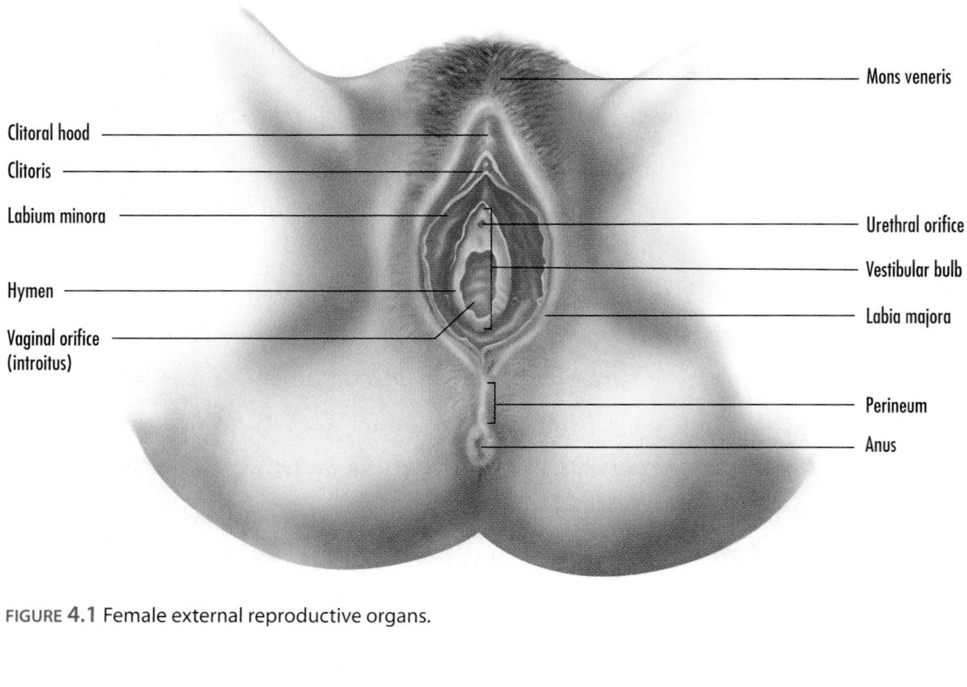

Both females and males have external and internal genitals, or reproductive organs. We begin with the external female genitals and progress inward.

The External Genitals

The external female genitals are the mons pubis, labia majora, labia minora, clitoris, vestibule, and urethral opening (Figure 4.1). All of these organs together are called the **vulva.**

The Mons Veneris
The **mons pubis** (also called the **mons veneris,** or **mount of Venus**) is the rounded, soft area above the pubic bone that becomes covered with hair at puberty. Since the mons contains numerous nerve endings, it can be sexually stimulated.

The Labia Majora
The **labia majora** (major lips) are two large folds of skin whose main function is to protect the external genitalia. Unless the labia majora are spread apart, the other external genitalia are not visible. The outer surfaces of the labia majora also grow hair after puberty, and the inner surfaces remain smooth. Within the tissue of the labia majora are smooth muscle fibers, nerves, and vessels for blood and lymph.

The Labia Minora
The **labia minora** (minor lips) are two folds of skin lying inside the labia majora. Loaded with blood vessels and nerve receptors, the labia minora and their upper part, the clitoris, are very sensitive to stimulation. During sexual

FIGURE 4.1 Female external reproductive organs.

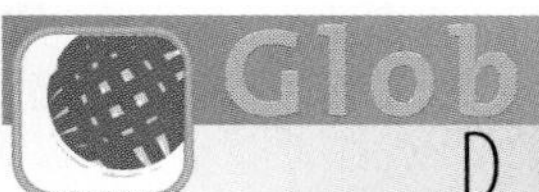

DIMENSIONS

Female Genital Mutilation in Various Parts of the World

Female genital mutilation has been used throughout the world as a means of diminishing sexual stimulation. The result, the argument goes, is that fewer women participate in sexual intercourse outside marriage and fewer women engage in masturbation. Female mutilation can take several different forms. The most simple form is *circumcision,* whereby the clitoral hood is removed. In a *clitoridectomy,* the clitoris itself is surgically removed. Genital *infibulation* is the most complex procedure: The clitoris and the labia minora are removed, and both sides of the vulva are scraped raw and then stitched together. When the tissue grows together, only a small opening remains through which urine and the menstrual flow pass. During these procedures, it is unusual for sterile instruments to be used. Most of the time razor blades or broken glass is used to do the cutting, without the benefit of pain-reducing medications or disinfectants. Therefore, as you might imagine, aside from causing psychological trauma, female mutilation can result in serious medical complications. The combination of infections, bleeding, and pain can cause shock, gangrene, and even death.

Female mutilation is common in some African, Middle Eastern, and Asian countries. In fact, one study found that 97% of married women in Egypt had had some form of genital mutilation performed on them (El Hadi, 1997)—this in spite of the World Health Organization (WHO) and the United Nations Children's Fund (UNICEF) 1980 joint plan to lobby leaders of countries in which female mutilation is common to work toward eliminating this practice. Since then, numerous other organizations and governments have also publicly opposed female genital mutilation, even though the tendency is to avoid interference in cultural practices of sovereign countries. In 1996, the Egyptian government outlawed female genital mutilation, although most Egyptian women are still circumcised. Grass-roots organizations, such as the Kenyan women's organization Maendeleo ya Wanawake, and Tostan in Senegal, have also sprung up around the world with the goal of eliminating female genital mutilation. These groups conduct educational campaigns encouraging women to break the generational cycle of female genital mutilation by preventing their daughters from experiencing it. Too often, however, these groups are met with indifference or outright defiance (African Awakening, 1998), because mothers believe that if their daughters do not observe such cultural practices, they will be outcasts, finding it difficult to marry.

arousal, blood fills the labia minora, causing them to spread, making the vagina more accessible. Within the labia minora lie **Bartholin's glands.** The glands slightly lubricate the labia during coitus (intercourse).

The Clitoris

The **clitoris** is the most sensitive structure in the female body. This small organ contains two spongy bodies, the **corpora cavernosa,** that have the capacity to fill with blood during arousal. (The penis, a similar organ, contains spongy bodies that react to arousal in a similar way.) During sexual stimulation, the corpora cavernosa fill with blood, causing the clitoris to become erect. Popular knowledge about the sensitivity of the clitoris has led males to seek out and stimulate it to arouse their female sexual partners. (Here is a case in which knowledge can have either a positive or a negative effect on sexual relationships. Men who carefully and delicately stimulate the clitoris may sexually arouse their partner, but those who rub incessantly will only irritate the clitoris and thereby irritate their partner. We discuss sexual-arousal techniques in more detail in Chapter 7.)

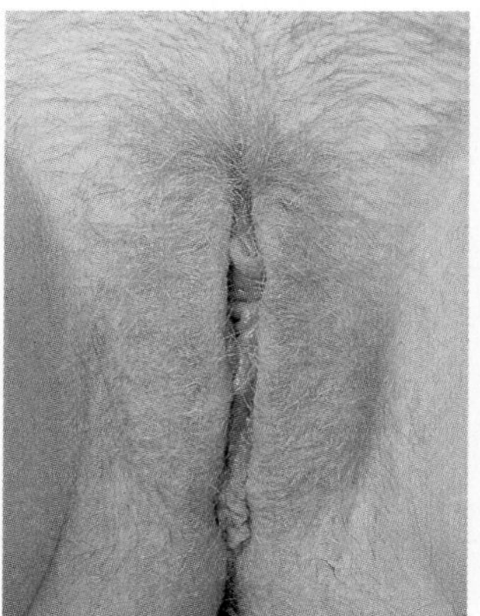
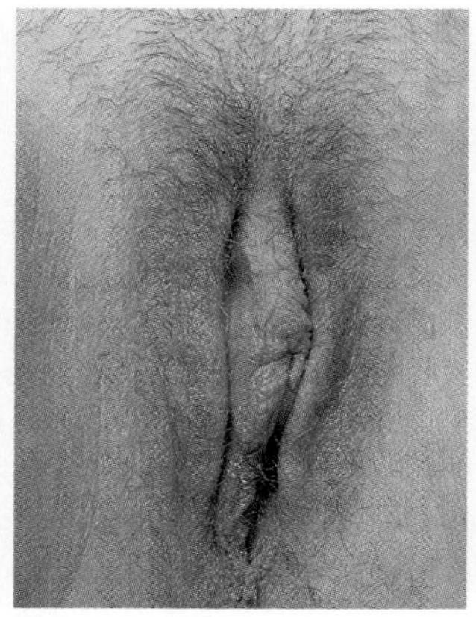
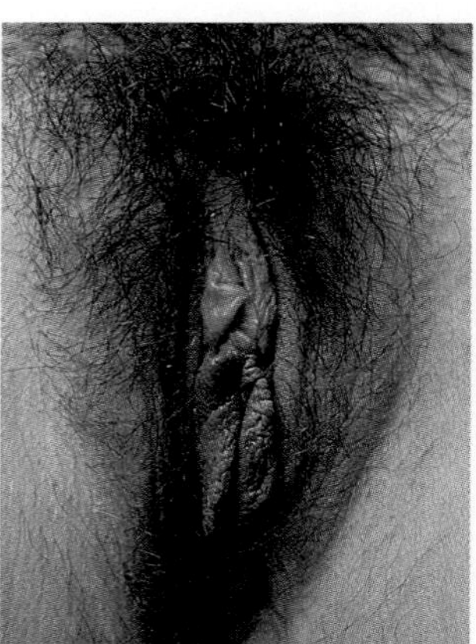

Many variations exist in the female external genitals.

clitoral hood
The skin covering the clitoris.

vestibule
The area containing the vaginal and urethral openings.

hymen
A thin connective tissue covering the opening of the vagina.

annular
Type of hymen that surrounds the vaginal opening.

septate
Type of hymen that bridges the vaginal opening.

cribriform
Type of hymen that creates a sievelike covering for the vaginal opening.

The clitoris is covered by the **clitoral hood.** As can be seen in Figure 4.1, the hood is attached to the labia minora. One function of the clitoral hood is to protect the glans of the clitoris. When we discuss the male reproductive organs, we will observe that the foreskin of the penis protects the glans penis in a similar way.

Knowing about the anatomy of the reproductive system offers guidance for sexual functioning, and the relationship of the clitoris, the clitoral hood, and the labia minora provides a case in point. During sexual intercourse, the clitoris retracts under the clitoral hood. Still, for many women the clitoris can be stimulated if the penis is positioned correctly. One position that will stimulate the clitoris is called "riding high." With the female lying on her back, the male places his penis into the vagina so that its upper shaft rubs on the clitoris. Another option is for the penis to be pressed, thrusting downward, on the lower part of the labia minora so as to create downward movement of the hood and its contact with the clitoris. Many women, however, require additional manual stimulation of the clitoris to cause orgasm during intercourse.

The Vestibule

When the clitoris is erect and the labia minora spread, the urethral and vaginal openings (called the **vestibule**) become visible.

The Urethral Opening

The urethral opening, where urine is excreted, is not generally considered a part of the reproductive system in females, although there is some evidence that women who do experience something akin to ejaculation do so through the urethra.

The Hymen

The **hymen,** a thin connective tissue containing a relatively large number of blood vessels, covers the opening of the vagina in women who have an intact hymen. The function of this tissue is unknown. Hymens vary in shape and size: A hymen may surround the vaginal opening (an **annular** hymen), bridge it (a **septate** hymen), or form a sievelike covering (a **cribriform** hymen) (Figure 4.2).

Normally all forms of hymens have openings that are large enough to permit menstrual flow or the insertion of a tampon or a finger but that are usually too small to permit an erect penis to enter without the hymen's tearing. Historically the presence of an intact hymen was considered proof that a woman had never had intercourse. But the hymen can be ruptured by accident or by normal exercise, as well as by intercourse, so a tear in the tissue

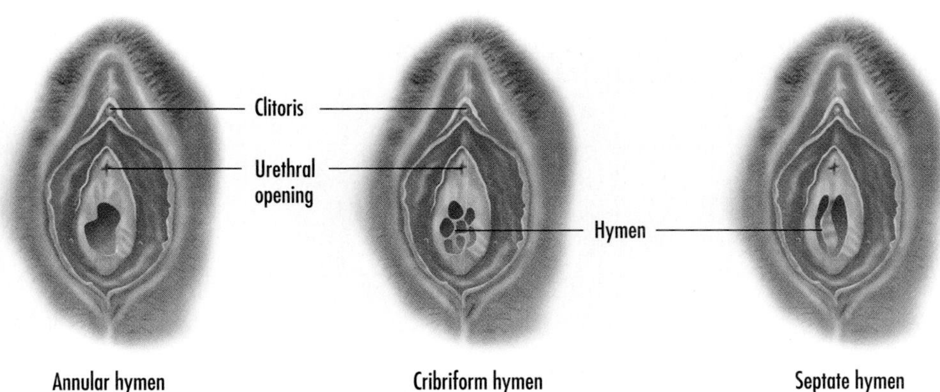

FIGURE 4.2 The various types of hymens.

is not a reliable indication that a woman is no longer a virgin. The rupturing of the hymen during first intercourse generally does not result in a great deal of pain and bleeding, although some people expect it to do so. Pain is usually related to muscular tension due to anxiety or to entry of the penis into the vagina before the vagina is sufficiently lubricated; care and attention can ordinarily prevent it. A few drops of blood may be noticeable.

The Internal Genitals

The female internal genitals consist of such structures as the vagina, uterus, fallopian tubes, and ovaries. These structures of the female internal genitalia, as well as relevant surrounding structures, are depicted in Figures 4.3 and 4.4.

The Vagina

The **vagina** is a hollow, tunnellike structure, about 4.5 inches (11.4 centimeters) long, that opens outward to the vestibule and at the opposite end into the uterus. The vagina has several reproductive functions: It surrounds the penis and receives its ejaculate during intercourse, serves as the route of exit for the newborn, and provides an exit for menstrual flow. When the vagina is empty, its lips and walls are in contact, but during childbirth the vagina can expand wide enough for the baby to pass through, and during intercourse it can both expand and close tightly enough on a penis to provide sexual satisfaction. Soft transverse folds in the vaginal wall enable the vagina to expand, and muscle fibers within the walls enable it to contract, as they do in orgasm. No muscles surround the vaginal entrance (the **introitus**); however, the **pubococcygeal** and **bulbocavernosus muscles** that support the vagina can be voluntarily contracted so as to intensify sexual responsiveness by forcing the vaginal walls to close on the penis. Exercises to help women develop greater control of these muscles (called **Kegel exercises** after their proponent) are frequently recommended by sexual counselors (Kegel, 1952). To learn to control the pubococcygeal muscles, try the following:

1. Insert a finger into the vagina and contract muscles in that area until you feel the vagina squeeze the finger.
2. Practice squeezing and then relaxing these muscles—first slowly, then rapidly.
3. Practice the preceding exercise about three times daily until you feel you have voluntary control of the pubococcygeal muscles.

vagina
A hollow, tunnellike structure of the female internal genitalia whose reproductive functions are to receive the penis and its ejaculate, serve as a route of exit for the newborn, and provide an exit for menstrual flow.

introitus
The vaginal entrance.

pubococcygeal muscle
A muscle that encircles the vagina and supports it.

bulbocavernosus muscle
A muscle that encircles and supports the vagina.

Kegel exercises
Exercises to help women develop greater control of muscles supporting the genitalia.

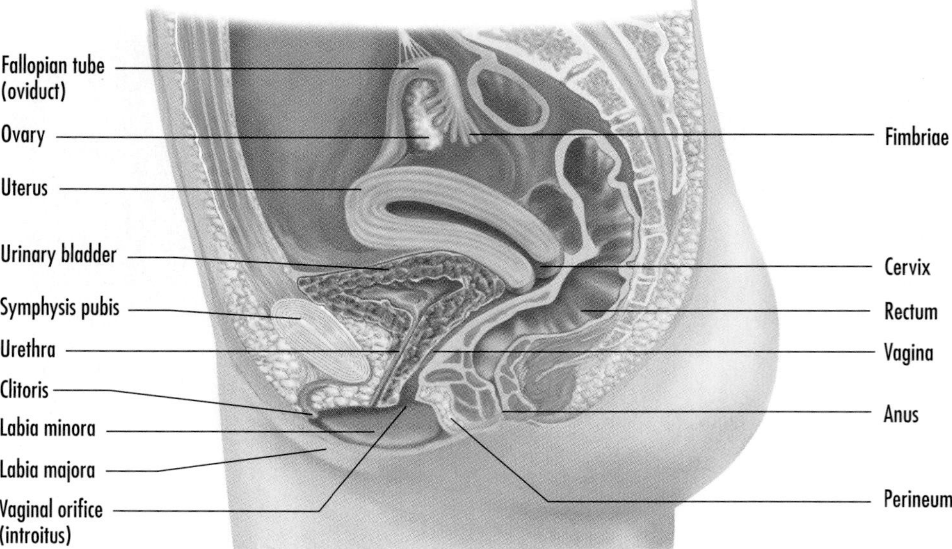

FIGURE 4.3 Organs of the female reproductive system.

The Grafenberg Spot

One would think that after centuries of studying the human body and its sexual nature there would be little room for disagreement regarding its function. Not so. The existence and the effect of the **Grafenberg spot (G spot)** provide a case in point.

The stimulation of an area along the anterior (front) wall of the vagina, several inches into the vaginal canal and just below the bladder, appears to be sexually exciting for many females. This area is known as the Grafenberg

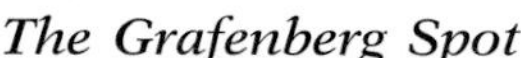

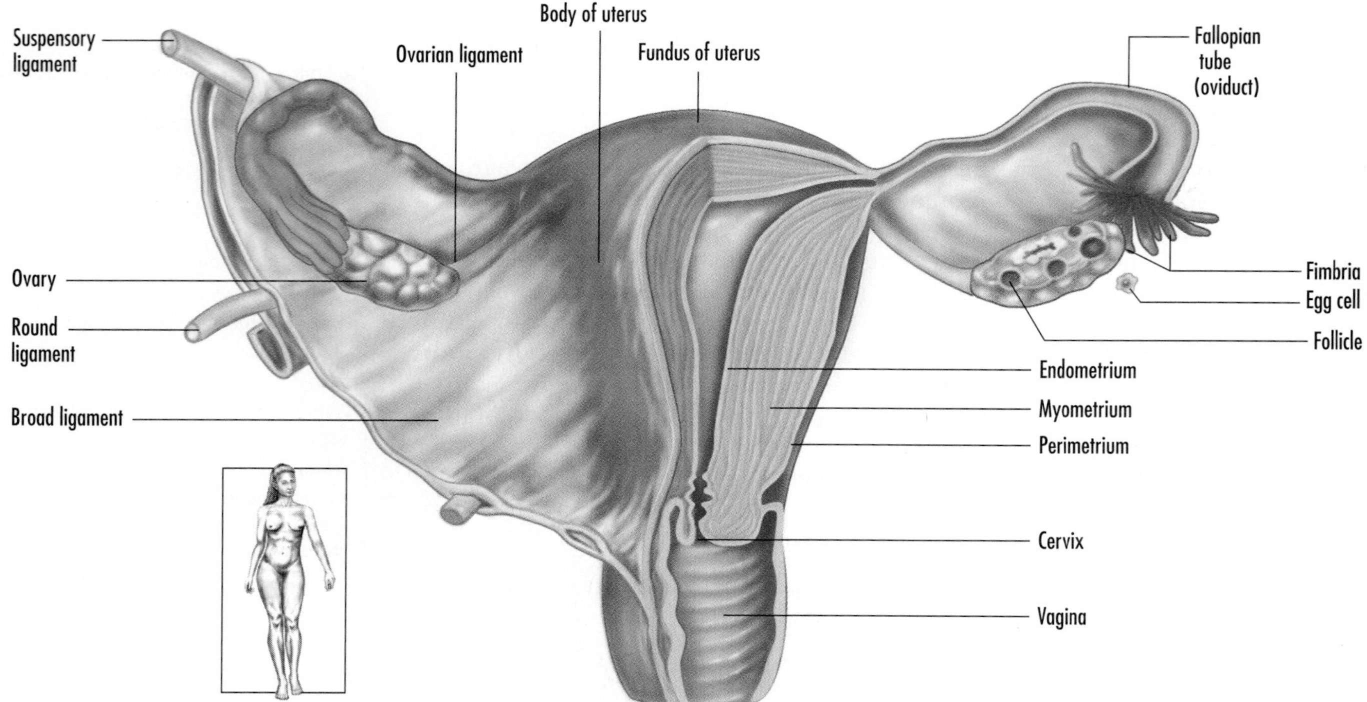

FIGURE 4.4 An anterior view of the female reproductive organs showing the relationships of the ovaries, fallopian tubes, uterus, cervix, and vagina.

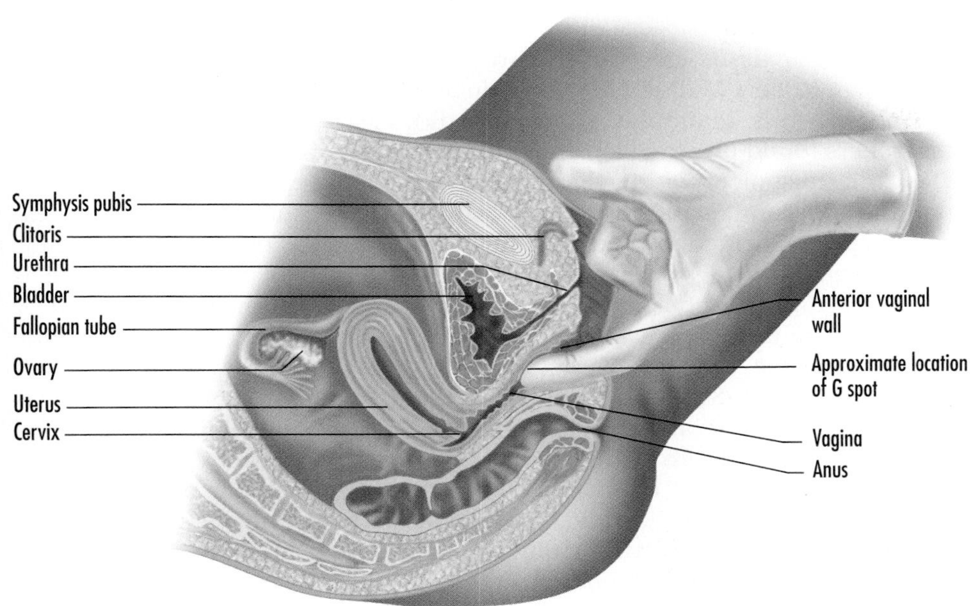

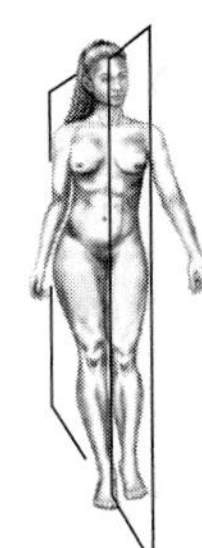

FIGURE 4.5 The location of the Grafenberg spot.

spot, named after Ernest Grafenberg, the gynecologist who first noted its erotic potential (Figure 4.5) (Grafenberg, 1950). The presence of glands in this area has been known for some time (Skene, 1880), and it is these glands—called **Skene's glands**—through which a type of ejaculate is expelled in some women when they experience orgasm by stimulation of the G spot (Grafenberg, 1950; Sevely & Bennett, 1978; Addiego, et al., 1981; Belzer, 1981; Perry & Whipple, 1981; Zaviacic, et al., 1988).

Others maintain that there is no one particular spot in the vagina that is more sensitive than others to stimulation. For example, the noted sexual therapist Helen Singer Kaplan believes there are many spots within the vagina that are sexually arousing, and the G spot is merely one of those (Kaplan, 1983). Masters and Johnson agree with Kaplan; they report that only 10% of the women they studied "had an area of heightened sensitivity in the front wall of the vagina or a tissue mass that fit the various descriptions of this area" (Masters, Johnson, & Kolodny, 1985). Although some women reported sensitivity in the front wall of the vagina, a study by Alzate and Londono (1984) could not locate a specific spot such as that described by Grafenberg. Heath (1984) found an area of erotic sensitivity and concluded that it is larger than previously described: about the size of the width of the middle two fingers and at least two-thirds the length.

To stimulate the G spot, two fingers should be inserted into the vagina. The fingers should be pressed deeply into the tissue of the anterior wall of the vagina between the posterior side of the pubic bone and the cervix. Initially a woman may report a slight feeling of discomfort, a pleasurable feeling, or a sensation of needing to urinate. This latter reaction is probably due to pressure on the bladder. After a short period the tissue may swell, and unpleasant sensations may be replaced with erotic sensations. Women who experience orgasms from stimulation of the G spot often report them to be intense. Perry and Whipple describe this orgasm as resulting in a more intense uterine contraction than orgasm from stimulation of either the clitoris or the vagina (Perry & Whipple, 1981). Other researchers do not agree that a "uterine orgasm" distinct from other orgasms exists (Masters, Johnson, & Kolodny, 1985).

Grafenberg spot (G spot)
An area located along the anterior wall of the vagina, several inches into the vaginal canal, that when stimulated in some women may result in sexual excitement and/or orgasm.

Skene's glands
Glands located along the walls of the vagina that are thought to be analogous to the male prostate gland and the site from which some women eject a fluid during orgasm.

uterus
A pear-shaped hollow structure of the female genitalia in which the embryo and fetus develop before birth.

cervix
The mouth of the uterus, through which the vagina extends.

os
The opening to the uterus.

corpus
The upper two-thirds of the uterus.

fundus
The upper end of the uterus, closest to the opening of the fallopian tubes.

perimetrium
The outermost layer of the uterus, sometimes termed the *serosa,* a very elastic layer, that allows the uterus to accommodate a growing embryo and fetus.

myometrium
The middle layer of the uterus, consisting of smooth muscle that aids in the pushing of the newborn through the cervix.

endometrium
The innermost layer of the uterus, to which the fertilized egg attaches and by which it is nourished as it develops before birth, which is partly discharged (if pregnancy does not occur) with the menstrual flow.

fallopian tubes (oviduct)
The routes through which eggs leave the ovaries on their way to the uterus, in which fertilization normally occurs.

ovary
A structure of the female genitalia that houses ova before their maturation and discharge and that produces estrogen and progesterone.

The Female Prostate

That glandular tissue exists in the area of the G spot is not debatable. The pathologist Robert Mallon (1984) conducted autopsies on women and found evidence of this glandular tissue, as did Heath (1984). Both of these researchers found prostatelike glandular tissue in the front wall of the vagina. When the substances within these glands were analyzed, they were found to contain fluids similar to those found in the male prostate. Hence, some sexuality experts have concluded that there are a female prostate (the Skene's glands) and a female ejaculate. Further evidence for a female ejaculate is offered by Addiego and colleagues (1981), who analyzed the fluid expelled by females at the time of orgasm and found it to contain an enzyme (prostatic acid phosphatase, or PAP) characteristic of semen. However, when Goldberg and associates (1983) studied this ejaculate, they concluded that it was similar to urine. Alzate and Hoch (1986) also found ejaculate secreted through the urethra. To complicate matters further, a study conducted by Belzer and associates (1984) concluded that the ejaculate obtained from women contained significantly more prostatic acid phosphatase than did their urine. Obviously, further study is needed to confirm the existence of a female ejaculate beyond any doubt.

That some women expel a fluid from the vagina during orgasm has been demonstrated. The prevalence of this phenomenon remains unknown. Whether this fluid is similar to that of the male prostate is a matter of much research and debate. What is not discussed or researched, however, is the concern expressed by the Boston Women's Health Collective (1998) regarding the possibility that the G spot orgasm will become a new "ideal" for the sexually liberated woman. It would indeed be unfortunate if this new ideal created pressure on women who do not experience erotic feelings when the Grafenberg spot is stimulated and, therefore, perceive themselves to be inadequate sexually. When the media popularize sexual information, as they did with the Grafenberg spot, often education is needed to remind the public about the many paths to sexual fulfillment. This is particularly true today.

The Uterus

At the top of the vagina lies the **uterus,** a pear-shaped hollow organ with muscular walls. Its function is to nurture the developing embryo and fetus. Except during pregnancy, the uterus is about 3 inches (8 centimeters) long, 3 inches wide at the top, and 1 inch (2.5 centimeters) thick. The uterus extends into the vagina at its **cervix;** the actual opening to the uterus in the cervix is called the **os.** The upper two-thirds of this cavity is called the **corpus,** and the top end is called the **fundus.** Most uteruses tilt forward (that is, they are *anteflexed*) over the bladder; approximately 20% tilt backward (*retroflexed*) (Figure 4.6). Women with retroflexed uteruses are more likely to experience discomfort during menstruation and may have more difficulty in inserting a diaphragm as a result of the angle of the cervix. Contrary to widespread belief, however, the ability to conceive is in no way affected by the position of the uterus.

The uterus consists of three layers. The outermost layer, the **perimetrium,** is very elastic, enabling the uterus to accommodate a growing embryo during pregnancy. The middle layer, the **myometrium,** consists of smooth muscles, whose ability to contract helps push the newborn through the cervix and into the vagina (which during childbirth acts as the birth canal). The innermost layer of the uterus is the **endometrium.** This layer is loaded with blood vessels and can therefore provide the nourishment necessary to sustain a developing fetus. It builds up and partly sloughs off as the menstrual flow in every menstrual cycle, unless fertil-

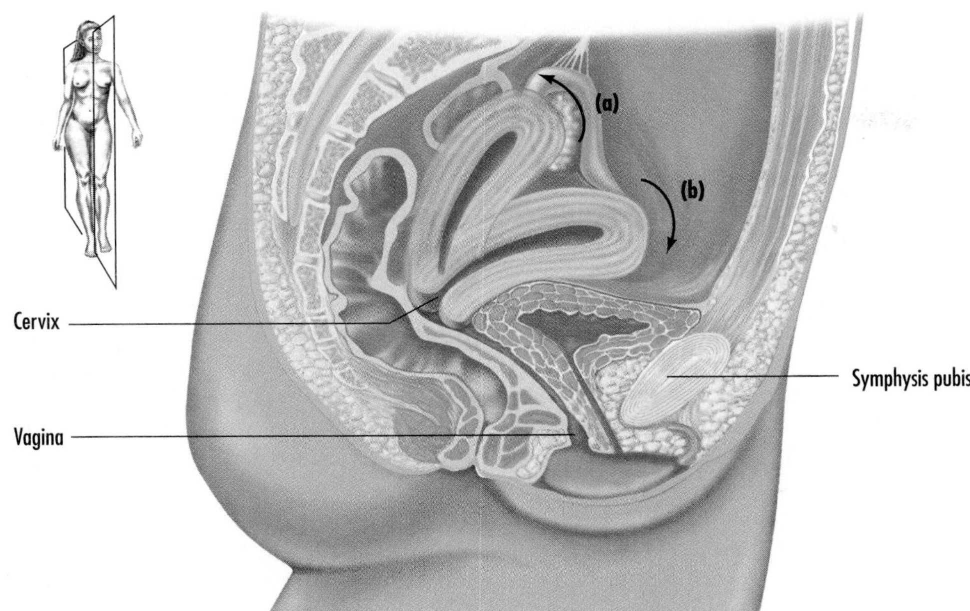

FIGURE 4.6 Various positions of the uterus: (a) anteflexed and (b) retroflexed.

ization takes place. Figure 4.7 depicts the anatomical relationships of the three layers of the uterus.

The Fallopian Tubes and the Ovaries

At the fundus, the uterus opens into the two **fallopian tubes** (we will use this more common name, although **oviduct** might be more appropriate), and at the other end of each tube is an **ovary,** the organ that produces and stores the *ova,* or eggs. When a female is born, each of her ovaries contains approximately 40,000 to 400,000 eggs. Every egg has the potential to be fertilized by a sperm to become an embryo. After the girl reaches puberty, one of these eggs is usually discharged through the wall of one of her ovaries during each menstrual cycle. The egg develops inside a capsule called a

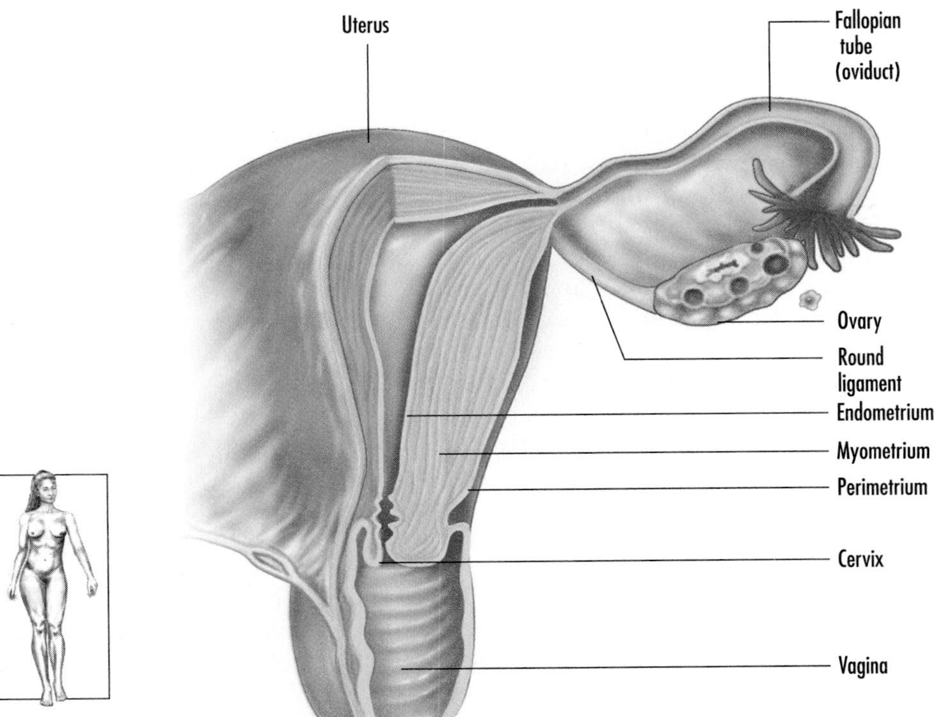

FIGURE 4.7 Layers of the uterine wall.

Graafian follicle
A part of the ovary from which a mature egg ruptures, allowing the corpus luteum to develop in the location where the egg was released.

corpus luteum
A yellowish structure that develops in the Graafian follicle at the discharge of an ovum and that produces progesterone and estrogen.

progesterone
A hormone secreted by the corpus luteum signaling the endometrium to develop in preparation for a zygote.

estrogen
A hormone produced by the ovaries whose level in the blood helps control the menstrual cycle.

fimbriae
The fingerlike ends of the fallopian tubes that catch the ova when they are discharged from the ovaries.

cilia
Hairlike structures that guide objects, such as ova, moving past them.

ectopic pregnancy
The attachment and development of the zygote in a location other than in the uterus.

mammary glands
Milk-secreting glands located in the female breast.

prolactin
A pituitary hormone that stimulates the production of milk from the mammary glands.

areola
The darkened part of the breast immediately surrounding the nipple.

Graafian follicle and is discharged when it has matured. The discharged egg, now matured and freed from its capsule and the ovary, is ready to be fertilized by a male's sperm. When the follicle ruptures to discharge its egg, the empty follicle, now a yellowish structure called the **corpus luteum,** secretes a hormone **(progesterone)** that signals the endometrium to prepare for a fertilized egg. Progesterone and **estrogen,** another hormone produced by the ovaries, play significant roles in menstruation, birth, growth, and aging.

When the ovum is discharged from the ovary, it is directed into the fallopian tubes. As shown in Figure 4.4, these tubes serve as routes for ova to reach the uterus. The newly released ovum is caught by the fingerlike end of the fallopian tube, called a **fimbria,** and is guided into the cone-shaped open end of the tube. If fertilization takes place, it usually takes place there.

Whether fertilized or not, the ovum continues on its journey through the tube, moved along in a sweeping motion by tiny hairlike structures called **cilia.** The destination of the fertilized ovum is the endometrium in the uterus, where it becomes attached and continues its development. An unfertilized ovum also travels to the endometrium, then disintegrates, and eventually is expelled through the vagina, along with some of the endometrium, in the process called *menstruation.* (Once an ovum is expelled, the menstrual cycle is completed. Soon an ovary will discharge another mature egg and the process will begin again.)

It should be noted that occasionally a woman may produce more than one egg per cycle, thereby becoming prone to multiple births. Fertility drugs, which may result in multiple births, are suspected of causing the maturation of several eggs per cycle. Sometimes the fertilized egg may attach in the abdominal cavity or the fallopian tube rather than in the uterus. This is termed an **ectopic pregnancy.** Ectopic pregnancies are discussed in Chapter 9.

The Breasts

Although the female breasts are not reproductive organs, they do have significance in sexual arousal and response, and they serve an important reproductive function in providing milk for the newborn infant. Each breast contains about 15 to 20 clusters of milk-secreting structures called **mammary glands** (Figure 4.8). Each of these mammary gland clusters has an opening to the nipple, where the milk ducts open. The stimulation of the newborn's sucking on the nipple causes the pituitary gland to secrete a hormone called **prolactin,** which in turn stimulates the production of breast milk.

Most of the breast is fat and connective tissue. Except for small muscles in the area of the nipple and **areola** (the darkened skin around the nipple), there are no muscles in the breast. Because the breast is muscle-free, exercises to increase breast size are ineffective. Over the years the breasts may hang lower than normal if the ligaments are stretched by lack of support or by jostling (for example, not wearing a bra while jogging).

The nipples—of men as well as women—are richly supplied with nerve endings that respond with pleasurable sexual feelings when stimulated. During sexual arousal the nipples become erect. The size of the breasts, or their shape, is not related to sensitivity. Women with either small or large breasts may be equally sexually stimulated by the fondling of the breasts. Though some have characterized our society as making a fetish of large breasts, preferences in breast size and shape vary from individual to individual. It should

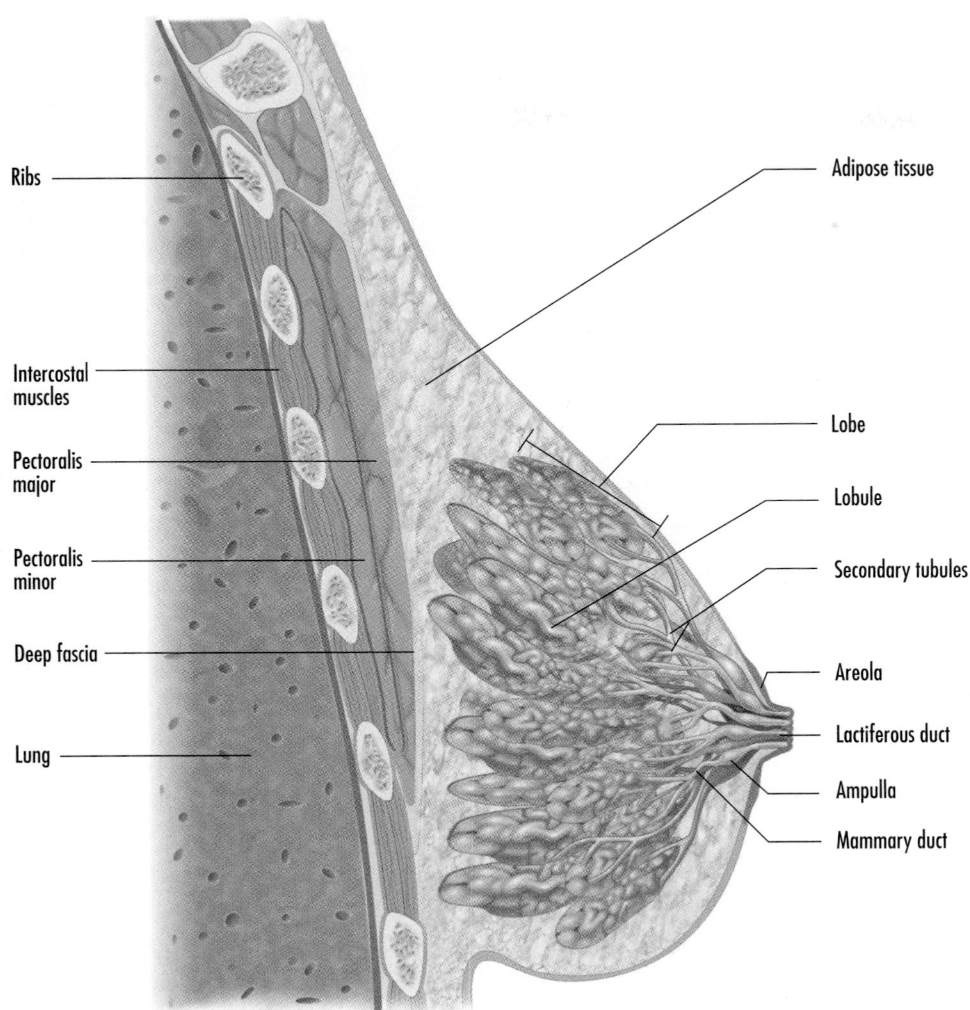

FIGURE 4.8 The female breast.

be noted, however, that although breast size varies, extent of glandular tissue is comparable in all women's breasts. Because the amount of glandular tissue is the same, women with small breasts produce the same amount of breast milk after childbirth as women with larger breasts and are therefore as successful breastfeeding their babies as are women with larger breasts.

Our society has so emphasized breast size that many women have their breasts reconstructed. In the past, liquid silicone was injected to enlarge the breast, but approximately 60% of women experienced problems such as infection, deformity, or exceptional hardness of the breast. More recently, silicone pouches containing saline solution have been implanted to reshape the breast. However, in 1992, in response to reported breakage of the pouches, the Dow Chemical Company, the largest manufacturer of silicone pouches, stopped manufacturing them and agreed to pay for their removal for women who so desired. However, the most recent research indicates that silicone implants are not the health issue previously thought. In a study of the research related to silicone breast implants, the Institute of Medicine (a subgroup of the National Academy of Sciences) found no convincing evidence that chronic disease was more likely to develop in women with silicone breast implants than women without implants (Reuters, 1999). Furthermore, during a lawsuit against breast implant manufacturers, a federal judge

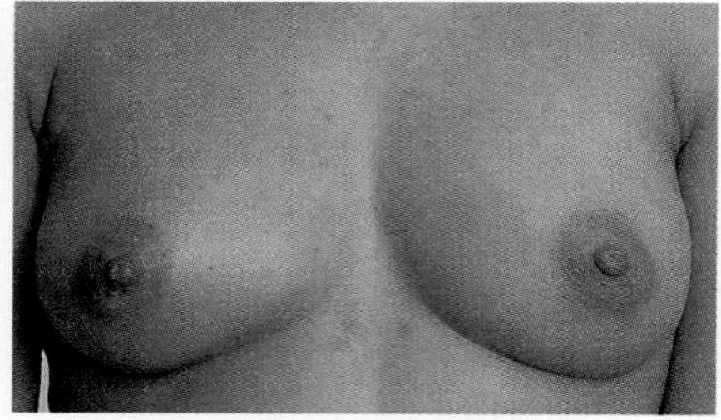
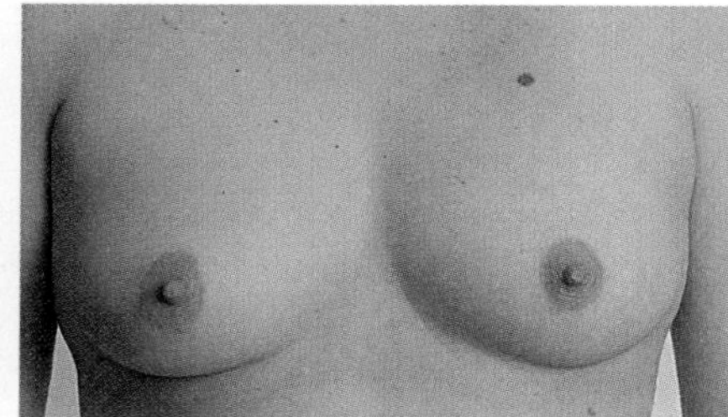
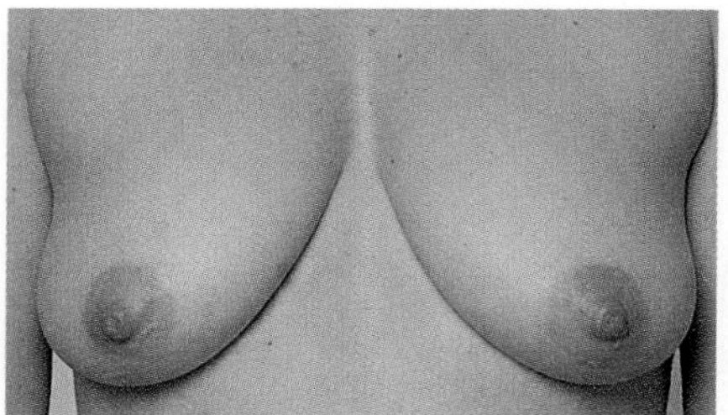

The size and shape of breasts vary among women.

appointed a panel of scientists to study the issue and report their findings to the court. The court-appointed panel found no convincing evidence that silicone breast implants cause disease of the immune system as alleged in the lawsuit (Schwartz, 1998). Silicone pouch implants are still regularly used in breast reconstruction for women who have had a radical mastectomy due to cancer of the breast.

We also need to be concerned about other health issues regarding the breast, such as cancer of the breast. (We discuss this in greater detail later in the chapter.) Suffice it to say here that women need to perform regular breast self-examinations and obtain periodic medical checkups by a health professional to make sure that any abnormalities are identified early, thereby increasing the likelihood that treatment will be successful and as noninvasive as possible.

Table 4.1 reviews the functions of the female reproductive organs.

hypothalamus
A structure in the brain that controls the pituitary gland and is directly connected by nerve pathways to various organs of the body.

releasing factors
Chemicals released from the hypothalamus that affect the function of various body parts.

hormone
A chemical substance secreted by a ductless gland, which is carried to an organ or tissue where it has a specific effect.

endocrine glands
Glands that secrete their products into the bloodstream.

pituitary
The "master gland," an endocrine gland located at the base of the brain that stimulates the other endocrine glands to produce their hormones.

gonadotropins
Sexual hormones secreted by the pituitary that stimulate the gonads to produce their hormones.

gonads
The male testes and the female ovaries, which produce gonadotropin hormones responsible for the development of secondary sexual characteristics.

follicle-stimulating hormone (FSH)
A hormone, secreted by the anterior portion of the pituitary gland, that "instructs" the ovaries to prepare an egg to be released from a follicle.

luteinizing hormone (LH)
A hormone, secreted by the anterior portion of the pituitary gland, that stimulates ovulation.

The Hormones

What happens at the sight of an attractive person of the opposite (or same) sex, perhaps in a skimpy bathing suit? If the stimulus is sufficiently interesting, it can result in the first stages of sexual response—for example, increased heart rate, vaginal lubrication, and erection of the penis or clitoris. How does the visual image result in these physical changes? The chain of events is rather complex. It starts with the **hypothalamus,** a structure in the brain that, either through direct nerve pathways or through chemicals called **releasing factors,** can instruct various body parts to function. The hypothalamus might be said to serve as a bridge between external stimuli and physiological responses. But let us go back to the bathing suit. Two things happen: (1) When the individual perceives the external stimulus as sexually exciting, the hypothalamus "tells" the pituitary gland to secrete its hormones, and (2) these chemicals stimulate the adrenal gland to secrete its hormones and the testes and ovaries to secrete their hormones. These secretions change the blood flow (producing vasocongestion), the heart rate, breathing, vaginal moistness, and so on.

These powerfully acting **hormones** are chemical substances that influence organs and tissues. They are produced by **endocrine glands,** which are glands that secrete their products into the bloodstream. The thyroid, for example, secretes a hormone that travels to the heart and increases the heart rate. The adrenal gland secretes the hormone adrenalin, which travels to the bronchial tubes of the lungs and dilates them. As we have just seen, the secretions of several glands are involved in sexual response.

The **pituitary,** a pea-shaped gland located at the base of the brain, serves as a sort of master gland to the others in the system. It stimulates the other

TABLE 4.1 **Functions of the Female Reproductive Organs**

Organ	Function
Ovary	Production of egg cells and female sex hormones
Fallopian tube	Conveying of egg cell toward uterus; site of fertilization; transport developing zygote to uterus
Uterus	Protection and sustaining of life of embryo and fetus during pregnancy
Vagina	Conveying of uterine secretions to the outside of body; receiving of erect penis during sexual intercourse; transport of fetus during birth process
Labia majora	Enclosing and protection of other external reproductive organs
Labia minora	Formation of margins of vestibule; protection of openings of vagina and urethra
Clitoris	Organ richly supplied with sensory nerve endings associated with feeling of pleasure during sexual stimulation
Vestibule	Space between labia minora that includes vaginal and urethral openings
Vestibular glands	Secretion of fluid that moistens and lubricates vestibule

glands to release their hormones. The front part of the pituitary secretes three sexual hormones, called **gonadotropins,** which act on or stimulate the **gonads** (the testes and ovaries). The gonads are also endocrine glands, and they produce their own hormones. The three gonadotropins are **follicle-stimulating hormone (FSH); luteinizing hormone (LH),** often called the **interstitial-cell-stimulating hormone (ICSH)** in males; and prolactin (produced only during pregnancy and breastfeeding). Once stimulated by these gonadotropic hormones, the gonads produce their own hormones: estrogens, progesterones, and androgens. The adrenal gland also secretes androgen directly.

In women estrogens and progesterones regulate the menstrual cycle, with estrogens important in producing vaginal lubrication. Although estrogens and progesterones have no known function in men, the presence of too much estrogen in the male body can lower interest in sexual activity and may result in enlargement of the breasts. **Androgens** affect the sex drive of both men and women: The presence of too much causes excessive sexual appetite, the presence of too little androgen decreases sexual interest. FSH stimulates cells in the seminiferous tubules (called **spermatocytes**) to produce sperm.

Despite the fact that hormones account for and influence sexual differences, males and females produce the same hormones. Estrogens and progesterones are considered female hormones and androgens male hormones, but both males and females produce all three. They do differ in the amounts they produce, however. For example, males have levels of the strongest androgen **(testosterone)** 10 times those of females, and females have significantly more estrogens than males. Obviously, too, males and females differ in the organs activated by the hormones. Long before we begin to think about hormones and our sexuality, hormones have already had significant effects.

Menstruation

At some time during puberty a girl reaches **menarche;** that is, she has her first menstrual cycle. Then, and cyclically thereafter unless she is pregnant, blood (actually the blood-enriched endometrium) is discharged (or flows) from her uterus through her vagina for several days. The Latin origin of the word **menstruation** is *mensis,* meaning "month," because the menses, or periods,

interstitial-cell-stimulating hormone (ICSH)
A hormone, secreted by the anterior portion of the pituitary gland in males, that stimulates the production of sperm.

androgens
Male sex hormones.

spermatocytes
Cells that develop through several stages to form sperm.

testosterone
The male sex hormone produced in the testes that is responsible for the development of male secondary sexual characteristics.

menarche
The time when a female begins her first menstrual cycle, usually at 8 to 16 years of age.

menstruation
The cyclical emission of the blood-enriched endometrium when pregnancy does not occur.

supposedly occur monthly. Actually they are not so predictable. Between menarche and menopause, when menstruation ceases, a woman's menstrual cycle may stabilize in a 28- to 30-day pattern (20- to 40-day cycles are also quite normal), or it may never stabilize. Cycles may vary in length from period to period, or they may be stable for a long time, fluctuate, and become stable again. Menstruation has been called the "curse," the "monthly sickness," and worse, but it is a normal physiological response to hormonal activity.

Menarche

The reason menstruation begins when it does is not exactly known. One hypothesis relates to the increase in body fat at puberty as a result of hormonal secretions (Frisch & McArthur, 1974; Fishman, 1980). Evidence for this hypothesis can be found in long-distance runners. Many women who jog long distances lose considerable weight. It is not uncommon for such women to experience secondary **amenorrhea;** that is, they no longer menstruate regularly. In fact, some experts estimate that as many as 50% of women runners experience a cessation of menstruation (Reynolds, 1987). In addition, women suffering from anorexia nervosa—a condition in which the woman is so preoccupied with being thin that she eats very little and loses a great deal of body weight and fat—often lose their periods. In truth, though, no one really knows why women joggers or anorexics cease to menstruate, and, at least for the joggers, there appears to be more going on than just a loss of body fat. Other studies have found that many thin female joggers continue to menstruate, and many heavier ones do not (Ullyot, 1986).

amenorrhea
The absence of menstruation in a woman who should be menstruating.

zygote
A fertilized egg.

proliferative phase
The first part of the menstrual cycle, during which FSH production is increased and the follicles are maturing.

secretory phase
The second part of the menstrual cycle, during which ovulation occurs and the production of LH stimulates the development of the corpus luteum.

menstrual phase
The part of the menstrual cycle during which the endometrial lining is sloughed off as the menstrual flow.

follicular phase
The part of the menstrual cycle during which menstruation occurs and the pituitary increases the production of FSH so the follicles mature: a combination of the menstrual and proliferative phases.

ovulation
The part of the menstrual cycle when the ovum is discharged from the ovary.

luteal phase
The same phase of the menstrual cycle as the secretory phase, which includes ovulation and the production of LH from the corpus luteum.

Menstrual Physiology

The menstrual cycle begins when the pituitary gland secretes two hormones: FSH, which stimulates the growth, or "ripening," of follicles in the ovary; and LH, which stimulates the ovary to release one egg, that is, to *ovulate.* Once the egg is released, the area from which it was released (the Graafian follicle) becomes a yellow body (corpus luteum). The Graafian follicle secretes the hormone estrogen, and the yellow body secretes progesterone and estrogen. Progesterone causes the lining of the uterus to thicken and store nutrients in preparation to receive, implant, and nourish a fertilized egg, called a **zygote.** If the egg is not fertilized, the yellow body degenerates and thus becomes unable to secrete progesterone any longer. The lack of progesterone is a signal to expel the unneeded endometrium. This tissue, gradually shed over the course of a few days, is the menstrual flow. The cycle is then ready to begin anew.

Phases of the Menstrual Cycle

Figures 4.9 and 4.10 depict the role of hormones in the menstrual cycle and its phases. The first phase is termed the **proliferative phase.** It is during this phase that FSH production is increased by the pituitary gland, which in turn stimulates the follicles in the ovaries to mature. The follicles then can produce estrogen, which causes the endometrial lining of the uterus to thicken and prepare for the implantation of the zygote. The pituitary then increases production of LH, in response to the elevated levels of estrogen in the bloodstream, causing one follicle to prepare to expel an ovum (the Graafian follicle), and the proliferative phase proceeds until ovulation.

The **secretory phase** of the menstrual cycle begins once ovulation occurs and entails continued secretions of LH, which stimulate the development of the corpus luteum. The corpus luteum secretes progesterone, causing further thickening and engorgement of blood of the endometrium. If implantation

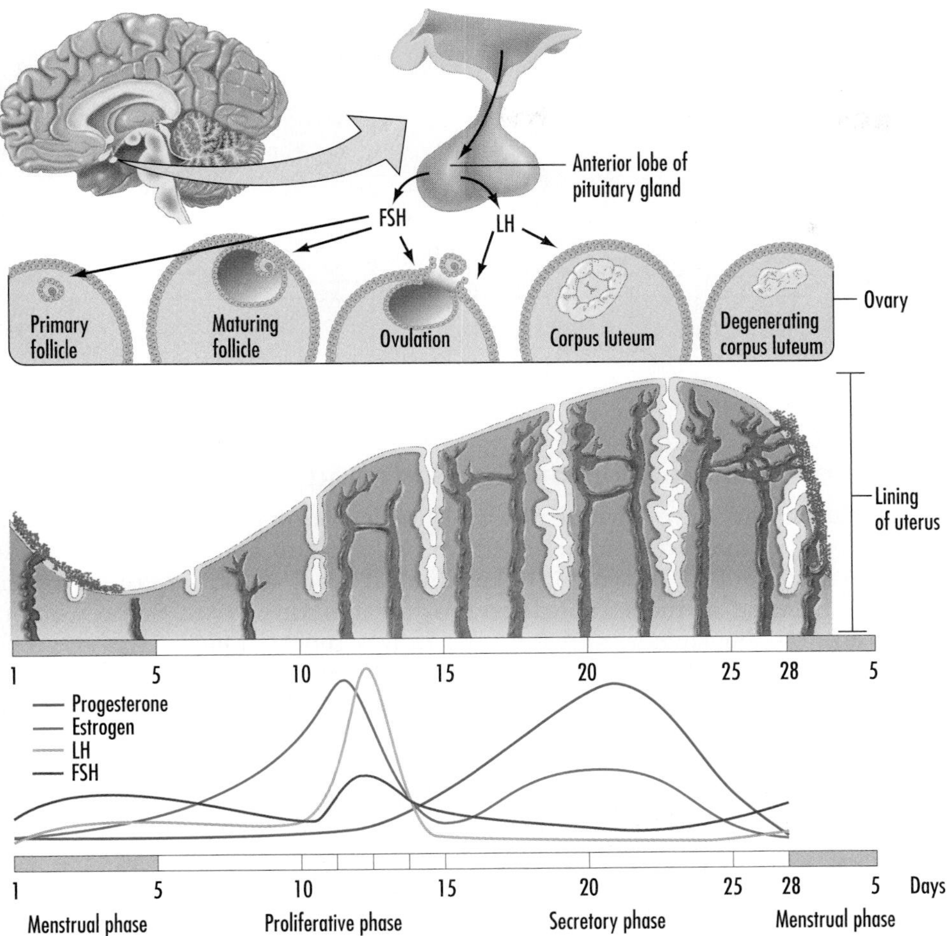

FIGURE 4.9 Hormones from the hypothalamus control the release of hormones from the pituitary gland, which in turn regulates production of ova and sex hormones from the ovaries. Note how the rise and fall of the hormone level is related to the building up and sloughing off of the uterine lining.

does not occur, the pituitary shuts down production of FSH and LH, causing degeneration of the corpus luteum. The result is a decrease in the secretions of estrogen and progesterone.

The next phase of the menstrual cycle is the **menstrual phase,** in which the endometrial lining of the uterus is sloughed off as the menstrual flow.

Some sexuality experts divide the menstrual cycle into three different phases: the **follicular phase, ovulation,** and the **luteal phase.** The follicular phase coincides with the menstrual and proliferative phases, ovulation is marked by the discharge of the ovum from the Graafian follicle, and the luteal phase is the same as the secretory phase. This categorization pertains to changes in the ovaries, whereas the previous categorization refers to changes in the uterus.

As noted in Figure 4.9, in a 28-day cycle ovulation occurs on day 14, with the menstrual flow lasting for 4 days. The great variation in the menstrual cycle—among women and even in any one woman—should be emphasized. The 28-day cycle, although often spoken of as *the* cycle, is not very common. Furthermore, in spite of menstrual cycles' differing in length, there is little difference in the luteal phase of these cycles. That is, regardless of the length of the menstrual cycle, once ovulation occurs, it basically takes 14 days until menstruation begins. For example, if a woman's cycle is 42 days long, she will ovulate on day 28, and 14 days later she will menstruate; if her cycle is 30 days long, she will ovulate on day 16 and will still menstruate 14 days later.

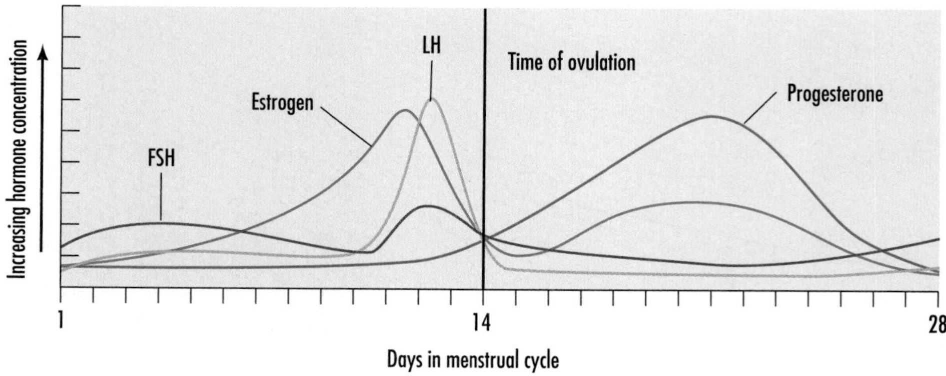

FIGURE 4.10 Changes in relative concentrations of hormones during ovulation and menstruation.

Effects of Menstruation on the Body and Mind

Menstruation can have several physical and emotional effects, which vary greatly from woman to woman and from one cycle to another. There is evidence that some 10% of women take time off from work, school, or other activities because of menstrual discomfort (Patterson, 1990). Some women report cramps, backaches, and pimples; others report none of these symptoms. Some women report feeling depressed, bloated, nervous, or weak, and others do not. Whether a woman experiences any of these effects—be they physical or emotional—may be a function of what she expects to experience. Evidence for this hypothesis does exist. For example, when researchers conducting studies of menstruating women inform the women of what the study is about, women report more of these symptoms than when they do not know what is being studied (Brooks, Ruble, & Clark, 1977; Ruble & Brooks-Gunn, 1979). Because many of these symptoms cannot be objectively measured, what a woman expects to feel may create a self-fulfilling prophecy. That is not to say women do not experience real discomfort; rather, the mind may affect the amount of discomfort experienced.

Stress researchers have determined that the mind–body connection is a real one. That is, with certain actual illnesses and diseases either the mind affects the body so as to prepare it to become ill or the mind changes the body in a way that makes the illness worse than it might otherwise be (Greenberg, 2002). Other factors that might influence menstrual symptoms include diets too high in saturated fats, a lack of regular exercise, and work in extremely cold environments (Greenwood, 1986).

The preceding discussion is not meant to negate the real physical and emotional effects of menstruation. For example, depending on one's age, and whether one has given birth to a child or not, cramping associated with menstruation can vary. Teenagers and perimenopausal women—those in the period between the beginning of menopause and the complete cessation of a woman's period—report worse cramping than is usual, whereas women who have given birth to a child report less cramping.

Menstrual Problems

Several conditions associated with menstruation require special attention. Among these conditions are dysmenorrhea, amenorrhea, and premenstrual syndrome.

Dysmenorrhea

Painful menstruation is termed **dysmenorrhea.** Many women experience some discomfort and pain during some menstrual cycles, and other women experience discomfort and pain regularly. More than 50% of women have periods so painful that they visit their physicians at some time during their life (Greenwood, 1986), and it has been estimated that 70% to 90% of menstruating women have some degree of menstrual problems on a regular basis (Reid & Yen, 1981). Women may experience severe abdominal cramping, a bloated feeling, headaches, backaches, and nausea. An estimated 10% to 15% of women experience menstrual pain each month severe enough to prevent normal daily function at school, work, or home (www.drkoop.com).

The cause of **primary dysmenorrhea**—that is, pain during menstruation—is not specifically known. Many health practitioners identify the cause as **prostaglandins,** substances produced by body tissues that act as hormones. Prostaglandins, found in unusually high amounts in women with dysmenorrhea, cause the muscles in the uterus to contract. This contraction causes pain and cuts off some of the blood supply (with its oxygen) to the uterus, thereby causing more discomfort (American College of Obstetricians and Gynecologists, 1985).

To treat primary dysmenorrhea, physicians sometimes prescribe antiprostaglandin medications such as Naproxen (Aleve), Anaprox, or Ponstel. These medicines inhibit the production of prostaglandins and relieve pain, dizziness, headache, nausea, vomiting, and irritability in many women. Many women who do not use prescription drugs find aspirin or ibuprofen helpful in relieving pain (these also somewhat inhibit prostaglandin production). Other remedies proposed for dysmenorrhea include eating more fish and vegetables and less animal fats and taking calcium, vitamin B, and magnesium supplements. Drinking plenty of fluids has also been recommended, because it seems that when the body is dehydrated, the hormone vasopressin is secreted. Vasopressin conserves bodily fluids, an effect that is not what a woman feeling bloated needs. Oral contraceptives can also help relieve menstrual pain by eliminating ovulation and thereby decreasing the amount of prostaglandin produced. In addition, placing a heating pad on the abdomen, lightly massaging the abdomen with the fingertips (effleurage), drinking warm beverages, taking a warm shower, doing waist-bending exercises, having an orgasm, and walking may alleviate some menstrual pain.

Secondary dysmenorrhea is painful menstruation caused by some other identifiable condition. For example, **endometriosis** (a condition in which endometrial cells attach and develop on some body tissue other than the uterus) can cause secondary dysmenorrhea, as can pelvic inflammatory disease, uterine tumors, and blockages of the opening to the uterus (the os). In these cases, treatment consists of finding and removing the cause of the menstrual pain, which may require surgery or medication.

The fear of pregnancy alone, for example, has been known to create enough anguish and anxiety in sexually active women to cause a cessation of menses. Fearing pregnancy, many couples wait with bated breath for the evidence that the woman is not pregnant—menstruation. A slight delay in her period (not unusual) makes the woman anxious about the possibility of an unwanted pregnancy. Her anxiety can then further delay menstruation or create amenorrhea. Thus a vicious cycle develops that only a pregnancy test or the menstrual flow can break. Any woman who has been sexually active and has missed more than one period should have a pregnancy test.

Amenorrhea

Amenorrhea is the absence of menstrual flow. If a woman has never menstruated and is 18 years or older, her condition is called **primary amenorrhea.** If menstruation ceases after menarche, the condition is called **secondary amenorrhea.** Amenorrhea may be caused by pregnancy, malfunctioning of the ovaries, cysts or tumors, disease, hormonal imbalance, poor nutrition, or emotional distress. It may also be caused by strenuous exercise of the sort done

dysmenorrhea
Painful menstruation.

primary dysmenorrhea
Painful menstruation, the cause of which is unknown.

prostaglandins
Hormonelike substances produced by body tissue that may cause dysmenorrhea.

secondary dysmenorrhea
Painful menstruation caused by some identifiable condition such as endometriosis.

endometriosis
The growth of the endometrium uterine lining at a location other than in the uterus.

primary amenorrhea
A condition in which a woman of age 18 years or older has never menstruated.

secondary amenorrhea
A condition in which a woman has ceased menstruating after menarche.

by runners and young dancers (Shangold, 1981). The causes of amenorrhea in physically active women are not known. Some experts hypothesize that exercising women experience a decrease in body fat that may contribute to the cessation of their periods, as it does in anorexic women. Lower body fat may interfere with production of the amount of estrogen needed to menstruate. Among female athletes, amenorrhea is quite common (Shangold, 1985), and it is suspected the cause is a combination of low body fat, the stress upon the body as a result of strenuous physical exercise, and the psychological stress associated with competition. Although the actual cause of amenorrhea in female athletes is difficult to determine, it does not follow that some physical condition does not exist in any one woman—athlete or not—that can be identified as the cause of her menstrual problem. It is advised that women whose menses cease consult their physicians to discuss any conditions or illnesses that are treatable.

Premenstrual Syndrome

Some women experience mood changes and other physical and emotional discomforts just before their menstrual periods. This condition is referred to as **premenstrual syndrome (PMS).** In fact, more than 150 disorders have been associated with premenstrual syndrome; some of the more common ones are depression, tension, anxiety, mood swings, irritability or anger, difficulty in concentrating, lethargy, weight gain, fluid retention, bloating, breast soreness, joint or muscle pain, nausea, vomiting, and headaches (Mayo Clinic, 1998a). It has been estimated that at some time during their reproductive years 40% of women experience PMS (Harvard Medical School, 1984; Mayo Clinic, 1998a; Reid & Yen, 1981).

premenstrual syndrome (PMS)
Marked mood fluctuation during the week before menstruation, accompanied by physical symptoms.

Premenstrual syndrome was described by Katharina Dalton, a leading researcher in the treatment of PMS, in *Once a Month* (1979): "Once a month with monotonous regularity, chaos is inflicted on American homes as premenstrual tension and other menstrual problems recur time and again with demoralizing repetition." Reading this, many women found solace in the fact that other women had similar experiences each menstrual cycle, whereas others, some researchers argue, were subjected to a suggestion that their cycles were illnesses of some sort with accompanying discomforts they might otherwise have considered quite normal. As a matter of fact, as we have previously noted, only about 10% of women have premenstrual discomfort that is severe enough to interfere with their normal functioning (Keye, 1983; Patterson, 1990). In any case, it is undeniable that many women do experience something akin to PMS fairly regularly (see Table 4.2).

TABLE 4.2 **Premenstrual Symptoms Reported by Women**

Summarizing previous research findings, Dr. Colleen Boyle and her colleagues from the Department of Epidemiology and Public Health, Yale University School of Medicine, reported that the following premenstrual symptoms occur in women:

Age (Years)	Breast Pain No. (%)	Back or Stomach Cramps No. (%)	Moodiness, Irritability, or Depression No. (%)	Weight Gain or Bloating No. (%)	Total N
20–29	57 (36%)	128 (81%)	121 (76%)	136 (86%)	158
30–49	158 (44%)	221 (61%)	266 (73%)	285 (79%)	362
Total	215 (41%)	349 (67%)	387 (74%)	421 (81%)	520

Source: Boyle, C. A., et al., Epidemiology of premenstrual symptoms, *American Journal of Public Health, 77* (1987), 349–350.

There is no laboratory test or other sure way to diagnose premenstrual syndrome. Doctors rely on the woman's menstrual history, often requesting that patients keep a diary of the onset, duration, and the nature and severity of symptoms for at least two menstrual cycles. If symptoms such as those cited are present in the week before a woman's period, subside as her period starts, and are absent the week after her period, she is diagnosed as having PMS. This diagnosis is important not only to determine the treatment to recommend but to help screen out other conditions commonly confused with PMS, such as contraceptive side effects, dysmenorrhea, eating disorders, substance abuse, depression, and other psychiatric disorders (Ransom & Moldenhauer, 1998).

There have been numerous theories about the causes of PMS. These are described in the following list, along with the recommended treatment based on the theory of causation.

1. *Prostaglandins.* As a woman's uterine lining begins to shed during the menstrual cycle, prostaglandins (hormones) are released into her bloodstream. As the prostaglandins build up, they cause the uterine walls to become tense and to contract, resulting in cramping. As with dysmenorrhea, antiprostaglandin medications are recommended, such as aspirin, acetaminophen (for example, Tylenol or Datril), or ibuprofen (Motrin, Advil, or Nuprin).
2. *Progesterone.* Progesterone builds up during the menstrual cycle, causing PMS symptoms. Antiprogesterone medications are recommended to alter the menstrual cycle (speeding or delaying the onset of bleeding).
3. *Natural opiates.* Women experience a drop in the level of the neurotransmitter beta-endorphin, which is manufactured in the brain the week before the menstrual flow. This neurotransmitter has been described as the body's natural opiate in that it alleviates pain and generally makes you feel good. Treatment involves administering the drug naloxone, which maintains high levels of beta-endorphins.
4. *State of mind.* The symptoms of PMS are the result of brain activity—that is, the mind. Moods, perceptions, thoughts, ideas, self-confidence, and self-image are "choreographed" by the brain premenstrually. Treatment, therefore, entails counseling and other means to help women change their states of mind.

Other treatments include the following:

1. Birth control pills to stop ovulation.
2. Medications such as injectable medroxyprogesterone acetate (Depo-Provera) to stop ovulation and menstruation temporarily in severe cases.
3. Antidepressants in lower dosages than usually prescribed for depression, such as fluoxetine hydrochloride (Prozac), sertaline hydrochloride (Zoloft), paroxetine hydrochloride (Paxil), and venlafaxine hydrochloride (Effexor), if symptoms are mainly emotional.
4. A vegetarian diet.
5. Naturopathic medicine that includes lifestyle and dietary changes and may consist of nutritional supplements, botanical medicines, homeopathy, Chinese medicine, acupuncture, hydrotherapy, manipulation, physical therapy, or minor surgery (Phalen, 2000).

late luteal phase dysphoric disorder (LLPDD)
A type of premenstrual syndrome in which mental and emotional symptoms occur the week before menstruation. This is the name given to that condition by the American Psychiatric Association.

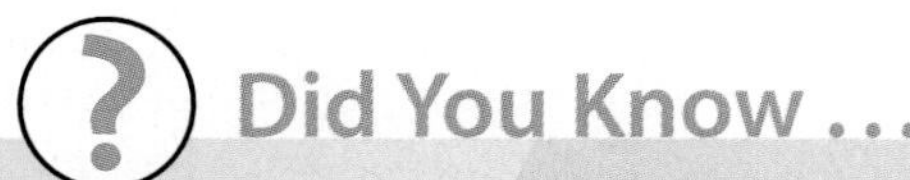

When the American Psychiatric Association included PMS in its *Diagnostic and Statistical Manual of Mental Disorders IV* as an illness, terming it **late luteal phase dysphoric disorder (LLPDD),** some people objected to the potential negative economic and social impact for all women. They believed it promoted a view of women as unreliable and unstable. However, others were grateful that women could then collect health insurance for treating PMS and that research would be focused on the condition.

In addition, the following is recommended (Mayo Clinic, 1998b):

1. Maintain a healthy body weight.
2. Lower the intake of salt and salty foods, especially before the period, to reduce fluid retention and bloating.
3. Avoid alcohol before the period to minimize depression and mood swings.
4. Avoid caffeine, such as in coffee, cola, and tea, to reduce moodiness, tension, and breast tenderness.
5. Increase the intake of carbohydrates such as breads, potatoes, cereals, vegetables, and rice.
6. Decrease the intake of simple sugars such as table sugar, syrup, brown sugar, honey, candy, and sweetened soda.
7. Reduce total fat intake, especially saturated fats, such as is found in marbled meats, cold cuts, butter, whole milk, and ice cream.
8. Eat smaller, more frequent meals rather than three large meals, do not skip meals, and try to eat at the same time every day.
9. Exercise regularly to enhance the sense of well-being.

Endometriosis

Sometimes tissue resembling the inner lining of the uterus (the endometrium) is found outside the uterus. This condition is known as *endometriosis*. Endometriosis is found most often on the lining of the pelvic cavity, the ovaries, the rectum, and the colon and in the uterus and on the bladder. Sometimes it is also found on the small intestine, liver, spleen, and lymph nodes. Endometriosis is, unfortunately, not an uncommon occurrence. In fact, it is estimated that 15% of all women of reproductive age have endometriosis (Koop, 1998). Although it can affect all women, endometriosis is most common among 25- to 30-year-olds, although it has also occurred in girls as young as 11 years of age.

The causes of endometriosis are not known, although there are several theories. One theory holds that pieces of the endometrium somehow find themselves in the fallopian tubes and are transported into the pelvic cavity. This is called *retrograde menstruation*. The endometrium pieces then adhere to one another to form adhesions, which cause pain. Another theory is based on the realization that in the early stages of fetal development there are but a few cells present and that these cells eventually differentiate into different tissue. This theory posits that perhaps cells outside the uterus, for some unknown reason, take on the function of cells in the endometrium. Still

Ethical DIMENSIONS

Should PMS Be Used as an Excuse for Socially Unacceptable Behaviors?

In 1980 and 1981, in two separate trials, British courts set free two women who admitted to murder because they were judged to suffer from PMS. In the first case, a barmaid, Sandie Smith, stabbed another barmaid during a fight. Testimony proved Smith had a history of violent outbursts that, when subsequently treated, were controlled with injections of progesterone. In the other case, Christine English purposely drove her car into her lover after an argument. English, too, was able to prove that she suffered from PMS and that she had menstruated a few hours after the murder. Both women were judged to have "diminished responsibility" and had their charges reduced to manslaughter. They were then released contingently on their getting treatment for their PMS.

Some people believe that PMS is so unsettling a condition that the physical discomfort and the emotional changes can understandably make a woman irritable, angry, hostile, and prone to do things she might not otherwise do. Given an incident to provoke such a reaction, even violent acts can be performed without the woman's really being responsible for them. These women should be encouraged to seek treatment for their illness rather than be regarded as criminals. They should be treated with compassion rather than imprisoned. Advocates of this position would contend that these women are not in control of their decisions and should, therefore, be excused for their actions.

Others argue that murder is never excusable. If women are allowed to offer PMS as a defense, then any ill person can use a similar defense. That would allow antisocial behavior to occur without any punishment or societal sanctions. Anarchy would result. Women, or other sick people, could (short of committing murder) sign contracts and not be held responsible for them, could steal items from stores and not be prosecuted for that theft, and could even sexually abuse children without fear of reprisal. Opponents of this PMS defense conceive of an unmanageable situation if PMS sufferers, or any other group of ill people, are not held accountable for their actions.

If you were a judge, would you rule that "diminished responsibility" was a justifiable defense for women who experienced PMS? What other behaviors would you allow to be excused by PMS? What other physical or emotional conditions would you allow to be similarly used to explain people's actions?

another theory argues that endometrial cells are transported through the bloodstream or through the lymph system to sites elsewhere in the body. Finally, some researchers believe that a breakdown in the function of the immune system resulting in an inability to destroy endometrium cells that manage to leave the uterus is responsible for endometriosis.

Women who acquire endometriosis usually experience a great deal of pelvic pain. This pain most often occurs just before or during menstrual bleeding, and usually abates after bleeding ceases. Pain may also be experienced in the lower back or lower abdomen and may be associated with urination. Fatigue and/or bloated feelings may occur, there may be blood in the urine and/or heavy menstrual bleeding, and diarrhea or constipation may result. In addition to causing these uncomfortable symptoms, endometriosis can lead to serious health consequences. For example, scar tissue can form and result in infertility. Or, adhesions can connect organs such as the uterus, fallopian tubes, ovaries, and intestines.

Endometriosis is treated in several ways, depending on the severity of the symptoms and the location of the tissue. Laparoscopic surgery—in which two small incisions are made in the abdomen through which is inserted a

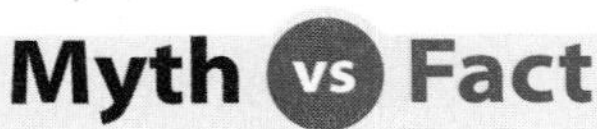

Myth: The menstrual cycle is 28 days long and does not fluctuate in length for any one woman.
Fact: The most prevalent menstrual cycle happens to be 30 days long. Even so, the cycle varies greatly from woman to woman and even for any one woman.

viewing instrument to perform the surgical cut—can be helpful in identifying the existence of endometrial tissue outside the uterus and determining its location. Then the tissue can be surgically removed before the procedure is completed. Sometimes the tissue has spread so extensively that the surgeon needs to open the abdomen to remove it rather than merely inserting a laparoscope. This procedure is called a *laparotomy.*

In addition to surgery, there are medications that result in lower levels of estrogen than normal and, therefore, alleviate much of the pain associated with endometriosis. Some of these drugs are synthetic hormones that stop the ovaries from producing estrogen, causing cessation of menstruation. These are known as *gonadotropin-releasing hormone analogues (GnRH analogues).* Another drug sometimes used is a synthetic hormone derived from testosterone (Danazol). More frequently, oral contraceptives are prescribed to prevent ovulation and reduce (when estrogen and progestin are used in combination) or eliminate menstrual bleeding. Finally, relief from pain may be obtained temporarily with ibuprofen or other analgesics (pain relievers).

The Menstrual Cycle and Sex

Many researchers have searched for a relationship between sexual interest and the time of the menstrual cycle. Findings of these studies have, for the most part, been contradictory. Some researchers report that women are more interested in sex just *before* menstruation (Kinsey, Pomeroy, & Martin, 1953), and others find them most interested *during* menstruation (Friedman, et al., 1980). Still others report the *middle* of the menstrual cycle to be the most sexually active (Adams, Gold, & Burt, 1978) or the time just *after* the menses to be when most sexual fantasizing occurs (Matteo & Rissman, 1984). Several other studies have not found the midcycle related in any way to heightened sexual arousal (Bancroft, 1984).

Some researchers describe two peaks during the menstrual cycle: just before menstruation and just after. Gold and Adams (1981) proposed an interesting explanation for why these parts of the menstrual cycle are associated with heightened sexual arousal. They suggest the anticipation of a lack of sexual intercourse while they are menstruating leads women to want to "get all they can" before they begin menstruating, and the actual deprivation during menstruation leads women to "want to make up for lost time."

When are women most sexually aroused? The answer to this question probably varies from one woman to another and, in addition to menstrual physiology, depends on such factors as one's lover, the setting, and numerous psychosocial factors such as the woman's comfort with her body, her level of self-esteem, and her religious and cultural beliefs regarding menstruation.

Myth vs Fact

Myth: Women are usually emotionally "low" premenstrually and emotionally "high" at ovulation.
Fact: This has not been conclusively determined. There are conflicting research findings and criticism of the methodology researchers have employed to answer this question.

Myth: Women's work activity needs to be adjusted during their periods.
Fact: Though this myth has been used to support job discrimination practices against women, there is no evidence that women cannot function normally in their jobs when menstruating.

Myth: Women should not swim or exercise as usual during their periods.
Fact: With the usual hygienic practices used by women, there are no known physical reasons for not exercising as usual. For some women, iron supplementation may be necessitated by the iron lost in the menstrual blood, but that precaution is a simple one.

Myth: Women's sexual desire is at a peak just before and just after menstruation.
Fact: For some women and for some cycles this may be true. However, sexual desire involves more than one's physical condition—the nature of the relationship, the setting, one's comfort with sexuality, one's health, and so on—so that expecting sexual desire to be determined solely by the menstrual cycle is unrealistic.

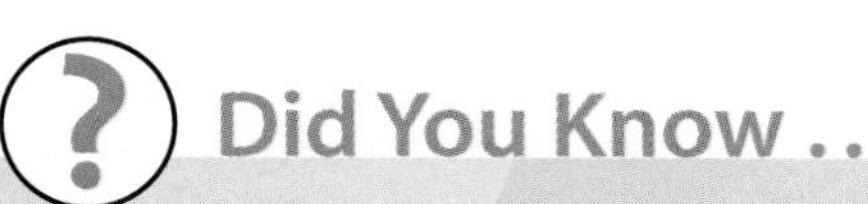

If a couple decides to engage in sexual intercourse when the woman is menstruating, they should realize that transmission of HIV is probably more likely at this time of the menstrual cycle than at any other. That is because of the blood present and the probability that some of that blood will have contact with an opening (albeit microscopic) into the body. If HIV is in that blood, it can infect the sexual partner. The "safer sex" practice of refraining from sexual intercourse while a woman is menstruating is usually overlooked. From the woman's perspective, participating in coitus while menstruating can facilitate HIV entry into her body.

Although there are no medical reasons to refrain from coitus during menstruation, many couples do so. At least one study found over half the men and women surveyed believed couples should not engage in sexual intercourse when the woman is menstruating (Research Forecasts, 1981). Some people refrain from coitus during menstruation because of religious taboos. For example, in Orthodox Judaism menstruating women are considered unclean and are supposed to sleep in a separate bed. When they are through menstruating, Jewish women are supposed to cleanse themselves in a ritual bath called a *mikvah*. Others refrain from sexual intercourse during menstruation because of the potential messiness. Still others refrain because of the physical discomfort they feel—bloating, cramping, or fatigue. And, finally, there are women who are ashamed of their menstrual flow and prefer to keep it a private matter not shared with anyone. A couple who refrains from sexual intercourse during menstruation should be comfortable with their decision, whatever the reason; likewise, a couple who decides to engage in coitus during this time should be comfortable with their decision.

A couple who decide to engage in sexual intercourse during the menstrual period can take several actions to make that experience as enjoyable as possible. First, they should discuss any concerns they may have, for example, the potential messiness or any religious inhibitions. Second, the woman can wear a diaphragm or cervical cap to hold back the menstrual flow. Because the menstrual fluid can sometimes irritate the penis, the man should wear a condom (a good idea anytime coitus occurs). With these simple actions, coitus during menstruation can be a positive and rewarding experience.

Pregnancy and Lactation

Because pregnancy and **lactation** (the production of breast milk) are discussed in detail in Chapter 9, only a brief discussion of the role played by hormones in these two processes is presented here. The hormonal involvement in both pregnancy and lactation is significant. A missed period usually indicates to a woman that her hormone level has changed because of pregnancy, but hormones are active in a pregnancy before the expected period is missed. Once conception occurs, the fertilized egg continues down the fallopian tube to become implanted in the endometrium, which has been enriched by earlier secretions of estrogen. Because the pituitary gland waits for the signal of diminished estrogen to continue the menstrual cycle (by releasing FSH) and because estrogen secretion continues rather than diminishes once fertilization occurs, the menstrual cycle is interrupted. Once the **placenta** (the organ that joins the fetus to the mother's uterus) develops, it too secretes a hormone, called **human chorionic gonadotropin (HCG).** The most frequently used means of testing for pregnancy is to check the woman's urine for the presence of this hormone. Throughout the pregnancy the placenta also manufactures large quantities of both estrogen and progesterone.

lactation
Production of breast milk.

placenta
An organ of interchange between mother and fetus, for the exchange of oxygen, nutrients, and waste through its cells.

human chorionic gonadotropin (HCG)
A hormone secreted by the placenta whose presence in a woman's urine is the most common medical method of determining pregnancy.

One to 3 days after the birth of the baby, the mother's breasts begin producing milk in preparation for breastfeeding. Milk production is a result of the effect of the sucking of the infant on the nipple, which also stimulates the pituitary to secrete the hormone *prolactin*. Prolactin, in turn, stimulates the development of breast milk. In addition, sucking on the nipple stimulates the pituitary to produce the hormone oxytocin, which is responsible for the breast's being able to eject milk.

Breastfeeding has many advantages. For example, nursing can provide the nutrients needed by the newborn and passes antibodies that provide protection from a variety of illnesses. In addition, breastfeeding helps the uterus

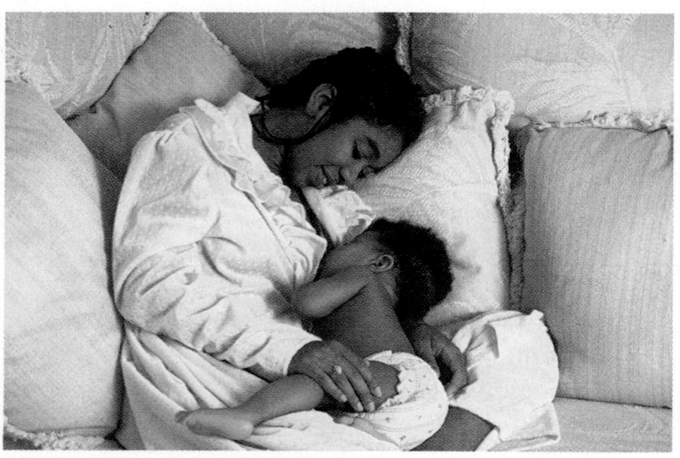

Breastfeeding can provide babies with necessary nutrients and antibodies to prevent disease. For the woman, breastfeeding can help her uterus return to its previous size and position sooner.

return to its previous size and location and helps to stop internal bleeding. As an added benefit, breastfeeding has some effectiveness as a contraceptive because high levels of prolactin inhibit ovulation. However, relying on breastfeeding as a means of contraception is not wise because it is much less effective than the other methods. Not to be overlooked are the savings in cost and the convenience that nursing provides. In addition to these tangible benefits associated with breastfeeding, there are psychological advantages. For example, some mothers may feel closer to their infants when they breastfeed. This feeling has been referred to as *bonding* or *attachment*. The American Academy of Pediatricians recommends that mothers breastfeed throughout the infant's first year of life.

Still, breastfeeding has several disadvantages. (It seems nothing is perfect!) If the new mother has ingested certain drugs or medications, these may be passed to the newborn through the mother's milk and be potentially damaging. Examples of such drugs are antibiotics, hormones in contraceptives, alcohol, and toxic substances ingested in foods. Also, cow milk ingested by the mother contains antibodies suspected of causing colic in breastfed babies. In addition, although breastfeeding is convenient in that a bottle need not be prepared, it does limit the flexibility of the mother. That is, she needs to be available to the infant when he or she is hungry unless she expresses milk and freezes it. Further, fathers can participate in bottle-feeding but not in breastfeeding. It is for this reason that some men prefer that their wives bottle-feed their babies. However, many families decide to use breastfeeding predominantly, but for the father or partner to offer the infant one bottle a day. Today well over half of the mothers in the United States breastfeed their babies.

Menopause

Usually between the ages of 40 and 55 years, women produce progressively less estrogen and progesterone, as an effect of aging on the ovaries. Whereas the pituitary continues to produce FSH and LH, the ovaries can no longer respond to these pituitary hormones as they once could. This decrease in estrogen and progesterone occurs over approximately a 5- to 10-year period and results in a cessation of menstruation. The period when these changes take place is called the **perimenopause,** or the **climacteric;** when menstruation has not occurred for a year, we call that **menopause.**

perimenopause (climacteric)
The period just before menopause when the production of estrogen and progesterone is decreasing, usually a 5- to 10-year period.

menopause
The time when a woman's menstrual cycle ceases, usually between 40 and 55 years of age.

hot flashes
Intermittent sensations of heat reported by menopausal women, possibly caused by decreased estrogen production.

Symptoms of Perimenopause and Menopause

About 80% of perimenopausal women report mild symptoms or no symptoms at all; only 20% report symptoms severe enough to cause them to seek medical attention (National Institute on Aging, 1986). The symptoms that perimenopausal and menopausal women experience can vary from headaches, dizziness, palpitations, insomnia, anxiety, depression, and weight gain to hot flashes and vaginal dryness. **Hot flashes** (sometimes referred to as *hot flushes*) are sudden waves of heat felt throughout the body, often accompanied by reddening, sweating, and, sometimes, dizziness (Willis, 1988). Some women experience hot flashes infrequently, whereas others may have them every few hours or so. They may last a few seconds or, in severe cases, a full 30 minutes. And some women never have hot flashes. Because hot flashes tend to occur more frequently at night, they often disturb sleep, causing the woman to awaken in a sweat. In particularly bothersome cases, they may contribute to insomnia. Hot flashes appear to be caused by hormonal fluctuations that affect the nerves that govern the dilatation or constriction of the blood vessels. When the blood vessels rapidly dilate in response to hormonal secretions, a sense of warmth may result. Another theory is that the temperature control mechanism in the brain's hypothalamus is affected by the decrease in hormonal production from the ovaries (Bates, 1981; Erlik, et al., 1981). Generally, hot flashes cease after 2 years, but in some cases they may last longer.

Vaginal dryness results from the lowered amount of estrogen in the vaginal walls, which causes shrinking and thinning and causes the vaginal mucosa to become thinner. The net result is that both the length and the width of the vagina become smaller and the vagina cannot expand during penile insertion as it once could. In addition, there is diminished vaginal lubrication during perimenopause and menopause. These changes can mean painful intercourse as well as an increased risk of vaginal infection (National Institute on Aging, 1986). Over-the-counter lubricants can be helpful in these cases.

A significant symptom caused by the decrease in estrogen production is the decalcification of the bones. **Osteoporosis** is the disease that results when enough calcium is lost in the bones to make the person susceptible to bone fractures and bending (for example, curvature of the back—sometimes called "dowager's hump" because it is common among older women). Women older than 50 years of age lose about 10% of their bone mass every 10 years (Kahn, 1984); the result is an increased risk of bone fractures. Women older than 60 years of age suffer from 10 times as many fractures of the forearm as do men (Elliott, 1979). It seems that osteoporosis occurs more frequently in white women who are fair skinned (especially blonds and redheads), who smoke cigarettes, who drink alcohol, who are physically inactive, who are underweight, and whose diet is low in calcium (Greenwood, 1985; National Institute on Aging, 1986). Osteoporosis can develop in men, too.

osteoporosis
A condition of weakened bones resulting from decalcification (loss of calcium) of bone that increases in the absence of estrogen and is of particular concern in postmenopausal women.

estrogen replacement therapy (ERT)
Treatment of women who have insufficient estrogen production (including menopausal women) with synthetic estrogen supplements.

Treatment for Menopause

As we have mentioned, only a minority of women have menopausal symptoms severe enough to make them seek medical attention. For those women there are several alternatives. One of the more controversial therapies considers menopause to be merely an estrogen deficiency and treats it by replacing estrogen. In fact, approximately 17 million women in the United States were taking hormones to relieve symptoms of menopause that included hot flashes, sleep disturbances, and vaginal dryness in 2002 (Redfearn, 2002). However, over the years **estrogen replacement therapy (ERT)** (alternatively referred to as *hormone replacement therapy, HRT*) has been controversial.

Estrogen supplements were used extensively until the 1970s, when it was found that their use increased the incidence of endometrial cancer. However, since then, progestin has been added, resulting in the sloughing of the endometrial lining and the virtual elimination of endometrial cancer. Subsequently, estrogen and progestin supplements were widely prescribed (Rosenberg, 1993).

It was believed that the benefits of estrogen replacement therapy included the elimination or diminishing of postmenopausal symptoms such as hot flashes and vaginal dryness. It was also thought to be protective against development of heart disease. In addition, estrogen replacement was said to add calcium to the bones, thereby increasing their density (Speroff, et al.,

1996; The Writing Group for the PEPI Trial, 1996). More dense bones are less susceptible to osteoporosis, which can lead to bone fractures. Other research seemed to indicate that estrogen replacement therapy prevented or delayed the onset of Alzheimer's disease (Tang, 1996; Waters, 1997; Wickelgren, 1997).

Research studies were unclear regarding the role of estrogen replacement therapy in the development of breast cancer. Early studies found that estrogen without progestin was connected to the development of breast cancer (Bergkvist, et al., 1989; Berkowitz, et al., 1985). More recent studies have also found that estrogen replacement increases a woman's risk for breast cancer and that the longer she takes estrogen, the greater the risk (Colditz, et al., 1995). However, other studies concluded that estrogen replacement had no relationship to the subsequent development of breast cancer (Risch & Howe, 1994). A long-term study conducted by the American Cancer Society of more than a million women concluded that 10 years after the onset of estrogen replacement there was actually a decrease in breast cancer risk (*USA Today,* 1998). Experiments are being conducted with new drugs to replace estrogen as a treatment for postmenopausal women; some studies indicate that these drugs reduce the risk of breast cancer. These drugs are called *selective estrogen receptor modulators* (SERMs). In the next few years they should be better understood.

Until recently, medical opinion appeared to weigh in on the side of estrogen replacement therapy for most women, that is, until more definitive studies concluded otherwise. The first of these was conducted by American Cancer Society researchers, who reported in the *Journal of the American Medical Association* (Rodriguez, et al., 2001) that women who had estrogen replacement for 10 years or more were found to be at increased risk of dying of ovarian cancer. That risk remained even after the cessation of the estrogen replacement. However, the study that really turned the tide against estrogen replacement therapy as routine treatment for menopausal women was conducted by the National Institutes of Health's Women's Health Initiative (WHI) (Writing Group for the Women's Health Initiative, 2002). In a study observing 16,000 women over 5 years it was concluded that ERT presented a significant risk to many women. Among the WHI study findings were the following:

- Postmenopausal women who took estrogen had a 60% higher probability of development of ovarian cancer than women who did not take estrogen replacement
- ERT actually increased the risk of development of heart disease rather than lowering it, as previously thought
- ERT increased the risk of experiencing stroke
- ERT increased the risk of development of breast cancer
- ERT decreased the risk of development of colorectal cancer
- ERT decreased the risk of hip fracture

In addition, a study of the emotional benefits of ERT found only women with hot flashes experienced improved emotional well-being (Hlatky, et al., 2002). For other women, there was no benefit to ERT and, in many cases, their emotional health actually worsened.

In spite of these findings, the controversy regarding the use of ERT for particular women continues. Part of the controversy relates to the findings of the WHI study. When observed more closely, the increased risk reported is relatively small. For example, whereas 30 of 10,000 women who do not take estrogen experience heart disease each year, 37 of 10,000 on ERT experience heart disease each year. That is an increase of only 7 women in 10,000. Although that risk is small, it does eliminate the rationale that ERT helps prevent heart disease in women. Likewise with stroke and breast cancer: ERT increases the risk of stroke each year from 21 per 10,000 women not on ERT to 29 of 10,000 on ERT. Breast cancer risk increases from 30 per 10,000 to 38 per 10,000. Colorectal cancer risk *decreases* from 16 per 10,000 to 10 per 10,000 each year; and hip fracture risk *decreases* from 15 per 10,000 to 10 per 10,000.

The WHI study has led to the recommendation that ERT not be prescribed as standard practice to postmenopausal women. That is because even though the differences are small, when they are totaled across the population, the amount of increased cases is dramatic. The guidelines are different, though, when individual women are concerned. That is because the benefits of ERT for any one woman may outweigh the small increased risk. For example, women who have osteoporosis and are at risk of hip fracture may decide, with their doctors, that the decreased risk of hip fracture associated with ERT is worth the increased risk of heart disease or breast cancer. Of course, a woman's age may also factor into this decision. It is with this reasoning that the predominant recommendation regarding ERT is that a woman and her physician consider the pros and cons, the benefits and risks, in light of the woman's particular circumstances before deciding whether to use ERT. For more information about ERT, visit the web site of the Association of Reproductive Health Professionals at www.arhp.org/hrtresources.

Other treatments for menopause disorders specific to preventing osteoporosis include sufficient physical exercise to strengthen the bones, a diet rich in calcium to slow bone decalcification, refraining from smoking of cigarettes and drinking of alcohol, and avoidance of carbonated soft drinks that contain high levels of phosphorus, which may contribute to a phosphorus–calcium imbalance associated with osteoporosis. Foods such as milk, sardines and salmon canned with bones, oysters, and dark green vegetables are recommended because they are all high in calcium.

Some physicians may also prescribe tranquilizers for women who have difficulty with the psychological aspects of menopause. It is unclear whether the depression some women report during menopause is a cause of that condition or is caused by other changes that usually occur during that stage of life (for example, children's leaving home, aged parents' needing more attention, or a woman's life's taking a new direction).

In addition to estrogen replacement therapy, other treatments for hot flashes have been recommended. These include sleeping near an open window or fan; taking black cohosh (an ancient Native American remedy for rattlesnake bites) in capsular form; and ingesting phytoestrogens such as soy or flaxseed, vitamin E, 40 mg of red clover, combinations of bioflavanoids and vitamin C, chaste tea, evening primrose, and licorice (Phalen, 2001), although a study of 29 other studies (called a *metaanalysis*) found that only black cohosh relieved hot flashes (Kronenberg & Fugh-Berman, 2002).

Treatment for vaginal dryness can include the use of lubricated creams, vegetable oils, or water-soluble jellies (such as K-Y or Lubifax) and suppositories (such as Replens) (Greenwood, 1985). In addition, it appears that regular masturbation or participation in sexual intercourse helps reduce vaginal soreness.

It would be unfortunate to close this section without citing the benefits and positive aspects of menopause. Because women can no longer conceive, the fear of pregnancy is removed, and lovemaking is often more enjoyable as a result. However, a woman who has ceased to menstruate has

change-of-life baby
A baby born to a menopausal woman who, in spite of not menstruating regularly, ovulated.

breast cancer
The second most common type of cancer in women.

breast self-examination (BSE)
A periodic self-care procedure that involves feeling the breast for any abnormalities that is recommended for every female once every menstrual cycle or every month after menopause.

not necessarily ceased to ovulate. So-called **change-of-life babies** have been known to surprise women just entering menopause who thought they could no longer conceive. Especially during perimenopause—when the menses occurs, however infrequently—caution is advised.

The anthropologist Margaret Mead talked of "postmenopausal zest" to describe the excitement, stimulation, and enjoyment that can result from menopause. If viewed in this way, the postmenopausal years can be rich with new opportunities and experiences. If its negative aspects become the focus, menopausal symptoms will probably increase, and psychological discomfort will result. It is up to a woman's friends, relatives, and colleagues at work to help her focus on the positive aspects of menopause rather than its less desirable components. In addition, many women now turn to support groups (for example, The Red Hot Mamas) or online forums to share strategies on ways to manage menopausal symptoms.

Hormone Therapy

Hormonal therapy for women is not limited to menopausal problems. Androgens, for example, are administered to transsexuals or genetic females being raised as males to promote the development of male secondary sex characteristics at puberty. Androgens can also be used to increase interest in sexual activity in women with sexual dysfunction (Kaplan, 1974), although the person's belief that the androgens will be effective is a factor here. Finally, androgen treatment seems to suppress cancerous growth in some breast cancer patients.

Sexually Related Diseases: Self-Care and Prevention

Some diseases are not transmitted by sexual activity but do affect sexual organs. These are termed sexually related diseases (SRDs). Advances in chemical and surgical treatment of diseases of the sex organs have improved 5- and 10-year survival rates and made restoration of function more attainable than ever before. Maintaining reproductive health means following safer sexual practices, paying attention to your body, monitoring it for certain signs, using the specialized health services available, and seeking information—from organizations and publications—on issues related to reproductive health. Successful treatment of SRDs generally depends on early diagnosis of potential problems.

The Female Reproductive System

Self-care and disease prevention activities for the female involve many of the sexual organs, including the breasts, cervix, uterus, ovaries, and vagina.

The Breasts

The most common breast disorders are cancer, cystic mastitis (mammary dysplasia), fibroadenoma, nipple discharge, and breast abscess. Most of these disorders occur only in women, but men are susceptible to breast cancer too.

Breast Cancer The breast is the second leading site of cancer in American women (the first is the lung) and the second major cause of cancer death. At the time of this writing, it is estimated that 211,300 new cases of breast cancer will have been diagnosed in women in 2003, and 1,300 cases will have been diagnosed in men (American Cancer Society, 2003). After increasing about 4% per year in the 1980s, breast cancer incidence rates have leveled off to about 112 cases per 100,000 persons. Still, 40,200 women and 400 men will probably have died of breast cancer in 2003. And yet, death rates from breast cancer continue to decline, especially among younger women. The 5-year survival rate for localized breast cancer increased from 72% in the 1940s to 97%

in 2003. If the cancer has spread regionally, however, the 5-year survival rate drops to 77%, and, if the cancer has spread to distant locations (metastasized), the survival rate drops to 23%. Sixty-seven percent of women diagnosed with breast cancer survive 10 years, and 56% survive 15 years.

No specific cause of breast cancer is known, but epidemiological studies have identified certain risk factors that predispose women to breast cancer. One of these risk factors is age. As women get older, the risk increases. The risk is also higher in women who have a family history of breast cancer, who experienced an early menarche or a late menopause, who recently used oral contraceptives or postmenopausal estrogens, and who never had children or had the first live birth at a late age. Other suspected risk factors are a diet high in fat, although a large-scale 1999 study calls this relationship into question (Holmes, et al., 1999); exposure to pesticides and other selected chemicals; alcohol consumption; weight gain; induced abortion; and physical inactivity. In addition, two new genes that appear to make women susceptible to breast cancer have been discovered, BRCA1 and BRCA2. However, only 5% to 10% of breast cancers are thought to be inherited, and only 5% of breast cancer patients were found to have the gene BRCA1 or BRCA2. One study found that 75% of women in whom breast cancer develops have no identifiable risk factor other than gender and age (Hortobagyi, McLelland, & Reed, 1990). This makes it especially important for all women to learn breast self-examination and to have regular breast examinations by a physician.

Breast self-examination (BSE) is among the most valuable self-care procedures women can adopt. Although medical specialists actively check for breast cancer in routine examinations, checking one's own breasts every menstrual cycle increases the chances of early detection. The technique is simple, and its value is immeasurable; if cancer is present, the earlier it is diagnosed, the better the chance for survival.

In April 1987 a committee of the United States Public Health Service (which had been established to recommend those medical procedures with demonstrated effectiveness and those without) caused concern among cancer prevention specialists by citing BSE as a procedure whose value had not been clearly shown. The committee was charged with reviewing the scientific evidence for many medical screenings and examination procedures and eliminating those that contributed to the increasing cost of health care. As such they decided that BSE was not employed by enough women and cancers not found in enough quantity to warrant public health campaigns to encourage women to perform the examination. Other cancer experts, who argued that BSE does not cost a woman any money and that it can uncover early treatable cancers, recommended that women ignore the committee's finding and continue doing monthly BSEs. Canadians have also waded in on this issue. The Canadian Task Force on Preventive Health Care (Baxter, 2001) studied the benefits and harms associated with breast self-examinations and found no evidence of effectiveness and evidence of harm. The harm included an increase in the number of physician visits for the evaluation of benign breast lesions and significantly higher rates of benign breast biopsy findings. As a result, the Canadian Task Force recommended that women not perform breast self-examinations. BSEs do have the potential for finding cancers early, while they can be treated the least invasively. Consequently, your authors encourage monthly BSEs.

For best results, perform the exam when the skin is wet or moist—after showering or after applying body lotion. Menstruating women should perform this test 1 week after their period; postmenopausal women should check their breasts at least once a month. All women should check their breasts visually in the mirror and by means of this exam. Consult a gynecologist if you find a lump, a thickening, or any other unusual feature.

Gender DIMENSIONS

Breast Self-Examination By regularly examining her own breasts, a woman is likely to notice any changes that occur. The best time for breast self-examination (BSE) is about a week after your period ends, when your breasts are not tender or swollen. If you are not having regular periods, do BSE on the same day every month.

1. Lie down with a pillow under your right shoulder and place your right arm behind your head.
2. Use the finger pads of the three middle fingers on your left hand to feel for lumps in the right breast.
3. Press firmly enough to know how your breast feels. A firm ridge in the lower curve of each breast is normal. If you are not sure how hard to press, talk with your doctor or nurse.
4. Move around the breast in a circular, up-and-down line, or wedge pattern (a, b, c). Be sure to do it the same way every time, check the entire breast area, and remember how your breast feels from month to month.

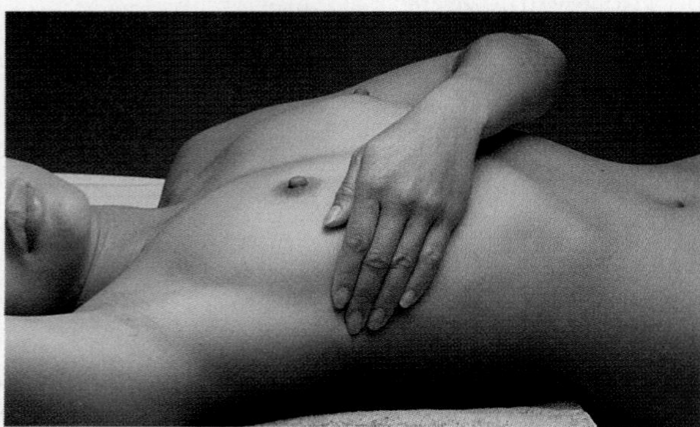

5. Repeat the exam on your left breast, using the finger pads of the right hand. (Move the pillow to below your left shoulder.)

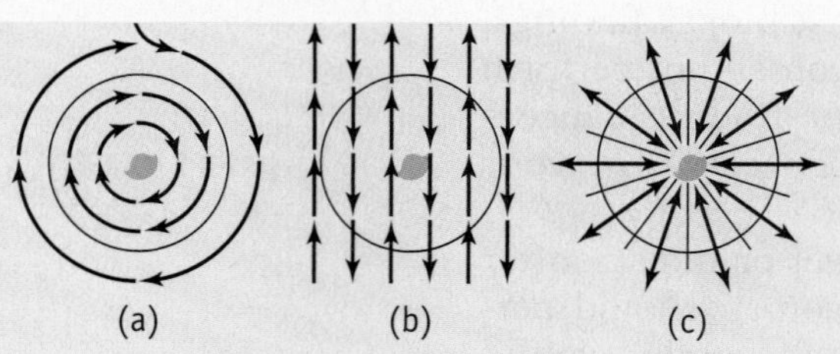

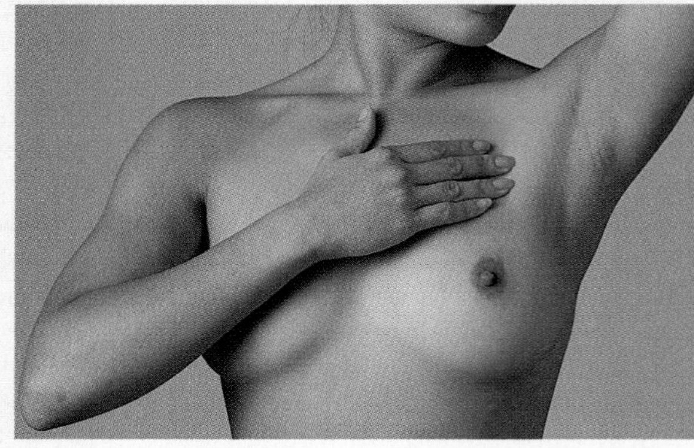

6. If you find any changes, see your doctor right away.
7. Repeat the examination of both breasts while standing, with one arm behind your head. The upright position makes it easier to check the upper and outer part of the breasts (toward your armpit). This is where about half of breast cancers are found. You may want to do the standing part of the BSE while you are in the shower. Some breast changes can be felt more easily when your skin is wet and soapy.

For added safety, you can check your breasts for any dimpling of the skin, changes in the nipple, redness, or swelling while standing in front of a mirror right after your BSE each month.

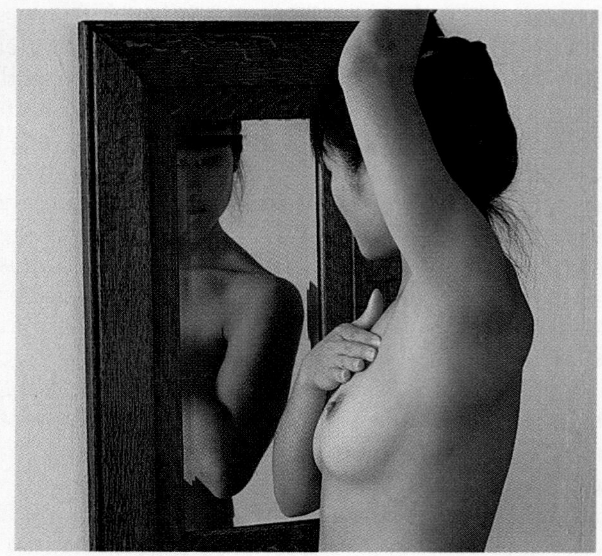

About 90% of all breast lumps are discovered by women at home rather than in a clinical setting; most are benign. The most common site is the upper outer quadrant of the breast. About 80% of patients with breast cancer report lumps. Much less often symptoms can include pain in the breast, discharge from the nipple, a change in the character of the nipple itself, and changes in the character of the breast.

As we have mentioned, in addition to performing BSE regularly, it is recommended that women have regular breast examinations by a physician. These examinations include both **clinical breast exams** and **mammography** screening, depending on a woman's age and medical history. A clinical breast exam is similar to BSE, except that it is conducted by a physician trained to detect any abnormalities. It is suggested that women aged 20 years and older have a clinical breast examination regularly, preferably every 3 years between ages 20 and 40 years and annually thereafter. The recommendations regarding mammograms are more complicated. A mammogram is an X ray of the breast that often allows physicians to detect breast lumps before they would be palpable by a physician (see Figure 4.11). It is agreed by medical experts that women older than age 50 years should have a mammogram annually; it is in regard to younger women that some disagreement prevails. A Consensus Development Conference of experts was organized by the National Institutes of Health in 1997 to arrive at a recommendation for mammography. That committee concluded that women between 40 and 49 years should consult their physicians regarding the intervals for mammography. In other words, there was some but not enough evidence that mammography between ages 40 and 49 years identified enough cancers or that, once identified, enough cancer deaths were prevented to justify such a recommendation. The National Cancer Institute went along with the Consensus Conference recommendation. However, the American Cancer Society disagreed; that organization still recommends that mammography should begin by age 40 years and between the ages of 40 and 49 years it should be performed every 1 to 2 years. The American Cancer Society reports that in 1995, 64% of women aged 40 to 49 years had had a mammogram within the previous 2 years, 53% of women aged 50 years and older had had a mammogram within the previous year, and 49% of women aged 65 years and older had had a mammogram within the previous year (American Cancer Society, 1995). Obviously, we have a long way to go in educating women about the need to get mammograms and the benefits they can expect.

When breast cancer is suspected, a **biopsy** is performed. In a **needle biopsy** a fine needle is inserted into the tumor and fluid or cells are withdrawn. If the lump dissipates as soon as fluid is obtained, the lump is confirmed as a cyst and generally no further procedure is needed. An **open biopsy** is a minor surgical procedure during which tissue of the tumor is removed and examined for possible cancer **(carcinoma).**

Patients who have breast cancer are classified in terms of stages. These stages are determined by the characteristics of the tumor and the lymph nodes and whether **metastasis**—spread of the cancer to other body sites—has occurred. Treatment naturally depends on the stage of the cancer. The treatment of breast cancer may involve **lumpectomy,** in which only the breast lump and lymph nodes under the arm are removed, usually followed by radiation therapy; **mastectomy,** in which the breast and lymph nodes under the arm are removed; **chemotherapy,** treatment with drugs; **radiation therapy;** and **hormone therapy.** There are three kinds of mastectomy: *simple mastectomy,* in which the whole breast is removed, sometimes along with lymph nodes under the arm; *modified radical mastectomy,* the most common form of mastectomy, in which the breast, many of the lymph nodes under

clinical breast exam
A breast examination conducted by a physician to detect any abnormalities.

mammography
An X ray of the breasts to detect any abnormality before it is visible or palpable.

needle biopsy
Insertion of a needle into a lump in a breast to see whether fluid (which indicates a cyst rather than a tumor) can be removed.

biopsy (open biopsy)
Usually referred to as an open biopsy, a minor surgical procedure during which tissue of a tumor is removed and examined for presence of cancer.

carcinoma
A type of cancer emanating from epithelial cells.

metastasis
Spread of cancer from a primary site to other parts of the body.

lumpectomy
Removal of a lesion, benign or malignant.

mastectomy
Removal of the breast and/or other tissue.
Simple: Removal of only the breast (sometimes with removal of lymph nodes under the arm).
Modified radical: Removal of the breast, lymph nodes, lining of the chest muscle, and sometimes part of the chest wall.
Radical: Removal of the breast, lymph nodes, and chest muscle.

chemotherapy
Use of chemicals (medication) to treat disease; may be oral, intravenous, intramuscular, or topical.

radiation therapy
A form of treatment for cancer that uses carefully directed radiation to destroy cancer cells.

hormone therapy
Form of treatment for cancer that uses hormones to combat cancer cell growth.

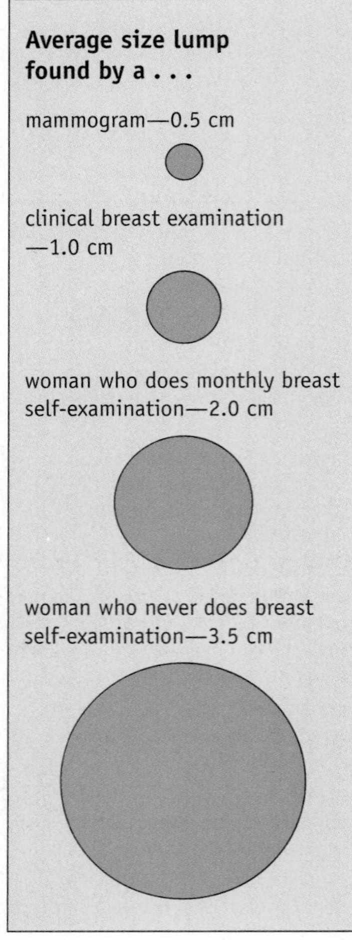

FIGURE 4.11 The sizes of breast masses detectable by mammography, physical examination, and self-examination illustrate the importance of screening mammography in the early detection of breast cancer.

the arm, the lining over the chest muscles, and sometimes part of the chest wall are removed; and *radical mastectomy* (also called the *Halstead radical mastectomy*) in which the breast, chest muscles, and all lymph nodes under the arm are removed. Radical mastectomy used to be the most frequently performed operation for breast cancer but now is used only when the tumor has spread to the chest muscles.

For patients with no lymph node involvement, hormone therapy may be prescribed as a preventative measure against recurrence of cancer. The most commonly used hormones are tamoxifen and special "designer estrogens," which may be administered for 5 years. There presently remains a question regarding the increased risk of development of cancer of the uterus for women on hormonal therapy. For early-stage breast cancer, long-term survival rates after lumpectomy plus radiation therapy are similar to survival rates after modified radical mastectomy, and, therefore, this less invasive procedure is being used more often—except for those women who choose not to experience the side effects of radiation and thus choose mastectomy.

We live in a society in which breast size and shape are mistakenly seen as contributing greatly to a woman's sexuality. Thus a woman who loses a breast through amputation can be devastated. Many women who have had mastectomies, whether or not they are sexually active, suffer feelings of loss, fear of rejection, and, of course, fear of the cancer's recurrence. Community support systems such as the Reach to Recovery Project of the American Cancer Society (ACS) and the Breast Referral Service, founded by Rose Kushner, who herself recovered from a mastectomy, give invaluable support to women in adjusting to the treatment of their cancers. The involvement of lovers or husbands and children is of great importance, because all of them, not just the woman, must adjust to her changed appearance and emotional sensitivity. Breast reconstruction after a mastectomy is also available. It offers a woman a more normal appearance and often eases her acceptance of the change in her body. This option should be discussed with the surgeon before breast surgery, if possible.

Reconstructive breast surgery can create a breastlike structure by using saline (salt) water encased in a silicone pouch that is implanted under a woman's skin and chest muscle. There has been some concern regarding the safety of breast implants in recent years. Implants were considered a medical product—not a drug—and are therefore not regulated by the Food and Drug Administration. At this point, the research is inconclusive. Some research seems to indicate that this concern is unwarranted (see pp. 119–120), although other studies did find health problems associated with earlier silicone implants. When introduced, silicone was injected directly into the breast tissue. That procedure resulted in development of lumps, infections, collapsed lungs, and pneumonia. However, this procedure was legislated out of existence and is no longer used. Another alternative, the silicone gel pouch, sparked concern that the pouch might rupture and the gel would leak out, or that the gel would leak out through the pouch's semipermeable membrane a little at a time. To be safe while studying the likelihood of this happening, silicone implants were taken off the market in 1992, except for use by mastectomy patients. Today, saline solution is used instead of silicone.

Cystic Mastitis Also called *chronic cystic mastitis, fibrocystic condition,* and *mammary dysplasia* (cell change), **cystic mastitis** is the most common breast condition. It is usually found in women 30 to 50 years of age. Because cystic mastitis is uncommon in postmenopausal women, it is believed to be related to estrogen activity. In cystic mastitis small and large cysts form in the breast tissues. The cysts are generally filled with fluid and may have to

cystic mastitis
Known also as fibrocystic disease, a condition characterized by fluid-filled lesions (cysts) that are tender and believed to be related to estrogen activity.

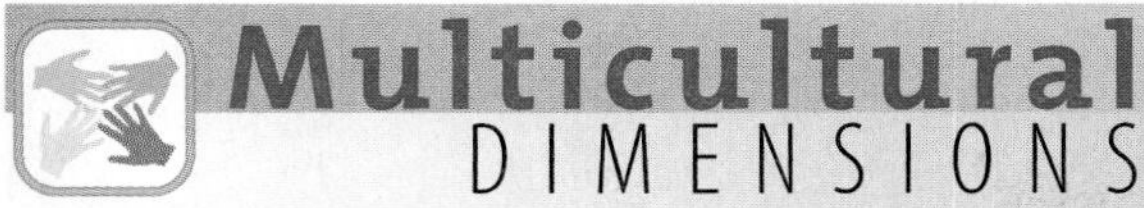

Multicultural DIMENSIONS

Breast Cancer More Deadly in African Americans Although breast cancer develops more often in white women, African-American women are more likely to die of it. Researchers and epidemiologists have been perplexed as to why. It was originally assumed that this difference was due to the disproportionately high number of black women who live in poverty, resulting in lack of access to health care. That, in turn, would lead to later diagnosis and, consequently, less effective treatment. However, having studied this dilemma for several years, scientists have concluded that, although poverty status plays a role (it is estimated that poverty accounts for approximately 50% of the cause), biology is significantly involved. Tumors in black women are just more virulent.

Evidence for this conclusion can be found in a study that compared black and white women who belonged to health maintenance organizations (HMOs) in which health care was readily available (access to mammograms and other medical care). Still, the black women HMO members had larger and more advanced tumors when diagnosed. The suspicion was that these tumors grew faster, and that is why at the time of diagnosis they were larger and more advanced.

Research also indicates that African-American women do not wait any longer to seek medical diagnosis when identifying a breast abnormality than do white women. Consequently, that is not a significant variable in the difference in tumor size or death rates between black and white women.

A review of research of breast cancer in black women published in the *New York Times* (Kolata, 1994) summarized what is known about this situation. Cited are several studies in which tumors in African-American women were found to be more actively dividing than those in white women, and more lacked hormone receptors and had tissue features indicative of unfavorable diagnosis.

Although it is wise for all women to perform breast self-examinations on a regular basis and to obtain regular medical examinations, given what we know about tumors in black women, it is particularly prudent for them to do so.

be drained frequently. Sometimes the cysts must be removed. Studies have concluded that "fibrocystic breasts" occur frequently in women and are not associated with significant increases in risk for breast cancer (Cady, 1986; Deckers & Ricci, 1992). One research report indicated a possible link between cystic mastitis and coffee, tea, cola, and chocolate consumption. On the basis of this study, some practitioners recommend that women decrease or eliminate the consumption of these products. But because this treatment approach has not been tested by using randomized double-blind studies, medical researchers and practitioners have questioned its validity (Cady, 1986).

Fibroadenoma **Fibroadenoma** is a benign (noncancerous) tumor that may develop in white women in their early 30s and in black women somewhat earlier (there are no data on other groups). The tumor is usually firm, round, and somewhat movable. Generally the treatment is surgical removal.

fibroadenoma
A benign (noncancerous) tumor that is firm, round, and somewhat movable.

Nipple Discharge A discharge from the nipples of women who are not nursing can be due to cystic mastitis, to a small benign tumor (called a *papilloma*) in a duct leading to the nipple, or to an uncommon condition *(ectasia)* in which the ducts of the breast enlarge and distend, allowing fluid to accumulate and escape. Occasionally the use of hormones—such as oral contraceptives and postmenopausal estrogen supplements—can cause nipple discharge, which should cease when the drugs are discontinued. Any discharge from the nipples should be checked by a physician.

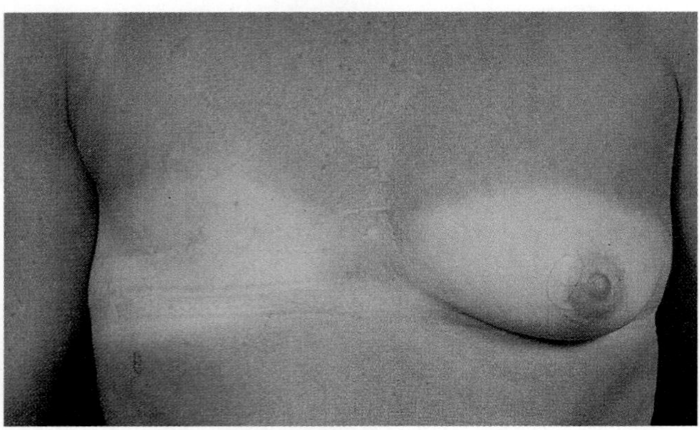

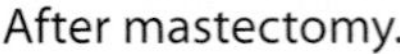

After mastectomy.

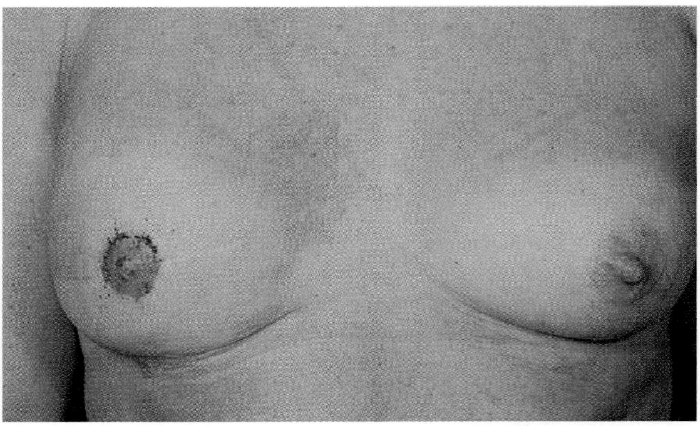

After reconstructive surgery after mastectomy.

breast abscess
Infection of the breast characterized by redness, swelling, and a painful or tender mass.

invasive cervical cancer
Cancer that has invaded a wide area of cervical tissue.

Pap smear
A test of the tissue of the cervix for cervical cancer (named after its founder, Dr. Papanicolaou).

Breast Abscess Generally **breast abscesses** (infections) are seen in nursing women, but they occur in nonnursing women as well and in either case should be treated by a physician. Redness, swelling, or a tender, painful mass is symptomatic of breast infection. If the infection is not stopped, an abscess can develop. These are usually treated by incision and drainage, antibiotics, or both.

The Cervix

Rates of **invasive cervical cancer,** which involves deep-tissue layers of the cervix and sometimes spreads to other organs, have decreased steadily over the past several decades. This decline is attributed to the increase in Pap smear screening, which leads to early detection and subsequent early treatment. Still, an estimated 12,300 cases of invasive cervical cancer probably have been diagnosed in 2003 with 4,100 deaths (American Cancer Society, 2003), in spite of a decline in death rate from cervical cancer on average of −1.5% per year since 1982. Cervical cancer death rates declined for African-Americans more rapidly than for whites. However, in 2003 the mortality rate for African-American women (13.6 per 100,000) was still more than one and one-half times as high as it was for white women (8.1 per 100,000).

Although the exact cause of cervical cancer is unknown, several factors can put you at risk. Among these are having your first intercourse at an early age, having multiple sex partners, having many pregnancies, having a mother who took diethylstilbestrol (DES) while pregnant with you, and having a sexually transmitted infection caused by the human papillomavirus (HPV).

The American Cancer Society recommends a **Pap smear** be performed annually with a pelvic exam in women who are, or have been, sexually active or who have reached the age of 18 years. After three consecutive annual exams have normal findings, the Pap test may be performed less frequently at the discretion of the woman and her physician. Pap smear screening is a simple procedure that involves swabbing a small sample of cells from the cervix, transferring these cells to a slide, and examining them under a microscope. Regular gynecological screening is advised for all women, particularly because early cell changes in the cervical tissue do not present symptoms a woman can recognize herself—although invasive cervical cancer sometimes does cause a bloody discharge between periods and/or bloody spotting after intercourse. Unfortunately, data indicate that not enough women are getting regular Pap tests. In a study presented in the National Health Interview Survey, it was reported that only two-thirds of women 18 years and older had had a Pap test in the previous 3 years.

Treatment for invasive cervical cancer generally consists of surgery and radiation, or both. Eighty-eight percent of patients survive 1 year after diagnosis, and 70% survive 5 years. When detected at an early stage, invasive cervical cancer is one of the most successfully treated cancers, with a 5-year survival rate of 92% for cancers that have not spread. Unfortunately, only 55% of invasive cervical cancer in white women and only 45% in African-American women are diagnosed at this stage. Again, this points to the value of getting a Pap test regularly.

At the time of this writing, it is estimated that 40,100 cases of cancer of the uterus, most often of the endometrium, will be diagnosed in 2003. Incidence rates of uterine cancer have varied since the mid-1980s. In 2003, the incidence rate for white women was 26.0 per 100,000, and 17.7 per 100,000 for African-American women (American Cancer Society, 2003). Although incidence rates are higher among white women than African-American women, the relationship is reversed for mortality rates. African-American women have mortality rates that are nearly twice as high as rates among white women (7.0 per 100,000 compared to 3.9 per 100,000) (American Cancer Society, 2003).

Estrogen is the major risk factor for uterine cancer. Women who choose estrogen replacement therapy to combat the effects of menopause, who are administered tamoxifen to prevent breast cancer or its recurrence, who experience an early menarche, who have a late menopause, who never have children, or who do not ovulate have been shown to be at increased risk. Some accommodations have been made, however, to decrease this risk. For example, some studies indicate that adding progesterone to estrogen replacement therapy can offset the risk of uterine cancer, and as a result this has become standard practice. Other risks for uterine cancer include infertility, diabetes, hypertension, and obesity. On the other hand, pregnancy and the use of oral contraceptives appear to provide protection against uterine cancer.

The Pap test is rarely effective in detecting uterine cancer early. It is with this realization that the American Cancer Society recommends that women older than 40 years have an annual pelvic exam and that women at high risk have an endometrial biopsy at menopause and periodically thereafter. Early warning signs include uterine bleeding or spotting; pain is a later symptom. Treatment, which depends on the stage of the cancer, consists of surgical removal of the uterus and/or ovaries, radiation therapy, hormonal therapy, and chemotherapy. The 1-year survival rate for endometrial cancer is 93%. The 5-year survival rate is 96% if the cancer is discovered at an early stage, when it is contained regionally. Survival rates for whites exceed that for African Americans by at least 15% at every stage.

The Ovaries

Ovarian cysts and tumors can occur when a female is any age. A cyst is an abnormal cavity that is filled with fluid. The most common ones are called **functional cysts;** these occur on the follicle or corpus luteum and are usually caused by the failure of the follicle to rupture and discharge the egg. Generally they are small and not particularly significant. They usually disappear spontaneously within a month or two.

Dermoid cysts are common in young women. They contain hard, fatty material, and sometimes remnants of teeth. These are believed to be embryonic in nature and are considered benign. Most ovarian cysts and tumors are usually benign, but if they cause symptoms such as pain, tenderness, and internal bleeding, they can require surgery. Because there is always the possibility

functional cyst
An ovarian cyst that occurs on the follicle or corpus luteum, usually caused by the failure of the follicle to rupture and release an egg.

dermoid cyst
A type of benign ovarian cyst commonly found in young women.

of future problems, such as malignancy, a woman should remain under medical supervision once cysts or tumors have been diagnosed.

Stein–Leventhal syndrome
Reproductive malfunction in women; a syndrome of endocrine origin that involves ovarian cysts, amenorrhea, and infertility.

ovarian cancer
Cancer of the ovaries that causes more cancer deaths than any other cancer of the female reproductive system.

douche
Cleansing of the vagina by inserting a nozzle that secretes a recommended cleansing substance, a controversial procedure.

toxic shock syndrome (TSS)
A syndrome caused by *Staphylococcus aureus* bacteria in which symptoms include high fever, nausea, vomiting, diarrhea, and a drop in blood pressure; a potentially fatal syndrome that has been linked with the use of superabsorbent tampons.

gynecologist
A physician specializing in women's reproductive health.

In the **Stein–Leventhal syndrome** the ovaries become enlarged and have cysts on them. Infertility and secondary amenorrhea also result. This syndrome, seen in women 15 to 30 years of age, is considered to be of endocrine origin. Once diagnosed it is treated by medication or by surgery. Both treatments attempt to reestablish regular menstrual cycling. Most patients respond to therapy, and frequently fertility is restored to normal.

Ovarian cancer killed an estimated 14,300 American women in 2003. In fact, ovarian cancer causes more deaths than any other cancer of the female reproductive system. An estimated 25,400 new cases of ovarian cancer were diagnosed in 2003, amounting to 4% of all cancers among women. One of the reasons ovarian cancer is so deadly is that its symptoms are "silent": That is, they are unnoticed until late in development. Rarely does abdominal swelling occur and even more rarely abnormal vaginal bleeding. Stomach gas, discomfort, and distention that cannot be explained by other causes may indicate a need to have a thorough medical examination with ovarian cancer in mind.

Risk factors include never having children, being older (ovarian cancer occurs more frequently in women in their 80s), and having had certain other cancers such as colon and endometrial cancers. As with all cancers, early detection is important. Pelvic exams are most valuable, because Pap tests rarely are effective in uncovering ovarian cancer. In 2000 a new technique using sonography was developed that has the potential of diagnosing ovarian cancer earlier than is presently possible. This new method, *transvaginal ultrasonography,* was able to diagnose stage 1 ovarian cancer in 59% of women, whereas other methods could only detect 30% of these stage 1 cancers (Sato, et al., 2000). Treatment can include surgical removal of one or both of the ovaries and/or the fallopian tubes (called a *salpingo-oophorectomy*) and the uterus *(hysterectomy).* If disease is detected early and the tumor is small, only the involved ovary is removed. This is especially important to young women who want to have children. Radiation therapy and chemotherapy are also used in the treatment of ovarian cancer. The 1-year survival rate from the time of diagnosis is 78%, and the 5-year survival rate is 50%. However, if cancer is diagnosed and treated early, the survival rate goes up to 95%. Unfortunately, only 25% of cases are detected in their localized stage. Five-year survival rates for women whose cancer has invaded the abdominal region of the body or has traveled to distant parts of the body are 79% and 28%, respectively.

The Vagina

Normal vaginal secretions are odorless, and the acidity of the vagina helps it to cleanse itself. Nevertheless, some women choose to cleanse the vagina by **douching**—that is, by rinsing with water or a vinegar and water solution. A vaginal douche, the value of which has been questioned, is not recommended and can be harmful if not done correctly. Damage can occur in two main ways: (1) Improper insertion of the douching material may actually damage the tissue, resulting in an increased chance of infection; (2) the chemical balance of the vagina can be altered, affecting contraceptive function. For instance, if a woman is using a spermicidal cream or other form of spermicide as a means of contraception, douching may destroy its effectiveness.

Smegma, a cheeselike substance secreted by the glans penis of males, may have effects on women's health. A female engaging in coitus with a male who has not washed away smegma could be subjecting herself to vaginal infections. There is also some concern that smegma may contribute to cancer of the cervix. It seems prudent, therefore, for sexually active women to make sure that their male sexual partners engage in the routine hygiene care necessary to remove smegma. Although it may be embarrassing, this may be a small price to pay for the prevention of vaginal infection and cervical cancer. Signs of sexually transmitted infections should also be given attention. Make sure to check your vulva routinely. See a health care provider if you have unusual discharges, abdominal pain, or open sores on your genitalia.

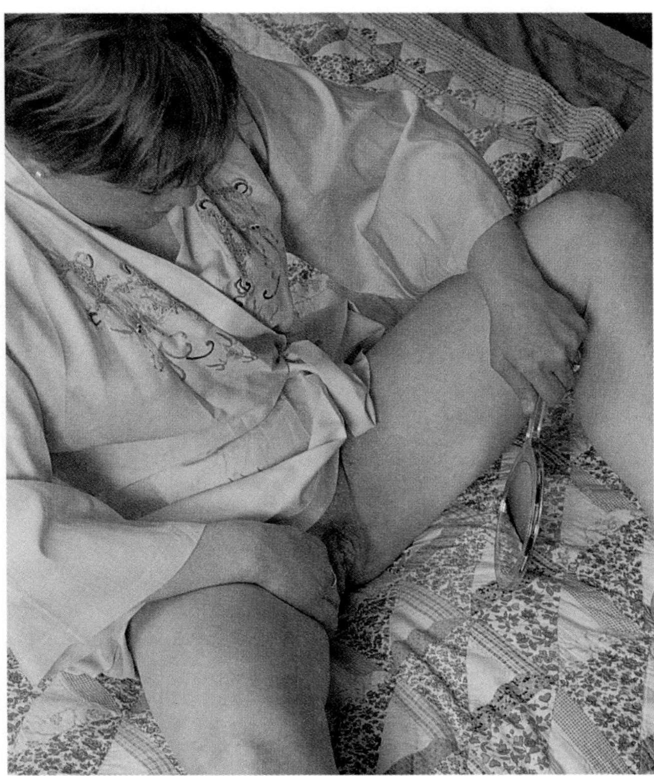

Sexual health begins with routine self-exams.

Toxic Shock Syndrome (TSS)

In the late 1970s several young women died of a previously little-known disease called **toxic shock syndrome (TSS).** The toxins that cause this syndrome are produced by the *Staphylococcus aureus* bacteria, which may grow in the vagina and are absorbed by the body. These toxins enter the bloodstream and cause high fever (above 102°F), nausea, vomiting, diarrhea, a rapid drop in blood pressure, and sometimes aching muscles and peeling skin on the palms and feet. The exact mechanism of transmission is unknown. The syndrome appears to be linked to the use of tampons—particularly those made of superabsorbent material. It is thought that the presence of the tampon in the vagina for a prolonged period (6 hours or more) may provide an environment conducive to proliferation of the toxin-producing bacteria. When some tampons are inserted into the vagina, small irritations of the vaginal mucosa may occur and promote entry of the bacteria.

It is recommended that superabsorbent tampons not be used because they pack the vagina tightly, prevent air circulation, and allow bacteria to proliferate. It has also been suggested that women using other types of tampons leave them in place for no longer than 2 hours and not use them at all during the night while sleeping.

TSS—which has a relatively high fatality rate (5%)—was originally reported by 3 in 100,000 women.

Toxic shock syndrome has been seen in both genders among postsurgical patients, burn victims, and patients with boils and abscesses. Nonmenstrual cases constitute about 13% of all reported cases. Experts do not know why certain body sites are affected more than others.

Care from Medical Specialists

All health-related specialists agree that you should report any unusual signs or symptoms related to the reproductive system to a specialist in women's reproductive health—a **gynecologist** or a gynecological nurse practitioner. Furthermore, the American College of Obstetrics and Gynecology recommends that women have a routine gynecological exam every year, even when no signs or symptoms appear. Routine checkups, usually conducted on a special table with the woman's knees up and her feet in stirrups, consist of the following procedures:

1. An inspection of the external genitals for any irritations, discolorations, unusual discharges, or other abnormalities.
2. An internal check for cystoceles (bulges of the bladder into the vagina) and rectoceles (bulges of the rectum into the vagina). The examiner also looks for pus in the Skene's glands and for the strength of the pelvic and abdominal muscles. He or she also tests

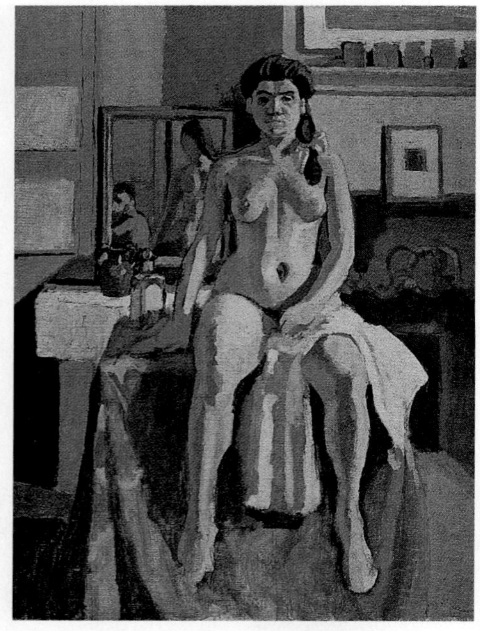

Henri Matisse's *Carmelina* depicts a young woman about to receive a gynecological exam. (You can see the doctor in the mirror.) The painting set off quite a furor when acquired by the conservative Museum of Fine Arts, Boston, in 1932. The museum's treasurer complained, "I shall never again be able to bring my wife to the museum!"

urine control by asking the patient to cough while checking to see whether urine flows involuntarily.

3. An inspection of the vagina and cervix by means of a **speculum,** a plastic or metal instrument that is inserted into the vagina to hold the walls apart during the examination (Figure 4.12). (At this point and throughout the remainder of the examination, if you are interested in seeing your genitals and watching the exam, ask the examiner to set up a mirror for you and to point out the various organs. If the examiner is not sympathetic to this request, you might consider looking for another practitioner.) The examiner will look for anything unusual, such as lesions (sores) or inflammation affecting the vagina or cervix. Next the practitioner will scrape a tiny amount of tissue from the cervix by using a small wooden instrument called a *spatula.* This tissue will be used for the Pap smear. *If requested by the patient,* the smear can also be tested for signs of gonorrhea.
4. A bimanual examination (Figure 4.13). By sliding the index and middle fingers of one hand into the vagina and pressing down on the abdominal wall from the outside, the examiner feels for the uterus, fallopian tubes, and ovaries to determine their position, their size, and the presence of pain or inflammation. The examiner may also examine the internal genitals by inserting one finger into the rectum and another into the vagina.
5. An examination of the breasts for lumps or thickenings.

FIGURE 4.12 Medical examination with speculum and spatula in place.

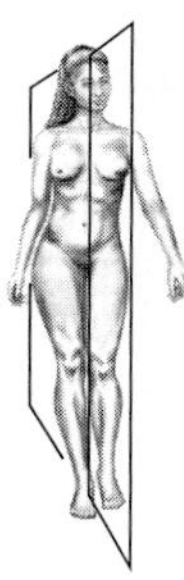

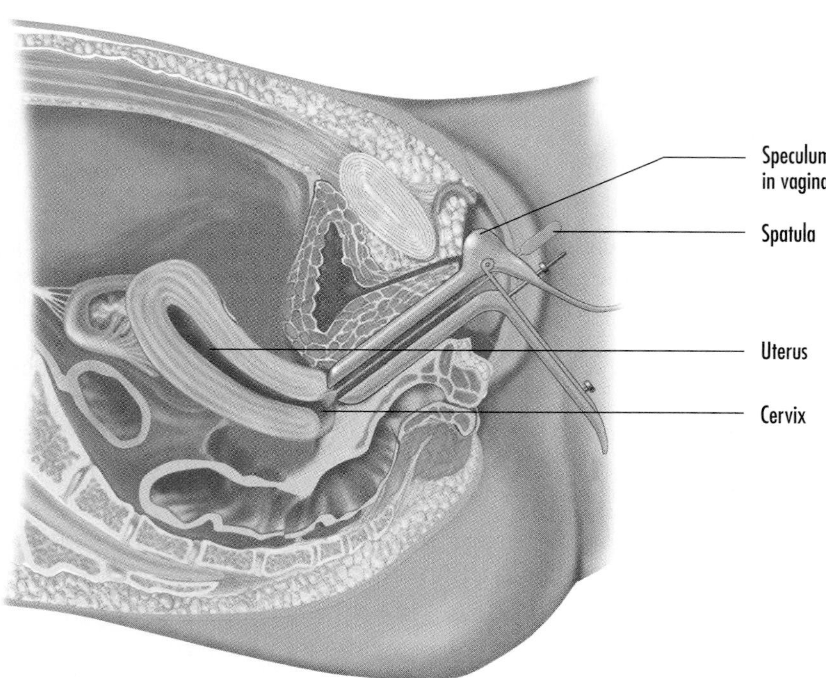

Two additional points should be noted about the routine gynecological exam. First, although the checkup may be uncomfortable, it should not be painful. Second, before beginning the physical examination, the practitioner should take a gynecological history. Noted on the history should be information regarding the regularity, flow, and any changes in the menstrual cycle; any pregnancies, miscarriages, or abortions; all birth-control methods used; the incidence of breast cancer in close female relatives; and whether or not the woman's mother took the drug DES during her pregnancy with the patient—that is, whether the patient is a "DES daughter." DES is a drug that was given in the 1940s and 1950s to women with a history of miscarriage. It is no longer used for miscarriages, because it has been found that vaginal cancer is more prevalent in DES daughters than in other women (Kaufman, 2000; Herbst, 1972), that DES sons may also experience higher than expected infertility rates (Gill, Schumacher, & Bibbo, 1977), and that women who took DES have breast cancer in greater numbers than non-DES women. If the patient's mother did take DES, a periodic **colposcopy,** a check for changes in the vagina and cervix, should be conducted. The examiner uses an instrument called a *colposcope* to view the vagina for abnormal tissue growth. The examiner might also perform a biopsy.

speculum
A metal (or plastic) instrument that is inserted into the vagina to hold the walls apart, allowing for medical examination.

colposcopy
An examination of the vagina and cervix using an instrument—a colposcope—in order to detect abnormal tissue growth.

Care from Organizations and Available Publications

For women, the ACS, the National Organization for Women, the March of Dimes, women's health centers and clinics, as well as local organizations of women who have had breasts removed due to cancer are but a few of the groups devoted to improving women's reproductive health. These groups function in various ways: Some publish written material, others lobby for legislation and funds, and still others provide social support for women with reproductive health problems. In addition, clinics conduct medical examinations, test and care for STIs, and offer premarital blood tests and other services for women.

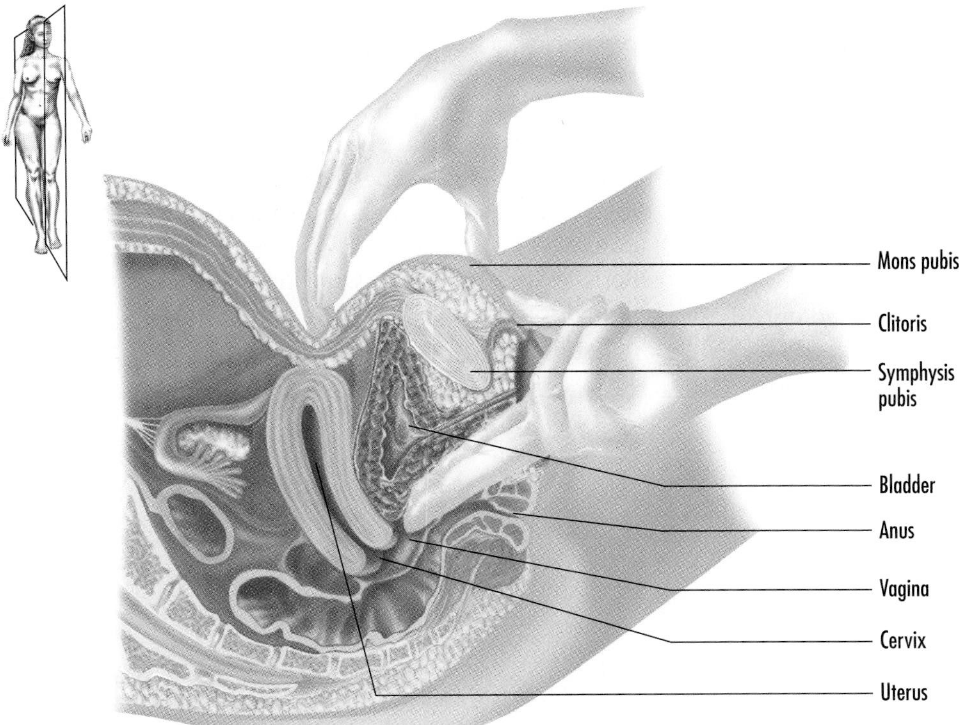

FIGURE 4.13 Bimanual examination.

Exploring the DIMENSIONS of Human Sexuality

Our feelings, attitudes, and beliefs regarding sexuality are influenced by our internal and external environments. Go to sexuality.jbpub.com to learn more about the biological, psychological, and sociological factors that affect your sexuality.

Biological Factors

When a sperm with an X chromosome meets an egg (all of which have X chromosomes), a female will develop. Biological factors continue to influence development throughout life.

- Genetic coding affects physical appearance, including height; coloration of skin, hair, and eyes; breast size; and many aspects of health.
- Female physical appearance changes at puberty, when the lean-body-mass-to-fat ratio changes from about 5:1 to about 3:1, signaling the body to commence menarche.
- Hormonal changes affect mood.
- At menopause, lower estrogen levels increase a female's risk for heart attack.

Sociocultural Factors

Sociocultural factors interact with biological factors to influence health.

- Socioeconomic status influences prenatal care and nutrition.
- Ethnic heritage influences health. Black women tend to get a more virulent form of breast cancer, resulting in a higher death rate. Jewish women are genetically at risk for scoliosis (curvature of the spine).
- Culture influences women's health. Fear of Western medicine prevents some immigrants from seeking treatment at early stages of a problem.
- Laws can affect what health insurance is required to cover. Because women are underrepresented in public office, their needs are sometimes overlooked.
- Media and ads that present ultrathin women as ideals can influence the eating patterns and health of women.

Psychological Factors

Psychological factors interact with other factors and can influence health.

- Women tend to have nearly twice the rate of depression of men.
- Teen women with low self-concept have a higher probability of having an unwanted pregnancy and birth.
- Expressiveness of emotions helps women stay mentally and physically healthy.
- Learned attitudes and behaviors about gender roles can prevent a woman from fulfilling her potential.
- Body-image problems in women can lead to long-term disorders, such as bulimia and anorexia nervosa.

CASE STUDY

The physiological development of a female starts when a sperm with an X chromosome fertilizes an egg. But socioeconomic status of the mother influences whether or not prenatal care is received, good nutrition will be available, and medical help will be sought. If the mother smokes, drinks, or abuses drugs during pregnancy, the fetus will be affected.

A woman's physiology is further altered during puberty and menopause. The increased fat content at puberty negatively affects many women's body image, and that in turn negatively affects self-concept.

Unable to control the changes taking place within her body, the pubertal girl sometimes resorts to controlling the one thing she can control: food intake. Dieting is common, but excessive food control, or self-induced vomiting after meals, can result in a serious eating disorder.

Discussion Questions

1. List and describe the parts of the female reproductive system, including external and internal genitalia.
2. Compare the roles of breasts as child nurturer and sexual organ.
3. Describe how hormones react to sexual stimuli and make a person aroused.
4. What physiological changes occur in a woman's body during the menstrual cycle? What are the resulting psychological effects?
5. How does a woman's body change at menopause? What can she do to prevent problems that result from menopause?
6. Describe the self-care and preventive medicine that a woman should practice to ensure her sexual health.

Application Questions

Reread the anecdote that opens the chapter and answer the following questions.

1. How could you use your understanding of the parts of the human body to improve your sexuality? Is such knowledge as important as the ability to communicate or to understand the diverse needs of a partner? Put another way, would an expert on sexuality be a better lover?
2. Describe how you feel when you look at anatomical drawings of genitalia. Do you feel sexually excited? embarrassed? bored? Explain why you feel that way.

Critical Thinking Questions

1. Some women argue that only another woman can really understand the feelings and sensations that a woman feels, that male gynecologists are likely to discount some female concerns, and that it is easier to talk with another woman than a man about their sexual health. Others may argue that medical competency and compassion are not limited by gender. Should a gynecologist be a woman? Explain your answer.
2. If you look at the women on TV, in movies, and in magazines, the pervasive image is clear: lean and busty. Yet the psychologist G. Terence Wilson, an eating disorder specialist, points out that a woman cannot be lean and have large breasts—it is not biologically possible. As a woman loses fat, her breasts reduce in size. Should a woman who finds herself lean and flat get breast implants or regain weight so her breasts will be larger? Explain your answer.

Critical Thinking Case

As discussed in the chapter, some researchers believe that onset of menarche occurs on the basis of body composition—namely, when a woman reaches a certain percentage of body fat. It also appears that amenorrhea (cessation of menstruation) occurs in women athletes with low body fat and in women with anorexia nervosa.

Consider the negative connotations associated with body fat in our society, especially as portrayed in the mass media. What reaction might prepubescent girls have to learning that they will gain body fat and then reach menarche? How could junior- and senior-high school students be taught in a positive manner about the body composition changes associated with the onset of menarche? Would such knowledge lead young girls to diet in order to prevent menarche?

One final question: A very athletic person in your dormitory tells you that she has heard about the relationship between body fat and amenorrhea. She tells you that she does strenuous aerobic exercise as a means of what she calls "natural birth control." What would you tell her?

Exploring Personal Dimensions

Taking charge of self-care and prevention greatly increases your chance of achieving sexual health and wellness. For the following statements, circle YES or NO. Then fill in the dates to help you keep track of your self-care activities.

I do breast self-examinations monthly.	YES	NO
My last breast exam was on _________.		
My next breast exam is due on _________.		
I do vaginal self-examinations on a regular basis.	YES	NO
My last vaginal exam was on _________.		
My next vaginal exam is due on _________.		
I have regular gynecological examinations.	YES	NO
My last gynecological exam was on _________.		
My next gynecological exam is due on _________.		
I have regular Pap smears.	YES	NO
My last Pap smear was on _________.		
My next Pap smear is due on _________.		
I have regular mammograms (if applicable).	YES	NO
My last mammogram was on _________.		
My next mammogram is due on _________.		
I keep track of my menstrual cycle.	YES	NO
My last period began on _________.		
My next period is due on _________.		
I practice safer sexual activities.	YES	NO
I understand that vaginal intercourse during menstruation increases the risk of transmitting HIV.	YES	NO
I have a family medical tree listing diseases.	YES	NO
I discussed my family's medical history with my doctor.	YES	NO

Sexuality Online

Go to the web component for *Exploring the Dimensions of Human Sexuality* at sexuality.jbpub.com for web exercises, additional resources related to this chapter, and student review tools.

Suggested Readings

Angier, N. *Women: An intimate geography.* Boston: Houghton Mifflin, 1999.

Barbach, L. *The pause: Positive approaches to menopause.* New York: Dutton, 1993.

Borysenko, J. *A woman's book of life: The biology, psychology and spirituality of the feminine life cycle.* New York: Riverhead Books, 1998.

Boston Women's Health Book Collective. *Our bodies, ourselves: For the new century.* New York: Simon & Schuster, 1998.

Landau, C., Cyr, M., & Morton, A. W. *The complete book of menopause.* New York: Perigee, 1994.

Love, S. M. *Dr. Susan Love's hormone book.* New York: Random House, 1997.

Minkin, M. J. & Wright, C. V. *What every woman needs to know about menopause.* New Haven, CT: Yale University Press, 1996.

Mortola, J. F. Issues in diagnosis and research of premenstrual syndrome, *Clinical Obstetrics and Gynecology, 35* (1992), 587–598.

O'Brien, P. M. Helping women with premenstrual syndrome, *British Medical Journal, 307* (1993), 1471–1475.

Reukauf, D. & Trause, M. *Commonsense breastfeeding: A practical guide to the pleasures, problems and solutions.* New York: Atheneum, 1988.

Rosenberg, L. Hormone replacement therapy: The need for reconsideration, *American Journal of Public Health, 83* (1993), 1670–1673.

Slade, M. Managing menopause, *American Health,* (December 1994), 66–69.

Steege, J. F. & Blumenthal, J. A. The effects of aerobic exercise on premenstrual syndrome in middle-aged women: A preliminary study, *Journal of Psychosomatic Research, 37* (1993), 127–133.

Steinberg, R. & Robinson, L. *Women's sexual health.* New York: Donald I. Fine, 1995.

CHAPTER 5

Male Sexual Anatomy and Physiology

FEATURES

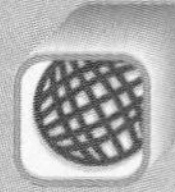

Global Dimensions
Male Genital Mutilation and Circumcision Practices

Ethical Dimensions
What Are a Dead Man's Rights?

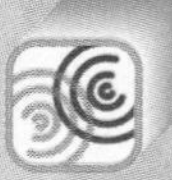

Communication Dimensions
Should Boys Be Taught About Masturbation?

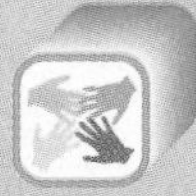

Multicultural Dimensions
Screening for Cancer

Gender Dimensions
Testicular Self-Examination

CHAPTER OBJECTIVES

1. Name and describe the parts of the male reproductive system to include the external and internal genitalia, including the pathway of the sperm.
2. Discuss the role of hormones in males as they enter puberty.
3. Cite various diseases that can affect the male reproductive system and the self-care procedures, as well as medical treatments associated with these diseases.

sexuality.jbpub.com

Global Dimensions: Male Genital Mutilation and Circumcision Practices
Prostate Cancer
Care from Organizations and Available Publications

INTRODUCTION

An economics professor recently told me that a father had come in to talk about his son's mediocre academic performance. The father asked for a second chance for his son, explaining that "too often he thinks with his other *head." Of course, this is not the first time I had heard this suggestion that men "think with their penises."*

The notion goes back to the fifth century. In the Greek comedy Lysistrata, *the women of the city decide to withhold sex from their men until all wars are ended. The men quickly put their civic pride aside in favor of their women—thinking with their "other heads," no doubt!*

However, today's man may think more about *his penis than* with *it. And the great obsession seems to be size. In the mid-1900s a national sex survey found that men thought the average length of a penis was 14 inches; women thought it was 12 inches. However, the average length is really about 6 inches!*

Magazines like Penthouse Forum *do not help, either. Chock-full of large appendages—10 inches here, 8 inches there, a "foot long" here, as "thick as his arm" there—the stories are meant to present fantasy, not reality.*

The writer Susan Minot provides an interesting perspective in her short story "Lust."

> *Tim's was shaped like a banana, with a graceful curve to it. They're all different. Willie's like a bunch of walnuts when nothing was happening, another's as thin as a thin hot dog. But it's like faces; you're never really surprised.*

As you will read in this chapter, for all the worry that men may feel, it is quite natural for men's penises to vary considerably, just as their faces do.

The Male Reproductive System

As females do, males have both external and internal genital organs. Figure 5.1 depicts a side view of the male external and internal genitalia, and Figure 5.2 shows a view from the rear. We begin our study of the male reproductive system with the external genitals.

The External Genitals

The male external genitals are the penis and the scrotum.

The Penis

The **penis** is a male sexual organ consisting of the root, the shaft, and the glans. As we have mentioned, penis size concerns many students, who often ask about the "average-size penis." As a *general* guideline, the average penis is about 2–5 inches long when relaxed (flaccid) and about 4–7 inches long when erect. When sexually aroused, the penis becomes stiff and enlarged (erect) because its tissues fill with blood. The penis shaft is attached to the body by its root. The head of the penis is called the **glans penis.** The glans contains the urethral opening, or **meatus,** where both seminal fluid (which contains sperm) and urine are passed. Marking the end of the glans is a raised ridge called the **coronal ridge,** or **corona.** The coronal ridge helps to form a seal with the walls of the vagina during sexual intercourse. Below the corona the body, or shaft, of the penis begins. Although the entire penis is sensitive and sexually excitable, the glans and corona are particularly sensitive; in fact, they are the most sensitive parts of the male anatomy.

Historically penis size has been a matter of fascination. The ***Kamasutra,*** an ancient Indian book on erotica, classified men according to penis size in

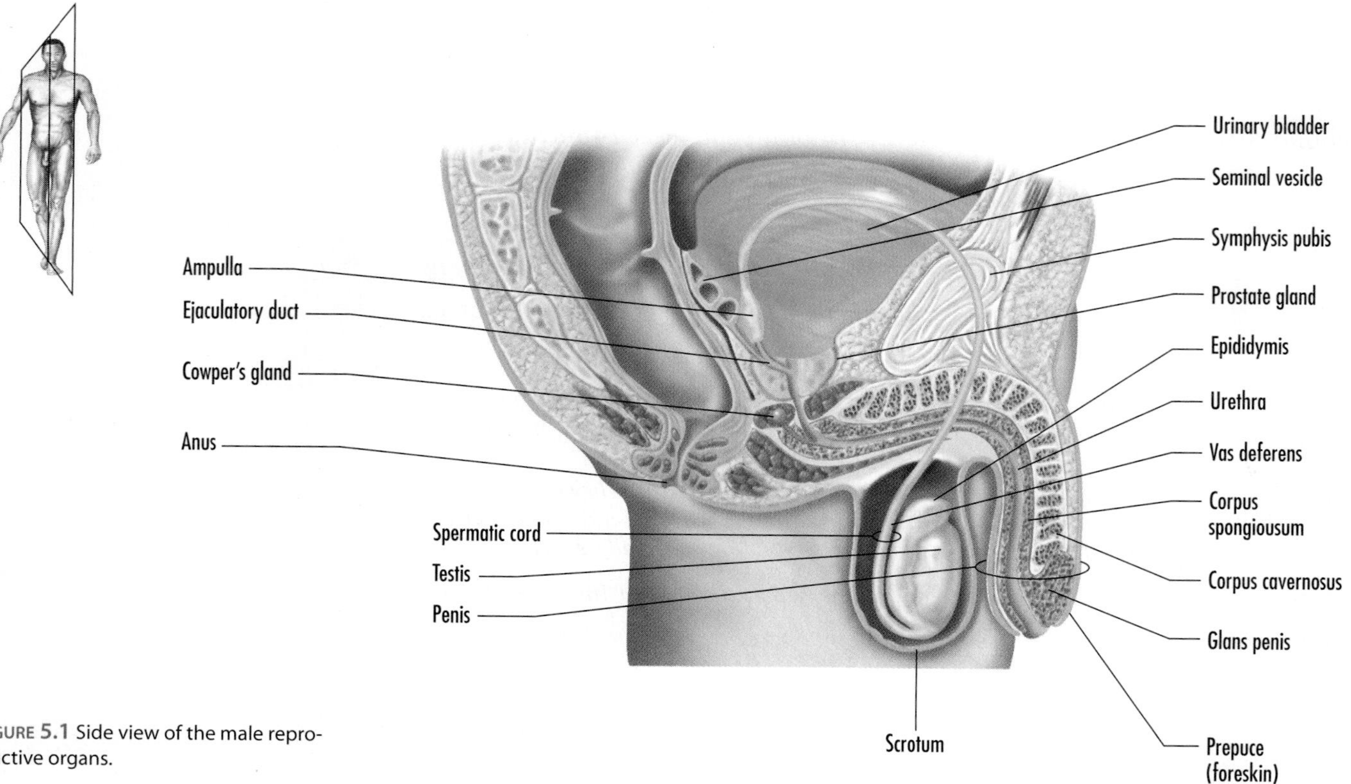

FIGURE 5.1 Side view of the male reproductive organs.

three categories: hare-men (erect penises of approximately 4.5 inches [11 centimeters]), bull-men (erect penises of approximately 6.75 inches [17 centimeters]), and horse-men (erect penises of approximately 9 inches [23 centimeters]). Other sources correlated penis size with personality traits or with the size of some other part of the body. Penises that are short when **flaccid** gain more size during **erection** than those that are longer when flaccid. Thus, although flaccid penises may differ significantly in length, erect penises are of similar lengths (Jamison & Gebhard, 1988). One way this has been described is that some men are "showers" and others are "growers" (Haffner & Schwartz, 1998).

Two contradictory views regarding penile size flourish in our time: "The larger the penis, the more satisfied the female" and "Women don't care about the size of a man's penis." It is not clear which is nearer the truth. Because the vagina adapts to the penis regardless of its size, some people have argued that size is unrelated to the sexual satisfaction of the female. However, part of our response to another's body is visual, and it seems reasonable to assume that if individual men have preferences for breasts of certain sizes and

penis
Structure of the male external genitalia consisting of the root, shaft, and glans; also contains the urethra, through which urine is excreted.

glans penis
The head of the penis.

meatus
The opening of the urethra in the head of the penis, where both seminal fluid and urine are passed.

coronal ridge (corona)
The raised ridge where the glans penis ends and the penile shaft begins.

Kamasutra
Ancient sex manual from India.

flaccid
The relaxed, unerected state of the penis.

erection
The extension of the penis and its engorgement with blood when the male is sexually stimulated.

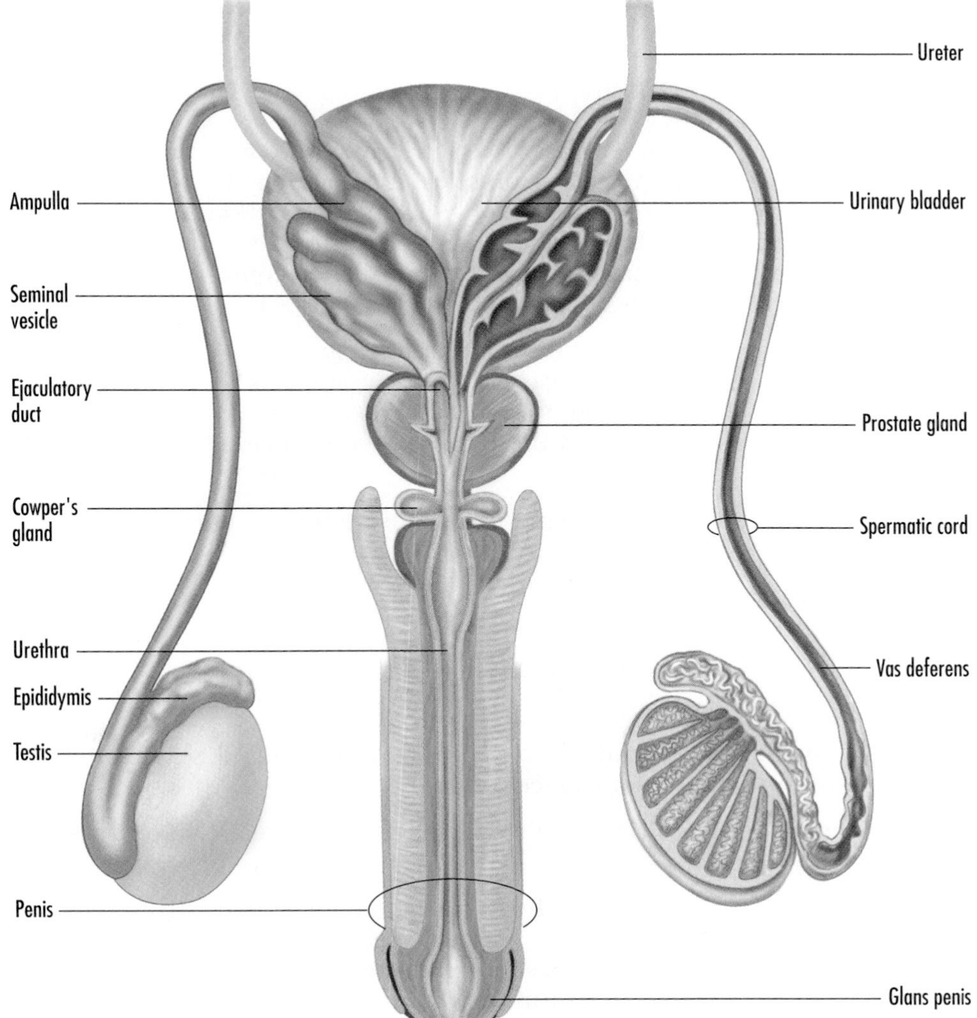

FIGURE 5.2 Posterior view of the male reproductive organs.

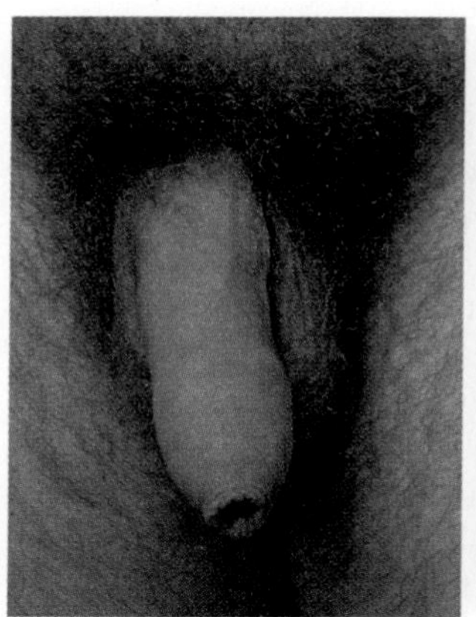
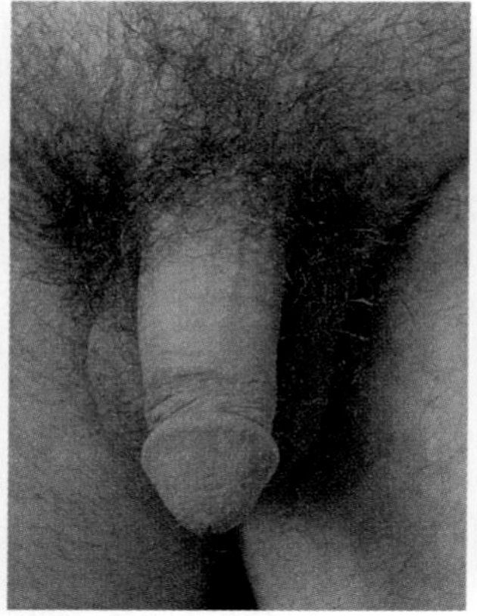
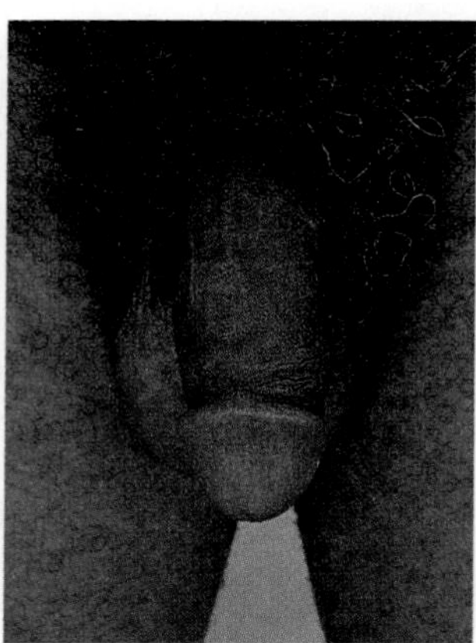

Many variations exist in the size and shape of the male genitals.

shapes, so individual women react differently to penises of different shapes and sizes. None of these preferences has anything to do with function unless it causes anxiety. The vagina contracts around the penis, regardless of its width or circumference. Furthermore, the inner two-thirds of the vagina has very little sensitivity. Both of these facts lead most authorities to conclude that penile width or length is unrelated to sexual satisfaction. Some women do, however, report preference for penises of a certain width or length. Whether these preferences are physiological or psychological is unknown at this time.

Just as women can strengthen the pelvic musculature with Kegel exercises, so can men strengthen the muscles surrounding the penis. Because these muscles are usually contracted only during ejaculation, they tend to be weak. By strengthening the muscles surrounding the penis, men may experience more satisfying orgasms and maintain better control of ejaculation. To do male Kegel exercises (Zilbergeld, 1978)

1. Identify the muscles you will be strengthening: Stop the flow of urine by squeezing these muscles. When the penis is flaccid and these muscles are squeezed, there is a slight movement of the penis. When the penis is erect and these muscles are squeezed, it moves up and down.
2. Start by squeezing and relaxing these muscles in 15 short bursts, twice a day.
3. When able, gradually increase the number of contractions from 15 at any one time to 60.
4. The next step is to contract these muscles for a slightly longer period, 3 seconds at a time.
5. After a while, you should be able to practice 60 long (3 seconds) and 60 short contractions twice a day.
6. You should start noticing results after 1 month of regular exercises.

Circumcision

The glans penis is covered by a **foreskin** (sometimes called the **prepuce**). For hygienic, cultural, or religious reasons, the foreskin is sometimes surgically removed. Removal of the foreskin—called **circumcision**—is more usual in the United States than in European countries. Circumcision takes place in the hospital approximately 2 days after birth or, if performed according

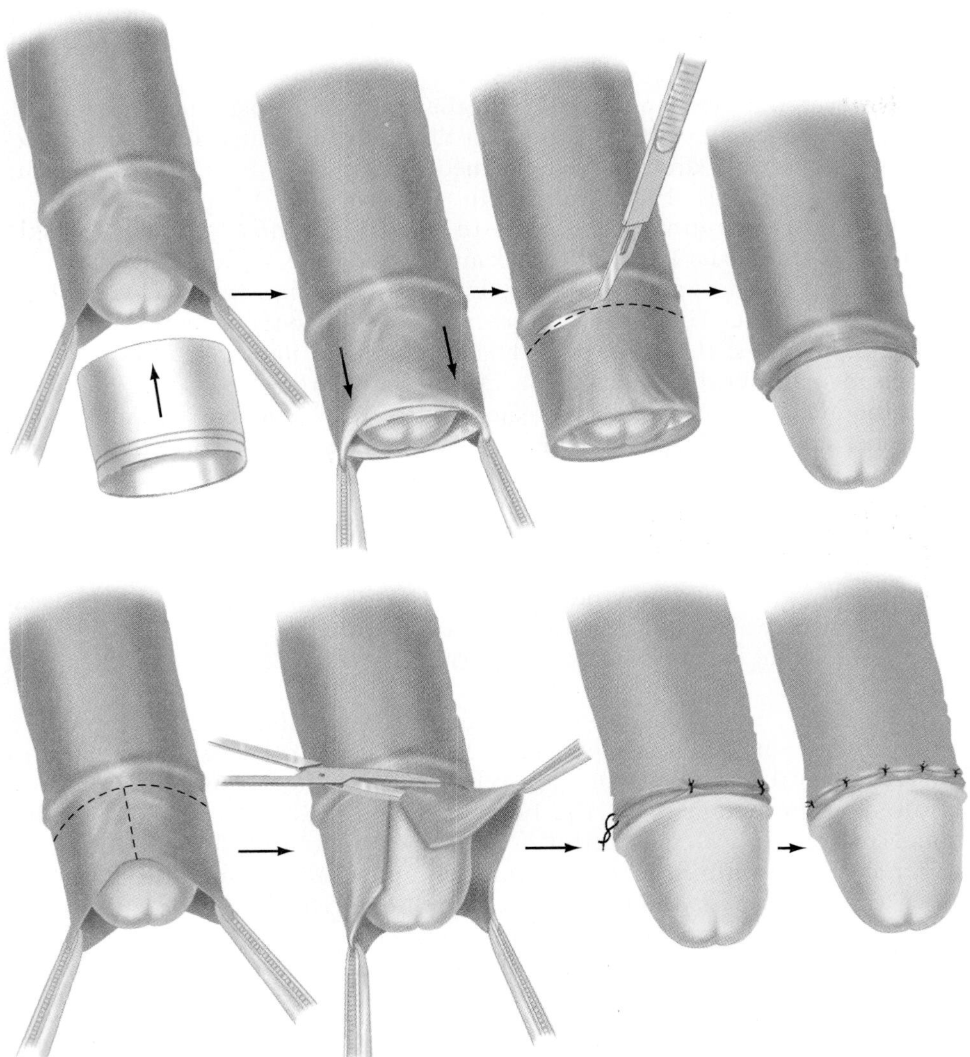

FIGURE 5.3 Methods of performing circumcision. (a) In this method, a piece of plastic is placed over the glans, and the foreskin is stretched over the plastic and trimmed off. (b) In this method, the foreskin is carefully cut "freehand" and then stitched.

to Jewish custom, 8 days after birth. In addition to Judaism, the Muslim faith requires circumcision. Figure 5.3 shows how circumcision is performed.

Hygiene also provides a rationale for circumcision. Several preputial glands—glands that secrete hormones only after puberty—are located in the foreskin and under the corona (Tyson's glands). These glands secrete an oily substance that, if not removed from under the foreskin, can combine with dead skin cells to form a cheesy substance called **smegma.** If this smegma is not regularly removed from under the foreskin, it becomes granular and irritates the glans penis, causing discomfort and possibly infection. Removing the smegma requires washing the glans penis. This becomes more difficult if the foreskin is not removed, because it has to be retracted manually to expose the glans.

Since 1971, the American Academy of Pediatrics (AAP) has released several statements noting that there is no medical reason for circumcision. As a result, circumcision rates in the United States dropped from a high of 95% of newborn males in the mid-1960s to an estimated 58% in 1987 (Rovner, 1990). However, in 1990, the Academy (Brower, 1989) reversed its position, citing advantages based on the work of Dr. Thomas Wiswell and colleagues (1985). Wiswell found that uncircumcised infants were 10 times more likely

foreskin (prepuce)
The covering of the glans penis, which is removed during circumcision.

circumcision
The surgical removal of the foreskin covering the glans penis.

smegma
A cheeselike substance secreted by the glans penis that must be removed from below the foreskin of uncircumcised males to prevent irritation and/or infection.

to have urinary tract infections than circumcised babies. Wiswell also reported that of 50,000 cases of cancer of the penis over a 50-year period, only 10 occurred in circumcised men.

However, not everyone agrees with the AAP's new position. For example, Smith and colleagues (1987) found no difference in rates of urinary infections, and other researchers have reached similar conclusions over the years (Samuels & Samuels, 1983; Wallerstein, 1980).

But another argument attempts to justify circumcision: The foreskin interferes with sexual stimulation because it serves as a barrier to the glans penis. There are no data to support this argument and, in fact, logic would indicate otherwise. The foreskin retracts when the penis becomes erect, and the glans penis is, therefore, able to be stimulated just as it is for the circumcised male. Furthermore, some people have argued the opposite: That is, if the glans is not usually protected by a foreskin, it may become insensitive because of its repeated contact with clothing. Therefore, the circumcised penis may, in fact, be *less* sensitive than the uncircumcised penis. Neither viewpoint is conclusive.

phimosis
Condition resulting when penile erection causes pain because the foreskin is too tight.

scrotum (scrotal sac)
A sac of skin that contains the testes and spermatic cords.

testes
Male gonads contained within the scrotal sacs that produce sperm cells and the male sex hormone testosterone. Singular form: testicle.

spermatic cord
The cord from which the testicle is suspended that contains the vas deferens (defined later), blood vessels, nerves, and muscle fibers.

Still other reasons have been offered to justify circumcision. For example, uncircumcised males may be at greater risk of penile cancer, and their female sexual partners may be at greater risk of vaginal infections, cervical cancer, genital warts, and other sexually transmitted infections. However, for every study that supports these concerns, there appear to be studies that refute them.

There are more reasons for not being circumcised. First is concern about the trauma the infant experiences. Because infants cannot be administered general anesthesia or pain-relieving narcotic agents, circumcision is often performed without the benefit of anesthesia. To respond to this concern, some physicians inject a local anesthetic directly into the penis in an attempt to diminish or eliminate the pain associated with circumcision. Another issue is the risk of infection, hemorrhage, emotional trauma, and other effects associated with any surgical procedure.

Yet, there is agreement among medical experts that when the foreskin is so tight that an erection hurts or pain is experienced during sexual inter-

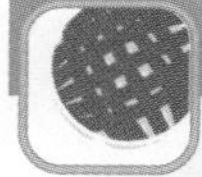

Global DIMENSIONS

Male Genital Mutilation and Circumcision Practices

Around the world and throughout history there have been many societies that have practiced male genital mutilation. For example, castration, the removal of the testes, was common in ancient Rome; eunuchs, castrated men, dressed as women and became priests. Islamic societies are forbidden by the Koran to castrate men. Yet they used men castrated by the Christians as keepers of the harem, because they posed no threat of engaging in sexual activities. In addition, boys were castrated in the Middle Ages in Europe in order to maintain their soprano singing voices after puberty.

In some societies in the Pacific, men are circumcised, but the foreskin is not totally removed; instead, it is slit lengthwise and folded back. This is called *supercision*. Sometimes the foreskin is stretched tightly over a piece of bamboo, and then the incision is made. Circumcision is often associated with entry into manhood in these cultures and is usually celebrated with a ceremony of some sort.

sexuality.jbpub.com

course, removal of the foreskin is recommended. This condition is known as **phimosis.**

To summarize, here are reasons parents might consider circumcision:

- They are Jewish or Muslim. Infant circumcision is part of these religious traditions.
- If the father is circumcised, parents might want their son's penis to be like his father's penis.
- Parents do not want to have to teach their sons to clean their foreskins.
- Circumcised men have a lower incidence of urinary tract infections.
- Some uncircumcised men have problems as they grow up, for example, pain during intercourse, requiring circumcision during adulthood. This is much more painful and dangerous than newborn circumcision.
- The rate of cancer of the penis, though extremely rare, is higher in uncircumcised men.
- Uncircumcised men may be more susceptible to sexually transmitted infections.

Here are reasons parents might not want to circumcise their son:

- Circumcision is not part of their cultural tradition.
- Circumcision is painful for infants.
- If the father is not circumcised, parents might want their son's penis to be like his father's penis.
- As with any surgery, circumcision poses some risks. In rare cases (less than two times in 1,000) infection or even damage to the penis occurs.
- They think circumcision is not natural. Boys are born with penises with foreskins; their intact penises should be left alone.
- Circumcision is done without the infant's permission. This should be an adult choice.
- The child is ill at birth. Circumcision should never be done on a sick or medically unstable infant.

The Scrotum

The other external structure of the male reproductive system is the **scrotum,** which is located below the penis. The scrotum is a sac of skin containing the **testes** and the **spermatic cords.** It comprises two layers, the outer layer, which is covered with hair and sweat glands, and the inner layer (called the *tunica dartos*), which contains muscle and connective tissue. This organ regulates the temperature in the testes by drawing them up toward the body when the body is cold and letting them hang lower, away from the body, when it is hot. As a consequence the temperature of the testes is always approximately 5.6°F (3.1°C) cooler than the internal body temperature. This temperature-control function is necessary for the production of viable sperm. The scrotum also contracts when the inner thigh is stimulated or when it is chilled. This effect, is due to the contraction of the cremasteric muscles located in the spermatic cord, which is known as the *cremasteric reflex.*

Myth vs Fact

Myth: Whereas females can strengthen their pelvic muscles, thereby exercising better control of their sexual response, there is not much males can do.
Fact: Males can strengthen their pelvic muscles also. They can perform Kegel exercises to strengthen the muscles surrounding the penis, thereby achieving more satisfying orgasms and maintaining better control of ejaculation.

Myth: There is no medical reason for males to be circumcised.
Fact: Recommendations regarding circumcision have changed over the years. More recently, it has been suggested that uncircumcised males may be at greater risk of penile cancer and that their female partners may be at greater risk of reproductive health problems. However, circumcision poses the risk of infection, hemorrhage, emotional trauma, and other conditions. Whether to be circumcised is a decision that needs a great deal of consideration.

Myth: Breast cancer affects women; men do not have to worry about contracting it.
Fact: Men can also contract breast cancer. In 2003 approximately 1,300 new cases of breast cancer were diagnosed, and 400 men died of it.

Myth: The ejaculate is made up predominantly of sperm.
Fact: The ejaculate, semen, consists mostly of seminal vesicle and prostate gland secretions. The volume of sperm is approximately the size of a pinhead.

Myth: A male with a small flaccid penis has much to worry about.
Fact: First, small flaccid penises tend to expand more during erection than do large flaccid penises. Second, the nerve endings in the vagina are in the outer third, making the length of the penis somewhat superfluous, at least as far as sexual satisfaction is concerned.

The Internal Genitals

The male internal genitals contain numerous organs housed within the penis, the scrotum, and the pelvis (refer again to Figure 5.1).

The Urethra

The **urethra** is a tube through the penis that begins at the bladder and ends at the meatus. Its function is to provide a route for both semen and urine to exit the body. **Urine** is a waste product of the body that is stored in the bladder until it is expelled through the urethra. **Semen,** which is discussed later in this section, contains **spermatozoa,** or **sperm,** as well as other substances.

The Corpora Cavernosa and the Corpus Spongiosum

In addition to the urethra, the penis contains three spongy bodies: two **corpora cavernosa** and the **corpus spongiosum,** which are structures filled with networks of blood vessels and nerves. It is these columns of tissue, which fill with blood during sexual arousal, that make the penis grow hard and erect. During ejaculation the muscle surrounding the corpus spongiosum (the bulbocavernosus muscle) contracts and forces semen outward through the urethra.

The Testes

As mentioned, the testes (Figure 5.4) are suspended in the scrotal sac by spermatic cords, the **vas deferens** (through which sperm leave the testes), blood vessels, nerves, and muscle fibers. The testes produce sperm (about 50,000 every minute) and **testosterone,** a male sex hormone generally responsible for male secondary sexual characteristics (for example, deep voice, facial hair, and body hair). Within each testicle are approximately 1,000 **seminiferous tubules,** which are responsible for producing sperm, in a process called **spermatogenesis.** The cells between the seminiferous tubules, called **interstitial cells,** produce testosterone.

Once sperm are produced in the seminiferous tubules, they travel through the **vasa efferentia** to the **epididymis,** where they are stored and nourished for up to 6 weeks.

The Pathway of the Sperm

A mature sperm is about 0.0024 inch (0.0060 centimeter) long, with a head, neck, midpiece, and tail. The normal sperm contains 23 chromosomes. Each sperm contains a sex chromosome that determines the sex of the offspring. Sperm can be stored for up to 6 weeks in the epididymis before proceeding up the vas deferens to the **ampulla** (an enlarged portion of the vas deferens). Here in the ampulla the sperm receive more nutrients from the **seminal vesicles,** two sacs, each about 2 inches (5 centimeters) long, that secrete a substance believed to activate the sperm's **motility** (ability to move spontaneously).

With sufficient sexual stimulation, the ejaculatory process begins. Fluid from the **prostate gland** mixes with the sperm and with the secretions of the seminal vesicles, further aiding sperm motility and prolonging sperm life. The prostate fluid is an alkaline medium that offsets the acidity in the vagina that would otherwise kill the sperm. The **Cowper's glands,** two pea-sized glands adjacent to the urethra, empty into the urethra another alkaline fluid, which serves to neutralize the acidity caused by the urethra's transport of urine. The Cowper's glands secretions are the tiny droplets that sometimes appear on the tip of the penis before ejaculation. This secretion may contain some sperm left over from a previous ejaculation; therefore, it can cause pregnancy to occur even if the penis is withdrawn before ejaculation.

Ejaculation itself is the expulsion through the penis of semen, the mixture in which the sperm are carried. Ejaculation results from muscular con-

urethra
The tube through which the bladder empties urine outside the body and through which the male ejaculate exits.

urine
The body-waste product stored in the bladder and eliminated through the urethra.

semen
The male ejaculate, which contains sperm and other secretions.

spermatozoa (sperm)
The mature male sperm cell.

corpora cavernosa
A spongy body in the penis that contains a network of blood vessels and nerves.

corpus spongiosum
A spongy body in the penis that contains a network of blood vessels and nerves.

vas deferens
The duct, through which sperm stored in the epididymis (discussed later) is passed, that is cut or blocked during vasectomy.

testosterone
The male sex hormone produced in the testes that is responsible for the development of male secondary sex characteristics.

seminiferous tubules
The structures located within the testes that actually produce the sperm.

spermatogenesis
The manufacturing of sperm in the seminiferous tubules.

interstitial cells
The cells (sometimes called Leydig's cells) between the seminiferous tubules, where testosterone is produced.

vasa efferentia
The duct through which sperm produced in the seminiferous tubules travel to the epididymis.

epididymis
The location where sperm are stored in the testes and where nutrients are provided to help the sperm develop.

ampulla
The enlarged portion of the vas deferens where sperm are provided nutrients from the seminal vesicles; also, the part of the fallopian tube of women containing the cilia.

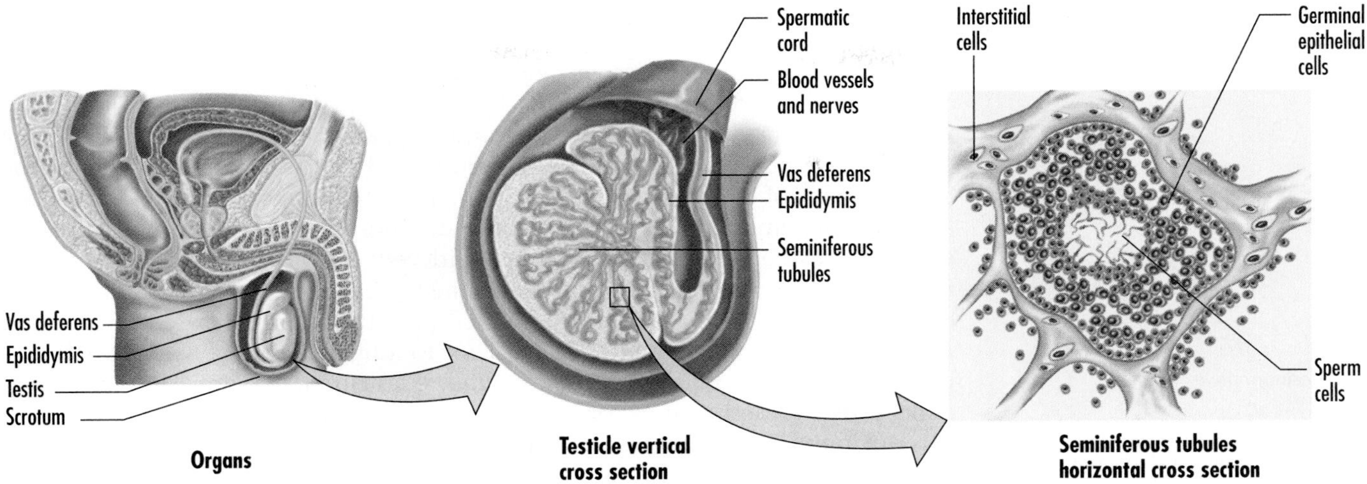

FIGURE 5.4 Testicle cross section.

tractions of the glands and ducts of the reproductive system. The expelling of semen is usually accompanied by **orgasm,** the climax of a growing complex of pleasurable sensations. Both the ampulla and seminal vesicles contract, as does the bulbocavernosus muscle surrounding the corpus spongiosum in the penis. The ejaculated semen contains sperm (the volume is about the size of a pinhead) and about a teaspoonful of secretions from the seminal vesicles, the prostate gland, and the Cowper's glands. Approximately 300 million sperm are expelled in a single ejaculation. According to some authorities, semen contain at least 20 to 35 million sperm per cubic centimeter in a male who is fertile—that is, able to fertilize an ovum.

During ejaculation a valve at the bladder's entrance closes to prevent urine from entering the urethra.

Table 5.1 reviews the functions of the male reproductive system.

seminal vesicles
Two sacs of the male internal genitalia that secrete nutrients to nourish sperm.

motility
The ability to move spontaneously, which is required for fertilization.

prostate gland
A structure of the male internal genitalia that secretes a fluid into the semen before ejaculation to aid sperm motility and prolong sperm life.

Cowper's glands
Two pea-sized glands adjacent to the urethra that secrete a lubricating fluid before ejaculation.

ejaculation
The ejection of semen from the penis during orgasm.

orgasm
The peak release of sexual tension, accompanied by sensory pleasure and involuntary rhythmic muscular contractions; ejaculation in the male.

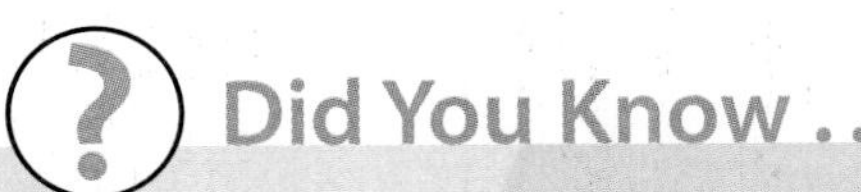

1. Testosterone causes bones to thicken and for this reason is sometimes administered to elderly people who have osteoporosis.
2. Excessive concentrations of sex hormones are metabolized primarily in the liver, with the products excreted in the bile and urine. Consequently, people with liver disorders experience the effects of excessive sex hormones (for example, the development of excessive body hair, development of breasts, or aggressiveness).
3. Sex hormones stimulate growth, thereby explaining the rapid growth that occurs during puberty. However, they also stimulate ossification (hardening) of the epiphyseal disks (a band of cartilage at the end of the bone), which causes bones to stop growing. Because estrogens produce greater effects on the disks than androgens, females stop growing earlier than males.

Hormones

At some time during puberty, boys become capable of reproduction. This capability is accompanied by the ability to ejaculate, although initially the male's ejaculate does not contain mature sperm. The cause of male reproductive capacity is the increased secretion of androgens, followed by the development of secondary sex characteristics. Accompanying male reproductive capacity, and also a result of increased androgen production, is a heightened interest in sex. This can be considered double jeopardy, because an increase in sexual appetite in a person newly capable of fertilizing an ovum can create problems—such as unplanned pregnancy or frustrated **libido.** The majority of both males and females seem to adjust to this new condition and pass through this phase of life unscarred. Unfortunately some do not, as evidenced by the high rate of pregnancy in unmarried teenage girls.

During puberty, increased testosterone level leads to growth of the penis, prostate, seminal vesicles, and epididymis. The reason males cannot ejaculate before puberty is that the prostate and seminal vesicles are not functional until they are "turned on" by the increased level of testosterone. Late-developing boys (15 to 16 years old) have been found to experience less sexual activity during adolescence than do early developers (Kinsey, 1948; Masters, Johnson, & Kolodny, 1982, p. 169). This difference has been attributed to the effect of testosterone on increasing the sexual appetite in males. No long-lasting effect on sexual behavior has been reported, however.

libido
Sexual desire, or drive.

male climacteric
Sometimes termed the "male menopause," which occurs at about the same age that women experience menopause, when men experience slightly decreased testosterone production and begin to question the directions in which their lives are headed.

midlife crisis
A time of life, usually between 40 and 50 years of age, during which men question the path their lives have taken and make plans for changing their goals.

Male Climacteric

Do men have an experience analogous to menopause (termed the **male climacteric**)? The answer to this question is not clear. There is evidence that at approximately the same age at which women experience menopause, some men experience what is called a **midlife crisis.** Men wonder about the meaning of their lives thus far and worry about what the future holds for them. They may become more people-oriented and less job-and-task-oriented (Sheehy, 1976, 1998). They may grow concerned about a diminishing interest in sexual activity and a reduction of sexual potency. Some men, to reas-

TABLE 5.1 **Functions of the Organs of the Male Reproductive System**

Organ	Function
Testes	
Seminiferous tubules	Produce spermatozoa
Interstitial cells	Produce and secrete male sex hormones
Epididymis	Stores and allows maturation of spermatozoa; conveys spermatozoa to vas deferens
Vas deferens	Conveys spermatozoa to ejaculatory ducts
Ejaculatory ducts	Receive spermatozoa and additives to produce seminal fluid
Seminal vesicles	Secrete alkaline fluid containing nutrients and prostaglandins
Prostate gland	Secretes alkaline fluid that helps neutralize acidic seminal fluid and enhances motility of spermatozoa
Cowper's gland	Secretes fluid that lubricates urethra and end of penis
Scrotum	Encloses and protects testes
Penis	Conveys urine and seminal fluid outside the body; acts as the organ of copulation

Ethical DIMENSIONS

What Are a Dead Man's Rights? An article in the *Washington Post* by Lawrence Proux (1997) reports that the center for Bioethics at the University of Pennsylvania has documented 25 cases in which sperm were taken from dead men and preserved by deep-freezing. Furthermore, a survey of 273 fertility centers in the United States identified 82 requests for taking sperm from dead men, of which 25 had been honored. It is possible to remove sperm up to 24 hours after death, and the person most often making the request is the widow. However, there also are records of social workers and even an intensive care nurse who made such a request.

Who has a right, if anyone at all does, to have such a request honored? Only the spouse, or a parent as well?

Should men have the right to decide whether they will have children and with whom, even after they are dead?

Should sperm taken from dead men be used by women unrelated to them, whose husbands do not produce viable sperm? Who else should have access to this sperm?

Should the sperm be sold and the proceeds go to the man's family? What should be done with the frozen sperm if the dead man's family decides not to use them?

These are tough decisions that should be guided by ethical principles, which you will study in Chapter 18.

sure themselves about their sexual capabilities, begin to date younger women or initiate extramarital affairs.

The hormonal evidence usually cited for this male climacteric is a decrease in testosterone production at about age 40 to 50 years (Masters, Johnson, & Kolodny, 1982). However, the decrease in the testosterone level is believed by many experts to be minimal, too insignificant to influence male behavior. Furthermore, middle-aged women face many of the same concerns and fears about the past and the future and put themselves through similarly agonizing self-examinations. In trying to decide what accounts for the midlife crisis, researchers' difficulties in distinguishing the psychological and sociological influences from clearly identifiable physiological and hormonal changes are practically insurmountable. In women, decreased estrogen production and increased FSH production, as well as a lack of menstrual flow, serve as irrefutable evidence of menopause. No similar evidence exists for a

Did You Know . . .

Androstenedione is the supplement that Mark McGwire made famous during his 70-home-run season. Touted as an artificial steroid, it was said to raise testosterone levels. But researchers at the University of Iowa found that it did not raise testosterone levels or increase strength. A side effect was lower levels of "good" cholesterol (high density lipoproteins), raising the risk of heart disease. Preliminary results of a further study by the Harvard researcher Hoel Finkelstein for Major League Baseball showed that androstenedione raised estrogen levels in men—and could result in breast enlargement!

Source: Body-building aid questioned, *CBSNews@aol.com* (June 3, 1999).

male climacteric. Still, most observers admit that males often go through a change of life—whether hormonally, psychologically, or culturally based—that deserves recognition and attention.

Hormone Therapy

Hormone therapy is also administered to men. For instance, testosterone supplements are sometimes administered to treat erectile dysfunction in older men (though testosterone levels are not low in all men who have trouble maintaining erection). Sometimes this treatment for erectile dysfunction is effective; other times it is not. The reason for this inconsistency is unclear; however, it is safe to say that the complex nature of sexuality makes it only partially responsive to hormone treatment. Testosterone supplements may not have much effect when personality, past experiences, the sexual partner, effectiveness in communication, setting, and so on, continue to have negative effects.

Self-Care and Prevention

Male reproductive care is as specialized as female reproductive care. Men should learn proper hygiene and methods of monitoring their reproductive health. When problems arise, males should consult their own medical specialists (internists or urologists). As with females, there are many organizations and publications that focus exclusively on issues of male reproductive health.

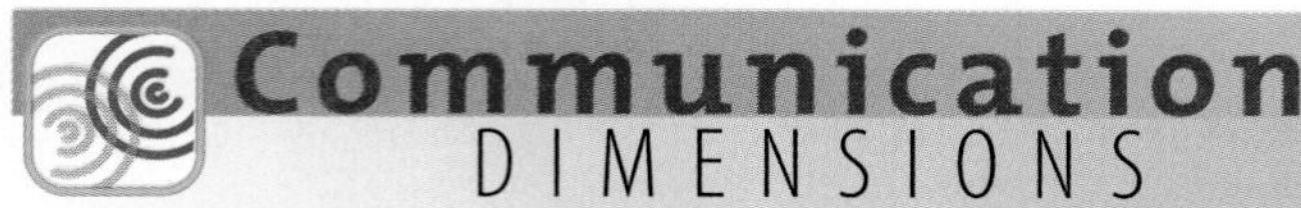

Should Boys Be Taught About Masturbation?

Discussing masturbation with preadolescents or adolescents is both sensitive and controversial. One way to present the information is to develop a list of common myths surrounding masturbation. While developing this list, the instructor must cautiously adhere to community and school standards and make sure the content of the discussion matches the age-appropriate level of the children being educated. A good resource identifying the developmental level at which various messages about masturbation ought to be directed is produced by the Sexuality Information and Education Council of the United States (National Guidelines Task Force, 1996).

This is a sample list of common myths about masturbation.

1. *Everyone masturbates.*
   On the contrary, some people never masturbate.
2. *When people marry or are in a committed relationship, they no longer masturbate.*
   Even some married people and those in committed relationships sometimes masturbate.
3. *Masturbation causes physical or mental harm.*
   There is no evidence of harm caused by masturbation, unless someone feels embarrassed, shameful, or guilty about masturbation.
4. *Masturbation is natural and therefore should be done in public.*
   Masturbation is a private matter and should, therefore, be done in private.
5. *All religions recognize masturbation as a natural sexual activity.*
   Some religions oppose masturbation and attempt to discourage their adherents from engaging in it.

Source: National Guidelines Task Force. *Guidelines for comprehensive sexuality education,* 2nd ed. New York: Sexuality Information and Education Council of the United States, 1996.

Breast Cancer in Men

Cancer of the breast occurs in men as well as women, although it is considered rare. An estimated 1,300 new cases of male breast cancer were diagnosed in 2003, and 400 men died of it that same year. Breast cancer is seen in men as early as their 30s. Although this cancer is rare, men are wise to examine their breasts for lumps. The procedure is the same for men and women.

Treatment for male breast cancer is similar to that of female breast cancer with one major difference: The psychological and emotional consequences of breast removal are not as significant for males as for females. Consequently, men seldom need counseling or a cosmetic means of disguising breast-tissue removal.

The Prostate

An important self-care procedure involves the prostate gland. The symptoms of **prostatitis** (inflammation of the prostate) are pain in the lower back, pain in defecation, pain during a rectal exam, and pus in the urine. Prostatitis usually affects younger men and can be cured with antibiotic drugs. If you experience these symptoms, consult a physician.

> **prostatitis**
> Infection of the prostate gland.
>
> **digital rectal examination (DRE)**
> A rectal examination whereby a physician inserts a finger into the rectum of a male patient to check for any abnormalities of the prostate.

An estimated 198,100 new cases of prostate cancer were diagnosed in the United States in 2001, and an estimated 31,500 men died of it that same year. Prostate cancer is the second leading cause of cancer death in the United States (lung cancer is the first). Between 1989 and 1992, prostate cancer rates increased dramatically, probably because of the use of a blood test developed to identify an antigen produced when prostate cancer is present. The blood test measures the presence of prostate-specific antigen (PSA). Since 1993, prostate cancer incidence rates have declined. It should be pointed out that prostate cancer incidence rates are nearly twice as high for African-American men as they are for white men. The reason for this difference is not known, but some experts have conjectured that diets high in fat and/or the presence of a gene that may make the prostate more susceptible to the effects of testosterone may be the cause (Squires, 1995).

There are several factors that place a man at risk of development of prostate cancer. One of these is age. As a man gets older he becomes more susceptible to prostate cancer, although the cancer may have been present at a younger age but not fully developed. More than 70% of prostate cancers are diagnosed in men who are older than 65 years of age. Heredity is suspected of playing a role in perhaps 5% to 10% of cases.

Signs and symptoms include weak or interrupted urine flow; the need to urinate frequently, especially at night; blood in the urine; pain or burning when urinating; and persistent pain in the lower back, pelvis, or upper thighs. However, some of these symptoms may be caused by an enlargement of the prostate, which is common as men age, without the presence of a tumor. This condition is called *benign prostatic hyperplasia (BPH)* and can be treated with medications. The only way to distinguish BPH from prostate cancer is by a medical examination that includes a **digital rectal examination (DRE)** and a PSA blood test. On June 12, 1997, the American Cancer Society published updated guidelines for prostate cancer screening (American Cancer Society, 1997). The guidelines state, "Both prostate specific antigen (PSA) and digital rectal examination (DRE) should be offered annually, beginning at age 50 years, to men who have at least a ten-year life expectancy, and to younger men who are at high risk." The reason a 10-year life expectancy is cited is that prostate cancer is usually a slow-growing cancer; thus it is thought prudent for men to refrain from having treatment if they are not expected to live long enough to benefit from that treatment. These

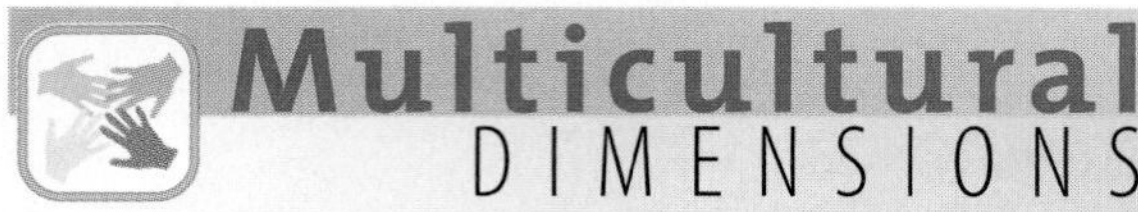

Screening for Cancer

Latinos enrolled in prepaid health insurance plans, such as health maintenance organizations (HMOs) and preferred provider organizations (PPOs), that do not charge patients for cancer screening are still less likely than white, non-Latinos to be screened for various cancers, including prostate cancer. It is hypothesized that cultural attitudes such as fatalism and machismo are to blame. As reported by the agency for Health Care Policy and Research (1994), Latinos feel less vulnerable to cancer and are unconvinced that early detection will make a difference to their survival. These culturally based attitudes are suspected of playing a role in the higher proportion of Latino versus non-Latino whites whose cancers, prostate cancer among them, are diagnosed in their later stages, after the cancer has spread to other parts of the body. As evidence of this conclusion, it is pointed out that Latinos are less likely than non-Latino whites (67% versus 80%) to have had at least one digital rectal examination and are less likely to have heard of digital rectal examination than non-Latino whites (89% versus 97%). One recommendation offered by researchers to alleviate this disparity in prostate cancer outcomes is to develop cancer-control messages in Spanish designed to encourage early detection and screening (Perez-Stable, Otero-Sabogal, & Sabogal, 1994).

men would likely die of some other condition before the prostate cancer killed them. An abnormal PSA test result is one with a value above 4 mg/ml, which would then lead to follow-up evaluation and subsequent procedures. These may include a biopsy of tissue extracted from the prostate gland.

If cancer is suspected, treatment consists of surgery, radiation, and/or hormonal therapy and chemotherapy if the cancer is in a late stage. However, because there is significant potential for serious side effects of these treatments (such as erectile dysfunction and/or incontinence), if the cancer is classified as low-grade and/or at an early stage, careful observation over a period without immediate treatment (called "watchful waiting") may be advised.

Eighty-five percent of all prostate cancers are diagnosed while still localized, and these patients have a 100% 5-year survival rate. During the past 20 years, the 5-year survival rate for all prostate cancers increased from 67% to 97%. Seventy-nine percent of men with prostate cancer survive 10 years, and 57% survive 15 years.

It is possible to perform a self-examination of the prostate, but to do so one should have a good understanding of the anatomy of the reproductive system. You should know where the prostate gland is located and what organs surround it. To perform the exam, lie on your side with your knees drawn up toward your chest and insert a lubricated finger gently and slowly into your anus. Gently feel for the prostate, which will feel like the fleshy part of the palm of the hand. If it feels too hard or if it feels different from your previous check, relate these signs to a urologist. As discussed, a medical specialist should examine the prostate gland yearly after a man is 50 years old, even if he performs prostate self-exam.

The Testes

testicular cancer
Cancer of the testicles; the most common form of cancer in men aged 29 to 35 years.

Testicular cancer is the most common form of cancer in men during late adolescence and early adulthood. Most cases occur in men aged 15 to 40 years. It is estimated that about 7,600 new cases of testicular cancer were diagnosed in 2003 and that 400 men died of testicular cancer that year. The testicular cancer risk is four times greater for white men than it is for African-American men. The rate has doubled among white Americans in the past 40 years and has remained the same for African Americans.

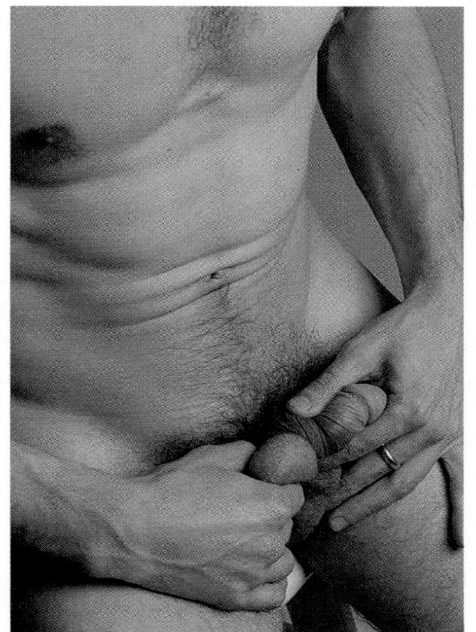

Sexual health begins with routine self-exams.

Among the risk factors for testicular cancer are undescended testes (cryptorchidism). Approximately 14% of cases of testicular cancer occur in men with a history of cryptorchidism. Other risk factors include a family history of testicular cancer, certain occupations (miners, oil and gas workers, leather workers, food and beverage processing workers, janitors, and utility workers), cancer of the other testicle, and infection with HIV. Testicular cancer is not related to injury or to vasectomy.

Treatment consists of surgery, radiation therapy, and/or chemotherapy. Surgery involves removal of the testicle. A cut is made in the groin, and the spermatic cord and the testicle are withdrawn from the scrotum through the opening. This procedure is called a *radical inguinal orchiectomy*. Depending on the stage of the cancer, some lymph nodes may also be removed. With only one testicle removed, the patient remains fertile. However, if two testicles need to be removed, the patient will no longer be able to produce sperm. Another side effect of the surgery is the possibility of damage to the nerves that control ejaculation. Damage to these nerves may also cause infertility. Men who still wish to have biological children can store sperm in a sperm bank for use after the surgery.

Treatment is highly effective if the cancer is diagnosed early. Ninety-five percent of stage 1 cancers can be cured, 90% to 95% of stage 2 cancers can be cured, and approximately 70% of stage 3 cancers can be cured. The lower the stage number, the earlier the cancer was diagnosed.

Self-examination of the testicles can lead to early detection of problems (see the accompanying Gender Dimensions feature). Any lumps, masses, or thickened areas may be symptoms of abnormality, not always cancerous; however, because the statistics show high incidence of malignancy of testicular tumors, medical diagnosis and consultation are imperative. As with other forms of cancer, early diagnosis increases your chance of survival.

The Penis

Penile discharges of pus, painful urination, itching, or sores or warts on the genitals may indicate the presence of a sexually transmitted infection. Also, as suggested earlier in this chapter, men should make sure that smegma is washed away daily to prevent irritation or infection in them and their partners. For circumcised males, keeping the penis smegma-free is easy, involv-

Gender DIMENSIONS

Testicular Self-Examination

To examine your testicles, first take a hot shower or bath so that the testicles hang farther outside the body than usual. Check each testicle in turn, rolling it gently between the thumb and the index and middle fingers to search for any small, hard lumps or swelling (testicular lumps are usually painless). The scrotal skin should feel firm but not too hard (somewhat like an earlobe). Call any lumps, swelling, hardness, or other unusual features to a physician's attention.

ing rolling only a little of the remaining foreskin out of the way during normal showering. Uncircumcised men have to be more careful, pulling back the foreskin and washing the glans and the inside of the foreskin.

Care from Organizations and Available Publications

Several organizations aid men in caring for their reproductive health: The American Cancer Society publishes brochures and pamphlets describing self-examinations of the breasts and testicles; local health departments operate clinics providing medical examinations, testing, and care for STIs, premarital blood tests, and counseling about birth control and sexual problems. Other organizations, such as the National Cancer Institute, keep track of the incidence and frequency of diseases related to reproductive health. And still other organizations, such as the Health Research Group, a nonprofit group devoted to studies to improve health care, conduct research to prevent and treat various conditions affecting the male reproductive system.

Exploring the DIMENSIONS of Human Sexuality

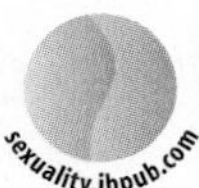

Our feelings, attitudes, and beliefs regarding sexuality are influenced by our internal and external environments. Go to sexuality.jbpub.com to learn more about the biological, psychological, and sociological factors that affect your sexuality.

Biological Factors

When a sperm with a Y chromosome meets an egg, a male offspring will develop. Biological factors continue to influence development throughout life.

- Genetic coding affects physical appearance, including height; coloration of skin, hair, and eyes; muscularity; and many aspects of health.
- Physiological changes result at puberty from the hormone testosterone, which in turn affects muscle development and body size. Testosterone also increases aggression and leads to increased rates of heart attacks.
- Toward middle age, testosterone levels begin to drop, resulting in decreased muscle mass, increased fat, and a reduced sex drive.

Sociocultural Factors

Sociocultural factors interact with biological factors to influence health.

- Laws affect what conditions health insurers must cover. Several states in 1998 passed laws requiring Viagra to be covered as a prescription.
- Religion may affect the decision as to whether to circumcise the penis.
- The cultural bias allowing men to be sexually permissive can compromise a man's sexual health and wellness.
- Ethnic heritage influences health; for example, African-American males tend to have higher levels of stress and heart disease than white males.
- Media and ads portray the ideal man with extreme muscularity, achievable only with tremendous work and, in many cases, illegal steroids.
- Family, neighbors, and friends often reinforce gender stereotypes.
- Behavior proscribed by society as illegal can influence health; for instance, a man can compromise his health by using anabolic steroids.

Psychological Factors

Biological and sociocultural factors combine to influence psychological factors.

- Body image and self-concept are enhanced for many men through exercise and competitive sports.
- In men who suppress their emotions, increased levels of stress can result.
- Learned attitudes and behaviors about gender roles can lead to unhealthy lifestyles for men.

CASE STUDY

The physiological development of a male starts when a sperm with a Y chromosome fertilizes an egg. More male than female pregnancies occur, but because male fetuses are weaker, a greater number of miscarriages result. Also, more male infants die than do female infants.

Socioeconomic status of the mother determines whether or not prenatal care is received, appropriate prenatal and postnatal nutrition is available, and medical help is sought. If the mother smokes, drinks, or abuses drugs during pregnancy, the fetus can be adversely affected.

A man's physiology is altered during puberty. The increased testosterone levels result in greater muscularity and a slimmer body. But testosterone also causes increased aggression.

Male gender roles are often hard for many men to uphold and can result in unhealthy behaviors. Repression of emotions also results in increased stress.

Discussion Questions

1. Name and describe the parts of the male reproductive system, including external and internal genitalia.
2. Explain how the increase and decrease of testosterone level affect the male reproductive system, including physiological and psychological effects.
3. Describe the self-care and preventive practices that a man should use to ensure his sexual health.

Application Questions

Reread the story that opens the chapter and answer the following questions.

1. The phrase "Most men think with their penis" clearly derives from the belief that hormones (physiology) control the man, and not vice versa. Do you believe this is correct? Or do sociocultural and psychological factors help balance a man's thinking?
2. The notion of penis size has generally been shown in research to be of little importance to women. Why does size continue to be a matter of jokes and of apprehension among men?
3. Can the male concern with penis size be compared to a woman's concern about her breast size? (After all, more than 100,000 women have breast enhancements each year.) If men could get relatively safe penis-enlargement surgery, do you believe that many would?

Critical Thinking Questions

1. In many schools throughout the country, sexuality education classes mention the concept of menstruation in a mixed-gender goup. But the real discussion of menstruation only occurs in the follow-up "girls only" groupings. Consider whether boys should be taught about menstruation. Without factual knowledge, how can boys comprehend the physical and emotional issues surrounding menstruation? How can they be prepared for safer sexual practices during menstruation if they have not learned about it? Finally, how would you explain menstruation to a group of fifth-grade boys?

Critical Thinking Case

Dad has not been feeling like himself lately. He is unusually tense and easy to upset. It may be due to his lack of sleep. He goes to bed at the same time he always has, but he wakes up often in the middle of the night to urinate. When you ask him about it, he says that he really does not excrete a great deal of urine, just enough to relieve the feeling of having to urinate. As you try to help Dad, answer the following questions.

1. What are some possible causes of Dad's waking up often in the middle of the night to urinate?
2. What would you suggest Dad do about his dilemma? How could you help facilitate his taking this action?
3. What other reproductive system health issues would you expect Dad to encounter as he gets older? What can he do to prevent or postpone the occurrence of these conditions? What can he do to respond to them as they arise?

Exploring Personal Dimensions

For Men Only

Taking charge of self-care and prevention greatly increases your chances of achieving sexual health and wellness. For the following statements, circle YES or NO. Then fill in the dates to help you keep track of your self-care activities.

I do testicular self-examinations monthly.	YES	NO
I did my last testicular exam on _________.		
My next testicular exam is due on _________.		
I have regular physician's examinations.	YES	NO
My last physician's exam was on _________.		
My next physician's exam is due on _________.		
My physician perfoms a digital rectal exam.	YES	NO
I practice safer sexual activities.	YES	NO
I have a family medical tree listing diseases.	YES	NO
I discussed my family's medical history with my doctor.	YES	NO

Sexuality Online

Go to the web component for *Exploring the Dimensions of Human Sexuality* at sexuality.jbpub.com for web exercises, additional resources related to this chapter, and student review tools.

Suggested Readings

Bechtel, S. & Roystains, L. *Sex: A man's guide.* Emmaus, PA: Rodale Press, 1997.

Belshin, L. E. *The complete prostate book: Every man's guide.* Rocklin, CA: Prima Publishing, 1997.

Bordo, S. *The male body: A new look at men in public and private.* New York: Farrar, Straus, & Giroux, 1999.

Butler, R. N. & Lewis, M. I. *Love and sex after 60.* Westminster, MD: Ballantine Books, 1993.

Levant, R. & Brooks, G. R. *Men and sex: New psychological perspectives.* New York: Wiley, 1997.

Milsten, R. & Slowinski, J. *The sexual male: Problems and solutions.* New York: Norton, 1999.

Morgentaler, A. *The male body: A physician's guide to what every man should know about his sexual health.* New York: Simon & Schuster, 1993.

Westheimer, R. *Sex for dummies.* Indianapolis: IDG Books Worldwide, 1995.

Zilbergeld, B. *The new male sexuality.* New York: Bantam Books, 1999.

I»N»T»E»R chapter FOCUS

Body Image

FEATURES

Gender Dimensions
Dissatisfaction with Body Parts

Multicultural Dimensions
Weight and Culture

Ethical Dimensions
To Train or Not to Train—That Is the Question

Gender Dimensions
Why Are Eating Disorders Mainly Found in Women?

CHAPTER OBJECTIVES

1 Discuss body image, its role in sexuality, and the way media have created impossible body-image ideals to emulate.

2 Describe how to improve one's self-image.

3 Describe the problems that poor body image causes for females and males, including eating disorders, muscle dysmorphia, steroid use, and cosmetic surgery.

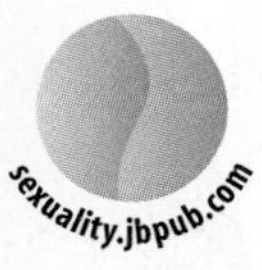

sexuality.jbpub.com

The Influence of the Media
Genetics: Building on Your Strong Points
Eating Disorders
Sports and Dieting

INTRODUCTION

If you had the privilege of knowing Marc Grabowski for some time, as one of your authors has, you would assume that he must have always been a confident young man. As a graduate of Boston University (class of 1999), with a double major in political science and philosophy, he works as a trainer at a local gym while applying to law schools. Not only that: The month before he graduated, he placed fifth in the National Physique Committee's New England Body Building Competition as a heavyweight. Marc appears to be a pillar of strength and confidence.

But as with most people, Marc's confidence and bodily self-assurance have been built up over many years. In fact, Marc had very low self-esteem when he started high school. Smaller and lighter than his friends, he was picked on constantly (called "Ostrich Boy" because of his long neck). As his self-image sank, Marc decided to do something about it. He started lifting weights in his basement at age 14 years. By the time he was 16 years old, he had joined a gym. To Marc and his male friends, weight and size mattered. Their perception was that gaining any weight—fat, water weight, anything—was great.

It was not only his friends who pushed the weight issue. Marc would look at magazines like Flex *and* Muscle & Fitness *and believe that he "could get like that": amazing abs or bulging biceps in 30 days! The articles focused on weight lifting but failed to mention nutrition, cardiovascular work, drugs (steroids), and muscle maturity. As Marc has learned, muscles take years to mature and grow dense in fibers so that they can stand out as hard as iron.*

Yet those magazines continue to peddle false dreams. As Marc puts it, "They'll intentionally deceive the readers just to sell magazines." Worse than that: As many others do, Marc injured himself, rupturing the capillaries in his chest, by following the training routines in such magazines. And when the cover-boy results do not appear, that is a further blow to one's self-esteem.

Having a better body image has made Marc's social life easier. "Like it or not, the first thing people notice about you is your physical appearance. In social situations, that can be an advantage. But that is balanced against professional situations, where the negative connotations of a large size have to be overcome." Although he readily admits to "hiding behind the weight,"

Marc also says he enjoys life more. "It's nice to hear someone say, 'you've gotten in great shape.'"

By the time he reached Boston University, Marc set a goal to be in a bodybuilding show by the time he graduated. Although his studies always came first, Marc began the final preparations and dieting in his senior year.

The diet is what does most people in. During the off-season, Marc ate 10,000 calories or more a day. But as the contest drew nearer, he began to diet. By the last month, all Marc ate were 7 to 10 pounds of chicken and six potatoes a day! (And, of course, he drank water.) The diet takes a physical toll by depleting energy. Marc had trouble staying awake while studying for and taking exams.

The strict diet also has psychological effects. He felt "totally miserable" for the final 2 months of dieting. Marc deliberately tried to avoid social situations when he got cranky. He did not date during his final semester of college—and that, he ironically points out, somewhat defeated the original purpose of bodybuilding!

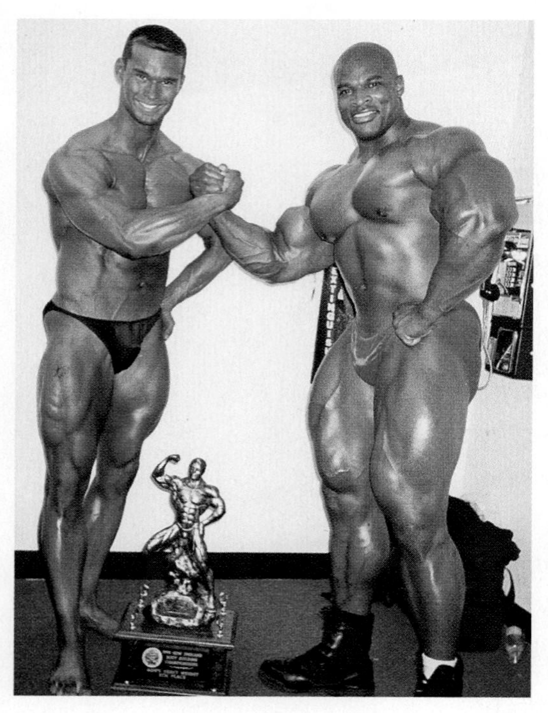

There is always a bigger fish in the water! Although in tremendous shape for a college student, Marc Grabowski is dwarfed by a "professional" bodybuilder. Here, Marc receives postcompetition congratulations from the 1998 Mr. Olympia, Ronnie Coleman.

By the show, Marc was down to 206 pounds, with an incredibly low 2.7% body fat. Within 24 hours after the show, he had regained back 18 pounds (mostly water) and he gained an additional 10 pounds over the next 6 days. Marc lost the weight for a specific event but had no problem regaining it. Marc feels comfortable at an off-season weight of about 250 pounds and a body fat percentage of 10%.

As a personal trainer, Marc enjoys seeing the day-to-day growth of his clients—both in muscle and in confidence. The psychological effects of training are clear to Marc: Not only do clients have better body images, but their increased confidence is also seen in their becoming more outgoing. Clearly, a positive body image can improve your self-confidence.

As you will see in this chapter, obtaining your desired body image can be good for you both physically and psychologically. However, as Marc's story should show, it is important to keep your true goals in mind and, as you do so, respect your body and its needs.

Source: Interview with Marc T. Grabowski, June 9, 1999.

Body Image

body image
The mental image we have of our own physical appearance.

Body image refers to the mental image we have of our own physical appearance. It is influenced by many factors—among them are weight, our weight distribution, our values about physical appearance, our concepts of a good physical appearance, our ethnic background, and what we see in others around us, what we hear through the media, and what we hear from others. We have previously discussed the importance of self-concept in relation to human sexuality. Self-concept is usually closely related to body image. A better body image contributes to a more confident individual; the better we feel about ourselves, the more likely we are to pursue a potential partner.

Body image also affects sexual behavior. People with a positive body image are more likely to be open to sexual expression that exposes the body. Those with a poor body image might be less likely to pursue sexual expressions that cause them to reveal themselves and make them feel uncomfortable. Societally imposed standards of sexual performance and appearance can also cause sexual behavior problems. For example, both women and men may become so concerned about their body image that they are too preoccupied to experience sexual pleasures and intimacy. Thus, they may avoid sexual encounters (Faith & Share, 1993).

Many interesting points about body image were presented in the findings of *Psychology Today*'s 1997 body image survey (Garner, 1997). Despite the concerns of feminists and other observers, body image issues seem to be growing in importance. Body image influences much of our behavior and self-esteem. It governs whom we meet and whom we select as life partners, as well as our day-to-day interactions and our comfort level. Despite this importance, there is a growing gulf between actual and preferred shapes. As individuals, we are growing heavier, but our body preferences are growing thinner.

Results of the *Psychology Today* survey indicated that 89% of the women wanted to lose weight, and 22% of the men wanted to gain weight. Some women also reported avoiding pregnancy because of a fear of what a pregnancy would do to their bodies. Sexual experiences affect our body image, and our body image affects our sexual experiences. For example, 40% of men and 36% of women said that unpleasant sexual experiences caused negative feelings about their body. However, 70% of men and 67% of women felt that good sexual experiences contributed to satisfactory feelings about their body. In addition, 23% of women considered sexual abuse very important in negatively shaping their body image. Finally, 93% of women and 89% of men wanted models in magazines to represent the natural range of body shapes.

Women seem to be more likely than men to have poor body image. In a study with more than 3,500 participants who were university employees and bank workers, men were more likely to be overweight than women. However, women were significantly more likely than men to perceive themselves as overweight, even when their weight was within the appropriate range for their height. Overall, female university employees were 3 times as likely, and female bank workers 10 times as likely as men, to see themselves inaccurately (Women up to 10 times more likely to have poor body image than men, 2001).

A growing number of researchers say that many men are also suffering from body image problems—and they are often reluctant to seek help (Morgan, 2002). Some say that binge eating has become as prevalent for college men as binge drinking—about 40% of them do it. One group of researchers

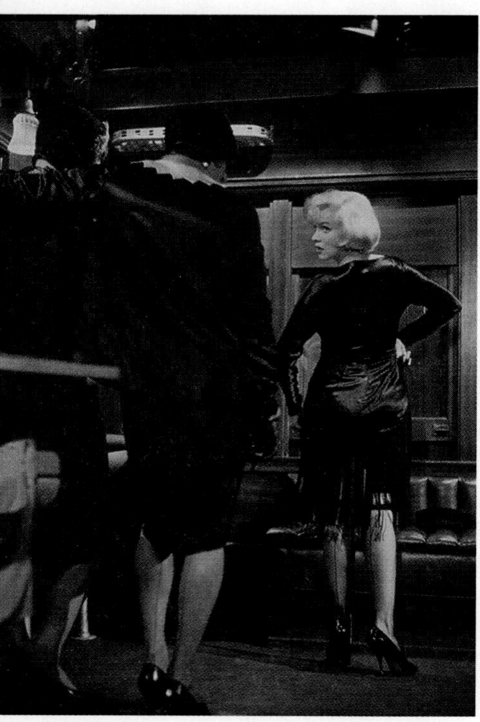

The ideal of the perfect female body has changed dramatically over the past several decades. When Marilyn Monroe sashayed away from Jack Lemmon and Tony Curtis in the movie *Some Like It Hot,* Lemmon quipped that she looks like "Jell-O on springs." Although a compliment in 1959, it would make most women cringe today.

has named severe body-image problems in men "the Adonis complex." It can include eating disorders and a disorder called *muscle dysmorphia,* in which men perceive their bodies as perpetually puny. Some researchers argue that almost half of all college men are dissatisfied with their body.

Body image can be a unique problem for physically challenged people, such as those who have any kind of physical difficulty, including changes in body contours due to accident or disease and changes in body functioning that might relate to sexuality. People with disabilities or disease may view themselves as flawed or unattractive.

Women with disabilities have shown a preoccupation with taking action to enhance their attractiveness (Nosek, 1996). For some, this means maintaining cleanliness and neatness; for others it means using makeup and fashionable clothes. One respondent reported that she used makeup and fashionable clothes to look "less disabled."

Depending on the type of physical challenge, various areas of concern need attention, including the feelings of loss of control over one's bodily functions, the inability to care for personal needs, the fear of being less of a person, and the feeling of being unacceptable. Education and counseling about body image are important and ideally should also involve the partners of challenged persons.

For many people, thinking about body image and how they would like to look imply becoming thinner. In recent years, however, there has also been a movement to acknowledge that there is a great range of beauty and attractiveness. For example, Emme became a well-known and sought-after size-16 supermodel. Also, *Mode,* a fashion magazine, was developed for women who wear average and large sizes.

For years the 11-inch-tall blonde, blue-eyed Barbie fashion doll represented the ideal American beauty—even though Barbie's stick-thin figure is impossible to achieve in real life. Now Barbie has some competition: the Emme doll. Based on supermodel Emme's size 14–16 figure, it is the world's first plus-size fashion doll. Emme hopes the doll will give girls the "emotional armor" to help them deal with poor body image. The doll is a vehicle for talking about health, fitness, anorexia, and obesity, she says (Mendelsohn, 2002).

The Elusive Perfect Body

What does the perfect body look like? The answer to that question will probably depend on the purpose we have in mind. Taking a look at successful female athletes gives us some excellent examples. The best swimmers tend to be relatively tall and look like a capital *Y* from the front, with wide, flexible shoulders; long arms and hands; a narrow waist; and lightweight legs. Swimmers get by with more body fat than other athletes because it lets them ride higher in the water. Top speed skaters, in contrast, are shorter and look rather average from the waist up. Farther down, however, we see heavily muscled legs with rather short thighs. At the same time, the female gymnast probably has a lean, petite frame; a fine-boned face; small breasts; and long arms. A body that excels in one athletic context can be a hindrance in others.

Of course most of us are not training to be Olympic athletes, but there is a lesson here for all of us. The bodies closest to "perfect" are, to a large extent, born that way. We must take what we have and develop and use it as best we can. We can make the most of the genetic gifts we do have. In the end, "the perfect body is the one that will allow you to do things you enjoy and allow you to live your life to the fullest—without compromising your health" (Barnette, 1993).

Gender DIMENSIONS

Dissatisfaction with Body Parts It is interesting to compare the feelings of men and women about specific parts of their body. Here are the percentages of 4,000 respondents who reported feeling dissatisfied with parts of their body:

	WOMEN	MEN
1. Overall appearance	56%	43%
2. Weight	66%	52%
3. Height	16%	16%
4. Muscle tone	57%	45%
5. Breasts/chest	34%	38%
6. Abdomen	71%	63%
7. Hips or upper thighs	61%	29%

Some respondents reported that body image and sexual experiences are related. For example, some said that as they feel less attractive, they have less desire for sexual activity.

Source: Garner, D. M. The 1997 Body Image Survey results, *Psychology Today, 30* (1997), 30–44.

Why Models Look So Perfect

A quick glance at the covers of major fashion and sports magazines—or at the ads therein—seems to bolster the argument that "some have it, some don't." These models, as well as those in many movies, seem too perfect to be real. Could these people look like that all the time? The answer is, of course, no. But they do look that way for the millisecond that the camera snaps.

Getting "the look" begins long before the photo shoot ever takes place. For example, months before a movie begins production, the director (and/or art director) hires a specific personal trainer who will get "the look" that the director wants. Workouts and diet are structured to transform the actor or actress. The look can be as specific as the "ripped-up" look of Linda Hamilton in *Terminator* and *T2* to the elongated calf muscles that the director wanted for Demi Moore in *Striptease*.

Still in preproduction, clothes, makeup, and lighting are chosen to enhance whatever qualities have been chosen (for example, Pamela Anderson's cleavage in *Barb Wire*). The day of shooting starts with hours of makeup application (sometimes over the entire body), hair styling, and clothes fitting. Ever wonder how clothes can fit so skintight on some people? No problem: The clothes are literally pasted on!

Production is the time when the camera rolls (or snaps). The art director makes clear what is desired from the photographer, who in turn adjusts lighting and the camera lens to make it happen.

Then the fun begins. During postproduction, any alterations at all can be made to the pictures. The same digital wizardry that put dinosaurs on the screen in *Jurassic Park* is available to the print world. You have probably heard that blemishes are covered, teeth are routinely whitened, wrinkles in clothes are deleted. But did you know that *Penthouse* routinely augments breast size? *Playboy* thinks nothing of slimming the waist and thighs of models. A knowledgeable source has told one of the authors that when photos of a playmate's rear end were not approved, the postproduction team put a new rear end on her!

To increase the sex appeal of female models, it is not uncommon for art directors to "stretch" legs to give them a longer, thinner look. Just think: You could go from being short and stocky to having the body of Cameron Diaz with a few clicks of a computer mouse!

Eventually, the picture that emerges is one that matches the art director's vision—not one that shows the person's real body. And that is not always good. To make the point that image retouching can go too far, the retouching artist Kathy Grove redid one of the most famous Depression-era photographs, Dorothea Lange's *Migrant Mother*. Grove's point is simple: Do not believe everything you see.

The Influence of the Media

A 1999 study found that all-too-perfect models who grace magazine covers send powerful—and often negative—signals to figure-conscious adolescent girls. More than two-thirds of girls in grades 5 through 12 said magazine photos influenced their notion of the ultimate figure.

Forty-seven percent said they wanted to lose weight because of those pictures. But only 29% of the 548 girls interviewed were actually overweight, according to the study, published in the March 1999 issue of the journal *Pediatrics* (Field, et al., 1999).

"Even among the girls who don't read the magazines, very frequently, they, too, felt influenced," said Alison E. Field, an epidemiologist at Brigham and Women's Hospital and the study's lead author. "It really does permeate society."

It is interesting to note that about one-third of the respondents were in elementary school. Even at that age, 50% reported reading fashion magazines at least two to five times a month. High-frequency magazine readers of any age were three times more likely to exercise and lose weight than infrequent readers and three times more likely to have unrealistic body expectations.

"Young girls reading magazines certainly compare their bodies to the models that they see in there and come away with sometimes unhappy feelings with the way they look," said Stephanie Dolgoff, executive editor of *Glamour*, which targets 18- to 35-year-olds.

For years, some people have criticized the Barbie doll for presenting children with standards for body size and appearance that are both unrealistic and unattainable for most females. Experts also have become concerned about the impact of the "GI Joe Extreme" action figure, which has a more muscular and defined body than past GI Joe figures. At issue is whether such dolls plant the concept of the ideal body in children's minds—a concept that usually cannot be achieved without using obsessive behaviors to lose weight and gain muscle.

Relatedly, beauty pageants are another way society defines its ideal of beauty, including weight and shape. Researchers computed the body mass

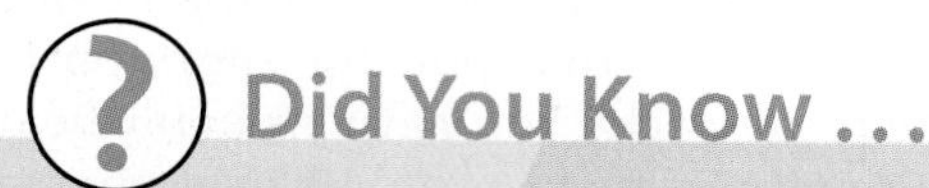

The average American woman is 5′4″ tall and weighs 144 pounds; the average model is 5′9″ tall and weighs 109 pounds. The average store fashion mannequin was size 8 in the 1980s; now it is size 4–6, and some are size 2. Even some of the thin mannequins are shown with large breasts—perhaps even mannequins get breast implants?

Source: Reported on *Good Morning America* Sunday, October 18, 1998.

index (BMI) (weight divided by the square of height) of winners of the Miss America Pageant from 1922 to 1999. There was a significant decline in the BMI over that time, placing an increasing number of winners in the range of undernutrition. Pageant winners' height increased less than 2%, but body weight decreased by 12% (Rubinstein & Caballero, 2000).

Even *Playboy* centerfold models have changed over time (Voracek & Fisher, 2002). A review of *Playboy* centerfold models' body measurements over a 50-year period showed that over time bust size and hip size decreased, while waist size increased. Body mass index and bust-to-hip ratio decreased, while waist-to-hip ratio, waist-to-bust ratio, and androgyny index increased. The study's authors concluded that shapely body characteristics of centerfold models have given way to more androgynous ones.

Interestingly, Bryla (2002) explored the effects of media on female image. She concluded that beyond media exposure, awareness and internalization of sociocultural ideals appear to be significant predictors of body image disturbance. In other words, looking at the effects of media on body image is not a simple matter.

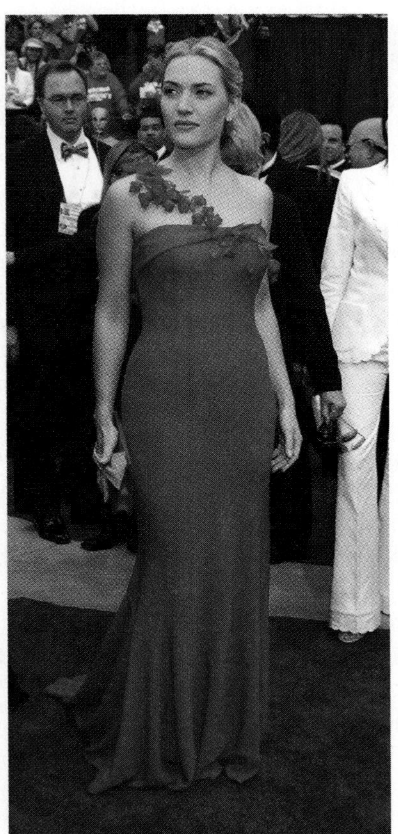

Anything is possible with photo retouching. The February 2001 issue of the U.K. edition of *GQ* magazine features a retouched image of the actress Kate Winslet. Famous for defending the appearance of fuller-figured women, Winslet has received attention not only for her acting, but also for the fluctuations in her weight. Winslet responded to the cover with shock, "I do not look like that," the actress, 27, told the *Daily Mail*. "And, more importantly, I don't desire to look like that." The controversy has highlighted how common it is for magazines to retouch photographs of models and celebrities, male and female. How do you think this practice affects the body image of young people?

Source: People (January 27, 2003).

Diversity and Body Image

In the past in the United States, the idea of beauty involved using the images of Barbie or Ken dolls or the like with the goal of creating some version of a white person. For example, it has been common for the winners of Latin American beauty contests to look "international": tall; not-too-dark hair; light skin; high, girlish bust; and long legs. Latinas often have to cope with the way the world would like to change them: if only the earrings were smaller, the makeup not so dramatic, the hair not so wild, the walk not so sexy, the hand gestures not so expressive, the emotions not so on-the-surface, and they were thinner (Fernandez, 1993).

Other examples related to diversity and body image are also apparent. For example, African-American adolescent females seem to be happier with their body and less likely to diet than are European-American adolescent females (Wilson, et al., 1996). A major problem for some African-American women who seek psychological help is their skin color. For Asian-American women, eye surgery is sometimes done so they will look more like whites.

However, as the result of pressure from groups interested in emphasizing the diversity of real life, products, methods, and goals relating to beauty have changed. Even plastic surgeons have learned a lot about working with people from diverse backgrounds.

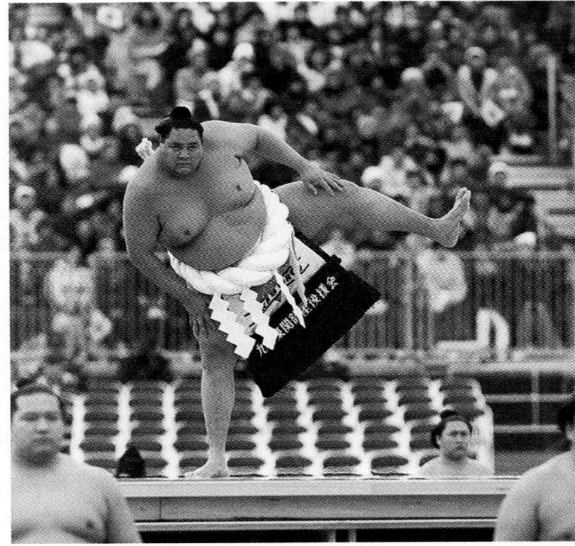

In Eastern cultures, the shape of a powerful body is that of a pyramid—with a strong base as the foundation. In Western culture the shape of a powerful body is that of an upside-down pyramid—broad shoulders and tapered waist.

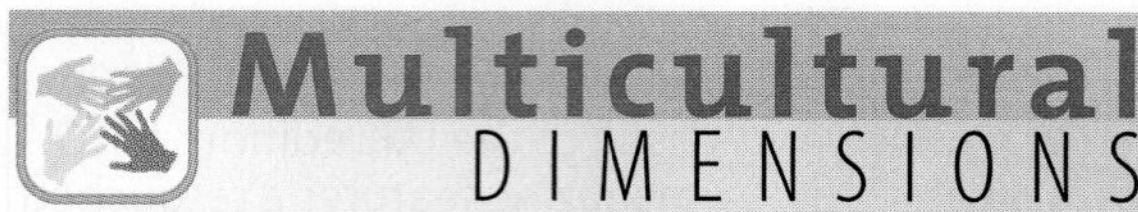

Weight and Culture

For many people in many cultures, body image is directly linked to body weight. The National Health and Nutrition Examination Survey (NHANES III), conducted by the Centers for Disease Control (CDC) in the early 1990s, found almost 35% of the U.S. population obese (they weigh at least 20% more than their ideal body weight). However, data from the study also suggest that the weight is not distributed evenly:

- The groups having the highest proportion of overweight people were African-American, Hispanic women (49%), and Mexican-American women (47%).
- Rates of obesity for white women had risen 9% to 33.5% since a similar study in the 1980s. Rates were up 4% for African-American women and 7% for Mexican-American women.
- White men showed a steep increase in obesity rates.

Some researchers have found that Puerto Ricans and immigrant Mexican women perceive a cultural environment that favors an overweight body image. Indeed, a pediatrician who had worked with Hispanics in Harlem told one of the authors about the "Gerber baby" syndrome: Hispanic mothers perceived the chubbiness of the "Gerber baby" (the infant pictured on Gerber baby products) as a sign of health and wealth. Thus, to fatten their children up, the mothers added Hershey's strawberry mix to their baby's formula—and, later, to the baby's milk. Although this practice created the desired image of a chubby child, it could have serious long-term health consequences.

Sources: Juarbe, T. C. The state of Hispanic health: Cardiovascular disease and health, in *Hispanic voices: Hispanic health educators speak out,* Torres, S., ed. New York: National League for Nursing, 1996; Bass, A. Record obesity levels found, *Boston Globe* (July 20, 1995), 1, 10; Elmer-Dewitt, P. Fat times, *Time* (January 16, 1995), 63–64.

Building a Better Self-Image

Given that none of us will be perfect, and given that we all have imperfections in our appearance, we can still look better and improve our body image. It may not always be easy, but small efforts can also make a huge difference.

When we feel good about the way we look, we are happier and likely to feel better about others. Many actions can help you improve your body image. Here are some examples (Bruess & Richardon, 1995):

1. Do not feel a need to apologize about every blemish you might see in your appearance. Chances are, others do not notice them anyway. None of us is perfect.

2. Be careful about basing your body image on what you see and hear in advertisements. They are carefully produced to send certain messages to sell products. Few people look and act the way the people you see in the ads do.

3. Attractive people are often judged by others to be more warm, interesting, friendly, considerate, and strong than those who are less attractive. In spite of our defects, we can do things to feel more attractive. For example, clothes, styles, and personal hygiene all affect attractiveness. What can you do to feel more attractive?

4. You should be free to be yourself; however, the message you send about your appearance and the ones you receive from others may not always be the same. For example, a female might not wear a bra because she wants to be comfortable; another person might interpret that as a desire to be sexy. What messages are you sending in the appearance you present?
5. The way you move your body (body language) can also indicate the way you feel about yourself. Watch what others do when they are nervous, happy, or sad. Use this information to control some of your body movements so they send messages you want to send.

Body image is important. People who feel good about themselves are more attractive to others than people who do not. Concentrate on your strengths. Do you have great hair? Eyes? Hands? Play them up. But remember your other strengths, too. Are you funny? Kind? Smart? You are more than just your looks.

Creating Your Optimal Body

Imagine that you are a personal trainer in a local fitness center. A center member gives you a magazine and says, "I want to look like the person in this picture, and I need you to help me do it!" What should you do?

If you are the one who wants to resemble a person in a magazine picture, it might be wise to remember that you need to optimize your own body. It does us no good to strive to be someone else. There may be qualities of other people—physical as well as others—that we want to obtain, but we cannot be exactly like another person.

Genetics: Building on Your Strong Points

A person who is 5′4″ tall may strive to be an Olympic basketball player, but his or her chance of success is not good; the 6′8″, 225-pound man will probably not make a good competitive gymnast. Although these examples are extreme, we need to keep them in mind when we consider what is possible and best for each of us.

Ethical DIMENSIONS

To Train or Not to Train—That Is the Question

A professionally prepared personal trainer knows how to help people develop the body to look the best it can. The trainer also knows that it is usually not possible to change the body type of a person drastically. So, what should a trainer who runs his or her own business and needs paying clients do when a person asks to look the way someone pictured in a magazine does? If the trainer agrees to help the person resemble the one in the picture, there will be false hopes created; however, you could argue that at least the person will improve his or her appearance and health—and probably body image as well. Or, should the trainer tell the client that there is no way he or she can look like the picture and explain how unrealistic expectations can cause a waste of money if he or she tries to obtain objectives that cannot be reached?

As we mentioned in the box on page 177, many people are not happy with the appearance of their body. Another study reported that about 40% of adult men and 55% of adult women are dissatisfied with their body weight. As many as 85% of first-year male and female college students desire to change their body weight. The primary cause of this concern is the value that society, in general, assigns to physical appearance (Williams, 1996).

Your Body Weight

Most often when we think of body weight, we think about what the scale says when we stand on it. Although this is useful information, if you are serious about reaching your optimal body weight, it would be worthwhile to learn more about some topics beyond the scope of this book: **body mass index (BMI)** and **body composition.** Knowing about these will help you understand your body weight better and have more realistic goals.

body mass index (BMI)
Weight in kilograms divided by the square of the height in meters.

body composition
The percentage of fat versus lean tissue.

What the scale says is not always the complete truth, and what we see is not always what we are. For example, sometimes overweight people see themselves as heavier than they really are. When they look in a mirror, they see a bigger abdomen, rear end, and thighs than they actually have. This body image may be hard to change, even if body weight decreases.

Other overweight people may see themselves as much slimmer than they really are. They often rationalize away their need to lose weight. However, some people see themselves as they really are. Those with realistic body images tend to have the greatest success with weight control.

Diet

The diet business is big business in the United States. At any given time 48 million adult Americans, including 60% of all adult women, are on a diet, and we spend over $36 billion annually on diet products (Bruess & Richardson, 1995). Despite the interest in diet products and services, few people have long-term weight control success.

To have any hope of long-term success with weight loss, our approach to diets must change. A "diet" must mean permanent changes in eating habits. Do not waste time on dieting if you are not committed to maintaining a healthy weight throughout your life. If you want to change your eating habits, you must pay close attention to the kinds and amounts of foods you eat. There is no substitute for well-balanced diets and a reduction in intake of calories—especially when combined with proper exercise habits.

Exercise

Exercise plays an important role in losing pounds and keeping them off: Researchers have compared the effects of weight loss by diet only and by exercise only. They found that the group who were only exercising lost a higher percentage of fat and had more success keeping off the weight than the group who were only dieting (Bruess & Richardson, 1995).

Moderate exercise suppresses appetite, rather than increasing it, as many people think. You might want to exercise just before a meal to take advantage of that effect. Another benefit of exercise is that it strengthens muscle tissue. Muscle tissue requires more calories than fat tissue does to maintain itself, so as lean muscle tissue increases, more calories are burned. This is important, because our resting metabolic rate accounts for about 70% of the calories we burn.

The ultimate goal of any weight-loss program should be the loss of body fat, not just body weight. Those who combine diet and exercise lose more fat and are more likely to keep it off. Exercise and sound eating habits result in a steady weight loss that can be maintained on a permanent basis if you maintain your exercise and dietary changes.

Issues Related to Trying to Be Perfect

Although we know it is impossible to be perfect, some people are so concerned about their body image that they run into problems, such as eating disorders, obsessive muscle dysmorphia, and complications of cosmetic surgery.

Eating Disorders

In the quest to be attractive and improve one's body image, some people are willing to pay a high price. It is common to want to look as good as we can, and many people attempt to control body weight by using various diets at some time during their lives. A fear of fat seems to drive some people to extreme forms of eating behaviors. Compulsive overeating (also called *binge eating*) and compulsive dieting are the behaviors known as *eating disorders*. Wardlow (1997) found that among female college athletes 15% of swimmers, 62% of gymnasts, and 32% of all varsity athletes showed disordered eating patterns.

Anorexia nervosa is a condition in which the individual severely limits calorie intake; it is sometimes described as self-induced starvation. The DSM-IV-TR criteria for anorexia are given in Table IF1.1. Anorexia can be fatal. Most people with anorexia are white females less than 25 years of age who are focused on a goal of extreme thinness and willingly starve themselves and overexercise to reach that goal.

> **anorexia nervosa**
> A condition in which the individual severely limits caloric intake.

Although this condition affects females 95% of the time, it may be more common than previously thought among college males. Most males with anorexia are men who depend on their thin physique for employment—such as models. Anorexia results in death in about 10% of all cases in both sexes.

TABLE IF1.1 DSM-IV-TR: Diagnostic Criteria for Anorexia Nervosa

A. Refusal to maintain body weight at or above a minimally normal weight for age and height (for example, weight loss leading to maintenance of body weight less than 85% of that expected; or failure to make expected weight gain during period of growth, leading to body weight less than 85% of that expected).

B. Intense fear of gaining weight or becoming fat, even though underweight.

C. Disturbance in the way in which one's body weight or shape is experienced, undue influence of body weight or shape on self-evaluation, or denial of the seriousness of the current low body weight.

D. In postmenarcheal females, amenorrhea, that is, the absence of at least three consecutive menstrual cycles. (A woman is considered to have amenorrhea if her periods occur only following hormone, for instance, estrogen, administration.)

Specify Type

Restricting Type: during the current episode of anorexia nervosa, the person has not regularly engaged in binge-eating or purging behavior (that is, self-induced vomiting or the misuse of laxatives, diuretics, or enemas)

Binge-Eating/Purging Type: during the current episode of anorexia nervosa, the person has regularly engaged in binge-eating or purging behavior (that is, self-induced vomiting or the misuse of laxatives, diuretics, or enemas)

Source: Diagnostic and Statistical Manual of Mental Disorders, Fourth Edition, Text Revision. American Psychiatric Assoc., 2000.

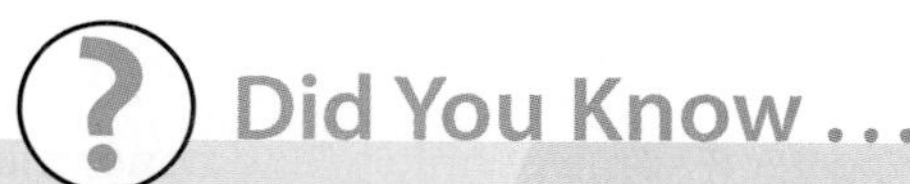

Did You Know . . .

How can you tell if someone you love has an eating disorder?

Here are possible warning signs:

1. Evidence of bulimia, such as laxatives on the dresser or vomitus in the toilet bowl.
2. Moaning about a fat behind by a person who is rail thin.
3. Hiding under baggy clothes.
4. An energy level so low that he or she sleeps much of the time.
5. The growth of baby-fine hair on arms and legs (as the shrinking body tries to keep warm).
6. Underweight by 15%.
7. Loss of menstrual cycle for 3 months.
8. Brittle nails and/or swollen joints.
9. A chronic sore throat and/or dental problems.
10. Bloating and other digestive complaints.

Source: Adapted from Gorman, C. Disappearing act, *Time, 152, no. 10* (November 2, 1998), 110.

Although the exact cause of anorexia is unknown, it seems to involve a combination of psychological and environmental factors. The female with anorexia might reject food in an attempt to avoid dealing with what she feels are society's demands that she become a superwoman. The severe weight loss can make the female resemble a young girl, in what some researchers feel is a conscious attempt to avoid dealing with issues related to intimacy and sexuality. People with anorexia might feel that their weight is the only factor they can control in a world where expectations of others seem difficult to fulfill. One of the most difficult to understand aspects of anorexia is self-perception. Regardless of how much weight has been lost, the person with anorexia still feels too heavy (Bruess & Greenberg, 2004).

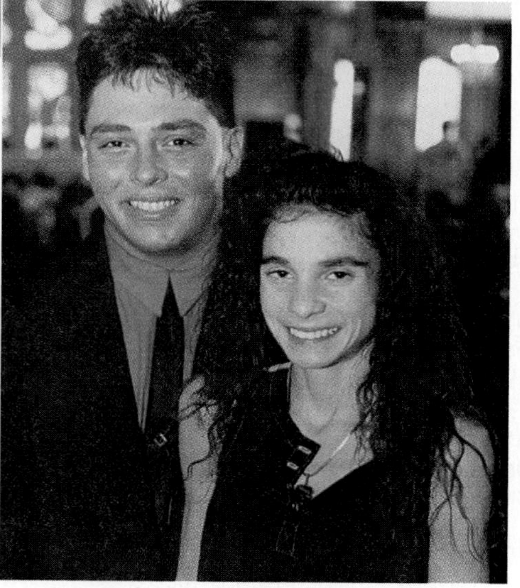

Many female athletes turn to some form of dieting to maintain an edge in competitions. The nationally ranked gymnast Christy Henrich took her dieting too far and struggled with anorexia nervosa for several years before she died of it in 1994. Here she is seen performing in the late 1980s (above) and just before her death in 1994 (right).

In a 1992 survey of collegiate athletes, 93% of the programs reported eating disorders among women. Fifty-one percent of the women's gymnastics programs reported eating disorders among team members, a far greater percentage than in any other sport. One world-class gymnast at a well-known university admitted that her entire team would binge and vomit together after meets. It was a "social thing." Christy Henrich, another world-class gymnast, was 4′10″ tall and weighed 95 pounds at the peak of her career. Believing that she was too fat, she got her weight down to 61 pounds and eventually died of multiple organ failure at 22 years of age. Shortly before that, she had reduced her weight to 47 pounds (Dying to win, 1994).

Bulimia nervosa is a condition in which the person periodically binges and purges, with an obsessive fear of becoming fat. Bulimia (insatiable appetite) has been confused with anorexia nervosa because periodic bingeing is common to both disorders; however, a number of the characteristics are different. People with bulimia are usually older than people with anorexia and may have been anorexic earlier. Whereas people with anorexia are obsessed with being thin, people with bulimia have an obsessive fear of becoming fat.

About 2–3% of the population have bulimia, and about 95% of these are females. People with bulimia tend to be close to normal weight and may appear to have normal eating habits. During their secretive eating binges, people with bulimia may consume 10,000 calories or more within a few hours. Afterward they try to purge the food through a variety of methods, including vomiting, laxatives, diuretics, and exercise. After bingeing and purging, the person with bulimia may feel depressed and discouraged about the behavior (Bruess & Richardson, 1995). The DSM-IV-TR criteria for bulimia are given in Table IF1.2.

Binge-eating disorder (BED) is an eating disorder characterized by recurrent binge eating but not by inappropriate weight-control behaviors. Persons with BED do not regularly engage in purging, and the majority are obese. They also may be referred to as "compulsive overeaters." The DSM-IV proposed criteria for BED are given in Table IF1.3.

bulimia nervosa
A condition in which the individual periodically binges and purges, with an obsessive fear of becoming fat.

binge-eating disorder (BED)
Eating disorder characterized by recurrent binge eating but not by inappropriate weight-control behaviors.

TABLE IF1.2 **DSM-IV-TR: Diagnostic Criteria for Bulimia Nervosa**

A. Recurrent episodes of binge eating. An episode of binge eating is characterized by both of the following:

(1) eating, in a discrete period of time (for example, within any two-hour period), an amount of food that is definitely larger than most people would eat during a similar period of time and under similar circumstances

(2) a sense of lack of control over eating during the episode (for instance, a feeling that one cannot stop eating or control what or how much one is eating)

B. Recurrent inappropriate compensatory behavior in order to prevent weight gain, such as self-induced vomiting; misuse of laxatives, diuretics, enemas, or other medications; fasting; or excessive exercise.

C. The binge-eating and inappropriate compensatory behaviors both occur, on average, at least twice a week for three months.

D. Self-evaluation is unduly influenced by body shape and weight.

E. The disturbance does not occur exclusively during episodes of anorexia nervosa.

Specify Type

Purging Type: during the current episode of bulimia nervosa, the person has regularly engaged in self-induced vomiting or the misuse of laxatives, diuretics, or enemas

Nonpurging Type: during the current episode of bulimia nervosa, the person has used other inappropriate compensatory behaviors, such as fasting or excessive exercise but has not regularly engaged in self-induced vomiting or the misuse of laxatives, diuretics, or enemas

Source: Diagnostic and Statistical Manual of Mental Disorders, Fourth Edition, Text Revision. American Psychiatric Assoc., 2000.

TABLE IF1.3 DSM-IV: Proposed Diagnostic Criteria for Binge-Eating Disorder

A. Recurrent episodes of binge eating. An episode of binge eating is characterized by both of the following:

(1) eating, in a discrete period of time (for example, within any two-hour period), an amount of food that is definitely larger than most people would eat during a similar period of time and under similar circumstances

(2) a sense of lack of control over eating during the episode (for instance, a feeling that one cannot stop eating or control what or how much one is eating)

B. The binge-eating episodes are associated with three (or more) of the following:

(1) eating much more rapidly than normal

(2) eating until feeling uncomfortably full

(3) eating large amounts of food when not feeling physically hungry

(4) eating alone because of being embarrassed by how much one is eating

(5) feeling disgusted with oneself, depressed, or very guilty after overeating

C. Marked distress regarding binge eating is present.

D. The binge eating occurs, on average, at least two days a week for six months.

E. The binge eating is not associated with the regular use of inappropriate compensatory behaviors (for example, purging, fasting, excessive exercise) and does not occur exclusively during the course of anorexia nervosa or bulimia nervosa.

Source: Diagnostic and Statistical Manual of Mental Disorders, Fourth Edition. American Psychiatric Assoc., 1994.

Treating Eating Disorders

Many approaches are used in the treatment of anorexia, but the prognosis is not good. Drug therapy is used in about 25% of the cases, and behavior modification in about 45%. A combination of approaches is also used. Most specialists recommend a period of hospitalization to ensure weight gain, and families are often involved in the therapy. The prognosis for people with anorexia is worse than for people with bulimia.

Overcoming bulimia requires establishing a normal eating pattern that eliminates dieting. Although people with bulimia can hide their disorder from others, they are more likely than people with anorexia to seek treatment; however, they might expect immediate results and become frustrated with therapy. Antidepressant drugs are used in the treatment of bulimia, as is psychological therapy. Antidepressant medication and psychological treatments can also reduce binge eating of BED patients.

Muscle Dysmorphia

Body image and goals related to it may change over time. Thus, as someone makes progress with weights, or in gymnastics or figure skating, the ideal of the perfect body image may become more "perfect." A perpetual chasing of the ideal can cause people to lose perspective about their actual body image. An example of this was given in the opening story of this chapter.

Gender DIMENSIONS

Why Are Eating Disorders Mainly Found in Women?

It seems clear that physical attractiveness is more important for women than men. This is because beauty is often a central aspect of femininity (girls learn early that being pretty draws attention to them), and women's self-worth is often tied to establishing and maintaining close relationships. They can improve their feeling of self-worth based on others' opinions and approval of them.

The ideal standard of physical attractiveness has become thinner over the past few decades. This makes it even harder for women to meet the standard, so they are more likely to resort to extreme ways to control their weight—such as rigid dieting and purging.

Even when men take extreme measures to control their weight, it is usually done to improve their athletic performance (such as with jockeys and wrestlers). Their goal of losing weight is secondary to their goal of performing well. For women, however, dieting to achieve an ideal weight is related to their self-evaluation.

Source: Adapted from Wilson, G.T., et al., Eating disorders, in *Abnormal psychology: Integrating perspectives.* Needham, MA: Allyn & Bacon, 1996, 370.

One disorder that afflicts bodybuilders is essentially the opposite of anorexia nervosa. Called **muscle dysmorphia,** it involves bodybuilders who, despite their extremely muscular bodies and tip-top shape, consider themselves to be puny (Brody, 1998). Weight lifting, for some people, can become a dangerous obsession (Bilger, 1998).

muscle dysmorphia
A disorder whereby a bodybuilder in top shape considers himself or herself to be puny.

Psychiatrists have found that as many as 10% of the men and 84% of women who are bodybuilders may have this "negative anorexia." For example, men who did not think they were well built could press the equivalent of their own body weight. Even though they recognized muscularity in others, their view of themselves was very negative (Cohen, 1997). Muscle dysmorphics with body weight well above 200 pounds are sometimes so ashamed of their "undersized" bodies that they rarely leave their homes, preferring instead to follow a regime of weight lifting in their basement, interrupted primarily for periodic protein consumption (Zorpette, 1998).

Goodale and associates (2001) used a mixed-gender sample of 323 college students to study muscle dysmorphia. She concluded that it is an increasingly common problem among athletes and nonathletes alike, that both men and women are susceptible to it, and that it has many similarities to established dieting disorders. For example, perhaps because of media glorification of lean and muscular physiques, those with muscle dysmorphia place undue emphasis on body weight and shape when judging their own worth.

Muscle dysmorphia does not usually involve the serious medical complications of anorexia, but it still can have significant effects. It is certainly normal for people who go to a gym to want to improve their physique and build larger muscles. The turning point from normal goals to muscle dysmorphia occurs when the quest for "massive" size takes over one's life, destroying career, relationships, and, ironically, self-esteem.

Sports and Dieting

Eating disorders may be the gravest health problem facing female athletes, affecting gymnasts, figure skaters, swimmers, distance runners, divers, and even tennis and volleyball players. According to a *Sports Illustrated* special report, the American College of Sports Medicine reported that "as many as 62% of females competing in 'appearance' sports (like figure skating and gymnastics) and endurance sports suffer from an eating disorder" (Noden, 1994). Given the importance that sport attaches to weight—and, in subjectively judged sports, to appearance—it is not surprising that eating disorders are common among athletes.

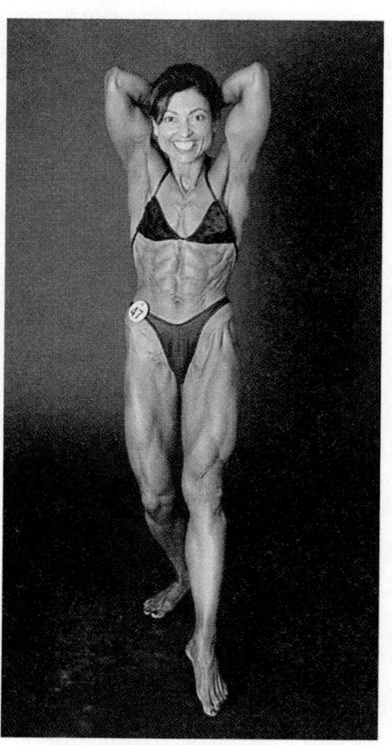

Fifteen years of consistent training has given 49-year-old Terri DeAngelis a body many people wish were their own. Terri is a positive role model for her personal-training clients, with whom she spends a good deal of time working on body-image problems and solutions. Although many may wish they had such great abs, how many people would actually be willing to pursue the diet and exercise regimen that made Terri's body what it is?

As we have mentioned, some sports, such as women's gymnastics, emphasize smallness. Vera Caslavska, who won the overall titles at the 1964 and 1968 Olympics, was a relatively normal-sized 5′3″ and 121 pounds. After she was upstaged in 1968 by the pixie Olga Korbut (4′11″ and 85 pounds), gymnastics was never the same (Noden, 1994). In 1976, the average woman on the U.S. Olympic team was 5′3″ and 105 pounds; by 1992 she was 4′9″ and 88 pounds (Noden, 1994).

But weight—and dieting—also play a major role in endurance sports. As an athlete's weight falls, his or her aerobic power increases. Put another way, it takes less energy to run if you weigh less; thus more energy can be expended on running faster. So, runners and swimmers also succumb to the need to diet to win.

Mary T. Meagher, former world-record holder in the 100- and 200-meter butterfly, states that "men grow into what they're supposed to be. They're supposed to be big and muscular. A woman's body naturally produces more fat. We grow away from what we're supposed to be as athletes" (Noden, 1994).

Steroid Use

steroids
Synthetic versions of the male hormone testosterone that promote tissue growth.

Steroids are synthetic versions of the male hormone testosterone. Steroid abuse is fast becoming a very serious problem among adolescent males, both athletes and nonathletes, who take large doses in an attempt to achieve much greater body mass quickly. In addition to potential to halt growth and bone development, steroid use can cause testicular shrinkage, increased cholesterol levels, infertility, decreased sexual drive, prostate cancer, kidney disorders, liver malfunction, aggression and violence, suicidal tendencies, and extreme moodiness. Steroids can also be psychologically and physically addictive.

Steroid abuse is a major problem among teenagers. A 1998 report found that 2.7% of Massachusetts middle-school athletes were using steroids (Begley & Brant, 1999). The National Institute of Drug Abuse reports that as many as a half-million Americans below 18 years of age may be abusing anabolic steroids to improve athletic performance, appearance, and self-image (NIDA, 1999). Steroid abuse is not limited to males: About 6.5% of adolescent boys and 1.9% of girls reported the use of steroids without a prescription (COHIS, 1999).

People may go to unhealthy extremes simply to look good. Goodale and coworkers (2001) reported that the most common reason male bodybuilders give for using steroids is to enhance looks.

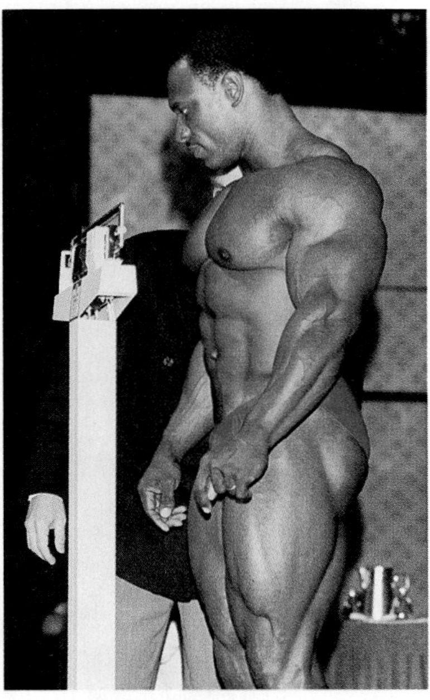

Many people look at eight-time Mr. Olympia Lee Haney only in terms of his muscles. But Haney keeps body image in perspective, placing God, family, and friends above business—and to Haney, bodybuilding was a business.

Women in endurance sports also take steroids. Steroids help a runner in two ways: A thin runner expends less energy in running; by speeding muscle recovery, a long-distance runner is able to recover faster, train more, and thus run faster.

The adverse effects of steroids in women include lowered voice, increased body and facial hair, male-pattern baldness, enlarged clitoris, decreased breast size, and changes in or cessation of menstruation. There are not sufficient studies of female steroid users to fully understand the extent to which a woman's body may be damaged and whether the effects are permanent.

In addition to the many adverse effects of steroids listed, there is a risk of HIV transmission through shared needles. Finally, anabolic steroids are illegal in the United States; their use carries stiff fines and possible imprisonment.

Some feel that a "male body ideal" has caused increasing numbers of males to develop an "Adonis Complex"—defined as a condition shared by millions of males who develop eating disorders, abuse steroids, work out compulsively, or otherwise obsess over their physical appearance. The taboo against overt male vanity inhibits men from seeking help for their disorders (Miller & Sharlet, 2000).

Makeovers and Cosmetic Surgery

If we pay attention to our favorite movie and TV stars, we see that they radically change their appearance from time to time. The makeover has become a powerful draw for many stars—they feel it can renew the spirit, save a career, and even mend the heart. Indeed, Hollywood may be in the grip of a redo revolution. Some stars like to re-create themselves, increase their confidence by showing that they can wear more than one style, and avoid being linked with a look created by a past role (O'Neill, 1998).

In our quest to create the perfect look, we may see the stars radically change theirs and decide we want to do it too. People today often view their body as increasingly malleable. Sometimes, they even want to use ways that look easy, such as liposuction, implants, and plastic surgery (cosmetic surgery).

liposuction
A technique for removing adipose tissue with a suction-pump device.

Liposuction is a technique for removing adipose (fat) tissue with a suction-pump device. A hollow suction tube, which is attached to a special vacuum, is inserted into small incisions in the skin. It is used primarily to remove and reduce areas of fat around the abdomen, breast, legs, face, and upper arms. Liposuction can be helpful for the removal of fat in particular areas, but it should not be viewed as a way to lose large amounts of fat or to change one's physique dramatically. Most people lose an average of only 3 pounds as a direct result of the procedure (Graham, 1997). According to the American Society of Aesthetic Plastic Surgery (2003), liposuction was the top cosmetic

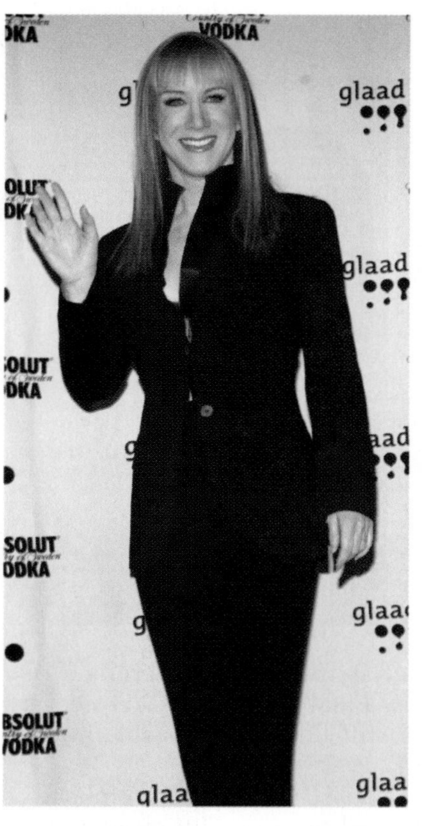

According to the American Society of Plastic Surgeons, liposuction is the most popular cosmetic surgery procedure for men and women, after rhinoplasty. Comedian and star of the television sitcom *Suddenly Susan* Kathy Griffin underwent liposuction in an attempt to drop from a size 4 to a size 2. Medical complications during and after the surgery, as she recounts in an article published by *Glamour* magazine, proved to be nearly fatal. Have you ever considered undergoing cosmetic surgery in pursuit of your ideal body? Do you think the benefits outweigh the risks?

surgical procedure in 2002, with about 373,000 performed. This was an 11% increase since 1997. Liposuction on a single location has an average total cost of $3,500, with a range of $2,000–$10,000, a cost not usually covered by insurance.

As liposuction has become more popular, the number of inexperienced practitioners has grown. If the procedure is to be done, it must be done by a skillful, trained professional. Even in the most skilled hands, liposuction is not risk-free. A few patients are left with scarring or rippling of the skin, and some need another procedure 6 to 12 months later to fix uneven results (Graham, 1997).

As we discussed in Chapter 4, breast implants have been around for quite a few years, but in the early 1990s a great debate surfaced about their safety. As of October 1998, Dow Corning, a maker of silicone-gel breast implants, agreed to compensate women who said they became unwell after the devices were implanted. Claims centered on the possibility of breast implants' causing systemic disease, potential ruptures or failure, and potential toxicity. Interestingly, this settlement, which affected more than 177,000 women, was reached even though studies of thousands of women turned up no solid evidence that implants caused ailments (Ault, 1998; Suhr, 1998). Manufacturers of breast implants have won the vast majority of breast implant verdicts in recent years, but the debate about their safety continues. To prevent the possible risks of silicone gel leakage, most breast implants now use saline (salt) solution in a silicone pouch.

cosmetic surgery
Surgery done for the sole purpose of improving the appearance.

rhinoplasty
Surgery done to change the shape of the nose.

Cosmetic surgery includes the procedures already mentioned, and there are also many other possibilities. Many people elect to have cosmetic surgery when a part of their body makes them self-conscious or uncomfortable. After surgery, many patients say they have a more positive self-image. Statistically, about 15–16% of the total number of cosmetic operations are done on men, and about 6% are done on African Americans—up from 4% in 1992 (Zimmer, 1998; American Society of Plastic Surgeons, 2003).

Another common procedure is **rhinoplasty** (surgery done to change the shape of the nose). It usually takes 1 to 2 hours, costs from $3,000–$12,000, and averages about $4,500. It is not covered by insurance unless the nose structure impedes breathing. As with any surgery, there can be undesirable results. The patient may not like the aesthetic result and want a revision, the newly formed nose may make breathing difficult, or fibrous scar tissue may form. In 2002 more than 354,000 rhinoplasty procedures were performed (Zimmer, 1998; American Society of Plastic Surgeons, 2003).

Breast augmentation was the second most frequent cosmetic surgical procedure (about 250,000 cases) performed in 2002, up 147% since 1997 (American Society of Aesthetic Plastic Surgery, 2003). The average total cost was $6,000.

More men are turning to implants to enhance their pectoral muscles (Miller, 2002). Putting in a pair of palm-size silicone discs can cost from

$4,000 to $10,000. It takes less than 2 hours and is usually performed in a doctor's office under general anesthesia. This is a relatively new procedure, but many experts feel there will be a lot more pectoral implants in coming years. In 2002 nearly 1 million American men elected to have cosmetic surgery.

The top 5 procedures may be listed differently depending upon the source. For example, one study listed the top 5 procedures for men as being nose reshaping, liposuction, eyelid surgery, hair transplantation, and breast reduction (Miller, 2002). The American Society of Plastic Surgeons (2003) listed the top 5 for men as being nose reshaping, liposuction, eyelid surgery, hair transplantation, and ear surgery. For women, the top 5 were breast augmentation, liposuction, nose reshaping, eyelid surgery, and face lift. The overall top 5 were nose reshaping, liposuction, breast augmentation, eyelid surgery, and face lift.

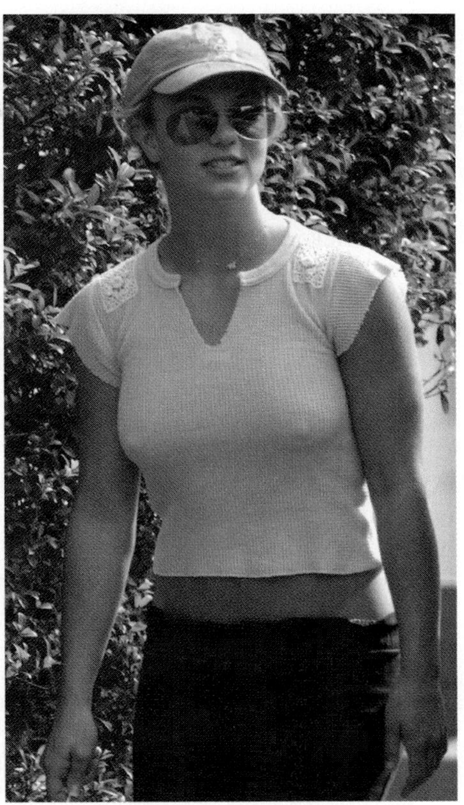

Young girls emulate superstars like Britney Spears, who in 1999 had breast augmentation surgery. In fact, according to the American Society of Plastic and Reconstructive Surgeons, 3,095 girls age 18 and younger had breast implants in 2002, up 19% from 2001 and up 59% from 1999. Breast augmentation surgery is the most common cosmetic surgery procedure for women, with 236,888 operations performed in 2002. Interestingly, most of the surgeries take place in California, Texas, and Florida—why do think that is the case?

Some women want breast implants; others want to have large, heavy breasts reduced in size. This procedure may not necessarily be considered cosmetic surgery, depending on the intention and the situation, because it may be performed to relieve physical ailments such as back and neck pain caused by large, heavy breasts. It involves removal of fat and breast tissue and may leave noticeable scars. The procedure may also affect the ability to breastfeed. It usually takes 2 to 4 hours and costs $5,000–$10,000, and may be covered by insurance if medical problems are associated with the size of the breasts. In 2002 about 115,000 breast reductions were performed on females, an increase of 147% since 1997 (Zimmer, 1998; American Society of Aesthetic Plastic Surgery, 2003).

tummy tuck
Extensive surgical procedure that removes excess skin and fat from the abdomen.

Whereas liposuction only removes fat, the **tummy tuck** is a more extensive surgical procedure that removes excess skin and fat from the lower abdomen and tightens the abdominal muscles. It usually requires a hip-to-hip lower-abdominal incision and takes 1 to 2 hours to complete if fat deposits are below the navel. If a more extensive procedure is needed, it can take 2 to 5 hours. It costs $5,000–$9,000, with an average total cost of $6,400, usually not covered by insurance (Zimmer, 1998; American Society of Aesthetic Plastic Surgery, 2003).

Other available procedures include face lifts, upper and lower eyelid reduction, and chin implantation. In short, we can have just about any part of our body altered if we are strongly motivated and have the means to pay for it. Because it is legal in most U.S. states for any physician to advertise him- or herself as a plastic or cosmetic surgeon, candidates for surgery must select a well-trained plastic surgeon for any type of cosmetic surgery.

Several trends indicate that cosmetic surgery will continue to be a growth industry. Younger people are getting more cosmetic procedures, people who have had cosmetic procedures tend to have others, men are becoming more "vain" and the number getting surgery has doubled since 1992, and the aging of the population is likely to result in more cosmetic surgery (Grant, 2001).

The top 5 nonsurgical procedures in 2002 were botulinum toxin injection (Botox) with 1.6 million procedures, up 2,356% since 1997; chemical peel (using a chemical solution to peel away the skin's top layers) with 1.4 million procedures, up 118% since 1997; collagen injection (to plump up creased or sunken facial skin or add fullness to lips) with 1.1 million procedures; microdermabrasion (mechanical scraping of top layers of the skin to soften sharp edges of surface irregularities) with 915,000 procedures; and laser hair removal with 855,000 cases. Overall, baby boomers aged 35–50 years had the most procedures (44%). Men and women aged 51–64 years had 25% of the procedures, those aged 19–34 years had 22%, and those 65 and older had 5%. Those age 18 and under had 3.5% of all cosmetic procedures (American Society of Aesthetic Plastic Surgery, 2003).

Finally, body piercing has been used by some people to enhance their body image. No longer a practice carried out in back rooms, body piercing is making its way into socially acceptable studios. Although many people have questioned the motivations behind body piercing, Myers (1992) reported that many who use body piercing are "sane, successful people." He reported that body piercing in the United States seems to function by giving people a strong sense of self and a connection with others by marking relationship events in commitment ceremonies, by enhancing people's feelings about their body, by providing the rush of the piercing experience, and by giving people a way to rebel against mainstream society. The most common places for body piercing are the face or ears; some people pierce their tongues, nipples, abdomen, and genitals. This practice is not risk-free; it sometimes produces infection.

Discussion Questions

1. Explain how media have created an unrealistic body image for women and men.
2. What strategies can be used to create a more positive body image?
3. What problems, both physical and psychological, occur when people try to make themselves more "perfect"?

Application Questions

Reread the story that opens the chapter and answer the following questions:

1. As do many teens, Marc had a poor body image. Teased by his friends ("Ostrich Boy") and haunted by the images in men's magazines, he turned to lifting weights. If you had a chance to talk to a group of 14-year-old boys, what advice would you give them on how to handle body-image issues? What about a group of 14-year-old girls?
2. One of the problems about weight lifting to improve body image is that you can "never be too big." The more muscle you gain, the more you strive for. Although Marc looks large by most people's standards, he is dwarfed in the photo with Mr. Olympia Ronnie Coleman. But as goals are set higher, workouts require more time in the gym, more sleep for recovery, and more time for eating properly. How is it possible to manage the desire for continued physical improvement without becoming obsessive?
3. Consider the changes in Marc's body image as he goes to law school, gets a job, gets married, has children, and so on. How might Marc's body image change across time? If he suddenly found himself divorced and single at age 40 years, should he hit the weights again?

Critical Thinking Questions

1. Because excessive weight has been linked to many health problems, why should we all not strive to be thin? Is it more harmful to diet excessively or to be obese?
2. You are an assistant college coach. An athlete returns from summer vacation, having put on 30 pounds of muscle. He says he spent the summer "lifting his ass off." You think he may have used steroids. Would you report him to the school's athletic director? (If he were found to have taken steroids, he could be expelled from school. However, if he continued to use steroids, he could suffer serious medical problems.)
3. Would your answer to question 2 be different if a female athlete returned in the fall with an additional 15 pounds of muscle? Explain your answer.
4. The noted eating-disorder psychologist G. Terence Wilson has stated that, biologically, women cannot be thin and have large breasts. Yet many women exercise and diet until they have low body fat and then have breast implants to compensate. Role models for the thin-yet-busty type include professional bodybuilders, many of the athletes on daytime TV exercise shows, and many actresses. How do such role models affect women?

Critical Thinking Case

Before attending college, your girlfriend Amanda ran cross-country and track. But with the pressures of college studies, part-time work, and your relationship, she has little time to exercise. She has started to worry more and more about the "freshman 15," the extra weight that many college freshmen gain. She often comments on how good the cover girls on fashion magazines look. That is not all: You have noticed she rarely eats when you go out. When you mention this, she says she is trying to help save money for a vacation. When you find over-the-counter diet pills hidden under her bed, she says, "Everyone takes them." When you tell her that someone heard her throwing up in the bathroom after meals, she flatly denies it. When you tell her she is looking "rather thin," she smiles and says, "Thank you."

You have read the DSM-IV diagnoses in this chapter and do not believe that she has an eating disorder. However, you are concerned about Amanda's physical health and psychological well-being. How could you help her to improve her body image?

Exploring Personal Dimensions

Body Image

How do you feel about the appearance of these regions of your body?

	Quite satisfied	Somewhat satisfied	Somewhat dissatisfied	Very dissatisfied
Hair	❑	❑	❑	❑
Arms	❑	❑	❑	❑
Hands	❑	❑	❑	❑
Feet	❑	❑	❑	❑
Waist	❑	❑	❑	❑
Buttocks	❑	❑	❑	❑
Hips	❑	❑	❑	❑
Legs and ankles	❑	❑	❑	❑
Thighs	❑	❑	❑	❑
Chest/breasts	❑	❑	❑	❑
Posture	❑	❑	❑	❑
General attractiveness	❑	❑	❑	❑

1. Which of your thoughts and actions enhance your body image?
2. Which of your thoughts and actions are detrimental to your body image?
3. What societal forces (expectations of friends and parents, advertising, celebrities and professional athletes, etc.) influence your body image most strongly?
4. What could you do to become more satisfied with your body image?

Sexuality Online

Go to the web component for *Exploring the Dimensions of Human Sexuality* at sexuality.jbpub.com for web exercises, additional resources related to this chapter, and student review tools.

American Society of Asethetic Plastic Surgery, 2003. [Online]. Available: http://surgery.org/statistics.html.

American Society of Plastic Surgeons, 2003. [Online]. Available: www.plasticsurgery.org.

CHAPTER 6

Gender Dimensions

FEATURES

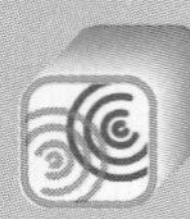

Communication Dimensions
Men Are from Mars; Women Are from Venus

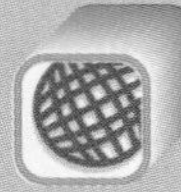

Global Dimensions
The Oppression of Women

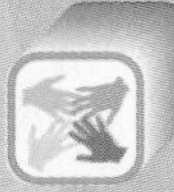

Multicultural Dimensions
How the Economy Affects Gender Equality

Gender Dimensions
Gender Equality on the College Campus

Ethical Dimensions
Extreme Sex Roles—The Price of Honor

Ethical Dimensions
Should Dad Dress As a Woman?

Gender Dimensions
Is There Gender Equality in College Sports?

CHAPTER OBJECTIVES

1. Describe the biological, psychological, and sociocultural differences between males and females.

2. Explain the effects of gender identity, sex roles, and sex stereotypes on sexuality.

3. Analyze how the women's movement has affected both females and males.

sexuality.jbpub.com

Gender and Health
Global Dimensions: The Oppression of Women
Ethical Dimensions: Extreme Sex Roles—Price of Honor
The Women's Movement

INTRODUCTION

When Mark attended college in the late 1970s, he thought all the talk about sex differences was bunk. Men and women appeared to share equal places in classrooms and in faculty positions. Women appeared to have the same opportunities as men in the outside work world. He and his classmates believed that the wage gap and glass ceiling were things that past generations dealt with. Those were the days.

But Mark still remembers one college guest speaker—a distinguished American composer. During his speech, the aging composer asserted that women were not good composers because their social upbringing left them devoid of technical skills. He told the stunned audience—among whom sat several prominent female composers—that boys take things apart and put things together, while girls play with dolls. Therefore, boys grow up with more technical abilities, which to him included the ability to orchestrate music. It seemed that everyone in attendance wrote off his comments as those of an elderly man from another era.

But as Mark joined the workforce, married, and had children, he began to witness more and more sex differences and biases. As the years passed by, the number of female friends who had experienced sexism in the workplace grew from none to all of them. *It became clear that women and men did communicate differently, manage differently, work differently, play differently.*

In Mark's marriage, gender roles have been reversed—because of work situations, not a deliberate decision. While his spouse works a managerial "nine-to-five job" (read, 7:00 A.M. to 6:00 P.M.), Mark writes and edits out of his home. He is responsible for raising two young children and for doing most household jobs. Because children cannot be ignored, he often has to put off work until they are in bed.

Mark has become keenly aware of the sex differences among parents. At his son's independent school, where most students' mothers do not have a job, he is one of the few fathers who take the child to school, go to parent–teacher conferences, and volunteer for various events. This creates quite a dilemma in friendships: While playing both the mother and father role, he really does not fit into either group. Mark also notes that teachers react differently to him: When several mothers voiced a complaint to a teacher, the teacher spoke to them directly; however, the teacher would only communicate with Mark in the presence of a senior administrator.

Suprisingly, sex biases exist even among medical professionals. At his son's first pediatric appointment, the male doctor's first question was a stern "Where is the child's mother?" Some years later, during a hospital emergency room visit, the doctors and nurses clearly listened to every small comment his spouse made—yet brushed off Mark's input as insignificant.

As Mark's experience shows, gender plays a role in many aspects of our lives—at home, at work, and in our social activities. We develop a sexual identity, which is the outgrowth of the interaction of biology—being male or female—and social learning. Society's expectations for the behavior of men and women are conveyed to the individual by a process called socialization, *which has a dominant influence on gender roles. As children model adults' behaviors, these sex roles are perpetuated, though traditional gender roles are changing as a broader range of behaviors is accepted by society.*

If someone asked you whether you were a woman or a man, your first thought would probably be, What a ridiculous question! You know what gender I am. Still, that question might lead you to ask other questions about gender, such as, How did I learn to act as a man or woman? To what extent is my masculinity or femininity natural, and to what extent is it learned? Are my personal characteristics determined or influenced by my gender? In this chapter we explore some of the forces that influence our conceptions of ***masculinity*** *and* ***femininity.***

masculinity
Those qualities characteristic of and suitable for boys and men according to the rules and expectations of a society.

femininity
Those qualities characteristic of and suitable for girls and women according to the rules and expectations of a society.

Gender Differences

When sex differences and similarities are considered, discussions often center on "nature versus nurture." Those who argue from a nature perspective attribute most characteristics to biological differences or similarities. Those who argue more for nurture believe that we become the way we are mostly as a result of social factors and learning. There are persuasive arguments on each side, and some people believe that a combination of nature and nurture makes us the way we are.

People learn attitudes and values and have their personal experiences in a "gendered world." All societies, however, do not deal with gender issues equally. Compared with less-industrialized societies, for example, modern Western societies are less gendered in terms of occupational roles, child care, clothing styles, and certain social and recreational activities (Tiefer & Kring, 1995).

We will discuss some sex differences related to attitude and behavior. Caution is needed when considering such differences, however, because there are

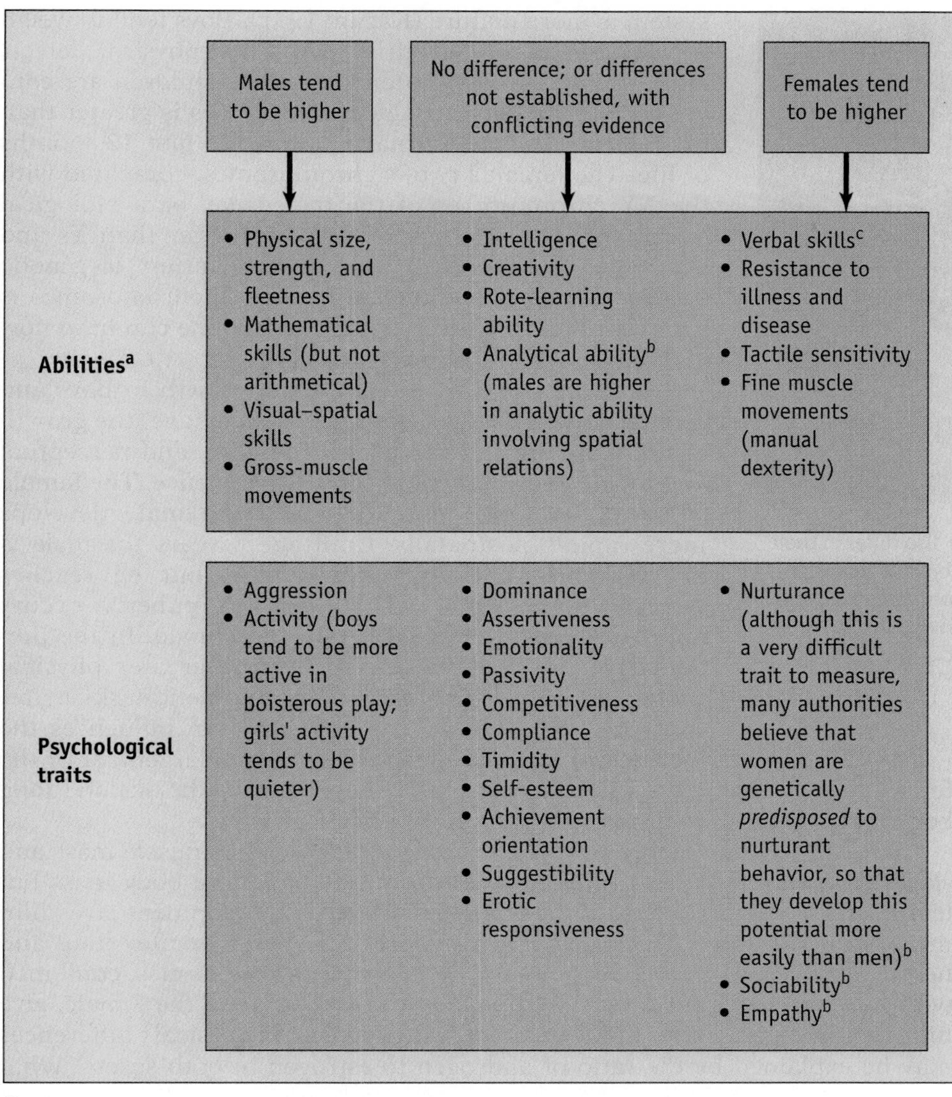

	Males tend to be higher	No difference; or differences not established, with conflicting evidence	Females tend to be higher
Abilities[a]	• Physical size, strength, and fleetness • Mathematical skills (but not arithmetical) • Visual–spatial skills • Gross-muscle movements	• Intelligence • Creativity • Rote-learning ability • Analytical ability[b] (males are higher in analytic ability involving spatial relations)	• Verbal skills[c] • Resistance to illness and disease • Tactile sensitivity • Fine muscle movements (manual dexterity)
Psychological traits	• Aggression • Activity (boys tend to be more active in boisterous play; girls' activity tends to be quieter)	• Dominance • Assertiveness • Emotionality • Passivity • Competitiveness • Compliance • Timidity • Self-esteem • Achievement orientation • Suggestibility • Erotic responsiveness	• Nurturance (although this is a very difficult trait to measure, many authorities believe that women are genetically *predisposed* to nurturant behavior, so that they develop this potential more easily than men)[b] • Sociability[b] • Empathy[b]

Notes
[a]Sex-linked abilities not indicated here are the four biological imperatives (gestation, lactation, and menstruation in the female, and sperm production in the male).
[b]These abilities and traits are especially controversial. Men tend to be superior in analyzing problems related to manipulating objects in space; some authorities find that more women than men are predisposed to being nurturant by their genetic programming—some judge emotions and expressions better than men.
[c]It is curious that although most writers, orators, and newscasters are men, girls score higher on tests of verbal ability, and remedial reading and writing programs enroll far more boys than girls. Either verbal ability in children is not related to later professional verbal skills, or cultural factors (opportunity and expectation) must explain this phenomenon.
Source: Sexton, L. *The individual, marriage, and the family,* 4th ed. Belmont, CA: Wadsworth, 1980.

FIGURE 6.1 Sex-linked differences in abilities and in physical and psychological traits.

many variations in these attitudes and behaviors. Overgeneralizing can result in inappropriate stereotypes. At the same time, extensive data suggest that, on average, each gender has an undercurrent, a melody, a theme (Fisher, 1992).

Developmental Differences

There is no question that males and females differ biologically in more than their physical structure and biological function (Figure 6.1). Developmentally girls are more advanced than boys at birth—that is, their central nervous

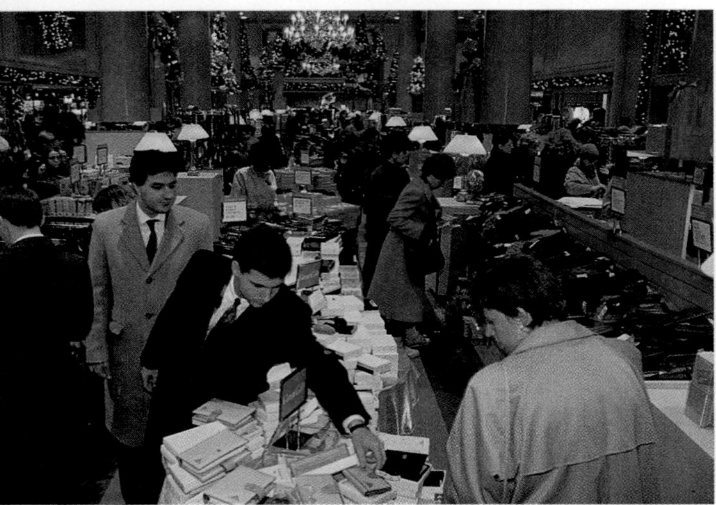

According to a 1998 study, men and women also differ in their reaction to holiday shopping. All 36 male subjects showed a dramatic increase in blood pressure when confronted with crowds and lines. But one in four females showed increased blood pressure. What physiological, psychological, and social factors would cause such a result?

system is more mature (Kagan, 1971). Boys tend to weigh more when born, but girls have fewer physical defects and a higher survival rate. More male children are conceived, but the miscarriage rate for males is greater than for females, and more males die in the first 12 months of life. The female's two X chromosomes, compared with the XY chromosomes of the male, may be a biological advantage. The X chromosomes are larger than Ys and can supply the female with a greater variety of genetic material. Even if one of the female's X chromosomes is a carrier of genetic defects, the second one can have normal genes that offset any genetic defect.

In infancy and early childhood, growth in boys and girls is similar. The development of language, the growth of body organs and the nervous system, and perceptual and motor development proceed in sequence. The female is more developed prenatally, but the male develops more rapidly postnatally. Until age 8 years the male is heavier and taller than the female, but he reaches puberty more slowly. The onset of puberty occurs approximately 2 years earlier in the female. In the preadolescent period the female, having greater physical maturity, can perform physical and athletic tasks better than the male. With menarche, estrogen influences the increase of **adipose** (fat) tissues and enlargement of the female pelvis. Eventually the estrogen prevents growth in the skeletal long bones, and height stabilizes for girls at about age 17 years.

adipose
Pertaining to fat tissue in the body.

When the male reaches puberty, androgen increases his muscle mass and skeletal development, and thus the adolescent boy has more body mass but less fat than the girl. This androgenic effect on male development gives him more strength and more speed. Furthermore, the male's greater lung and heart capacity and greater capacity for oxygen transport to tissues, combined with his predisposition toward being taller and heavier than the female, give him more power. Harris (1976) states, "The degree of [physical] differences may be explained by the ratio of androgen to estrogen in both sexes." What that means for an individual's physical activity is not fixed. Harris goes on to point out, "Training, coaching, and experience can alter one's inherent capacity for physical performance."

Sex and Abilities

Eleanor Maccoby and Carol Jacklin (1974) examined much of the research on the influence of sex on abilities. They found that, until early adolescence, boys and girls have similar verbal abilities. At 11 or 12 years of age, however, females have greater abilities in language and verbal tasks, whereas males perform better than females in visual–spatial tasks. This visual–spatial difference in performance persists into adulthood (see Figure 6.2).

More recently, it has become clearer that, on average, girls speak sooner than boys. They use more words and are more grammatically accurate. By age 10 years, girls are better at foreign languages. They also excel at verbal reasoning, written prose, verbal memory, pronunciation, and spelling. Although there can be a wide range of differences, on average, women show more verbal skills than men (Fisher, 1992).

Whether boys have more highly developed mathematical abilities than girls is still debated. Certainly boys' mathematical skills increase rapidly at adolescence and into adulthood, whereas girls experience no such rapid jump,

(a) Problem-Solving Tasks Favoring Women

Women tend to perform better than men on tests of perceptual speed, in which subjects must rapidly identify matching items—for example, pairing the house on the far left with its twin:

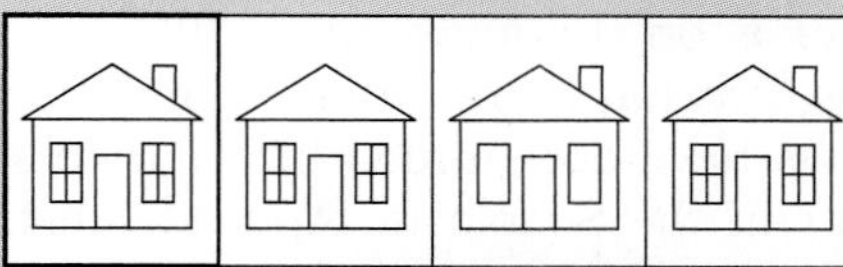

In addition, women remember whether an object, or a series of objects, has been displaced:

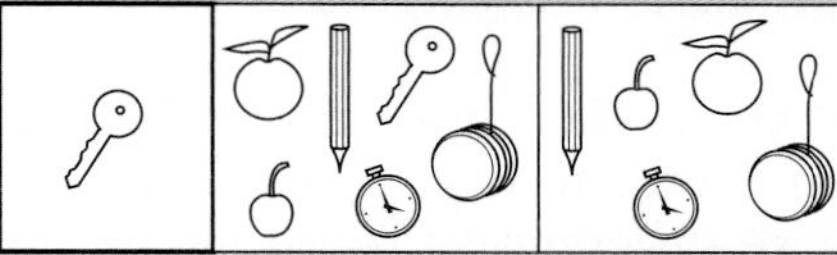

On some tests of ideational fluency, for example, those in which subjects must list objects that are the same color, and on tests of verbal fluency, in which participants must list words that begin with the same letter, women also outperform men:

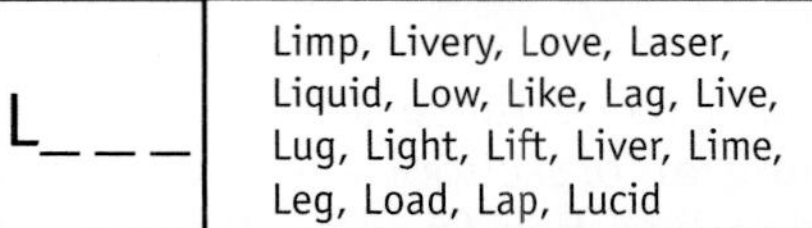

Women do better on precision manual tasks—that is, those involving fine-motor coordination—such as placing the pegs in holes on a board:

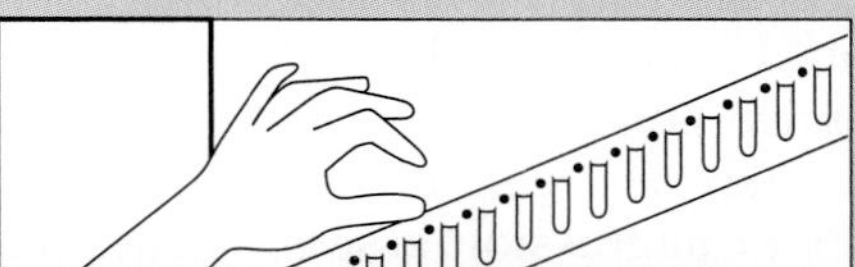

And women do better than men on mathematical calculation tests:

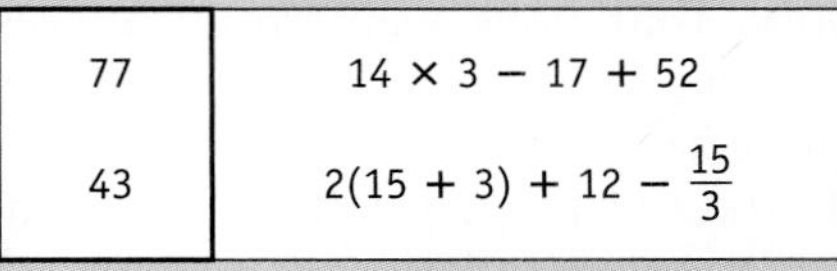

(b) Problem-Solving Tasks Favoring Men

Men tend to perform better than women on certain spatial tasks. They do well on tests that involve mentally rotating an object or manipulating it in some fashion, such as imagining turning this three-dimensional object:

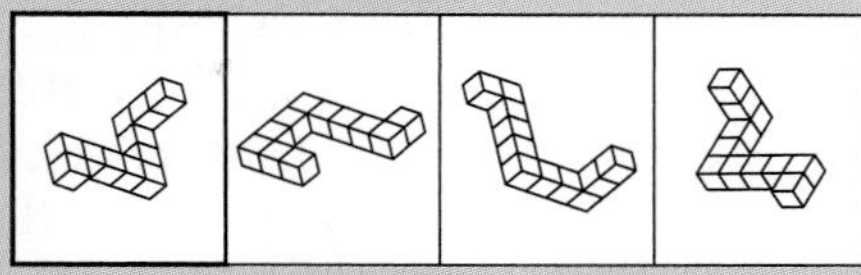

or determining where the holes punched in a folded piece of paper will fall when the paper is unfolded:

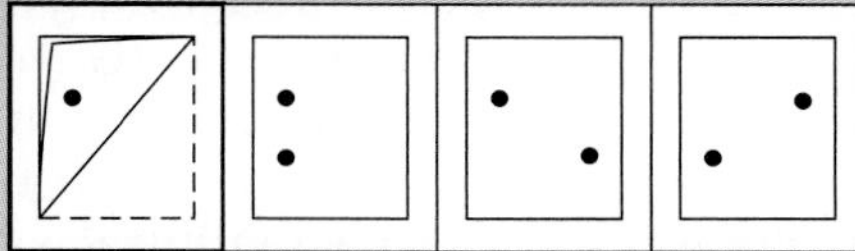

Men also are more accurate than women in target-directed motor skills, such as guiding or intercepting projectiles:

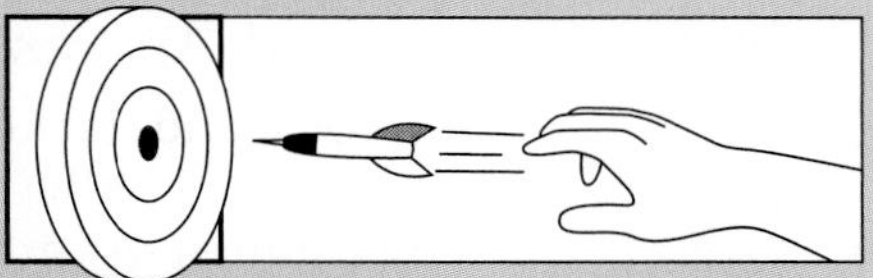

They also do better on disembedding tests, in which they have to find a simple shape, such as the one on the left, once it is hidden within a more complex figure:

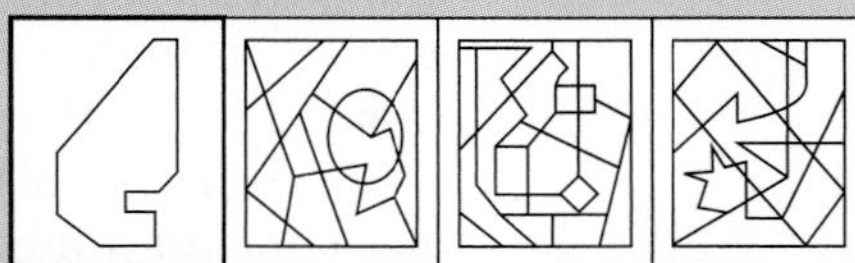

And men tend to do better than women on tests of mathematical reasoning:

1,100	If only 60% of seedlings will survive, how many must be planted to obtain 660 trees?

FIGURE 6.2 Problem-solving tasks for women and men. Research suggests that some problem-solving tasks may demonstrate gender-related performance differentiation.
Source: Kimura, D. Sex differences in the brain, *Scientific American, 267* (1992), 188–195.

but historically mathematics was perceived as a masculine area of study in which girls were not expected or encouraged to excel. Further, mathematics was viewed as necessary to so-called male careers and not particularly useful or necessary for female careers. Because many females were raised to believe that they cannot or should not succeed in this subject area, their performances on math measures tend not to be high or, if high, have been neither developed nor regarded as a source of pride, pleasure, or opportunity. Beginning in the 1970s, however, there were indications that females' perceptions of their ability to master mathematics were changing. A study found an increase in the number of females enrolling in mathematics courses. This rise could in turn lead increasing numbers of women to enter the engineering and science fields, breaking down the belief that these career areas are "unfeminine" (Girls interested in mathematics is on the increase, 1980).

It does seem that men, on average, excel at higher mathematical problems (not at arithmetic). Seventh-grade boys have done much better than seventh-grade girls on mathematical problems in the Scholastic Aptitude Test. In the United States, 75% of the PhDs in math are awarded to men (Fisher, 1992).

Whatever the cause, in tests of 12th graders' cognitive abilities, boys outnumber girls by five to four in both the top 10% and the bottom 10% of performers with girls bunched in the middle. Similar results occur with other examinations (Guyot, 2001).

Does this mean that biology is destiny when it comes to these abilities? No, because even though each gender seems to have specific abilities, there are also cultural explanations for these differences. These include teachers' assumptions and their treatment of students, parents' attitudes toward their children, the perception of society that math has been for males, each gender's self-perception and ambitions, and social pressures on adolescents—just to name some possibilities.

Sex and Aggression

Maccoby and Jacklin (1974) found boys to be more aggressive both physically and verbally than girls, beginning at preschool age. Male aggression, they claimed, is aimed at other males rather than females. Rape would seem to be an obvious exception, but Maccoby and Jacklin did not include it in their study. Boys and men remain aggressive into their college-age years, but with maturity this trait diminishes. The researchers found that even though some parents believe boys to be more aggressive than girls, these parents do not place a high value on aggression. In fact there is evidence that boys are punished more than girls for aggressive behavior.

Hyde (1984) also reported that there are gender differences in aggression. After an analysis of 143 studies of aggression assessing the magnitude of gender differences, she found that, for all types of aggression, males were more aggressive than females.

In a study of aggressiveness in Japan, the Philippines, Mexico, Kenya, India, and New England, it was found that boys were more aggressive in each culture. Nurturing is often considered to be the female counterpart to male aggressiveness. Many women of every ethnic group and culture around the world show more interest in infants and more tolerance of their needs. Some people would like to attribute this female nurturance to learned behavior, but it seems there is also a biological foundation (Fisher, 1992).

Domestic violence in the United States continues to be a major problem. Whereas most forms of violence have decreased in recent years, acts of violence against women by a male intimate or acquaintance have remained constant and may be increasing (May, 1998). A lot of men know they are bigger and stronger than their female counterparts on the job or at home, and they apparently see nothing wrong with using this difference to their advantage.

Tavris (2002) provided a different view related to female aggression. She pointed out that many recent authors have written about hidden and formerly secret female aggressiveness. She said that girls are not sweeter than boys, but just as bad, sexual, and aggressive—maybe even meaner, given the ruthless and sneaky ways they control each other. For example, our culture refuses girls access to open conflict, and it forces their aggression into nonphysical, indirect, and covert forms. Girls use backbiting, exclusion, rumors, name calling, and manipulation to inflict psychological pain on targeted victims. Boys, in short, resort to physical aggression; girls, to "relational" aggression.

Anger and aggression are learned behaviors and are characteristic of humans. Traditionally they have been viewed as more appropriate for males than for females; however, as we move toward humanism and less-defined parameters of what is male and what is female, we must reevaluate our cultural acceptance of these behaviors.

Sex and Health

There also appear to be differences in males' and females' health attitudes and behavior. Taking action to prevent health problems is more common among women than men. Men tend to rely on their spouses for social support related to their health, but women are more inclined to turn to friends and their children. Women report an average of 13.5 days per year when illness required a reduction in usual activity, but men report only 6.7 such days. In general, women live longer than men, but they also experience more health problems and make more extensive use of health services (Kandrick, Grant, & Segall, 1991).

Only a minority of patients prefer a medical care provider of a particular sex, but when there is a preference, males show less sex preference than females. Women do have a clear female preference in the fields of general practice and gynecology, because of the intimate nature of the clinical intervention. Men with a preference wanted male surgeons, neurologists, and internists. Both men and women preferred female social workers, nurses, obstetricians, and midwives (Kerssens, Bensing, & Andela, 1997).

Females are significantly more likely than males to receive prescriptions for antibiotics (Sayer & Britt, 1997). It is hard to know whether this occurs because physicians are more likely to prescribe antibiotics for females or because females request them more frequently.

Also, sex-role identity is related to an individual's decision whether to engage in behaviors that affect health. College males with an androgynous gender-role identity (meaning they scored above the median on psychological tests for both masculinity and femininity) engaged in healthier behaviors more often than males scoring above the median in only masculine or feminine psychological characteristics (Baffi, et al., 1991).

Another sex issue related to health is that most health insurance plans provide coverage for prescription drugs, but many plans exclude coverage for prescription contraceptives (Arndorfer, 1998). This can result in an extra financial burden on women and also make it more likely that some will use less-effective contraceptive methods—making unwanted pregnancy more likely.

On an international level, Guptka (2001) pointed out that power imbalance increases HIV risk. For example, in many societies there is a culture of silence surrounding sexuality that dictates that "good" women are expected to be ignorant about sexual behavior and passive in sexual interactions. This makes it difficult for women to be informed about HIV risk reduction and, even if informed, to be proactive in negotiating safer sexual activity. In addition, the traditional norm of virginity for unmarried females increases young women's risk of infection, because it restricts their ability to ask for information about sexuality because of fear that they will be thought to be sexually active. In cultures in which virginity is highly valued, some young women practice alternative sexual behaviors, such as anal intercourse, to preserve their virginity. These behaviors may place them at increased risk of HIV. Accessing treatment services for STIs can be highly stigmatizing for women. Finally, using barrier methods as safer options for sexual activity can be a dilemma for women in societies in which motherhood is considered to be a feminine ideal.

Some people think health care delivery and research benefit men at the expense of women. They feel that heart disease has been studied more in men and that women have been excluded in major national clinical studies. Others feel that women have benefited from medical research, as shown by improvements in breast cancer research as well as developments in laparoscopic surgery and ultrasound that were initially used on women's bodies (Daniel & Levine, 2001).

There are also some sex differences related to sexual satisfaction and health. Although both males and females rate sexual satisfaction as very important to a person's quality of life, if there are sexual problems 57% of the women thought that women would be blamed most often. Only 37% of the men said that. Among women, 81% feared that a physician would blame sexual problems on a "head" problem, whereas this concerned only 60% of the men (Recer, 1999).

Males and females show similar degrees of physical and emotional satisfaction with their sexual partnerships. For example, 46.6% of men and 40.5% of women reported they were extremely physically satisfied with their partner. Extreme emotional satisfaction was reported by 41.8% of males and 38.7% of females. These similarities exist even though 75% of males and only 28.6% of females reported they always had an orgasm during sexual activity. There were also no real differences in the number of men (90.2%) and women (87.5%) who reported themselves to be in excellent or good health (Laumann, et al., 1994).

gender role
Complex groups of ways males and females are expected to behave in a given culture.

It has even been proposed that **gender-role** expectations may relate to the expression of depressive symptoms. For example, among college students it has been found that females reported more emotional symptoms of depression than males. However, males reported more withdrawal and physical symptoms of depression than females (Oliver & Toner, 1990).

Kluger (2003) reported that twice as many women as men suffer from depression and twice as many men suffer from alcoholism. Similarly, women tend to be more prone to anxiety disorders, and men are more likely to have conditions stemming from impulsiveness and violence.

In recent decades it was found that men with a history of heart disease were two to four times more likely than females to die later of sudden cardiac death. However, now women heart attack survivors are becoming almost as likely as men to succumb to sudden cardiac death. This gender gap has narrowed a great deal (Sudden cardiac death gender gap closing in on women, 2002).

Men lead women in 12 of the 15 causes of death in the United States and die an average of 5.4 years earlier than women. In 1920 the difference was just 2 years. Although some of this gender gap may be due to biological differences, many experts now believe that much of the gap is due to inattention to men's health—from society and from men themselves. For many years there has been special attention given to women's health, but there has been no similar emphasis on men's health. There has not been a government Office of Men's Health to match the similarly named office for women. In addition, women are more likely than men to get routine preventive care; men give up on treatment plans and discontinue medications sooner than women do; men tend to see themselves as invulnerable to pain; and men's stoic attitude may further harm health by magnifying the effects of stress (Why men die younger than women, 2002).

An interesting gender twist related to nutrition has occurred. Supermarket aisles are filling up with nutrient-rich female-friendly treats (Winters, 2001). There was a nutrition bar called "Luna" decorated with silhouetted dancing girls and packed with ingredients that women are supposed to need. It quickly became the top-selling bar in natural food stores. Then there was a line of breakfast cereals from Zoe foods produced by a woman who wanted to make granola for women who were like her menopausal mother. General Mills produces Harmony cereal for women, and Quaker has a Nutrition for Women oatmeal. These new foods have in common that they are supposed to have nutrients that benefit women in particular. Manufacturers are trying to appeal as much to women's emotional needs as to their dietary ones. In reality, the basic laws of nutrition still apply to both men and women.

Sex and Dating

When it comes to dating, females assume that many males will attempt to deceive them, but males do not seem to feel that females will deceive them. Females are especially sensitive to the possibility of deception if males are attempting to persuade them to participate in sexual behavior. Females, who bear the greater risk in reproduction, are more cautious about mating (Keenan, Gallup, & Goulet, 1997).

What is the effect of sex on emotional reactions to termination of a romantic relationship among college students? Women tend to feel more joy and relief than men, men and women are equally likely to blame themselves for break-ups, women are more likely than men to blame their partner, and men are more likely to distract themselves with other activities, such as work or sports (Choo, Levine, & Hatfield, 1996).

Communication DIMENSIONS

Men Are from Mars; Women Are from Venus

John Gray, the author of the bestseller *Men Are from Mars, Women Are from Venus,* explains one reason why men and women may sometimes be frustrated in communicating with each other. He says women expand, and men contract. By this he means that women are likely to expand a topic, whereas men want them to get to the point. For example, he says that generally when a man speaks he has already silently mulled over his thought until he knows the main idea he wants to communicate. Then he speaks. A woman, in contrast (according to Gray), does not necessarily speak to make a point; speaking assists her in discovering her point. When she explores her thoughts and feelings out loud, she figures out where she wants to go.

For example, a man may want to pull away and take a little time to mull over his thoughts so he knows what he wants to say. However, a woman may find greater clarity by expanding and sharing. When she begins sharing, she is not necessarily aware of where it will take her, but she is confident it will take her where she needs to go. For her, this is a process of self-discovery.

It is important for both men and women to understand these potential differences. Mutual support, and some nurturing, can go a long way toward improving communication.

Source: Gray, J. *Men, women and relationships.* New York: Harper Paperbacks, 1996.

Two issues related to sex and dating are frequency of sexual behavior and number of partners. Common sense would indicate that, on average, heterosexual men and women would have equal numbers of sexual partners. However, males consistently report more partners than females do. Is this because men are inclined to exaggerate sexual experience, and women to minimize it? Because people have faulty memories? Or because women and men view sexual activity differently? For example, some research on sexual satisfaction has assumed that coital orgasm was the goal for both partners. A focus on the male sex drive may have created a different perspective among males and females, and even a sense among women that they fall short sexually (Miller, 1999).

Power is fundamental to both sexuality and gender. Typically, men have been more powerful in relationships. Therefore, in sexual behavior male pleasure often supersedes female pleasure and men have greater control than women over when, where, and how sexual behavior takes place (Gupta, 2001).

The nature of intimacy can also be a factor related to male–female relationships. Women often derive intimacy from talking and may express disappointment if men do not verbally share their problems, express their emotions, or listen to theirs. Men are more likely to define emotional closeness as working or playing side by side (Fisher, 1992).

One interesting development related to dating, at least among some successful women, is the lesser boyfriend (Tan, 2001). Some women, such as Julia Roberts, Jennifer Lopez, and Ann Heche chose less successful beaus. Today's modern woman often works and is financially independent. Some feel this is true female empowerment. Therefore, women can make a choice among men based on personality, as opposed to making a choice only within the group of men who earn as much or more. Also, in the case of celebrities, his career is not as important as hers, so when they go out, she gets all the attention. Interestingly, Jennifer Lopez changed her mind, was divorced, and in 2003 she and Ben Affleck were considered by many to be Hollywood's hottest couple.

Other Gender Issues

Segell (1989) asked men and women what they talk about when they get together with their closest friends. Men reported work issues, sports, and goals for the future as the top three topics, in that order. However, for women the top three were children, personal problems and self-doubts, and work issues.

Goleman (1998) reported on differences in what disturbed men and women. Qualities that disturbed women most about men were sexual demands (making her feel sexually used or trying to force sexual behavior), condescension (making her feel inferior or stupid), and emotional constriction and excess (hiding his emotions; drinking or smoking too much). Qualities that bothered men about women most were sexual rejection (being unresponsive to sexual advances; being a sexual tease), moodiness, and self-absorption (fussing over appearance; spending too much money on clothes).

Schwartz (1998) felt that the most important fact about today's men and women is how similar they have become. Similarity, however, introduces some new challenges: issues of equity (fairness between men and women), independence (survival has become less dependent on a lifetime, or even a part-time, union), and sexual desire (the sexual ability of men and women has been extended for many years).

The father's role at home is under negotiation. Research shows that when men take an active role in the details of running a home and raising children, they develop emotional sensitivities, avoid boastful and threatening behavior, and include women in community decision making. Increasing men's involvement in family work thus has the potential to increase women's public status and reduce men's propensity for violence (Coltrane, 1998).

Helen Fisher (Males, Females, and Evolution, 2001) mentioned other gender differences. She said men usually want to cut straight to the point; they do not like getting distracted by side issues. Women have a more contextual view of the world and see issues as part of a larger whole. Also, young males often take many more risks than young females do. Scientists think this may be linked to differing levels of a chemical in the brain. In addition, females are more likely than males to bear grudges, sometimes for a very long time.

Gender and the Workplace

It seems that men and women may even have different approaches to situations in which they are going to be evaluated, such as for job performance. Men may be more likely to respond to the competitive nature of such an evaluation and therefore develop a self-confident approach that leads them to deny the value of others' evaluations. Women, however, may be likely to approach such situations as opportunities to gain information about their abilities (Roberts, 1991).

Employment history may be another factor in gender-role attitudes. Employed women have been found to be less traditional in their views of women's appropriate roles than women who are not employed (Coverdill, Kraft, & Manley, 1996).

Christie Hefner, the chief executive officer of Playboy Enterprises, pointed out that gender is a factor in leadership styles, but there are as many leadership differences among women as there are differences between men and women. She reported seeing highly autocratic women leaders and also very participatory, nurturing men leaders (Hefner, 1996).

An extensive study showed that women scored higher on orientation to production and getting results, and men scored higher on strategic planning and organizational vision. Women were seen as operating with more energy, intensity, and emotional expression; men were seen as more low-key and quiet through the control of emotional expression. Women were rated higher on people-oriented leadership skills, whereas men were rated higher on business-oriented leadership skills by bosses and peers (Do men and women lead differently? 2000).

Many people have assumed that women would rather work with and be supervised by other women, but some studies (Sachs, 2001) indicate that women can be each other's worst enemies on the job. According to such studies, women often betray and undermine one another; they damage other women's career aspirations; and they often fail to support other women—even actively undermining their authority and credibility. One theory is that for two women to forge a positive relationship, their self-esteem and power must be kept "dead even." When one woman gets more power, it sets off tensions and leads to hostility and sniping. One-third of the women in these studies said they would prefer a male boss.

Because more than half the women with babies younger than 1 year are in the workforce, increasing numbers of them want to breastfeed their infants. In response, more companies are meeting this need by setting up a private room and a work schedule so mothers can pump their breast milk (Luscombe, 2001). Some companies provide a private room, a hospital-grade pump, a carrying case for discreet transport of the pumping paraphernalia and expressed milk, plus bottles and access to a refrigerator. One company, Cigna, in which 80% of the workforce is female, saved about $240,000 a year in health care expenses for breastfeeding mothers and their children and another $60,000 through reduced absenteeism. This does not include the incalculable goodwill of happy new parents. In 2001 Illinois became the fourth state to enact legislation protecting a woman's right to express milk at work.

The relationship between salaries of men and salaries of women has long been of interest to some people. U.S. Census Bureau statistics indicate that in 2000 nearly 4.6 million men and 925,000 women were paid $100,000 or more (Thomas, 2001). Median earnings were $30,132 for men compared to $18,996 for women. That means the typical male worker received $158.62 for every $100.00 earned by a female. It is difficult to interpret the meaning of these data accurately, however, without knowing more about years of experience, academic preparation, levels of responsibility, and other variables that may influence salary levels.

Differences of salaries of men and women do not necessarily indicate that wage discrimination is rampant. For example, women tend to work fewer hours than men and women tend to make educational and occupational choices that will give them flexibility if they interrupt their careers for child rearing—even though they may earn less. Women without children make about 95% as much as men with similar jobs and experience (What gender gap? 2001).

Some men say the work atmosphere turns very chilly when they seek time off to care for infants or take their kids to doctors' appointments (Grimsley, 2002). A man in Maryland was awarded $665,000 after a long legal battle to protest the state's refusal to grant him parental leave to care for his ailing wife and their infant daughter. He said he was told, "God made women to have babies," and he should not ask for leave to care for his wife and daughter.

Although barriers to success in the workplace have frustrated women, conditions are changing. In 1900, most of the 21% of white women who were employed were confined mainly to textile and garment factories; almost all of the 41% of black women who had jobs were agricultural workers or servants. Today, many women wield power in small business. In the United States, nearly as many people work for women-owned businesses as are employed by Fortune 500 companies worldwide. Small businesses are often founded by women who have left corporations because they felt that the glass ceiling (an inability for women to be promoted to higher administrative levels) was impeding their progress. Today, 49% of the professional, managerial, and administrative workforce is women—and 86% of all Fortune 500 companies have at least one woman board member (Wellington, 1998).

Sex and Advertising

Many aspects of society contribute to our thinking about masculinity and femininity. For example, characters in MTV commercials, and those in music videos, are often stereotyped. Signorielli and associates (1994) found that female characters appeared less frequently, had more beautiful bodies, were more physically attractive, wore more sexy and skimpy clothing, and were more the object of another's gaze than their male counterparts.

Sex roles have been depicted in television commercials for many years. The authoritative male voice is still used in more than 90% of commercials. Since the 1950s, there has been a change in the images of women in commercials but not in men's images. Women are shown significantly more as representing managerial and professional occupations. They are much more likely to be pictured in job-related activity and in more diverse occupations than in the past. In contrast, images of men have changed little. There has been only a slight increase in the images of men parenting and a decrease in the images of men portrayed performing housework. It seems that commercial imagery has done little to change traditional expectations for men (Allan & Coltrane, 1996).

Sex bias in medical advertising may be one factor contributing to different treatment of women and men by physicians. Significantly more male than female patients were found in medical advertising. The facial expressions of men were likely to be serious or neutral, whereas the facial expressions of women were more often judged to be pleasant. These stereotypical portrayals may contribute to physicians' being less likely to take the symptoms of women, compared to those of men, seriously (Leppard, Ogletree, & Wallen, 1993).

Have there been changes in masculine and feminine traits over time? An analysis of 59 studies done since 1973 indicates that women have increasingly reported masculine-stereotyped personality traits as characteristic of themselves. These changes may be the result of a cultural shift whereby women's work and professional roles have changed since the studies began (Twenge, 1997).

The behavior of men and women around us merges with cultural beliefs and values to form our personal views of gender. Do all men think about women and other men the same way? Or all women think about men and other women the same way? Of course not. From a sociopsychological perspective, gender is an arbitrary, ever-changing, socially constructed set of attributes (Worden & Worden, 1998).

Myths About Male–Female Differences

Socialization determines a great deal of what many people choose to see as "naturally" masculine or feminine. People look at the ways many women and men and girls and boys *do* behave and conclude that those are the only ways in which females and males *can* behave. Countless myths explain real or apparent differences in male–female feelings, attitudes, aptitudes, and behavior.

Gender Identity, Roles, and Stereotypes

Once a baby is delivered and "It's a boy!" or "It's a girl!" rings out, social influences go to work to form the baby's gender identity and mold his or her future role. Each society has a set of rules for how its males and females should behave. Boys and girls learn early to conform to these established behavior standards and take on their accepted roles. Psychologists have tried to explain how children do this in terms of psychoanalytical, social-learning, cognitive-developmental, and gender-schema theories.

According to psychoanalytical theory (explained by Sigmund Freud), appropriate gender typing means that boys grow to identify with their fathers and girls with their mothers. Identification is completed as children resolve the **Oedipus complex** (sometimes called the *Electra complex* in girls). From roughly age 3 to 5 years, children supposedly develop incestuous wishes for the parent of the other gender and see the parent of the same gender as a rival. This is resolved when the child eventually identifies with the same-gender parent and develops behaviors typically associated with that gender. Today the psychoanalytical theory of gender-role development is not widely accepted.

Myth vs Fact

Myth: Females lack achievement motivation compared to males.
Fact: There are no differences here. Females have just as much achievement motivation as males.

Myth: Females have lower self-esteem.
Fact: Self-esteem is influenced by many factors. A person's gender, however, has no effect on self-esteem.

Myth: Females are better at learning roles and simple repetitive tasks.
Fact: The ability to learn roles and simple repetitive tasks is not influenced by gender.

Myth: Males are more analytical.
Fact: There is no difference in analytical skills between males and females.

Myth: All men think about women the same way. (Or all women think about men the same way.)
Fact: It is incorrect to conclude that all people of a certain gender think the same way about anything.

Myth: Females are more social than males.
Fact: The interest in being social, or the ability to be social, does not vary by gender even though it certainly can vary from one individual to another.

Myth: Females are more affected by heredity than males.
Fact: We are all influenced by our heredity, but our gender makes no difference in this situation (except that a few diseases are specific to one gender or the other).

Myth: Males are more affected by environment than females.
Fact: Everyone is influenced by the environment, but we are not affected more or less because of our gender.

Oedipus complex
A development stage in which the boy wants to possess his mother sexually and sees the father as a rival (similar to the female *Electra complex*).

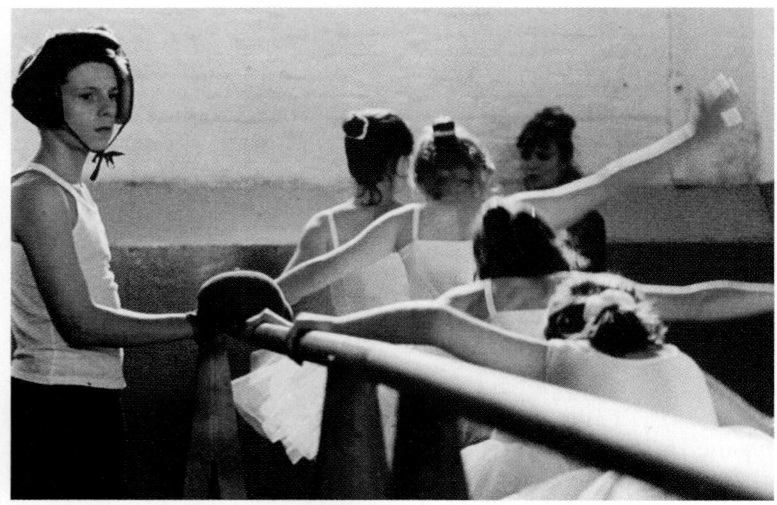

Billy Elliot is the story of a young boy who wants nothing more than to become a ballet dancer, despite the expectations of his father and the other residents of the tough mining village in which he lives, who would like him to pursue boxing and other "manly" activities. Much like his character in *Billy Elliot,* Jamie Bell, who plays Billy, had a difficult time growing up as a young man who wanted to pursue a talent in dancing. Both Billy and Jamie nevertheless pursued their talent, despite opposition and embarrassment, and eventually gained recognition and fame. What about all of the other young men and women who, because of society's expectations, did not pursue their dreams and goals? Is it healthy to impose such gender-based expectations on children?

In social-learning theory, the development of gender-typed behavior is explained in terms of processes such as observational learning, identification, and **socialization.** Children learn what is deemed masculine or feminine by observing, experimenting, and being rewarded for certain behaviors.

In cognitive-developmental theory, children form concepts about gender and then make their behavior conform to their gender concepts. This is called **gender typing.** By about age 7 to 8 years, **gender constancy** develops in most children. They realize that gender does not change even if the appearance and actions of people change. When children learn that gender is permanent, they independently try to act the way boys or girls "should act," because of an internal need for their behaviors to be consistent with what they know.

Gender schema theory indicates that children develop a grouping of mental representations about male and female personality traits, physical qualities, and behaviors. Once they develop a gender schema, they begin to judge themselves according to traits considered relevant to their genders. By doing this, they blend their developing self-concepts with the gender schema of their culture. Many associations can be made between gender and other qualities, such as strength and affection. Traditionally, strength has been viewed as a masculine trait and affection as a feminine trait. Other gender distinctions may be viewed as important—such as men's being sexually assertive and women's being sexually passive, or men's being in leadership positions and women's being placed in lesser positions.

socialization
The process of guiding people into socially acceptable behavior by providing information, rewards, and punishments.

gender typing
The process whereby children develop behavior that is appropriate to their gender.

gender constancy
The concept that people's gender does not change—even if they change their dress or behavior.

gender schema
A grouping of mental representations about male and female physical qualities, behaviors, and personality traits.

gender identity
The awareness and acceptance of one's gender.

Gender Identity

Gender involves more than just a biological component; it also includes the biological, social, and cultural norms and something called **gender identity.** Gender identity is one's self-image as a female or a male; it is the attachment one has to one's role. Societal and cultural factors are thought to exert more influence on gender identity than the biological component. At the very least, gender identity should be considered a biopsychosocial process—it is a result of interaction of biological, psychological, and social factors.

Masculinity and femininity are not innate or instinctive. The masculinity or femininity of gender identity needs a healthy human brain in which to take root. However, the developing brain is shaped by the environment in which it grows and from which it takes its mental nourishment (Money, 1988). In this way the biological foundation is shaped by psychological and sociological influences.

Because each society defines its roles for males and females and perpetuates behaviors through gender-role socialization, boys are given reinforcement for behaving in a "masculine" way, and girls receive reinforcement for exhibiting "feminine" behaviors. Should either gender engage in cross-sex conduct, such behavior is labeled gender-role-inappropriate; when each sex

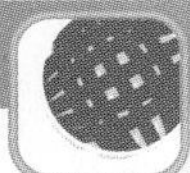

Global DIMENSIONS

The Oppression of Women

Until September 1996, Afghan women, particularly those living in cities, were highly involved in public life. They wore contemporary clothing, participated in government, and worked in all professions. In 1996, an extremist Islamic militia called the Taliban overtook two-thirds of Afghanistan and stripped females of their most basic rights.

If a woman lived in a house, the windows had to be painted black, as did all but the front windows of a car she might occupy. She could go out of the house only in the company of a close male relative.

Women could not work as doctors, nurses, or midwives and could not be treated by male doctors. Women with serious illnesses could die untreated. Women could not work outside the home, attend school, or even, for fear of terrible punishment, wear shoes that made noise when they walked. Parents could not teach their daughters to read. The Taliban did all this in the name of extremist Islamic views unique to itself; their treatment of people had nothing to do with traditional Islamic beliefs.

Mavis Leno, wife of Jay Leno, a member of the board of directors for the Feminist Majority Foundation, chaired a national campaign to demand an end to the Taliban's oppressive treatment of women.

Another example of oppression of women became public in 2001. First a hardline militant group in Kashmir announced they would throw acid at women who did not wear veils and the traditional *burkah,* a long black cloak that covers a woman from head to toe. Later it was announced that women not wearing the veil would be shot. To prevent trouble, the heads of girls' schools and women's colleges asked their students to dress conservatively and to wear no makeup (Overland, 2001).

Even after American troops invaded Afghanistan, many Afghan women were still mistreated. They continued to be abused, harassed, and threatened all over Afghanistan. For example, a team of 90 women from the Ministry of Religious Affairs harassed women in Kabul's streets for "un-Islamic behavior" such as wearing makeup and, in some instances, followed them home to castigate their parents or spouses (We want to live as humans, 2002).

Source: Extreme Taliban laws oppress Afghan women, *USA Today* (October 28, 1998), 25A.

behaves as the society deems normal, that behavior is labeled gender-role-appropriate and is rewarded.

Gender roles differ markedly from society to society. For example, Arapesh women do all the routine carrying, because their heads are thought to be stronger, and the men share the care of children. Both Samoan men and women do heavy gardening, fishing, cooking, and handiwork. Societies in various parts of the world have directed the socialization of their children so that (intentionally or unintentionally) women will be kept "in their place." For example, mythology has been used to maintain female subordination; women have been secluded during menstruation so they would not "jeopardize" the well-being of the community; women have been excluded from sacred public rituals and high-status economic roles; a preference for male children has been common; and sexist humor and ridicule have been used (Layng, 1989). Many societies discourage any deviation from the prescribed gender roles; others, such as ours, are now working toward flexibility and individualism in a wide variety of behaviors.

The expectation that people will exhibit certain characteristics and/or behaviors dictated by the customs and traditions of the society is called **stereotyping.** Expecting individuals to behave in particular ways because they are male or female is referred to as **gender-role stereotyping.** There

stereotyping
The expectation that individuals will exhibit certain characteristics or behaviors.

gender-role stereotyping
Expectation that individuals will behave in certain ways because they are male or female.

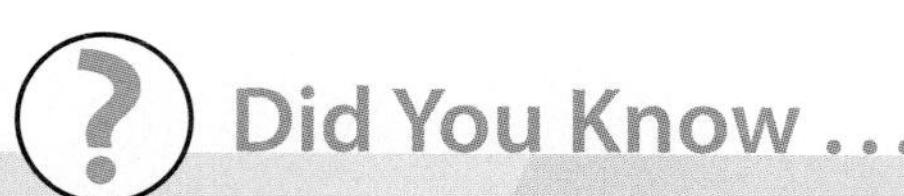

Gender differences are everywhere, even in the decision of whether to enter college or the workforce out of high school. According to a study released in June 1999 by the American Association of University Women, women were more likely than men not to attend college because of their credit-card debt or lack of scholarships and other college aid. Other barriers to college cited in the study were the need to care for children and lack of support from spouses. But men who go straight from high school into the workforce tend to do so because they were "never that interested" in college (McQueen, 1999).

are still many rigid, unyielding traditional attitudes about gender-role behaviors that make it difficult for people to express themselves and for society to implement change. Stereotypical images of people do not take into account individual differences. Until recently the stereotypical woman or wife in our society was passive, quiet, and concerned primarily with home, husband, and children; the stereotypical man was gruff, strong, unfeeling, and concerned mostly with work and money. The danger of such stereotypes is that people take them seriously and act on them, turning a blind eye to the qualities, capabilities, and interests of individuals—frequently denying even their own. People often believe that those who deviate from stereotypes are not as good as those who conform to them. Thus, one who accepts as true the stereotypes described might look down on a woman who cared about work or a man who chose to stay home with his children. People become boxed in not only by social pressure to conform closely to the stereotype, but also by rigid customary practice (such as promoting men but not women in business and professions, hiring women but not men to nurse and teach small children, or paying men more than women, regardless of their responsibilities), as well as by law. The assumptions behind such stereotyped behavior are being challenged today, and laws are being changed as well, but popular assumptions and attitudes are slow to change and are still passed on.

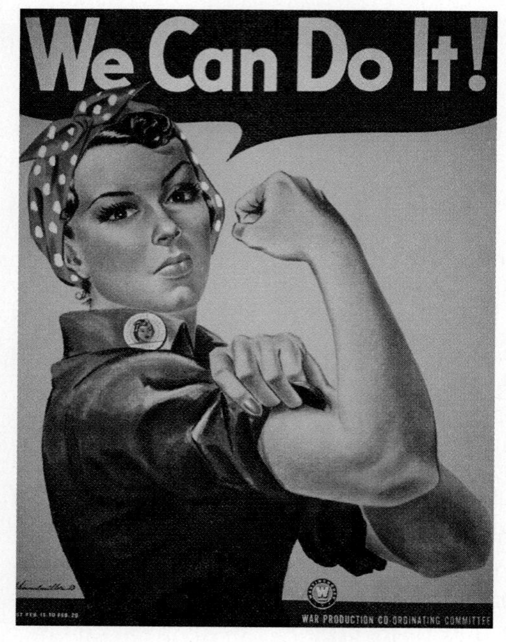

During World War II, Rosie the Riveter was part of the U.S. government's public relations campaign to get women into the workforce. Rosie shows off a strong bicep but still has a perfect manicure.

Teaching Gender Roles and Stereotypes

Gender roles are taught throughout the life cycle, but parents probably have the greatest effect, especially when children are very young. Very early on, parents reinforce the behaviors deemed acceptable to their child's gender with such remarks as "What a good, sweet girl!" or "What a big, strong boy!" accompanied by smiles and nods of approval. There is no doubt that most, if not all, of the forces of socialization in our culture—parents, teachers, peers, movies, television, and books (targeted at children and adults)—encourage different behaviors in boys and girls. The resulting sets of traits are what we call *masculinity* and *femininity*. Let us look briefly at a few examples of how gender roles and stereotypes are taught.

The Influence of Schools

School personnel pass on social stereotypes in a number of ways. For example, if teachers feel that boys are naturally more aggressive or that girls are naturally more passive, how will this attitude influence the way they treat their students? If gender-role stereotyping

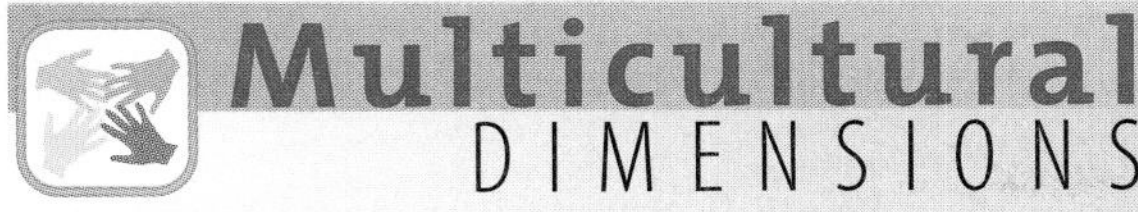

Multicultural DIMENSIONS

How the Economy Affects Gender Equality Relations between men and women are influenced by race, class, and sexuality; however, the most pressing issue for men and women of color, especially those who are poor and working class, is the economy. While both the employment rates and real wages of men are down, women are working in greater numbers, and their wages are on the rise.

For working-class African Americans, Latinos, and Native Americans, the effect of these changes has been harsh. The decline in employment for men has caused an increase in domestic violence, alcohol abuse, and other problems associated with joblessness. However, the increase in women's employment and economic resources is not enough to allow most to support a family; nor has it been accompanied by available, affordable child care.

These changes not only challenge the expectations traditionally associated with gender but also are reshaping families along distinctive racial and class lines. For example, although families maintained by single women have become a permanent feature in all racial and class categories, this type of family is most prevalent among people of color and the poor.

Among whites, the chief cause of the increase in households headed by women is women's growing economic independence. But the growth in African-American households headed by women partly reflects the employment problems of African-American men.

In addition, for all immigrant groups, life in the United States leads to increased rates of single parenthood and divorce.

The economic challenges facing poor and working-class African-American, Latino, and Native American men and women constitute the most pressing issue in relations between the sexes today. This is because racial and ethnic discrimination, combined with economic difficulties, make these groups extremely vulnerable to shifts in the economic and social climate.

Source: Dill, B.T. Economic disparity is key for all minorities, *The Chronicle of Higher Education, 45, no. 6* (October 2, 1998), B7–B8.

exists in teachers' expectations, it can lead to biases in how they treat and evaluate their students. In a study sponsored by the American Association of University Women, it was found that girls and boys received very different treatment in the classroom. Among other results, it was found that teachers called on and encouraged boys more than girls; that boys who called out answers without being recognized were generally not penalized, but girls were reprimanded for the same behavior; and that boys were more likely to receive praise for the content of their work and girls for its neatness (Kantrowitz, 1992).

In another study, Sadker and Sadker (1985) found that teachers praise boys more than girls, give boys more academic help, and are more likely to accept boys' comments during class discussions. It was also clear that boys dominated classroom discussions. The researchers studied the classroom for gender-role stereotyping and found the following:

1. While girls sat patiently with their hands raised, boys waved their hands frantically when they wanted to say something during the discussion.
2. Boys were eight times more likely to call out an answer or offer a comment than were girls.
3. When children called out answers or comments without being called on, boys' responses were accepted more than were girls'.

4. Teachers tended to call on students of the same gender during a discussion. This tendency was even more pronounced when calling on boys.

5. Students were divided by gender and sat in separate areas of the room. This pattern may exacerbate the tendency to call on the same gender in a discussion.

sexism
The prejudgment that because of gender a person will possess negative traits.

If teachers believe in stereotypes, they may expect one sex to excel more than the other in certain subjects, they may encourage one sex more than the other, or they may favor one sex in terms of attention and/or extra help. They may even intentionally or unintentionally promote **sexism,** which is a prejudgment that because of gender a person will possess negative traits. Teachers can help promote the healthy sexual development of children if they provide equal opportunities for girls and boys, do not impose gender stereotypes, and do not use sexist language. Although young children are busy establishing their own identities, and many may exhibit stereotypical behavior, it is the role of the teacher to encourage learning and responsible behavior that does not discriminate (Brick, 1994).

School materials can also influence gender-role stereotyping. For example, in preschool picture books there has been a trend toward depiction of greater gender equality. At the same time, however, female characters are more likely to be shown as dependent or submissive, and males as independent and creative. Many subtle traditional expectations still exist (Oskamp, Kaufman, & Wolterbeek, 1996).

Gender DIMENSIONS

Gender Equality on the College Campus

In 1997 the New England Council of Land-Grant University Women created a document entitled *Vision 2000,* which was a call to high-level university administrators to ensure full and equitable participation by women in New England universities. The gender-equality goals in the document were intended to

1. Foster faculty and administrative accountability for gender equality in curriculum and pedagogy
2. Implement diversity initiatives
3. Promote family-friendly policies (affordable and available child care, flex time, and parental leave policies)
4. Encourage women's academic and career development
5. Establish and support strong women's centers
6. End sexual harassment of and violence against women
7. Correct inequities in hiring, promotion, tenure, compensation, and working conditions for women employees

Critics of *Vision 2000* claim that it is a plot by women's studies faculty to stifle academic freedom—that they will determine gender-equality standards and impose them on recalcitrant faculty. They worry that feminist "indoctrination" of students will lower academic standards and destroy academic debate. Others feel that it is time to ensure gender equality in higher education. They point out that there are fewer women faculty members overall and they are concentrated in lower ranks, less well-paid career tracks, and part-time and non–tenure track positions.

Are the goals of *Vision 2000* needed at your college or university? How is your institution dealing with each of the seven areas listed? What else might have to be done on your campus?

Sources: Vision 2000, New England Council of Land-Grant University Women, February, 1997. Available: http://www.umass.edu/wost/articles/vision2k/whole.htm; Ferguson, A. Gender equity on the college campus, *Boston Globe* (Feb. 23, 1997), 27.

Some people claim bias still exists in achievement tests. Language in the tests has often referred to males and their environments. Women were disproportionately shown to be homemakers, and men to be engaged in directive, leadership, achieving roles. Boys were described in action terms; girls were described in helping or more passive terms. A strong bias against nontraditional behavior in both sexes has been evident in many tests.

Even at the college level, educators need to be sensitive to the influence of the classroom environment. It has been thought that female students participate less often and less assertively than male students in college classrooms and that the professors' discriminatory behaviors are partly responsible. Crawford and MacLeod (1990) found, however, that males did seem to participate more but that the gender differences were not due to professors' discrimination. Female professors were more likely to create a participatory climate for all students, and this climate, of course, results in a better classroom environment for female students as well. The most important influences on student interaction are the class environment in general, the class environment for the individual student, and specific positive and negative professor behaviors.

Teachers, books, and tests are powerful forces, but it is important to stress that gender stereotypes are perpetrated by other factors as well. Children take to the classroom notions of gender roles formed through the influence of parents and peers.

The Influence of Parents and Peers

In most cases, as soon as a child is born, interaction between parents and child begins—interaction that differs according to the gender of the child. Traditionally, a girl is thought to be fragile, to need protection, and to have needs that revolve around personal appearance and development. A boy is seen as tough, physically active, and unemotional. Children perceive these expectations, which tend to define their reality. Because the mother is usually the primary caregiver, the female child finds it easier to learn her appropriate gender role than does the male child. The female internalizes feminine behavior and is rewarded for her identification. The male may be in a bind. He may not have a constant role model because his father may not be around as much as his mother. He frequently learns from the mother's telling him that boys "don't do" certain things. Thus boys may learn to be anxious about gender-role identity.

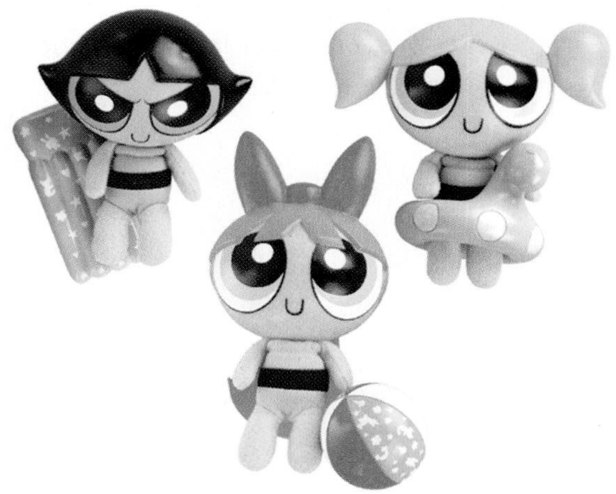

The television cartoon *Powerpuff Girls* is often cited as providing good role models for little girls, showcasing strong female characters capable of rational thought and conflict resolution. The trio work together to defeat their oppressors without resorting to actual violence, using instead cunning wit and strength. In its portrayal of all females as strong and capable, the show turns the standard ideas of gender roles upside down without sacrificing the female identity. Why do you think television producers have traditionally been reluctant to create children's programs that feature girls or women as action heroes? Why do you think there has been a recent proliferation of female action heroes in children's and adults' television and film?

It seems that increasing numbers of parents try to prevent teaching gender-role stereotypes to their children, but this can be hard to achieve. They may act differently toward a child, depending on its gender, even if they do not intend to do so. For example, if a boy is asked to participate in sports or help his father with outside chores while a girl is asked to wash dishes or clean her room, this pattern sends messages about expected gender roles.

What children observe at home in regard to sex roles also sends important messages. For example, even when both parents work outside the home in managerial or professional jobs, the redistribution of roles within the family has not yet clearly or completely occurred. Societal expectations and behavioral norms are the likely reason for this (Duxbury & Higgins, 1991). American women—even those employed full time—continue to work more hours than do their husbands on household tasks, and there is little evidence that men's proportionate share of family work has changed much in recent years (Blair & Lichter,

Ethical DIMENSIONS

Extreme Sex Roles—the Price of Honor

News of an interesting ethical situation related to female sexual behavior was reported in 1999 from Jordan. In 1998, Sirhan, a 35-year-old man, was proud to say that he had murdered his younger sister. She had reported to the police that she had been raped. Sirhan said, "She committed a mistake, even if it was against her will. Anyway, it's better to have one person die than to have the whole family die from shame." To Sirhan, it was more ethical to kill his sister than to suffer from the shame that would have sullied his "male honor."

For centuries, Arab men have engaged in "honor killing"—the intrafamily killing of errant females. Honor killing has its roots in the crude Arabic expression "A man's honor lies between the legs of a woman." For Arab women, virginity before marriage and fidelity afterward are considered musts. Men are expected to control their female relatives. If a woman strays, it is widely believed, the dignity of the man can be restored only by killing her. In Jordan the 25 or so cases of honor killing documented every year make up a quarter of all homicides there.

Forbidden sexual activity is not always the issue. Marrying or divorcing against the family's wishes can also provoke murder. The law winks at honor killers. If a man catches his wife or a close female relative in the act of adultery and kills her, he is exempt from punishment.

Running away is next to impossible for women, because Arab societies are close knit, and few women have the means to live alone. "Rafa," 20 years old, was locked up in prison to protect her after her uncles and brothers vowed to murder her for having a 3-day affair with a coworker. She said, "With the mistake I made, I deserve to die."

Honor killing has started to receive media attention, and a hotline has been created by the Jordanian Women's Union for women in distress. However, honor killings are hard to combat because of the extremely strong feelings related to male and female gender roles in Jordan.

Source: Beyer, L. The price of honor, *Time, 153, no. 2* (January 18, 1999), 55.

1991). Many social scientists feel parents are very influential in regard to establishing gender roles (Fagot, Leinbach, & O'Boyle, 1992).

The question of whether or not we can, or want to, raise "gender-neutral" children has been debated. Some argue that it not only is possible but also can result in more positive self-esteem. They say that children raised with gender-neutral expectations will have a more open, positive view of the world in general. Others argue that gender and gender-role expectations are tied very closely to familial and cultural expectations. They feel that gender-specific role fulfillment is vital to certain cultures, ensuring the survival of important cultural traditions (Can we raise "gender-neutral" children? 2003).

The peer group is also an important influence in learning about sex roles. Even early in life, children choose members of their own sex as playmates most of the time. This segregation by gender continues into the school years and helps contribute to sex-typing in play activities that help prepare children for adult roles (Moller, Hymel, & Rubin, 1992).

The influence of peers becomes increasingly important by late childhood and early adolescence. Conformity can be viewed as being very important, and behaving according to traditional gender roles promotes social acceptance by peers (Martin, 1990). Those who do not behave in ways accepted by the peer group are likely to be pressured and even ridiculed.

There is no question that biology is important. There are biological factors that tilt males and females in different directions related to their interests and behavior, but numerous social factors influence the way the biological tilts can be redirected (Baldwin & Baldwin, 1997). In other words, regarding the nature versus nurture debate, biology does matter; however, the way we are treated and what we learn can drastically influence our expression of gender roles.

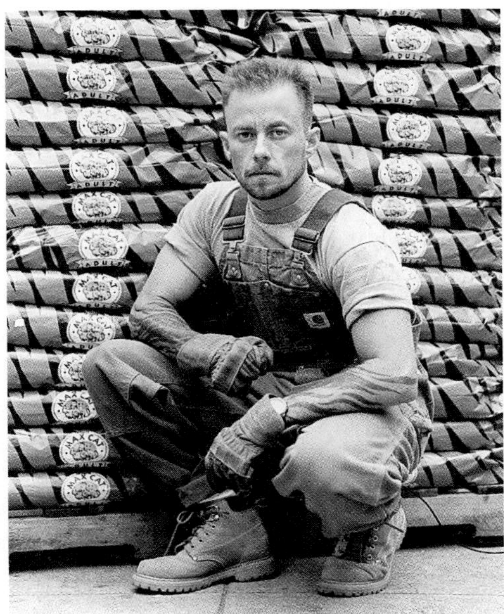

Although female-to-male transsexuals may be more rare than male-to-females, some women can feel just as uncomfortable with their gender as men. Loren Cameron (above) comments that early in his life, he felt great discomfort with being female, but once he made the commitment to change his gender, he became proud of the body image that he was creating.

Gender Identity Difficulty—Transsexualism

There are some people who experience **gender dysphoria.** They believe they are trapped in the body of the "wrong sex." They feel they are not really the gender indicated by their genitals. Sometimes the term *gender dysphoria* is used interchangeably with the term **transsexual.** Other times the term *transsexual* is used to refer to people who wish to have, or have had, their genitals surgically altered to conform to their gender identity. Therefore, an anatomically male transsexual feels that he is a female but that some quirk of fate provided him with male genitals. He wants to be socially identified as the female he believes himself to be. He does not derive sexual excitement from cross-dressing, as is the case with a transvestite, but views himself as a female. (We will discuss transvestism in In Focus: Atypical Sexual Behavior.)

Transsexualism, which is a gender orientation, is not to be confused with homosexuality, a sexual orientation. Some transsexuals are homosexual, and some are heterosexual. Unless a transsexual chooses to tell another person, an observer will probably not know whether homosexual or heterosexual behavior is being practiced.

Estimates of the number of transsexuals vary widely. Some experts say the numbers range from 1 in 100,000 to 1 in 37,000 for males and from 1 in 400,000 to 1 in 100,000 for females. This amounts to about 25,000 transsexuals in the United States (Selvin, 1993). In the 1960s and 1970s, when the medical procedures for changing the genitals of a transsexual were developed, about three of every four people who wanted their gender changed were men. More recently, this ratio has narrowed to about one to one, and many now think the incidence of transsexualism is similar among males and females (Pauly, 1990).

According to the International Foundation for Gender Education (2003), more modern estimates indicate that 1 in 10,000 or even 1 in 1,000 people are transsexuals. It is estimated that about half of these are female-to-male and half are male-to-female transsexuals. However, the International Foundation emphasizes that this is a very rough estimate.

There is no clear understanding of either the causes or the nature of transsexualism (Money, 1994). Some theorists believe the causes relate to early parent–child relationships related to gender roles of mothers and fathers and the ways that parents treated a child. Others focus on hormonal imbalances that influenced the brain during prenatal development; however, no one knows for sure.

Gender-Reassignment Surgery

The idea of gender reassignment is controversial, and psychotherapy has not been very useful for most transsexuals. Surgery is part of gender reassignment, but, because it is irreversible, professionals usually require that the transsexual live publicly as a member of the other sex for a year before undergoing surgery. During this time it is easier for the person or the medical personnel to change their minds. Surgery is not something to be taken lightly, and it is usually done only after careful screening of the individual.

A lifetime of hormonal treatment is also necessary. Male-to-female transsexuals take estrogen. It causes fatty deposits to develop in the breasts and hips, inhibits beard growth, and softens the skin. Female-to-male

gender dysphoria
Feeling trapped in the body of the "wrong" sex.

transsexual
A person whose gender identity does not match her or his biological sex; also a person who wishes to have, or has had, his or her gender surgically altered to conform to his or her gender identity.

Ethical DIMENSIONS

Should Dad Dress As a Woman? Should Dad Participate in His Child's Field Trip While Dressed As a Woman?

In Saint Louis, most of the kids on a fourth-grade field trip did not notice or did not care that a classmate's father was dressed as a woman, in jeans, a sweater, and nice shoes. Most of the teachers were equally untroubled. However, one parent spotted the "cross-dressing" dad and alerted some friends. As a result, one school board member proposed a new policy that would require parent chaperones to wear "gender-appropriate" clothing for school functions.

The father described had dressed as a woman at work for years, kept his hair long, worn slacks and blouses, and used a name that could be either male or female. He had actively participated in his daughters' education and in their schools while in women's attire with no previous problems.

Some people argue that it is ethical to require parents to wear "gender-appropriate" clothing at school functions. Others argue that it is not ethical to do this because it violates the parents' rights to dress as they please—particularly because to qualify for sex-change surgery individuals must first go through a prolonged period of transition when they present themselves in public as the gender they want to become.

What do you think?

Source: Simon, S. After Dad dresses as woman, field trip controversy still boils, *The Birmingham News* (January 6, 2003), 4B.

transsexuals take androgens, which promote deepening of the voice, masculine hair distribution, large muscles, and loss of fatty deposits in the breasts and hips. The clitoris may also grow larger.

It is not possible to construct internal genital organs or gonads, so gender-reassignment surgery is mostly cosmetic. Male-to-female surgery is usually more successful because it is easier to construct a vagina than a working penis. The vast majority of transsexuals who undergo surgery are happy with the outcome. Gender-reassignment surgery is done in only a few places in the United States, is very expensive, and is usually not covered by health insurance policies. Indeed, only 2,500 such operations have been performed in the United States since 1953. Clearly this is something to be done only with extensive counseling and medical support.

A special case of potential gender-reassignment surgery relates to the question of what should be done with intersex infants—those born with ambiguous or mixed genitalia and chromosomal structures. It is estimated that every year in the United States about 65,000 babies are born with ambiguous genitalia. Some people believe that feminizing surgery should be done at birth to ensure that the baby will be able to function later as an adult woman. Others feel that children should remain intact until they are older and decide for themselves what, if anything, to do about their ambiguous genitalia (Should parents surgically alter their intersex infants? 2003).

The Influence of Sex Stereotypes on Sexuality

As you can see, sex-role stereotyping limits self-expression and personal growth and development, and that limiting in turn affects sexuality. When individuals define masculinity and femininity for themselves, they express personal beliefs through gender-role behaviors. The traditional definitions are confining, emphasizing as they do conventional conformity to long-existing gender-role norms. We have referred particularly to males' being socialized toward initiating, aggressive, and directive behaviors and females' being socialized toward receiving, passive, and compliant behaviors. In descriptions of anatomical function, for example, the vagina has tended to be described as receiver, not for sexual pleasure but for reproduction. The penis is often described in terms of insertion based on need, dominance, and desire. Thus again, men initiate and women are passively receptive.

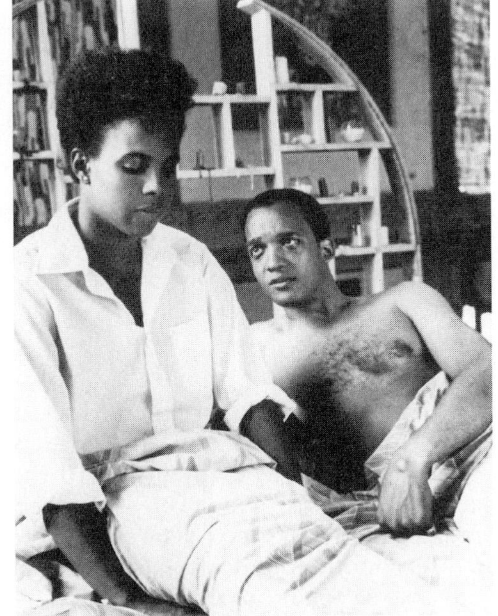

Movies often find humor in reverse-gender situations. In *She's Gotta Have It,* Spike Lee spins a tale of Nora Darling, a young woman from Brooklyn who is carrying on three simultaneous sexual relationships. Although each man wants Nora to commit to him, she defies being "owned" by only one man. Although humorous in a movie, reverse-gender situations in real life are not always so pleasing to the participants.

The pressure to conform to socialization has provoked in both sexes anxieties that we are only now beginning to discuss freely and reevaluate. The emphasis on the macho aspects of male performance tends to obliterate consideration of men as sensitive, gentle, nurturant, and intimate beings who can relate to adult partners on a variety of levels. The emphasis on the passivity of women has long neglected consideration and acknowledgment of them as full sexual beings with the same needs as men for expression and fulfillment.

There are implications here for a person's social abilities. For example, Quackenbush (1990) found that androgynous males (those with a blending of so-called psychological masculine and feminine characteristics) reported the greatest degree of comfort and confidence in dating and social–sexual situations. Thus, a blending of social competencies appears to ensure effective social functioning. As one example of this blending, the capacities to assert oneself and empathize with others are important social interaction skills.

Each sex needs to be able to express feelings heretofore defined as either masculine or feminine. Both sexes need to be directive and sensitive in order to function effectively. Women need to make decisions in parenting, in controlling their careers, and in their sexual behavior. Men need to accept responsibility for parenting, be comfortable as receivers as well as givers, and accept that sharing intimacy and intimate acts does not mean loss of control.

Many men and women in our society still differ in their expectations for interpersonal relationships. Some women still expect assertive, in-command, successful men; some men still expect supportive, helpful, receiving women. Stereotypes of the dominant male and the submissive female continue to influence the interpersonal dynamics between the sexes. Both sexes have been socialized into these expectations, and socialization probably accounts for more of these distinctions than does biology.

Sex roles may also influence marriage rates among women. Among young women who expect to complete a 4-year college degree or more, believing that wives should be homemakers leads to lower rates of marriage; however, among young women with low educational expectations, believing that wives should be homemakers leads to higher rates of marriage (Barber & Axinn, 1998).

Men have often learned to equate sexual activity with the fulfillment of their needs for support, tenderness, and the feeling of being loved. Women have often not been taught that receiving sexual pleasure has value. Mixed feelings about what they really feel and what society tells them they are supposed to feel can confuse both sexes.

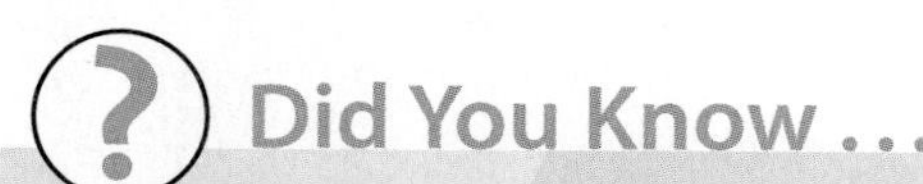

Did You Know . . .

Even in personal advertisements in a newspaper, gender differences for desired companion attributes were consistent with traditional gender-role stereotypes. Relative to the opposite sex, women emphasized employment, financial, and intellectual status, as well as commitment. Men emphasized physical characteristics. Also, considerably more men than women placed ads (Davis, 1990).

Gender differences related to sexual behavior and expectations have been found among adolescents in grades 8–10. Boys initiated sexual intercourse earlier than girls, but by grade 10 the girls' rates of sexual intercourse surpassed the boys'. However, girls were less likely to intend to have sexual intercourse in the next year than were boys. Girls reported higher intention to use condoms and also felt more pressure than boys to engage in sexual intercourse (Nahom, et al., 2001).

The popular press suggests that men and women may always have problems because they are so different. Examples often given are in communication (she wants more talk; he wants more action); intimacy (she needs to relax to participate in intimate sexual behavior, but he needs to participate to relax); division of household labor and child care (she says she does more; he talks about how much he does); and money and careers (she says he does not value her job as much as his; he notes that he makes more money) (Blau, 1994).

Related to communication, the following are some of the ways to close the gender gap (Blau, 1994):

- **G**et honest before you get angry: Something deeper than dry cleaning or dishwashing is probably bothering you.
- **E**stablish systems for sharing chores and child care.
- **N**egotiate the division of labor and the division of love.
- **D**o not get locked into your role: Try swapping responsibilities on occasion.
- **E**xpress your emotional needs and expectations and really listen to your partner.
- **R**eview the cultural messages of your childhood to help understand the conflicts inherent in your new roles.
- **G**ive each other time to change: Do not monitor or criticize.
- **A**ccept your differences and applaud each other's strengths.
- **P**rotect your intimate time together.

Men and women seem to be different in their reactions to their first sexual intercourse experience (Guggino & Ponzetti, 1997). Women were more likely to report that their first sexual experience left them feeling less pleasure, satisfaction, and excitement than men were. In addition, women felt more sadness, guilt, nervousness, tension, embarrassment, and fear. If guilt feelings do emerge as a result of first sexual intercourse, the likelihood of future sexual dissatisfaction is greatly increased (Moore & Davidson, 1997).

There is increased thinking that similarities between men and women, particularly in the human struggle for intimacy, far outweigh differences. Healthy couples appear to transcend traditional gender roles, and the roles, such as pursuer and distancer, are interchangeable. There is no one definition of an intimate, healthy relationship. Love and respect are essential in a good relationship (Worden & Worden, 1998).

In terms of human sexual expression, both partners need the freedom to be self-disclosing, intimate, and communicative. Restrictive definitions of roles serve only to repress the joy, pleasure, and emotionally fulfilling responses of sexual intimacy. And perhaps equally important is the fact that gender-role stereotyping also restricts personal fulfillment in nonsexual relationships between men and women.

The Possibilities of Androgyny

According to legend, there once were three kinds of humans—the male, the female, and the androgyne. All humans had two sets of arms and legs. The males and females had two faces and two sets of genitalia of the same gender. The androgynes each had one masculine face and one feminine face, one set of female genitalia, and one set of male genitalia. This group of humans had tremendous strength and an arrogant nature, which offended the gods.

Zeus, to punish them, split the androgynes in half and remade them as hemipeople. Thus, men and women have lost their other half and seek it in other people.

The word **androgynous** originated from the story of the androgynes. An androgynous person is one who has a combination of masculine and feminine characteristics—one who exhibits some traits of both masculinity and femininity as defined by the society. Thus an androgynous male might be nurturing, in addition to providing, and an androgynous female might be assertive as well as soft-spoken. The idea of androgyny can serve as a means of doing away with gender-role stereotyping. Many people feel that they must conform absolutely to society's notions of maleness and femaleness, especially in the ways they acknowledge and express (or repress and deny) their feelings. In conforming, they lose the opportunity to express themselves as individuals. But if, as a society, we were to view people as androgynous, then all of us might consider the expression of a variety of emotions appropriate for everyone. A significant benefit would be that people who expressed their true feelings, unswayed by the demands of gender-role stereotypes, would experience a greater depth of sexual intimacy with their partners than would those concerned solely with how manly or womanly they appear.

androgynous
Exhibiting a combination of masculine and feminine traits as defined by the society.

The concept of androgyny has been around a long time. For example, in 1975 Sandra Bem, a noted proponent of androgyny, indicated that stereotypical gender roles were restrictive and unhealthy. She described androgynous people, by contrast, as flexible and healthy. She felt that rigidity in gender-role expectations was reflected in inflexible responses in real-life situations. To test her theory, Bem developed the Bem Sex Role Inventory. She gave a group of men and women a list of personality characteristics—some traditionally masculine (assertiveness, ambition, independence), some traditionally feminine (dependence, sensitivity, gentleness), and some neutral (friendliness, likability)—and asked the subjects to rate the accuracy of each term in describing them. Participants were then placed in situations that tested masculine and feminine behaviors such as nurturance, responsiveness to a troubled person, and conformity. Men who had described themselves as having masculine traits were not comfortable with "feminine" activities, and women who had described themselves as having feminine traits were not comfortable doing "masculine" tasks. But androgynous men and women were able to function in all situations (Bem, 1975).

It should be noted that not all studies are supportive of the androgyny concept. In one study, although androgynous workers reported greater satisfaction with their jobs than other workers, they also reported more job-related stress (Rotherham & Weiner, 1983). Another study found androgynous males to be less emotionally healthy than masculine males, to have fewer drinking problems, to be less introverted, and to feel more in control of their behavior (Jones, Chernovetz, & Hansson, 1978). Yet many experts and numerous studies tend to agree that freedom from stereotypical gender roles allows for greater health and life satisfaction.

Sex-role stereotypes can be burdensome even—indeed especially—to those who do not accept them. Both genders have placed a high value on traditional masculine traits, but women have long been denied fulfillment in those terms. Instead, women have traditionally gained recognition on the basis of their ties with others (predominantly the males in their lives) as daughters, wives, and mothers. Whereas men's successes have been measured in terms of power, money, and social standing, women's successes have been measured in terms of mothering, nurturing, and affiliation with the successful man or men in their lives. Women who do seek fulfillment in traditionally nonfeminine ways—creating their own styles of behavior—often encounter much resistance, both fierce and subtle. Those who reject the historical gender-role stereotypes and assume more assertive, commanding traits often are not accepted.

Stereotypes of masculinity burden men, too. Males who express nurturant, gentle traits may find themselves criticized and perhaps ridiculed by other men and even by some women. The roles of men are being critically examined, and a variety of strategies are being proposed to create change. Men have been accused of being resistant to a change in women's roles, reluctant to share or give up power that has been theirs historically, and unwilling to accept the "threat" of egalitarian relationships. Many men may well resist role change, but to accuse men in general of being uncaring, unfeeling, and unwilling to implement personal and social change deprives both genders of the opportunity to achieve gender-role change.

Interesting studies have related leadership to androgyny. Some studies have shown the gender-stereotypic expectation that women lead in an interpersonally oriented style and men in a task-oriented style, but other studies do not show these differences. It has also been found that women tended to adopt a more democratic or participative, and a less autocratic or directive, style than men (Eagly & Johnson, 1990). In other studies it has been concluded that both "consideration" (often thought to be feminine) and "structuring" (often thought to be masculine) behaviors are necessary for effective leadership. It was suggested that increased awareness of the androgynous nature of effective leadership behaviors might weaken the biases in favor of male leaders (Cann & Siegfried, 1990).

On a related note, male supervisors in a large government agency indicated that they would not treat female employees differently from male employees. Male coworkers, however, reported that they treated other male coworkers more favorably than female coworkers. Supervisors, as compared with male coworkers, reported more favorable attitudes toward female workers (Palmer & Lee, 1990). It is interesting that the managers seemed closer to the concept of androgyny than the coworkers.

As a final note about androgyny, it has been pointed out that although the ideal of androgyny has proved quite workable in the workplace, it is not so workable within the family. Popenoe (1993) expressed concern that insufficient consideration has been given to the risks of going too far down the path. He indicated that parental androgyny is neither feasible, because of inherent biological differences that have significance for parenting, nor desirable. He pointed out that some gender differentiation is important for child development, and probably for marital stability.

The Women's Movement

In recent decades we have seen social upheaval that has changed our society in a variety of ways. Patterns of sexual behavior have been affected, for example, by contraceptive technology, abortion, and sterilization. Divorce has become more acceptable, and changes in leisure pursuits, delays in pregnancy, and the acceptance of intentional childlessness all offer women a greater diversity in lifestyle. But perhaps the single most important effect has been the women's movement. The ability of women to explore their potential has never been as great as at this time. Economic independence, control over reproduction, and choices in relationships and lifestyle have given women freedom from domination by men and the opportunity for self-direction as individuals. Statistics illustrate the increasing inroads into the labor force being made by women as they seek to achieve economic independence and/or to supplement the family's income.

There were at least four groups who converged in the 1960s to help create the modern women's movement. First, there were those, such as Eleanor Roosevelt, who used John F. Kennedy's Presidential Commission on the Status of Women to reveal pervasive sexism in American society and law. Second, there were those who were from the civil rights movement, broadening the definition of equality to include women. The third group, working-class women, turned to feminism and the women's movement in their struggle for the Equal Pay Act of 1963. The fourth group was made up of white, middle-class suburban women, who found themselves stifled by gender stereotypes (Kerber, 1999).

The women's movement probably also is responsible for increased attention to victims of sexual assault and other forms of violence. A better understanding of aggressive behavior, improved methods and services for assault victims, and greatly increased education on these topics are all evidence of this increased attention. In addition, the public discussion of sexual harassment thoughout recent years must be at least partially attributed to the women's movement. There is also a growing body of literature about many issues related to gender.

With the change in the present and potential status of women have arisen new pressures and anxieties about role redefinition and intimate relationships. Women are more informed about their physiology and their right not only to expect sexual fulfillment and satisfaction but also to initiate or refuse sexual behavior. For many, traditional values concerning virginity, self-sacrifice for children, lifelong commitment to marriage, and the support role of women are giving way to new modes of commitment. These changes can be seen as giving both women and men a chance to explore a number of alternatives. For whatever reasons, however, it seems that college students may have more traditional views of maleness than of femaleness. When more than 400 undergraduate students were asked to describe their concept of maleness and femaleness, concepts of maleness were framed more stereotypically than were concepts of femaleness (Hort, Fagot, & Leinbach, 1990). Perhaps the women's movement has helped make changes in concepts of femaleness, but not of maleness.

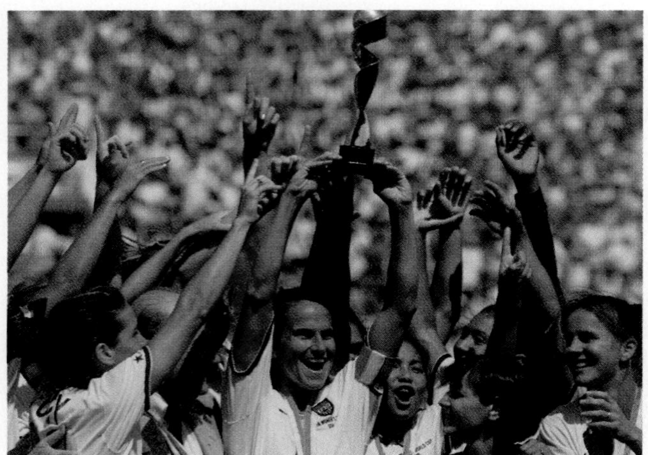

In July 1999, the United States women's soccer team won the gold medal at the World Cup competition. The team members, as well as their sponsors, used the opportunity to underscore the vast achievements that women have made in sports—as well as society in general.

Of course, the women's movement has not erased all male–female differences; nor has it totally changed everyone's opinions. For example, after reviewing prime-time television programs for all networks, Davis (1990) concluded that few changes had been made in the portrayals of women since the 1970s. Despite educational and occupational advances of women, gender differences in the realm of work and family experiences remain substantial. Marriage and parenting continue to be positively associated with work involvement and rewards for men, but they are related to persistent employment disadvantages for women (Cooney & Uhlenberg, 1991). According to one study, well-educated people do not seem to support efforts to reduce gender inequality as much as less well-educated people. In fact, women with employed husbands are less supportive of efforts to reduce gender inequality than women without a male wage earner. Women in general, however, are more likely than men to perceive gender inequality and more supportive of efforts to combat gender inequality (Davis & Robinson, 1991).

Some people feel true female empowerment has been shown recently by women (notably some movie stars) who have chosen as partners men who are less successful than they are. Because many modern women work outside the home and are financially independent, they are empowered enough to make a choice among men based on their personality, as opposed to making a choice only among men who earn as much or more. His career is less important than hers, so when they go out she gets all the attention (Tan, 2001).

Helping women achieve sexual equality requires an updated model of sexual behavior that encompasses women's needs, abilities, problems, and preferences. This new model should start from the premise that men and women have a right to complete and accurate information about the ways their bodies function sexually. The model should help women see that sexual behavior can be as exciting and rewarding for them as it is for men. The model should not be competitive with men, but it should help women to broaden their sexual agendas, play to their own sexual strengths, and take into account their unique needs and capabilities (Chalker, 1994).

As are women, men are questioning stereotypical scripts for masculinity in larger numbers. This questioning holds the promise of far greater freedom to explore and express their full humanity. Just as there are many different factions in the women's movement, there are also different factions in what can be lumped together as the "men's movement." On the "partnership" side are men who are working for gender equality, the reduction of male violence, and the promotion of more satisfying relationships. On the other side are those men openly working against equality, either denying that there is inequality or claiming women should be, and want to be, dominated by men (Eisler, 1995).

The Institute for Women's Policy Research (Overview of the status of women in the states, 2001) reported that gains in education and income and an increased presence in politics helped women boost their economic and social status. Yet, even states rated highly in their report must progress in order for women to gain equality with men. The institute looked at political participation, employment and earnings, economic autonomy, reproductive rights, and health and well-being in all states. Detailed results can be seen at the institute's web site at www.iwpr.org.

In 2003 an interesting gender-equity issue arose within the sport of golf. In Virginia a 17-year-old girl won the high school boys' golf tournament. However, she won playing from tees set closer to the hole than the tees the boys used. The rules had been changed 4 years earlier to allow girls to compete with this advantage. Earlier, a woman professional golfer won a tournament to qualify to play in a men's professional tournament. She, too, had competed from tees set closer to the hole. It was later ruled that when she played in the men's professional tournament she had to play from the same tees as the men. It is controversial whether or not females should be required to play from the same tees as the men if they are going to compete against men. Bowen (2003) said that once females play against males they should play by the same rules. If a female is racing against a male in the 100-meter run, for example, she should not be able to start 20 meters ahead just because she is a female. It will be interesting to see how this issue is resolved in the coming years.

The Sexuality Education and Information Council of the United States has the following position statement on gender equality and equity:

> *Gender equality and equity are fundamental human rights. Women and girls should be protected from gender-based violence, including sexual, physical, and psychological abuse. They should have equal access to paid employment, credit, education, and job training. There should be universal access to age-appropriate information and education about sexuality, gender roles, contraception, and sexually transmitted diseases (STDs), including HIV/AIDS. Gender stereotyping in educational curricula, the mass media, and other public communications should be eliminated. All sexual relationships should be governed by principles of equity, consent, and mutual respect, with men and women having mutual responsibility for contraception, parenting, and child care.*

Many people were surprised when a female Kansas state senator said she was opposed to women's suffrage (Bullers, 2001). Senator Kay O'Connor said that she does not support the 19th Amendment, which guarantees women the right to vote, and that if it were being considered today she would vote against it. She said, "Men should take care of women, and if men were taking care of women (today) we wouldn't have to vote."

Social and economic inequities still exist. However, overall, American women are on a slow and uneven road to equality. Gains in education and income and an increased presence in politics have helped women boost their economic and social status in recent years (Overview of the status of women in the states, 2000).

Gender DIMENSIONS

Is There Gender Equality in College Sports?

Since 1972, Title IX of the Education Amendments has forbidden sex discrimination at institutions receiving federal funds. One important, and still controversial, part of this legislation relates to college sports. After more than 30 years of living with Title IX, there are still many viewpoints about it. Some people believe that men have been penalized for having a higher interest in athletics than women. They point to the fact that in some cases men's sports have been cut to comply with Title IX. Others believe that Title IX has not hurt men's sports, and it has greatly helped women's athletic opportunities. Efforts continue among athletic officials, college administrators, and legislators to see how to deal best with Title IX and its implications (Gender equity in college sports: 6 views, 2002).

Exploring the DIMENSIONS of Human Sexuality

Our feelings, attitudes, and beliefs regarding sexuality are influenced by our internal and external environments. Go to sexuality.jbpub.com to learn more about the biological, psychological, and sociological factors that affect your sexuality.

Biological Factors

- Chromosomes (XX or XY) determine biological gender.
- Primitive gonadal tissues differentiate into prenatal ovaries or testicles.
- At puberty, sex hormones cause emergence of primary and secondary sexual characteristics. Sex hormones continue to act throughout one's lifetime.
- Testosterone plays a role in aggression; estrogen has been linked to heart attack prevention.
- Most medical studies have been completed on men, and findings have been assumed to be the same for women, without taking into account gender differences in hormones and chemical makeup.

Sociocultural Factors

- Sex-role orientation begins at birth. Children are treated differently according to social standards for gender.
- Family, neighbors, friends, and teachers influence our thinking about gender through their actions.
- Ethnic groups pass down sex-specific heritages and sex roles.
- Mass media are often sex-biased, portraying men and women in traditional, stereotypical roles.

Psychological Factors

- Expressiveness and communication style differ between sexes, as men withhold feelings and women express them openly.
- Women suffer more from self-esteem issues relating to body image, as they attempt to live up to the biologically impossible "Barbie" standard.
- In a society where men are presented with greater opportunities, motivation and possibility of achievement are harder for women.

CASE STUDY

Your sex plays a major role in how you perceive the world—and how the world perceives you. Sex plays a pervasive role in many areas that define our self-concept, including career opportunities. Men and women communicate in different styles, and express emotions differently. Physiological differences play out in health—women do live longer, but are sick more often.

Sex roles are influenced by virtually all social and cultural aspects, including religion, ethnic heritage, family traditions, peers, and even the mass media.

In sexuality, a "double standard" still exists, as men are encouraged to be and women are discouraged from being sexually active.

Discussion Questions

1. Of the many differences between the sexes, which do you feel are the most important nonbiological differences? Explain your answer. In your own college or university, are male and female students treated differently? Give specific examples.
2. Compare and contrast the feelings of males and females toward sexuality. Then discuss how the genders can bridge those differences.
3. How can women achieve sexual equality with men without becoming competitive? Does such a change need to begin with women—or with men?

Application Questions

Reread the story that opens the chapter and answer the following questions.

1. Is the writer androgynous? Explain why or why not.
2. What conflicts has the author experienced from his "reversed" gender role?
3. Is there any merit to the composer's comment that gender play during childhood influences abilities later in life? What other factors probably influenced the development of women composers?
4. As a student, how do you view the future of sex roles? How will life experiences affect your view of sex roles?

Critical Thinking Questions

1. Consider the expression "Candy is dandy, but liquor is quicker." Explain the gender bias of the expression. What type of tensions might such thinking create between the sexes?
2. As you read in the text, Christie Hefner, CEO of Playboy Enterprises, discussed the role of female managers in the *Media Studies Journal* (Spring/Summer 1996). Consider Hefner's statement. Is there a sex bias in the United States toward the male management style? What other reasons might explain the lack of women in high-level executive positions and on boards of directors?
3. Michael Jackson is often cited as an androgynous person. Why does the popular press believe this? Is it true?

Critical Thinking Case

Because of physiological differences, men and women often have slightly different medical symptoms. The same seems true for psychological problems. For example, school-aged boys who act out in class are often considered for the *DSM-IV* diagnosis of Attention-Deficit/Hyperactivity Disorder. Boys who receive treatment can learn to do quite well in school. However, girls have been socialized not to act out in class; they tend to have different symptoms and are less often diagnosed. That difference puts those young girls at a disadvantage, leading to poor scholastic achievement and low self-esteem.

In adulthood, depression is diagnosed in women nearly twice as often as in men. Research from the 1990s suggests that when men are faced with negative emotions, they distract themselves through drinking or sports. Women, in contrast, tend to focus attention on the negative mood. If such focus intensifies the negative mood, a woman would be more prone to a diagnosis of depression.

1. Should separate diagnostic manuals for psychiatric disorders be written for men and women? Explain your answer.
2. Should psychiatrists focus their training on one gender? Or should training be generic? Explain your answer.

Exploring Personal Dimensions

Female–Male Differences and Similarities

Females and males respond in similar ways to sexual stimulation. However, in some ways they also respond dissimilarly. To assess your knowledge of these similarities and differences, determine whether each of the following statements describes a response that is similar or dissimilar for females and males. Then place a check mark to indicate your answer. The correct answers appear at the conclusion of the statements.

Similar	Dissimilar	
——	——	1. Erection occurs.
——	——	2. When a sexual fantasy occurs, hormones are secreted.
——	——	3. Testosterone is produced by the body.
——	——	4. During sexual excitement, the nipples become erect.
——	——	5. Sex flush appears during the excitement phase of the sexual response cycle.
——	——	6. Males and females can have multiple orgasms without requiring a rest period.

Correct Answers

1. Similar. Both the penis and the clitoris become engorged with blood and become erect.
2. Similar. Hormones in both genders activate various body parts in response to sexual stimulation.
3. Similar. Testosterone is produced in the interstitial cells of the testes in men and in the ovaries of women (although in a small amount).
4. Similar. Although nipple erection is more obvious in women, it occurs in men too.
5. Dissimilar. In men, sex flush occurs during the plateau phase, whereas in women it occurs during the excitement phase.
6. Dissimilar. Whereas women have the capacity to be multiorgasmic, males generally need to experience a refractory period before subsequent orgasms.

Sexuality Online

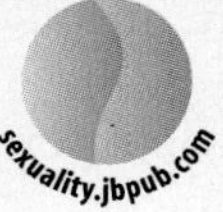

Go to the web component for *Exploring the Dimensions of Human Sexuality* at sexuality.jbpub.com for web exercises, additional resources related to this chapter, and student review tools.

Suggested Readings

Dixon, J. A. & Foster, D. H. Gender, social context, and backchannel responses, *The Journal of Social Psychology, 138* (February 1998), 134–136.

Doyle, J. *The male experience.* Dubuque, IA: Brown & Benchmark, 1991.

Elkins, R. On male femaling: A grounded theory approach to cross-dressing and sex-changing, *The Sociological Review, 41* (February 1993), 1–29.

Feminist Majority Foundation. Available: www.feminist.org.

Freund, K. & Watson, R. J. Gender identity disorder and courtship disorder, *Archives of Sexual Behavior, 22* (February 1993), 13–21.

Global perspectives on gender, sexual health, and HIV/AIDS, *SIECUS Report, 29, no. 5* (June/July 2001), 1–32 (entire issue devoted to these topics).

Hill, C. A. Gender, relationship stage, and sexual behavior: The importance of partner emotional involvement within specific situations, *Journal of Sex Research, 39, no. 3* (August 2002), 228–240.

Midence, K. & Hargreaves, I. Psychological adjustment in male-to-female transsexuals: An overview of the research evidence, *The Journal of Psychology, 131* (1997), 602–614.

Milkie, M. Contested images of femininity: An analysis of cultural gatekeepers' struggles with the "real girl" critique, *Gender and Society, 16, no. 6* (December 2002), 767–792.

Overview of the status of women in the states. Institute for Women's Policy Research (2001). Available: www.iwpr.org.

Pines, A. M. Gender differences in romantic jealousy, *The Journal of Social Psychology, 138* (February 1998), 54–71.

Simon, R. W. Gender, multiple roles, role meaning, and mental health, *Journal of Health and Social Behavior, 36, no. 2* (1995), 182–194.

CHAPTER 7

Sexual Response and Arousal

FEATURES

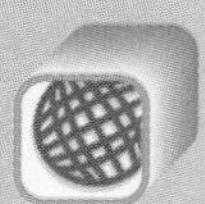
Global Dimensions
Aphrodisiacs and Tigers: A Strange Mix

Gender Dimensions
Male–Female Differences in Sexual Response

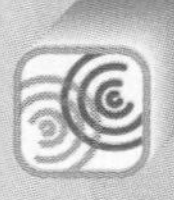
Communication Dimensions
Discussing Sexual Desires

Ethical Dimensions
Should Sexual Enhancements Be Used to Increase Sexual Arousal?

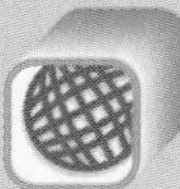
Global Dimensions
Age of First Intercourse

CHAPTER OBJECTIVES

1. Describe the role of the brain in sexual response, including the hormones involved and the role they play.
2. Describe the four phases of the Masters and Johnson sexual response cycle, as well as other theoretical models of sexual response.
3. Describe the physiology of orgasm in both males and females, differentiating between the different types of orgasm.

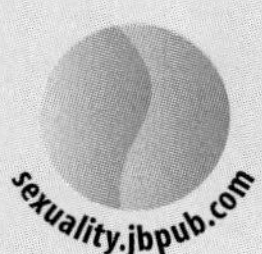

sexuality.jbpub.com

The Brain and Sexual Response
Aphrodisiacs
The Masters and Johnson Sexual Response Cycle

INTRODUCTION

Brian was sitting in his social studies class paying more attention to the attractive Tanya than to the teacher's lecture. Since he had entered high school he found himself more and more interested in girls, whose presence distracted him from his school work at times that were inappropriate. It was during one of these times that his social studies teacher asked Brian to identify a particular geographical region on the map in the front of the room. This was a problem for two reasons, both related to Tanya. First, Brian had no idea where that geographical region was, and, second, Brian's infatuation with Tanya and the accompanying fantasies resulted in Brian's having an erection. Now, erections are not something that high school students, or anyone else for that matter, choose to display before peers, so, understandably, Brian was embarrassed. What was he to do?

This has happened to many high school males, who somehow manage to use textbooks to shield their erections or find some excuse to delay walking to the front of the room until "it is safer." Some high school girls and older females also experience sexual excitement that results in an erection, in this case of the clitoris. Yet, they are not as vulnerable as males to being exposed because clitoral erection is not evident through women's clothes. Women also experience vaginal lubrication when sexually excited, but this too is not readily identifiable when one is dressed.

If this reaction has happened to you, perhaps you wondered whether you are "normal"—you are. Perhaps you discussed this concern with your close friends. Most of us probably did not discuss it with our parents. That would have been too embarrassing. Maybe you read about these reactions in a magazine or saw them depicted in a movie. Unfortunately, too many young people rely on these sources for information about sex—and magazines and movies often relay misconceptions and misinformation. But how were you to know that? Where else could you go? Whom else could you speak with?

This chapter provides the information you may have wondered about since that time when your body first responded sexually. Included is a description of the typical human sexual response and the means of eliciting that response. Our goal is to help you establish and maintain a satisfying and effective sexual relationship when you decide you are ready for one. We begin with the study of the usual human sexual response.

Sexual Arousal and Response

When unaroused, the penis is flaccid; the skin of the scrotal sac is wrinkled, thin, and loose; and the testes hang down from the body. In females, the labia are thin and enclose the vestibule, the clitoris extends from under the clitoral hood, the inner part of the vagina remains elongated, and the nipples of the breast are not erect.

After sexual excitement diminishes, these structures return to their prearoused state. This takes some time, which varies from person to person.

Sexual pleasure and satisfaction are both psychologically and physiologically based. Without the subjective feeling of pleasure, physiological arousal will not occur. For example, if you dislike the body odor of your partner, it will be difficult for you to develop an erection if you are a male or lubrication of the vagina if you are a female. As we shall soon see, pleasurable sexual stimulation will lead to an identifiable sexual response cycle. Knowing what this response cycle is can help you view your sexuality as a normal part of your functioning, for it suggests that sexual responses can be understood, predicted, and studied in the same way that other physiological processes can. Furthermore, learning to discern and distinguish your own bodily responses can enable you to pay attention, tell your partner about your responses, and thus increase your enjoyment.

How the Mind and Body Control Sexual Response

When a person becomes sexually aroused, several different parts of the body work together to create the psychological feeling of arousal and the accompanying physiological reactions. When Brian fantasized about Tanya, his brain, glands, nervous system, circulatory system, and reproductive system were only some of the bodily parts involved. Before we discuss the particular response to sexual stimulation, let us look more closely at what happens between the body and mind on such occasions.

The Brain: The Master of the Body

As with most vital functions, the brain is a key player during sexual arousal (Greenberg, 2002). It is the brain that interprets the stimulation—be it visual, olfactory, or other—and begins the process of "activating" other body parts.

The brain includes two major components: the **cerebral cortex** (the upper part) and the subcortex (the lower part). Figure 7.1 shows the structures of the brain and their locations. The subcortex includes the cerebellum (coordinates body movements), the medulla oblongata (regulates heartbeat, respiration, and other such basic physiological processes), the pons (regulates the sleep cycle), and the diencephalon. The diencephalon has many purposes, including the regulation of the emotions. It is made up of the

cerebral cortex
The part of the brain called the *gray matter* that controls higher-order functioning such as language and judgment.

limbic system
The part of the brain referred to as the "seat of emotions," which produces emotions in response to physical and psychological signals.

reticular activating system (RAS)
A network of nerves that connect the cortex and the subcortex—the connection between mind and body.

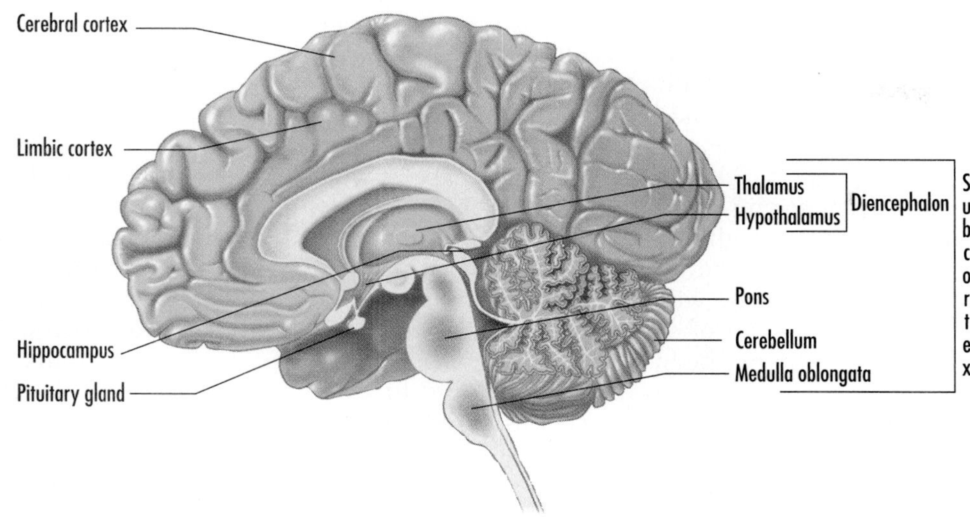

FIGURE 7.1 Many areas of the brain are involved in interpreting and determining each person's reaction to sexual stimulation.

thalamus and hypothalamus. The thalamus relays sensory impulses from other parts of the nervous system to the cerebral cortex. The hypothalamus, a key structure in sexual arousal, is the primary activator of the autonomic nervous system, which controls basic body processes such as hormone balance, temperature, and the constriction and dilation of blood vessels.

The **limbic system,** called the "seat of emotions," consists of the thalamus and hypothalamus (the diencephalon) and other structures important in sexual arousal. The limbic system is connected to the diencephalon and is primarily concerned with emotions and their behavioral expression. The limbic system is thought to produce such emotions as fear, anxiety, and joy in response to physical and psychological signals.

The cerebral cortex (called the *gray matter*) controls higher-order abstract functioning, such as language and judgment. The cerebral cortex can also control more primitive areas of the brain. When the diencephalon recognizes fear, for instance, the cerebral cortex can use judgment to recognize the stimulus as nonthreatening and override the fear.

Last is the **reticular activating system (RAS).** In the past, cortical and subcortical functions were considered dichotomized; that is, human behavior was thought to be a function of one area of the brain or the other. Now, brain researchers believe there are neurological connections between the cortex and subcortex that feed information back and forth. This network of nerves, the RAS, can be considered the connection between mind and body. The reticular system is a kind of two-way street, carrying messages perceived by the higher-awareness centers to the organs and muscles and also relaying stimuli received at the muscular and organic levels up to the cerebral cortex. In this manner, a sexually stimulating touch can generate physiological responses.

The Brain and Sexual Response

When you encounter a sexual stimulus of whatever kind, this message is passed to the brain via nerves. Once reaching the brain, the message passes through the reticular activating system either from or to the limbic system and the thalamus. The limbic system is where emotion evolves, and the thalamus serves as the switchboard, determining what to do with the incoming messages. Next, the hypothalmus is activated and, in turn, activates the autonomic nervous system and the endocrine system through messages sent via nerves or substances released into the bloodstream.

All of this is generalized, of course. No two people are exactly the same, so no two people should be expected to react in exactly the same manner to sexual stimulation. First, what one person finds sexually arousing, another might not. As a result, one person might experience erection or vaginal lubrication when seeing pictures of people engaged in sexual activities, whereas another person might be "turned off" by this material. Second, because of illness or injury, some typical responses may be precluded for some people. For example, a male with a spinal cord injury might not be able to achieve an erection in spite of what might usually be sexually arousing for others. Furthermore, some people have little control over apparently involuntary responses; however, other people are able to exercise some control. For example, although ejaculation is considered an involuntary response to sexual stimulation, we know that people can learn to control (that is, delay) ejaculation should they choose to. So, in general, there is a great deal of variation in sexual response, even though there are certain typical means of reacting to sexually stimulating stimuli.

The Autonomic Nervous System

The autonomic nervous system consists of the sympathetic nervous system and the parasympathetic nervous system. These "subnervous systems" connect to various parts of the body through nerves. Consequently, as sexually arousing stimuli are experienced, messages are sent via the nerves to body parts, instructing them to react. The heart rate increases, muscles tense, perspiration occurs, and the mind starts racing. In addition, certain arteries are instructed to open (dilate) and allow more blood to flow through. That is why, for instance, the penis and the clitoris become erect. Arteries in these structures dilate, allowing blood to flow to the area; the nerves instruct veins to constrict, thereby holding the blood in that one place. The result is erection. The increase of blood to the genital area, called *engorgement,* also creates pressure on the walls of the vagina, resulting in vaginal lubrication. Furthermore, muscles also contract as a result of messages sent through the nerves that make up the autonomic nervous system. For men, for example, contractions of the Cowper's gland, the seminal vesicles, and the prostate gland result in fluids' being secreted into semen; contractions of the abdominal muscles and the muscles surrounding the reproductive organs are experienced by women.

The Role of Hormones in Sexual Arousal

The endocrine system is responsible for the secretion of hormones that travel to various body parts, instructing them how to behave. For example, when you are "stressed out," hormones are deposited into the bloodstream by the pituitary, adrenal, thyroid, and other glands and transported around the body, resulting in an increase in heart rate, muscle tension, blood pressure, and perspiration.

Sexual arousal works similarly. When you encounter a sexually arousing stimulus, your endocrine system is activated; hormones are secreted, and changes occur in your body. That is what happens when someone fantasizes about a sexual experience. The fantasy translates into a sexual response that depends on the release of hormones that target certain body parts and bodily functions.

As we discussed in Chapters 4 and 5, sexual hormones are produced in the testes and ovaries. Testosterone, an androgen produced predominantly in the interstitial cells of the testes in men and in the ovaries in women (although a small amount is also produced in the adrenal glands), affects sexual interest, or *libido.* The more testosterone, the greater the interest in sex. Conversely, the less testosterone, the less interest in sex. As discussed in Chapter 6, Islamic societies once used castrated men to watch the women in the harem because their lowered interest in sex made them no threat to the women.

Recognizing the influence of testosterone on sexual interest, and in an attempt to enhance sexual satisfaction, some people turn to chemical aids. One of these "aids" is the substance used by the baseball player Mark McGwire during his record-breaking home run season. Popularly referred to as "andro," androstenedione is marketed as a dietary supplement; thus it is not regulated by the U.S. Food and Drug Administration (FDA). Athletes employ androstenedione to help them recover from weight-training workouts. Chemically, androstenedione is a steroid hormone "and a near cousin of testosterone" (How experts view andostenedione, 1998). The association with testosterone was enough to convince some people to use it to enhance sexual satisfaction. The problem with doing so is twofold: (1) The amount of testosterone may not be sufficient for the desirable effects, and (2) its use may result in harmful side effects, especially over the long term. Among other potential side effects, steroid use can lead to liver cancer, mood swings, hair growth, masculinization in women, and atrophied testes in men. In spite of these problems, androstenedione's possible effects on sexual arousal seem to override good judgment for some people hell-bent on making their sex lives ever richer.

Aphrodisiacs: Seeking the Ultimate in Sexual Pleasure

An *aphrodisiac,* named after the Greek goddess Aphrodite, the goddess of love, is any substance that arouses sexual desire and/or enhances sexual response. For centuries people have searched for a safe and effective aphrodisiac without much luck. This search has led to "Spanish fly" *(canthardin),* which results in irritation of the urinary tract. Now, is that sexually arousing? It has led to substances to make one "horny," such as ground-up rhinoceros horns or elephant tusks, which just do not work. Oysters, clams, and even the testicles of bulls ("prairie oysters") have been tried without the desired effect.

Even substances that are toxic have been ingested in the hope of enhancing sexual desire and response; *amyl nitrate* is one of these substances. Amyl nitrate is designed for use by heart patients to reduce chest pain. Its container is "popped" open when chest pain occurs; thus the containers are often called "poppers." Amyl nitrate became popular among some gay men as an aphrodisiac because it facilitated anal intercourse by relaxing the anal sphincter muscle. Although it does dilate blood vessels in the brain and genitals, resulting in warmth in the abdomen and pelvis, facilitating erection, and possibly prolonging orgasm, it is also associated with disturbing side effects. For example, amyl nitrate can cause dizziness, headaches, and fainting and can even result in death in extreme cases.

Bupropion (acquired under the brand name Wellbutrin) and L-dopa are other substances that have been ingested for their aphrodisiac effects. Bupropion is an antidepressant drug, and L-dopa is a drug used for treating patients with Parkinson's disease. Both of these drugs act on the brain receptors that produce dopamine and so can increase libido. However, unsupervised use of a drug that affects the brain is dangerous; it must be monitored by a physician and prescribed for a specific medical purpose.

Alcohol and *marijuana* have also been ascribed aphrodisiaclike qualities. However, if they work at all, they diminish judgment and make people feel less stress about sex. That may be good, or that may be bad. A decrease in inhibitions may result in high-risk sexual behaviors (such as vaginal or anal intercourse without a condom) that may transmit a sexually transmitted infection (STI) or cause an unwanted pregnancy. Furthermore, alcohol is a central nervous system depressant that can interfere with sexual arousal rather than enhance it. Marijuana can distort perceptions and make one

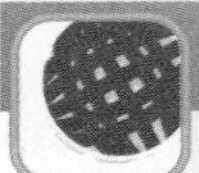

Global DIMENSIONS

Aphrodisiacs and Tigers: A Strange Mix Some of the most expensive aphrodisiacs in the world are made from parts of male tigers. The most prized and valuable aphrodisiacs are made from the tiger's penis—often made into a soup! Less expensive "love potions" are made from everything else down to the tiger's crushed bone. Such aphrodisiacs are extremely popular, predominantly in Asian countries.

The net result is that the last several thousand of the world's tigers are endangered—and all for naught. As with many other aphrodisiacs, no physiological sexual response results from ingesting tiger parts.

To help debunk the myth of the tiger as aphrodisiac, the Wildlife Conservation Society hired a Singapore ad agency to create the ad shown here. The TV ad (intended for an Asian audience) shows mating tigers. The voice-over reads, "The last 5,000 tigers in the world are being killed. All because some men believe that eating tiger penis will give them legendary sexual prowess. Perhaps they too can make love for a full 15 seconds."

What psychological effects might such an "aphrodisiac" have in a country where there is a long-standing cultural belief that it works? Might the ability to pay a great deal of money for such an aphrodisiac have a psychological boosting effect? Will the ad help to "destroy the myth," as it claims? Explain your answer.

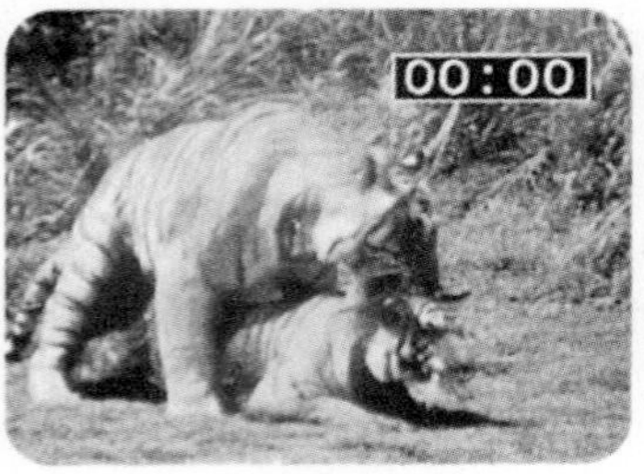

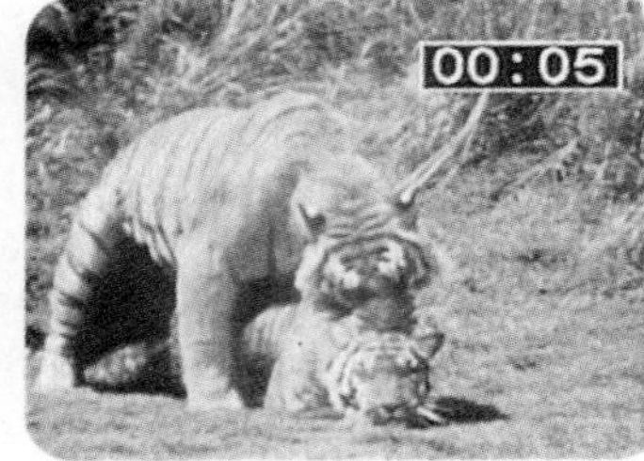

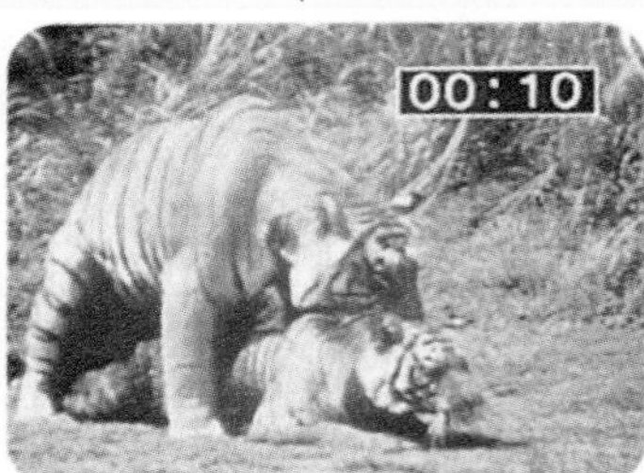

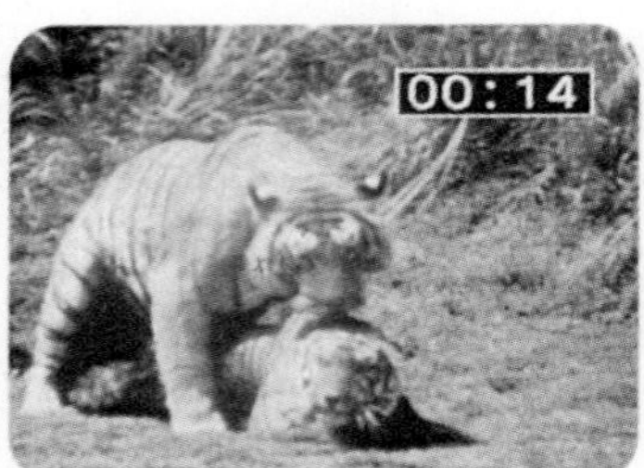

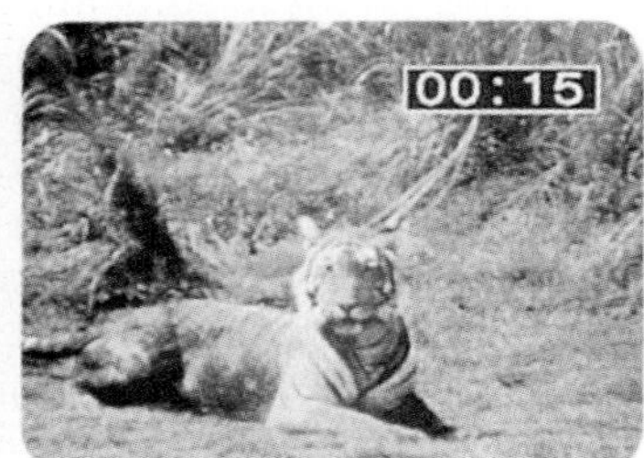

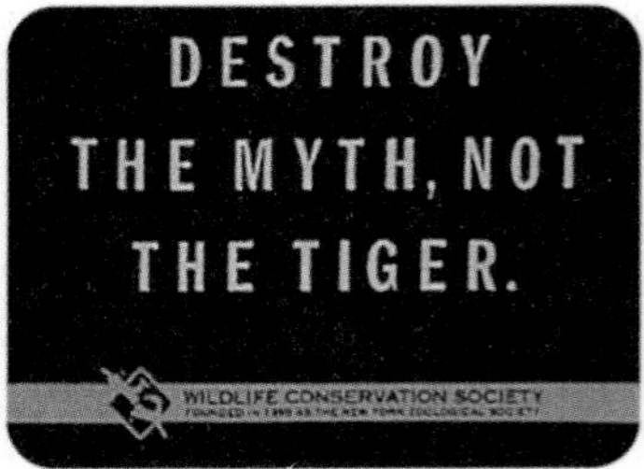

think that the sexual experience continued longer than it really did. Both of these substances can lead to problems in the short run and over prolonged use; in addition, marijuana is illegal.

One substance that appears to have potential as an aphrodisiac is *yohimbine hydrochloride,* from the sap of a West African tree, the yohimbine tree. Yohimbine has been reported to aid some men with erectile dysfunction to achieve and maintain an erection for a long-enough period to engage in sexual intercourse (Rowland, Kallan, & Slob, 1997). However, it does not work for all men with erectile dysfunction, and whether it enhances the sexual response of other men is unknown.

Even drugs that inhibit sexual desire have been the focus of researchers for many years. These drugs are called *anaphrodisiacs.* For years, rumor has had it that one of these substances, *potassium nitrate,* known as *saltpeter,* is

Did You Know . . .

Researchers (Rubenstein, 1991) asked 5,000 readers of *American Health* magazine, admittedly a biased sample, what they might do to feel more sexually attractive and to respond better sexually. Just over half the women (58%) and almost half the men (49%) surveyed said they would be willing to exercise 1 hour a day to be better lovers, but relatively few of either the women (9%) or the men (12%) would take an aphrodisiac. To enhance their sexual response, 61% of the women and 55% of the men listened to music while engaged in sexual intercourse at some time during the month before the survey, and 19% of the women and 23% of the men watched an X-rated videotape during coitus. What was surprising is that 38% of the women and 34% of the men watched television during intercourse.

Source: Data from Rubenstein, The American health sex survey, *American Health* (December 1991), 56–57.

used by the military to diminish the sexual desire of soldiers and is used in summer camps to control the "raging urges" of teenagers. However, all that potassium nitrate does is increase the need to urinate; some people obviously think that is enough to interfere with sex.

Yet some drugs do interfere with sexual response. These tend to be central nervous system depressants such as opiates (such as heroin), tranquilizers, antihypertensive medications, antipsychotic and antidepressant drugs (such as Prozac), and, surprisingly to many people, nicotine, which constricts blood vessels and decreases vasocongestion in the genitals.

The Masters and Johnson Sexual Response Cycle

The research of Masters and Johnson (1966) revealed a great deal about human sexuality. One of their major contributions was their description of the four phases of the human sexual response.

Excitement Phase

During the first phase of the Masters and Johnson **sexual response cycle,** the *excitement phase,* sexual stimuli result in a number of specific changes in the bodies of men and women. Heart rate, blood pressure, and muscle tension all increase. Blood engorges the abdominal area, resulting in an increase in penile and clitoral erection, as well as an increase in size of the labia minora, vagina, and nipples. The testes move closer to the body, and the scrotal skin thickens and tightens during the excitement phase. In addition, vaginal lubrication occurs, and the labia majora spread and separate so as to make the vestibule more accessible. Some of these structures also deepen in color as a result of the increased blood to the area. The engorgement of blood is also responsible for the darkening of the skin on the chest and breasts called the *sex flush.* Although the sex flush occurs in both genders, it is more common in women. It also occurs in all ethnic groups, although it may be more evident in whites than in people of color.

sexual response cycle
The sequence of physiological and psychological reactions as a result of sexual arousal.

transudation
The process of vaginal lubrication resulting from engorgement of blood that creates pressure that forces moisture to seep from the spaces between the cells.

Transudation is the process resulting in vaginal lubrication. When a female is sexually aroused, blood flows into the area surrounding the walls of the vagina in a process called *vasocongestion.* The pressure of the increased blood causes a seepage of moisture from the spaces between the cells. This moisture crosses the vaginal lining, first appearing as droplets. Eventually the fluid builds up in sufficient quantity to moisten the entire inner walls of the vagina. The amount of moisture may even be enough, depending on the woman's position, to leak out of the vagina and lubricate the labia and introitus.

The excitement phase may be short or last for several hours. The longer it lasts, the more variability occurs. For example, changes in the penis and the vagina vacillate over time during an extended excitement phase, so that the penis may occasionally become less erect, and vaginal lubrication may diminish periodically as well. The exciting aspect of excitement (pun intended) is the great variability among people. Some respond quickly; others need more time. Some favor moving to the next phase quickly; others desire more time. Some focus on their own reactions and feelings and satisfaction; others are more concerned with the partner's satisfaction. Furthermore, any one person may experience the excitement phase differently from one sexual encounter to another.

Plateau Phase

The second phase of Masters and Johnson's sexual response cycle is called the *plateau phase*. During the plateau phase, excitement becomes enhanced. Heart rate quickens, blood pressure rises, muscle tension increases, and breathing is faster. In men, Cowper's gland secretions may result from muscular contractions. The penis becomes fully erect, and the testes move closer to the body cavity. In women, the clitoris retracts under the clitoral hood; the inner two-thirds of the vagina fully extends, forming a "tenting" effect and creating a receptacle for semen; and the outer third of the vagina engorges with blood, forming the orgasmic platform. Although the plateau phase usually lasts but a few minutes, there are reports of more intense orgasms by people who have purposefully extended the plateau phase. And yet, orgasm is not the necessary follow-up to plateau. Although for men the loss of erection is unlikely once plateau is reached, in women as we shall soon see, reaching the plateau phase may be sufficient for sexual satisfaction.

Orgasm Phase

The *orgasm phase* for males consists of two stages: the *emission stage* and the *expulsion stage*. During the emission stage, muscular contractions of the vas deferens, the seminal vesicles, and the prostate gland create a buildup of semen in the urethral bulb located at the base of the penis. At the same time, the external urethral sphincter contracts, holding in the semen. Concurrently, the internal urethral sphincter contracts, thereby preventing semen from entering the bladder (a condition known as *retrograde ejaculation*) and urine from entering the urethral bulb where the semen has accumulated. The accumulation of semen in the urethral bulb creates a sensation of imminent and inevitable ejaculation, which usually lasts only a few seconds. Soon the second stage, expulsion, occurs.

During the expulsion stage, the **internal urethral sphincter** remains contracted, so urine and semen do not mix. However, the **external urethral sphincter** relaxes, and muscles surrounding the urethral bulb and the urethra contract, with the result that the accumulated semen is expelled from the urethral opening. Although there is some variation from one person to another, males generally experience intense sensations during the first couple of contractions and less sensation during later contractions. The degree of sensation appears also to be related to the amount of semen expelled.

In women, the orgasm phase also consists of muscular contractions and intense sensations. The pelvic muscles that surround the vagina, in particu-

internal urethral sphincter
The valve that prevents urine from entering the urethra and sperm from entering the bladder during ejaculation.

external urethral sphincter
The valve that closes during the emission stage, resulting in a buildup of semen, and that opens during the ejaculation stage, allowing semen to be expelled.

sex flush
A darkening of the skin of the neck, face, forehead, or chest during sexual stimulation.

myotonia
Muscle tension occurring during sexual arousal.

hyperventilation
Deep and rapid breathing that occurs during sexual excitation.

tachycardia
An increase in heart rate that occurs during sexual activity.

vasocongestion
Increased blood flow to an area of the body; which occurs in the pelvic area during sexual arousal.

Gender DIMENSIONS

Male–Female Differences in Sexual Response

There are many similarities and many differences in how males and females respond to sexual arousal. Masters and Johnson found the following similarities in the response cycle of men and women:

1. *Nipples.* Both males' and females' nipples become erect and wider in diameter when sexually stimulated.
2. *Sex Flush.* Males and females both experience a darkening of the skin of the neck, face, forehead, or chest during sexual stimulation, known as the **sex flush.** This darkening of the skin is a result of the accumulation of blood in these areas.
3. *Muscle Tension.* Commencing during the plateau phase and involving the legs, arms, abdomen, neck, and face, muscle tension **(myotonia)** appears in both sexes. During orgasm, muscles of the abdomen, chest, and face are also tensed. After orgasm, during the resolution phase, there is a release of all muscular tension in both sexes.
4. *Breathing.* During sexual excitation, both sexes experience deep and rapid breathing, called **hyperventilation.**
5. *Heart Rate.* Heart rate increases from a normal resting rate of about 72 up to 180 or more beats per minute during orgasm are not unusual in either sex. Such an increase is termed **tachycardia.**
6. *Blood Pressure.* Blood pressure rises in both males and females during sexual excitation.
7. *Perspiration.* Approximately one-third of both males and females perspire after orgasm.
8. *Blood Flow.* Increased blood flow to the pelvic area results in clitoral and penile erection and vaginal lubrication. This increased blood flow is termed **vasocongestion.**
9. *Orgasm.* During orgasm there is a rapid contraction of muscles in both sexes, with a relaxing of the muscles after orgasm.

The following listing describes the differences in the sexual responses of males and females:

1. *Nipples.* Whereas females are most likely to experience nipple erection during the excitement phase, males usually experience it during the plateau phase. Further, female nipple erection appears to disappear soon after orgasm (although this is an illusion caused by the swelling of the areolae), whereas male nipple erection is often obvious long after.
2. *Sex Flush.* Whereas males experience sex flush only in the plateau phase, in females sex flush can occur either late in the excitement phase or in the plateau phase. And though it may occur on the neck, forehead, and chest of both males and females, the sex flush occurs over the lower abdomen, thighs, lower back, and buttocks of females only.
3. *Muscle Tension.* In females muscular tension causes an increase in the length and width of the vagina and expansion of the diameter of the cervix; in males it causes elevation of the testes: that is, they are moved closer to the body by the contraction of muscles supporting them.
4. *Breathing.* Hyperventilation has different effects on males and females. After orgasm, males must wait for hyperventilation to diminish before being able to have another orgasm or even to achieve another erection; this period while breathing slows is referred to as a *refractory period.* Females, however, may have another orgasm before hyperventilation subsides—that is, without a refractory period and without entering a resolution phase. Consequently some females are capable of many orgasms in a short period.
5. *Blood Pressure.* Blood pressure increases somewhat more in males than in females. In males systolic blood pressure has been found to increase 40 to 100 mm Hg and diastolic blood pressure 20 to 50 mm Hg during sexual stimulation. In females the increase ranges from 30 to 80 mm Hg systolic and 20 to 40 mm Hg diastolic.
6. *Perspiration.* In men, sweating is usually limited to the soles of the feet and palms of the hands. Women are more likely to perspire over the back, thighs, chest, and sometimes the trunk, head, and neck.
7. *Orgasm.* Women are more likely than men to be multiorgasmic. Further, orgasm for the woman usually lasts longer than for men. The disagreement about female ejaculation was discussed in Chapter 4; it is sufficient to say here that, at the very least, female ejaculation does not occur as often during orgasm as does male ejaculation.

orgasmic platform
The narrowing of the outer third of the vagina during orgasm caused by contractions of the muscles in that area.

refractory (recovery) period
The time needed by males for recovery between orgasms.

multiple orgasms
Orgasms that occur without the need for a refractory, or recovery, period.

lar those that make up the **orgasmic platform,** contract 3 to 15 times, each contraction lasting less than 1 second. Other weaker and slower contractions follow. In addition, uterine contractions occur, beginning from the top of the uterus and proceeding downward.

In both males and females, other changes occur during orgasm. For example, heart rate increases dramatically, blood pressure rises, and breathing becomes rapid and shallow. Muscles throughout the body contract, and perspiration is evident. And an intense, pleasant psychological feeling associated with the release of sexual tension afforded by orgasm occurs.

Resolution Phase

During the *resolution phase,* there is a return to the unaroused state. In males, there is a decrease in the size of the penis as the erection is lost. This occurs in two stages: The first lasts about 1 minute as the blood exits the corpora cavernosa; the second takes several minutes as the blood leaves the corpus spongiosum. This is a result of the opening of the veins in the penis, which allows blood to be removed from the area. The testes become smaller and move down from the body cavity, and the scrotal skin becomes thinner and looser.

In women, muscles relax, and the uterus, vagina, and labia return to their unaroused positions and color. As a result of the uterus's returning to its unaroused position, the cervix lowers into the seminal pool. If sperm is present in the seminal pool, the cervix is likely to have contact with them, and fertilization is possible. If one is trying to become pregnant, then the woman should lie on her back after intercourse to encourage this contact. Of course, the best way to prevent pregnancy if engaging in sexual intercourse is to use some method of contraception.

In addition to the preceding changes, during the resolution phase the clitoris returns from under the clitoral hood and the sex flush dissipates. In both males and females, heart rate, blood pressure, and breathing rate return to normal, and muscle tension decreases. Males then experience a **refractory (recovery) period** during which they are incapable of another orgasm. This period may be only several minutes for young males but is usually longer in older males. Females, however, are capable of having **multiple orgasms** before needing to recover.

Each of us, male and female, progresses sequentially through the preceding four phases if we experience orgasm. Clearly, many body processes are involved during sexual activity, and each phase of the response affects the body somewhat differently. Even if we do not reach the orgasmic phase, we may pass through the earlier phases. For example, you may be engaged in sexual stimulation and quickly reach the excitement phase. The plateau stage may occur next, but—just your luck—the telephone rings and your excitement dissapates when you find out a loved one needs your help.

In studying the sexual response cycle in males and females, Masters and Johnson found both startling differences and amazing similarities. Knowing how females and males compare and contrast sexually is important to reinforcing the notion that we all have much in common while still preserving our differences.

If any of these responses is new to you, do not be surprised. You probably do not know everything about your digestive functions or nervous system, for instance, so why would you know everything about your sexual responses without studying them? The next time you are sexually aroused (either physically or by thoughts or fantasies), stop for a moment and attempt to identify the responses just discussed—or reflect now on some past sexual experience. Remember, no two of us are exactly alike. Consequently you may not experience all the sexual responses as we have described them. This is to be expected. Generally, though, you will find that your sexual responses are similar to the ones described.

Figure 7.2 depicts the typical male sexual response according to Masters and Johnson. Males start with the excitement phase, move to the plateau phase, proceed to have an orgasm, and then either move through the resolution phase, in which they return to the prearoused state, or to a refractory period (a part of the resolution phase), during which they recover from the orgasm and prepare themselves for another orgasm. Masters and Johnson found this pattern to be standard, although men report variations on this model.

Females were described by Masters and Johnson as being more varied in their sexual responses. Figure 7.2 also shows this variability. Pattern (a) is similar to the male pattern with a progression from excitement to plateau to orgasm and then resolution, except that it depicts a female's ability to have multiple orgasms without a refractory period. Pattern (b) shows the woman's progressing from excitement to an enhancement of this excitement during the plateau phase and then moving directly to resolution (bypassing orgasm). This pattern implies that women may be sexually satisfied without experiencing an orgasm. Pattern (c) depicts another possible female sexual response cycle in which there is no definitive plateau phase but a rapid escalation to orgasm and a very quick resolution.

Figures 7.3 and 7.4 summarize changes that occur in males and females during the four phases of the Masters and Johnson sexual response cycle.

Other Theoretical Models of Sexual Response

Two other models descriptive of the human sexual response are particularly noteworthy. These models are the product of years of experience in sexual counseling and therapy.

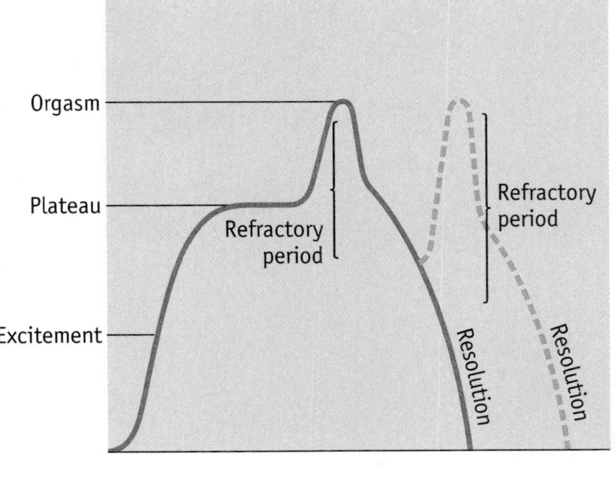

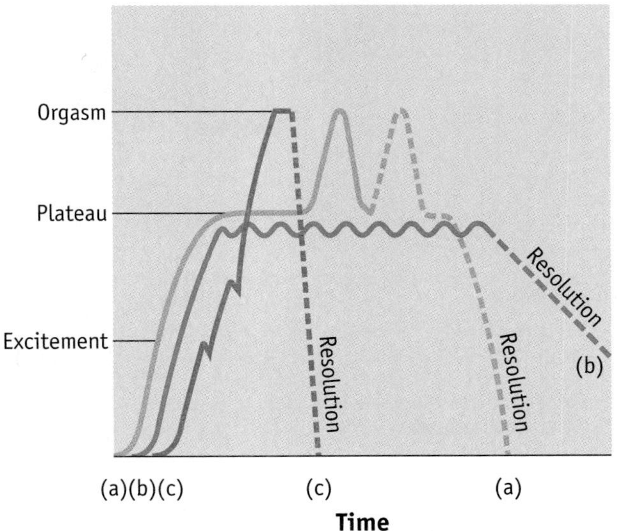

FIGURE 7.2 According to Masters and Johnson, the male sexual response cycle (a) is much more predictable than is the female response cycle, and (b) females can have a similar response to males—that is, moving through the four phases and experiencing orgasm—or can maintain the plateau phase without orgasm. Females can also be multiorgasmic without experiencing a refractory period.

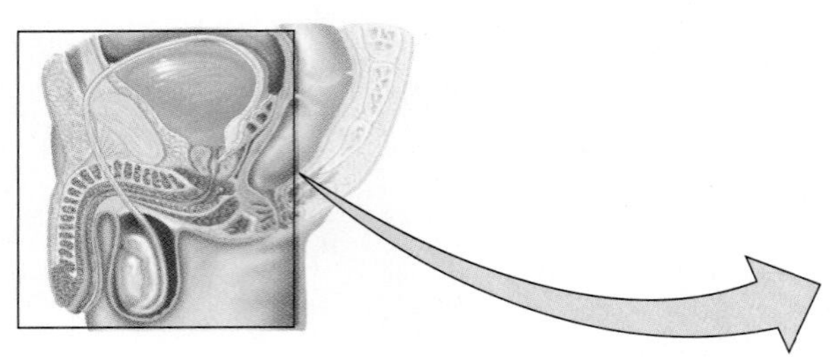

(a) Unaroused State

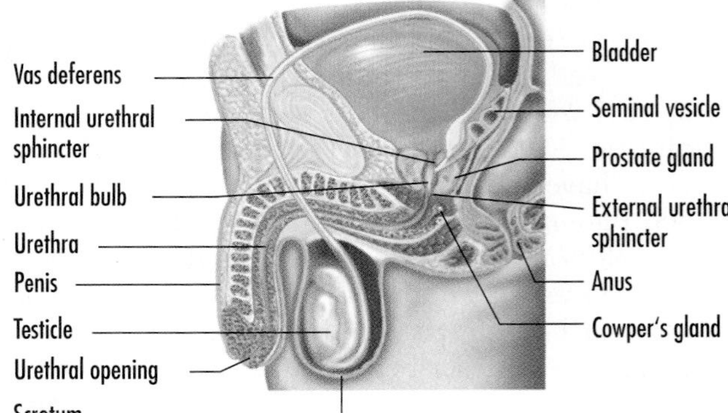

(b) Excitement Phase

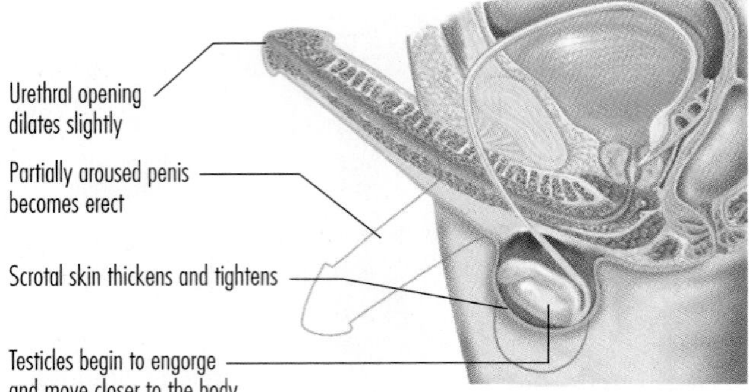

(c) Plateau Phase

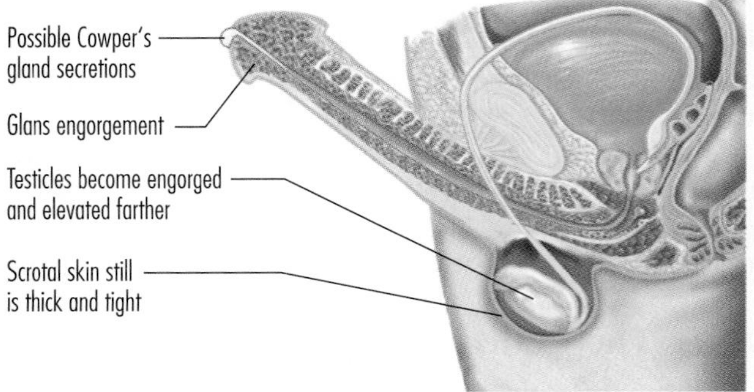

(d) Orgasm Phase: Emission Stage

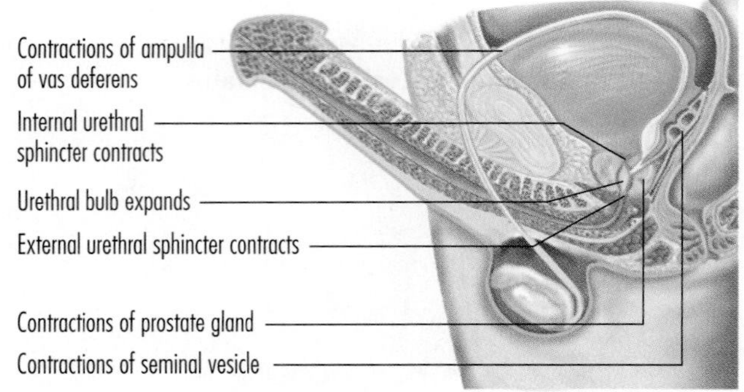

(e) Orgasm Phase: Expulsion Stage

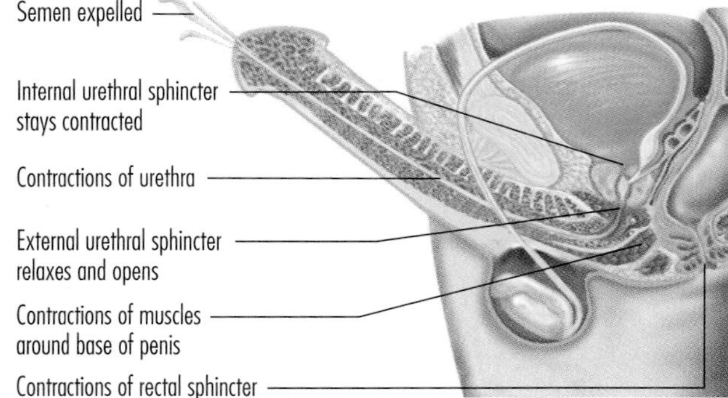

(f) Resolution

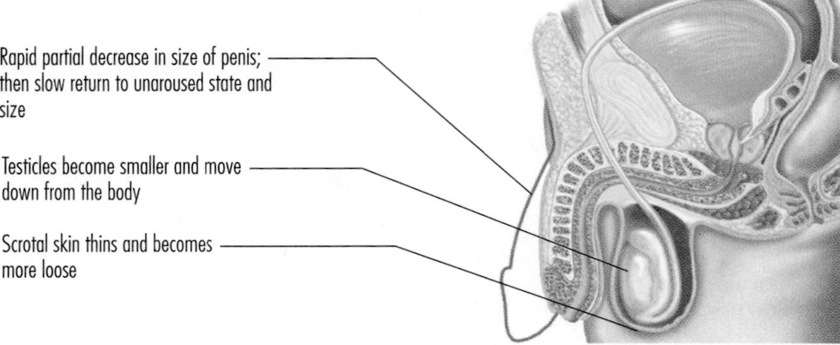

FIGURE 7.3 Male sexual response cycle, in detail.

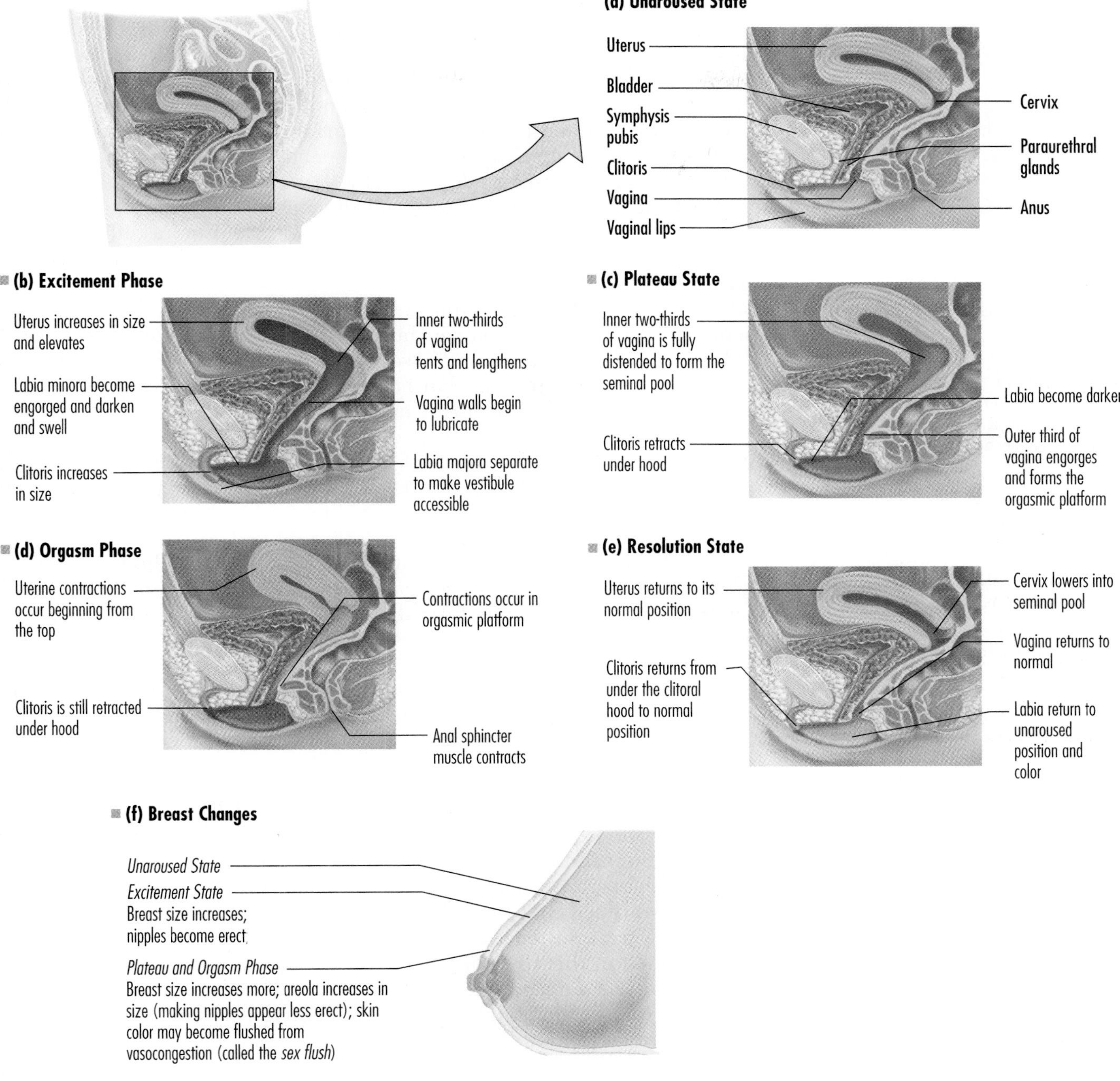

FIGURE 7.4 Female sexual response cycle, in detail.

Kaplan's Triphasic Model

Originally, the noted sex therapist Helen Singer Kaplan (1974) proposed a biphasic model of the human sexual response. That model conceptualized sexual response as having two identifiable phases. The first phase involved vasocongestion of the genitals, and the second phase consisted of the reflexive muscular contractions of orgasm. Kaplan argued that the two phases were each controlled by a different part of the nervous system: vasocongestion, by the parasympathetic nervous system, and orgasm, by the sympathetic nervous system (both are components of the autonomic nervous system). Furthermore, she explained, different structures are involved in each of these phases: the blood vessels for vasocongestion and the muscles for orgasm. Kaplan gave other justifications for the biphasic model, but space limits our discussion to the justification that derived from Kaplan's observations in her professional practice. Kaplan noted that the interference with vasocongestion resulted in erection problems in the male, whereas different sexual dysfunctions (premature ejaculation and retarded ejaculation) were the result of orgasm impairment. In some females, normal vasocongestion and sexual excitement were experienced in spite of the presence of orgasm problems. Because problems with vasocongestion were quite different from and mutually exclusive with problems with orgasm, Kaplan believed the biphasic model to be valid.

Over the years Kaplan's biphasic model evolved into a triphasic one. Kaplan (1979) now conceptualizes human sexual response as consisting of a **desire phase,** an **excitement phase,** and a **resolution phase.** During her practice as a sex therapist Kaplan has found that sexual dysfunctions fall into one of these three categories and that these categories are separate and distinct (that is, it is possible to function well in one or two phases while having problems in another). The unique component of Kaplan's triphasic model is the desire phase—a psychological prephysical sexual response stage. Masters and Johnson's model ignores this part of the sexual response.

desire phase
The first stage of the sexual response cycle, as described in Helen Singer Kaplan's model, which consists of psychologically becoming interested in sex before any physical changes occur.

excitement phase
The second stage of Kaplan's model of sexual response, which consists of physiological arousal and changes and, possibly, orgasm.

resolution phase
A stage of the sexual response cycle consisting of a return to the prearoused state.

Sexual desire is not always present during sexual activity, however. Sometimes a person may engage in sexual activity to satisfy his or her partner rather than because he or she feels the desire. A speaker in one of our sexuality classes described how when his wife complains of some ache or pain (or the proverbial headache) when he is interested in sex, he asks where she feels bothered. When he finds the spot, he gently massages that area, soon turning the massage into a sensual experience. Shortly, he relates, the desire phase is reached.

Zilbergeld and Ellison's Model

Another model of human sexual response consists of five components. The therapists Bernie Zilbergeld and Carol Ellison (1980) were concerned that Masters and Johnson's model ignored the cognitive and subjective aspects of the sexual response, while focusing exclusively on the physiological aspects. They argued that the subjective elements of sexual desire and sexual arousal were omitted from the Masters and Johnson model. *Sexual desire* is defined in this five-component model as the frequency with which a person wants to engage in sexual activity; *sexual arousal* is defined as how excited one becomes during sexual activity. The five components of this model are as follows.

1. Interest, or desire
2. Arousal
3. Physiological readiness (for example, erection or vaginal lubrication)
4. Orgasm
5. Satisfaction (one's evaluation of how one feels)

As with Kaplan's model, Zilbergeld and Ellison's model allows for sexual dysfunctions that pertain to desire although other responses may be normal. Consequently, this component can be isolated from the other components for treatment by a sex therapist. One might describe the triphasic and the five-component models as being more inclusive of the psychological aspects of the sexual response, whereas the Masters and Johnson model is more concerned with the physiological aspects.

Erotic Stimulus Pathway

An important contribution to our knowledge of sexual response is that of the Erotic Stimulus Pathway (ESP) theory of David M. Reed (Haffner & Stayton, 1998). The ESP theory enhances our understanding and ability to treat sexual dysfunctions. Reed divides the sexual response cycle into four phases that correspond to those of Kaplan and Masters and Johnson. For many people, these phases are learned developmentally. Figure 7.5 compares the Masters and Johnson model with the Reed model.

In the *seduction phase* a person learns how to get aroused sexually and how to attract someone else sexually. Seduction translates into memories and rituals. For example, adolescents may spend much time on personal appearance, choice of clothes, and mannerisms, all of which can enhance positive self-esteem if the adolescents like the way they feel. If the adolescents feel good about the way they look and feel, then attracting another person will be much easier. As the adolescents get older, these positive feelings are translated into sexual desire and arousal. These seductive techniques are stored in memory and can be activated later on in life.

In the *sensations phase,* the different senses can enhance sexual excitement and ideally prolong the plateau phase. The early experiences of touch (holding hands, putting arms around a loved one) become very important. The sense of vision (staring at a loved one, holding an image of him or her when absent) is a way of maintaining interest and arousal. Hearing the loved one in intimate conversation or over the telephone becomes very important. Hearing the sounds of a partner responding to sexual stimulation can be titillating. The smell of the loved one, either a particular scent he or she wears or the sexual smell, produces additional excitement. Finally, the taste of a food or drink or the taste of the loved one becomes important to memory and fantasy. All these senses extend the excitement into a plateau phase, which makes one want to continue the pleasurable moment over a longer

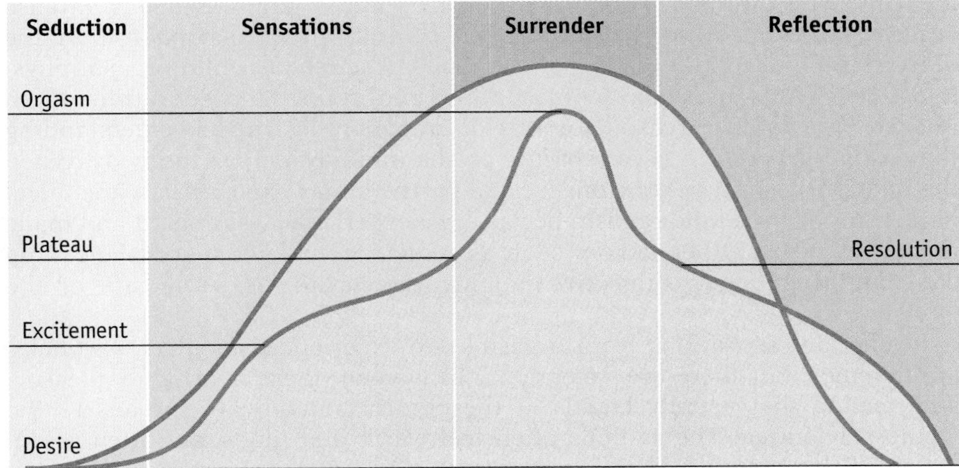

FIGURE 7.5 Sexual response curve.
Source: Masters, et al., 1966; Kaplan, 1979.

period. These seduction and sensation experiences are the psychological input to the physiology of sexual response. They are the precursors to sexual climax and orgasm.

In the *surrender phase,* orgasm is a "psychophysiological surprise." The psychodynamic issues surrounding orgasm are power and control. Persons with orgasmic dysfunction may be in a power struggle with themselves or with their partners or with the messages received about sex. Overcontrol or undercontrol can affect orgasmic potential and the ability to allow all of the passion to be expressed.

In the *reflection phase,* meaning is given to the experience. Whether the sexual experience is interpreted as positive or negative may determine the desire for subsequent sexual activity—at least with that sexual partner, under those circumstances, or with those behaviors. Recognize, though, that not every sexual experience can be, or should be, a "10." As the authors have heard it expressed, "Sometimes sex is a four-course gourmet meal, and sometimes it's like having cereal for dinner. Most of the time it's like having hamburgers or chicken. When it's cereal, you have to remember that there are better times ahead."

Orgasm

Our nonsexual lives tend to be goal oriented. We may have goals to graduate from college, to become established in a good career, or to live in a large house. It should be no surprise that goal orientation has invaded our sexual lives as well. For too many of us, orgasm becomes the goal of almost all of our sexual behavior. We forget about the pleasure that can be derived from sexual activity that does not lead to orgasm, and we forget that the communication and the quality of our relationships can be enhanced through sexual activity that does not result in orgasm. The question "Did you come?" tends to be as much a part of the sexual experience as removing one's clothes.

Orgasmic Sensation

The feelings that accompany orgasm are quite different from the physiological responses and may even contradict what we know is occurring physiologically. For example, women may experience a physiologically intense orgasm (a dozen or so measurable muscular contractions) but report the orgasm to be of mild intensity, or they may experience a mild orgasm physiologically (four muscular contractions) but report the sensation of an intense orgasm. The reason for this discrepancy lies in the understanding that sexual experience is interpreted by the mind as well as the body. When the relationship is a healthy one, sexual partners may experience a great deal of pleasure from a mild orgasm because the experience was shared and made them feel closer. Other factors such as mood, expectations, and the setting can also affect one's subjective judgment regarding the intensity of the orgasm.

Generally, sensations from orgasms are experienced similarly by males and females, but there are exceptions. In women, there is a highly pleasurable feeling that usually begins at the clitoris but quickly spreads to the whole pelvic area. The genitals often feel warm and tingly, and then a sensation of throbbing in the lower pelvis may be noticed. In men, the experience is also highly pleasurable. They usually experience warmth, pressure, and sometimes a throbbing during the moment when they have reached the "point of no return" (that is, ejaculatory inevitability), at which point men

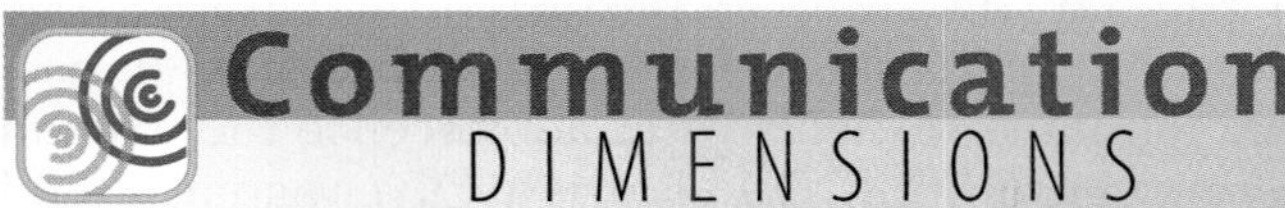

Communication DIMENSIONS

Discussing Sexual Desires Communicating sexual desires is embarrassing for many people. After all, sex is not something we are taught to talk about openly. The irony for many of us is that we are taught at a very young age that sex is so "dirty" that we should save it for someone we love. Does not make much sense, does it? Of course, sex is not dirty, although it may make sense to refrain from certain sexual activities altogether and to engage in others only when you are ready. When the time is right, if we could share what we find sexually arousing with a partner, we would be that much more satisfied. To help you along in this process, we have prepared the following guidelines. We recognize, though, that not all of you have chosen to engage in sexual activities with a partner. Still, these guidelines will be useful if and when you decide the time is right for you to do so.

- Speak about what you like sexually at times in which you are not engaged in sexual activity. This allows for a conversation that can be more rational than one carried on while emotions are running high.
- Be specific. State what you like and how you like it, what you dislike and why you dislike it.
- Ask your partner to do the same. Let your partner know that you want to please him or her as well as yourself. If your partner realizes you are concerned about his or her pleasure, he or she will be more likely to be concerned about your pleasure.
- During sex, let your partner know how you feel about what he or she is doing. Reinforce the behaviors you like by letting him or her know they are pleasing.
- Do not hesitate to refrain from any sexual activity you find unpleasant, uncomfortable, or distasteful. When doing so, explain your reasons to your partner.

Remember, you can have a more satisfying sexual relationship, when you are ready to do so, by being able to communicate freely about sex and what you find pleasurable and what you find displeasing.

cannot prevent ejaculation. In many men, ejaculation itself is experienced as a sensation of pumping.

The similarity of male and female orgasms was vividly demonstrated by two studies involving college students (Proctor, Wagner, & Butler, 1974; Wiest, 1977). In these studies, students wrote descriptions of their orgasms, and these descriptions were analyzed by a group of experts. The experts could not distinguish between the male and female descriptions, and the researchers concluded that males and females experience similar sensations as a result of orgasm. Although males and females do not generally differ in the sensations they report accompanying orgasm, orgasms *do* differ. That is, an individual may experience an orgasm today that is either more or less intense than one yesterday, and one person may experience orgasms generally more intensely than another person. These differences are not a function of gender; rather, a less pleasurable experience may be a result of guilt, shame, embarrassment, an uncomfortable setting, frustrations with the sexual partner, hostility, distrust, low self-esteem, or other factors.

Controversies About Orgasm

Several controversies surround the topic of orgasm.

Types of Orgasm

First, experts disagree about the types of orgasms that exist. In the early 1900s, Freud theorized there were two different types of female orgasm: the clitoral and the vaginal. He viewed the clitoral orgasm as an immature sex-

Myth vs Fact

Myth: It is easy to tell when a male has an orgasm because the ejaculate gives it away.
Fact: Although it is usually true that a male will ejaculate during orgasm, this is not always the case. Males may have an orgasm without ejaculating.

Myth: During the plateau phase of the Masters and Johnson sexual response cycle, conditions remain pretty much the same.
Fact: Although Masters and Johnson chose to call the second phase of the sexual response cycle the *plateau phase,* changes do occur. What occurred during the excitement phase is intensified during the plateau phase.

Myth: Whereas women can be multiorgasmic, men cannot.
Fact: Although it occurs relatively infrequently, some men do report needing very little time before being able to have another orgasm.

Myth: Males and females differ tremendously in their responses to sexual excitation.
Fact: There certainly are many differences between males and females in their responses to sexual excitement. Still, there are many similarities as well.

Myth: The clitoris can be stimulated easily during sexual intercourse.
Fact: Relatively early in the sexual response of women, the clitoris retracts under the clitoral hood. Therefore, it is not easily accessible to touch and/or stimulate unless the clitoral hood is purposefully pulled back.

ual response that women outgrew. Because he considered the clitoris to be a stunted penis, Freud believed the clitoral orgasm was an expression of masculine sexuality rather than feminine sexuality. If at adolescence the woman had not transferred her erotic focus from the clitoris to the vagina, Freud believed that psychotherapy was in order. When Freud's theory was operationalized, surgical removal of the clitoris **(clitoridectomy)** was actually performed on girls who were too clitorally focused, as determined by their masturbating by stimulating the clitoris.

Masters and Johnson's (1966) research identified but one type of orgasm. Regardless of the point of stimulation—clitoris or vagina—and regardless of the method of stimulation—penile insertion or vibrator—Masters and Johnson reported the same physiological occurrences during orgasm. However, Masters and Johnson did report a difference in the sensations of orgasm that depended on whether they were a result of coital or noncoital activities. They found orgasms from coitus to be less intense than orgasms from noncoital means. This finding was validated by Hite (1976), who found the clitorally stimulated orgasm to be more intense than the orgasm from coitus. Hite also found the coital orgasm to be more diffused throughout the body than was the locally intense clitoral orgasm.

To complicate matters further, other researchers (Singer & Singer, 1972) have reported three distinct types of orgasms: vulval, uterine, and blended. Singer and Singer included emotional satisfaction as a consideration in their research. **Vulval orgasm** is the same as the orgasm described by Masters and Johnson and includes contractions of the orgasmic platform; however, the vulval orgasm is not sexually satiating, and therefore another orgasm can be experienced immediately. A **uterine orgasm** can occur only in the presence of vaginal penetration and involves a woman's holding her breath just before orgasm and then exhaling when the climax occurs. In contrast to the vulval orgasm, the uterine orgasm is sexually satiating and is therefore usually followed by a refractory period. The **blended orgasm** is a combination of these two; that is, there are contractions of the outer third of the vagina as well as breath holding. These researchers make it clear that no one form of orgasm is better than another, just different.

How many forms of orgasm are there? As with other areas of human sexuality, there is disagreement. The important point is that orgasm can be conceptualized as merely a physiological reaction to sexual stimulation or as a complex of interactions between partners (the setting, the mood, and a host of other variables). To consider an orgasm as solely a bodily reaction is to ignore the interactive nature of the human mind and the human body and the impossibility of separating them. Without a mind to realize that sexual stimulation is, in fact, stimulating, there is no orgasm.

Recognizing Orgasms

At the beginning of the sexuality classes we teach, we ask students to write questions they would like answered before the semester ends. A common question asks how a man can recognize when his female partner is faking an orgasm. The women in the class are astute enough to know that when their male partners ejaculate, they experience orgasm. What they do not usually know is that sometimes orgasm can occur without an ejaculate—for example, in men with disease of the prostate or in prepubescent boys. Men, however, want to know how to recognize that their partners are sexually satisfied.

This question has several implications that deserve some attention. First, it expresses a concern for the woman's sexual satisfaction. On the

Ethical DIMENSIONS

Should Sexual Enhancements Be Used to Increase Sexual Arousal?

How far should people be allowed, or encouraged, to go in their search for sexual satisfaction and sexual arousal? Some people argue that anything that does not negatively affect another person is appropriate to enhance sexual arousal. They believe the use of X-rated videotapes, sexually explicit written material, and erotic clothing is within the bounds of acceptability. They also suggest that engaging in sexual relations with a number of different people can provide the experience necessary to reach one's sexual potential. Further, any physical barriers to sexual arousal should be eliminated at any cost. So if a man has blockage of the penile arteries, he should undergo bypass surgery to provide the penis with the blood it needs to become erect. And if there is damage to the penis as a result of an accident, options should include Viagra, artificial penises, surgery to implant rods in the penis to provide an erection, or penis transplantation (from someone who has recently died—similar to heart, kidney, and other organ transplantation).

Others believe that enhancing sexual arousal is appropriate, but only within certain limits. They argue that sexually explicit material is pornographic and/or obscene. Its use is unacceptable for any reason, and it should be outlawed. Furthermore, altering the body "merely" for sexual purposes goes against nature, is therefore "unnatural," and should not be tolerated. Sexual arousal should be enhanced through improving the relationship between the couple, and that can be accomplished only in a marriage, and one in which the spouses remain sexually faithful to each other. Only then, advocates of this view argue, can the couple engage in "lovemaking" as opposed to "sexmaking," because sex without love can never achieve the level of arousal that sex with love can.

What do you think? What is appropriate and what is inappropriate when trying to enhance sexual arousal?

surface, that appears to be healthy; however, it is our experience that when asked by men, this question is more related to a man's ego than to a woman's satisfaction. That is, if the male can "give" the woman an orgasm, he must be a good lover. Another interpretation of this question could be that men are afraid their female sexual partners might fake orgasms. A woman may fake an orgasm to meet her partner's expectation, to feed her partner's ego, to end the sexual encounter, to present herself as "normal," or to meet the "goal."

Beyond the fact that faking an orgasm is dishonest and deceitful, it may lead your partner to think that something unsatisfying to you was great and should be repeated the next time. However, if what a partner does is pleasurable but does not result in a climax, that might be enough. If so, why not tell your partner? Sexual activity can be enjoyed for itself without being directed toward the goal of orgasm.

Men are also prone to faking orgasms if they are unable to achieve one. When a man has been drinking alcoholic beverages, for example, and cannot reach the orgasmic phase, he might feel threatened by how this may be interpreted by his partner. Will his partner think he is less than a real man? Will his partner think he is sexually dysfunctional? Will his partner think he does not find him or her sexually attractive? Some men believe it is easier to fake an orgasm than to allay these fears.

Whether a man or woman fakes orgasm regularly, the person would be well advised to discuss the situation candidly with his or her partner. Such

clitoridectomy
Surgical removal of the clitoris.

vulval orgasm
An orgasm in a female that includes the contractions of the orgasmic platform, which is not sexually satisfying and, as a result, allows another orgasm to occur almost immediately.

uterine orgasm
An orgasm in a female that can occur only in the presence of penile penetration and that involves a woman's holding her breath just before orgasm and then exhaling when the climax occurs.

blended orgasm
An orgasm in a female in which there are contractions of the muscles in the outer third of the vagina as well as breath holding; a combination of the vulval and uterine orgasms.

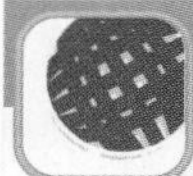

DIMENSIONS

Age of First Intercourse A study by the London International Group (1998) found that men and women worldwide are starting to engage in sexual intercourse at ever earlier ages. The study queried 10,000 sexually active adults from 14 developing and developed countries. The average age at first intercourse was 17.4 years (down slightly from the previous year's 17.6 years). However, there was a great deal of variability from country to country. For example, the average age at first intercourse in the United States was 15.8 years, whereas it was 19.0 years in Hong Kong. Differences also occurred in the frequency of intercourse. Whereas the average adult reported engaging in coitus 112 times a year, French and Americans reported more frequent intercourse (151 and 148 times per year, respectively) than did men and women from Hong Kong and Thailand (77 and 69 times per year, respectively). In addition, 40% of Americans wanted coitus more often, whereas only 7% of Mexicans expressed that desire.

a discussion can often result in a closer relationship and the understanding that setting up sexual performance goals is self-defeating. Some women do not reach orgasm, some have an orgasm once during intercourse, and some are multiorgasmic. Some men do not reach orgasm, some have an orgasm once during intercourse, and some are multiorgasmic (although some recovery time between orgasms is necessary). For people of either gender who do not reach orgasm, pleasure from coitus can still be attained. Rather than asking, "Did you come?" we should ask, "What did I do that you liked?" "How can I pleasure you more?" "How can we feel more intimate?" "How can we improve our relationship?"

Simultaneous Orgasm

Another question students often ask is how they and their partners can achieve an orgasm together. Unfortunately, some couples have as an ideal a choreographed orgasmic release, timed so that it occurs at the same time for both partners. Not only is this difficult to achieve, but concentrating on this goal detracts from the enjoyment of the coital experience. As long as each person is satisfied, the exact timing of the orgasm is of no particular importance. Although simultaneous orgasm is an undeniably exciting event, it is only one of a wide range of satisfying sexual patterns.

Exploring the DIMENSIONS of Human Sexuality

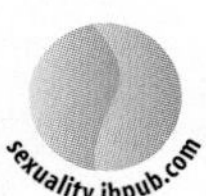

Our feelings, attitudes, and beliefs regarding sexuality are influenced by our internal and external environments. Go to sexuality.jbpub.com to learn more about the biological, psychological, and sociological factors that affect your sexuality.

Biological Factors

- Sexual arousal and response are physiological reactions to sexual stimuli.
- Masters and Johnson showed that some aspects of the human sexual response cycle are similar in men and women; however, differences exist.
- The body releases hormones when a person is sexually stimulated.
- Physical disabilities, injuries, or illness may alter the ability to respond to sexual stimuli.
- Male testosterone levels decline with age, affecting sexual response.
- Drugs, alcohol, and some aphrodisiacs may alter sexual response.

Sociocultural Factors

Biological factors are influenced by sociocultural and psychological factors. For example, some people are turned on by pornography; others are turned off.

- Religious beliefs influence our feelings about sexuality in general.
- Culture and ethnic heritage influence what we find sensual or attractive.
- Media and ads influence the types of sexual stimulation to which we react.
- Family, neighbors, and friends provide information about and influence our sexuality.
- Ethical decisions must be made regarding how far you and your partner are willing to go to achieve sexual arousal.

Psychological Factors

- Our feelings toward our partner influence the sexual response derived.
- Our level of experience influences our response to sexual stimuli.
- Learned attitudes and behaviors include discovering the stimuli to which we respond.
- Body image influences our self-concept. The better we feel about ourselves, the sexier an image we portray to others.

CASE STUDY

Although the human sexual response cycle is a physiological pattern, many factors influence the ways individuals actually experience the stages. Physical differences, including age, illness, injuries, and disabilities, may alter the response. Illicit drugs, alcohol, and aphrodisiacs also may alter the physical sensation we experience. Some drugs, such as Viagra, may enhance the response cycle.

The stimuli that we react to differ with culture and ethnic group, media exposure, even hygiene. Education and religious beliefs may also have an effect; a person who feels guilty about sexuality may have a more repressed reaction.

Finally, our self-image and our feelings about our partner greatly influence sexual response and arousal. Many people believe that happy times—experiencing a loving relationship, being successful professionally, and so on—make for better sex.

Discussion Questions

1. Describe the reaction of the mind and body when one is aroused by a sensual stimulation. How might artificial hormones or aphrodisiacs alter the response cycle? How would alcohol or other mood-altering drugs affect the cycle?
2. Compare and contrast the Masters and Johnson human response cycle with the models of Kaplan, Zilbergeld and Ellison, and Reed. Why does the Masters and Johnson model continue to attract the most attention?
3. Explain how understanding types of orgasms and recognizing orgasms could lead to a better sexual relationship.

Application Questions

Reread the story that opens the chapter and answer the following questions.

1. Assuming that Brian and Tanya start dating, what visible signs of sexual arousal (aside from erection) might Tanya detect in Brian? What might Brian detect in Tanya?
2. Do you think Brian's feelings about Tanya might differ if he met her after gym class and she reeked of sweat? Explain.

Critical Thinking Questions

1. Laurie Cabot, a well-known practicing witch, often suggests that love potions or spells do work. She writes that a "spell is a thought, a projection, or a prayer." Thus, Cabot implies that the psychological effort that you put into a spell can produce a physiological response. Given this idea, would a love potion work? Put another way, would the extra attention you lavish on someone make that person more attracted to you?
2. The drug Viagra positively affects sexual response, especially in older men. However, increased sexual response is accompanied by higher blood pressure and a faster heartbeat—which has resulted in heart attacks and dozens of deaths. Explain why 30 million U.S. males have been willing to take the risk. Also consider why their partners would want them to risk their health for sexual pleasure.
3. *Baywatch* was one of the most-viewed TV shows in the world, with more than 1 billion viewers per week. Apply what you learned in the chapter to explain why.

Critical Thinking Case

It has been argued that too much emphasis is placed on orgasm and not enough on the total sexual experience, including talking and nongenital touch. Because sexual intercourse is a way of expressing love for another, the argument proceeds, the emphasis during the experience should be on the total relationship, the love expressed, whole-body sensations, and the feeling of closeness. Concentrating exclusively or primarily on the orgasm is self-defeating and narrows one's experience of sexuality.

In contrast, some people believe that sexual intercourse (or mutual masturbation or oral–genital sex) certainly includes all of the above but, in addition, has a culmination—orgasm. This culmination is so satisfying and, given effective sexual therapy, so available that it should be sought. Although sexual intercourse and other modes of sexual expression can be satisfying without orgasm, an orgasmic conclusion certainly adds to the experience and satisfaction.

What do you think? Why?

Exploring Personal Dimensions

Sexual Stimuli

Once the senses encounter sexual stimuli, the brain takes over, deciding how to respond. Which of the following sexual stimuli do you find arousing? If you have a partner, which does your partner find arousing? More importantly, with which stimuli do you share sexual arousal?

	YOU		**YOUR PARTNER**	
SIGHT				
Sexually explicit videos	Y	N	Y	N
Sexually explicit magazines	Y	N	Y	N
Romantic movies	Y	N	Y	N
Books	Y	N	Y	N
Lingerie	Y	N	Y	N
Skin	Y	N	Y	N
TOUCH				
Satin sheets	Y	N	Y	N
Leather	Y	N	Y	N
Massage	Y	N	Y	N
Scratching	Y	N	Y	N
SMELL				
Perfume (or cologne)	Y	N	Y	N
Flowers	Y	N	Y	N
Scented candles	Y	N	Y	N
TASTE				
Kissing	Y	N	Y	N
Oral sexual activities	Y	N	Y	N
Whipped cream	Y	N	Y	N
SOUND				
Whispering	Y	N	Y	N
Moaning (or groaning)	Y	N	Y	N
Music	Y	N	Y	N
Silence	Y	N	Y	N

What other sexual stimuli can you think of?

Sexuality Online

Go to the web component for *Exploring the Dimensions of Human Sexuality* at sexuality.jbpub.com for web exercises, additional resources related to this chapter, and student review tools.

Suggested Readings

Barbach, L. G. *For yourself: The fulfillment of female sexuality.* New York: New American Library, 1991.

Barker, T., ed. *The woman's book of orgasm: A guide to the ultimate sexual pleasure.* Secaucus, NJ: Citadel Press, 1998.

Bechtel, S. *The practical encyclopedia of sex and health: From aphrodisiacs and hormones to potency, stress, vasectomy and yeast infection.* Emmaus, PA: Rodale Press, 1993.

Bechtel, S. *Sex: A man's guide.* Emmaus, PA: Rodale Press, 1997.

Eisler, R. *Sacred pleasures: Sex, myth, and the politics of the body.* San Francisco: HarperCollins, 1995.

Haffner, D. & Schwartz, P. *What I've learned about sex: Wisdom from leading sex educators, therapists, and researchers.* New York: Perigree Books, 1998.

Lopiccolo, J. & Heiman, J. *Becoming orgasmic: A sexual and personal growth program for women.* Englewood Cliffs, NJ: Prentice Hall, 1988.

McCarthy, B. & McCarthy, E. *Male sexual awareness.* Berkeley, CA: Publishers Group West, 1998.

Pietropinto, M. Sensuality scale: Test your responses, enhance your desire, *Self* (July 1990), 104–107, 152.

Quadango, D. M. The menstrual cycle: Does it affect athletic performance? *The Physician and Sports Medicine, 19* (1991), 121–124.

Reinisch, J. *The Kinsey Institute: New report on sex.* New York: St. Martin's Press, 1990.

Schnarch, D. *Passionate marriage: Sex, love, and intimacy in emotionally committed relationships*. New York: Norton, 1997.

Sprecher, S. & McKinney, K. *Sexuality.* Newbury Park, CA: Sage Publications, 1993.

Torgovnick, M. *Primitive passions: Men, women, and the quest for ecstasy.* New York: Random House, 1996.

CHAPTER 8

Contraception

FEATURES

Ethical Dimensions Should Schools Provide Abstinence-Only Sex Education?

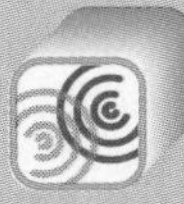
Communication Dimensions Talking About Condom Use

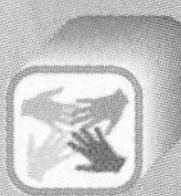
Multicultural Dimensions Ethnic Differences in Condom Use

Gender Dimensions Gender Equality in Contraception Use

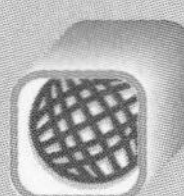
Global Dimensions Contraception in Russia

CHAPTER OBJECTIVES

1. Discuss the reasons to use contraceptives, ways to choose a contraceptive, and the difference between theoretical and user effectiveness.

2. Evaluate the nonprescription methods of contraception, including the effectiveness, the reversibility, and the advantages and disadvantages of each. Explain why some have higher rates of user effectiveness than others.

3. Evaluate the prescription methods of contraception, including the effectiveness, the reversibility, and the advantages and disadvantages of each. Explain why some have higher rates of user effectiveness than others.

4. Discuss the viability of future contraceptive methods.

sexuality.jbpub.com

Ethical Dimensions: Should Schools Provide Abstinence-Only Sex Education?
Emergency Contraception
Norplant
The Future of Contraceptives

INTRODUCTION

Throughout life, people's use of and need for contraceptives change. The case history of Susan presents a typical contraceptive user. During her first sexual encounter at age 18 years, Susan's high school boyfriend used withdrawal.

During her freshman year at college, she began a steady sexual relationship with Jack. Because she was in a monogamous relationship and did not have to worry about sexually transmitted infection (STI) transmission, Susan began to use oral contraceptives (the pill). After she had difficulty remembering to take her pill every day, Susan switched to injectable medroxyprogesterone acetate (Depo-Provera). Every 3 months she would receive her birth-control shot at a clinic.

After she and Jack broke up, she was abstinent for a year—the most foolproof method of contraception available. Susan graduated from college and was fitted with a diaphragm; she also used condoms with her two partners.

By age 25 years she married Stephen and had levonorgestrel (Norplant) inserted into her upper arm. The Norplant releases a steady stream of contraceptive into the reproductive system and is effective for up to 5 years. After about 5 years, she had the Norplant removed. At her doctor's suggestion, she switched to a non-hormone-based contraceptive (foam and condoms) for 3 months before trying to conceive a child.

After the birth of her first child, she was fitted with an intrauterine device (IUD). Two years later it was removed when she planned to conceive a second child. After the birth of their second child, Stephen had a vasectomy. After several follow-up tests to assure that no sperm were left in his ejaculate, Susan and Stephen enjoyed monogamous, unprotected sex.

Five years later, Susan and Stephen divorced. As one of her first acts as a newly divorced woman, Susan had a laparoscopy—a method of female sterilization. Although she could not become pregnant, she also began to practice safer sex and insisted that her partners wear latex condoms.

In other words, it is possible for a woman to use nearly every contraceptive method available during her more than 30 years of fertility. The method may change, depending on where she is in the life cycle.

This chapter reviews the currently available methods of contraception, their effectiveness, and their advantages and disadvantages.

Contraception

contraception
Means of preventing pregnancy.

theoretical effectiveness
The ability of a method of contraception to prevent pregnancy as measured by researchers in controlled laboratory settings.

user effectiveness
The ability of a method of contraception to prevent pregnancy as actually used at home by people not being monitored.

Contraception is the prevention of conception. You may already have thought hard about the consequences of such decisions as whether or not to become pregnant, have an abortion, or adopt a child. If you have considered or do consider such matters, you will understand how significant contraception can be to your life. Many babies are born each year to mothers who are too young or too emotionally immature to raise them well, or to mothers who are too old to carry a fetus to term without a high probability of a birth defect. Many pregnant teenagers and their sexual partners never finish their schooling because of the need to support and care for their child. Some couples who marry in response to pregnancy are soon divorced. Married couples who have already raised children may find yet another pregnancy a threat to their economic and psychological health. Managing this financial burden, as well as dealing with the time and energy necessary to care for an infant, can be as harmful to them—though perhaps in different ways—as to teenagers. But clearly the economic burden a child entails can present problems for people in various age groups and income levels.

Contraceptive and condom use should be routine for sexually active young people and adults unless they are seeking pregnancy *and* they are in a mutually monogamous relationship. Yet, too many people use contraception inconsistently or ineffectively. The result is that almost 60% of all pregnancies in the United States are unintended, a higher rate than in all other developed countries (Institute of Medicine, 1995).

There are many reasons people give for not using a contraceptive method. They include the following:

1. It could not happen to me.
2. I feel guilty (or immoral) if I plan in advance.
3. I am too embarrassed to buy contraceptives.
4. Someone may find out I am using contraceptives (parents, for instance).
5. Once I used contraceptives, I could not stop myself from participating more.
6. It was not a planned experience.
7. It (pregnancy or coitus) has not happened yet, so it will not happen.
8. It is not natural to use contraceptives.
9. It ruins the fun.
10. I am too lazy.

11. I could not imagine myself having a child (pregnancy is beyond my comprehension).

12. I experience coitus too infrequently to be concerned with contraception.

Ask yourself these questions as you read this chapter: Am I ready to have sexual intercourse? Am I committed to avoiding pregnancy myself or preventing a partner's pregnancy at this time? Am I committed to avoiding passing on a sexually transmitted infection? Am I committed to using a contraceptive method every time I have intercourse? Is my partner? If the answer to any of these questions is no, ask yourself another question: What will I do when a pregnancy occurs? Remember, almost 9 in 10 heterosexual couples who do not use a contraceptive method become pregnant within a year.

Contraceptive Effectiveness

We begin our discussion of contraception methods with a warning: The effectiveness of each method is difficult to determine precisely, so you should consider the rates cited for each method as being *approximations only*. Also note that for each method we provide both rate of theoretical effectiveness and rate of user effectiveness. **Theoretical effectiveness** is the ability of the method to prevent pregnancy as measured by researchers in controlled laboratory settings. It represents perfect use every time. In contrast, **user effectiveness** is the ability of the method to prevent pregnancy when used at home by people not being monitored. It represents typical use.

In the latter setting, mistakes are often made—for example, a condom may be put on incorrectly. Consequently, user effectiveness is always lower than theoretical effectiveness. A good contraceptive method is one that limits the gap between the way it is prescribed to be used and the way it is actually used. As can be seen in Table 8.1, there is usually a vast difference between these two measures of contraceptive effectiveness.

TABLE 8.1 **Contraceptive Effectiveness**

Methods	Theoretical Effectiveness	User Effectiveness
Abstinence	100%	?
Periodical abstinence	91–99%	75%
Withdrawal	96%	81%
Male condom	97%	86%
Female condom	95%	79%
Spermicide	94%	76%
Oral contraceptives	100%	95.5%
Depo-Provera	99.7%	99.7%
Norplant	99.7%	99.7%
IUD	97–99%	98–99%
Diaphragm	94%	80%
Cervical cap	91%	80%
Tubal ligation	99.9%	99.9%
Vasectomy	99.9%	99.8%
No method	15%	15%

Source: Hatcher, et al., 1998.

Use is measured by the number of women in 100 who will not become pregnant during the first year of use of the particular method. Table 8.1 shows the effectiveness of varied methods of contraception.

Contraception Versus Safer Sex

Couples today need to discuss how they will prevent both pregnancy and transmission of sexually transmitted infections (see Chapter 14). Many of the most effective methods of preventing pregnancies—oral contraceptives, hormonal implants, sterilization—provide *no* protection against sexually transmitted infections. The IUD, which is highly effective at preventing pregnancies, actually increases the likelihood of STIs. The male condom provides the best protection available against sexually transmitted infection but has a lower rate of effectiveness against pregnancy. There are three ways to achieve maximal effectiveness against both sexually transmitted infections and pregnancies relative to sexual intercourse: Abstain from all types of intercourse, use condoms and a spermicide together, or use a condom and a hormonal contraceptive together. Because sexually transmitted infections pose a threat to the future fertility and health of college students, and because abortion is legal if an unplanned pregnancy occurs, many experts recommend that if only one method is used, it should be a condom.

Nonprescription Methods

Abstinence

abstinence
Avoidance of any type of sexual intercourse.

penetrative behaviors
Any behavior whereby penetration occurs—for example, penile–vaginal intercourse, oral sex, or anal intercourse.

People define **abstinence** in different ways: For some it means no sexual contact of any kind; for others it means no **penetrative behaviors,** including penile–vaginal intercourse, oral sex, or anal intercourse. Many adolescents, young adults, and adults choose to abstain. People choose abstinence for a variety of reasons:

- Their religion teaches that sexual intercourse is appropriate only in marriage.
- They are not in a loving, committed relationship.
- They do not have a partner.
- They want to avoid the risk of pregnancy or sexually transmitted infection.
- The relationship they are in is not ready for the intimacy of intercourse.
- They are not ready for intercourse.
- They are ill or their partner is ill.
- They or a partner have been exposed to a sexually transmitted infection.
- They feel that a sexual relationship would complicate their life.

Choosing abstinence does not necessarily mean forgoing sexual pleasure. There are many ways to give and receive sexual pleasure without the risks of sexual intercourse. These include deep kissing, massages, fondling, dancing, masturbating alone, masturbating together, and showering together.

However, for these activities not to end in intercourse, couples must communicate their desire not to have sexual intercourse in any form and must agree to stick to sexual limits.

Effectiveness
Abstinence is the only 100% effective method of fertility control and STI prevention—if the couple or individual is truly committed to remaining abstinent. Actual user effectiveness rates are unknown. One wit has said that vows of abstinence fail much more frequently than condoms do; people say that they are practicing abstinence but have intercourse. Communication and commitment are essential. One researcher estimates that actual failure rates for abstinence may be as high as 31% in the first 17 months alone (Haignere, 1999).

Reversibility
Abstinence does not affect fertility.

Advantages and Disadvantages
Abstinence is an excellent method of fertility control and STI prevention. It is free, you always have it with you, there are no side effects, and no one's parents will be upset if you use it! It is 100% effective but only if you use it every time and only if your partner is equally committed to its use. Just as with any method, one should occasionally reconsider whether it is still the method of choice. And be sure to choose another method of birth control, before you decide to stop using it!

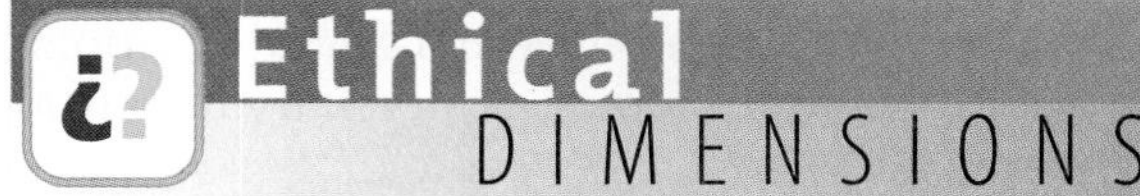

Should Schools Provide Abstinence-Only Sex Education?

In September 1996, the U.S. Congress passed the Welfare Reform Act, in which they approved a little-noticed $50 million appropriation to

1. teach young people the social, psychological, and health gains to be realized by abstaining from sexual activity
2. teach abstinence from sexual activity outside marriage as the expected standard for all school-age children
3. teach that abstinence from sexual activity is the only certain way to prevent out-of-wedlock pregnancy, sexually transmitted infections, and other associated health problems
4. teach that a mutually faithful monogamous relationship in the context of marriage is the expected standard of human sexual activity
5. teach that sexual activity outside the context of marriage is likely to have harmful psychological and physical effects
6. teach that bearing children out of wedlock is likely to have harmful consequences for the child, the child's parents, and society
7. teach young people how to reject sexual advances and how alcohol and drug use increases vulnerability to sexual advances
8. teach the importance of attaining self-sufficiency before engaging in sexual activity (SIECUS, 1998)

All 50 state health departments are using this money. Proponents of the program say that abstinence until marriage is the only acceptable sexual behavior. They believe that giving contraceptive information to teenagers gives them a mixed message and encourages them to have sexual intercourse. They say that it is immoral to give young people any support if they are sexually active.

Opponents of the program believe that it will deny young people lifesaving contraceptive and STI-prevention information. They point out that there are no evaluations in the professional literature that indicate that abstinence-only programs are effective (Kerr, 2000). They also argue that this program is immoral in denying information to the more than half of America's teenagers who have sexual intercourse.

What do you think? Is there an abstinence-only-until-marriage program in your area? Is there a comprehensive sexuality education program? What do young people need? What were you taught?

Withdrawal

Withdrawal is probably the oldest contraceptive method on record. In the Bible, Onan practices withdrawal, or **coitus interruptus,** so as not to impregnate his dead brother's widow. To practice withdrawal, the couple has vaginal intercourse until the man feels that he is about to ejaculate. He withdraws his penis and ejaculates away from the woman's vulva.

Effectiveness

Many people assume that withdrawal is an ineffective method of contraception. However, many contraceptive experts believe that withdrawal is an underrated method. It is about as effective as most barrier methods. If it is used perfectly, 96% of women will not become pregnant in a year. And even in a year of typical use, 81% of women will not become pregnant. In studies of heterosexual couples among whom the man was infected with HIV and the woman was not, withdrawal cut the HIV transmission rate by at least half (Hatcher, et al., 1998).

Many people have been taught that preejaculate fluid might contain sperm. However, preejaculate fluid is a lubricating solution produced by the Cowper's glands (see Chapter 5) that contains *no* sperm. A previous ejaculation could leave a small number of sperm within the urethral lining, which if mixed with the preejaculate fluid could pose a small risk of fertilization. However, the few small studies that have been done have not found the presence of sperm in preejaculate fluid. It is believed that normal urination removes these sperm (Hatcher, et al., 1998).

To quote the authors of *Contraceptive Technology* (Hatcher, et al., 1998), "Withdrawal is a considerably better method of contraception than no method at all." If the man does not withdraw in time and the woman is at a fertile point in her cycle, emergency contraception should be considered (covered later in this chapter).

Advantages and Disadvantages

Withdrawal is free, always available, and relatively easy to use. It has no medical side effects, and it offers some protection against sexually transmitted infection.

The major disadvantage to withdrawal is that some men, particularly young men, do not recognize impending ejaculation and thus ejaculate inside their partner, putting her at risk of pregnancy. Some couples report that withdrawal interrupts sexual pleasure, because the woman enjoys feeling the man ejaculate inside her, and that the man must monitor his reactions during intercourse instead of simply enjoying himself.

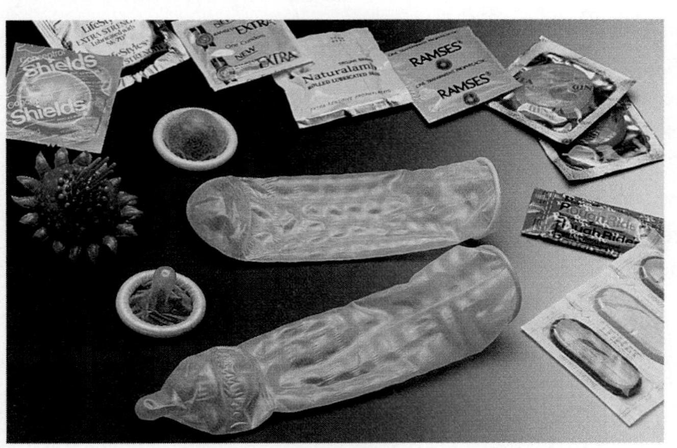

A wide variety of condoms are available in various colors, sizes—even flavors. Only latex condoms have been shown to prevent transmission of STIs and HIV; animal skin condoms do not. Condoms should be used in every act of intercourse, from start to finish.

Male Condom

Condoms are one of the oldest contraceptive methods, dating back to 1350 B.C., when Egyptian men put sheaths on the penis before intercourse. In the 18th century, Colonel Cundum invented penile sheaths using dried animal intestines. In the 19th century, after rubber was vulcanized, condoms began to be mass produced (Hatcher, et al., 1998).

Today most condoms are made of **latex,** a synthetic form of rubber. About 5% of condoms are made from the intestines of lambs; these are known as *skin* or *lambskin condoms.* Skin condoms, because they are more porous than latex condoms, do not provide protection against many sexually transmitted infections and are not recommended.

Communication DIMENSIONS

Talking About Condom Use

You are on your third date in a nice restaurant with a new friend. You are attracted to each other; on the last date, you spent a pretty hot half hour kissing and touching each other. You are pretty sure that you are ready to have intercourse and are hoping that your new friend feels the same way. But how do you know? And, how do you bring up condom use?

The waiter just delivered dessert. Dinner is coming to an end. Your date says, "Hmmm, do you want to come back to my room?" You say, "I think there are a few things we need to talk about first."

Here's how a successful discussion about condoms with a new partner might go.

> CHRIS: I really like you. I've been fantasizing a lot since our last date about us having sex.
>
> PAT: Me, too. But, it's important to me that we use condoms and practice safe sex.
>
> CHRIS: Of course. I always use condoms. And because I was hoping you were interested too, I bought some today.
>
> PAT: I bought some today, too! How about we skip dessert?

But of course, it is not always that easy (although it should be). Chris might have said, "I hate condoms." Here are some ways that Pat might answer.

1. "Not with me you won't. I've learned how to make condom use really fun. I hope you want me to show you."
2. "I'm really sorry to hear that. I would never have sex with someone unless he used a condom."
3. "Tell me which condoms you've used. Maybe we can try a different brand or type."
4. "Well, it looks as if we have an important decision to make. We can agree not to have any kind of intercourse and just mess around. Or, we can just be friends. But, I won't have intercourse with you without a condom."

Condom use with a new partner is essential until you have both been tested for sexually transmitted infections and have decided to be monogamous. Remember, "A man who doesn't want to use a condom with you, probably didn't use one with his last partner either" (Haffner & Schwartz, 1998).

In 1997, the U.S. Food and Drug Administration (FDA) approved the first condom made of **polyurethane,** a type of plastic. Initial studies show that polyurethane condoms are as effective as latex condoms but more comfortable to use. Some users have said that they enhanced sensitivity.

There are more than 100 brands of condoms available in the United States today. The U.S. Centers for Disease Control and Prevention provide the following directions for the consistent and correct use of condoms. Individuals who use condoms to prevent unwanted pregnancies and STIs must understand the meaning of *consistent* and *correct* condom use.

CONSISTENT USE

- Use a condom with every act of sexual intercourse, from start to finish, including penile–vaginal intercourse, oral intercourse, and anal intercourse.

CORRECT USE

- Store condoms in a cool place out of direct sunlight (not in wallets or glove compartments). Latex will become brittle as a result of changes in temperature, rough handling, and age. Do not use damaged, discolored, brittle, or sticky condoms.
- Check the expiration date.

withdrawal
Removing the penis from the vagina before ejaculation.

coitus interruptus
The Latin term for *withdrawal,* which means "interrupted intercourse."

condom
A sheath that covers the penis.

latex
A synthetic rubber.

polyurethane
A type of plastic.

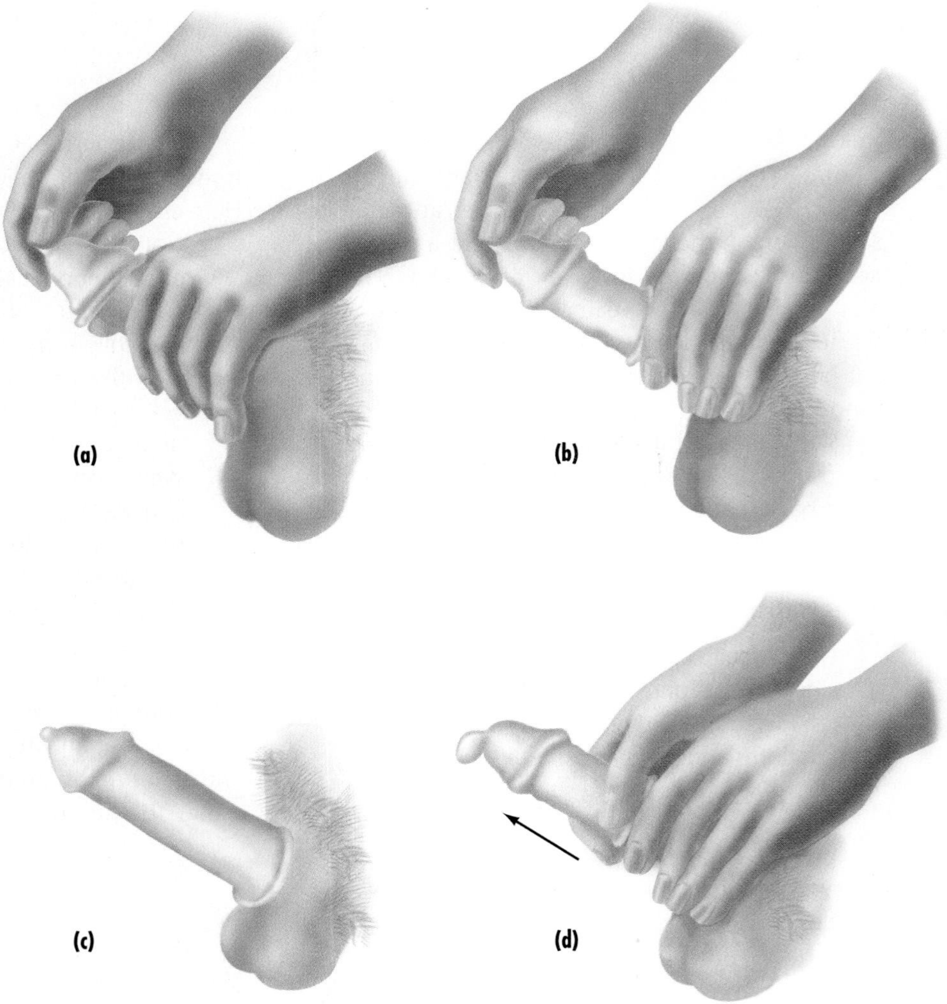

FIGURE 8.1 If you have never used a condom before, you should practice before the first time you use one during sexual intercourse. To put a condom on: (a) Put on the condom by pinching the reservoir tip and unrolling it all the way down the shaft of the penis. (b) Be sure that there are no air bubbles, which could cause the condom to break. (c) The condom should have extra rubber at the top and should be unrolled to the very base of the penis. (d) After ejaculation, be sure to withdraw the penis with one hand holding the rim of the condom so that it does not accidentally slip off or leak.

- Carefully open the condom package—teeth or fingernails can tear the condom.
- Use a new condom for every act of sexual intercourse.
- Put on the condom after the penis is erect and before it touches any part of a partner's body. A man who is uncircumcised must pull back the foreskin before putting on the condom.
- Put on the condom by pinching the reservoir tip and unrolling it all the way down the shaft of the penis from head to base (see Figure 8.1). If the condom does not have a reservoir tip, pinch it to leave a half-inch space at the head of the penis in which semen can collect after ejaculation.
- Withdraw the penis immediately if the condom breaks during sexual intercourse and put on a new condom before resuming intercourse. When a condom breaks, use spermicidal foam or jelly and speak to a health care provider about emergency contraception.
- Use only water-based lubrication. Do not use oil-based lubricants such as cooking/vegetable oil, baby oil, hand lotion, or petroleum jelly—these will cause the condom to deteriorate and break.

- Withdraw the penis immediately after ejaculation, while the penis is still erect; grasp the rim of the condom between the fingers, and slowly withdraw the penis (with the condom still on) so that no semen is spilled.

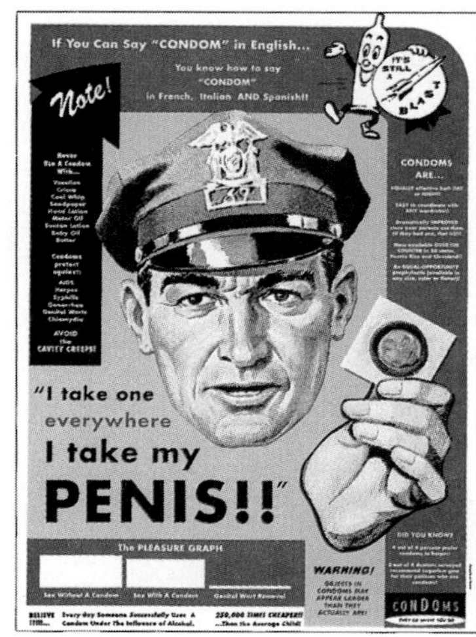

Humor is often used to convey serious messages, as seen in this poster from the King County (Washington) Health Department. Which of the ideas conveyed in the poster hit home with you?

The prevalence of AIDS has renewed interest in condoms. Experts advocate sexual abstinence, monogamy with an uninfected partner, or the use of a condom to prevent the spread of HIV. Latex and polyurethane condoms when used correctly can both prevent sperm from entering the vagina and microorganisms that might cause an STI from entering through tiny tears in the vagina or on the penis. As mentioned, animal skin condoms do not offer this protection and should *not* be used for the prevention of STIs.

Condom sales have increased dramatically in recent years. Since the early 1990s, Americans have purchased more than 450 million condoms each year (Hatcher, et al., 1998).

School personnel in particular have taken some unusual actions in an attempt to encourage their sexually active students to use condoms. At the high school level, some schools have decided to install condom vending machines in their rest rooms or have condoms available in the nurse's office or school clinic. Several colleges have done likewise. For example, the University of Virginia decided that allowing students to buy cigarettes (products harmful to their health) from vending machines while not providing the opportunity to purchase condoms (products that could protect sexually active

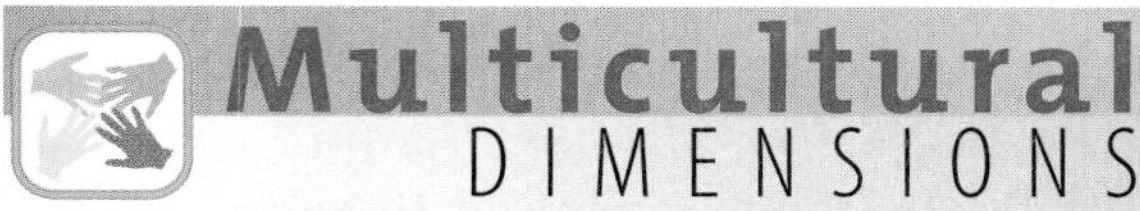

Ethnic Differences in Condom Use Condom use has increased dramatically among teenagers, but they tend to use them inconsistently. According to the 1995 National Survey of Adolescent Males, 9 in 10 teen boys who had intercourse had used condoms some time in the past year. However, there are significant ethnic differences in condom use.

African-American teen boys use condoms most frequently. Sixty-eight percent of sexually active African-American teen boys used a condom at last intercourse. Sixty-two percent of sexually active white teen boys did so, but only 48% of sexually active Hispanic boys had used condoms at last intercourse (MMWR, 1998).

Birth control use also varies by ethnicity. One in four white teen girls had used oral contraceptives at last intercourse, but only one in six African-American girls and one in seven Hispanic girls had.

There are many theories to explain these differences, but there is no definitive research. Many supposed ethnic differences are really related to socioeconomic status. In the United States, people of color are much more likely to live in poverty than whites. Therefore, white teen girls may have better access to prescription methods of birth control than teenage girls of color, and they may receive more education about contraceptive methods. African-American and Hispanic girls may have less information and may have heard more myths about the pill.

Cultural differences may affect condom use. Young African-American men may be encouraged to carry and use condoms to demonstrate their manhood. Conversely, some Latino men may give young men the message that "real men don't use condoms."

And unfortunately, many young people living in poverty, who are proportionally more likely to be young people of color, do not have the motivation to avoid childbearing or sexually transmitted infections that will affect them in the future. Many poor young women believe a baby will give meaning to their life. And as a young man in inner-city New York once said to one of us, "Why should I care about a disease that might kill me 10 years from now? Most of the men I know don't live until their mid-20s, or they are living in prison."

students from illness and disease) from vending machines did not make sense. Consequently, they converted some cigarette vending machines to dispense condoms (U-Va. dorm machines to sell condoms, not cigarettes, 1998).

Effectiveness

Condoms are very effective: Only 3% of couples using a condom correctly and for every act of intercourse become pregnant in the first year of use. It is 86% effective in typical users. The major reason condoms fail is that people forget to use them for each act of intercourse. Condoms are also highly effective at preventing the spread of HIV, gonorrhea, chlamydia, and trichomoniasis (CDC, 2001).

Advantages and Disadvantages

Advantages of condoms include the following: They are relatively inexpensive, they are easy to obtain, they do not require a visit to the doctor, they may help a man control ejaculation, they provide protection from sexually transmitted infections, and they have none of the unhealthful side effects associated with some of the other methods of contraception. Finally, condom use takes some of the burden of birth control off women. As the women's movement works toward female–male equality, more and more women seek to share the practice of birth control with their partners.

The major disadvantage is that many men complain that condoms reduce sensitivity and spontaneity. Trying different brands can improve sensation, and putting the condom on as foreplay can make it more fun.

Female Condom

female condom
A sheath worn inside the vagina.

spermicide
Chemical compound that immobilizes or kills sperm on contact.

The newest vaginal barrier is the **female condom** (Figure 8.2). The female condom appeared on the market in the United States in 1993. There is currently only one brand of female condom on the market. The Reality Female Condom is a loose-fitting sheath made of polyurethane with rings on both ends. One ring covers the cervix; the other ring remains outside the vagina and partially covers the vulva.

The female condom is like the male condom in that it can be used only for one act of intercourse. It is unlike the male condom because it can be inserted up to 8 hours before intercourse, although it may not be comfortable for everyday wear. Female and male condoms should *not* be used together because they can stick together and dislodge each other.

Effectiveness

The female condom has effectiveness rates similar to those of the diaphragm and cervical cap. For perfect users, it is 95% effective in preventing pregnancies. In typical users, studies have found it to be 79% effective. As noted by the Planned Parenthood Federation of America: Although it is not as effective as the condom, the female condom is a valuable option for women who want to prevent sexually transmitted infection or unintended pregnancy (Planned Parenthood Federation of America, 2003).

Advantages and Disadvantages

Most users in the preliminary studies were pleased with the method. They felt that it was easy to use and that it interfered with physical sensation less than male condoms and provided an important woman-controlled alternative to male condoms. Other users reported that it was awkward to use, was messy, and made oral–genital contact difficult and unpleasant.

Spermicides

A **spermicide** kills and/or immobilizes sperm on contact, thereby preventing their movement toward an egg (Figure 8.3). Spermicides may be foams, gels, films, suppositories, creams, or jelly foams. Foams and creams are placed

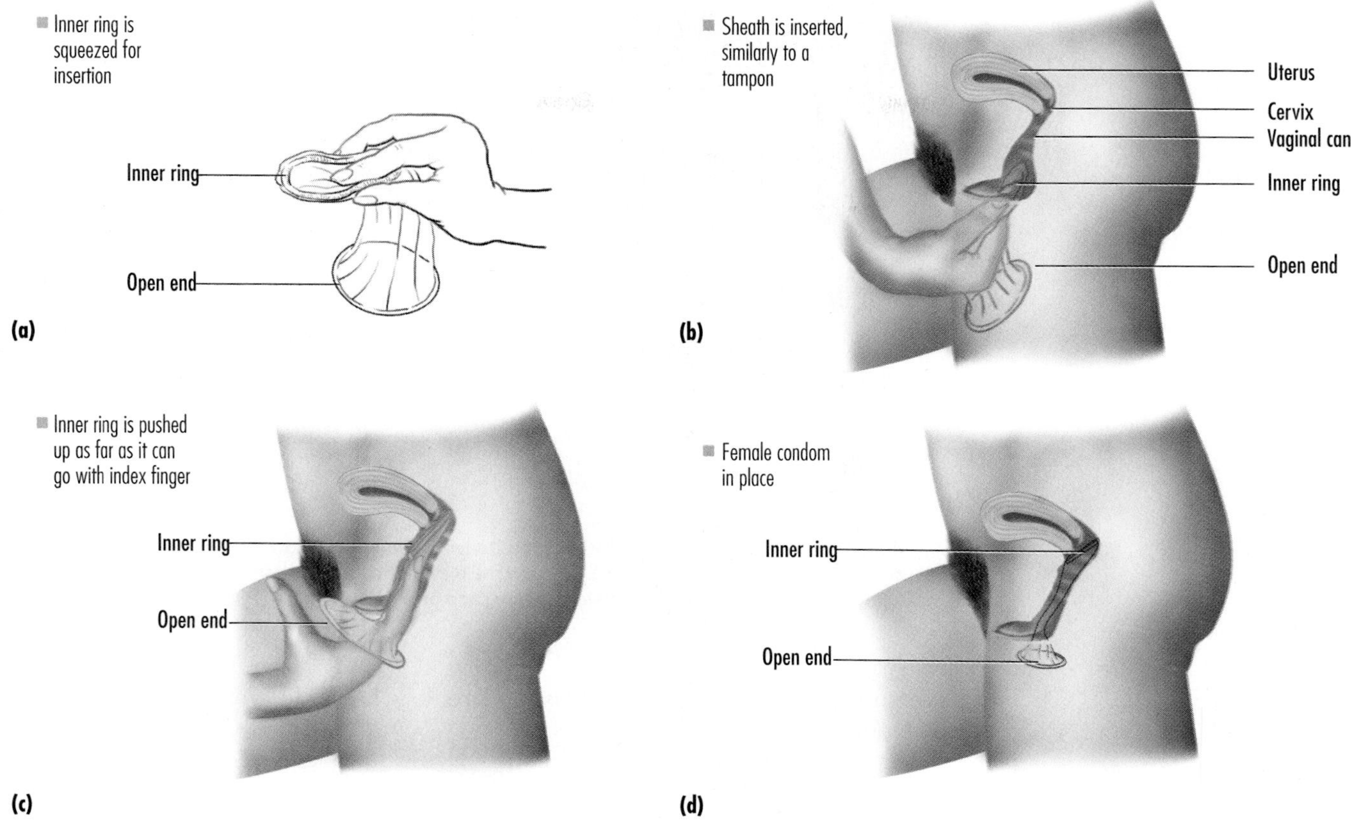

FIGURE 8.2 To insert and position a female condom, (a) squeeze the inner ring for insertion; (b) insert sheath as you would insert a tampon; (c) push inner ring as far as it can go with index finger; (d) the condom is now in place.

against the cervix by means of a plastic applicator. Spermicidal films (small squares coated with spermicides) and suppositories are inserted manually high into the vagina. Most spermicides must be inserted within 1 hour of intercourse, and some are not effective for the first 10 to 15 minutes after insertion. Users should read the packet insert instructions carefully.

Effectiveness

The theoretical effectiveness rate of spermicides is relatively high: 94% of women using spermicides perfectly will not become pregnant in 1 year. However, they have the lowest user effectiveness rate (about 76%) of any method, including withdrawal. In studies, almost one-quarter of women who relied on spermicides exclusively became pregnant in 1 year (Hatcher, et al., 1998). As for condoms, this ineffectiveness is probably due to inconsistent use of spermicide with every act of intercourse or incorrect use (for example, putting it in too soon or too late). However, the good news is that using condoms and spermicides *together* provides contraceptive protection almost as effective as that of oral contraceptives. The bad news is that few couples use both methods simultaneously.

Reversibility

Spermicide use has no effect on future fertility.

Advantages and Disadvantages

There are many advantages to spermicide use. They are easy to use, are available at drug stores and supermarkets without a prescription, and do not have any serious side effects. They are an important backup method to

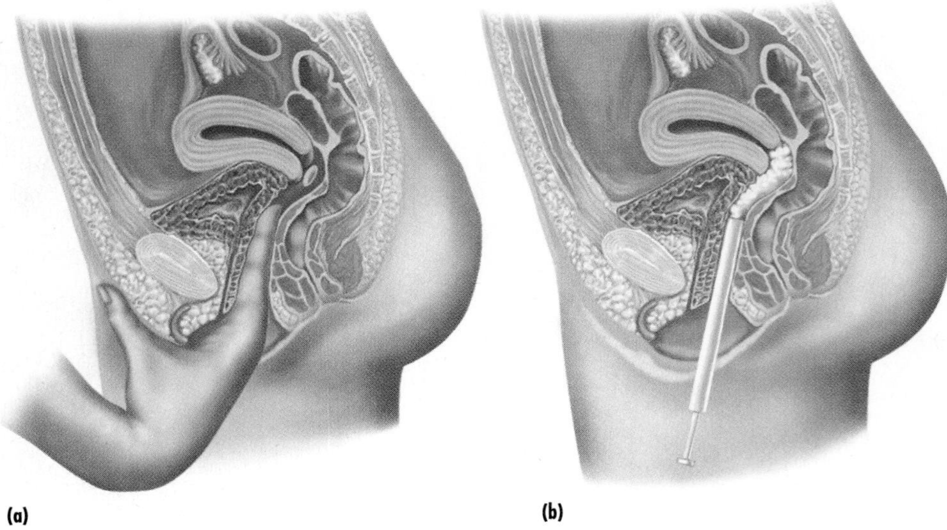

FIGURE 8.3 (a) Read the instructions for use of suppositories carefully and follow them. Be sure to wait the proper time for the suppository to dissolve. (b) Insert the plastic applicator into the vagina as far as possible to make sure that the foam covers the cervical opening and press the plunger.

have on hand if a condom slips or breaks. They do not require partner involvement.

Until recently, family-planning counselors would have said that the only disadvantage to spermicide use was its low effectiveness rate in actual users. However, studies in 2000 suggested that **Nonoxynol 9,** the major spermicidal agent used in most products, may also cause lesions and ulcers in the vaginal walls. This may make women more prone to HIV infection. In a 1999 interview, Penelope Hitchcock, head of the STI branch of the National Institute of Allergy and Infectious Diseases, advised women to avoid products with Nonoxynol 9 at that time (Kaiser Daily Reproductive Health Report, 1999). Nonoxynol 9 also should not be used alone to prevent the spread of HIV (Gayle, 2000).

Nonoxynol 9
The major spermicidal ingredient.

natural family planning (NFP)
Calculation of a woman's fertile times and abstention from intercourse on fertile days.

fertility-awareness methods
Methods used to determine fertile days.

fertility-awareness-combined methods
Calculation of a woman's fertile times and use of a barrier or withdrawal on fertile days.

Natural Family Planning

You may have heard this riddle: Q: What do you call people who practice rhythm? A: Parents.

Natural family planning (NFP) is also known as **fertility-awareness methods,** or the *rhythm method.* There are several fertility-awareness methods: the *calendar method, ovulation method,* and *symptothermal method.* Each of these methods is based on the identification of the days in the woman's menstrual cycle when she is most likely to be fertile and the avoidance of intercourse during those days (natural family planning) or use of a barrier method or withdrawal during those days **(fertility-awareness-combined methods).**

There are many types of spermicides available, including foams, gels, films, suppositories, creams, and jelly foams.

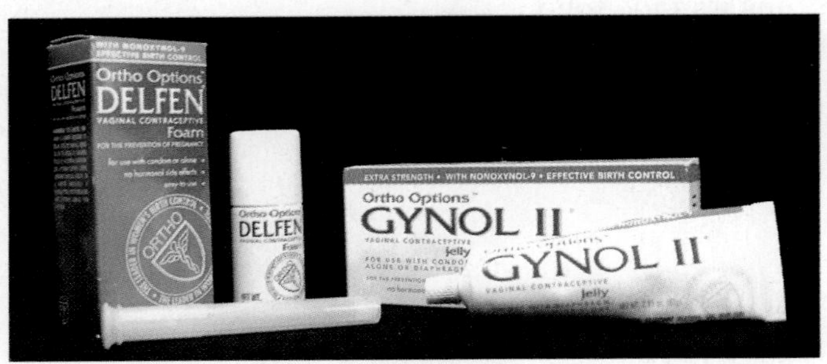

Fertility-awareness methods are based on the knowledge that there are only about 6 days in a cycle during which a woman can become pregnant. The ovum lives less than 1 day; sperm can live up to 5 days inside the woman's genital tract (Hatcher, et al., 1998).

People interested in using these methods need to see a trained educator for help in learning to observe, chart, and recognize the woman's fertility signs and patterns. It is estimated that it requires 4 to 6 hours to learn fertility-awareness methods so that they can be used effectively (Hatcher, et al., 1998). For that reason, detailed instructions are not included in this text.

People using the **calendar method,** first developed in the 1930s, keep track of the woman's menstrual cycles for several months and then, with the help of a trained person, determine which days she is most likely to ovulate. It is the least effective of the fertility-awareness methods; even with perfect use, there is a 9% chance of becoming pregnant.

Ovulation methods are much more effective. Women can chart their **basal body temperature** or their cervical secretions or both. Basal body temperature is a person's temperature upon awakening. Temperatures usually drop immediately before ovulation and then rise sharply during and after ovulation (Figure 8.4). Thus, a woman takes her temperature by using a specially calibrated **basal body thermometer** before she gets up each morning. The temperature is then charted on a monthly graph, and after 3 days of elevated temperature, it is considered safe to have intercourse without the risk of pregnancy.

Cervical secretions can also be monitored and charted. After menstruation, cervical secretions are scant. As estrogen levels increase, cervical mucus becomes thick and cloudy. When estrogen peaks at midcycle, the secretions become clearer, stretchy, and slippery. In fact, at ovulation, the mucus can be stretched 2 to 3 inches between the thumb and forefinger. After ovulation, the secretions become thick again, and some women may notice a cervical mucus plug. At this point, it is considered safe to have intercourse without worrying about pregnancy.

calendar method
Charting of the length of a woman's periods for several months to determine the days she is most likely to be fertile.

ovulation methods
Observation of signs of ovulation to calculate fertile days.

basal body temperature
A woman's body temperature immediately upon waking.

basal body thermometer
A special thermometer used to measure changes in basal body temperature.

cervical secretions
Normal fluids from the cervix that change consistency during the month.

Gender DIMENSIONS

Gender Equality in Contraception Use

During most of human history, contraception was a male responsibility. The only methods available were the condom and withdrawal. Oral contraceptives became available in 1961, and many women were elated. They could now control contraceptive use and thus their risk of becoming pregnant. The pill was effective, was easy to use, and did not require partner participation. Many men who came of age during the 1960s and 1970s never thought much about contraception.

In the 1990s, the HIV/AIDS epidemic and the epidemic of sexually transmitted infections once again shifted the responsibility. Men who are not in monogamous committed relationships now have to use condoms on a regular basis. But many women are unwilling to rely on condoms for pregnancy prevention because they are only 86% effective in preventing pregnancies in typical users. Some men are unwilling to use condoms once they find out that their partner is using the pill. And many men do not like to use condoms, claiming that they reduce sensitivity and sensation.

Heterosexual couples today need to negotiate how they will prevent an unwanted pregnancy *and* how they will protect themselves against sexually transmitted infections. Couples need to discuss who has primary responsibility for contraception. They need to address such questions as, Who will buy the condoms? Who will pay for contraception? Should the man accompany the woman to the clinic visit? And, perhaps most important, what will they do if an unplanned pregnancy occurs?

There are ways that couples can share the responsibility for contraceptive and condom use. Men can remind their partners to take their pills or check their IUD strings. They can learn to insert the diaphragm or female condom as part of foreplay. Women can learn to place the condom on the man's penis as part of foreplay. Contraceptive use and safer sex practices can truly be a shared responsibility.

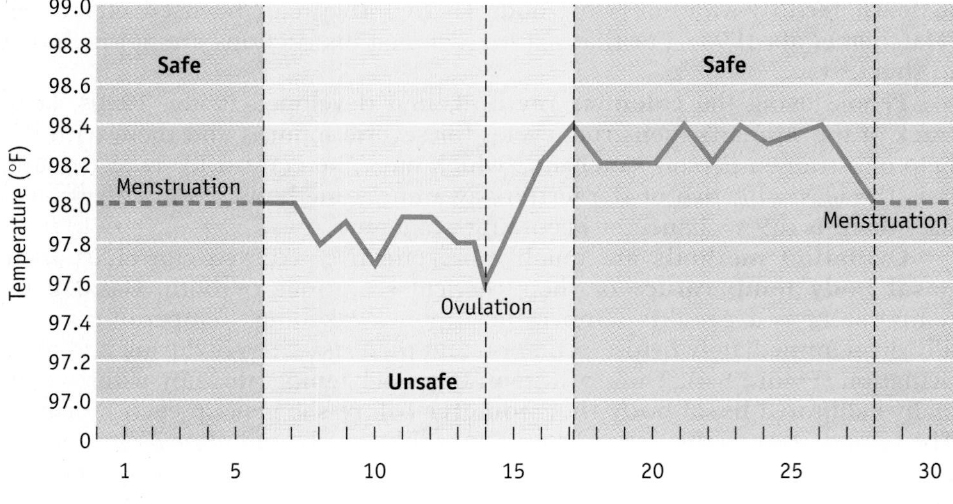

FIGURE 8.4 The basal body temperature method of contraception involves charting a woman's body temperature each morning to determine when unprotected sexual intercourse is safe. Once the basal body temperature has risen for 3 consecutive days, she can assume that ovulation has taken place and that the rest of the days in that menstrual cycle are safe for unprotected intercourse.

The **symptothermal method** involves checking both basal body temperatures and cervical secretions and charting them to identify fertile and nonfertile times. When this method is used perfectly, only 2% of women become pregnant, making it as effective as the most effective prescription forms of contraception.

Commercially available ovulation-prediction kits are not currently recommended for contraception. However, they may be helpful for women who are trying to conceive.

symptothermal method
A combination of natural family-planning methods, in which both temperature and signs of ovulation are observed and charted.

oral contraceptive (OC)
A daily pill taken to prevent ovulation.

combined pill
Oral contraceptive containing estrogen and progestin.

minipill
A progestin-only pill.

Effectiveness

Natural family-planning methods can be highly effective methods of contraception. If they are used perfectly, only 1% to 9% of women using these methods in a year have an unintended pregnancy. The symptothermal method is the most effective natural family-planning method; using a calendar alone is only 81% effective. Fertility-awareness methods can also be used effectively to help couples become pregnant.

Reversibility

Natural family-planning methods stop preventing pregnancies as soon as they are discontinued.

Advantages and Disadvantages

Fertility-awareness methods have many advantages. They are an excellent way for men and women to learn about their own fertility. They require both partners' involvement, they are free, and they may alert women to the need for some kind of medical attention. Their primary disadvantage is that they provide no protection against STIs, and the couple must be vigorously committed to abstaining from intercourse during fertile times. If the couple is not rigorous about charting cycles or has intercourse during fertile periods, pregnancy is likely to occur.

Prescription Methods

Oral Contraceptives

There are several different types of **oral contraceptives (OCs).** In fact, since oral contraceptives were introduced, there have been 56 brands that included 33 unique formulations in the United States alone. These different pills can be categorized into two general classifications: *combined pills* and progestin-only pills (sometimes referred to as *minipills*), and multiphasic formulations.

The **combined pill,** used since the 1960s, contains both estrogens and progestin (synthetic progesterone). To use the combined pill, a woman ingests the first pill in the packet and takes a pill each succeeding day. Most packets contain 28 pills, but some contain only 21. The 28-pill packets contain 7 pills that have no benefit other than convenience: That is, the woman need not remember to stop taking her pills and then resume taking them 7 days later—as is required if using the 21-day packets. Usually menstruation occurs on the 23rd or 24th day (2 or 3 days after the last pill containing a hormone is ingested).

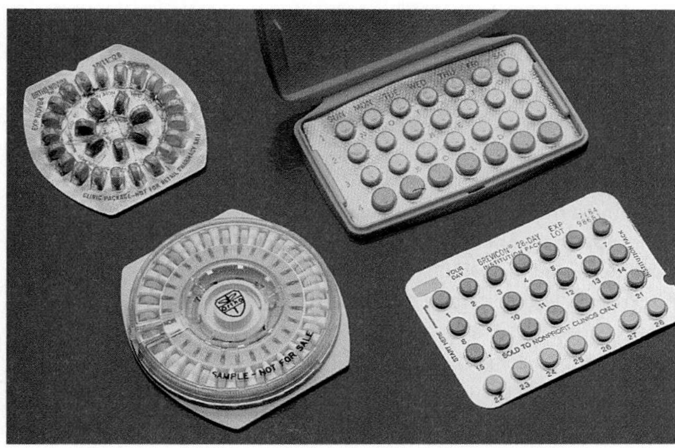

Although oral contraceptives are effective in preventing pregnancy, they offer no protection against STIs or HIV. For protection against pregnancy and STIs, try combining the use of oral contraceptives and latex condoms.

The combination pill's estrogen signals the brain's hypothalamus to prevent the pituitary gland from producing FSH and LH; the progesterone also inhibits LH production. Ovulation is suppressed. This suppression mimics the changes that occur in pregnancy.

The progestin-only pill was introduced in 1972. In spite of its lack of estrogen (high dosages of which were found to be related to physical complications), the **minipill** never achieved a great deal of popularity, and the percentage of women using it remains relatively low to this day. To use this type, a woman takes a pill on the first day of menstruation and every day thereafter. Because progestin is included in every pill, the hormone is ingested daily. With minipills, approximately 40% of women still ovulate (40% do not ovulate, and 20% sometimes ovulate). However, even if fertilization occurs, the progestin inhibits implantation. Moreover, the progestin causes the cervical mucus to inhibit to some degree the sperm's movement and ability to penetrate the ovum. Minipills are appropriate for women who cannot use estrogen.

The chemical composition of oral contraceptives has changed over the years in response to research on their effects and side effects. The typical amount of estrogen in early birth control pills was 0.1 milligram (mg). In 1968, fewer than 1% of the estimated 54 million retail prescriptions for oral contraceptives contained less than 0.5 mg of estrogen. In 1988 approximately 82% of the estimated 57 million retail prescriptions for oral contraceptives contained less than 0.5 mg of estrogen (Gerstman, et al., 1991). In the 1970s it was found that use of the higher-dosage pills (more than 0.5 mg) was related to cardiovascular complications. Today those higher-dosage pills are still available and used by women with specific medical problems such as uterine bleeding and endometriosis. However, most oral contraceptives using estrogen now contain between 0.20 and 0.35 mg (Schwartz and Gabelnick, 2002).

Regardless of which pill is used, a backup method of contraception should be employed for the first 7 days of pill use and as a precaution if a pill is forgotten for 2 or more days in a row. If a pill is forgotten one day, that pill should be taken immediately and the next pill taken as regularly scheduled. A backup method should also be used any time a woman uses antibiotics, such as tetracycline or penicillin, which reduce the effectiveness of the pill.

It is a good idea for a woman using oral contraceptives to have regular medical exams. Most physicians require a visit 3 or 6 months after a woman starts OCs, followed by an annual exam thereafter. There is no medical reason for a woman to "take a break" from pill use.

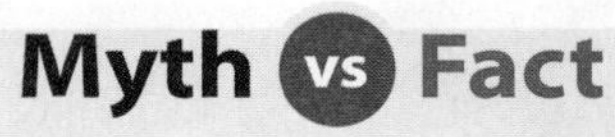

Myth: Birth control pills cause cancer.
Fact: Birth control pills are very safe. Although there may be a slightly increased risk of breast cancer among women using the pill, the pill is protective against other cancers such as uterine, ovarian, and endometrium cancer. Thus, women using the pill are less likely to contract cancer than women who have never been on the pill.

Myth: You need to take a break from the pill.
Fact: Women can stay on oral contraceptives as long as medical side effects do not develop. There is no need to take a break.

Myth: All condoms protect against sexually transmitted infections.
Fact: Only latex and polyurethane condoms protect against sexually transmitted infections. Animal skin condoms provide no protection against sexually transmitted infections.

Myth: Condoms protect against all sexually transmitted infections.
Fact: Condoms are highly effective at preventing the spread of such diseases as HIV infection, syphilis, and gonorrhea. They do not provide protection against genital warts, crabs, or lice, which can be transmitted through contact with the pubic hair or other parts of the genitals that are not covered by the condom.

Myth: Withdrawal is not a method of birth control.
Fact: Withdrawal is about as effective as barrier methods. It is much better than using nothing.

Myth: Once a person has had intercourse, he or she can no longer practice abstinence.
Fact: Abstinence is always a choice. Many teens, college students, and adults choose abstinence even though they have already had sexual intercourse.

Effectiveness

Apart from abstinence, sterilization, and hormonal implants, oral contraceptives provide the most effective means of preventing pregnancy. Only 1 in 1,000 women using oral contraceptives becomes pregnant in 1 year of perfect use. Among typical users, for example, some who forget to take their pills as directed, as many as 5% become pregnant in the first year.

The minipill is slightly less effective in preventing pregnancy: 0.5% of women (1 in 200) become pregnant in the first year. Minipill users have more breakthrough bleeding but fewer serious side effects.

It cannot be overemphasized that oral contraceptives provide *no* protection from sexually transmitted infections. Unless you are in a 100% monogamous relationship with a partner who has been tested for STIs and HIV, a condom must be used for each act of intercourse.

Reversibility

Some women who have been on the pill may require slightly more time to become pregnant than women using other methods. Therefore, clinicians generally recommend that women plan 3 months off the pill before they begin to try to conceive. However, oral contraceptive use does not affect future fertility.

Advantages and Disadvantages

Birth control pills have been reported as being 99.5% effective as actually used and 99.9% effective if used correctly all the time (Hatcher, et al., 1998). Besides being effective, the pill does not necessitate interrupting sexual activity. An added benefit for some women is that it helps to regulate the menstrual cycle. Birth control pills are available in the United States only by prescription from a physician, because they have other effects as well. For example, the combination pill may enlarge the breasts, may reduce acne, often eliminates mittelschmerz (a sensation of abdominal pain that sometimes occurs during ovulation), and reduces menstrual cramps. For estrogen-related problems with the combination pill, the progestin-only pill is recommended, because it contains no estrogen, and its low progestin dosage is thought to reduce adverse effects that progestin might otherwise cause.

Combined pills are very safe. In addition to protecting a woman against pregnancy, they lower a woman's risk of ovarian cancer, uterine cancer, breast masses, and ovarian cysts. They also lessen menstrual blood loss, cramps, and acne. Their primary disadvantage for sexually active college students is that they provide *no* protection against sexually transmitted infections, including HIV.

Symptoms can develop after use of the pill, even after some time. Abdominal pain, chest pain, shortness of breath, headaches, eye problems such as blurred vision, and severe leg pain are examples of such symptoms. If any of these is encountered, call the doctor. Other possible side effects exist. For example, the combination pill has been associated with a greater risk of circulatory system diseases, including heart attacks and strokes. If a woman is obese, diabetic, or hypertensive, the risk of circulatory system diseases is greatly increased. These women should use a different method (Hatcher, et al., 1998). Smoking is also a factor. The American College of Obstetricians and Gynecologists (ACOG) found that, among approximately 10 million users of oral contraceptives, 500 women die each year. The death rate would even be lower if heavy smokers, especially those older than 35 years, did not take the pill. This death rate is about 10 times lower than a woman's chance of death from an automobile accident or from childbirth. In addition, women with liver function problems, hypertension, circulatory problems, heart disease, breast cancer, asthma, varicose veins, or migraine headaches should avoid using oral contraceptives (Hatcher, et al., 1998).

There has been considerable debate over the years about whether oral contraceptive use can lead to breast cancer. In 1996 an analysis of more than 54 studies showed a slightly increased risk of breast cancer for current users (Collaborative Group on Hormonal Factors in Breast Cancer, 1996). However, since then oral contraceptive use has been correlated to a small increased risk of breast cancer. Current OC users have a small increased risk when compared to nonusers. This risk declines after OC use is discontinued; by 10 years post pill use, the risk is no higher for women who have never taken the pill (Collaborative Group on Hormonal Factors in Breast Cancer, 1996). Still, because OC use results in a 50% decrease in ovarian and endometrial cancers, fewer pill users die of cancer than nonusers (Coker, et al., 1993).

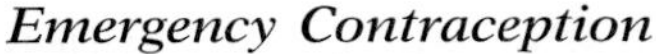

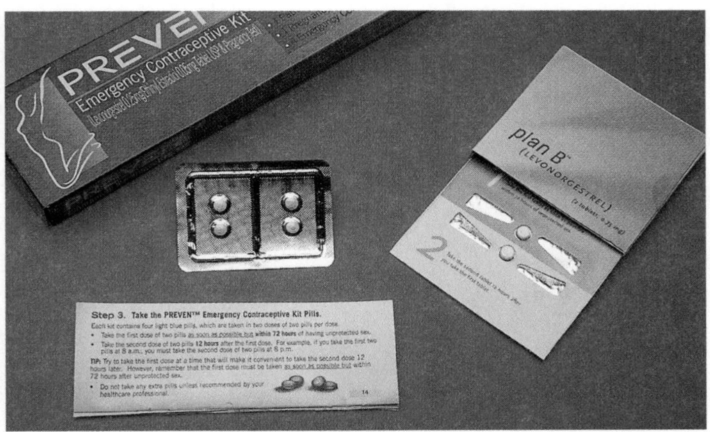

Plan B and Preven, both often referred to as the "morning-after pill," are the two primary brands of emergency contraceptives on the U.S. market. In recent years, there has been a movement toward making emergency contraceptives available without prescription, though this proposal has encountered much opposition and controversy regarding effectiveness and safety.

Emergency Contraception

Condoms sometimes slip or break; women forget more than two contraceptive pills in a row; the man ejaculates too close to the vulva even though he withdraws; a couple vowing abstinence has intercourse anyway. For all these cases, **emergency contraception** is now available. In addition, emergency contraception is available in cases of rape or incest.

The most commonly prescribed method of emergency contraception is to take 2 oral contraceptive pills within 72 hours of unprotected intercourse. One pill is taken as soon as possible after unprotected intercourse; the other is taken 12 hours later. The most frequent side effects are nausea and vomiting; many clinics and doctors prescribe an antinausea pill along with the first pill. These side effects last no more than 48 hours after treatment.

Some university clinics offer emergency contraception as part of their reproductive health services. If they do not, there is a toll-free number that has been set up in the United States to help women find clinics and doctors who will prescribe emergency contraception. It is 1-888-NOT-2-LATE. The American College of Obstetricians and Gynecologists estimates that emergency contraception could reduce by half the number of unintended pregnancies in the United States (ACOG, 2001).

emergency contraception
The use of oral contraceptives after unprotected sex has occurred at midcycle.

abortifacient
A medical method that causes an embryo or fetus to die.

Effectiveness

Emergency contraceptive pills prevent pregnancy by delaying or preventing ovulation and possibly altering the lining of the uterus so that it is inhospitable to implantation. Contrary to the claims of some antichoice proponents, they are not an **abortifacient** and do not end an established pregnancy. This may be why they are only 74% effective.

Advantages and Disadvantages

The advantage to emergency contraception is that it is the only method available if unprotected intercourse has occurred when fertility is likely. Emergency contraception should not be used as a regular method of contraception. It is significantly less effective than other methods, and its long-term use has not been studied. It also provides no protection against sexually transmitted infections.

The Contraceptive Patch

In December 2000, Johnson and Johnson applied for approval to market the first contraceptive patch. In March 2003, the patch became available to women seeking a method of contraception that released a steady delivery of hormones over time. In a short time it became the second most popular form of nonoral birth control in prescriptions and sales (Long, 2002).

Similar to the use of the nicotine patch, users wear it on the lower abdomen, buttocks, or upper arm. The patch is about the size of a matchbook and delivers a combination of estrogen and progesterone. Each patch is used for 7 days, then removed and discarded. Patches are worn for 3 weeks, followed by a patch-free week to allow menstruation to occur. The primary side effects of the patch are headache, nausea, and site reactions, which were experienced by 20% of users in clinical trials (Contraception patch, 2001). The patch is approximately as effective as birth control pills. It is 99.7% effective when used perfectly; for typical use it has a 92% user effectiveness rate (Long, 2002).

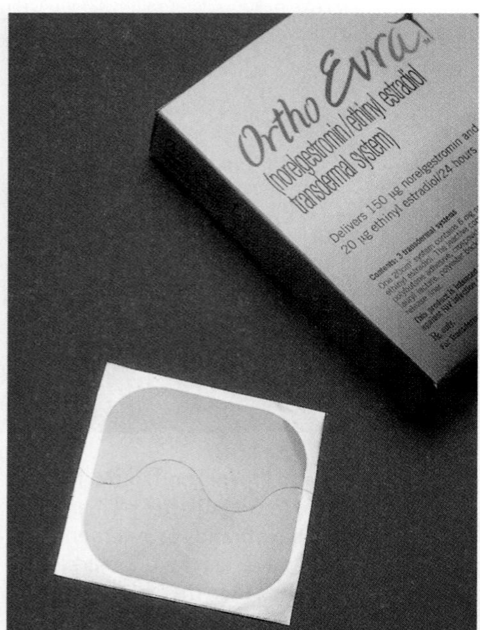

Ortho Evra is the first birth control patch approved by the FDA. Though the patch contains hormones similar to those in birth control pills, the patch needs to be changed only once a week, minimizing the margin of error and subsequent decreased effectiveness that is often the case with oral contraceptives.

Depo-Provera

Depo-Provera is another form of a progestin-only contraception method. It is a shot that is given every 12 weeks. Depo-Provera suppresses ovulation by inhibiting production of FSH and LH.

Effectiveness

Depo-Provera is even more effective than the pill. In 1 year, only 0.3% of women using Depo-Provera become pregnant. And because it is an injection, there is no chance that a typical user can use it incorrectly, unless she does not return in 3 months for her next shot. Many couples prefer Depo-Provera because its use is not related to intercourse activity.

Reversibility

Fertility may resume immediately after 13 weeks has passed since the last injection. However, studies show that women generally do not conceive for an average of 10 months after the date of the last shot (Hatcher, et al., 1998).

Advantages and Disadvantages

Depo-Provera is easy for a woman to use, simply requiring that she return to the clinic every 3 months. It is not used during coitus, and it is one of the most effective methods of preventing pregnancies.

Depo-Provera has few practical disadvantages. Women do need to have injections every 3 months, which may be difficult for some to schedule. Some women report minor weight gain, and many report changes in their periods. Some women have no periods on Depo-Provera; some have frequent bleeding. Spotting between periods is common in the first months of use. The major disadvantage to Depo-Provera is that it provides no protection against sexually transmitted infections.

In October 2000, the Food and Drug Administration approved a new injectable contraceptive that is being marketed under the trade name Lunelle. An injection like Depo-Provera, it contains both progestin and estrogen, whereas Depo-Provera has only progestin. It is given as a once-a-month intramuscular injection. Women on Lunelle have a monthly period and need to visit their health provider each month. Fertility resumes in 4 months after discontinuation as compared to approximately 10 months with Depo-Provera. Less than 1% of women who use Lunelle become pregnant in their first year of use. Lunelle is recommended for women who are good candidates for birth control pills but have trouble remembering to take them every day (Contraception and family planning: FDA approves use of Lunelle, the "injectable pill," 2000).

Depo-Provera
An injectable progestin-only contraceptive.

Norplant
The brand name of contraceptive hormonal implants containing levonorgestrel.

Norplant

In 1990 the FDA approved hormonal implants as a means of contraception. Marketed under the brand name **Norplant,** these implants consist of six matchstick-size capsules containing levonorgestrel, a progesteronelike synthetic hormone. Levonorgestrel prevents ovulation and causes endocrine dysfunction—no egg, no fertilization. It also thickens the cervical mucus.

Norplant is surgically implanted by a physician in a simple procedure, using a needle to insert the implants under the skin of the upper arm. This procedure usually takes approximately 15 minutes. Once in place, the implants release a low continuous dosage of levonorgestrel and remain effective for up to 5 years. Removal is minor surgery and may require more than one visit to the doctor.

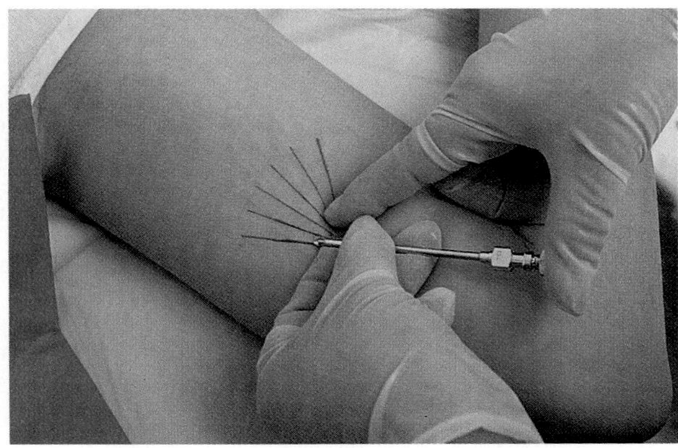

Once in place, hormonal implants are the easiest method of contraception to use. They also remain effective for up to 5 years.

Effectiveness

Studies of more than a half-million women in many countries have led researchers to conclude that Norplant is 99.7% effective in preventing pregnancy, making it the most effective method of contraception to date. There is no difference between the typical and perfect user effectiveness rates, because Norplant cannot be used incorrectly.

Reversibility

Once the Norplant is removed, conception can occur immediately. The median time to conception after the Norplant is removed in a woman who is trying to conceive is approximately 1 month (Hatcher, et al., 1998).

Advantages and Disadvantages

The advantages of Norplant are many, not the least of which is its actual use effectiveness rate. Once in place it can be forgotten; the woman need take no other actions. Furthermore, should a woman want to become pregnant at a later date, the implants can be removed in a minor surgical procedure and fertility usually returns during the woman's next menstrual cycle. And although the initial cost for the implants may be higher than that of some other methods of contraception, the total cost over its 5-year lifespan would be less than the cost of oral contraceptives.

As with all means of contraception, implants have their disadvantages. Some women may have difficulty affording the initial cost. Medicaid does cover Norplant insertions, but the Norplant Foundation provides a free set for low-income women who are not covered by Medicaid.

Some women are not good candidates for Norplant. Implants are more effective in women who weigh less than 110 pounds and are significantly less effective in women who weigh more than 154 pounds. Norplant use can also lead to menstrual irregularities such as prolonged bleeding and more frequent bleeding (Keenan, 1991). Furthermore, although the safety of Norplant has been tested, and it does not contain any estrogen, the World Health Organization recommends that women with unexplained vaginal bleeding or breast cancer not use these implants. In addition, anywhere from 2% to 8% of women using Norplant experience minor side effects that lead to implant removal. Among these side effects are menstrual irregularities and amenorrhea, ovarian cysts, headaches, acne, weight change, and hair growth. Depending on the study, between 76% and 95% of Norplant users continue with the method after the first year.

Finally, as for other hormonal methods of contraception, Norplant provides *no* protection against sexually transmitted infections. Women using

Norplant who are not in committed monogamous relationships must also use condoms to prevent STIs.

Given these advantages and disadvantages, one physician who is an expert on women's health recommends that implants be considered if (Patterson, 1990a)

1. You are interested in long-term contraception.
2. You are unable to use pills containing estrogen.
3. You have used barrier methods—for example, the diaphragm, spermicides, condom, cervical cap—and have become dissatisfied with them.
4. You have difficulty remembering to use your method.

Unfortunately, Norplant is no longer being marketed. In 2000, its manufacturer, Wyeth, became concerned that specified lots of Norplant might be ineffective because of a manufacturing error and, consequently, advised health care professionals to stop providing implants from those lots. In addition, Wyeth advised women who already had implants from those lots to use a barrier or hormonal contraceptive method to ensure protection from pregnancy. After conducting further tests, though, Wyeth concluded there was no problem with those lots and that women need no longer use a backup method of contraception. Unfortunately, the damage was already done to Norplant's reputation, and, citing "limitation in product component supplies," Wyeth decided not to reintroduce Norplant to the market (Wyeth, 2002).

Intrauterine Devices

intrauterine device (IUD) Synthetic device that is inserted into the uterus to prevent the sperm from fertilizing the ovum.

Intrauterine devices (IUDs) are synthetic devices that are inserted by a medical provider into the uterus to prevent pregnancy (Figure 8.5). Currently, only two IUDs are available in the United States: the Paragard Copper-T 380A and the Progestasert Progesterone T. The Paragard IUD can remain in place for 10 years, while the Progestasert IUD must be replaced every year (SIECUS, 2003).

No one really knows how IUDs prevent pregnancy, but a number of theories have been proposed:

1. They prevent sperm from fertilizing ova.
2. They immobilize sperm.
3. They change the environment in the fallopian tubes and in the uterus.

Current research does not support the theory that IUDs act as abortifacients.

IUDs are a highly effective method of birth control and are an excellent choice for women who have already had children and are in mutually monogamous relationships. They are generally not appropriate for teenage or college women because they increase the risk of sexually transmitted infections. The risk of pelvic inflammatory disease (PID) increases sixfold as a result of exposure to an STI after IUD insertion. In fact, IUD labeling states that nulliparous women (women who have not had a child) are not candidates for the IUD because of this increased risk of PID and subsequent infertility (Hatcher, et al., 1998).

In the United States in 1978, 20% of widowed, divorced, or separated women aged 15 to 44 years who used some method of contraception used an IUD (National Center for Health Statistics, 1978). However, with reports of its potential side effects—pelvic inflammatory disease, perforated uterus, ectopic (tubal) pregnancy, pregnancy complications (stillbirths, birth defects, low birth weight), and infertility—the number of women who used IUDs in

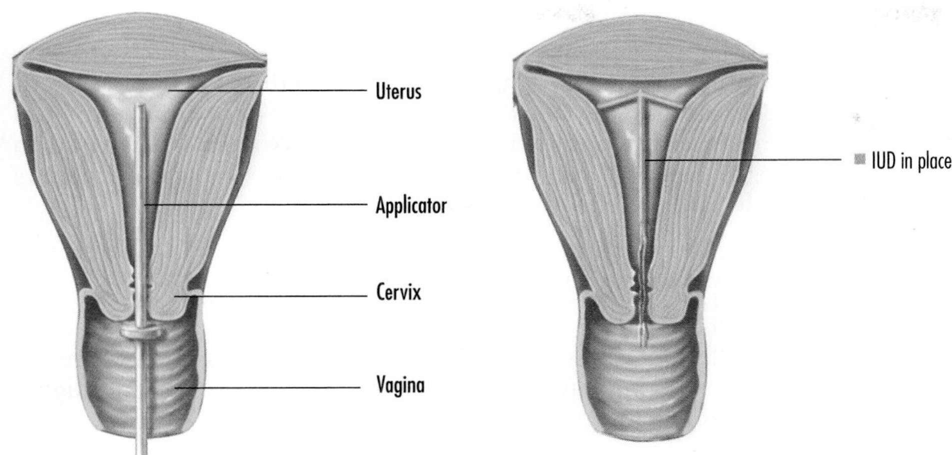

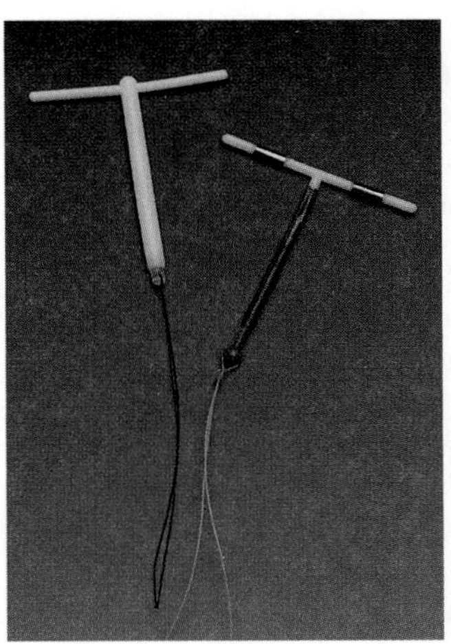

FIGURE 8.5 The IUD is inserted past the cervix into the uterus. Before insertion, the length of the uterus is measured with an instrument called a *sound*. Upon insertion, the arms of the IUD gradually unfold. Once the inserter is removed, the threads attached to the IUD are clipped to extend into the vagina through the cervical opening.

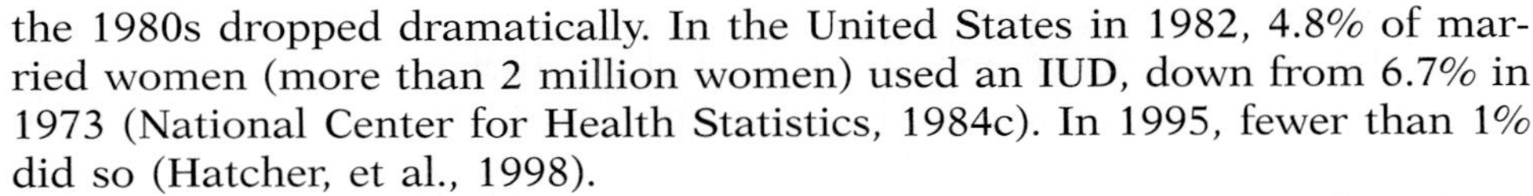

the 1980s dropped dramatically. In the United States in 1982, 4.8% of married women (more than 2 million women) used an IUD, down from 6.7% in 1973 (National Center for Health Statistics, 1984c). In 1995, fewer than 1% did so (Hatcher, et al., 1998).

In 1986, the manufacturer of the most widely used IUDs in the United States (G. D. Searle and Company) removed them from the market because of concern over pending lawsuits. Ever since the A. H. Robins Company urged physicians in 1980 to remove their Dalkon Shield IUD from women because of health complications, IUDs have been viewed with suspicion. By 1985, Robins had paid more than $520 million in lawsuits and was forced to seek protection under Chapter 11 of the Bankruptcy Code. By 1985, IUD sales accounted for less than 2% of the $1 billion contraceptive industry (Hantula, 1986). After G. D. Searle removed its IUDs from the market, IUDs were virtually unavailable, except Progesterone T. The one remaining IUD available in the United States was the Progestasert, manufactured by Alza Pharmaceuticals.

In this instance, the public attitude toward litigation interfered with the availability of a contraceptive choice. But other factors have been involved as well. As one professional publication stated, "Prohibitive costs of liability insurance, the costs of developing new products, the amount of time before the Food and Drug Administration grants approval and the costs involved in getting such approval are among the reasons for limited contraceptive choices" (Special report on contraception, 1986).

In 1988, GynoMed Pharmaceutical Inc. marketed the Copper-T 380A IUD, thereby giving women greater choice in deciding which IUD to use. To limit litigation, GynoMed developed information packages to ensure its IUD users gave informed consent to their use and insertion by reading the information inserts and signing a consent form. The physicians were also asked to sign forms attesting to receiving the information packages and to informing their patients about the benefits and risks associated with the Copper-T 380A. Nevertheless, the IUD is a highly effective method, which is easily inserted and removed.

In December 2000, the Food and Drug Administration approved a new 5-year IUD that is marketed under the name Mirena. It had been available in Europe for more than 10 years and had been used by 2 million women worldwide before its U.S. approval. It works by releasing levonorgestrel into the uterus. How the local release of levonorgestrel prevents pregnancy has yet to be fully explained. The 1-year failure rate for Mirena is only 0.1%, the lowest failure rate of any contraceptive method (FDA approves 5-year IUD, www.sexhealth.com).

Myth vs Fact

Myth: Providing birth control to young people encourages them to have sexual relationships.
Fact: There are no studies that indicate that young people who have access to family-planning methods are more likely to have sexual intercourse. They are more likely to use contraception.

Myth: You can borrow a friend's diaphragm in a pinch.
Fact: Diaphragms are fitted to an individual woman. You cannot borrow another woman's diaphragm.

Myth: If you roll on the condom the wrong way, reverse it and put it on the right way.
Fact: Microscopic tears can occur when you roll on a condom. Throw it out and start with a new one.

Myth: There is nothing you can do but hope and pray if you forget to use your method.
Fact: If you forget to use a method, there is emergency contraception available. It must be used within 72 hours of the act of unprotected intercourse. Call a provider near you or 1-888-NOT-2-LATE.

Effectiveness
The IUD is one of the most effective contraceptive methods. It is 97% to 99% effective in preventing pregnancy. There is only a 1% difference in theoretical and user effectiveness rates, because the woman does not control the use of the IUD once it is inserted (Hatcher, et al., 1998). Women are advised to check the strings to assure the IUD is still in place; not doing so accounts for the minor difference in effectiveness rates.

Reversibility
Once the IUD is removed, fertility resumes immediately.

Advantages and Disadvantages
The IUD is an excellent method for adult women in mutually monogamous relationships who have completed childbearing. In addition to being highly effective, it is easy to use and has no systemic side effects.

A major advantage of the IUD is that once inserted it remains in place, so planning before intercourse is unnecessary. (When it is in place, a string attached to the IUD emerges through the cervix. The woman feels for the string to make sure the IUD is present, because it is possible for it to pass out of the uterus with the menstrual flow or at other times. The device can also be removed by a physician by means of this string.) Another advantage is the IUD's high level of effectiveness.

The IUD's high rate of effectiveness is unfortunately offset by complications: As mentioned, the IUD can increase the chance of pelvic infection, especially in women with multiple sexual partners. This is one of the reasons IUDs are not recommended for teenage women or women who have not had children and plan to do so. IUDs can also be unknowingly discharged (in 2% to 10% of first-year users), and thus pregnancy can result. They can cause especially heavy menstrual flow, particularly in the first several months after insertion. Finally, there is a tiny chance that conception will occur with the device in place. This situation presents a dilemma. If the IUD is removed, a 25% chance exists that the pregnancy will end spontaneously, a result that may not be satisfactory to a person who is opposed to abortion. But if the device is kept in place, the result is likely to be an ectopic pregnancy, serious infection, blood poisoning, bleeding, or premature labor (Hatcher, et al., 1998).

A major disadvantage to the IUD is that it actually increases the likelihood of becoming infected with a sexually transmitted infection. This is especially true in the first month after insertion. Women who desire to have children in the future are not good candidates for the IUD. If they do choose the IUD, they must also use condoms.

Diaphragm

diaphragm
Shallow rubber cap that covers the cervix and prevents sperm from entering the uterus.

When in place, the **diaphragm** prevents the sperm from traveling through the uterus and up the fallopian tubes to fertilize an egg, and it holds spermicide against the cervix (Figure 8.6). The diaphragm is a shallow rubber, or synthetic rubber, cap surrounding a flexible metal ring that covers the cervix.

Diaphragms are available in several sizes and styles. Because the diaphragm's purpose is to prevent sperm from going beyond the vagina, its size and shape are very important. If the diaphragm does not fit exactly right, a chance exists that sperm can bypass this barrier. Clearly, using someone else's diaphragm is a poor idea. Diaphragms are fitted by physicians or gynecological nurse-practitioners and refitted after women give birth or gain or lose a significant amount of weight. Fit should also be checked during the yearly gynecological exam, and the diaphragm should be replaced every 2 years.

The diaphragm must remain in place for at least 6 hours after intercourse, and spermicide must be added for *each* act of intercourse. This combination of requirements, besides increasing effectiveness, allows the male and female to share the responsibility for contraception. (Diaphragms should be removed at least once every 24 hours to reduce the risk of toxic shock syndrome.)

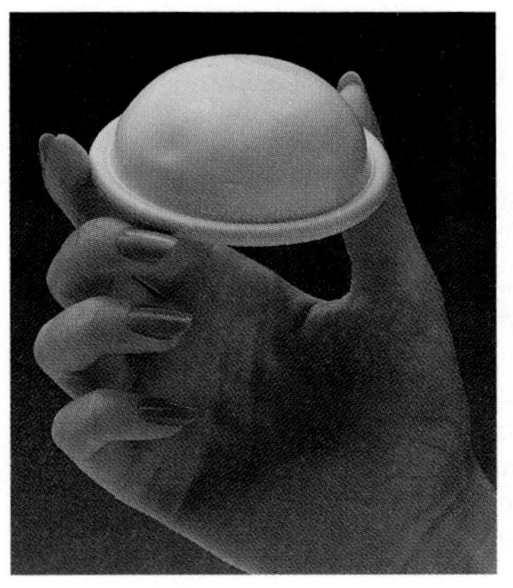

Effectiveness

When inserted properly and used with spermicide, the diaphragm is theoretically 94% effective and 80% effective as actually used. Some studies suggest that spermicides may prevent some STIs, and thus the diaphragm may help prevent STIs. Other studies indicate that they may cause abrasions in the vaginal walls that could increase susceptibility to STIs.

Reversibility

The diaphragm does not affect fertility (except when it is in place).

Advantages and Disadvantages

The major advantages of the diaphragm are that it is highly effective if used correctly and consistently, is easy to learn to use, and has no systemic side effects. Some couples make diaphragm insertion part of foreplay. The man can insert it into the woman's vagina before intercourse.

One disadvantage of the diaphragm is that it must be inserted before intercourse and inserted properly, requiring the woman or couple to plan

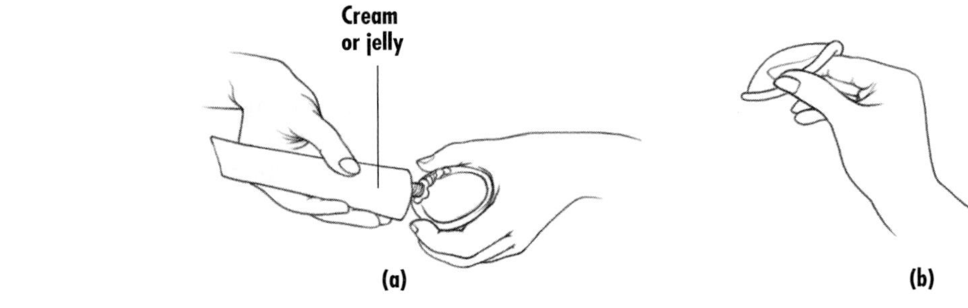

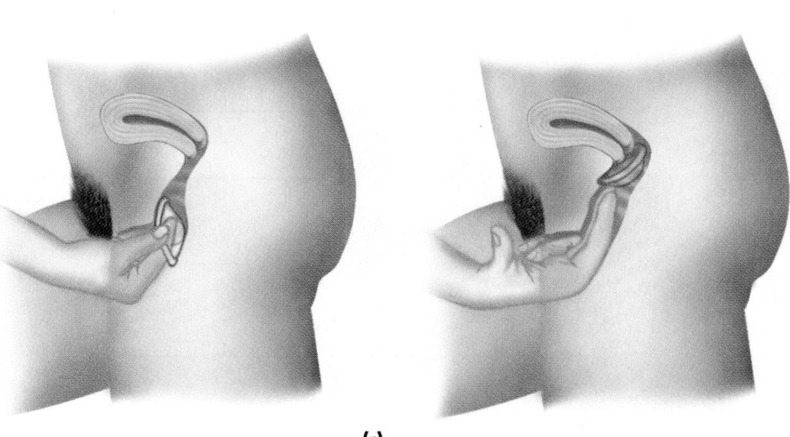

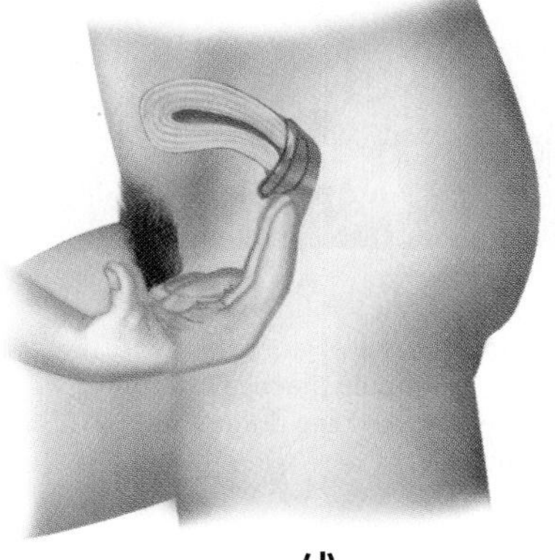

FIGURE 8.6 Procedure for inserting a diaphragm: (a) Before inserting the diaphragm, coat the rim and cup with a spermicidal cream or jelly. (b) Squeeze the rim of the diaphragm together between your thumb and index finger. (c) Insert the diaphragm into the vagina with the rim facing up and push it toward the small of your back. As you let go of the diaphragm, it will spring open. Continue to guide it to your cervix with the tips of your fingers. (d) Be sure to check that the diaphragm completely covers the cervix.

ahead. Some women are not comfortable touching their genitals and therefore find diaphragm use uncomfortable. Diaphragms provide only limited protection against certain STIs, so condoms must also be used to prevent STI transmission. In addition, some users may experience an increased risk of urinary tract infections. Oil-based lubricants should not be used with diaphragms as they erode the rubber.

Cervical Cap

cervical cap
Shallow rubber cap, smaller than a diaphragm, that covers the cervix to prevent sperm from entering the uterus.

The **cervical cap** is a rubber, plastic, or metal cap that covers the cervix and holds spermicidal cream or jelly. It is similar to, but smaller than, the diaphragm; is meant to stay in place longer; and is slightly less effective than the diaphragm (Figure 8.7). In 1988, the FDA approved the sale of cervical caps in the United States, although they have been used in Europe for decades.

At first glance the cervical cap appears to be both safe and effective (Smith & Barwin, 1983). In addition, the cervical cap can be left in place for 48 hours. However, the cap must be removed during menstruation to allow the menstrual flow to leave the body.

Although the cap is made in different sizes, not all women can use it because of the variation in shapes and sizes of cervixes. Cervical caps are not available from all medical providers. A women's health clinic is more likely to stock caps than a private physician. When people use the cap, they should *not* use oil-based lubricants (such as petroleum jelly, cocoa butter, cold cream, or mineral or vegetable oils), which tend to deteriorate the rubber in the cap.

Effectiveness

Overall, the cervical cap and the diaphragm have similar rates of effectiveness. The cervical cap is 91% effective theoretically, but user rates are 80%. The cap is much more effective in women who have never been pregnant (nulliparous women). The cap is 80% effective for nulliparous women com-

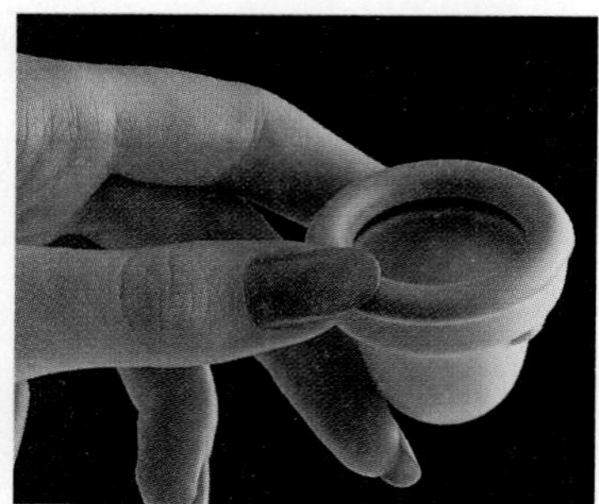

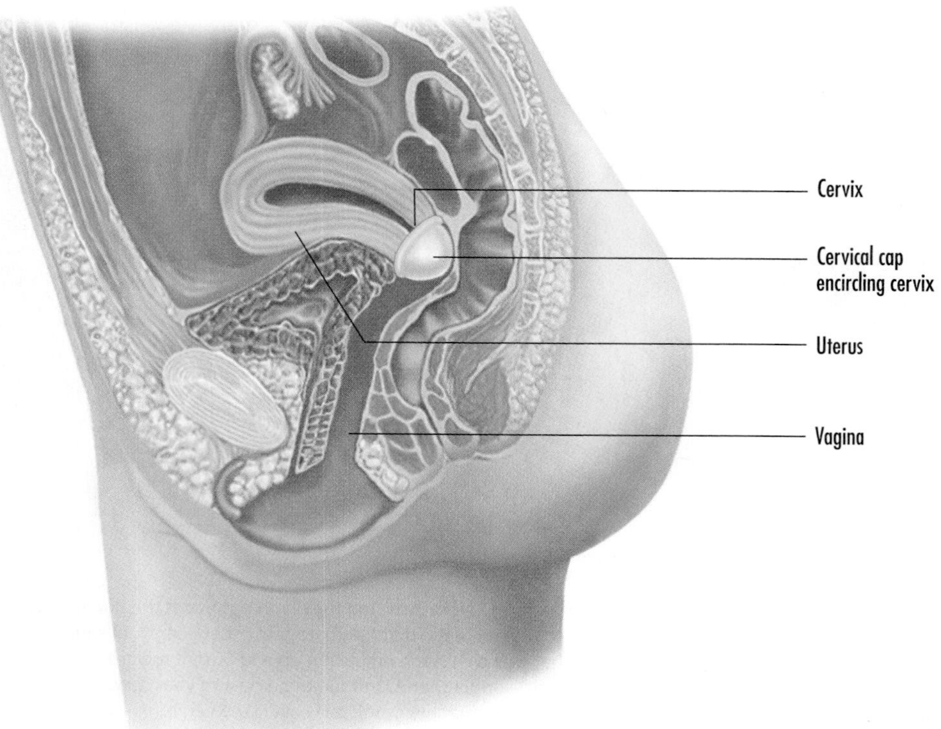

FIGURE 8.7 It is important that your cervical cap is always inserted correctly. You should practice inserting before using the cap during sexual intercourse.

pared to only 60% in women who have been pregnant. As with the diaphragm, spermicide used with the cervical cap may provide some protection against some sexually transmitted infections, but it may increase susceptibility to others. In nonmonogamous couples, condoms should also be used to prevent STI transmission.

Reversibility
The cap does not affect fertility (except when it is in place).

Advantages and Disadvantages
The cap is easy to use and has no systemic side effects. Many women like the fact that it can be kept in place for up to 48 hours and that spermicide use for additional acts of intercourse is optional.

There are also disadvantages associated with use of the cap. Some studies have found slightly higher than expected precancerous cervical abnormalities in cap users (Cervical cap precautions, 1989), though other studies have not been able to verify this finding. As a result, the FDA requires labeling that instructs women planning to use the cervical cap to obtain a Pap smear before being fitted. Women who have had an abnormal Pap smear result or who have cervical cancer are advised not to use the cap. In addition, the cervical cap may occasionally irritate the cervix, may cause an unpleasant odor or vaginal dryness, and has the potential for becoming dislodged during coitus. It can also cause toxic shock syndrome if it is not removed regularly.

NuvaRing

A vaginal ring that provides hormonal protection from pregnancy was approved by the Food and Drug Administration in 2001 and became available in 2002 (Organon, 2002). NuvaRing emits 0.015 mg of ethinyl estradiol (the estrogen component) and 0.120 mg of etonogestrel (the progestin component) daily for 21 days. In contrast, low-dose estrogen contraceptive pills contain 0.005 mg more estrogen, and other contraceptive pills contain 0.015 mg more estrogen. Whereas the diaphragm and cervical cap must be positioned correctly to provide maximal protection, NuvaRing need not. It cannot be inserted incorrectly, and it has a timer as a reminder when it needs to be replaced. The hourglass-shaped timer shows the number of days the ring will remain effective and beeps on the 21st day. Even if it is not removed immediately, protection remains for another week. NuvaRing is not recommended for use by women who smoke cigarettes, nor for those who have heart disease or are prone to circulatory diseases such as blood clots. NuvaRing costs approximately $39 in pharmacies and requires a prescription to be purchased.

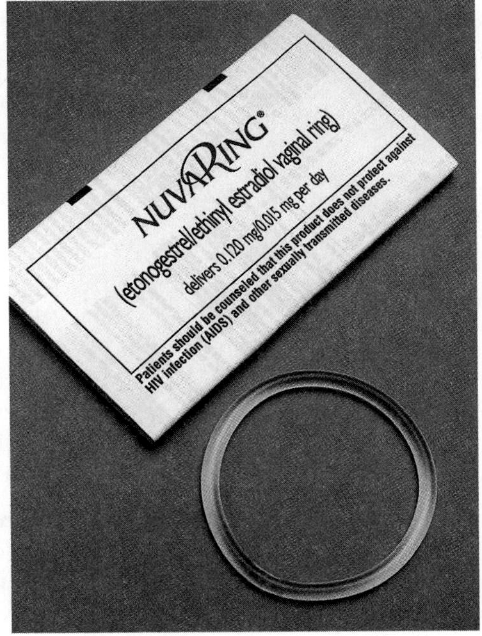

NuvaRing is a flexible, transparent, odorless ring that is about as big as a silver dollar and is inserted into the vagina, where it continuously releases low doses of estrogen and progestin that prevent pregnancy. Heralded for its convenience, NuvaRing leaves even less room for error than the contraceptive patch.

Effectiveness
NuvaRing is an effective hormonal contraceptive with many advantages. It has a theoretical and user effectiveness rate between 98% and 99%. The characteristic that once it is in place there is nothing else to do (contrasted, for example, with oral contraceptives, which require remembering to take a pill) greatly enhances its effectiveness as used.

Reversibility
NuvaRing is reversible once removed.

Advantages and Disadvantages
NuvaRing contains less estrogen than even the low-dose oral contraceptives, thereby decreasing the risks associated with synthetic estrogens. In addition, the ring does not require any daily action, as

does taking a pill each day. All that is required is replacement of the ring after 21 days. Consequently, its user effectiveness rate is quite high. Furthermore, the vast majority of women cannot feel the ring when it is in place and report being satisfied with this method of contraception.

As with all methods of contraception, there are also disadvantages associated with NuvaRing. The risk of synthetic estrogen is not eliminated; it is merely reduced. Therefore, as advised by the manufacturer, smokers and those susceptible to blood clots should not use the ring. Further, 14% of users experienced vaginitis (Redfearn, 2002), and 25% of men felt the ring during intercourse, although most reported they did not perceive that to be a problem. The manufacturer suggests removing the ring during intercourse if a partner finds that it causes a problem. It can be removed for up to 3 hours without losing its effectiveness. Another disadvantage of the ring for women who are uncomfortable touching their genitalia is the need for the user to insert it manually through the vagina. These women may prefer another contraceptive method that does not entail touching the genitalia. In addition, NuvaRing does not offer any protection against sexually transmitted infections. Finally, the monthly cost of the ring ($39) is approximately $9 higher than the monthly cost for oral contraceptives and, at the time of this writing, is not covered by health insurance companies.

Permanent Methods

Sterilization

Sterilization is a form of contraception that renders a person biologically incapable of reproducing. Men and women both may choose to be sterilized—made infertile—because they have all the children they want or because they do not want to have children. Women in ill health, perhaps those with serious heart conditions, may choose to prevent life-threatening pregnancies and births. Couples may choose not to have children if their genetic makeup, when passed to their offspring, would be likely to result in birth defects (for example, sickle-cell anemia or Tay-Sachs disease).

sterilization
A procedure that makes a person biologically incapable of reproducing.

vasectomy
Cutting or cauterizing of the vas deferens to prevent sperm from being ejaculated; a means of sterilization.

Individual methods of sterilization for men and women are described shortly. More than 15 million people rely on sterilization as their contraceptive method. Each year approximately a million people undergo sterilization procedures (Hatcher, et al., 1998). Sterilization has not always been so popular. In 1980, 99 million couples were using sterilization worldwide. By 1995, this number had climbed to 223 million couples (EngenderHealth, 2003). In the United States in 1982, 23% of women using a contraceptive method chose sterilization, whereas by 1995, 28% were using sterilization. Male sterilization rates have remained steady between 1982 and 1995, at 11% of those using a method of contraception choosing sterilization (National Center for Health Statistics, 2002).

Effectiveness

Male and female sterilization is highly effective. In the first year after sterilization, only 1 woman out of every 1,000 sterilized becomes pregnant, and only 1 in every 1,000 sterilized men causes a pregnancy.

Reversibility

According to Hatcher and colleagues (1998, p. 545), "Reversal of the sterilization procedure is expensive, not readily available, requires major surgery, and results are not guaranteed." In other words, although sterilization may be reversible, it should be considered a permanent method.

Advantages and Disadvantages

Sterilization is only for people who are certain that they do not want more children and who are fertile. Both female and male sterilizations have the same advantages. They are permanent, highly effective (99.9%), are cost-effective, lack side effects, do not interfere with intercourse, and are very safe. Their primary disadvantage is they provide no protection against STIs.

Male Sterilization

In men, sterilization entails interruption of the vas deferens in a procedure called a vasectomy (Figure 8.8). Vasectomy became popular as a method of contraception in the late 1960s and early 1970s. In 1971, a peak of 701,000 vasectomies were performed in the United States (Association for Voluntary Sterilization, 1982). The interest in vasectomy was a result of several factors, including concern about the health hazards of the oral contraceptive and extensive promotion by several national organizations (Association for Voluntary Sterilization, Planned Parenthood Federation of America, and Zero Population Growth). In addition, the medical community announced its support for vasectomy as a contraceptive method that was safe and effective.

In the early 1980s, the number of vasectomies performed declined, as a result of the publicity received by a couple of research studies. The mass media picked up on two studies involving vasectomized monkeys that found these monkeys had a greater degree of atherosclerosis (clogged arteries) than nonvasectomized monkeys (Alexander & Clarkson, 1978; Clarkson & Alexander, 1980). The hypothesis this research generated concerned the

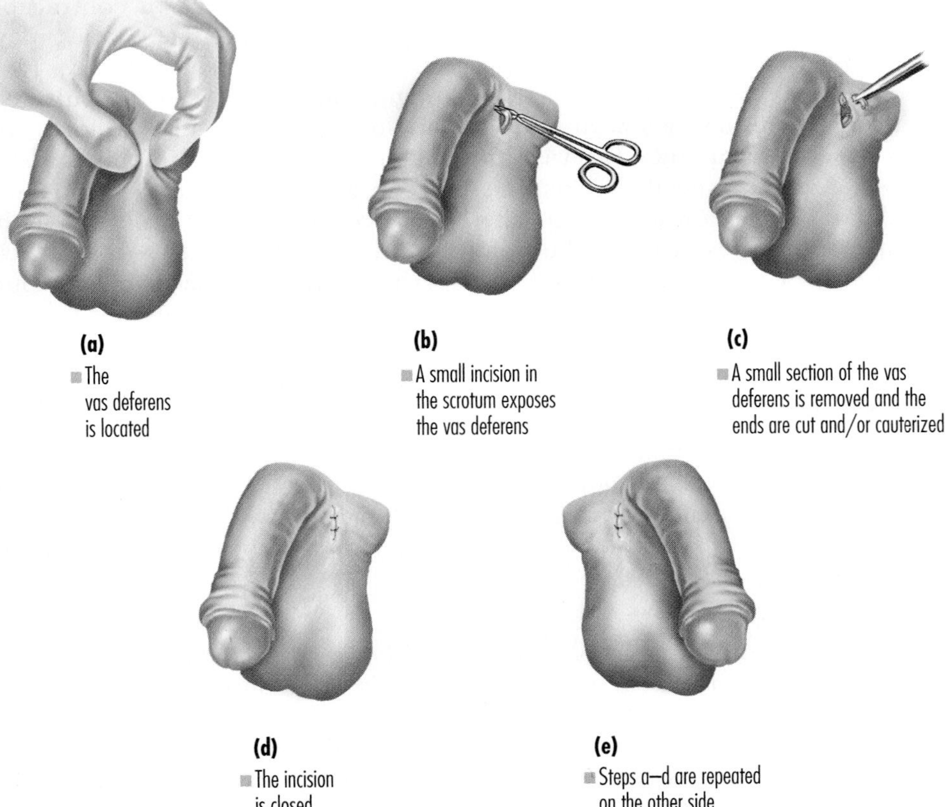

FIGURE 8.8 Vasectomy.

development of antisperm antibodies that formed certain immune complexes that circulate and accumulate on the walls of the arteries. The fear that heart disease would develop in vasectomized men decreased the number of vasectomies. Subsequent research, however, has not found any increased risk of heart disease in men who undergo vasectomy (Hatcher, et al., 1998).

Vasectomy is a simple, minor surgical procedure that takes about 30 minutes. A small opening is made in the scrotum, and the vas deferens is severed. This severing blocks sperm from entering the ejaculate, because it has no route out of the testes. Clips and plugs can also be used to interfere with the vas deferens passageway; the most widely used technique involves cutting the vas and sealing off its ends (by suturing or cauterization). Vasectomies are done under local anesthesia and require minimal care afterward. Vasectomized men are instructed to avoid hard work or strenuous exercise for several days, to wear a scrotal support for a week, and to take mild painkillers for postoperative discomfort. As soon as the man feels ready, he may resume sexual intercourse.

Unlike female sterilization, a vasectomy does not provide immediate infertility. Sperm may still be stored in the urethra or elsewhere in the reproductive tract and may not be expelled for 10 weeks or more. The amount of time required to expel this sperm depends partly on the frequency of ejaculation. For this reason, men are asked to return to the physician 6 to 8 weeks after the vasectomy with a semen specimen to be tested for the presence of sperm. Until the absence of sperm is verified, a condom, diaphragm, or other method of contraception is required to prevent conception. Usually two consecutive negative sperm analysis results are required before a backup method of contraception is no longer necessary.

Vasectomy is still considered to be a permanent means of contraception; however, with new microsurgical techniques, some vasectomies may be reversed in a very expensive procedure called a vasovasectomy. Two problems exist with these reversals, though. The first is the difficulty of repairing tissue that has been unused and closed off for a time. In fact, the longer the interval since the vasectomy, usually the more difficult it is to reverse. Second, even if the vas deferens can be opened, there is no guarantee that conception will occur. There may, for instance, be problems with the sperm as a result of antibody formation. Statistically, 81% to 98% of vasectomies can be reversed so that sperm appears in the ejaculate, but only about half of reversals (depending on which studies one reads) result in a pregnancy.

vasovasectomy
Reversal of a vasectomy, so that sperm can be ejaculated.

minilaparotomy
Female sterilization procedure that involves a small incision in the abdomen through which the fallopian tubes are pulled so they can be blocked.

ligation
The tying of the fallopian tubes to prevent the sperm–egg union.

laparoscopy
Female sterilization procedure that involves inserting a narrow viewing instrument—a laparoscope—through an incision in the abdomen and then performing ligation or applying clips or rings to block the fallopian tubes.

open laparoscopy
Female sterilization procedure during which a small incision is made in the abdomen through which a special tube (cannula) is inserted and around which the skin is sutured.

Female Sterilization

Female sterilization takes several forms; their goal is to prevent the egg from moving down the fallopian tube to be fertilized by a sperm. Female sterilization procedures include the minilaparotomy, laparoscopy, open laparoscopy, vaginal approaches, and transcervical methods (Minilaparotomy and laparoscopy, 1985).

Minilaparotomy

A **minilaparotomy,** sometimes called a *minilap,* requires a small incision just above the pubic hairline. An instrument is then inserted into the cervix to move the uterus and pull each fallopian tube into the incision. Part of the tube is taken out of the incision, where it is blocked by **ligation,** clips, or rings and then replaced in the abdomen. This procedure takes about 20 minutes, and the woman can usually leave the medical setting in 2 or 3 hours. Because the incision is very small (about 3 cm), few complications develop.

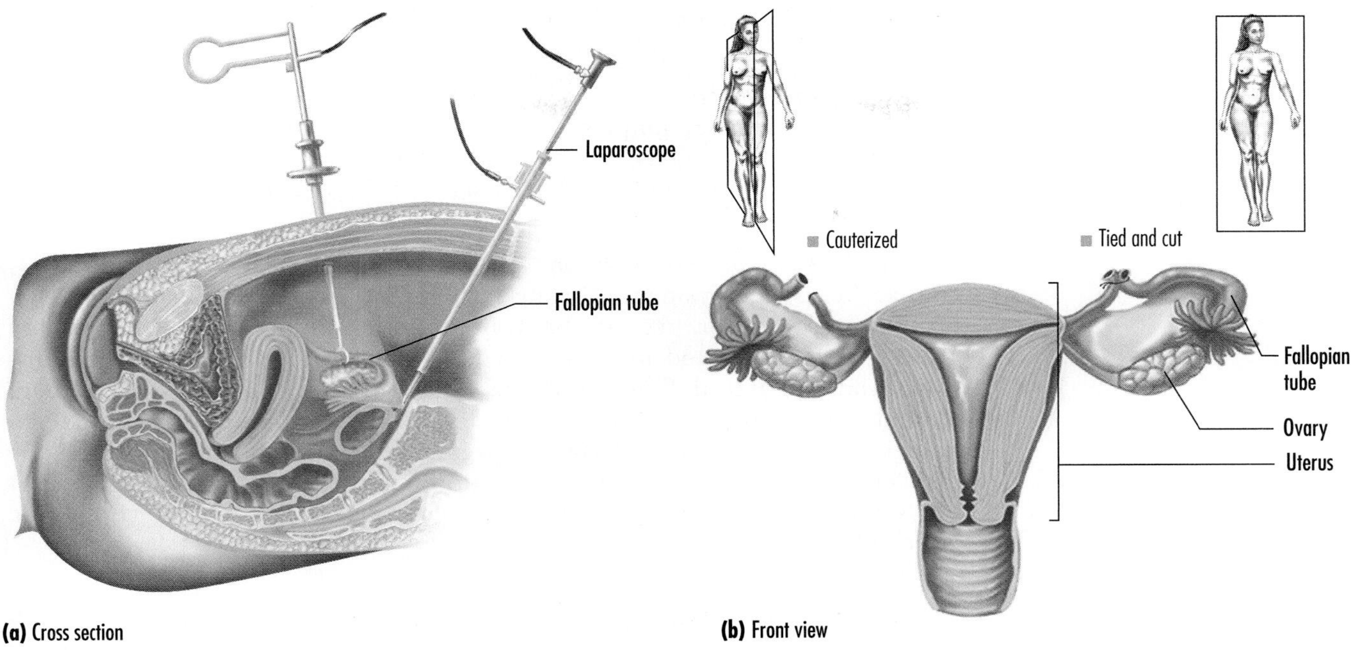

FIGURE 8.9 Female sterilization by laparoscopic ligation. (a) Cross section: The tubes are located using a laparoscope and cut, tied, or cauterized through a second incision. (b) Front view: The tubes after ligation.

Laparoscopy

A **laparoscopy** involves inserting into the abdomen a narrow stainless steel tube with fiber-optic cylinders that transmit light (Figure 8.9). This tube is called a *laparoscope*. Two types of laparoscopes can be used. With one, the physician can insert forceps and other instruments through the tube itself; therefore, only one incision is necessary. With the other type of laparoscope, two incisions are required because the tube does not permit other instruments to be inserted through it. Ligation by electrocoagulation (high-frequency electrical current) or application of clips or rings can take place during this procedure to prevent the passage of the egg.

Open Laparoscopy

Open laparoscopy was designed to minimize the chance of bowel or blood vessel injury. A small incision is made, through which a special tube (cannula) can be inserted and around which the skin is sutured. The instruments can be passed through the cannula. Because the physician can look into the abdomen during the insertion of the cannula, it is less likely that damage to the bowel or blood vessels will occur. This procedure has not been widely used because there are no well-controlled studies that clearly outline its advantages, and it takes slightly longer than a laparoscopy.

Vaginal Approaches

Two types of vaginal female sterilization techniques have been used: *culpotomy* and *culdoscopy*. Both of these procedures involve a small incision (3 cm) made in the wall of the vagina behind the cervix. The fallopian tubes are then pulled through the incision into the vagina, where they are occluded by ligation, clips, or rings. The minilaparotomy has been so successful and has had so few complications that culpotomy and culdoscopy are not often used. These techniques result in more pelvic infections, they are more difficult to perform, and they result in higher pregnancy rates than the minilap. They should only be done by highly skilled surgeons in exceptional cases.

Transcervical Methods
Other sterilization techniques that do not involve surgery are undergoing testing. These techniques occlude the fallopian tubes through the cervix; however, the potential for infection exists, and these techniques are used only experimentally.

Nonsurgical Female Sterilization
Quinacrine is a permanent, nonsurgical method of female sterilization that is not approved for use in the United States. Small pellets containing quinacrine are inserted into the uterus through the cervix; the pellets dissolve and the liquid flows into the fallopian tubes and obstructs them (Quinacrine sterilization, 2002). According to the Reproductive Health Technologies Project, the World Health Organization has called for halting the distribution of quinacrine for sterilization "until further scientifically rigorous safety and efficacy testing is done under ethical guidelines" (Emerging issues of the Reproductive Health Technologies Project, 2002).

Reversibility
As with male sterilization, female sterilization should generally be considered irreversible. Although surgical techniques can be successful in opening up the fallopian tubes, highly skilled surgeons and modern microsurgical equipment are required and are very costly. Furthermore, some experts report only 50% to 70% of women who undergo reversal surgery eventually conceive (Minilaparotomy and laparoscopy, 1985), whereas others report

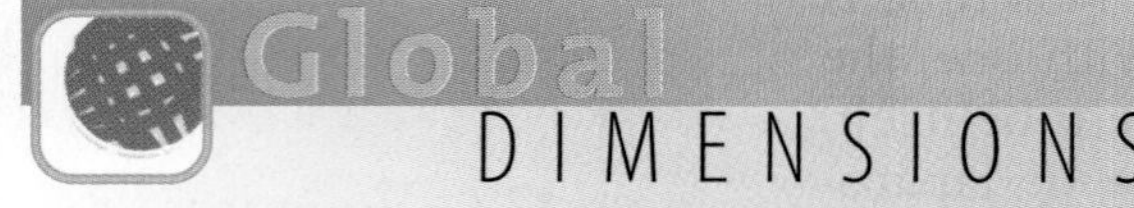

Contraception in Russia

In the United States, oral contraceptives and sterilization are the most popular methods of contraception. In other countries, women rely on a different combination of methods.

In 1998, the All-Russia Centre for Public Opinion and Market Research conducted a contraceptive prevalence study in three urban areas in Russia. They were surprised to discover that knowledge about modern contraceptives was extensive among Russian women. Ninety-seven percent of the Russian women were familiar with the condom, oral contraceptives, and the IUD, and 94% knew where to obtain them. A majority of women knew about female and male sterilization.

The IUD was the most popular method among Russian women. As many as 35% of women had an IUD. Condoms were used by only about 1 in 10 women, and oral contraceptives were used by less than 1 in 10 women. Only 2% of Russian women in these cities had been sterilized.

Russian women had very high rates of abortion. More than half the survey participants had had at least one abortion, and slightly more than one-quarter had had at least two. Nearly three-quarters of women aged 30–44 years had terminated a pregnancy with a medical abortion.

The researchers concluded that the use of modern contraceptives is now widespread in urban areas of Russia and that most women want small families. However, the rate of unplanned pregnancies is still unacceptably high, and the majority of these pregnancies end in abortion.

Source: Mahler, K. Rates of modern method use are high among urban Russian women who typically want small families, *Family Planning Perspectives, 30, no. 6* (November–December 1998), 293–294.

only between 0% and 60% reversal is possible for ligations, 0% to 75% for clips or rings, and 0% for electrocoagulation (Belcastro, 1986).

Several other factors also affect the reversibility of female sterilization. For example, the longer the section of the fallopian tube remaining after sterilization, the more likely reversal will be successful. The site of the blockage has some affect on reversibility, as do the type of procedure used, the age of the woman, and the interval since the sterilization procedure was conducted. Another factor to consider is the greater chance of ectopic pregnancies—women who have had reversal surgery are three times as likely to have an ectopic pregnancy as other women (Hatcher, et al., 1998).

The Future of Contraceptives

Research to find better methods of contraception continues. The perfect method of contraception, which will probably never exist, would:

1. Be 100% effective
2. Be very inexpensive (or even free)
3. Have no side effects
4. Be reversible
5. Involve no remembering to do something
6. Be convenient (not messy)
7. Prevent sexually transmitted infections
8. Be religiously and morally acceptable
9. Not interrupt sexual behaviors

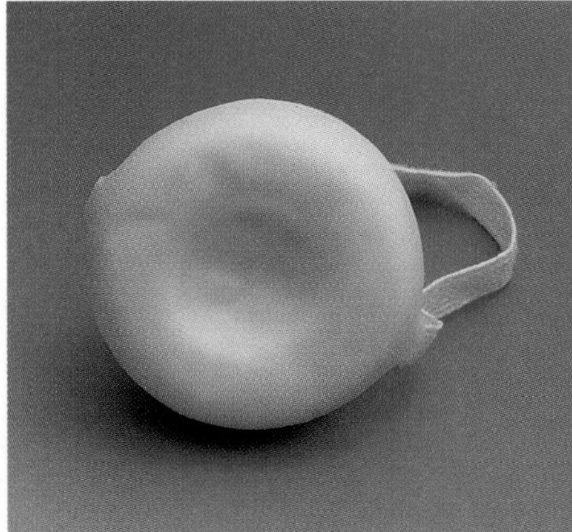

The Today Sponge, a contraceptive sponge, was reintroduced to the U.S. market in 2003.

During the 1990s, several new methods were approved for use in the United States. These included the female condom, nonlatex male condoms, Norplant, Depo-Provera, and Lunelle. New research continues, most involving extensions and improvements of current methods. The contraceptive methods now being researched include the following:

1. *Male contraceptive implants:* In 2001, clinical trials began on a male contraceptive implant. One hundred and twenty male volunteers in the United States and Europe received implants that contained the hormone etonogestral. This hormone is thought to prevent the production of sperm. If these trials prove safe and

Did You Know . . .

The contraceptive sponge is coming back! In March 1999, Allendale Pharmaceuticals purchased the rights to manufacture and market the Today Sponge, which was the most popular over-the-counter contraceptive for women before it was taken off the market in 1995.

The Today Sponge had been pulled from the market after the original manufacturer refused to add a water purification system that the FDA required. There was never any problem with Today Sponge's safety, just with the factory, according to the FDA.

effective, it is possible that male contraceptive implants will be available as early as 2005 (Male contraceptive implant, 2001).

2. *Implanon:* Implanon is a single-rod progesterone implant, only about 4 cm long, that inhibits ovulation while impeding motility in the reproductive tract. A small dosage of the same progesterone that is in the vaginal ring is released constantly. Implanon, designed to be used for 3 years, will include a device to allow women to insert and remove it easily. In clinical trials, no pregnancies were reported in more than 53,000 menstrual cycles (Long, 2003).

3. *Jadelle:* Manufactured by Wyeth, the former manufacturers of Norplant, this two-rod implant system continually releases progesterone to inhibit ovulation. The rods are 4.3 cm long and must be inserted and removed by a trained clinician. Jadelle was determined to be as effective as Norplant in its first 3 years of use (Sivin, et al., 1998). Potential side effects are similar to those of Norplant and include periodic breakthrough bleeding.

4. *Lea's Shield:* Lea's Shield is a cervical cap that allows the release of cervical fluids and air. Elliptical in shape and made of silicone rubber, it is slightly larger in its posterior portion so as to allow for a good fit on the cervix. The shield acts as other barrier methods do. Although it is being manufactured in only one size that fits all users, the shield requires a prescription. Reported to be comfortable and easy to use, the shield can be washed and used for up to 1 year. It is currently available in Germany, Austria, Switzerland, and Canada; however effectiveness data are limited (FDA approves Lea's Shield, 2002).

5. *Essure:* This method of birth control causes sterility without surgical anesthesia or incision and does not result in any visible scar. Passed through the vaginal canal and uterus, a small metal ring is inserted into the fallopian tubes. In 3 months an occlusion occurs, thereby blocking the sperm–egg union. Essure has been 99.8% effective in clinical trials (Long, 2002).

Exploring the DIMENSIONS of Human Sexuality

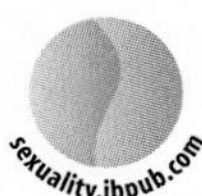

Our feelings, attitudes, and beliefs regarding sexuality are influenced by our internal and external environments. Go to sexuality.jbpub.com to learn more about the biological, psychological, and sociological factors that affect your sexuality.

Biological Factors

- Gender may affect contraceptive decision making. Males have only the option of condoms or vasectomy available; women have to deal with the fact that only they can become pregnant.
- STIs and HIV can be prevented only through strict use of latex condoms, abstinence, or 100% monogamy.
- Natural family planning relies on using physiological cycles and changes to monitor ovulation.
- Hormones such as estrogen and progesterone prevent the pituitary gland from producing FSH, without which the ova do not develop in the ovaries.

Sociocultural Factors

- Socioeconomic status affects contraceptive availability and use.
- Laws and government regulations limit contraceptive approval and availability.
- Religion affects contraceptive decisions, limiting some couples to natural family planning.
- Media and ad information can affect both contraceptive choice and brand choice.

Psychological Factors

- Experience may determine the contraceptive you choose.
- Emotions often get in the way of practicing contraceptives and safer sex.
- Learned attitudes and behaviors affect your willingness to negotiate contraceptive use and practice safer sex.
- Your self-concept may influence whether or not you negotiate contraceptive use with your partner or simply accept what your partner desires.

CASE STUDY

When choosing a method of contraception, you must consider the effectiveness, side effects, convenience, cost, and protection from STIs and HIV. However, your partner's willingness to use the same method also comes into play, because contraceptives are ineffective if not used properly over time.

Many factors influence your contraceptive use. Legally, the federal government regulates which contraceptives you can buy in the United States. Socioeconomic status also is a factor, because most contraceptives are neither free nor covered by all types of health insurance. Also, people of higher socioeconomic status have greater access to prescription contraceptive methods and are more likely to receive more education about contraceptive methods.

Religion also plays a role in contraceptive choice, because some religions only officially sanction natural family-planning methods. Communication skills also are involved, as you negotiate your contraceptive use with a partner.

Discussion Questions

1. List six key considerations in choosing a contraceptive method, and rank their relative importance. What method did you use to rank their importance?
2. Describe the nonprescription methods of contraception. Discuss the relationship issues that affect the choice of these methods.
3. Describe the methods of contraception requiring prescriptions. What types of information should be disclosed to a doctor when making a selection?
4. Discuss the varied methods of female and male sterilization. Should the possibility of reversibility be part of the decision process?

Application Questions

Reread the chapter-opening story and answer the following questions.

1. Discuss how Susan altered her contraception use in light of her changing lifestyle. What other contraceptive methods could she have used at each point? What suggestions would you have for her?
2. If Susan had a family history of diabetes, high blood pressure, or breast cancer, how would her choices of contraceptive be altered?
3. Consider Stephen's decision to have a vasectomy. Although it may have seemed the perfect method for him at the time—married, monogamous, finished with childbearing—it also leaves him without the ability to father more children, should he remarry. In light of this, should men routinely postpone sterilization until a later age—just in case? Or have sperm frozen for the future?

Critical Thinking Questions

1. Assume that you began a relationship with a partner who wanted to use natural family planning because of religious conviction. What advantages and disadvantages would that hold for you from a contraceptive and safer sex standpoint? Answer this question from both male and female viewpoints.
2. The prescription methods of birth control are all female-based. What role, if any, should the male partner have in the decision to use these methods?

Critical Thinking Case

Ben and Allie, both age 25 years, had been dating for 6 months and using latex condoms as their contraception method. Because their relationship was monogamous and increasingly dedicated, they had talked about switching to a different method but had never taken the time to discuss the options and how they would fit their lifestyle.

Then one evening, a condom broke. Allie pulled out the calendar on which she mapped her period, but the news was bad: It was right around the time of ovulation. Although committed to one another, they were not prepared to face the possibility of parenthood.

First consider what Allie and Ben should do immediately. Then outline some options for the couple's future, so that they do not face this situation again.

Exploring Personal Dimensions

Choosing a Contraceptive

There is no such thing as a 100% safe, 100% convenient, 100% easy-to-use contraceptive. Every contraceptive has advantages and disadvantages. People need to weigh these advantages and disadvantages for themselves.

Some questions that people need to ask themselves are as follows:

1. *Effectiveness.* What are the relative effectiveness rates for each method considered? How important is it to prevent pregnancy now? Is using abortion as a backup acceptable to you and your partner, or is an unplanned pregnancy acceptable at this time?
2. *Side effects.* Are you a good candidate for this method? Will you experience adverse side effects? Do you have a medical condition that should prevent you from using this method?
3. *Convenience.* Is this method easy for you to get? Is it easy to use? Will you use it every time?
4. *Cost.* Can you afford it? Does your campus health center provide it? Does your insurance cover it?
5. *STI protection.* Are you in a monogamous relationship? Are you sure? Do you have more than one partner? Do you know your partner's HIV status? Are you willing and committed to using a condom in addition to this method?
6. *Partner.* What does your partner think about this method? Will he or she want to use it every time? Do you want contraception to be a shared responsibility, or is it yours alone?

Sexuality Online

Go to the web component for *Exploring the Dimensions of Human Sexuality* at sexuality.jbpub.com for web exercises, additional resources related to this chapter, and student review tools.

Suggested Readings

Boston Women's Health Collective. *Our bodies, our selves.* New York: Simon & Schuster, 1998.

Hatcher, R. A., Trussell, J., Stewart, F., Cates, W., Stewart, G. K., Guest, F., & Korval, D. *Contraceptive technology,* 17th rev. ed. New York: Ardent Media, 1998.

Robert Hatcher. *A pocket guide to managing contraception.* Atlanta: Bridging the Gap Foundation, 1999.

The Planned Parenthood women's health encyclopedia. New York: Planned Parenthood Federation of America, 1998.

CHAPTER 9

Conception, Pregnancy, and Birth

FEATURES

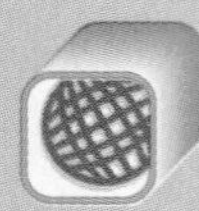
Global Dimensions
Childbearing Rituals

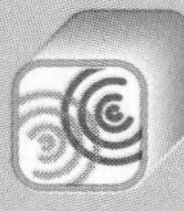
Communication Dimensions
Communicating About Pregnancy

Gender Dimensions
Fathers and Childbirth

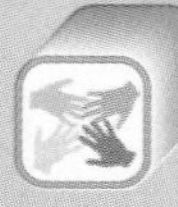
Multicultural Dimensions
Differences in Infant Mortality

Ethical Dimensions
Surrogate Mothers

CHAPTER OBJECTIVES

1. Explain what happens during the process of conception and implantation.
2. Explain what happens developmentally to the mother and embryo and fetus during the three trimesters of a pregnancy.
3. Describe the concept of prenatal care, and discuss the options for birth attendants and place of birthing.
4. Explain the many behaviors that can affect pregnancy outcomes, including use of drugs, diseases, and Rh incompatibility.
5. Identify maternal health problems that may be experienced during pregnancy.
6. Describe the physical and emotional reactions common during the three stages of giving birth.
7. Cite the causes of infertility, and describe various methods of treating it.

sexuality.jbpub.com

Birthing Alternatives
Nutrition and Weight Gain
Breastfeeding

INTRODUCTION

Mary was in her late 30s when she and her husband, Rich, decided to have another child. For a while, they did not expect to be successful. Month after month of unprotected intercourse resulted in no pregnancy. They began to think they might have waited too long.

Finally, all their efforts paid off. Mary's period was late, and an at-home pregnancy kit confirmed their hopes. Mary immediately set up a doctor's appointment to confirm the pregnancy. When she received the positive results, she set up a series of prenatal care appointments with her obstetrician.

At the first appointment, Mary checked out well. The doctor wanted her to have a sonogram at 15 weeks—just as in her previous pregnancies. But, because Mary was now older than 35 years, the doctor also wanted her to undergo amniocentesis to check the fetus for potential congenital abnormalities.

Mary had the sonogram at about 15 weeks and was told everything was fine. She had amniocentesis during the 16th week of pregnancy. The doctor called and scheduled an appointment to discuss the results, and Mary and Rich knew that prospects were not good.

The doctor explained that the test detected abnormal results, which could indicate a number of conditions—including mental retardation of the child. The doctor explained the problems of raising a mentally challenged child to the stunned couple and suggested they discuss whether to continue the pregnancy.

Mary and Rich pondered what to do. They believed this would be their last chance to have a child. And Mary, although very much in favor of a woman's right to choose to have an abortion, did not want to do so.

Although Mary and Rich knew in their hearts from the start that they wanted the baby, they were both still nervous as the due date neared. Mary went into labor. Because of the questions raised by the amniocentesis, the baby was to be delivered in an operating room; extra support staff stood by just in case.

The attending obstetrician delivered the baby and announced, "The first one is a bouncing baby boy." Now Rich and Mary were really stunned—what do you mean, "the first one"? Within a few minutes, the fraternal twin was delivered. Both children were born without any birth defect.

At the first follow-up appointment with her doctor, Mary wanted to know why she was not told she was pregnant with twins. The doctor said that during the sonogram, the one child must have been hidden behind the other. Because there was no indication of twins, the amniocentesis abnormalities were not attributed to a twin pregnancy.

In spite of Rich and Mary's experience, most conceptions and birth deliveries proceed as planned. Still, others result in unique circumstances, as did Rich and Mary's. In this chapter we discuss the usual and the unusual aspects of conception, pregnancy, and birth.

Creating a New Life

After the man ejaculates, the sperm move through the cervical mucus into the uterus, reaching the fallopian tube within about 5 minutes. Propelling movements of the uterus and fallopian tubes help the sperm to move. Also prostaglandin, a hormone found in semen, may intensify uterine contractions—not felt by the woman—and shorten the sperm's travel time. Sperm stay alive in the female reproductive tract for 24 to 72 hours. During the first 24 hours after ejaculation, they are at a peak level of health and fertility. The egg's peak fertile period lasts 8 to 12 hours, though an egg can be fertilized for up to 24 hours after ovulation (Creager, 1992).

conception
The union of the sperm and ovum; also called *fertilization.*

conceptus
The fertilized ovum; the product of conception.

zygote
A fertilized egg.

embryo
The developing fetus during the 2 months after conception.

Most frequently the millions of sperm in the ejaculate meet an egg in one of the fallopian tubes. For egg and sperm to unite, at least one sperm must penetrate the transparent outer layer of the egg. The sperm secretes an enzyme, hyaluronidase, that dissolves this outer layer, allowing the sperm to enter and fertilize the egg. The union of the egg and the sperm is called **conception,** and the product of that union is called a **conceptus.** At this point the sex of the potential offspring has already been determined by the absence or presence of a Y chromosome in the sperm. It is also possible, though not certain, that the number of offspring has been determined (more than one conceptus may have been conceived).

Implantation

Once the egg is fertilized, the conceptus is known as a **zygote.** The one cell of the zygote begins to divide even as it travels down the fallopian tube on its way to implant itself in the uterus. One cell divides into two cells, the two become four, and so cell division continues. By a week after conception, the zygote is a hollow ball of 100 cells. At this point it is termed a *blastocyst.* Now two layers of cells begin to form. The inner layer of cells will become the **embryo;** the embryo is the zygote from the time of implantation through the first 8 weeks of development. The outer layer of cells, called *trophoblasts,* secretes enzymes that erode the uterine lining so that the blastocyst can attach itself to the endometrium 7 or 8 days after fertilization (Figure 9.1). After implantation these trophoblasts and other cells proliferate and eventually form

Although many sperm cells may reach the egg cell, usually only one will fertilize it.

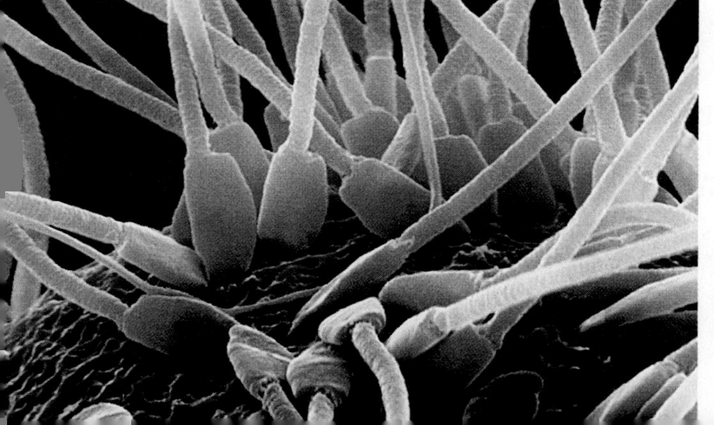

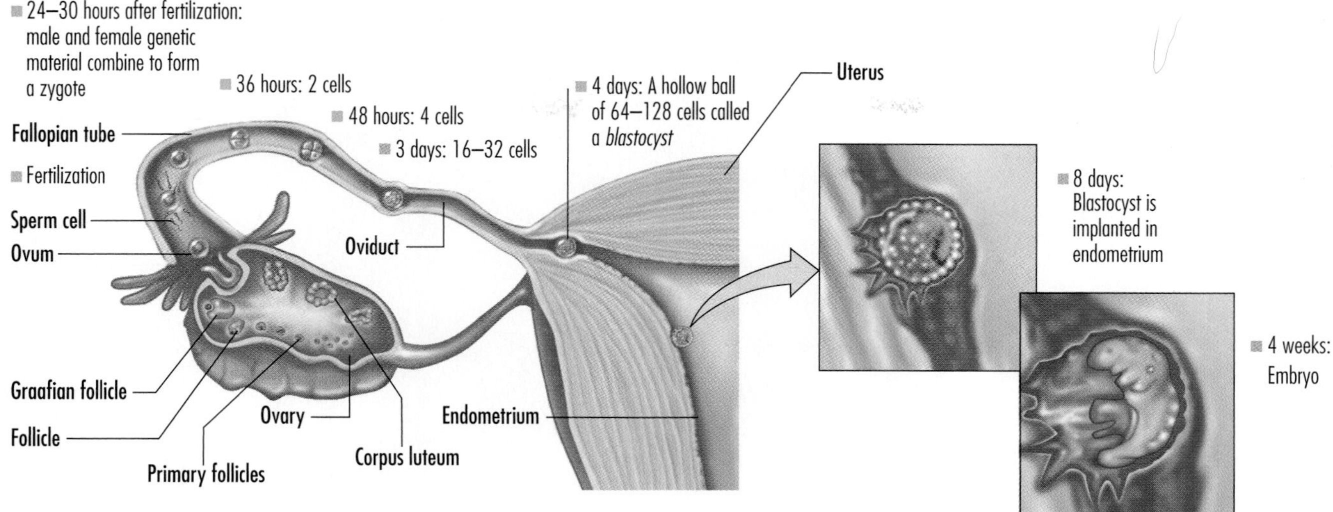

FIGURE 9.1 Following the ovum from ovulation through fertilization and implantation. After being ruptured from the ovary, the ovum is fertilized within the fallopian tube. It then travels to the uterus, where, as a blastocyst, it is implanted on the endometrium (lining) of the uterus.

the placenta, the umbilical cord, and the amniotic sac, a membrane filled with **amniotic fluid,** which surrounds the developing child by the end of the eighth week and absorbs shocks (Hole, 1990).

Immediately after implantation, the embryo begins receiving nourishment from the endometrial tissue of the mother. Progesterone acts on this tissue to produce the necessary nutrients—glycogen, proteins, lipids, and some minerals. The embryo is nourished from this source for 8 to 10 weeks until the placenta has developed sufficiently to take over.

The **placenta** is a disc-shaped organ that attaches to the uterine wall and is connected to the fetus by the **umbilical cord.** Together the placenta and the umbilical cord (which is attached to the baby at the navel and to the mother at the placenta) form the lifeline between the mother and the fetus. Nutrients, oxygen, and chemicals pass through the walls of the placenta to the fetus. Waste from the fetus is returned to the mother's blood. The placenta, which by the end of the pregnancy will reach a diameter of 8 inches (about 20 centimeters), contains two sets of blood vessels (Figure 9.2). Fetal circulation occurs within the fetus and the inner part of the placenta, while the mother's circulation flows in the walls of the uterus and the uterine side of the placenta. The fetus's blood flows through two umbilical arteries to the placenta and back from the placenta to the fetus by one vein. One important function of the placenta is to keep the blood systems of the mother and child separated from each other. It does this even though the placenta has *permeability,* that is, it allows some substances to pass between mother and fetus. Throughout the pregnancy, besides allowing nourishment and waste to pass between mother and child, the placenta helps to keep bacteria away from the fetus and allows antibodies (disease fighters) to cross to the fetus. These antibodies make the baby immune to diseases to which the mother is immune for about 6 months after birth.

As the embryo develops, the placenta secretes the hormone **human chorionic gonadotropin (HCG).** This hormone is detectable through blood tests 8 days after fertilization, just as the blastocyst is implanting, and its presence confirms pregnancy. HCG reaches its maximal level 7 weeks after fertilization and its lowest level about 9 weeks later (16 weeks after

amniotic fluid
The fluid inside the amniotic sac in which the fetus floats, it acts as a shock absorber, maintains the fetus at a constant temperature, and serves as a nutrient.

placenta
An organ of interchange between mother and fetus; oxygen, nutrients, and waste are exchanged through its cells.

umbilical cord
The lifeline between mother and fetus, which contains two arteries and one vein. Food, oxygen, and chemicals are transported to the child through the arteries, and waste is returned to the mother through the vein.

human chorionic gonadotropin hormone (HCG)
The hormone that appears in the blood and urine, providing evidence that a pregnancy has occurred.

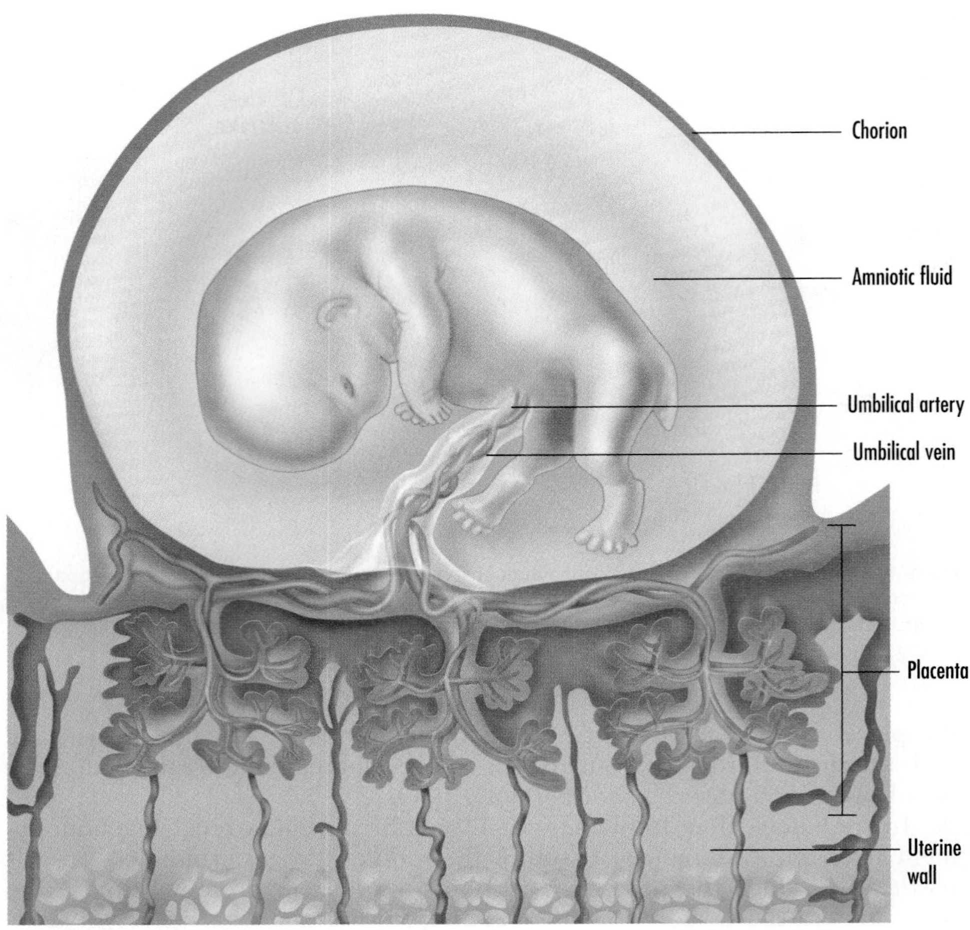

FIGURE 9.2 The embryo and placenta as they appear during the seventh week of development.

fertilization). The function of HCG is to keep the corpus luteum of the ovum alive so that it can continue to secrete estrogen and progesterone. Estrogen and progesterone maintain the uterine endometrium, which nourishes the early pregnancy. By about the 11th week of pregnancy, the placenta itself secretes enough progesterone and estrogen to maintain the pregnancy, and the corpus luteum dies.

Pregnancy

In the preceding section we focused on the developing zygote almost as if it were a being apart. But the development of a new person involves physiological changes in two human beings: the forming fetus and the mother. Let us back up now to account for the change in a woman after an egg is fertilized within her body.

After conception a woman is in a state of pregnancy, which lasts for the time the fetus takes to develop. This period can vary, but the time span from the last menstrual period to the birth of the baby is usually 9 calendar months (10 lunar months, 40 weeks, or 280 days). Most women deliver their babies within 2 weeks of the predicted date, sometimes called the **expected date of confinement (EDC).** About 4% deliver on the exact date. The EDC is calculated by a formula called *Nagele's rule:* Establish the first day of the last normal menstrual period, add 7 days, and subtract 3 months from this

expected date of confinement (EDC)
Due date for normal pregnancy that is usually estimated by Nagele's rule.

ectopic pregnancy
The development of the zygote in a location place other than the uterus.

pelvic inflammatory disease (PID)
Infection of the reproductive organs, particularly the uterus, fallopian tubes, and pelvic cavity.

date. The date is the EDC. Nagele's rule is based on a 28-day cycle, however, and, as we have noted, not all women have this cycle. Therefore, a medical practitioner will calculate each patient's EDC to the best of his or her ability, adapting the rule as necessary (Hale, 1978). At the point at which the fetus has the optimal chance for survival outside the uterus, the pregnancy has reached term, or completion.

Ectopic Pregnancy

An **ectopic pregnancy** is characterized by implantation of the blastocyst in a site other than the uterus. The rate of ectopic pregnancy has increased fivefold since 1970 and is now the main cause of maternal morbidity (illness) and mortality in the first trimester (Peterson, et al., 1997).

Women 30 years of age and older and African-American women are at a greater risk for ectopic pregnancy. It has been hypothesized that rates are higher for African-American women because they also have higher rates of **pelvic inflammatory disease (PID)** (Nederlof, et al., 1990).

Several major risk factors that are believed to predispose one to an ectopic pregnancy have been identified (Coste, Job-Spira, & Fernandez, 1991). These include PID, sexually transmitted infections (STIs), previous ectopic pregnancies, pelvic surgery, previous use of an intrauterine device (IUD), use of either an IUD or oral contraceptives at the time of ovulation, and maternal cigarette smoking at the time of conception.

It is essential that an ectopic pregnancy be diagnosed quickly. According to the Centers for Disease Control, all women should be aware of the signs and symptoms of ectopic pregnancy (Ectopic pregnancy—United States, 1987, 1990). Women of reproductive age should seek medical advice immediately if they experience pelvic and abdominal pain and a lack of menstruation accompanied by vaginal spotting or bleeding. These symptoms indicate the possibility of ectopic pregnancy. Ultrasound can confirm the presence of an ectopic pregnancy by 6 weeks' gestation, facilitating treatment that is the least destructive and costly.

Confirming Pregnancy

The signs of pregnancy known long before our current methods of testing were available are divided into three categories: presumptive, probable, and positive. Because many of the signs and symptoms of pregnancy may also be attributed to other conditions, medical practitioners proceed with caution to avoid a wrong conclusion. Emotional, endocrine, or systemic conditions can cause symptoms identical to the early signs of pregnancy.

Presumptive Signs

Presumptive signs and symptoms are those that may indicate pregnancy but that may occur when a woman is not pregnant. The presumptive signs and symptoms include missed menstrual periods, nausea and vomiting, a tingling feeling in the breast *(mastodynia)*, increased urinary frequency, some weight gain, fatigue, a rise in the basal body temperature, some skin changes, slight abdominal enlargement, and some vaginal discoloration and discharge. It is important to note that not all pregnant women experience all these symptoms.

Probable Signs

Probable signs and symptoms include the presumptive symptoms plus enlargement of the abdomen and the uterus, some painless uterine contractions, *ballottement* (at 16 to 20 weeks, bimanual examination gives the physician an impression that a floating object is in the uterus), and *uterine souffle*

Myth vs Fact

Myth: The peak period for sperm and egg to be fertilized is 1 week after they are released.
Fact: The peak period for sperm is about 24 hours after ejaculated, and the peak period for the egg is approximately 12 hours after release.

Myth: The egg is fertilized by the sperm in the uterus.
Fact: The egg–sperm union occurs in the fallopian tube.

Myth: Obstetricians are very accurate at predicting the date of delivery.
Fact: Only approximately 4% of women actually deliver on the expected date of confinement; most women do deliver within 2 weeks of their predicted due date.

Myth: To protect the fetus, pregnant women should refrain from exercising during their pregnancy.
Fact: Pregnant women can exercise without causing harm to the fetus. However, they should follow the exercise guidelines of the American College of Obstetrics and Gynecology.

Myth: As long as drugs are available over the counter, a pregnant woman can feel safe taking them.
Fact: All drugs have the potential to cause harm to fetuses. Therefore, pregnant women should refrain from taking all medications without the advice of their doctors.

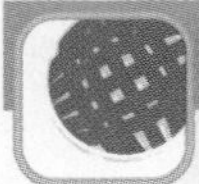

Global DIMENSIONS

Childbearing Rituals Ceremonies and rituals associated with childbearing have been developed in most societies, focusing on life-cycle events, including childbirth. Rules or prescriptions for the roles of mother and father vary among cultural systems. For example, many cultures prescribe that fathers be isolated from the processes and activities of pregnancy and birth. Another type of ritual, however, encourages men to participate in the birth of their offspring. This ritual is the *couvade,* practiced by some South American tribes. In this ritual, the husband, in a setting separated from his pregnant wife, mimics the childbearing process of his mate. At the same time his wife indicates the onset of labor and retreats to the care of selected women in the community, the husband goes to a hammock and proceeds to go through the motions of childbirth. This practice, according to the culture practicing it, attracts evil power to the husband, thus luring it from the mother, ensuring the safe delivery of the newborn (Aamodt, 1978).

Although the dominant culture of the United States does not hold such specific beliefs, it encourages men to participate more intimately than previous generations in the childbearing cycle. This "couvade ritual" involves classes for childbearing in which fathers are trained and prompted to take part in pregnancy, labor, delivery, and care of the newborn. . . . Trethowan and Conlon (1965) coined the term "couvade syndrome" to describe paternal bodily symptoms during pregnancy. . . . In interviews of American men, Munroe and Munroe (1971) found reports of sympathetic symptoms of pregnancy including nausea and vomiting, syncope, lassitude, leg cramps, weight gain, and backache, during the period of the wife's pregnancy. . . . Such findings of paternal symptomology are confirmed cross-culturally.

What do you think is the underlying physiology associated with this reaction?

Source: Sherwen, L. N. The pregnant man, in *Psychosocial dimensions of the pregnant family.* New York: Springer Publishing, 1987, 162–164. Used with permission from Springer Publishing Company, Inc., New York 10012.

(a rushing sound, which the physician hears through a stethoscope placed on the woman's abdomen). Uterine souffle in pregnant women is caused by blood filling placental blood vessels and spaces.

Positive Signs

What are conventionally called the positive signs of pregnancy are not present until the 17th week after conception. There are three of these signs, any one of which can confirm a pregnancy: fetal heartbeat, which can be monitored at 17 to 18 weeks; active fetal movement, at about the fifth month or between the 20th and 24th weeks; and palpation of the abdomen, by which the practitioner can detect the fetus. X ray would reveal a fetal skeleton, but this procedure is rarely used, because it can harm the developing fetus.

Women today do not need to wait months to confirm a pregnancy, and for the health of both the woman and the developing fetus it is best not to do so. Echography or ultrasonography (which measures sound waves as they pass through tissues of various densities, each returning its own echo) can be done as early as 4 weeks, and laboratory tests on urine and blood samples can now be done as early as 8 days after conception.

Pregnancy Tests

Pregnancy is confirmed by the presence of the hormone HCG, which is present in the blood and urine if a pregnancy exists. Currently the most frequently used laboratory test has the intimidating name of *beta subunit HCG radioimmunoassay.* This test measures the HCG in a blood sample and can confirm pregnancy, as mentioned earlier, about 8 days after conception occurs.

Two other laboratory pregnancy tests currently in use are the slide test and the test tube test. The slide test is a urine test that can be performed 2½ weeks after a missed menstrual period. Results are obtainable in about 1 or 2 minutes. The test tube test is performed, at the earliest, 2½ weeks after a missed menstrual period. In both the slide and tube tests, urine is mixed with a chemical reagent. The slide test is less sensitive and the blood test more sensitive to the presence of HCG.

Home pregnancy testing is also available. Commercial test kits that measure the presence of HCG in urine can be used as early as the day menstruation should have started. When used according to directions, they are considered to be quite accurate. The problem is that accurate use of a test by an inexperienced person can be difficult. Nervousness, possible misreading of directions, and improper handling of the kit's components can lead to inaccurate results. Often people feel the tests should be repeated. This can increase the cost considerably and still does not guarantee accurate findings. If one has a choice, a professional laboratory procedure is preferred. Professional testing is done by private, health-department, clinic, and hospital laboratories.

Fetal Development

Prenatal development is commonly regarded as having two stages: the **embryonic stage** (from the Greek *embryo,* "to swell"), which lasts 2 months, and the **fetal stage** (from the Latin *fetus,* "the young one"), which lasts from the beginning of the third month—when the fetus begins to look human—to birth (Figure 9.3). The 9-month pregnancy, however, is commonly viewed as consisting of three 3-month developmental periods called **trimesters.**

embryonic stage
The stage of prenatal development that includes the first 8 weeks of pregnancy.

fetal stage
Period from the ninth week of pregnancy to birth.

trimester
A 3-month period of the 9-month pregnancy, which is typically divided into three trimesters.

fetus
The developing child from the ninth week after conception until birth.

The First Trimester

During the first trimester, weeks 1 through 12, most of the embryo's physiological systems and body parts begin to form. At the end of the first month, the embryo is about 0.25 inch (0.6 centimeter) long. By this time, three cell layers have formed: the *ectoderm* (outer layer), from which the skin, sense organs, and the nervous system will grow; the *mesoderm* (middle layer), from which the muscular, circulatory, and excretory systems will form; and the *endoderm* (inner layer), from which the digestive system, glandular systems, and lungs will develop.

At the end of the second month, the embryo is about 1¼ inches (3 centimeters) long and weighs 1/30 ounce (0.9 gram). The head represents almost half the embryo's total bulk. Facial features such as eyes, ears, nose, lips, and tongue are visible, and the forehead is prominent because of the brain size (Figure 9.4).

When the third month begins, as mentioned, the developing child is called a **fetus.** At the third month the fetus, afloat in the amniotic fluid, is 3 inches (7.6 centimeters) long and 1 ounce (2.8 grams) in weight. It can move, but its motions are not yet felt by the mother. The fingers and toes have nails, and the genitals can be seen as male or female. By the end of the first trimester, the fetus is a miniature human. During the next two trimesters organs mature and general growth occurs.

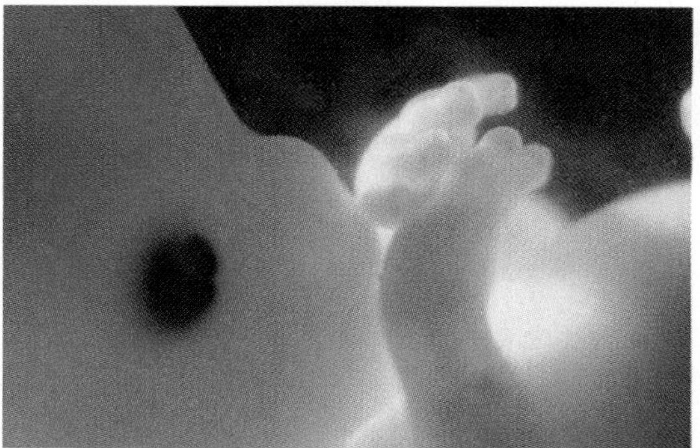

By the beginning of the eighth week of development, the embryonic body has recognizable human features.

The Second Trimester

During the fourth month, the first month of the second trimester, the greatest amount of fetal growth occurs. The fetus is now 6 inches (15 centimeters) long, the lower body is growing increasingly larger, and the head is

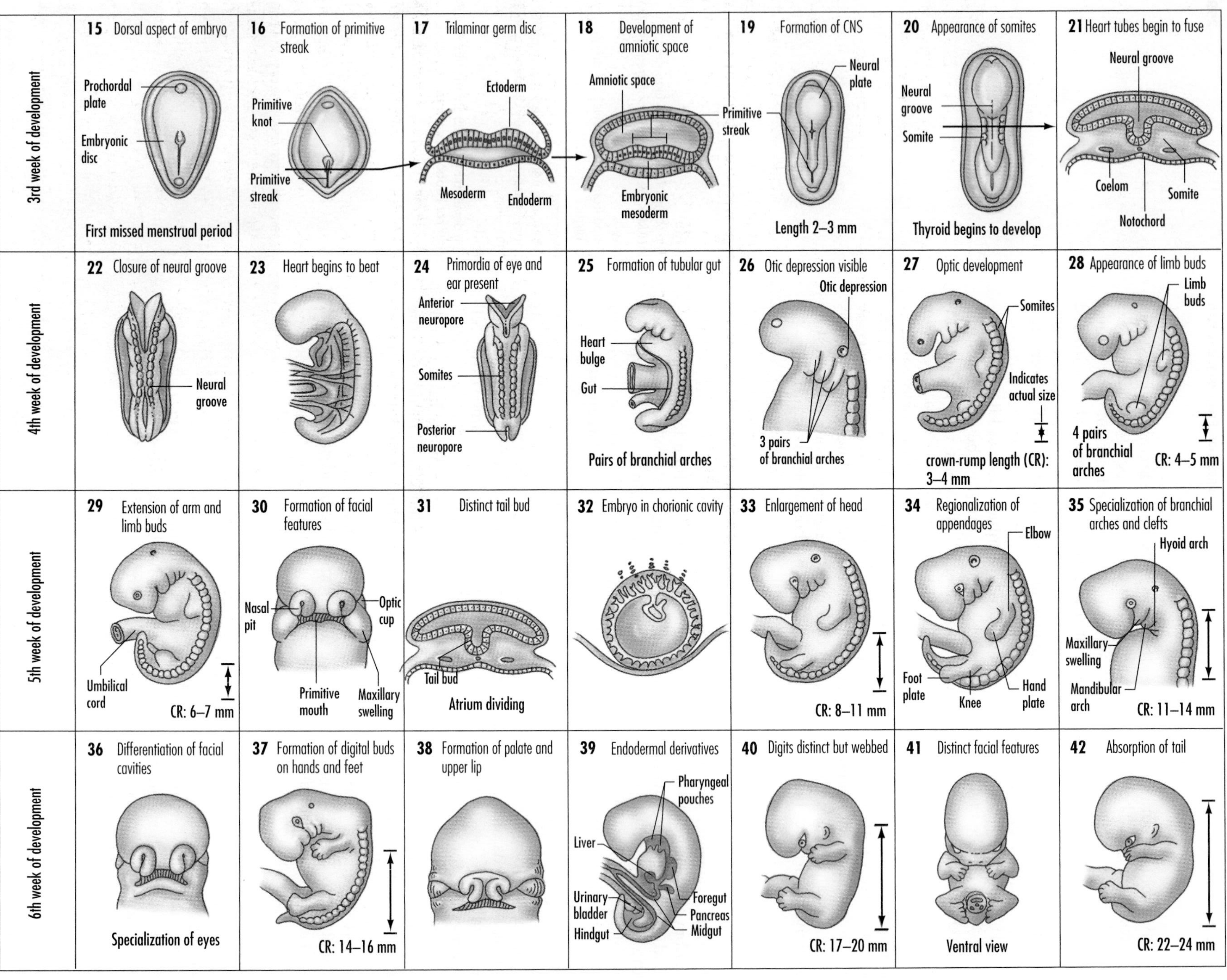

FIGURE 9.3 Major changes in fetal development from the third week after conception through the 10th week.

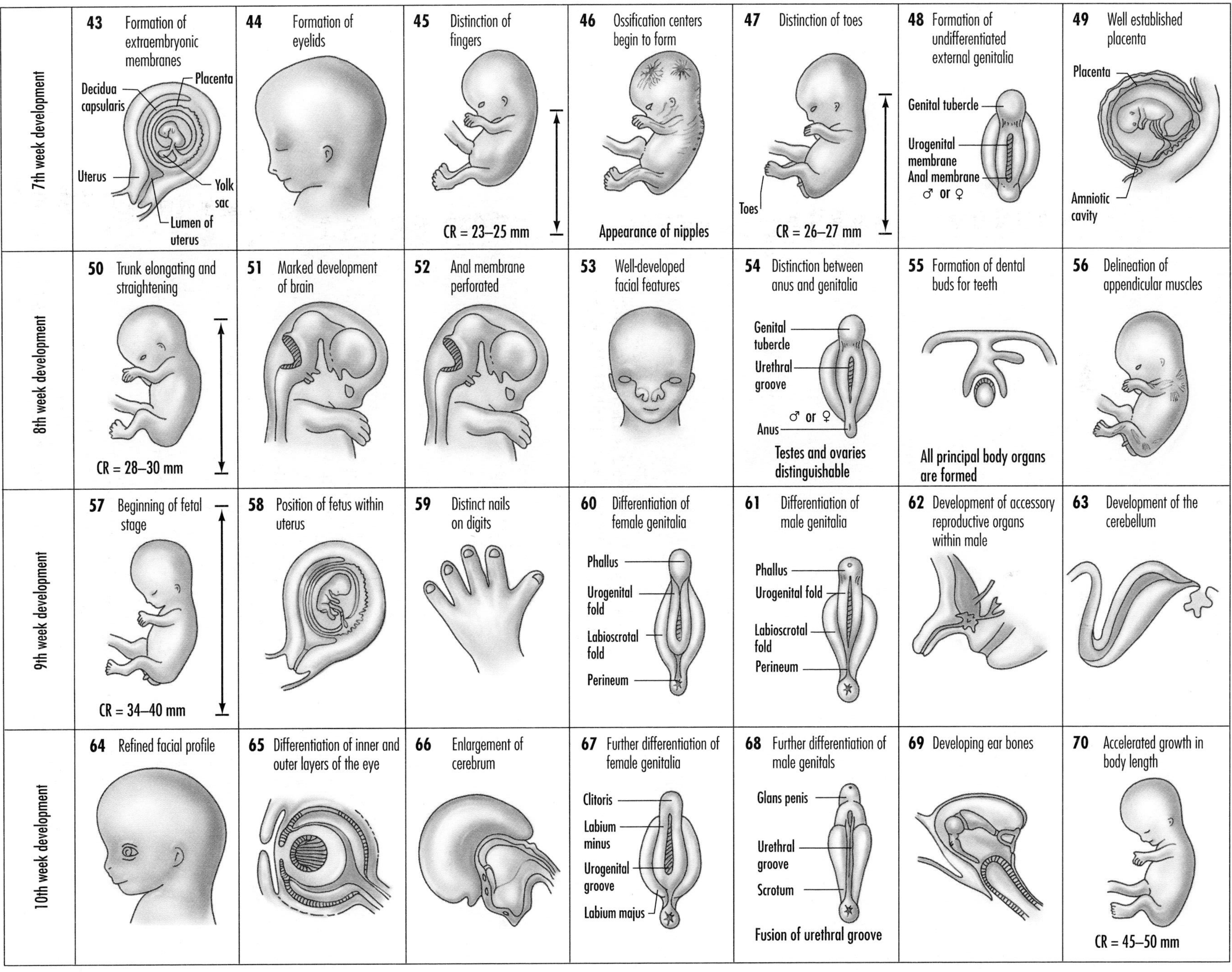
7th week development
43 Formation of extraembryonic membranes
Placenta
Decidua capsularis
Uterus
Yolk sac
Lumen of uterus
44 Formation of eyelids
45 Distinction of fingers
CR = 23–25 mm
46 Ossification centers begin to form
Appearance of nipples
47 Distinction of toes
Toes
CR = 26–27 mm
48 Formation of undifferentiated external genitalia
Genital tubercle
Urogenital membrane
Anal membrane
♂ or ♀
49 Well established placenta
Placenta
Amniotic cavity
8th week development
50 Trunk elongating and straightening
CR = 28–30 mm
51 Marked development of brain
52 Anal membrane perforated
53 Well-developed facial features
54 Distinction between anus and genitalia
Genital tubercle
Urethral groove
♂ or ♀
Anus
Testes and ovaries distinguishable
55 Formation of dental buds for teeth
All principal body organs are formed
56 Delineation of appendicular muscles
9th week development
57 Beginning of fetal stage
CR = 34–40 mm
58 Position of fetus within uterus
59 Distinct nails on digits
60 Differentiation of female genitalia
Phallus
Urogenital fold
Labioscrotal fold
Perineum
61 Differentiation of male genitalia
Phallus
Urogenital fold
Labioscrotal fold
Perineum
62 Development of accessory reproductive organs within male
63 Development of the cerebellum
10th week development
64 Refined facial profile
65 Differentiation of inner and outer layers of the eye
66 Enlargement of cerebrum
67 Further differentiation of female genitalia
Clitoris
Labium minus
Urogenital groove
Labium majus
68 Further differentiation of male genitals
Glans penis
Urethral groove
Scrotum
Fusion of urethral groove
69 Developing ear bones
70 Accelerated growth in body length
CR = 45–50 mm

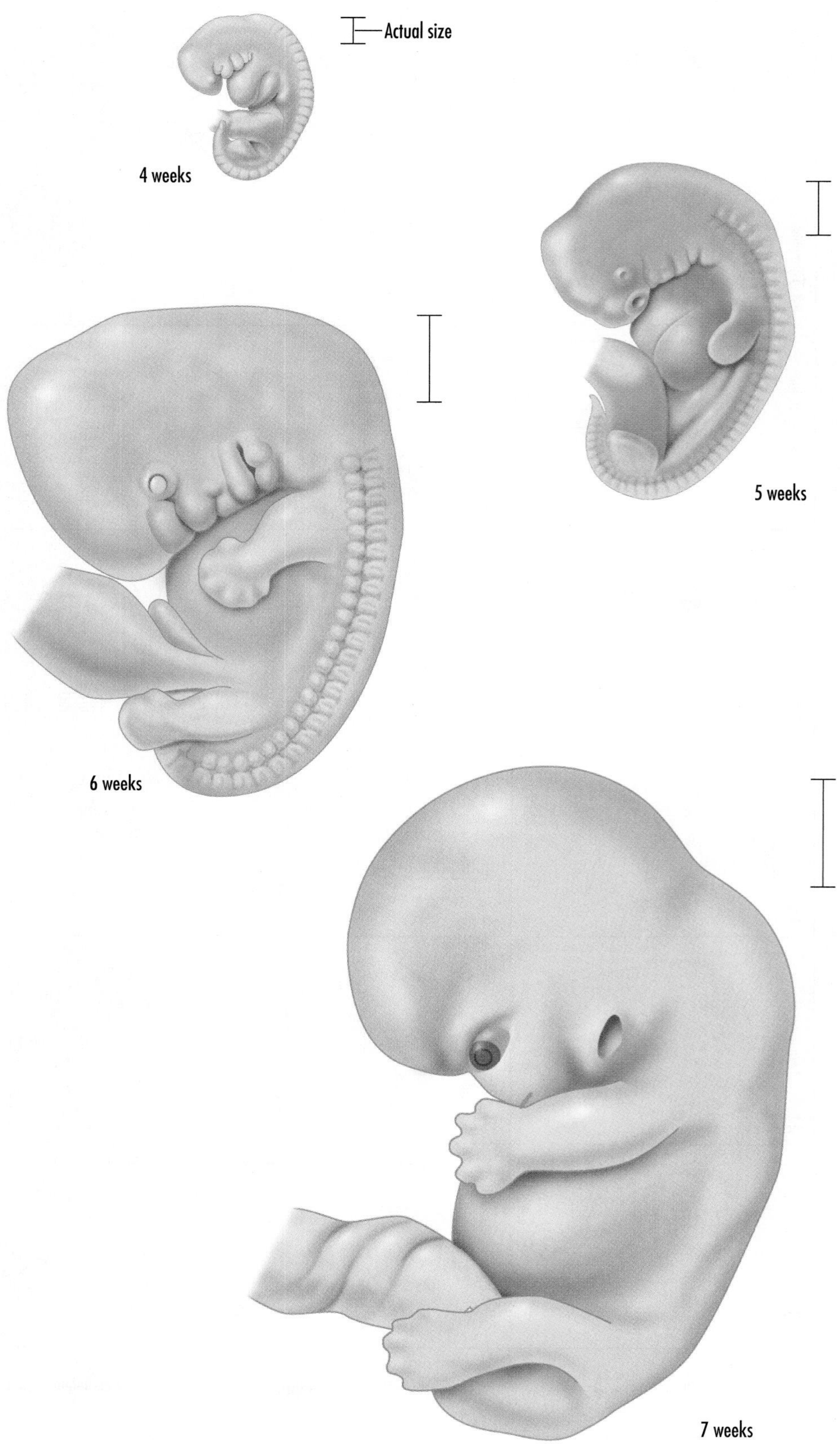

FIGURE 9.4 In the fifth through seventh weeks of development, the embryonic body and face start to develop a humanlike appearance.

now one-third the length of the body. The fetus moves and can suck, and its motion, called **quickening,** is felt by the mother. During the fifth month, the halfway point of the pregnancy, the fetus weighs about 1 pound (454 grams) and is about 12 inches (30 centimeters) long. It sleeps and wakes and has a preferred body position. During the sixth month the fetus grows about 2 inches (5 centimeters) and gains another pound. By this point the fetus's eyes are formed, it is sensitive to light, and it can hear uterine sounds. The skin is wrinkled and covered with fine hair. Though development is well under way, a baby born at this stage probably would not survive. By the end of this trimester, refinement of body features has occurred, movement is stronger, and further growth has been achieved.

quickening
Movements of the fetus felt by the mother; usually occurs about the fourth month of pregnancy.

The Third Trimester

During the period of the third trimester the baby positions itself more or less for birth. The most common fetal position, or *presentation,* is head down (Figure 9.5).

As a fat layer is laid underneath the skin, the fetus takes on a more babylike form. By the end of the seventh month, it is generally agreed, the baby can live outside the uterus, although babies have survived when born much earlier and cared for in neonatal intensive care units. By the end of the eighth month, the fetus weighs about 5 pounds and 4 ounces (2,384 grams)

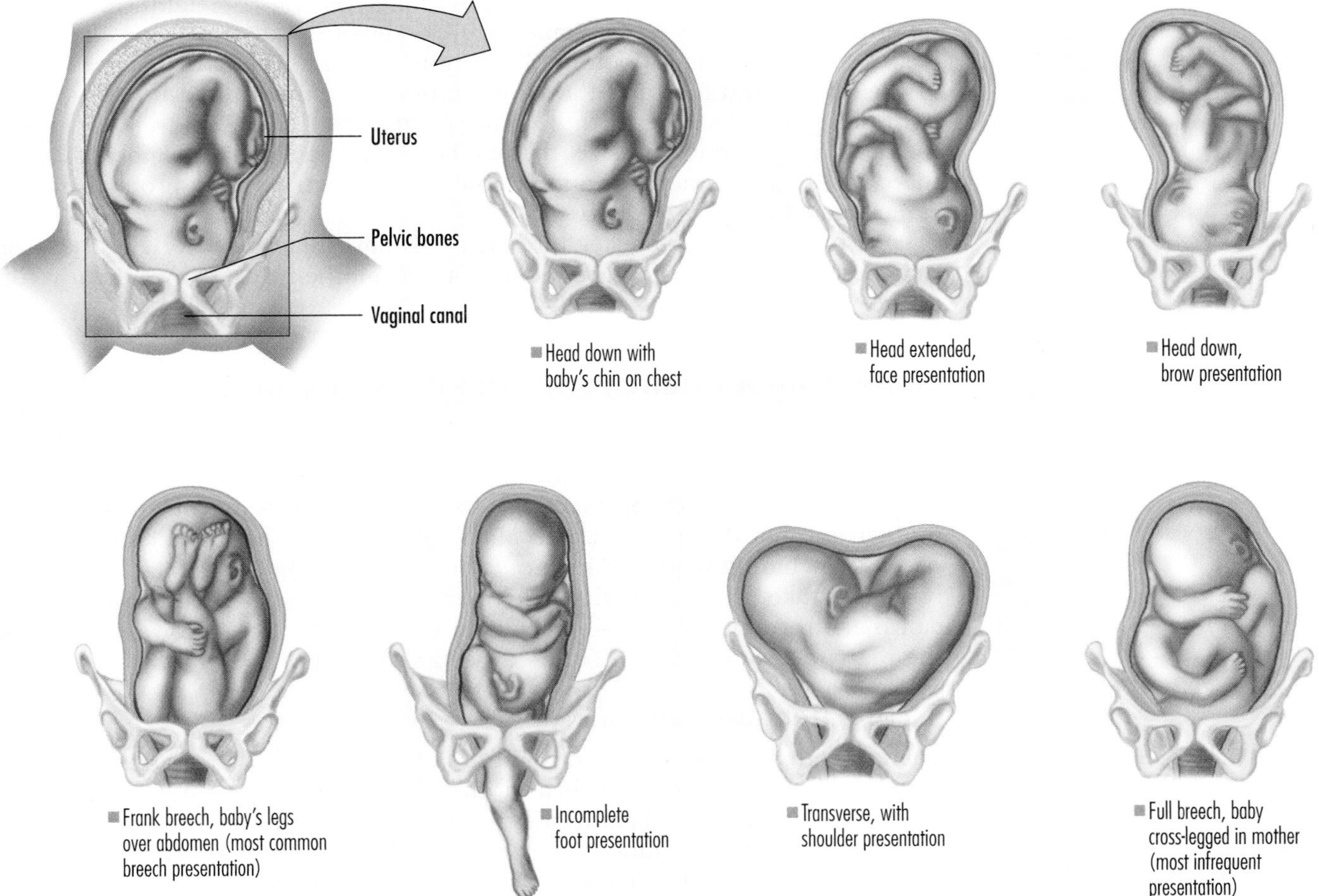

FIGURE 9.5 Fetal positions.

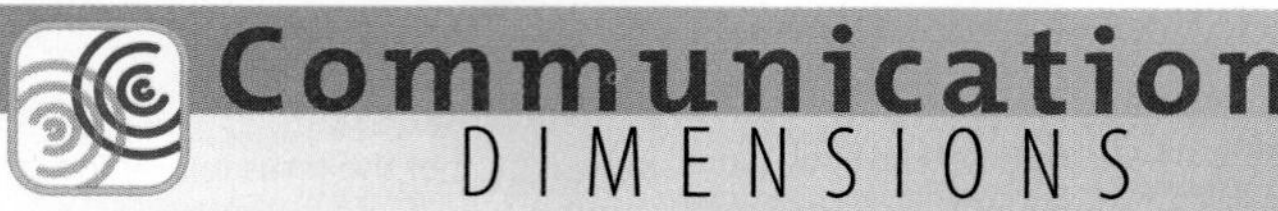

Communicating About Pregnancy Although it is not routinely discussed, most women do not have an easy time with pregnancy: morning sickness, continual tiredness, and new physical sensations may bring about momentary feelings of "Did I do the right thing?" This is balanced against society's view of happy pregnant women, who work until the last days of pregnancy and always smile.

From our experience, pregnant women who talk to other women who have been pregnant gain a great sense of relief. They find that their experience is not unique. Few women go through a "perfect" pregnancy. Ironically, women who have been pregnant usually wait for the pregnant woman to discuss an issue before opening up about their experience.

But pregnant women who talk to those who have not had children (a group that includes men) are often chided for their complaining. One pregnant woman recently said that after she had morning sickness at work—every day for weeks on end—most colleagues would smile and remind her of how "lucky" she was. Any complaining during lunch or breaks was met with reproachful glares—how dare she have a negative thought about the fetus inside her! She soon learned to keep her feelings to herself.

Explain why people have such a hard time talking about pregnancy. Is it because it is the result of sexual activity? Or because of the special roles that young children play in our society?

and is about 20 inches (51 centimeters) long. During the eighth and ninth months, skin redness lessens and wrinkles begin to disappear as the fetus begins to gain about 1½ pound (227 grams) a week. The nails reach the end of the fingers and toes and the fetus's actions become limited because of its tight fit in the uterus. As birth becomes imminent, in the 38th to 40th weeks, the head is 60% of its full size, the fine body hair has about disappeared, and the skin becomes smoother and is now covered with a waxy protective substance called the *vernix caseosa*.

During this last trimester the fetus will have reached a weight and size that prepare it to live independently of the mother. The baby is ready for delivery and birth.

Bearing a Healthy Infant: Prenatal Choices

Staying as healthy as possible is the pregnant woman's chief responsibility to her developing child. Pregnancy is a time of great change: Both physical and psychological factors affect the health and well-being of an expectant mother and her developing child. Many choices must be made by expectant parents, including whom to seek out for advice during pregnancy, where the birth will take place, and what health-enhancing lifestyle modifications they can make throughout the pregnancy. In the sections that follow, we discuss the many decisions facing today's expectant parents.

Birth Attendant Options

Even though pregnancy is a normal physiological event, there is still no question that a woman's general health affects not only her own experience of pregnancy but also the health of her developing child. The best advice for a healthy pregnancy is supervision by a health practitioner trained to give prenatal (prebirth) care. Thus, the selection of a health professional who will advise during the pregnancy and serve as the birth attendant during labor and delivery is an important decision that should be made by the expectant parents early in the pregnancy.

In the United States all physicians are trained in medical school in the procedures involved in pregnancy and birth. Generally, however, the family-practice specialist (a newer term for general practitioner) and the **obstetrician** are the primary providers of pregnancy care. The obstetrician has had specialized advanced training in this area. Many women physicians specialize in obstetrics, and a considerable number of pregnant women purposely seek women obstetricians. Some women feel that a female physician is more empathetic and understanding of the variety of body changes that occur during pregnancy and delivery. There is the possibility that the female physician has experienced parturition (the process of giving birth), and many pregnant women find this reassuring and relaxing.

There has been an increased interest in **midwifery** in the United States. Historically, American midwives were laypeople who helped with birth deliveries. Today nurse midwives are registered nurses (RNs) who receive advanced training in childbirth processes. Many states require nurse midwives to pass a national certification exam given by the American College of Nurse Midwives in order to be licensed.

Nurse midwifery is a good choice for families who consider birthing to be a natural process that does not require highly technological interventions (Otis, 1990). Nurse midwives routinely practice in freestanding birth centers and in hospitals. Some nurse midwives work with an obstetrician present at the delivery; some work alone but have an affiliation with an obstetrician who is on call for problem deliveries. Some nurse midwives assist in home deliveries with a physician present or on call.

Increasingly couples are planning their deliveries, making decisions that suit them, and choosing birth attendants and facilities to match their needs.

obstetrician
A physician who specializes in the care of pregnant women and the process of childbirth. Because these physicians are also gynecologists, they are often referred to as obstetrician–gynecologists or OB–GYNs.

midwifery
The practice by nonphysicians of assisting in the process of pregnancy and childbirth. Lay midwives are not trained health care professionals; nurse midwives are registered nurses who have received advanced training and often certification in the techniques of the birthing process.

Birthing Alternatives

To receive the kind of care they want before, during, and after delivery, future parents should investigate the birthing alternatives available in their area as soon as possible. Often the choice of a birth attendant is tied to the setting in which that birth attendant chooses to or is allowed to practice. Currently in the United States there are three major settings where labor and delivery typically occur: hospitals, the home, and freestanding birth centers. Each setting has advantages and disadvantages that should be considered by prospective parents.

Hospital Birth

Not many years ago most babies were born in hospital delivery rooms with the mother heavily drugged and the father barred from participating. Nowadays expectant parents often have a wide range of choices regarding the kind of delivery they will experience in the hospital setting.

Perhaps the most marked change is the increased participation of fathers in the birth of their children. Even in traditional births fathers are now allowed to be present in the delivery rooms of many hospitals, and in less conventional setups fathers often participate—perhaps by helping to hold the newborn as it emerges from the birth canal or by cutting the umbilical cord (under guidance, of course). This trend reflects a new appreciation for the role of fathers in child rearing. Although long considered "women's work," childbearing and raising are increasingly being recognized as joint undertakings, involving father and mother equally. The benefit of this new trend is that fathers share openly not only in the work and responsibility of parenting but in the joys and satisfactions as well. Many believe that this form of "male liberation" results in sounder father–child relationships and that strong father–infant bonds begin, as do mother–child bonds, at the moment of birth.

Most traditional hospital maternity facilities consist of separate rooms for labor, delivery, and recovery. Physicians, usually obstetricians, serve as the primary birth attendant, with assistance from nurses. Emergency equipment and trained personnel are quickly accessible should the need arise. **Analgesics** and **anesthetics** are options typically available only in this setting. High-risk pregnancies especially benefit from technological advances found in the hospital setting.

Although traditional labor and delivery rooms are still the standard in many hospitals, some hospitals provide the option of a more homelike birth setting for their clients. Typically this takes the form of a **birthing room,** which is attached to a labor and delivery suite and is often run by nurses and nurse midwives. The birthing room is decorated in a homelike style, often including soft lighting, wallpaper, a rocking chair, and a private bath. Mothers labor, deliver, and recover in one room with a support person, such as a spouse or other family member, present. Regulations regarding the use of a birthing room vary from one hospital to the next, and not uncommonly birthing rooms are used only for low-risk pregnancies. Couples interested in using a hospital birthing room need to find out whether this option is available at local hospitals and whether they are likely candidates for its use.

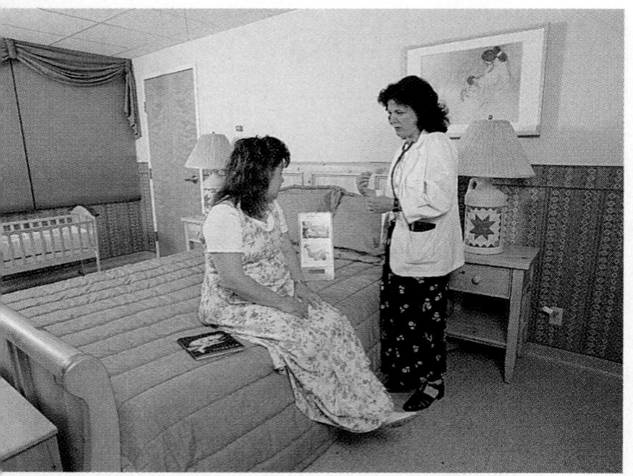

(a)

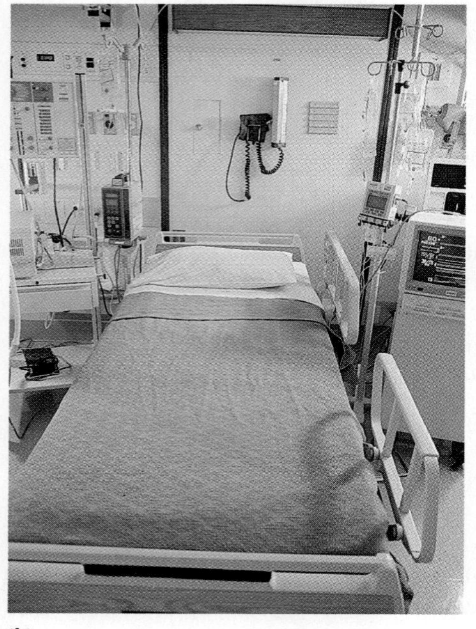

(b)

Many hospitals now offer a birthing room alternative (a) in addition to the traditional hospital delivery room (b).

Home Birth

Home birth with a nurse midwife is another birth alternative that is growing. Home birth is an option for only the healthiest women, and nurse midwives are trained to screen out women who might be at risk of complications during labor and delivery. Home birth candidates are watched closely during pregnancy for signs of possible risk. Nevertheless, the safety of home birth is debated in this country (Sussman & Levitt, 1989; Toussie-Weingarten & Jacobwitz, 1987).

If a couple chooses the home birth option, the midwife or physician—though relatively few physicians support home birth—goes to the couple's home and delivers the baby in a previously selected room. Children and other family members may be present. Currently only about 1% of women in the United States choose to have their babies at home.

Freestanding Birth Centers

The birth center is a birthing alternative available to prospective parents that represents a compromise between the traditional hospital delivery, characterized by medical intervention, and the controversial option of home birth. Birth centers are facilities that offer a homelike birth experience outside a hospital setting. Most birth centers are licensed by the state and are often run by nurse midwives. Typically, birth centers limit their clientele to low-risk pregnancies. Women are monitored throughout the pregnancy by a nurse midwife and may be referred to a hospital for delivery if complications arise during the prenatal period. Some emergency equipment is available in birth centers, and most birth centers are located in close proximity to a hospital for ready access if medical care is needed. It has been estimated that as many as 15% to 20% of women who begin delivery at a birth center are transferred to a hospital setting to complete the delivery (Toussie-Weingarten & Jacobwitz, 1987).

Prenatal and postnatal care are provided by the birth center's staff, and this continuity of care is a major benefit offered by birth centers. Freestanding birth centers are family oriented, encouraging family participation throughout the prenatal period. Couples are active participants in designing their personal birth plan, and family members are allowed to stay near the mother during labor and delivery.

Additionally, the infant remains with the mother after delivery. Although birth centers have increased in popularity and availability, they are not available in every city or even every state. It is estimated that there are nearly 135 birth centers in the United States, primarily in Florida, Pennsylvania, Texas, and New York (Kolander, Ballard, & Chandler, 1999). Couples who wish to use a birth center must investigate the availability of this birth alternative in their community.

Nowadays it is acknowledged that childbirth is an emotional experience as well as a physical one—and not just for the mother and child but for the father as well. The many birthing options available reflect this perspective and make responsible decision making by expectant parents increasingly important (Sussman & Levitt, 1989).

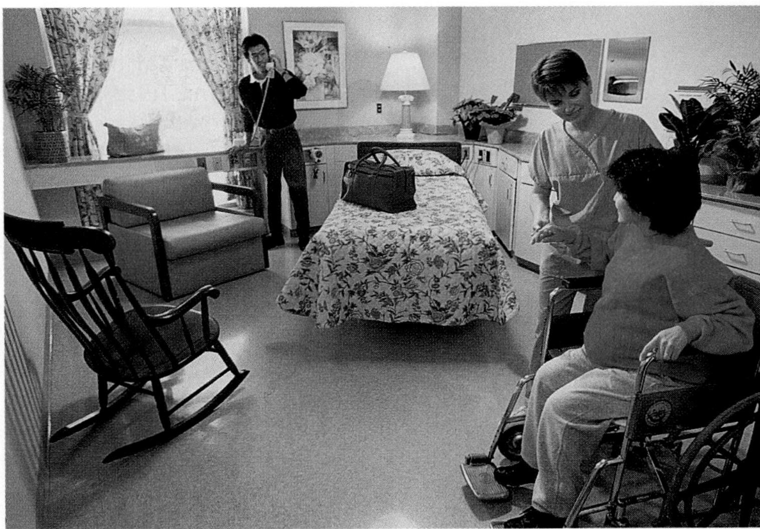

Many hospitals have built plush birthing centers to attract patients to this highly profitable area. Consumers have many options to choose from and should shop around and ask people they know for referrals before making a final selection.

Prenatal Care

Traditionally, **prenatal care** consists of monitoring fetal development, screening for high-risk pregnancy, and educating those involved about pregnancy and childbirth. For most normal pregnancies 10 to 12 prenatal care visits, beginning by the 6th to 10th week of pregnancy, are optimal. For a high-risk pregnancy more frequent visits may be necessary. Studies show that the risk of very low birth weight increases when women do not receive comprehensive prenatal care (Sable & Herman, 1997).

The prenatal evaluation begins, as most medical visits do, with the taking of a personal health history, relevant social and emotional factors, employment of the parents, conditions of their work environment, and the stability of their relationship itself. The practitioner is usually interested in knowing what sort of support system the woman and her new child will have, for many factors—both medical and nonmedical—can affect the well-being of a pregnant woman and her child. Additionally, a series of laboratory tests is usually completed at the first prenatal examination. These laboratory tests normally include examination for hemoglobin levels, glucose or protein in the urine, evidence of a current syphilis infection, antibodies for rubella (German measles), and blood type and Rh determination (discussed shortly). An examination of the cervix is also done at this time.

A family history is taken as well. Is the woman on her own—and thus possibly facing much stress and financial anxiety—or does she live with the baby's father? Is the father involved in the pregnancy? Is the baby wanted or unwanted? Was the pregnancy planned or unexpected? All these factors can place stress on the mother, and thus they have a bearing on her prenatal care. The medical practitioner overseeing her care will—or should—take an interest in these matters from the start. On the basis of this medical and social history, the practitioner will also determine how much information the expectant parents lack, what sort of guidance they need to adapt to the pregnancy, and, of course, what sort of delivery they favor. When pregnancy is concerned, the practitioner–client relationship is unique. If the couple, and particularly the mother, feel misgivings about their first choice, seeking another practitioner early in the pregnancy is highly advisable.

analgesics
Substances that decrease pain locally, such as topical creams.

anesthetics
Substances that elicit unconsciousness and thereby relieve pain.

birthing room
A homelike birth setting now available in some hospitals.

prenatal care
Care given to an expectant mother before the birth of her child that typically consists of monitoring fetal development, screening for high-risk pregnancy, and providing education for pregnancy and childbirth.

Nutrition and Weight Gain

Maternal nutrition directly affects fetal growth and development. The developing fetus depends on the mother for nutrition and can deplete her supply of necessary nutrients. For example, the mother usually needs iron supplements to prevent anemia. Iron is a major component of hemoglobin, which carries oxygen to the cells of both mother and baby. Protein influences tissue building in both the mother and baby and contributes to maintaining a healthy placenta and uterus. Vitamins ensure better resistance to infection, influence energy level, and aid in the absorption of calcium. Calcium is needed by the mother to prevent muscle irritability and by the baby to allow bone growth. Trace minerals, such as zinc and cobalt, build enzymes that influence chemical actions. The food intake of the mother fuels the development of the baby and directly influences the baby's weight gain (Table 9.1).

In 1990, the National Academy of Sciences published a report, *Nutrition During Pregnancy.* In it they suggest that food—not supplements—is the pre-

TABLE 9.1 Daily Dietary Allowances Recommended by the Food and Nutrition Board

		Lactating	
Dietary Allowance	Pregnant	First Six Months	Second Six Months
Protein (g)	60	65	62
Fat-Soluble Vitamins			
Vitamin A (μg RE)	800	1,300	1,200
Vitamin D (μg)	10	10	10
Vitamin E (mg (α = TE) TE)	10	12	11
Vitamin K (μg)	65	65	65
Water-Soluble Vitamins			
Vitamin C (mg)	70	95	90
Thiamine	1.5	1.6	1.6
Riboflavin (mg)	1.6	1.8	1.7
Niacin (mg NE)	17	20	20
Vitamin B_6 (mg)	2.2	2.1	2.1
Folate (μg)	400	280	260
Vitamin B_{12} (μg)	2.2	2.6	2.6
Minerals			
Calcium (mg)	1,200	1,200	1,200
Phosphorus (mg)	1,200	1,200	1,200
Magnesium (mg)	300	355	340
Iron (mg)	30	15	15
Zinc (mg)	15	19	16
Iodine (μg)	175	200	200
Selenium (μg)	65	75	75

RE = retinol equivalents

TE = tocopherol equivalents

NE = niacin equivalents

Source: Excerpted with permission from *Recommended dietary allowances,* 10th ed. © 1989 by the National Academy of Sciences. Published by National Academy Press, Washington, DC.

ferred source of the recommended daily allowances (RDAs) of nutrients needed for a healthy pregnancy. The major exception to this recommendation is iron supplementation. Because adequate amounts of iron cannot be consumed through food sources, a low-dose daily supplement of 30 mg of ferrous iron is recommended. The report recommends that all pregnant women have their diet assessed for nutrient content. Prenatal nutrition counseling is also essential. Only women who do not ordinarily consume an adequate diet and those women who are in a high-risk group (those carrying more than one fetus, heavy cigarette smokers, and alcohol and drug abusers) would be advised to take a daily multivitamin–mineral supplement.

There has been great controversy over this report. The drug companies that market vitamin supplements for pregnant women have taken a stand against the report (NIH panel rejects vitamin supplements, 1990). Additionally, some public health nutritionists have pointed out problems in implementing such recommendations (Brown & Story, 1990). Often, routine prenatal care does not include nutritional assessment and counseling. Additionally, current research indicates that "the consumption of an adequate diet by pregnant women in the United States, as assessed by the RDAs, appears to represent the exceptional rather than the usual case" (Brown & Story, 1990). Both sides agree, however, that it is important for pregnant women to meet the current RDAs. If they cannot meet their needs through food choices, supplementation may be appropriate. This is a decision that should be made in conjunction with one's physician or nurse midwife.

In the past it was the fashion in prenatal care to place pregnant women on strict regimens to prevent them from gaining more than about 20 pounds. Obese patients were even put on weight-reduction programs. New attitudes suggest that dieting during pregnancy can be harmful in that breakdown of fat produces toxic substances (called *ketones*) that can impair the mental and physical development of the fetus. Current recommendations for a healthy weight gain during pregnancy vary with the prepregnancy weight of the mother (National Academy of Sciences, 1990). Those mothers who were considered by their physician to be at a normal weight before conception should gain between 25 and 35 pounds. Those women who were underweight should gain slightly more (28 to 40 pounds); those who were overweight before pregnancy should gain less weight (15 to 25 pounds) (Figure 9.6). As has been implied in this discussion, extra nutrients are needed in pregnancy, and a wide variety of foods is needed to provide them.

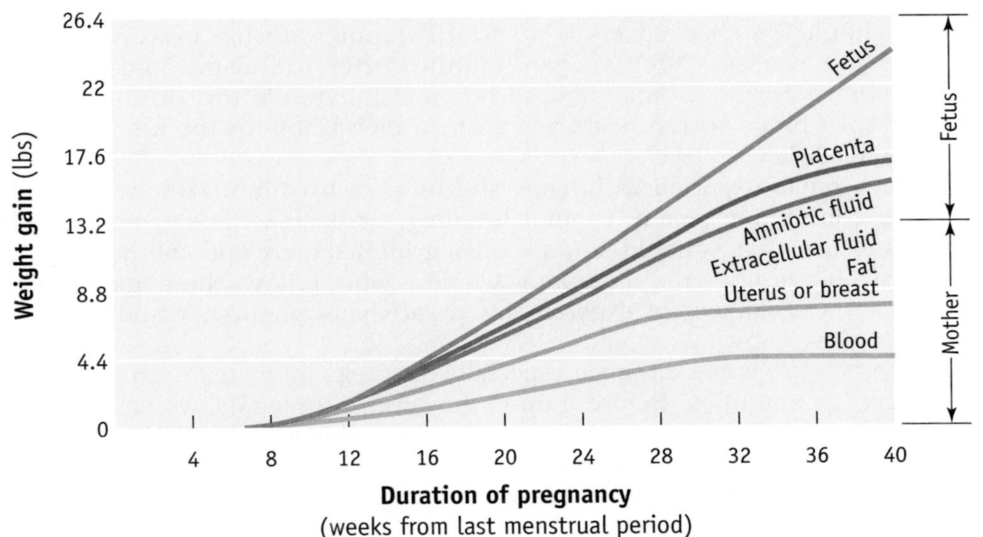

FIGURE 9.6 Pattern and components of maternal weight gain during pregnancy.

Exercise During Pregnancy

The safety of aerobic exercise during pregnancy has been questioned (Wight, 1986). Special concern has been voiced about the effects of such exercise on the developing fetus, especially in respect to potential fetal distress, intrauterine growth retardation, fetal malformations, and prematurity (Artel & Wiswell, 1986). Studies to date indicate, however, that "the incidence of complication in infants born to exercising women does not appear to be increased" (Wallace & Engstrom, 1987). It has been suggested that women who exercise during pregnancy benefit from a greater sense of well-being and control over their changing bodies. Other benefits include a lessening of the physical discomforts of pregnancy and an enhanced postpartum recovery (Bergfeld, et al., 1987).

To ensure the safety of both the mother and the developing infant, pregnant women should follow the exercise guidelines of the American College of Obstetrics and Gynecology (ACOG) (Sussman & Levitt, 1989). Before exercising during pregnancy a woman should consult her physician or nurse midwife. There are certain conditions, such as cardiac disease, a history of three or more spontaneous abortions (miscarriages), or abnormal bleeding, that are contraindications to exercise during pregnancy. If a woman has been sedentary before her pregnancy she should not attempt to take up a strenuous aerobic exercise program. A walking program or a program designed specifically for pregnant women would be most appropriate in this case. For those women who wish to continue their aerobic exercise program while pregnant, certain modifications should be made. The most important modification is time: Regardless of her level of fitness, a pregnant woman should not exercise aerobically for longer than 15 minutes at a time. Strenuous activity lasting longer than 15 minutes significantly raises maternal core body temperature and may lead to nervous system damage in the fetus. A pregnant woman who plans to exercise in more than one 15-minute interval should cool down for 5 to 10 minutes between intervals (Sussman & Levitt, 1989).

It is recommended that pregnant women exercise regularly (three to five times a week) and avoid outdoor exercise on hot, humid days. Regular intake of fluids during exercise, as well as consumption of adequate calories daily (usually an additional 200 to 300 calories), are essential for maintaining a safe exercise program. Pregnant women should not start or stop exercising suddenly; gradual warm-up and cool-down periods of 5 to 10 minutes are recommended. Proper clothing, especially a support bra and good athletic shoes, should be worn during exercise sessions. The pulse should be checked every 10 to 15 minutes during exercising and should not exceed 140 beats per minute. After exercising and cooling down, the pregnant woman should lie on her left side for 10 minutes to help return blood to the heart and restore blood flow to the uterine area (Sussman & Levitt, 1989).

If a woman experiences fatigue, shortness of breath, dizziness, nausea, uterine contractions, pain, vaginal bleeding, or decreased fetal movement during exercise, she should stop exercising immediately and call her physician or nurse midwife. Pregnant women who follow these guidelines improve their chances of experiencing a satisfying pregnancy and delivering a healthy baby.

Exercise programs designed especially for pregnant women can be found in many communities. Before joining, however, a pregnant woman should check to make certain that the program follows the ACOG exercise guidelines just described. For women in communities without such programs, ACOG has developed videotape programs that can be used at home.

Threats to Having a Healthy Infant

Mothers- and fathers-to-be often worry about whether their baby will be born healthy. In our technological society we are exposed to a larger number of risks to healthy pregnancy than ever before. Exposure to chemicals and radiation at the work site and in the home, lifestyle factors such as cigarette smoking and other drug use and abuse, and exposure to infectious agents are just some of the factors currently posing a risk to bearing healthy children. Although the great majority of infants are born healthy, both public health professionals and parents-to-be have legitimate concerns about infant morbidity and mortality.

In 1998, the National Center for Health Statistics reported an infant death rate of 7.3 deaths per 1,000 births in the United States. This represents a significant decrease from the 1988 rate of 10.1 deaths per 1,000 births. Still, compared with other developed countries, the United States ranks 25th in infant deaths. Additionally, the U.S. infant death rate is twice as high for African-Americans as for whites.

Birth defects are the leading cause of infant mortality and the fifth leading cause of years of potential life lost in the United States. It is estimated that approximately 80,000 infants are born with a major birth defect in this country every year. Approximately 8,000 of these infants die during the first year of life. The vast majority, however, must cope with a range of defects throughout their lives.

A new branch of research called **teratology,** which searches for the cause of birth defects, has emerged in recent years. Presently teratologists estimate that 5% to 6% of birth defects are caused by chromosomal defects, another 8% to 10% are caused by mutant genes, and about 6% to 10% are related to environmental causes such as toxic chemicals and drugs (Dowie, 1990). For the remaining 70% the cause is unknown.

teratology
The study of causative factors of birth defects.

Birth defects are one of the important causes of infant death in the United States; the second leading cause of infant deaths is low birth weight. Low birth weight, which is considered to be a birth weight of less than 5½ pounds, and very low birth weight (less than 3 pounds, 4 ounces) substantially increase an infant's chances of dying during the first year of life. This is especially true for African-Americans, for whom low birth weight is the leading cause of infant death in the United States (Lynberg & Khoury, 1990).

There are two types of low birth weight. The first involves infants who are born prematurely (before 36 weeks of gestation) and are thus underweight. A second type of low birth weight is known as *intrauterine growth retardation* (IUGR). These infants are born full term, but they are underdeveloped. Risk factors associated with low birth weight include younger (less than 18 years) and older (greater than 45 years) maternal age, high parity (having given birth to a large number of babies), poor reproduction history (especially a history of low birth weight), low socioeconomic status, low education levels, late or no prenatal care, low pregnancy weight gain, low prepregnancy weight, smoking, and substance abuse (Healthy People 2010, 2000).

Research into the causes and prevention of birth defects and low birth weight is greatly needed. Yet there is much we already know about preventing these conditions. Reducing these risk factors is the focus of our attention here.

Drugs and Other Substances

Any drug taken by a pregnant woman can potentially pass through the placenta to the fetus. If the drug (whether medically prescribed or self-prescribed) affects the mother in some way, it will also affect the developing baby. A danger of taking drugs during pregnancy is that an adult dose can be an overdose for a fetus. The liver of the fetus cannot metabolize drugs as can the adult liver, and the unchanged drug can affect the fetus differently from the mother. Furthermore, drugs can alter the metabolism of the mother, influence hormones in the bloodstream, and affect placenta functioning.

Over-the-Counter Drugs

Many Americans are polydrug users. *Over-the-counter drugs (OTCs),* sold legally without a prescription, are widely used for self-medication purposes. The use of many OTCs causes special concerns for pregnant women. Because of the extensive number of OTCs available, it is beyond the scope of this chapter to provide a complete review. The safest course of action for pregnant women is to avoid self-medication and OTC drugs until their use is approved by the physician or midwife acting as birth attendant.

Cigarette Smoking

Cigarette smoking has been identified as the "most toxic harmful exposure during pregnancy" (Werler, Pober, & Holmes, 1986); unquestionably it is harmful to the unborn baby. In general, smoking during pregnancy is associated with lower birth weights, higher rates of spontaneous abortion, structural changes in and decreased functioning of the placenta, and higher perinatal mortality rate (the perinatal period encompasses the time from 28 weeks of pregnancy to 1 to 4 weeks after birth). After birth, the infants of mothers who smoke are at a greater risk for childhood illnesses, especially respiratory disorders (Opp, 1990).

Infants born to smoking mothers weigh an average of 7 ounces less than infants born to nonsmoking mothers (Sussman & Levitt, 1989). As we mentioned, infants weighing less than 2,500 grams (5 pounds, 8 ounces) at birth are classified as low birth weight infants and have greater mortality rates. Between 20% and 40% of all low birth weight infants are born to women who smoke during pregnancy (Opp, 1990). The cause of low birth weight in infants of smoking mothers, although not proved, may be oxygen deprivation. Because carbon monoxide combines more readily with hemoglobin (oxygen carriers in the blood) than does oxygen and because cigarette smokers inhale carbon monoxide, the hemoglobin may be transporting more carbon monoxide and less oxygen than normal to the fetus. It is also possible that nicotine reduces placental blood flow, because it is a powerful constrictor of blood vessels, thereby lowering birth weight. The cyanide in smoke might also cause vitamin depletion. To detoxify the cyanide, the mother's body uses more vitamin B_{12} and essential sulfur amino acids, thus depriving the fetus of these nutrients. If smoking is stopped during the first 4 months of pregnancy, birth weights have been shown to approximate those of infants born to nonsmokers (Werler, Pober, & Holmes, 1986).

Marijuana

The research needed to establish the effect of a mother's marijuana use on the fetus is currently under way. Preliminary results suggest that there are many potential dangers involved in using marijuana while pregnant.

Tetrahydrocannabinol (THC), the primary psychoactive agent in marijuana and other cannabinoids, can pass through the placental barrier (Sussman & Levitt, 1989) and affect the ability of the placenta to function (Opp, 1990). Whether this causes any long-term effects on the fetus is not known.

Animal studies have indicated that marijuana is a teratogen (an agent capable of causing birth defects) (Sussman & Levitt, 1989). Many researchers who specialize in the study of birth defects now cautiously assume that any substance capable of causing birth defects in animals is potentially hazardous to humans as well (Dowie, 1990).

One study of marijuana use in pregnancy, the Ottawa Prenatal Prospective Study, has collected data from more than 700 pregnant women in the Ottawa, Canada, region since 1978. Preliminary findings indicate that infants born to mothers who regularly smoked marijuana during pregnancy have a marked decrease in response to a light repeatedly directed at their eyes. Additionally, regular heavy use of marijuana during pregnancy has been shown to heighten tremors and startles in the exposed infants. These findings may indicate either neurological dysfunction or drug withdrawal in infants exposed to marijuana in utero (Fried, 1986).

Alcohol

It is estimated that 20% of pregnant women in the United States drink alcohol while they are pregnant (Serdula, et al., 1991). Percentages of pregnant drinkers are even higher among some groups of women, such as smokers (41%) and the unmarried (35%). Though the overall percentage of pregnant women who consume alcohol appears to be decreasing significantly, this trend is not seen in women with a high school education or less, or in younger women (age 18 to 24 years).

According to Sterling Claren, a teratologist at Seattle's Children's Hospital, alcohol may account for up to 20% of all mental retardation in the United States (Dowie, 1990). To date, there is no consensus as to the amount of alcohol necessary to damage a fetus. Nevertheless, studies of the offspring of women considered to be alcoholic (that is, women who have about five drinks a day) show that alcohol consumption in pregnancy can cause fetal impairment to varying degrees. A particular pattern of deformity with mental impairment that occurs in offspring of these heavy drinkers has been labeled the **fetal alcohol syndrome (FAS)** (Jones & Smith, 1973a). Infants suffering from FAS may have unusual facial features, such as small eye slits; deep epicanthic folds (a fold of skin from the eyelid to the inner corner of the eye, giving it a slanted effect); upturned nose; a thin, flattened upper lip; and a flattened or decreased groove in the upper lip. They may also have heart defects, dysfunctions of the central nervous system, or growth deficiency. Growth and mental deficiencies appear to persist into adulthood (Mulvihill, 1986).

fetal alcohol syndrome (FAS)
Impaired psychological and physical characteristics common in infants born to alcoholic women.

No safe level of alcohol consumption during pregnancy has been established. In fact, a review of studies concluded that even small amounts of alcohol ingested during pregnancy resulted in offspring who were slightly shorter and weighed slightly less than children of mothers who did not ingest alcohol during their pregnancies (Fackelmann, 2002). Although it is problematic extrapolating research findings in animals to humans, it is still worth noting that rat pups exposed to alcohol in utero were more likely to have breast cancer as adults than rat pups not exposed to alcohol in utero. The surgeon general of the United States recommends that pregnant women avoid use of alcohol during any stage of pregnancy, because it can increase the risk of prematurity, low birth weight, and congenital defects.

Cocaine

The Centers for Disease Control and Prevention (2003) report on the prevalence of cocaine use, and this report is not reassuring. In fact, cocaine use starts at a young age. For example, 7.2% of ninth graders reported having used cocaine at least once in their lives. This figure increased as students got older so that by their senior year in high school, 12.1% report having used cocaine at least once. And, contrary to some people's stereotype of the typical cocaine user, white Americans report using cocaine twice as much as do African Americans, although African Americans have more cocaine-related emergency room episodes. In 1995, for instance, there were 142,164 cocaine-related emergency room visits, of which 40,899 were of white Americans and 76,714 were of

African Americans. Cocaine use by pregnant women is associated with higher rates of miscarriage, low birth weight, stillbirth, birth defects, premature labor, and long-term mental defects in the child exposed to cocaine in utero (Cocaine, 1987; Sussman & Levitt, 1989). Babies born to cocaine-using mothers may be born with an addiction to cocaine themselves and be subjected to a range of health risks, even death. We call these babies *crack babies,* named after crack cocaine, which is smoked rather than snorted. Research also indicates that the testes may be damaged in male fetuses exposed to cocaine, and both male and female infants may have chromosomal abnormalities caused by such exposure (Cocaine and pregnancy, 1991). Further research is needed to determine the effects of cocaine on the developing fetus.

Heroin and Other Narcotics

The common narcotics (or opiates) in use today are heroin, morphine, codeine, paregoric, hydramorphone hydrochloride (Dilaudid), laudanum, meperidine, and a synthetic narcotic, methadone. With the exception of heroin, which is outlawed, these drugs are used in medical practice for specific reasons under close supervision. For the discussion of drugs and pregnancy, we are referring to deliberate drug abuse—the street-drug use or abuse of narcotics.

Use of and addiction to heroin and the other opiates in a pregnant woman result in a narcotized fetus who must go through withdrawal. The mother's withdrawal from heroin while pregnant can lead to fetal death (Sussman & Levitt, 1989). Rapid withdrawal of the mother during the first trimester may result in miscarriage and result in life-threatening fetal distress if done during the third trimester. The experience of withdrawal after birth is very stressful for a newborn infant.

Heroin use during pregnancy has also been associated with jaundice, respiratory distress syndrome, low birth weight, growth retardation, birth defects, and infant death (Sussman & Levitt, 1989).

Steroids

Steroids are prescribed drugs such as sex hormones and other specific chemicals (cortisol and prednisone) used to treat kidney inflammations, joint inflammation, and tissue damage caused by rheumatic fever and other serious diseases. They can cross the placenta and cause fetal distress.

Diethylstilbestrol (DES)

DES is a synthetic nonsteroid estrogen first prescribed in the 1950s to prevent miscarriage. In 1971 it was discovered that DES caused a specific vaginal cancer in some female offspring of women who took the hormone during their pregnancy before the 18th week of gestation. Additionally, approximately 35% of exposed women exhibit benign vaginal epithelial cell changes. There is also a risk of problems with fertility and pregnancy. Male offspring are possibly vulnerable to infertility and prostatic problems.

Birth Control Pills

Studies of children of women who took oral contraceptives during pregnancy (before the pregnancy was known) have led medical experts to suspect that the pill increases the risk of heart and limb defects. Women who take oral contraceptives are advised to discontinue them for a few months before they attempt to conceive to ensure that the body's hormones are in natural balance before a pregnancy begins (Sussman & Levitt, 1989).

Diseases

Certain diseases can be passed from mother to fetus, but their significance varies with the stage of pregnancy. No matter how severe or how innocuous a disease might be in the pregnant woman, the effect on the fetus depends on the stage of fetal development at the time. Common diseases that can be transmitted to the fetus with harmful consequences follow.

German Measles (Rubella)

The disease rubella is most harmful to the fetus in the first trimester (the effect is almost nil after the third or fourth month). Common effects on the infant include hearing loss or deafness, eye defects, mental retardation, and behavioral problems. Death sometimes occurs shortly before or after birth (March of Dimes, 1986). To prevent rubella and its effects, it is recommended that women who have not had rubella be vaccinated well before they decide to conceive. Additionally, vaccines should be given to children at 15 months of age, because children are the major sources of rubella infection of pregnant women (Creager, 1992).

Diabetes

Diabetes is an insulin deficiency that affects sugar metabolism and that can influence fetal weight and complicate delivery. Infants of diabetic women may have a high birth weight (10 pounds or more) and a higher than average mortality rate.

Acquired Immune Deficiency Syndrome

Acquired immune deficiency syndrome (AIDS) is a viral disease characterized by depression of the immune system and the presence of certain opportunistic infections and malignancies. A fetus can become infected when the human immunodeficiency virus (HIV) crosses the placenta of an infected woman or during the birth process, when the infant might have contact with the mother's infected blood during delivery. It is currently estimated that about 26% of infants born to HIV-positive mothers will also be HIV-positive and may contract AIDS. However, with the administration of zidovudine, formerly azidothymidine (AZT), in the mother during pregnancy and in infants shortly after birth, this number can be decreased to 8.3% (Kolander, Ballard, & Chandler, 1999).

Syphilis

The STI syphilis is a common cause of stillbirth and can infect a fetus when the spirochetes cross the placenta. The infected fetus may show signs of syphilis at birth or may appear normal until adolescence, when signs of late syphilis appear. The fetus is unaffected if the mother receives penicillin before the fourth month.

Gonorrhea

This STI affects the eyes as the baby passes through the vagina and can, by transmission through the placenta, eventually cause a form of arthritis.

Herpes Genitalis

Herpes genitalis is an STI caused by the herpes simplex virus (HSV). If blisters are present on the genitals of the mother at the time of delivery, the virus can be absorbed by the baby, causing encephalitis, inflammation of the brain, and possible death. Less commonly, the fetus may be infected through the placenta while still in utero. A woman with a history of genital herpes will be followed closely from 32 weeks of gestation until delivery. If herpes lesions are present on her genitals, delivery will be by cesarean section.

Chlamydia

The STI chlamydia is caused by the intracellular parasite *Chlamydia trachomatis*. Infants born to mothers with chlamydia infections have a 70% chance of acquiring either inclusion conjunctivitis (an eye infection) or chlamydial pneumonia during delivery. All pregnant women should be screened for chlamydia at their first prenatal visit. The infection is easily treated with erythromycin stearate.

Genital Warts

Genital warts, another STI, are caused by the human papillomavirus (HPV). Infected mothers may transmit HPV to the fetus in utero or during the birth process (Fletcher, 1991). Genital warts have been found in children born to HPV-infected women. More common in infected infants, however, is respiratory papillomatosis, which causes hoarseness and respiratory distress. This is a lifelong illness that often requires multiple operations. If a pregnant woman has genital warts that are large, they may interfere with the birth process, requiring a cesarean delivery. Because of HPV's long latency period, many women may not know they are infected. Unfortunately, reliable screening tests are expensive and not routinely employed (Division of Sexually Transmitted Diseases, 2002).

Rh Incompatibility

Rh factor
The presence of Rh agglutinogens (antigens) in the blood, which indicates that a person is Rh-positive, whereas its absence designates the person as Rh-negative.

amniocentesis
Withdrawal by syringe of amniotic fluid to determine the presence of fetal abnormalities.

sonogram
A diagnostic picture revealing the fetal outline. In ultrasonography, sound waves are bounced off the fetus. With a scanner, the image is then projected onto a computer screen, revealing whether or not certain defects are present.

chorionic villi sampling (CVS)
A technique for prenatal detection of genetic defects that involves removal of some of the villi growing on the outer surface of the chorion and examining their chromosomes.

The **Rh factor** is a substance in the blood of about 85% of the population. If the Rh factor is present, the person's blood type is Rh positive (Rh+); if it is not present, the blood type is Rh negative (Rh−).

A problem in pregnancy exists when an Rh− mother is pregnant with an Rh+ child, a child who has inherited the positive factor from the Rh+ father. The mother's body develops anti-Rh agglutinins, antibodies to the presence of the Rh+, similar to the antibodies that fight disease. These anti-Rh antibodies enter the fetus and cause its red blood cells to clump together; that is, agglutinate. During the first such pregnancy, the mother's body does not develop many agglutinins. However, in subsequent pregnancies her body develops the anti-Rh agglutinins rapidly, and the babies of these pregnancies may be born anemic and jaundiced, with red blood cells and hemoglobin below normal. Treatment is accomplished by transfusion of the newborn infant with Rh− blood to stop the destruction of the red blood cells. In time the Rh− cells are replaced with the Rh+ cells that the baby's body normally makes. However, this condition can be prevented if the woman is administered the drug RhoGAM within 72 hours after a delivery or an abortion. RhoGAM neutralizes antibody formation.

Testing for Disorders

Amniocentesis is the drawing of fluid from the amniotic sac for the purpose of diagnosing fetal abnormalities (Figure 9.7). The procedure cannot be safely performed until the 16th week of pregnancy. A **sonogram,** or ultrasound, picture is taken to show the outline of the fetus so that the needle used will not touch the baby. Under sterile conditions and using a local anesthetic, a physician inserts a long needle through the abdominal and uterine walls into the amniotic sac and withdraws up to 20 milliliters (2/3 ounce) of fluid. The fluid, which contains cells sloughed off by the fetus, is analyzed for a variety of fetal abnormalities. The test analysis takes 10 days or longer. Chromosomal disorders, genetically induced metabolic disorders, sex-linked diseases, and genetics-linked inherited conditions can be determined by this procedure. Maternal age older than 35 years carries a higher risk of chromosomal disorders (such as Down's syndrome), and amniocentesis is recommended for these pregnant women. The sex and exact age of the fetus can also be determined by means of this procedure, although amniocentesis is rarely performed for these reasons alone because it always entails some risk to the fetus. Even though the procedure is performed under sterile conditions, there is always the risk of introducing infection into the uterine environment, inducing miscarriage, or damaging the fetus.

A newer technique for prenatal detection of genetic defects, **chorionic villi sampling (CVS),** has been approved by the Food and Drug Administration. The procedure is performed ideally at 8 to 10 weeks into the pregnancy.

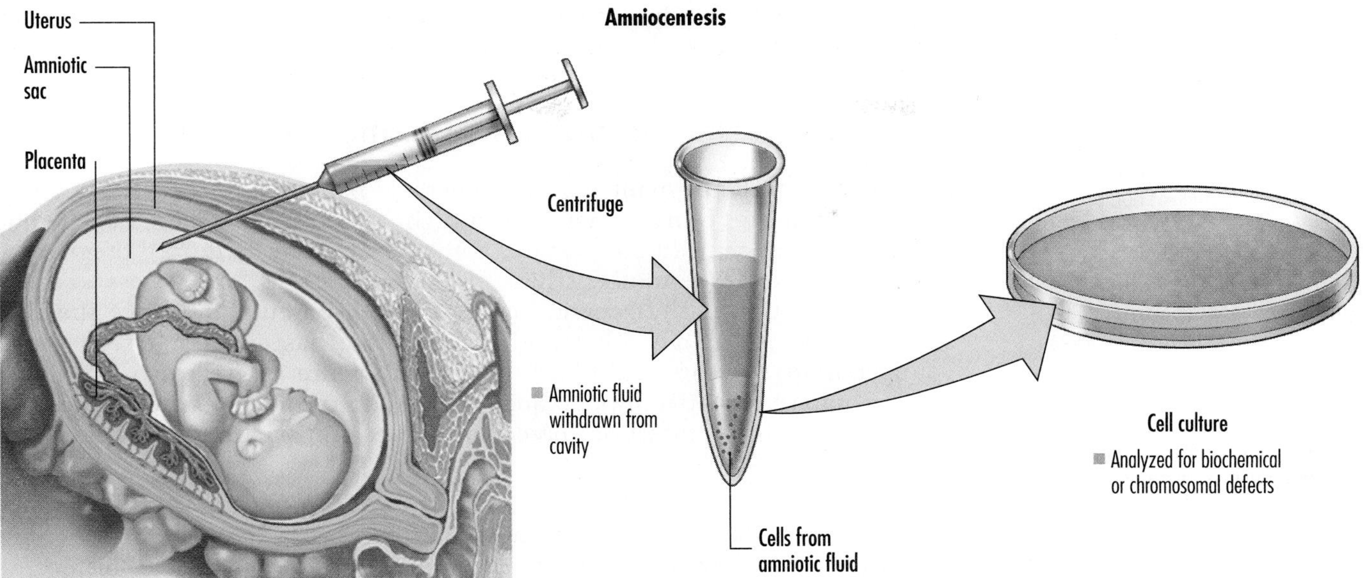

FIGURE 9.7 Amniocentesis is a test for fetal abnormalities that involves withdrawing amniotic fluid and inspecting the cells contained within it.

The chorion is the outermost protective covering of the growing embryo. The villi are threadlike, vascular (containing blood) protrusions growing on the outer surface of the chorion. In the procedure a plastic catheter is passed through the vagina into the uterus to these villi. Ultrasound is used to guide the insertion of this catheter. About 30 milligrams (0.001 ounce) of tissue is suctioned and then studied. Chromosome analysis can be done the same day; that is a significant advantage over the 2- to 3-week wait often required of amniocentesis analysis, particularly if pregnancy termination is desired. Also, if an abortion is needed, a first-trimester abortion is less risky to the mother than is one done in the second trimester. However, certain defects, such as neural tube defects, cannot be detected by this technique. If such a problem is suspected, amniocentesis must be performed (Goosens, et al., 1983). In a study comparing CVS with amniocentesis it was concluded that CVS is a safe and effective technique for early diagnosis of genetic abnormalities (Lewis, 1990). Nevertheless, CVS does carry a slightly higher risk of miscarriage than amniocentesis (1.3% and 0.5%, respectively).

Another prenatal screening test is available for detection of fetal abnormalities early in pregnancy. Maternal serum alpha-fetoprotein (MSAFP) testing is a blood test, performed at 15 to 18 weeks of pregnancy, to detect neural tube defects such as spina bifida (an open spine) and anencephaly (lack of higher brain structures) (Lewis, 1990). Abnormal levels of MSAFP also indicate several other conditions, such as twin pregnancy, ventral wall (heart) defects, Down's syndrome, and fetal demise (Healthy People 2000, 1991). This test, however, is a screening test that detects *potential* problems; it is *not* a diagnostic test that can confirm these conditions with certainty. Abnormal levels of MSAFP are an indication that a diagnostic test such as amniocentesis should be performed. MSAFP could be an important screening test for pregnant women aged 35 years and older. If such a pregnant woman, who would normally be placed in a high-risk category, had the MSAFP test and it indicated a low risk for fetal abnormalities, it could spare her from having amniocentesis (with its inherent risk of miscarriage) (Lewis, 1990). Currently, the American College of Obstetrics and Gynecology recommends that MSAFP screening be offered to all pregnant women early in prenatal care. MSAFP must be administered within the 15th to 18th week of gestation in order to be effective.

Maternal Health Problems During Pregnancy

About 20% of all pregnant women and their babies are "at risk." When a practitioner deems a pregnancy to be a high-risk one, the label indicates that the mother and/or child could suffer some adverse effects during pregnancy, labor, or delivery. The mother's health, economic status, and access to medical care, as well as the genetic history of both parents, influence the risk status of the pregnancy. The mother's age, too, has a major effect: those younger than 18 years and older than 40 years are at greatest risk. About 60% of maternal deaths in pregnancy and childbirth in the United States are due to hemorrhage, infection, preeclampsia, eclampsia, and convulsions.

Hypertension

Blood pressure that is above normal while the heart is contracted or relaxed, or both, is the condition called *hypertension*. Women who have a history of hypertension or who become hypertensive in pregnancy need attentive medical supervision, but their condition by no means precludes a successful pregnancy.

Hypertensive conditions induced by a pregnancy have been traditionally called the **toxemias of pregnancy.** Despite the term, however, these conditions are not caused by toxins—poisons—circulating in the blood, as some people believe. Toxemias are also called *preeclampsia* and *eclampsia*. **Preeclampsia** is pregnancy-induced hypertension accompanied by swelling of the face, neck, and upper extremities. These body parts swell when tissues retain too much fluid. Proteinuria, an abnormal amount of protein in the urine, is another symptom of preeclampsia. The term **eclampsia** refers to the preeclampsia events, plus convulsions or coma, and can be fatal. At present the causes of preeclampsia and eclampsia are unknown.

It is important to state that edema—the swelling of the tissues—does not always indicate an abnormal condition in pregnancy. In fact it is quite common among pregnant women. There is more than one type and cause of edema in pregnancy.

Nausea and Vomiting

Although the exact cause is unknown, the nausea and vomiting common to early pregnancy are thought to be caused by hormonal changes. **Morning sickness** is the usual term applied to these conditions, because the nausea often occurs early in the day and dissipates relatively quickly. Small meals, avoidance of strongly flavored foods, and eating of toast and jelly before moving around in the morning are suggested. As the body adjusts to the pregnancy, the nausea and vomiting disappear.

Severe, continuous vomiting in pregnancy (*hyperemesis gravidarum*) can be serious. Dehydration, loss of electrolytes, and dietary insufficiency can result and threaten the pregnancy. Bed rest and sedation are frequently necessary, and, in extreme cases, hospitalization and intravenous feeding are required. The treatment usually includes a search for the physiological or psychological causes, because most practitioners favor limiting the use of medication in pregnancy.

Hemorrhoids

Hemorrhoids are varicose veins of the anal area. They are caused by the same pressures that create varicose veins in the legs. The increased flow of blood to the pelvic area during pregnancy results in added pressure of blood flow,

toxemias of pregnancy
Hypertensive conditions, subdivided into preeclampsia and eclampsia.

preeclampsia
Pregnancy-induced hypertension; swelling of the face, neck, and upper extremities; and excess levels of protein in the urine.

eclampsia
Pregnancy-induced hypertension accompanied by swelling of the face, neck, and upper extremities, plus convulsions or coma, which may be fatal.

morning sickness
The condition of nausea and vomiting that is common in early pregnancy; thought to be caused by hormonal changes.

chloasma
A yellow to brown patch of skin pigmentation that may appear on the faces of pregnant white women; sometimes referred to as the "mask of pregnancy."

Braxton-Hicks contractions
Weak and slow uterine contractions that occur during the last few months of pregnancy.

parturition
The process of giving birth.

labor
The process of expelling a child by uterine contractions, dilation of the cervix, and bearing-down pressure.

delivery
The stage of childbirth characterized by the expulsion of the infant and the placenta.

contraction
The shortening or tension of uterine muscles during labor.

true labor
Characterized by regularly spaced contractions of the uterus, thinning and dilation of the cervix, and a descending of the presenting part of the fetus into the vagina.

dilation
In childbirth, the gradual opening of the cervix during labor.

which stresses the inelastic veins. In an effort to accommodate the increased blood flow, the veins are stressed, resulting in swelling, pain, and bleeding. The usual treatment employs sitz baths (a bath in which only the hip area is immersed) and topical creams. A pregnant woman who has hemorrhoids should tell her practitioner and allow him or her to prescribe treatment.

Other Conditions

A number of conditions frequently associated with pregnancy, although not serious, are often irritating. **Chloasma,** or the "mask of pregnancy," is a usually yellow to brown patch of skin pigmentation that appears on the faces of white women. The mask is thought to be caused by hormonal action that increases the number of pigment cells. Estrogen and progesterone can also produce these skin changes, as can ultraviolet light. When the pregnancy ends, the chloasma disappears.

Stretch marks, also more common in white women than in others, are visible white streaks in the skin of the abdomen and breasts, which enlarge during pregnancy. They are thought to be caused by a weakening of fibers in the tissue under the skin. It is believed that some people have a predisposition to this condition. In most instances stretch marks do not disappear, although they may fade or lighten in time.

Hair loss sometimes occurs because of an increase in hormone production. It is temporary when it does occur and as long as no significant health problems exist, normal growth recurs within 6 months after delivery.

Reddish branchlike vascular "spiders" in the neck, chest, face, and arms are due to high estrogen levels and vascular weakness. Small capillaries under the skin surface break, and uneven streaks become visible on the surface. These streaks also fade, but in some women they do not disappear completely.

During the last few months of a pregnancy, weak and slow contractions of the uterus occur. Known as **Braxton-Hicks contractions,** these contractions become more frequent as the pregnancy proceeds. Some researchers consider this a means through which the uterus practices for labor.

Childbirth

Parturition, derived from a Latin term meaning "to produce," is the process of giving birth. It begins with **labor**—contractions of the uterus, a gradual opening of the cervix, and purposeful bearing down by the woman—and ends in **delivery**—the expulsion of a child and the placenta. Sometimes women experience what is called *false labor.* False labor, common in late pregnancy, is characterized by brief uterine **contractions,** sometimes accompanied by mild back and abdominal pain and involving no changes in the cervix. **True labor** is characterized by (1) regularly spaced contractions of the uterus that gradually gain in intensity, (2) thinning and **dilation** (gradual opening) of the cervix, and (3) descent of the presenting part of the fetus into the vagina (Figure 9.8). The presenting part of the fetus is that part of its body that can be felt through the cervix during a vaginal examination. Usually the cervix begins to soften and dilate a few days to a few weeks before the actual delivery time.

Labor

Labor takes place in three distinct stages—at least from an obstetrician's point of view. Stage I is the period from the onset of labor to the point at which the cervix is fully dilated; that is, when the cervix is opened to 4 inches (10 centimeters) across. The average length of the first stage in a first pregnancy is

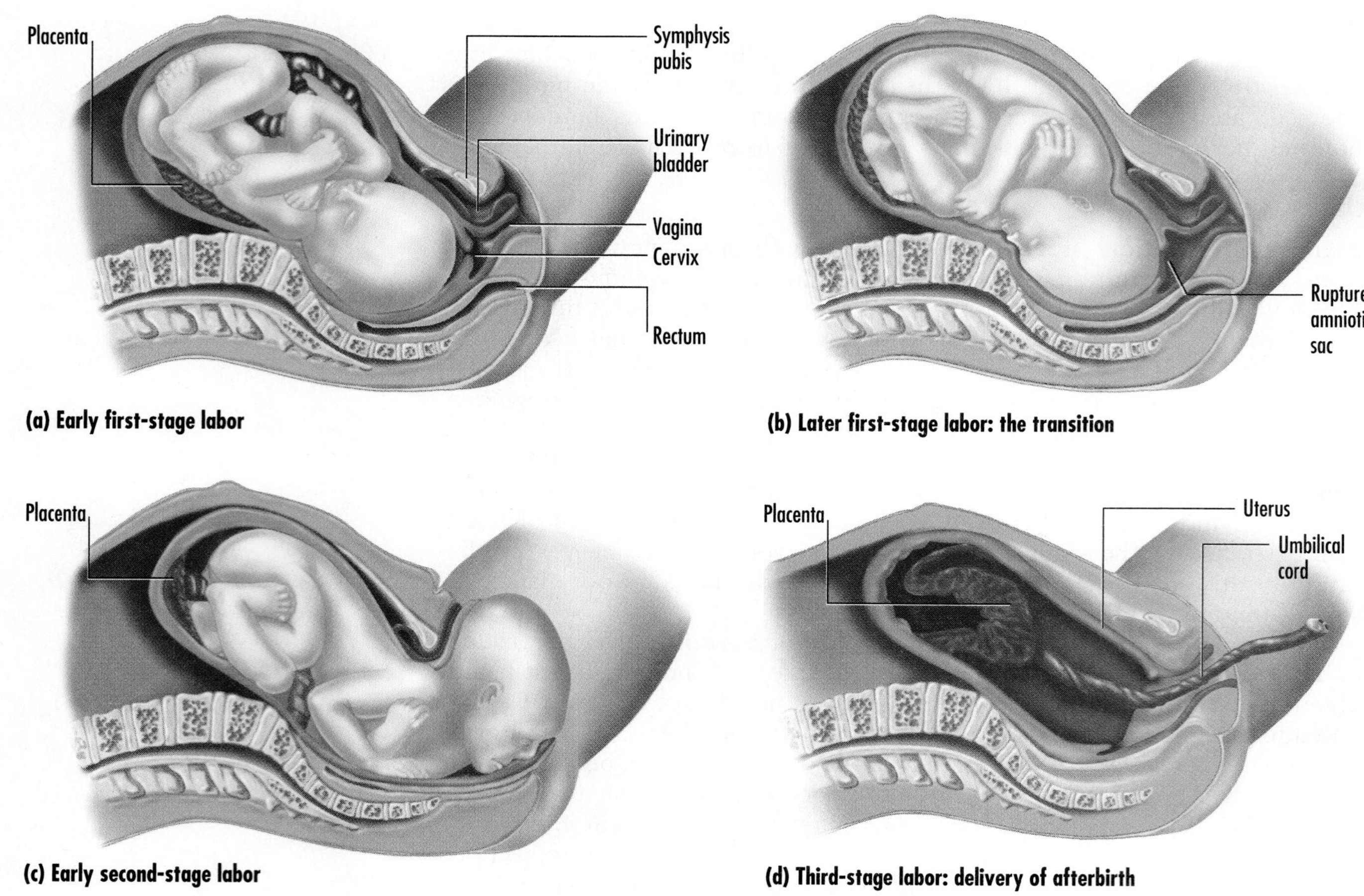

FIGURE 9.8 Childbirth: The stages of labor. (a) First stage: The cervix is dilating. (b) Late first stage (transition stage): The cervix is fully dilated, and the amniotic sac has ruptured, releasing amniotic fluid. (c) Second stage: The birth of the infant. (d) Third stage: Delivery of the placenta (afterbirth).

8 to 12 hours, but it often lasts up to 20 hours. Stage II is the period from full cervical dilation through the birth of the child. This stage can last from a few minutes to 2 hours in a normal delivery, though the longer time is most common. Stage III is the period from the infant's birth to delivery of the placenta, or **afterbirth** (usually taking up to 1/2 hour).

Labor usually begins with the first of the contractions that will mark the whole of the first stage. Often the contractions are irregular at first and of unequal length. But in true labor, they eventually occur in a settled pattern: for example, contractions of 30 to 40 seconds occurring every 2 to 3 minutes. Along with the onset of contractions a **bloody show** occurs—the disintegration of the mucus plug at the cervix. Usually the **amniotic sac** (the "bag of waters") ruptures spontaneously near the beginning of labor, experienced as either a rush or trickle of fluid through the vagina. Sometimes, however, contractions increase, but the amniotic sac remains unruptured; in such cases the attending physician or midwife breaks the sac. In some situations in which labor is overdue or dilation is progressing poorly, the drug oxytocin (Pitocin) is used to start labor or to increase the frequency of the contractions.

The medical attendants monitor the heartbeat of the fetus regularly by placing a stethoscope on the mother's abdomen, and they perform vaginal examinations periodically. In addition, an **electronic fetal monitor** is used to assess fetal heart rate. The doctor attaches an electrode to the woman's

Gender DIMENSIONS

Fathers and Childbirth

One of us vividly remembers driving his wife to the hospital when she went into labor and being met by a very accommodating nurse. She took us immediately into the labor room, an area in which women could scream and shout and kick. The comfort I was able to offer my wife was not immediately acknowledged—she had other things on her mind—but was nonetheless helpful and appreciated in retrospect. Yet, when it came time for her to deliver our son, my wife was wheeled into the delivery room and I was escorted to the waiting room. That was how it was done in those days.

Since then, more and more fathers are accompanying the mothers of their babies into the delivery room and observing the birth. Some even view the birth through a camera lens as they try to capture the moment for posterity. In this way they feel involved in all phases of childbirth and, some research indicates, develop a greater sense of closeness—bonding—with their children as well as with their spouses.

However, although this trend may be welcomed by most men, it also places a burden on others. Akin to the pressure on women to work outside the home or to have a "natural childbirth delivery," the one-model-fits-all approach ignores those men who prefer not to be in the delivery room. Some men may feel squeamish about medical procedures and fear fainting during the delivery, and others may feel uncomfortable observing their partners in pain. What types of accommodations could a hospital or birthing center provide for fathers who do not feel comfortable attending a delivery?

abdomen, and electrocardiographic impulses are transmitted to paper, giving a tracing (a reading) of the fetal heartbeat. Fetal heart rate can be influenced by such conditions as uterine contractions, problems with the placenta, and problems with the umbilical cord.

If anesthesia is used to reduce or eliminate the pain of contractions, it is administered late in the first stage or in the second stage. We discuss some of the choices women have regarding anesthesia later in the chapter.

Delivery

It is considered good medical practice for the physician or midwife to control the delivery to prevent a too sudden or too forceful ejection of the baby. The goal is to prevent injury to the central nervous system of the baby or injury to the mother's perineum, the area between the vulva and the anus.

Sometimes there is a need to enlarge the vaginal opening to permit the baby to pass through and to prevent the mother's tissue from tearing. In this event an incision is made into the perineum, a procedure called an **episiotomy.** Although in the past episiotomy was performed routinely in all hospital births, recently many physicians and midwives have been challenging the need for routine episiotomies, making the incision only when absolutely necessary.

The usual delivery is divided into three phases: delivery of the head, of the shoulders, and of the body and legs. **Crowning** is the presentation of the baby's head at the vaginal opening, or introitus. In a **breech delivery,** the baby presents the hip, body, shoulder, and the head in that order. Though rare, a breech delivery can be hazardous to the mother or baby, or both, for several reasons. The membranes can rupture prematurely, predisposing the mother to infection; because the buttocks of the baby do not conform to the contours of the lower uterus, labor can be prolonged; manipulation of the baby is more involved than in a head presentation, and lacerations may occur in the cervix, vagina, and

afterbirth
The delivery of the placenta.

bloody show
The expelling of the mucus plug (often streaked with blood) that has closed off the cervix during pregnancy.

amniotic sac
A fluid-filled membrane that surrounds the developing infant in the uterus.

electronic fetal monitoring
A technique used during labor whereby a physician places an electrode on the woman's abdomen to monitor the fetal heart rate for signs of fetal distress.

episiotomy
Incision between the vulva and anus to enlarge the vaginal opening at the time of birth.

crowning
The presentation of the baby's head at the vaginal opening.

breech delivery
A delivery in which the infant is born with another body part first, rather than head first. This form of delivery can be hazardous for both mother and infant.

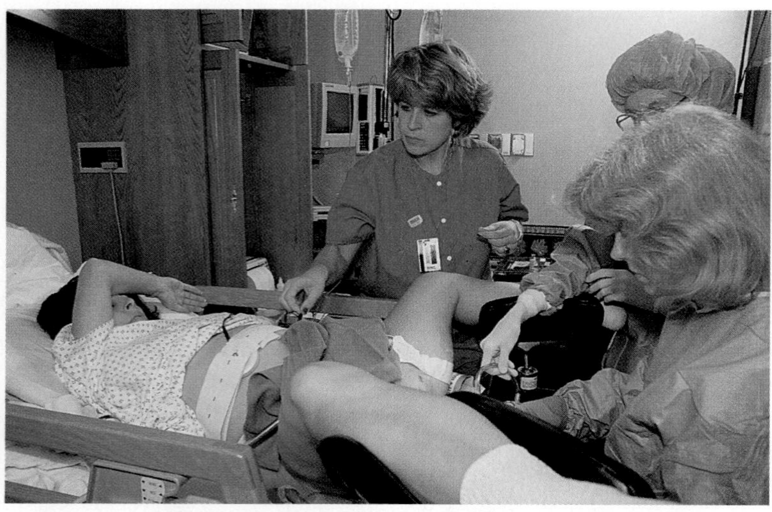

(a) In stage I of labor, the mother and baby are monitored electronically and helped by the attending staff.

perineum, possibly causing infection or hemorrhage. A breech delivery can be hazardous to the baby in that the umbilical cord may separate or be compressed between the baby and the inner wall of the uterus, depriving the baby of oxygen; intracranial hemorrhage can occur because of stress on the head as it is delivered last; and injuries to the head, neck, and upper arms can also occur during manipulations of delivery. Each breech delivery is managed according to its need.

Under certain conditions in which resistance inhibits the normal delivery mechanism, a forceps delivery may be necessary. Such conditions include the mother's exhaustion, cardiac or pulmonary problems, or illness; fetal distress; or certain obstetrical conditions (as certain positions of the baby's head). The forceps is a tool designed to deliver the baby's head and is used to gain traction and to rotate the baby. Forceps must be used carefully, however, because they exert force and can cause fetal damage.

After delivery of the baby, the umbilical cord is clamped and cut.

Delivery of Placenta

The third stage, delivery of the placenta and the membranes, usually occurs about 5 minutes after the baby is born. When the placenta emerges—again through contractions of the uterus—the doctor or midwife examines it carefully to be sure it is completely smooth. If the placenta is not smooth, it is likely that some placental tissue has remained in the uterus. Any tissue left behind may cause uterine bleeding or infection. If contractions stop before the placenta is expelled, manual techniques or injection are used to facilitate its delivery. If an episiotomy has been performed, it is repaired after the placenta is delivered.

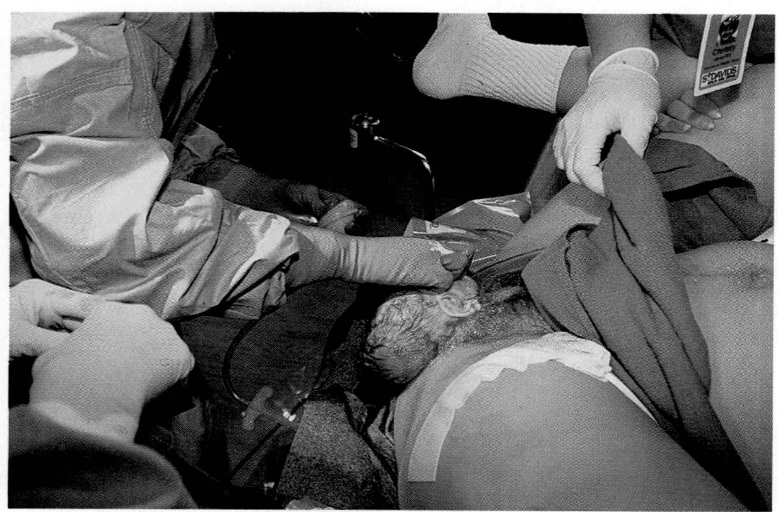

(b) During stage II of labor, the child is born, with the head appearing first.

Drugs Used in Childbirth

Expectant parents must grapple with the question of whether drugs will be used during delivery. Decisions about drugs in childbirth require some homework, because many kinds of drugs are available, all having different effects. Anesthetics inhibit perception, not just of pain but of touch and all other sensations, in the mother. General anesthetics not only affect the mother but also cross the placental barrier and reach the fetus. Most are central nervous system depressants and can act as such on the fetus. Some general anesthetics are used in pain-reducing concentrations, in which case they are less powerful depressants. These are usually inhaled. Among them are continuous nitrous oxide and enflurane.

Whereas general anesthetics put the individual to sleep, local anesthetics and local and

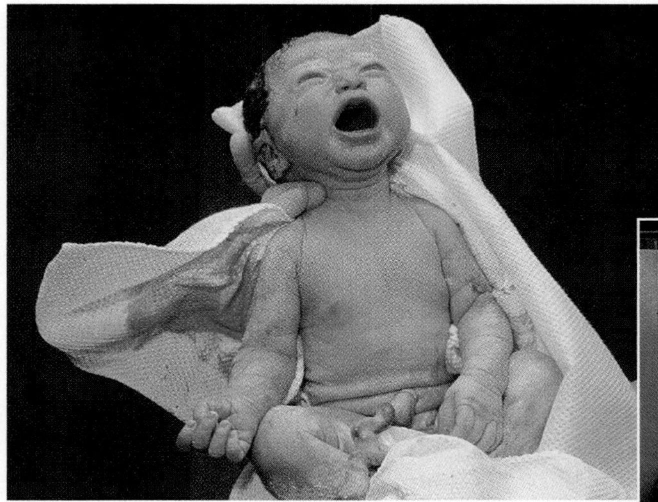

(c) The baby, 1 minute old, with umbilical cord.

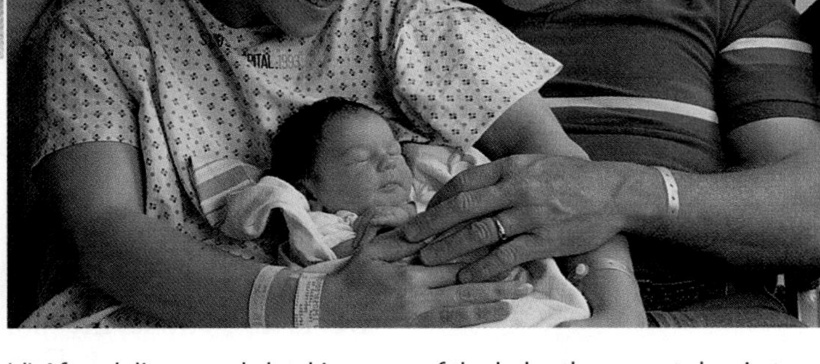

(d) After delivery and checking over of the baby, the parents begin to bond with their newborn child.

regional analgesics (reducers of pain perception) inhibit feelings and sensations in specific parts of the body. They can be used to reduce pain without placing the fetus in jeopardy. Hypnosis is an example of what is called an **obstetrical analgesia,** a nondrug pain reliever.

A local anesthetic injected around the nerves in a given spinal area reduces sensory feeling in a specific area of the body. A local anesthetic is generally administered during the later part of the first stage of labor and during all of the second stage. Single or multiple injections are administered via a catheter into the spinal area. Drugs commonly used for local pain relief include tetracaine, lidocaine, and bupivacaine. Different areas of the pelvic region are anesthetized by different procedures. **Saddle blocks,** or **epidural blocks,** anesthetize the area of the buttocks, perineum, and inner thigh (the area that literally sits on a saddle). In a **paracervical block,** injections are given at positions around the cervix.

Drugs have been used successfully and safely during labor for many years. Therefore, their use is not cause for alarm. Still, as with all drugs, there are potential risks, though minimal. Spinal anesthesia, for example, can cause headache, nausea and vomiting, and a drop in blood pressure. A reduction in blood pressure can reduce the oxygen supply to the baby and can change the fetal heartbeat.

Because pregnancy is a 9-month experience, expectant parents have plenty of time to discuss alternatives. Talks with the physician or midwife, with friends who have used different methods, and, most important, with each other will yield a well-thought-out decision.

Natural Childbirth

Drug-free childbirth has gained support in the latter part of the 21st century, particularly as the adverse effects of some drugs on the newborn have been discovered. This mode of giving birth is **natural childbirth**—or *prepared childbirth,* as it is sometimes called, because it involves education and practice. Electing to have a natural delivery often means that both parents are more involved in the pregnancy than they would be in a more traditional approach.

obstetrical analgesia
A nondrug pain reliever used in delivery (e.g., hypnosis).

saddle, or epidural, block
An anesthetic used during childbirth that blocks pain sensations in the buttocks, perineum, and inner thigh.

paracervical block
An anesthetic used during childbirth that blocks pain sensations in the pelvic area, in which injections are given at positions around the cervix.

natural childbirth
Drug-free childbirth; sometimes called *prepared childbirth.*

Did You Know . . .

In March 1999, the federal government ordered doctors and hospitals to stop demanding cash payments from poor women for epidurals to relieve pain in childbirth. Previously, women who could not pay cash for the epidural injection were offered weaker forms of pain relief. Doctors had complained that Medicaid reimbursements for pain relief treatment were too low, and thus women who had lower socioeconomic status were forced to suffer.

Within the natural childbirth movement, a number of specific options exist. The movement began early in the 1930s with Dr. Grantly Dick Read, an English physician. He developed a method of childbirth with no anesthetics or analgesics and published his approach in *Childbirth Without Fear.* At the heart of his method were techniques for relaxing tension to reduce the pain of labor. In 1950 a Russian named Velvoski published a work on his theory of psychoprophylaxis, which was taken up in France by Fernand Lamaze. Psychoprophylaxis is based on the premise that with the aid of a supportive coach (usually a husband, but any concerned, interested adult friend can play this role), a woman who has positive attitudes can reduce the stress and tension of parturition and relax the pelvic muscles. The objective is to reduce the pain of labor to the point where painkilling drugs become unnecessary. Exercise and breathing techniques are integral to what has come to be called the **Lamaze method.** The woman and her coach attend classes together once a week for approximately 6 to 8 weeks before the expected delivery date. Both adults participate in the birth process, with the coach guiding the mother in performing the exercises appropriate to the stage of labor.

With this approach the woman receives both emotional support and coaching, particularly during the delivery itself. As was noted earlier, an effort to include the father has many advantages, particularly regarding his relationship to the newborn. Because some men may feel frightened or uncomfortable at the prospect of being present at a birth, a couple must discuss the option thoroughly. Does the man eagerly look forward to participating? Is the woman willing to undergo a natural birth without her partner present and perhaps with another coach? As do most other aspects of reproductive behavior, the natural childbirth option requires free and open communication between partners.

The **Bradley method** is another natural childbirth program, started in the Denver area in the 1960s by Dr. Robert Bradley, a gynecologist and obstetrician. The Bradley technique has gained popularity in recent years. It is similar to Lamaze, but couples start to take classes much earlier in the pregnancy. As with the Lamaze method, breathing is used to help the woman release tension and relax. But an abdominal breathing technique is emphasized rather than the chest breathing of Lamaze.

The **Leboyer method** is related to natural, drug-free childbirth, but its focus is on the environment the newborn enters rather than on labor. The idea is to make the external environment as much as possible like the uterine environment so the newborn is not shocked by a rush of extreme sensations—cold air, harsh lights, loud noises—upon being born. In this method birth takes place in a darkened room, the people present speak in hushed tones, and the baby is immediately immersed in a tepid bath and stroked gently. Mother–infant bonding—the forging of a relationship through living and prolonged body contact—is given great emphasis in the Leboyer method. The baby is put to the mother's breast soon after delivery as part of this bonding process. The father's presence is encouraged in this method as well. The Leboyer method has many strict adherents, but others also draw freely from the method without using the full program.

Though natural childbirth can be extremely satisfying, it is important to realize that natural methods are not suited to every pregnancy. The mother's health, as well as her pain threshold, will influence the decision. It is particularly important for expectant parents to realize that even when they have made the decision to have a drug-free delivery, the woman may decide during labor that she needs something for pain. In such a case the mother may be given a mild tranquilizer. Women ought not to feel guilty about asking for drugs in labor. Natural childbirth is not a contest!

Lamaze method
An approach to childbirth in which exercise and breath control are central to reducing anxiety and discomfort.

Bradley method
A psychoprophylaxis approach to natural childbirth, which includes breathing and relaxation techniques.

Leboyer method
A method of natural childbirth that focuses on the external environment into which an infant is born, which attempts to imitate the uterine environment and encourages bonding immediately after birth.

cesarean section (C-section)
Surgical intervention to deliver the fetus, placenta, and membranes through an incision in the walls of the abdomen and uterus.

Cesarean Section

Cesarean section (C-section) is the delivery of the fetus and placenta through an incision in the walls of the abdomen and uterus. The procedure is performed when a delivery through the vagina would be of risk to mother or to baby. Presently, the most common reasons for C-sections are difficulty in delivery, repeat cesarean births, breech presentation, or fetal distress (Wolfe & Jones, 1991). C-sections are also performed if the mother has an STI that can be transmitted to the baby during a vaginal delivery, if the baby is too large to pass easily through the vaginal canal and opening, and if a vaginal delivery will cause potential harm to the mother because of certain illnesses (such as diabetes). In 2001, C-sections accounted for 24.4% of all deliveries in the United States (Stein, 2002). This is an all-time high and a jump of 7% from 2001. Some experts perceive the increased rate of C-sections as beneficial. They point to the possibility of fetal and maternal death from childbirth, and ruptured uteruses. The effects of labor and delivery on women's bodies are also reasons C-sections have increased. In particular, this concern revolves about "pelvic floor" disorders, such as muscles', ligaments', and other tissues' being stretched and damaged, resulting in urinary and/or fetal incontinence. "Twenty to 30 percent of women become incontinent after a single vaginal delivery," states the director of female pelvic medicine and reconstructive surgery at Loyola University Medical Center in Chicago (Stein, 2002). If C-sections can prevent these disorders, all the better, they argue. In addition, C-sections may alleviate anxiety because women know they do not have to endure hours of painful labor and delivery. Finally, C-section rates have increased, proponents argue, because women are having babies at older ages, thereby having more complications, and the increase in weight of Americans in general has led to an increase in the number of overweight mothers who carry bigger babies, for whom vaginal delivery is much more risky.

On the other hand, opponents of the increasing use of C-sections argue it is the result of obstetricians' being concerned about malpractice lawsuits. That is one reason, these opponents argue, that women who have had previous C-sections are increasingly finding that their doctors and hospitals refuse to participate in a vaginal delivery with them. In addition, fees are higher for C-section deliveries than they are for vaginal deliveries, and those suspicious of physicians believe this fee structure difference is one of the prime reasons for the high number of cesarean sections. Furthermore, those opposed to increases in C-section deliveries point out the risks of any surgery. These risks can be avoided, they believe, if a woman has vaginal delivery. As with many issues of sexuality, the appropriate use of cesarean sections is a matter of debate at the current time.

There are disadvantages to having a C-section. It is expensive; the mother needs a recuperative period that may interfere with her caring for her baby; there is scarring of the uterus; and there is the possibility, though slight, of hemorrhage or infection. It must be pointed out, however, that many babies and mothers would die without surgical intervention. Cesarean intervention is an alternative delivery method to be considered in certain complicated situations.

Premature Birth

When a child is born before the normal gestation period is completed but still has a chance of surviving, its birth is regarded as **premature.** It is estimated that about 12% of all babies born in the United States are premature. A premature infant is usually between 28 and 34 weeks' gestation, although some are as young as 24 weeks. These infants generally weigh less than 5.5 pounds (2,500 grams). Of the 250,000 "preemies" born annually, about 100,000 weigh less than 3.3 pounds (1,500 grams).

Prematurity is caused by many factors. One common cause is a maternal age below 16 years or above 40 years. Other causes include maternal malnutrition, cigarette smoking and alcohol consumption, inadequate prenatal care, and a history of a previous premature delivery.

The premature baby is born before some of its body systems can perform adequately. The respiratory system in particular is immature in these babies. They may forget to breathe and may have difficulty in moving the air through the respiratory tract. Sometimes their lung surfaces are unable to work with the necessary amounts of oxygen needed for survival because of immaturity of the lungs. These infants are usually placed in incubators, which are special cribs with controls to monitor temperature and oxygen levels. Because oxygen is necessary to sustain life, on the one hand, and because an excess of oxygen can cause eye damage (retrolental fibroplasia [RLF]), on the other hand, oxygen levels must be carefully controlled. A device has been developed that, when put on the baby's skin, can measure blood oxygen levels continuously.

Premature infants often have difficulty swallowing and digesting food, so they require special intravenous feedings. Small amounts of breast milk are fed to the baby as he or she begins to mature, both for nutrition and for the antibodies provided by the milk. Chemical tests that can detect some metabolic problems are used in the monitoring techniques.

Neonatal intensive care is the name given to the medical specialty of premature infant care. It is costly because it requires the talents of trained specialists and special equipment. Given this care, however, most premature babies develop normally and catch up to their peers somewhere between the end of the first year and the third year. The investment to child, family, and ultimately society certainly justifies the time and costs involved.

premature
Type of birth in which an infant is born before the complete term of gestation but late enough in the pregnancy that it has a chance to survive.

neonatal intensive care
A medical specialty that focuses on the care of premature infants.

oxytocin
A pituitary hormone that stimulates the breasts to eject milk so that breastfeeding may occur after childbirth.

colostrum
The yellow fluid secreted by the breasts just before and after childbirth until milk production begins.

letdown
The tingling sensation in the breasts when milk is forced out about 30 to 60 seconds after the infant begins to suckle.

bonding
A sense of close emotional attachment.

Breastfeeding

To ready the breasts for producing milk, glandular tissue and ducts proliferate during pregnancy as a result of the placenta's secretion of estrogen, progesterone, and lactogen. These developments account for the increase in breast size in pregnancy. Large amounts of estrogen and progesterone secreted by the placenta prevent milk production before birth, but after the placenta is delivered, both estrogen and progesterone levels drop significantly, and the level of the pituitary hormone prolactin rises. Prolactin secretion activates the breast cells to produce milk. A second pituitary hormone, **oxytocin,** acts as a stimulant for the breasts to eject milk.

Twenty-eight to 48 hours after delivery, the lactation process begins. For the first 3 or 4 days a thin, yellowish liquid called **colostrum** is secreted by the breasts. Colostrum is a high-protein substance containing many antibodies. Actual milk production begins between the fourth and seventh days, and by the seventh day mature milk production begins. The infant's sucking stimulates nerve cells in the nipples; the brain receives the message and stimulates the pituitary to secrete oxytocin, which in turn stimulates ejection of milk from the breasts. When the milk is forced out, the mother feels a tingling sensation known as a **letdown** about 30 to 60 seconds after suckling begins. This feeling is produced by a neurogenic reflex that is necessary for adequate milk supply to reach the infant. Continued milk supply is dependent on sucking. The infant's demand regulates the breasts' supply. When the baby sucks longer, the breasts produce more milk to meet the increased demand. When the baby sucks less, milk production decreases.

Breastfeeding benefits the baby by providing a diet of balanced, uncontaminated nutrients and antibodies against disease. The breastfeeding mother benefits too. Nursing helps the uterus to return to its nonpregnant shape and postpones the return of menstruation (although it is not a sufficient contraceptive by itself). In addition, breast cancer rates are lower for mothers who breastfeed. A study of more than 50,000 women from 30 different countries found that each year a mother breastfed reduced her risk of breast cancer by 4.3% (Collaborative group, 2002). But probably most important, breastfeeding encourages the close attachment, or **bonding,** of infant and mother. Perhaps not incidentally breast milk is less expensive than formula milk. Because of these multiple benefits, the American Academy of Pediatrics and the U.S. federal government recommend breastfeeding over formula feeding. Support for breastfeeding mothers is provided by organizations such as La Leche League and numerous books and articles. Such support is necessary in view of the inconvenience that accompanies breastfeeding, especially for employed women, and because some people regard it as old-fashioned or improper in public.

Some women do not produce sufficient milk to breastfeed. This may be the case with mothers who smoke cigarettes, for example. Others may not want to breastfeed because it is inconvenient or for other reasons. These women can also bond with their babies by holding them closely while bottle feeding. If inconvenience is the only issue, mothers can use a breast pump to extract milk that is stored for use by fathers or caregivers during bottle feeding.

Sexual Activity During Pregnancy and After Delivery

Some, perhaps many, pregnant couples are afraid to have intercourse for fear of hurting the fetus. The frequency and kinds of sexual activity that are safe during and after pregnancy are determined both by personal preference and by health. A woman with no medical problems can continue to have the kind of sexual and sensual life she had before pregnancy (Figure 9.9). Even for healthy women, though, changes in body size and sense of comfort might dictate alterations in sexual habits. In advanced pregnancy some couples tend to replace intercourse with manual stimulation.

When certain physical conditions are present, however, coitus might add risk to the pregnancy. For example, when spotting, bleeding, pain, or past history of spontaneous abortion is present, a medical practitioner should decide whether intercourse is permissible. In healthy women, orgasmic contractions are not harmful to the fetus and will not initiate labor.

Sexual feelings can change during pregnancy. A woman's desire may be influenced by her personal involvement with the baby late in pregnancy, her

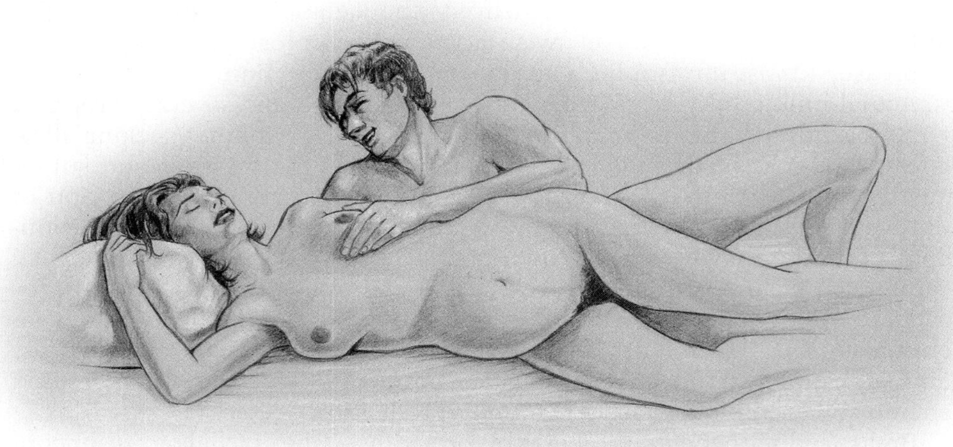

FIGURE 9.9 Pregnancy need not mean the end of sexual intercourse.

individual personality, her attitudes about sexuality, her feelings about her physical appearance, and so on. Here again, the necessity for free-flowing sexual communication, both trustful and honest, cannot be stressed enough.

Intercourse after delivery depends on many factors: whether there were complications during and after delivery, whether a C-section was performed, and of course, whether the woman is comfortable, particularly after a diffi-

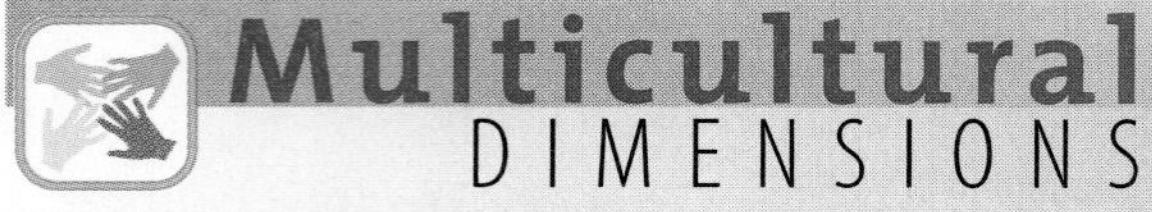

Multicultural DIMENSIONS

Differences in Infant Mortality Infant mortality comprises deaths occurring within the first year of life. In 2002, the U.S. government published the most current infant mortality rates (National Center for Health Statistics, 2002). The good news was that the infant mortality rate continued to decline, as it had over many years. Whereas in 1983 it was 10.9 per 1,000 live births, in 1999 the infant mortality rate was 7.0 per 1,000 live births.

The bad news was that the infant mortality rate for African Americans was still much higher than that for other subgroups in the population. In 1999, the white infant mortality rate was 5.8 per 1,000 live births, but the African-American infant mortality rate was 14.0 per 1,000 live births. The reasons for the high rate among African Americans are many and varied; poverty is foremost. Poverty rates are proportionately higher among African Americans than among whites. Consequently, African Americans cannot as readily afford health care, proper nutrition, and other services and behaviors that are conducive to birth of healthy babies. For example, whereas 85% of white mothers began prenatal care during the first trimester, only 74% of African-American mothers did. And, though only 3.3% of white mothers began prenatal care either during the third trimester or not at all, 6.7% of African-American mothers began prenatal care late or not at all.

To respond to this infant mortality rate gap between African-American and white Americans, communities have instituted educational campaigns encouraging early prenatal care, particularly targeted at African-American populations. Some of these programs rely on public service advertisements in newspapers, on signs on buses, or as messages over radio or television. Other programs employ women who live in the targeted communities to identify pregnant women, meet with them, and encourage them to see a health care provider. Still other programs employ a combination of these and other methods in conjunction with free or low-cost health care to help pregnant moms be healthier and deliver healthier children.

cult delivery. Most obstetricians prefer that couples delay intercourse until after the first postdelivery examination, which usually takes place 4 to 6 weeks after delivery. This is to be sure that the vulva has healed if there was a tear or an episiotomy and to allow time to discuss the choice of a method of birth control.

Couples should be sure to resume contraception before sexual intercourse after childbirth. Despite the fact that breastfeeding delays the return of menstruation, that alone is not a dependable form of birth control.

Hormonal Influences on Prenatal Development: Becoming Male or Female

The process of becoming a male or a female is a complicated one, involving chromosomes and hormones. As we have mentioned, a key influence on sex determination is the presence or absence of a Y chromosome.

Normal Sexual Differentiation

In the uterus, the fertilized egg always develops as if it were going to be female. If a Y chromosome is present, however, a male develops. Although the process by which the Y chromosome results in the development of testes is not completely understood, it appears that the body produces a substance called *H-Y antigen* that initiates this process. The testes then begin to form where ovaries might have otherwise been. If no Y chromosome is present, ovaries develop instead. This process of gonadal development, termed *sexual differentiation* (Figure 9.10), does not start until the beginning of the second month after conception.

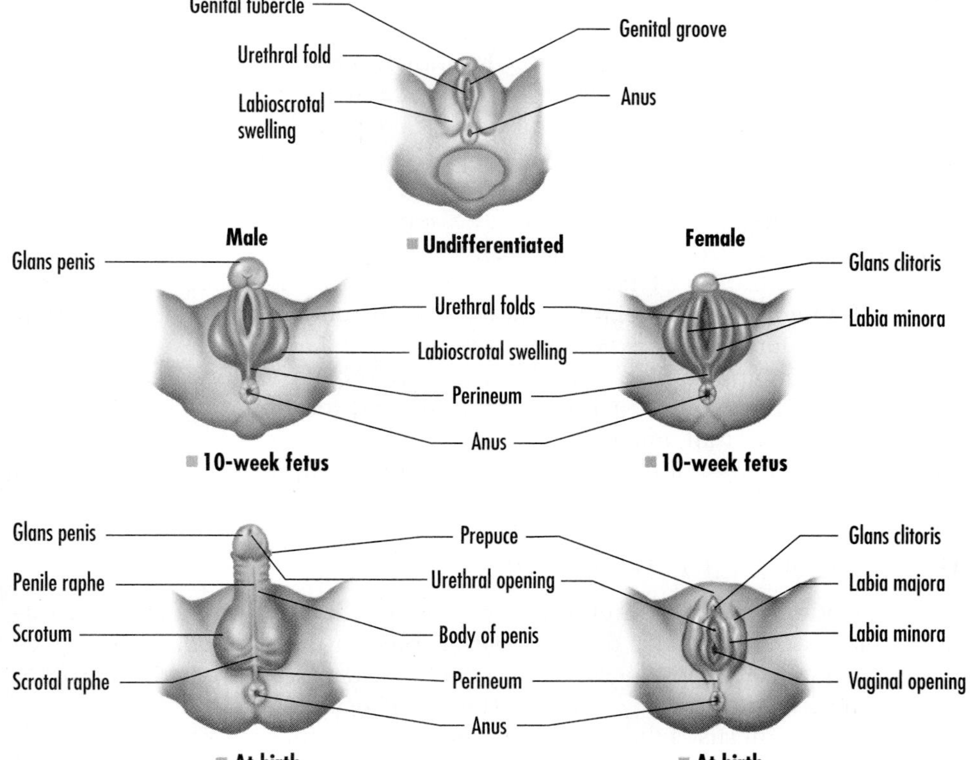

FIGURE 9.10 Prenatal development of external genitalia.

TABLE 9.2 **Homologous Structures**

Female	Male
Clitoral glans	Penile glans
Clitoral shaft	Penile shaft
Clitoral hood	Penile foreskin
Labia majora	Scrotum
Labia minora shaft	Bottom of penile
Ovaries	Testes
Bartholin's gland	Cowper's gland
Skene's gland	Prostate gland

Gonadal development is significant because the gonads produce their own hormones, which, in turn, affect the development of other structures in the reproductive system. For example, the fetal testes produce testicular hormones (androgens) that instruct the body to develop the vas deferens and other male reproductive structures. In addition, the fetal testes produce a "defeminizing hormone" called *Mullerian inhibiting hormone (MIH)* (or *Mullerian inhibiting substance [MIS]*), which prevents the reproductive tissue from forming a uterus and fallopian tubes. In females the absence of testicular hormones allows the tissue to form female reproductive structures (the labia, uterus, fallopian tubes, and others).

The tissue from which the reproductive organs develop is part of one of a pair of embryonic ducts. One of these, the *Mullerian duct,* develops into the female reproductive organs. The other, the *Wolffian duct,* develops into the male reproductive organs after the Mullerian duct degenerates as a result of MIH secreted from the testes. By the fourth month after conception, the gender of the fetus is clearly identifiable by the external genitalia.

The presence or absence of androgens determines whether a particular piece of tissue becomes a penis or a clitoris, a prostate gland or a Skene's gland, a Cowper's gland or a Bartholin's gland, or a scrotum or a labia majora. Structures that develop from the same tissue in this way are called **homologous** structures (see Table 9.2).

homologous
Organs that differ but that developed from the same tissue, for example, the glans penis and clitoris.

hermaphroditism
A condition in which a person has reproductive organs of both sexes.

infertility
The inability to reproduce.

The differentiation of the male and female brain is called *brain dimorphism.* Although this is a relatively new scientific endeavor, we do know that brain differentiation may extend into the first few days or weeks after birth. Interestingly, it appears that brain differentiation is *ambitypic;* that is, it allows for the coexistence of both masculine and feminine nuclei and pathways in some, if not all, parts of the brain. What this means is that the female can demonstrate masculine behavior and the male can demonstrate feminine behavior.

Abnormal Sexual Differentiation

The description of sexual differentiation assumes that everything goes according to plan, and it usually does. However, once in a while something goes wrong. In fact, it is possible for the genetic sex, or *genotype* (the chromosomes), the gonadal sex, or *phenotype* (testes or ovaries), and the internal sexual structures (uterus, fallopian tubes, prostate gland, and vas deferens) to differ. For example, a person with two X chromosomes can have a penis and an empty scrotum (no testes), two ovaries, a uterus, and fallopian tubes—yet still feel and act male. Conversely, it is possible for a female to grow up feeling feminine but have an X and a Y chromosome, two testes, and some internal male sexual structures (Money, 1987a).

This latter condition, in which an X and a Y chromosome are present but the tissues are insensitive to the testosterone produced by the fetal testes, is called the *testicular feminizing syndrome.* This is the most common form of **hermaphroditism,** a condition in which organs of both genders are present. A hermaphrodite can also be formed by the secretion of an excessive level of androgen from the adrenal gland of a female fetus. This condition is called *adrenogenital syndrome.* In addition, hermaphroditism has resulted from administration of a synthetic hormone (progestin)—a practice that is now banned but was previously used to prevent miscarriages.

Some experts differentiate between true hermaphrodites and *pseudohermaphrodites.* True hermaphroditism, which is very rare, is characterized by the presence of both ovarian and testicular tissue (sometimes called *ovotestes*). Pseudohermaphrodites have gonads that match their chromosomes (testes if they are XY or ovaries if they are XX), but their other reproductive structures may be mixed. This is a much more common form of hermaphroditism. Either type of hermaphroditism is treated with hormonal therapy, surgery, and counseling.

Other problems with sexual differentiation can be traced to the chromosomes. For example, in a condition called *Turner's syndrome,* which is caused by the presence of only one X chromosome (instead of two), the female fetus may be born with swollen hands and feet, be sterile, and remain short. In another condition, *Klinefelter's syndrome,* caused by an XXY genetic makeup, boys appear normal until puberty but then do not develop the normal secondary sex characteristics (discussed later) and often require testosterone injections throughout life.

Still another problem associated with sexual differentiation is called an *inguinal hernia.* The testes descend into the scrotum through a structure called the *inguinal canal.* This normally occurs by the seventh month of fetal development. If the inguinal canal does not close properly after the testes descend or if it opens up afterward, it is possible for the intestine to move down the canal and enter the scrotum. An inguinal hernia can be corrected surgically.

If the testes do not descend down the inguinal canal, as occurs in about 2% of male newborns, the condition is called *cryptorchidism* (more commonly called *undescended testes*). Usually the testes will descend during early childhood or by puberty. If they do not, however, either surgery or hormonal therapy is necessary for two reasons: (1) Testes in the abdomen are at too high a temperature to produce viable sperm, and if they are left undescended, infertility is likely to result; and (2) there is a greater risk of testicular cancer if testes are left undescended.

Infertility

Infertility, or the inability to reproduce, can cause great emotional anguish for people who want children. This unhappiness, accompanied by tension, frustration, and even resentment, can damage the health and the marriages of infertile couples. The situation may be further complicated by an inability or unwillingness to adopt a child. It is important to add, however, that while adoption may relieve the stress of wanting to raise children, it may not eliminate the stress related to infertility.

More than 5 million people of childbearing age experience infertility. Primary infertility is defined as inability to conceive despite having unprotected intercourse for at least 1 year. Secondary infertility is defined as inability to conceive despite having unprotected intercourse for at least 1 year and having previously conceived (Hatcher, et al., 1998). It is estimated that 10% to 15% of couples experience primary infertility.

Women and men can both contribute to infertility. Infertility is caused by the woman's problem in 35% of cases; by the male's problem in 35% of the cases; by both the woman and the man in 20% of cases. In 10% of cases, there is no discernible reason for the infertility.

Causes of Infertility

Among the leading causes of infertility in women are untreated gonorrhea and chlamydia infections. These may cause tubal occlusion in women and chronic cervicitis, both of which produce subfertility. In men, these diseases, if untreated, can cause epididymitis, leading to blocked sperm ducts and poor semen quality. Sexually active college students can help protect themselves from infertility by using condoms, practicing safer sex behaviors, and getting regular testing for STIs.

STIs are not the only diseases that affect fertility. About 1% of men become infertile after mumps. People with sickle-cell disease have higher infertility rates. Several drugs may inhibit sperm production or sperm function, including antimalarial drugs, antihypertensives, and calcium channel blockers. Such recreational drugs as narcotics or barbiturates can inhibit ovulation in women. Cigarette smoking and alcohol use are associated with both poor sperm quality in men and lower rates of conception in women.

¿? Ethical DIMENSIONS

Surrogate Mothers Some couples who attempt to conceive children cannot. In some cases, the cause is a lack of viable sperm. In other cases, the problem is a blockage of the fallopian tubes, which prevents the sperm–ovum union. In still other cases, the woman does not produce an ovum to be fertilized or, because of some medical condition, cannot carry a fetus in her uterus until delivery. In the latter circumstance, the woman's ovum can be fertilized by her partner's sperm outside the womb and implanted in the uterus of another woman, a *surrogate womb*. However, when a woman does not produce ova for fertilization, sometimes another woman's egg is fertilized by her partner and develops in that other woman's uterus. Upon delivery, the baby becomes the child of the father and his partner rather than of the father and the woman whose eggs and uterus were used for 9 months or so. The woman whose eggs and uterus were used is the biological mother, referred to as a *surrogate mother*.

When surrogate motherhood occurs without complications, it provides for everyone's needs. However, every once in a while, circumstances requiring creative solutions develop. For example, what do you think should happen if the surrogate mother does not want to give up the child after delivery? (Maybe she develops an attachment to the baby, or her situation has changed and she now wants a child of her own.) What should happen if the father and his partner do not want to accept the baby? (Maybe the baby has a birth defect, the couple has separated or divorced, or they just changed their minds about wanting children.) Each of these situations has actually occurred. What is your opinion?

Age is a factor in infertility for women and men. The older the woman is, the more likely she is to be infertile. Women are most fertile in their mid-20s; by the time a woman is 40 years old, she has a 50% decreased fertility rate and a two to three times greater chance of miscarriage (Toner & Flood, 1993). Conversely, a man's age does not seem to affect his sperm until his mid-60s (Gallardo, et al., 1996).

Exposure to toxic substances may be one of the causes of infertility when there is no discernible anatomical cause. Lead, toxic fumes, and pesticides appear to contribute to infertility by reducing sperm count, lessening sex drive, and increasing chances of miscarriage.

Finally, in some couples, a lack of knowledge about anatomy, physiology, and reproduction leads to infertility. These couples may not know when conception is most likely to occur, they may not have intercourse frequently enough to conceive, and they may not know how to time intercourse. The ovum is alive for less than 1 day; sperm can live as long as 5 days inside the woman. Couples must have intercourse before ovulation to maximize the possibility of pregnancy.

Treatment for Infertility

Infertility can be successfully treated. At least half of people with infertility who receive treatment are ultimately able to conceive. About 5% of couples who are infertile become pregnant without any treatment (Jones & Toner, 1993).

Fertility may be enhanced with some simple techniques. For example, having the woman lie on her back for an hour after coitus to aid sperm in traveling up, rather than out of, the vagina or even having more frequent intercourse, especially near the time of ovulation, can be enough to allow some couples to conceive. In addition, the man-on-top coital position increases the chances of conception because the cervix drops into the seminal pool. Placing a pillow under the woman's buttocks may also help prevent sperm from escaping out of the vagina. Identifying the time of ovulation and having sexual intercourse near that time can enhance the chance of conception as well, because the ovum is available for impregnation for only a short period. Trying to conceive often, in the most conducive position to conception, cannot result in pregnancy if there is no egg to fertilize.

For many couples, these simple techniques are not enough. Other procedures have thus been developed to enhance fertility. In all cases, however, the first step is an examination to determine why a couple is unable to conceive. At present several basic infertility screening procedures are used in this examination phase:

1. *Semen analysis.* The man is asked to masturbate and collect the ejaculate in a container. The ejaculate is then examined to determine the number of sperm present, the sperm's motility, and the amount of fructose (nourishment for the sperm) in the semen.

2. *Basal body temperature (BBT) recordings.* The woman is required to record her body temperature (with an oral or BBT thermometer) daily. The decrease in estrogen production as ovulation nears causes the basal temperature to drop about 0.3 degree. When ovulation occurs, basal temperature rises about 0.6 degree as a result of the corpus luteum's production of the hormone progesterone. Thus a physician can determine whether ovulation is occurring normally by monitoring the basal temperature.

3. *A fuller evaluation of ovulatory function.* A *biopsy* (microscopic examination of excised tissue) of the endometrium is performed. The secretions that progesterone produces in the endometrium are studied to provide further information regarding the normality of the woman's ovulation.
4. *Tubal patency tests.* Dye is projected through the fallopian tubes and observed by X ray to detect any blockage; also called *hysterosalpingogram.*
5. *Postcoital examination.* Two to 4 hours after the couple has had sexual intercourse, the cervical mucus is examined microscopically. The physician checks for several conditions of the cervical mucus that can be fatal to sperm (for example, too much viscosity or too little salt). The sperm are counted and their ability to travel determined, because the more motile the sperm, the greater is the likelihood of conception.
6. *Hormone monitoring.* Several ovulation prediction kits are currently sold over the counter. These kits measure the level of luteinizing hormone (LH), the hormone causing ovulation midway through the menstrual cycle. Urine tests can also be used to measure the amount of progesterone during various phases of the cycle. Other hormones (such as prolactin, thyroid hormones, and follicle-stimulating hormone [FSH]) can also be monitored.
7. *Cervical mucus evaluation.* The cervical mucus can be evaluated for its elasticity, its nature just before ovulation (it should be thin, watery, salty, and stretchy), and the presence of cells, debris, and proper pH level (degree of acidity or alkalinity).
8. *Ultrasonography.* High-frequency sound waves are transmitted and reflected by internal organs and structures. From the resulting pattern, detailed outlines of the reproductive system can be obtained.
9. *Hysteroscopy.* The uterus is expanded with carbon dioxide gas or liquid and is observed through a hysteroscope—a long, narrow, illuminated instrument that is inserted through the cervix into the uterus. Abnormalities such as polyps, fibroids, and adhesions can be identified in this manner.

These screening procedures determine the cause of infertility in approximately 85% of cases. (In the remaining 15% the cause of infertility is unknown.) Once the cause or causes are determined, treatment can be prescribed. Cessation of ovulation can be restarted through hormone therapy or by increasing body fat through nutritional therapy. Blocked fallopian tubes can be cleared through microsurgical techniques. Artificial insemination (projecting sperm from a male donor into the female's vagina by mechanical means) can be used when the male is not fertile. To aid women whose fallopian tubes are irreparably blocked, physicians in special clinics can unite the partner's sperm and ovum outside the woman's body. The fertilized egg is then allowed to develop in a petri dish and is implanted in the woman's uterus to create a pregnancy. This procedure, known as *in vitro fertilization,* and artificial insemination are discussed in detail in the next section.

Assisted Reproductive Technologies

During the latter part of the 21st century, advanced reproductive technologies (ARTs) have been developed to assist infertile couples in conceiving. The first American baby conceived in vitro was born in December 1981. Since then, technologies have become increasingly sophisticated in resolving infertility. The most common ART techniques are in vitro fertilization and gamete intrafallopian transfer.

In Vitro Fertilization

In vitro fertilization (IVF) has incorrectly been labeled the "test-tube baby" procedure. This is actually a highly sophisticated medical procedure, "which involves removing a ripened egg or eggs from the female's ovary, fertilizing it with semen, incubating the dividing cells in a laboratory dish, and then replacing the developing embryo in the uterus at the appropriate time" (Clapp, 1998). The woman's eggs can be used, or donor eggs can be used. The man's sperm can be used, or donor sperm can be used.

The success rate for IVF is not high. The birth rate per egg retrieval was 22.3% in 1995 (Clapp, 1998). Clinics are trying to improve the success rate by retrieving and fertilizing multiple eggs or transferring multiple embryos. As a result, multiple birth rates with IVF are as high as 20%. In the 1997 case of Bobbie McCaughey, seven embryos were transplanted, resulting in the birth of septuplets. In addition, women who become pregnant with more than one child through in vitro fertilization or gamete intrafallopian transfer (discussed later) have a twofold higher risk of development of preeclampsia than women who become pregnant spontaneously (Lynch, et al., 2002).

IVF raises numerous ethical issues. In some cases, women find out that all the embryos have begun to develop into fetuses, and they choose to have a procedure called *selective abortion,* whereby one or more of the fetuses are aborted to give the remaining fetuses a better chance to develop. In many clinics, more eggs are harvested than needed for a single cycle and are fertilized. These embryos are then frozen so that they can be used for future IVF procedures. However, in some cases, couples have divorced before the transfer of the embryos, and so couples have fought over these embryos as part of a divorce settlement. In a few widely publicized cases, embryos have been implanted after the man has died. Is the child in that case born to a married couple, or should he or she be considered an out-of-wedlock child? And, should insurance companies and Medicaid pay for IVF? In most cases, they do not. The procedure is expensive—nearly $10,000 per cycle. Should IVF be available only to well-to-do couples?

Gamete Intrafallopian Transfer

In gamete intrafallopian transfer (GIFT), rather than transplantation of an embryo into the uterus, an ovum is transferred to one or both fallopian tubes during laparoscopy. Fertilization occurs in the tube, as it does naturally, and the embryo implants in a regular conception cycle. It is an option only for women with open fallopian tubes. GIFT has a slightly higher pregnancy rate than IVF: Nearly 27% of egg retrievals result in a live birth (Adamson, 1998). However, there is a higher tubal pregnancy rate for using GIFT.

Artificial Insemination

About 20,000 babies yearly are produced by **artificial insemination.** There are two types of artificial insemination: *artificial insemination by a donor (AID)* and *artificial insemination by the husband (AIH).* Artificial insemination by the husband is generally attempted when the husband has one of a

artificial insemination
Introduction of semen into the uterus by noncoital means.

number of problems, such as a misplaced urinary meatus, impotence, or low sperm count. The semen is collected from the husband by masturbation or immediately after coitus. Either the specimen is collected by the couple and then taken to the clinic, or the man masturbates at the clinic. The sperm are then introduced into the woman's uterus by means of a syringe or by placement of the semen in a cervical cap fitted against the cervix.

Artificial insemination by a donor other than the husband is done when there is no husband or in cases where the husband produces no sperm (a condition called *azoospermia*), has a sperm count too low to ensure fertilization *(oligospermia)*, has sperm that are not viable enough for insemination, or has a combination of the last two conditions. The donor is screened for health factors and is matched to the husband in physical appearance and genetic background, though generally his identity is unknown to the receivers. For legal reasons, if the husband can produce even a minimal amount of sperm, some physicians mix his semen with that of the donor before inseminating the woman. Because in some states the question of legal paternity arises when AID is used, mixing sperm can help ensure the husband's status as father, because it cannot be disproved. In states that have no legal guidelines or statutes regarding paternity in such cases, lawyers encourage husbands to legally adopt children produced through AID.

Artificial insemination allows people to experience natural parenthood, even when they are unable to conceive through intercourse. And with AID, mothers at least are the biological parents of their offspring. Furthermore, many single women who are physically, emotionally, and economically capable of being mothers are unwilling to be impregnated through intercourse but are willing to be artificially inseminated. Obviously although artificial insemination offers the option of parenthood to many to whom it was barred, it also raises many questions of a moral nature—for example, whether it is fair to a child to bring it into the world with no known biological father.

Exploring the DIMENSIONS of Human Sexuality

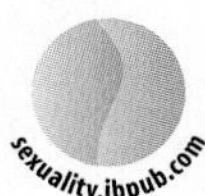

Our feelings, attitudes, and beliefs regarding sexuality are influenced by our internal and external environments. Go to sexuality.jbpub.com to learn more about the biological, psychological, and sociological factors that affect your sexuality.

Biological Factors

- Hormones create gender differentiation during the second month of prenatal development.
- Physiological cycles and changes in the fetus take place at an extremely fast pace.
- Physical appearance of the mother changes (for example, clearer skin) as hormonal changes take place.
- Parents' genetic characteristics determine many attributes of their children, such as height and hair color.

Sociocultural Factors

- Socioeconomic status influences infant and maternal health, because poor people have less access to prenatal care than well-off people do.
- Laws restrict access to abortions during the third trimester.
- Religion, culture, and ethnic heritage influence many beliefs about pregnancy, childbirth, and parenting.
- Media and ads may influence the choice of where to have a child or whether to have a midwife or physician.
- Family, neighbors, and friends who have children can provide invaluable advice and assistance to new parents.

Psychological Factors

- A pregnant woman's emotions can swing wildly because of hormonal shifts. The postpartum period can be associated with mild depression.
- Experience counts in pregnancy; subsequent infants go through labor faster and breastfeed more readily.
- Self-concept usually increases as a result of the responsibility of caring for another person.
- Learned attitudes and behaviors are often exhibited by pregnant couples.
- A woman's body image can suffer if she views herself as "getting fat" rather than as "carrying a child."

CASE STUDY

Pregnancy is a time of wonder and joy. For first-time parents, the world is forever changed after their infant is born. But even the degree of responsibility and emotional attachment to the child is influenced by many dimensions.

Biological age of the mother plays a factor. Teen pregnancies tend to have more medical complications for both mother and child. And risk of Down's syndrome increases with age: from 1 in 885 births at age 30 years, to 1 in 109 births at age 40 years, to 1 in 32 births at age 45 years.

Socioeconomic status plays a role in the health care of children. Parents on the low end of the socioeconomic scale lack parental and infant care, as well as the education and resources for raising healthy children.

Social pressure about child rearing is exerted by grandparents as well.

When disposable diapers were introduced, Pampers advertised them as "easier." But grandparent pressure—"What was wrong with the diapers we used on you?"—caused many parents to return to cloth diapers. Pampers had to change their marketing strategy from being easier to being better for the baby.

Working parents tend to rely on a far-flung network of day care providers, friends, family, and peer parents for emotional and practical advice. Without such support, the emotional impact of raising a child can be overwhelming.

Discussion Questions

1. Explain the process by which life begins, citing as much detail as possible.
2. What are the characteristics of fetal development that differentiate the three trimesters?
3. What can a pregnant woman do to increase the chance of having a healthy pregnancy and child?
4. Describe how varied drugs and diseases can threaten infant health.
5. What maternal problems may occur during pregnancy? And what can be done to alleviate some of these problems?
6. Differentiate the three phases of labor and methods of reducing the pain of labor.
7. Describe the benefits of breastfeeding an infant.
8. Is sex safe during pregnancy? Explain the situations in which it is or is not.
9. Compare and contrast the prenatal undifferentiated and gender-differentiated external genitalia, including the hormones that create the genders.
10. Explain the most common causes of infertility and the methods to treat such problems.

Application Questions

Reread the chapter-opening story and answer the following questions.

1. The Rich and Mary story underscores how the many dimensions of human sexuality play into our decision making. Although Mary believed in the social and ethical right of women to have abortions, her personal convictions and the psychological desire for another child led her to continue her pregnancy. What would you have done in Rich and Mary's situation? Which of the dimensions of human sexuality mentioned here would influence you?
2. The Rich and Mary story also underscores the fact that medical personnel often work with less than perfect information—they did not know she was carrying twins! If you had been in their situation, where could you find more information on analyzing amniocentesis test results? Would you pursue such avenues?

Critical Thinking Questions

1. A premature baby born at 24 weeks' gestation (5½ months), weighing about a pound, can be saved—at a cost of more than $300,000. But that is just the start. Many "preemie" children continue to have problems in school, requiring special-education programs. Choose a side and debate for or against saving children born more premature than 35 weeks. (*Note:* This question was submitted by a parent of two premature babies to provoke discussion.)
2. Hospitals have found that birthing centers are enormously profitable ventures. In major cities, hospitals compete for patients by having birthing rooms designed to look like homes with extra amenities and "freebies" (such as a champagne breakfast the morning after).

Yet to maintain profits, patients are sent home as soon as state laws allow—usually after a 2-night stay. Do patients benefit from such an arrangement—or is it simply a business deal for the hospitals?

Critical Thinking Case

For many years, there had been concern that too many cesarean birth deliveries were being performed in the United States. At its peak in 2001, the U.S. cesarean rate of nearly 25% of all births was higher than that of other industrialized nations. Interestingly, the data indicated that the increase in the cesarean rate did not contribute to the decline in infant mortality rate (Shearer, 1993). Making matters worse, maternal morbidity and mortality rates are higher in cesarean deliveries than in routine vaginal deliveries (Petitti, 1985). As a result, as one of the Year 2000 national health objectives, the U.S. Department of Health and Human Services recommended lowering the cesarean rate to no more than 15 per 100 births. In the Year 2010 national health objectives, the Department of Health and Human Services sought to decrease the rate of C-sections in women giving birth for the first time from 18% of live births to 15%, and from 72% of women giving birth who had a prior C-section to just 63%.

In 1999 24% of all deliveries in the United States were by C-section. It had previously been thought unwise and unhealthy for women who had a previous cesarean delivery to attempt a vaginal birth. The concern was for tearing of the tissue and possible infection for the baby. The standard practice was "Once a cesarean, always a cesarean." However, it was found that, barring complications, many women who had a cesarean delivery could deliver vaginally the next time without endangering their or their baby's health. As a result, the vaginal birth after previous cesarean (VBAC) rate had increased by 29% between 1991 and 1995. In 1998, 28% of women who had previously had a C-section and delivered again had a vaginal delivery.

Are the high rates of C-sections the result of the current medicolegal climate in the United States, which causes physicians to perform C-sections more often than in the past to protect themselves against a lawsuit?

Is the fact that C-sections earn the obstetrician more money a factor in the decision to perform them?

Given the increased risk to the mother of a cesarean delivery, and the evidence that it has little effect on infant mortality rate, is the relatively high rate of cesarean deliveries ethical?

Exploring Personal Dimensions

How Much Do You Know About Pregnancy and Birth?

For each of the statements that follow, indicate whether you think the statement is true or false. The correct answers and explanations appear after the questions.

True ____ False ____ 1. Pregnant women should stop exercising as soon as they discover they are pregnant.

True ____ False ____ 2. Once a woman has had a C-section, she should have C-sections for subsequent deliveries to prevent tearing of the abdominal tissue.

True ____ False ____ 3. The use of midwives has decreased in recent years.

True _____ False _____ 4. Breastfeeding is covered by the Pregnancy Discrimination Act, which guarantees that working women may breastfeed.

True _____ False _____ 5. Teen birth rates have increased recently and are of significant concern.

True _____ False _____ 6. In terms of a newborn baby's health, the length of time before its mother becomes pregnant again does not matter.

Answers and Explanations:

Each of the statements above is false.

1. Pregnant women are encouraged to continue exercising if they exercised before becoming pregnant. Some studies have suggested that exercise during pregnancy helps make the labor and delivery easier and shorter, promotes earlier recovery after delivery, and reduces the chance of C-sections. However, women who have not maintained an exercise regimen before becoming pregnant should not begin after becoming pregnant. Rather, they should exercise by adopting a mild walking or swimming program or consulting an expert on exercise and pregnancy for other activities that will be beneficial for them and their fetuses.
2. There is no reason why, as a matter of routine, women who have had one C-section need to have C-sections for subsequent pregnancies. C-sections need only be performed if the woman has an STI that can be transmitted during childbirth, if the baby is too large to pass through the vaginal opening, or if the stress of the delivery has the potential to cause harm to the mother.
3. Contrary to popular belief, the proportion of women who use a nurse-midwife rather than an obstetrician to deliver their babies is increasing. Whereas in 1975 only 1% of births were attended by a midwife, in 1995, 5.5% of births were facilitated by midwives (Stewart, 1998).
4. Many women have been fired or discriminated against for breastfeeding at work. However, the courts have failed to interpret the Pregnancy Discrimination Act as protecting these women. To correct this situation, legislation was introduced in the U.S. House of Representatives in 1998 to encourage employers to provide support for working mothers who choose to breastfeed their infants (Legislation would provide opportunities for working moms to breastfeed, 1998).
5. Birth rates for teenagers have actually decreased in recent years. Between 2000 and 2001, the birth rate for teens declined by 6%. Between 1991 and 2001, the teenage birth rate has declined by 26% (Martin, et al., 2002). This decline does not mean that teen birth rates are not too high and are not a national problem, for they are.
6. Research has shown that a short interpregnancy interval is a risk factor for infant mortality. Two explanations have been offered to explain this finding. The *maternal depletion hypothesis* suggests that at least 1 year between the birth of one child and subsequent conception is essential to restore maternal nutritional resources necessary for a successful pregnancy. The postpartum stress hypothesis states that caring for an infant can be so stressful that the physical or emotional strain can interfere with the growth of the fetus. In any case, a 1-year interpregnancy interval is recommended (Klerman, Cliver, & Goldenberg, 1998).

Sexuality Online

Go to the web component for *Exploring the Dimensions of Human Sexuality* at sexuality.jbpub.com for web exercises, additional resources related to this chapter, and student review tools.

Suggested Readings

American College of Obstetricians and Gynecologists. *You and your baby: Prenatal care, labor and delivery, and postpartum care.* Washington, DC: American College of Obstetricians and Gynecologists Patient Education, 1994.

Brownlee, S. The baby chase: Millions of couples have fertility problems, and many high-tech remedies. But who minds the pricey clinics they turn to? *U.S. News and World Report* (December 1995), 84–90.

Epps, R. P., ed. *The American Medical Women's Association guide to pregnancy and childbirth.* New York: Dell Books, 1996.

Iovine, V. *The girlfriends' guide to pregnancy.* New York: Perigee, 1997.

Klerman, L. V., Cliver, S. P., & Goldenberg, R. L. The impact of short interpregnancy intervals on pregnancy outcomes in a low-income population, *American Journal of Public Health, 88* (1988), 1182–1185.

MacDorman, M. F. & Singh, G. K. Midwifery care, social and medical risk factors, and birth outcomes in the USA, *Journal of Epidemiology and Community Health, 52* (1998), 310–317.

Reynolds, K. *Pregnancy and birth: Your questions answered.* New York: DK Publishing, 1997.

I»N»T»E»R chapter FOCUS

Unexpected Pregnancy Outcomes

FEATURES

Ethical Dimensions
Should Intact Dilation and Evacuation (D & E) Be Banned?

Communication Dimensions
Debating the Abortion Issue

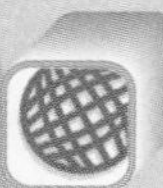

Global Dimensions
A Worldwide Preference for Boys

Gender Dimensions
Baby "Richard"

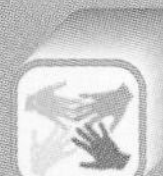

Multicultural Dimensions
International Adoptions

CHAPTER OBJECTIVES

1. Discuss abortion issues, including abortion procedures, legal history, and current attitudes toward abortion.

2. Describe the various types of adoptions and the laws surrounding them, including closed and open adoptions, agency adoptions, independent adoptions, and adoption by relatives.

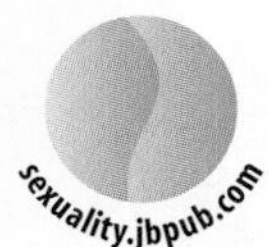

sexuality.jbpub.com

Global Dimensions: A Worldwide Preference for Boys
Emotions and Abortion
Multicultural Dimensions: International Adoptions
Foster Care and Adoption

INTRODUCTION

Too many pregnancies are unplanned and unwanted. The dilemma this causes for some men and women is eloquently described by the author Anna Quindlen (1988, 209–212).

> *It was always the look on their faces that told me first. I was the freshman dormitory counselor and they were freshmen at a women's college where everyone was smart. One of them would come into my room, a golden girl, a valedictorian, an 800 verbal score on the SATs, and her eyes would be empty, seeing only a busted future, the devastation of her life as she knew it. She had failed biology, messed up the math; she was pregnant. That was when I became prochoice.*

Quindlen then describes the birth of her own son.

> *It was the look in his eyes that I will always remember, too. They were as black as the bottom of a well, and in them for a few minutes I thought I saw myself the way I had always wished to be—clear, simple, elemental, at peace. My child looked at me and I looked back at him in the delivery room, and I realized that out of a sea of infinite possibilities it had come down to this: a specific person, born on the hottest day of the year, conceived on a Christmas Eve, made by his father and me miraculously from scratch.*
>
> *Once I believed that there was a little blob of formless protoplasm in there and a gynecologist went in there with a surgical instrument, and that was that. Then I got pregnant myself—eagerly, intentionally, by the right man, at the right time—and I began to doubt. My abdomen still flat, my stomach roiling with morning sickness, I felt not that I had protoplasm inside, but, instead, a complete human being in miniature to whom I could talk, sing, make promises. Neither of these views was accurate; instead, I think, the reality is something in the middle. And that is where I find myself now, in the middle—hating the idea of abortions, hating the idea of having them outlawed.*
>
> *For I know it is the right thing in some times and places. I remember sitting in a shabby clinic far uptown with one of those freshmen, only three months after the Supreme Court had made what we were doing possible, and watching with wonder as the lovely first love she had had with a nice boy unraveled over the space of an hour as they waited for her to be called, degenerating into sniping and silences. I remember a year or two later seeing them pass on campus and not even acknowledge each other because their conjoining had caused them so much pain, and I shuddered to think of them married, with a small psyche in their unready and unwilling hands. . . .*
>
> *I don't feel all one way about abortion anymore, and I don't think it serves a just cause to pretend that many of us do. For years I believed that a woman's right to choose was absolute, but now I wonder. Do I, with a stable home and marriage and sufficient stamina and money, have the freedom to choose abortion because a pregnancy is inconvenient just now? Legally I do have the right; legally I wanted always to have that right. It is the morality of exercising it under those circumstances that makes me wonder. . . .*
>
> *I have taped on my VCR a public television program in which somehow, inexplicably, a film is shown of a fetus* in utero *scratching its face, seemingly putting up a tiny hand to shield itself from the camera's eye. It would make a potent weapon in the arsenal of the antiabortionists. I grow sentimental about it as it floats in the salt water, part fish, part human being. It is almost living, but not quite. It has almost turned my heart around, but not quite my head.**

Many people are surprised to learn that most pregnancies are unintended. Yet, that is the case. When an unintended pregnancy occurs, decisions are required. Should the pregnancy be terminated? If so, which method of abortion should be used? What are the legal, moral, and health implications of this decision? Should the fetus be brought to term and a baby born? If so, should the child be raised by the biological parents? Should it be placed for adoption? If placed for adoption, should adoption be arranged through an agency or through a relative? What are the legal and moral implications of this decision? This chapter explores the alternatives presented to people who experience an unintended pregnancy.

Abortion

For unplanned pregnancies, the first decision to be made is whether or not to continue the pregnancy. Sometimes the woman or the couple decide to allow the pregnancy to continue, but something goes wrong and the fetus stops developing. Such natural cessations of the pregnancy are called **spontaneous abortions,** or miscarriages. Abortions requiring intervention to end the pregnancy are technically called **induced abortions.**

Abortion is safest in the earliest weeks of pregnancy. If a woman thinks she is pregnant and does not want to continue the pregnancy, she should perform a home pregnancy test or go to a clinic as soon as she misses a period.

Abortion Procedures

Vacuum Aspiration

Almost all abortions in the United States are performed during the first trimester of pregnancy, using a surgical procedure called **vacuum aspiration.** It is a surgical procedure that uses suction equipment to evacuate the contents of the uterus. It can also be used in the first weeks of the second trimester. Ninety-seven percent of the abortions performed in the 1990s used this method.

Manual vacuum aspiration (MVA) is a variation of vacuum aspiration that can be used from the detection of pregnancy to up to 12 weeks since the last menstrual period (LMP). In contrast to traditional vacuum aspiration procedures, it uses nonelectric suction instruments. The procedure takes 5 to 15 minutes, and the woman usually leaves the clinic within 2 hours.

Medical Abortions

Medical abortions are relatively new procedures that use drugs to induce abortion, including **mifepristone** or **methotrexate** in combination with **misoprostol.** Mifepristone was discovered by a French pharmaceutical company in 1978 and was previously known as RU 486. (*RU* refers to Roussel Uclaf, the French pharmaceutical company.)

Mifepristone blocks the hormone progesterone, which is needed to maintain a pregnancy. A woman who is no more than 49 days LMP takes mifepristone at a clinic visit. She returns to the clinic 2 days later and takes misoprostol, a prostaglandin that causes uterine contractions. In 92% of the cases, the pregnancy is terminated (Spitz, et. al., 1998; World Health Organization, 2000).

In the fall of 2000, mifepristone was approved by the U.S. Food and Drug Administration (FDA).

Methotrexate blocks folic acid and prevents cell division. A woman who is no more than 49 days past her last missed period receives an injection of methotrexate at a clinic and swallows misoprostol pills 2 to 7 days later. This combination is 92–94% effective in terminating pregnancy (Okie, 2000).

Currently, in the United States, methotrexate medical abortions are available only on an "off-label" basis. When drugs are approved by the U.S. FDA, their safety and efficacy are judged to warrant their use for specific conditions. Often, however, physicians discover other uses for those drugs and prescribe them for these other purposes. This practice, termed *off-label use,* is perfectly legal. Methotrexate is currently approved by the FDA for use by physicians for unruptured ectopic pregnancies, psoriasis, and rheumatoid arthritis (Hatcher, et al., 1998). Although approved for these conditions, it is used off-label by physicians for medical abortions. However, RU 486, mifepristone, was approved by the FDA for use in medical abortion on September 28, 2000.

Women who choose a medical abortion should understand that there is a 4% to 8% chance they will need to return for a surgical abortion. Still, many women consider medical abortions as easier and more natural than a surgical procedure (Harvey, Beckman, & Satre, 2001). Ninety-six percent of women in clinical trials of mifepristone would recommend the procedure to others, 91% would choose it again, and 88% said it was very or moderately satisfactory (Winikoff, et al., 1998).

Dilation and Evacuation

During the second trimester of pregnancy, **dilation and evacuation (D & E)** is the abortion procedure used. It involves dilating the cervix, scraping the walls of the uterus, and removing the endometrial lining with suction. In very rare cases (less than 1% of all abortions) a saline or prostaglandin solution is injected into the uterus to induce premature labor.

The vast majority of abortions are performed early in pregnancy. Fifty-eight percent occur within the first 8 weeks, 20% between weeks 9 and 10, and 10% between weeks 11 and 12. Thus, 88% of abortions are performed during the first trimester of pregnancy (Cates, Grimes, & Schulz, 2003). Only 1.5% are performed at 21 weeks or more, and only 0.04% are performed in the third trimester (Alan Guttmacher Institute, 1997). The procedure used during the third trimester is called an *intact D & E* and has been dubbed by opponents of legal abortion as a "partial birth abortion." This procedure is required when the fetus is too large for the other abortion procedures to be performed safely and effectively (see the box on page 346).

The Law and the Debate

Because abortion is an issue debated by citizens, ruled on by the judiciary, and legislated by elected representatives—not to mention its being a major decision for people who become directly involved in unplanned pregnancies—it is a topic that needs the fullest possible study and consideration.

For more than 3 decades, abortion has been vehemently debated in the political sector. Although in vitro fertilization, contraception, and sterilization all have their controversial aspects, none of them generates the political, religious, and emotional heat that abortion does. Some people believe induced abortion to be murder of a baby, whereas others see it as a medical intervention into a biological process. Some people feel that the question of when life begins is central to this debate: Is it at conception, at some point

spontaneous abortion (miscarriage) The natural termination of a pregnancy.

induced abortion Purposeful termination of a pregnancy.

vacuum aspiration Surgical procedure that uses a suction tube to evacuate the contents of the uterus, which can be used through the first weeks of the second trimester.

manual vacuum aspiration (MVA) A variation of vacuum aspiration that uses nonelectric suction instruments and can be used from detection of pregnancy through 12 weeks.

medical abortion A procedure that uses drugs to induce abortion.

mifepristone A drug that blocks the hormone progesterone, which is needed to maintain a pregnancy.

methotrexate A drug that blocks the hormone progesterone, which is needed to maintain a pregnancy.

misoprostol A prostaglandin that causes uterine contractions.

dilation and evacuation (D & E) Surgical procedure that involves dilating the cervix, scraping the walls of the uterus, and removing the endometrial lining with suction.

Ethical DIMENSIONS

Should Intact Dilation and Evacuation (D & E) Be Banned?

Intact dilation and evacuation is performed late in the second trimester when, in the judgment of the physician, it is deemed the best means of abortion—that is, the most effective and safest. Some reasons for this type of abortion are concern for the health of the pregnant woman, late determination of birth defects in the fetus, or the woman's delay in seeking abortion as a result of fear of letting others know that she is pregnant. Objections have been raised to this method of abortion because it is performed at or near viability of the fetus. Those opposed to abortion at any time in any form are understandably opposed to D & E. However, even some Americans supportive of a woman's right to abortion during the first trimester and through the second trimester until the fetus could live outside the womb are disturbed by abortions occurring so late in the pregnancy. In their desire to secure support for their position, opponents have dubbed D & E "partial birth abortion," attempting to have D & E viewed as the interference with the birth of a live baby, rather than the termination of a pregnancy.

Those opposed to placing restrictions on the type of abortion allowed argue that the most qualified person to make this decision is the physician. Therefore, they believe a ban on any type of abortion procedure would limit physicians' options at a time when performing it would be most effective and safest. Opponents to restrictions also believe that once restrictions are allowed, Right to Life supporters will use them as a wedge to introduce more restrictions, eventually eroding a woman's right to abortion.

In 1997, Congress passed a law banning D & Es. However, President Clinton vetoed that law, and Congress could not muster the votes required to override the veto. The following year, Congress again passed a similar law, but it was again vetoed by President Clinton. However, this time the House overrode the veto. Once the bill arrived back in the Senate, the veto was sustained, thereby preventing the legislation from becoming law.

In June 2000, the U.S. Supreme Court ruled in *Stenberg v. Carhart* that bans on intact D & E abortion were unconstitutional. That has not stopped proponents of these bans, however. Since the Supreme Court ruling, legislation banning D & E has been proposed in 11 states, although none has been approved (Sonfield, 2001). However, in 2003, the House again passed a ban on D & E and, with a sympathetic Senate and a conservative president (George W. Bush), it was believed that this time the ban would become law. Opponents, though, were sure to test the constitutionality of that law in the courts.

Do you believe D & E should be banned as an abortion procedure? Why do you believe as you do?

when the fetus could (with help) exist outside the uterus, or at birth? But a person's view of when life begins is only one factor in shaping his or her attitudes on whether induced abortion is morally acceptable. Another central issue is whether the individual woman has the right to make a decision so basic to her own life or whether the government has that right and power. Other attitudes also enter into the debate, for instance, attitudes regarding world population, religious issues, women's "place," political power, poverty, public and private child care, and the degree of responsibility people should assume for their sexual behavior.

At this writing political groups generally typed prolife are actively supporting candidates who are totally opposed to abortion. Their goal is to pass legislation making abortion illegal or even to pass a constitutional amendment prohibiting abortion in the United States. Groups labeled prochoice, however, believe that women should have the right to decide for themselves what they will do with their bodies. Consequently they oppose legislative restrictions on the availability of abortion to women who choose that option, and they wish to uphold the Supreme Court decision of 1973, which established the current legal status of abortion in the United States. The Court ruled (in *Roe v. Wade*) that abortion should be available to women during the first trimester (the first 3 months) of pregnancy. The decision is made by the pregnant woman and her physician. With regard to abortion during the second trimester, the Court ruled that the states can develop the regulations they deem necessary to maintain the pregnant woman's health. In the third trimester the states can limit or prohibit abortions if the mother's health is not in jeopardy.

ABORTION KILLS CHILDREN
ABORTION KILLS CHILDREN
KEEP ABORTION LEGAL
BOSTON STUDIOS

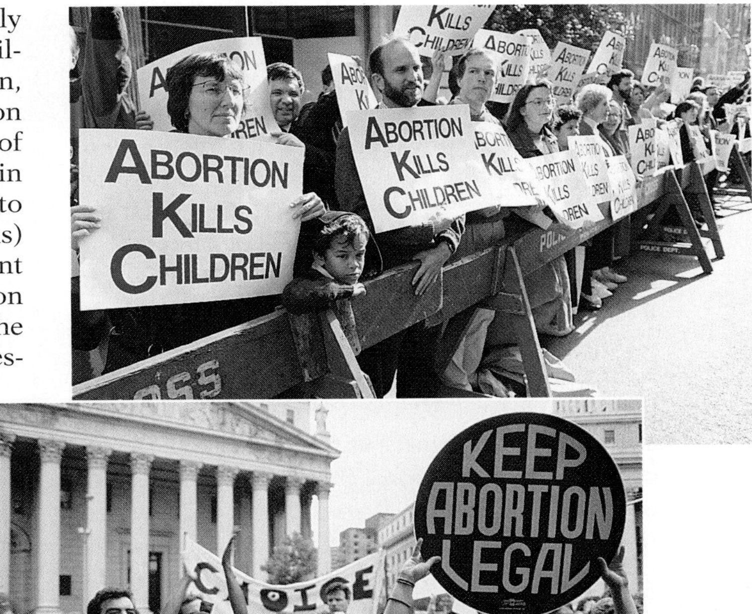

Both sides of the abortion issue attempt to show their strength in numbers with annual marches on Washington coinciding with the anniversary of *Roe v. Wade*. The marches do not happen on the same day, to minimize conflict as well as to accommodate the huge influx of people to Washington.

In 1983 the Supreme Court reaffirmed its 1973 decision and stated that the government could not interfere with abortion unless such interference was clearly justified by "accepted medical practice." In effect this ruling prohibited governmental interference even into the second trimester and invalidated state laws that required abortions during the second trimester to be performed in a hospital.

However, in 1989 a court made more conservative by new presidential appointments revisited this issue. They decided in *Webster v. Reproductive Health Services* that a Minnesota law requiring physicians to test fetuses to determine whether they could survive outside the womb before performing abortions was constitutional. That opened up the possibility that other regulations of abortion would be reviewed positively by the Court. Subsequently, two other cases were taken before the Supreme Court and decided in 1990. In *Hodgson v. Minnesota,* the Court rejected a law requiring a physician to notify both parents of a minor before an abortion could be performed. The rationale for this ruling was that some minors either do not live with both parents or have abusive or otherwise uncaring parents. The Court made it clear that if this law included a judicial bypass (in which a judge could approve the abortion if the parents were not the ones most appropriately notified), this law would be considered constitutional. In fact, in *Ohio v. Akron Center for Reproductive Health,* the Court held that a similar law that required notification of one parent and that did include a judicial bypass was constitutional.

In 1992, the Supreme Court reaffirmed the constitutionality of states attaching regulations to abortions, although they also reaffirmed the right of a woman to have an abortion if she chooses. In *Planned Parenthood of Southeastern Pennsylvania v. Casey,* the Court ruled that Pennsylvania could require a woman seeking an abortion to receive counseling; to wait 24 hours before an abortion could be performed; if a minor under 18 years old, to obtain a parent's informed consent or a judge's approval. The Court also ruled that a physician had to keep detailed records of abortions and reasons for performing late-term abortions. However, the Court refused to overturn *Roe v. Wade,* as many opposed to abortion had hoped a conservative Court would do.

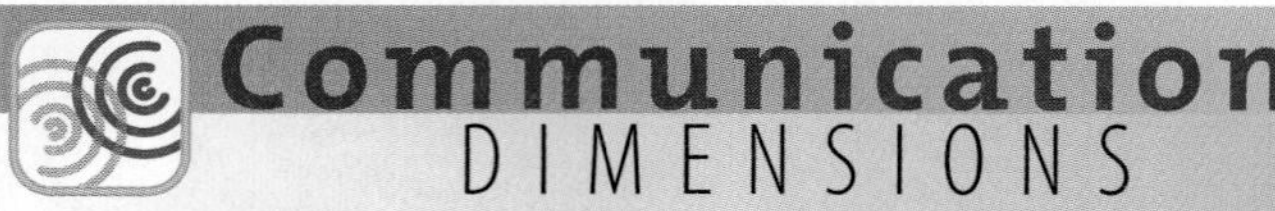

Debating the Abortion Issue Because of the intense emotions associated with abortion, as well as the moral and ethical implications, prochoicers and prolifers tend to talk past one another. This is unnecessary, however, because there are many points on which they can agree, and others that they can understand better. In summarizing polls of Americans on the issue of abortion, *USA Today* (1996) reported wide agreement among people who make up the "great middle." Most people believe in personal choice. Fifty-nine percent opposed a constitutional amendment to ban abortion except to save the life of the mother. Eighty-eight percent believed abortion should be legal if the mother's life is endangered, 82% if the woman's physical health is endangered, 77% if the pregnancy was caused by rape or incest, and 64% during the first 3 months of the pregnancy. Still, there was agreement that there ought to be limits. Seventy-four percent favored a waiting period, 86% favored informed consent, 74% favored parental consent for minors, 70% supported spousal notification, 71% favored a partial-birth abortion ban, and 82% believed abortion should be illegal during the last 3 months of pregnancy.

And yet, in arguing their positions, the two sides often take extreme positions. For example, extreme prolifers emphasize late-term abortions, whereas these abortions constitute only approximately 1% of all abortions. However, extreme prochoicers oppose any restrictions on abortion through all three trimesters of pregnancy.

The result is a figurative, and too often a literal, shouting match rather than a conversation, and this form of communication can unfortunately lead to extreme actions. The National Abortion Federation reports that between 1977 and 1998, there were more than 1,700 attacks on abortion providers (Abortion worker shootings, 1998).

Is this an effective way of communicating? Is this the way to resolve an ethical dilemma? How might groups such as clergy, citizens, or politicians work together to employ communication techniques that require listening as well as speaking?

In 1980 the Court made a decision that profoundly affected the availability of legal abortions. It ruled that the federal government could refuse to fund abortions for the poor, even though it funded other health care (the Hyde Amendment). The consequence of this action has been to prohibit poor women from obtaining safe abortions—the same abortions that middle- and upper-class women can receive by paying for them—with Medicaid funds. People who oppose abortion acknowledge that an inequity exists between poor and affluent women regarding the availability of abortion, but they view this circumstance as leaving the fetuses of more wealthy women unprotected by law. Some states have taken on the financial costs of abortion for poor women who are denied federal assistance by the Hyde Amendment.

Current Laws on Abortion Services

People who oppose legalized abortion have unsuccessfully tried to outlaw abortion services completely. However, they have been successful at limiting the availability of abortion under many circumstances.

For example, in October 1998 the U.S. Congress passed a $500 billion appropriations bill, which contained many restrictions on abortion. The bill prohibited

- Abortion coverage for workers insured by the federal government
- Abortions for women in federal prisons

- Abortions in overseas military hospitals
- Federal or local funding of abortions in the District of Columbia
- Medicaid funding of abortions, which primarily affects women with disabilities and low-income women
- Abortions through the Indian Health Service
- Federally supported embryo research

Many states have also passed laws limiting abortion services (Table IF2.1). These include laws limiting public and private funding for abortion, parental consent laws, waiting periods, and bans on certain procedures.

Who Has Abortions?

The Alan Guttmacher Institute monitors abortion laws and the characteristics of those having abortions (Alan Guttmacher Institute, 2000). They report that less than half (49%) of all pregnancies of American women are unwanted and that half of these are terminated by abortion. What surprises some people is that almost half (47%) of women who have an abortion have had a previous abortion, and 55% have had a previous birth.

Fifty-two percent of abortions are performed for women younger than 25 years. One-third of abortions are performed for women aged 20 to 24 years, and teenagers have 20% of all abortions. Of women who obtain abortions, two-thirds intend to have children in the future.

White women obtain 60% of all abortions, although proportionately more minority women obtain abortions. African-American women are more than three times as likely as white women to have an abortion, and Hispanic women are almost twice as likely.

Religion plays a role as well. Women who report no religious affiliation are more than four times as likely to obtain an abortion as other women. Although, among specific religions, Catholic women are 29% more likely to obtain an abortion than are Protestant women; the rate of abortions among Catholic women is comparable to the average of all American women.

Marital status is another variable associated with abortion. Two-thirds of abortions are obtained by women who have never been married.

There are three primary reasons women give for seeking an abortion. Three-quarters say that having a baby would interfere with their work, education, or other responsibilities. Approximately two-thirds say they cannot afford a child. And half say they do not want to be a single parent or are having problems with their husband or partner. Approximately 14,000 abortions occur because women have become pregnant as a result of having been raped. In addition, some abortions are performed for health-related reasons.

The Safety of Abortion

Abortion is an extremely safe procedure. Less than 1% of abortion patients experience a major complication. Of these, the primary risks are pelvic infection, hemorrhaging, or unintended major surgery. For abortions performed during the first 8 weeks of pregnancy, 1 death occurs per 530,000 abortions. The risk rises as the pregnancy progresses to 1 death per 17,000 during weeks 16 to 20, and 1 death per 6,000 after 20 weeks (Alan Guttmacher Institute, 2000). In comparison, the risk of death associated with childbirth is 10 times greater than that associated with abortion. Furthermore, there is no effect on subsequent pregnancies or births in women who have had the most common abortion procedure (vacuum aspiration) within the first 12 weeks.

TABLE IF2.1 Major State Abortion-Related Policies in Effect

State	Protect clinic access	Require abortion reporting	Require parental involvement in minors' abortion decisions	Require mandatory delay after state-directed counseling	Require state-directed counseling without mandatory delay	Restrict private- and/or public-employee insurance coverage	Restrict state funding for Medicaid recipients to rape, incest, or threat to mother's life	Restrict abortion after viability or a specified point in pregnancy
Number of restrictions	15	44	32	15	8	15	31	40
Alabama		X	X				X	X
Alaska					X			
Arizona		X						X
Arkansas		X	X				X	X
California	X				X			X
Colorado	X	X				X	X	
Connecticut	X	X			X			X
Delaware		X	X				X	X
Florida		X					X	X
Georgia		X	X				X	X
Hawaii		X						
Idaho		X	X	X		X		X
Illinois		X				X		X
Indiana		X	X	X				X
Iowa		X	X				X	X
Kansas	X	X	X	X			X	X
Kentucky		X	X	X		X	X	X
Louisiana		X	X	X			X	X
Maine	X	X			X		X	X
Maryland	X		X					X
Massachusetts	X	X	X			X		X
Michigan	X	X	X	X			X	X
Minnesota	X	X	X		X			X
Mississippi		X	X	X			X	
Missouri		X	X			X	X	X
Montana		X						X
Nebraska		X	X	X		X	X	X
Nevada	X	X			X		X	X
New Hampshire							X	
New Jersey								
New Mexico		X						
New York	X	X						X
North Carolina	X	X	X				X	X
North Dakota		X	X	X		X	X	X
Ohio		X	X	X		X	X	X

TABLE IF2.1 **Major State Abortion-Related Policies in Effect—cont'd**

State	Protect clinic access	Require abortion reporting	Require parental involvement in minors' abortion decisions	Require mandatory delay after state-directed counseling	Require state-directed counseling without mandatory delay	Restrict private- and/or public-employee insurance coverage	Restrict state funding for Medicaid recipients to rape, incest, or threat to mother's life	Restrict abortion after viability or a specified point in pregnancy
Number of restrictions	15	44	32	15	8	15	31	40
Oklahoma		X	X				X	X
Oregon	X	X						
Pennsylvania		X	X	X		X	X	X
Rhode Island		X	X		X	X	X	X
South Carolina		X	X	X			X	X
South Dakota		X	X	X			X	X
Tennessee		X	X				X	X
Texas		X	X				X	X
Utah		X	X	X			X	X
Vermont		X						
Virginia		X	X		X	X	X	X
Washington	X	X						X
West Virginia			X					
Wisconsin	X	X	X	X			X	X
Wyoming		X	X				X	X

Source: Alan Guttmacher Institute, Major state abortion-related policies in effect, 2001. Reprinted with permission. Available: http://www.agi-usa.org/pubs/abort_law/sum_1b.html.

Although there has been some concern raised about the psychological health of women as a result of experiencing an abortion, there is little evidence that women are negatively affected. In a study of more than 5,000 American women, those who had had an abortion actually had higher self-esteem and greater feelings of self-worth and capability than women who had not had an abortion (Russo & Zierk, 1992). Interestingly, women with a greater number of births or at least one unwanted birth had lower self-esteem than other women did.

Attitudes About Abortion: Changing and Unchanging

Since *Roe v. Wade,* attitudes toward abortion have been evolving, and many studies have attempted to identify Americans' attitudes. Most of these studies, though, asked only a few questions, leaving the interpretation of the results unclear (Cook, Jelen, & Wilcox, 1993). In 1989, CBS News and the *New York Times* conducted a national poll on abortion attitudes that included a wide variety of questions on abortion. Table IF2.2 presents the results of that survey. As noted in Table IF2.2, more than three-quarters of Americans agreed that abortion should be legal if the woman's health were endangered, if the pregnancy resulted from the woman's being raped, or if the fetus had

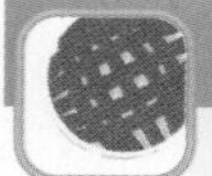

Global DIMENSIONS

A Worldwide Preference for Boys

Around the world, on average, there are 105 boys born for every 100 girls born. Yet in China, there are 111 boys born for every 100 girls. Why is China so different from the rest of the world? Unfortunately, it is not.

Throughout the world, especially in densely populated countries, there are many reasons that boy babies are preferred, most based on long-term gender bias. China has no social security system, leaving elders vulnerable. In a country where couples are encouraged to have only one child, boys are presumed to be more valuable, because they are able to work and support their parents as they age. Either girls are not able to earn enough money to support their parents, or they are married off and assume duties with their new families. This situation is exacerbated as China becomes a more capitalistic country requiring men to travel for business purposes, while women are expected to stay at home. Men's travel earns money and makes them still more valuable in the eyes of many Chinese parents.

So the preference is for boy babies, but what is done to ensure that more boys will be born than girls? The shocking answer is female infanticide. When a Chinese woman delivers a baby, the village midwife sometimes prepares a bucket of water in which, if it is a girl, the baby's head is submerged before she starts to breathe. In India, where boy babies are preferred to girl babies for many of the same reasons as in China, female infanticide takes on a slightly different form. Pregnant Indian women have amniocentesis to determine the gender of their fetus. If the fetus is a girl, they undergo an abortion. Although the Indian authorities attempted to outlaw the use of amniocentesis for this purpose, the populace became outraged and refused to change this practice.

Looking at the female infanticide practices from the eyes of Western culture, experts have concluded that until gender equality is achieved around the world, female infanticide will be difficult to eradicate. Along with female genital mutilation (discussed earlier in this book), female infanticide may be culturally based. Some people believe that Western culture should refrain from interfering with the practices of other cultures. Others believe that in this case interference is warranted. What do you believe?

a serious defect. Americans were less sure that abortion should be legal if desired for economic or social reasons. Approximately half of the respondents agreed abortion should be legal if the family were not able to afford the child, if the woman were unmarried, or if the birth would cause the woman to drop out of school. Only a little more than one-third believed abortion should be legal if the birth would interrupt a career. However, 70% agreed that the government should not ban abortion, and almost 60% agreed that it should be legal if the doctor agreed to it.

The CBS/*New York Times* poll was repeated in 1998 (*New York Times*, 1998). According to this study, whereas in 1989 41% of Americans believed abortion should be legal (generally available), in 1998 only 32% supported that point of view. In 1989, 41% of respondents believed that abortion ought to be difficult to obtain. That percentage increased to 45% in 1998. In 1989, 19% thought abortion ought not be legal under any circumstances. In 1998 that number changed to 22%. Americans are still overwhelmingly in support of abortion being available when the pregnancy poses a risk to the woman's health, if the pregnancy is a result of rape, and if the fetus has a serious defect. In 1998, only 25% believed abortion should be available if

TABLE IF2.2 **CBS/*New York Times* Abortion Attitude Poll Results**

Questions	1989 Percentage Agreeing	1998 Percentage Agreeing
Should abortion be legal if the		
Woman's health is endangered	91	88
Woman is raped	87	NA
Fetus has serious defect	76	75
Family cannot afford child	51	43
Woman is married but does not want more children	NA	39
Woman is unmarried	51	62
Woman does not want to marry the father	50	38
Birth would force school dropout	48	42
Birth would interrupt career	37	25
None of the above	6	NA
All of the above	31	NA
Abortion should be		
Generally available	41	32
Difficult to obtain	41	45
Not available	18	22
Government should not ban abortion		
Agree	70	60
Depends	4	NA
Disagree	26	NA
Reasons abortions occur are not serious enough		
Agree	41	49
Abortion should be permitted during		
First trimester	NA	61
Second trimester	NA	15
Third trimester	NA	7

NA, Not available.

pregnancy interrupted a career (down from 35% in 1989), and 62% opposed abortion simply because the woman was unmarried (up from 51% in 1989). Finally, Americans still want the government out of abortion. In 1998, 60% said the government should not get involved in the legality of abortion, more than three-quarters opposed the idea of a constitutional amendment banning abortion, and 60% believed that the *Roe v. Wade* decision was a good one.

Some new information was uncovered as well. For example, in 1998 support for abortion was dependent on when the abortion occurred. Sixty-one percent favored a woman's right to abortion during the first trimester. Only 15% supported abortion during the second trimester, and 7% were supportive during the last trimester. Also, 80% of the 1998 respondents supported parental consent and waiting periods before abortions could be performed.

Availability of Legal Abortion

It is becoming increasingly difficult for a woman to have an abortion in the United States. According to a study by the Alan Guttmacher Institute, more than 84% of counties in the United States do not have an abortion provider (Henshaw & Van Vort, 1994). And most OB–GYN residency programs do not require doctors to know how to do a first-trimester abortion: Only 12% of such programs require this training, and 30% offer no first-trimester training (MacKay & MacKay, 1995).

Further, many abortion clinics are picketed on a regular basis. In many cities, college students volunteer as escorts at local abortion clinics in order to assure that women can use the clinic without interference.

Violence has also plagued many abortion clinics. From 1996 to 1997, the number of arsons doubled and bombings tripled against abortion clinics (National Abortion Federation, www.prochoice.org/index.html). There were 18 women's health clinic arsons or bombings in 1997 and 1998 (Feminist Majority Foundation, 1998). Abortion providers have been murdered at the clinics they work at in Florida and Massachusetts. On October 23, 1998, an obstetrician was murdered in his home by a sniper because he provided abortions. Since the 9/11 terrorist attacks, more than 500 reproductive health clinics and women's rights organizations have received false anthrax threats (Alan Guttmacher Institute, 2001).

Thirty-one states have passed laws requiring that adolescents have parental consent for abortion. Fourteen states have passed laws requiring a woman to have to make more than one visit to a clinic to have an abortion, insisting on a "waiting period." Twenty-eight states have passed laws banning certain types of abortion procedures. Only 16 states have passed laws to address harassment and violence against abortion providers (SIECUS, 1998).

Public and Private Funding for Abortion

The patchwork of state laws concerning public funding for abortion services is complex. As a result of the Hyde Amendment, the use of federal Medicaid funds for abortion is prohibited except in cases in which the woman's life is in danger. The amendment was expanded in 1993 to include situations in which the pregnancy resulted from rape or incest. Each state establishes its own abortion funding policy related to state revenues. In 1998, 15 states funded abortion in their state medical assistance programs in all or most circumstances. Eleven states ban insurance coverage for abortion unless women pay an extra premium.

Emotions and Abortion

The emotional reactions to abortion are varied. Some women feel guilty, depressed, angry, and ashamed. Others feel none, or just a limited extent, of these feelings. The same range of emotions may apply to male partners as well.

Religious and moral beliefs; reactions of the medical staff, relatives, and friends; and the strength of the relationship between the partners all affect emotional responses (Moseley, et al., 1981). In addition, the earlier the abortion is performed, the lower the emotional cost. Perhaps the lack of humanlike features of the conceptus is what influences this finding. Realizing this, a film was developed by opponents of abortion and shown widely in the United States. Entitled *The Silent Scream,* this film is a 28-minute depiction of an abortion using ultrasound visualization. The viewers see a 12-week-old fetus being aborted by vacuum curettage and supposedly screaming in pain. The narrator, Dr. Bernard N. Nathanson, makes one feel that abortion is akin to infanticide because, he argues, "The unborn child is just another human being . . . all the rest of his human functions are indistinct from any of ours." Many physicians and others have taken issue with Dr. Nathanson. For example, the American College of Obstetricians and Gynecologists responded to *The Silent Scream* with a statement that there is no scientific evidence to support the assertion that a 12-week-old fetus feels pain. Others have argued the following points (Spake, 1985):

1. The cerebral cortex of a 12-week-old fetus is insufficiently developed to feel pain.
2. Fetal movements are the result of reflexive action rather than "frantic activity" away from "the abortionist's instruments."
3. Because the mouth of the fetus cannot actually be identified in the film, and because there is no air inside the fetus's lungs, the "scream" is no scream at all.
4. The fetal model used by Dr. Nathanson as he narrates is much larger than a 12-week-old fetus. In addition, many of the "fetuses" shown in the film are not fetuses but rather stillborn, premature infants.

The Silent Scream is but one example of the extreme emotion associated with the issue of abortion. Abortion facilities have been bombed, and staff and patients have been targets of harassment. Reputable abortion facilities provide counseling before the abortion to help the woman, alone or with her partner, make sure that she does indeed want an abortion performed—it is usually considered the best of several bad choices. In addition they provide counseling after the abortion to lessen the emotional costs associated with this decision. These functions are difficult to perform

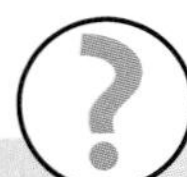

Did You Know . . .

On January 22, 2001, President George W. Bush reinstated the Global Gag Rule. This policy restricts foreign nongovernmental agencies that receive funds from the U.S. Agency for International Development from

- Providing legal abortions, except in the case of rape, incest, or endangerment of the woman's life
- Lobbying their governments to legalize abortion or to decriminalize abortion
- Providing advice or information regarding the availability of abortion and referring women to another clinic that offers abortion services
- Conducting educational campaigns regarding abortion

Consequently, health care organizations need to decide whether to give up needed funds for family planning and other reproductive services or to give up their rights of free speech and to provide their patients with complete and accurate medical information.

Do you think this rule is wise policy? If so, why? If not, why not?

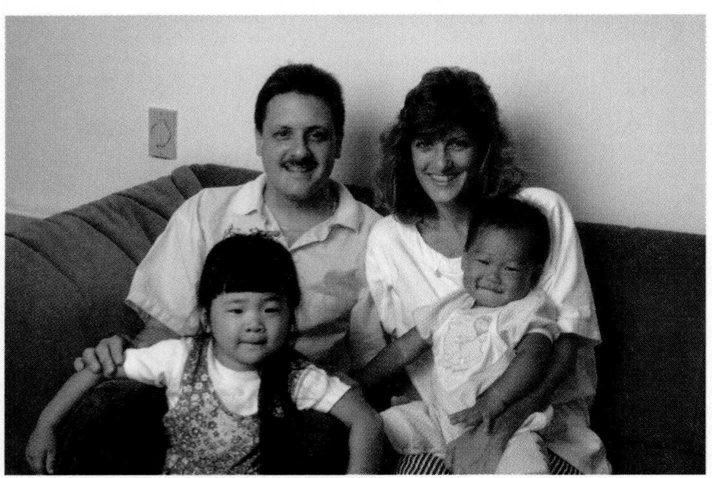

For many reasons individuals or couples may choose to adopt. International adoptions are among many options available.

well in the face of bomb threats, actual bombings, arson directed at abortion facilities, or picketing and/or harassment of patients seeking services at these facilities. Furthermore, some professionals choose not to subject themselves to this type of treatment and therefore refuse to work at abortion facilities. Of course, some refuse to work there because of their own moral objections as well.

Adoption

Another response to an unwanted pregnancy is delivery of the baby, followed by adoption placement. Women who are unwed and choose not to raise a baby or who do not have the financial resources necessary to raise a baby often select adoption as an alternative for providing a good life for their babies.

Types of Adoptions

There are two basic types of adoption (Kolander, et al., 1999). *Closed adoptions* are confidential; there is no contact between the birth parents and the adoptive parents. The identities of the birth parents and adoptive parents are kept secret. *Open adoptions* allow contact between the birth parents and the adoptive parents. In fact, the birth parents may even select the adoptive parents. Contact can occur regularly or intermittently throughout the child's upbringing.

Although there have been some highly publicized cases of birth parents' seeking to reverse them, adoptions are legally binding and irreversible after a limited period. Birth parents sign "relinquishment papers" after the baby is born, and, unless both birth parents have not signed these papers, the courts have refused to reverse adoptions.

Adoptions are arranged in three ways: agency adoption, independent adoption, and adoption by relatives (Planned Parenthood, 1998). In the case of *agency adoption,* the parents relinquish their baby to an adoption agency. These agencies are licensed by the government and may offer a number of services. They provide counseling, handle legal matters, make hospital arrangements for the birth, select adoptive parents, and refer the mother to agencies if financial assistance is needed. Usually, though not always, adoptions arranged through agencies are closed adoptions. Adoption agencies can be located through contacting most religious organizations, or by writing to the National Council for Adoption at 1930 17th Street, NW, Washington, DC 20009 or phoning them at (202) 328-1200. They accept collect calls from pregnant women.

In *independent adoptions,* the birth parents select the adoptive parents and relinquish the baby into their care. Independent adoptions are often arranged through a physician or a lawyer and, in some states, by independent adoption centers. Independent adoptions are usually open adoptions and, although not legal in all states, are supervised by a lawyer, who usually represents both sides. However, it is often recommended that the birth parents and the adoptive parents have separate legal representation to protect them from being exploited. Often, the adoptive parents agree to pay

Gender DIMENSIONS

Baby "Richard" In June 1990, Daniella Janikova and Otakar Kirchner, both immigrants from what is now Slovakia, conceived baby "Richard" (his name has been changed to protect his identity). However, before Richard's birth, Otakar returned to his country with a former girlfriend, leaving Daniella in the United States. Before the delivery, Daniella arranged to place Richard for adoption. Daniella was then introduced to the "Warburtons," a pseudonym for a family interested in adopting Daniella's baby. Daniella signed the necessary forms to arrange for the Warburtons to adopt Richard. However, under Illinois law, the father has to agree to an adoption. When Daniella was asked for the name and address of the father, she refused to give it, falsely stating that he had abused her. Richard was born on March 16, 1991.

A few days after Richard's birth, Otakar received a call informing him that Richard had died. One month later, however, he learned that the baby was alive, and soon he returned to Daniella. Otakar then hired an attorney, who started legal proceedings for the return of his child. Subsequently, he and Daniella were married.

The Warburtons, however, contested the return of Richard, and a Cook County Circuit Court judge ruled the adoption valid, declaring Otakar unfit largely because he had not filed a petition within 30 days of the birth (as required in Illinois) and because the prior testimony of Daniella alleged that he was abusive. However, when this decision was appealed, the Illinois Supreme Court in June 1994—after Richard had been living with the Warburtons for more than 3 years—overturned the adoption, stating that Otakar was led to believe that Richard had died and, therefore, could not have been expected to pursue his parental rights in a timely fashion.

After several appeals to the United States Supreme Court proved unsuccessful, Otakar and Daniella took custody of Richard on April 30, 1995. At the time of the wrenching transfer, Richard appealed to his adoptive mother, "I'll be good. Don't make me leave. I'll be good."

This case, tragic as it was for all parties, was decided on the rights of the father to agree to adoption of his biological offspring. That right is protected even if the biological mother chooses to place the child for adoption and, apparently, even if the child has been living with adoptive parents for many years.

the medical costs associated with the pregnancy and may even agree to pay for living expenses during that time. At the birth of the baby, the adoptive parents sign a "take into care" form that allows the adoptive parents to take the baby to their home while the state investigates their ability to raise the baby. This investigation usually takes 6 to 8 weeks. At any time while this investigation is occurring, either set of parents can change their minds. At the end of the investigation, the birth parents sign "relinquishment papers." Independent adoption can be facilitated by the Independent Adoption Center at 319 Taylor Boulevard, Suite 100, Pleasant Hills, CA 94523. Their telephone number is (800) 877-OPEN.

Adoption by relatives is used when the birth parents want the child to stay in the family. Even so, these adoptions require the approval of the courts. As in other adoptions, the relative is investigated by the state to determine ability to provide care for the child. Once the adoption is approved, the birth parents have no more rights pertaining to the child than they would in any other form of adoption.

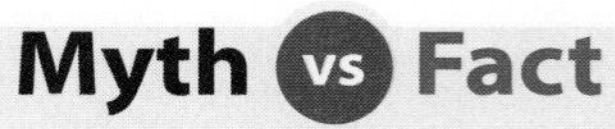

Myth: Most abortions are performed late in the pregnancy.
Fact: Ninety percent of all abortions are performed during the first trimester. These abortions are usually performed by vacuum aspiration.

Myth: Abortion is a dangerous procedure.
Fact: The risk of death during childbirth is 10 times greater than it is during abortion procedures. Furthermore, less than 1% of abortion patients experience a major complication.

Myth: Late-term abortions result in partial birth of the baby.
Fact: Opponents of abortion have labeled late-term abortion "partial birth abortion." This is a political tactic rather than an accurate description of late-term abortions. The correct term for these abortions is dilation and evacuation (D & E).

Myth: Adoptions have to be coordinated through an adoption agency.
Fact: Adoptions can be arranged independently, although these adoptions require court approval. In addition, adoptions can be arranged with relatives, although, again, they require court approval.

Myth: The withholding of the names of the birth parents (confidentiality and anonymity) is guaranteed by agencies and courts that arrange adoptions.
Fact: There is a debate taking place in our society regarding the rights of the birth parents versus the rights of the child. Several states have passed or are considering legislation to unseal adoption records.

Contemplating Adoption

Adopting a child is a decision that requires a great deal of consideration. So does the decision to give a child up for adoption. Planned Parenthood of America suggests that anyone considering giving a child up for adoption ask these questions:

1. Can you accept your child living with someone else?
2. Will going through pregnancy and delivery change your mind?
3. Are you willing to get good prenatal care?
4. Are you choosing adoption because abortion scares you?
5. Will the child's father approve of adoption?
6. Is anyone pressuring you to choose adoption?
7. Are you confident your child will be treated well?
8. Can you not be jealous of the adoptive parents?
9. Do you care what other people will think?
10. Do you respect women who place their children for adoption?

Someone contemplating placing a child for adoption may want to discuss these questions with her partner, clergy, professional counselor, or a trusted relative or friend.

Foster Care and Adoption

For parents who are not ready to decide between placing a child for adoption and parenting, many cities and counties provide temporary residences for their children. This arrangement is termed *foster care.* To arrange for this option, the birth parents must sign a legal foster care agreement that allows another family to care for the child. Often, foster care agreements specify the frequency of visits between the child and birth parents that will be allowed, the duration of stay with the foster care family, the amount of money the birth parents will have to provide the foster care parents for caring for their child, and the number and frequency of visits to a professional counselor (usually a social worker). Although foster care arrangements and regulations vary from state to state, if the foster care agreement is violated, the birth parents can lose the child permanently.

Foster care is also provided for children who are taken from their birth parents for abuse, neglect, or other behavior that precludes them from being able to raise their children and places their children at risk. Children placed in foster care permanently are eligible for adoption, and, in fact, that is the goal of state agencies that supervise foster care arrangements.

The U.S. foster care system includes more than 500,000 children, of which 126,000 are eligible for adoption. Fortunately, more and more of these children are being adopted. In 1995, 20,000 children in the foster care system were adopted. That number increased to 28,000 in 1996 and to 31,000 in 1997. In 1997, the U.S. Congress passed the Adoption and Safe Families Act, designed to speed up adoption of children in the foster care system. That legislation provided bonuses of $4,000 to states for every child in the child protective system for whom they arranged adoption. For particularly difficult cases—such as older children or those with disabilities—states were provided $6,000 for each adoption. To further the goal of arranging for adoptions of children in foster care, in November 1998 President

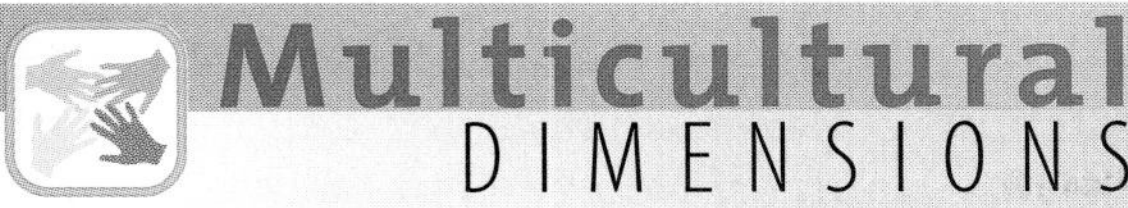

International Adoptions Many children from other countries are adopted by Americans. These adoptions may be the result of humanitarian concern of people who see children orphaned by war or widespread disease or difficulty in locating the type of American child they wish to adopt. These international adoptions, though, can be very costly. After travel and other expenses are considered, international adoptions can run as high as $30,000. Table IF2.A shows the numbers of international children adopted by Americans in comparison to the numbers of children adopted by citizens of developed countries. It is evident from this table that Americans adopt a greater number of international children than all of the other developed countries.

Given that there are American children waiting to be adopted, should the federal government discourage international adoptions? If so, what will happen to children orphaned by war or abused or neglected in other countries? Or should people wanting to adopt children be supported wherever those children come from?

sexuality.jbpub.com

TABLE IF2.A International Adoptions by Country

By Americans in 1998	
TOTAL: 15,774	
Russia	4,491
China	4,206
S. Korea	1,829
Guatemala	911
Vietnam	603
India	478
Romania	406
Colombia	351
Cambodia	249
Philippines	200
Others	2,050

By Canadians in 1998	
TOTAL: 2,222	
China	901
India	178
Russia	160
Haiti	156
Romania	91
Others	738

By French in 1998	
TOTAL: 3,777	
Vietnam	1,343
Colombia	294
Romania	178
Madagascar	174
Russia	156
Others	1,632

By Germans in 1996	
TOTAL: 1,567*	
Russia	150
Romania	130
India	130
Bosnia and Yugoslavia	90
Brazil	89
Turkey	72
Others	832

By Britons in 1998	
TOTAL: 258**	
China	129
Guatemala	27
India	22
Romania	17
Russia	13
Thailand	13
Others	37

*Includes international children who already were in Germany.
**Between 1993 and 1998 Britons adopted a total of 1,159 children from abroad.
Sources: U.S. State Department; Associated Press; national government agencies.

Clinton announced a plan to create an Internet site that would carry photographs and information about these children (Vobejda, 1998). The hope was that it would facilitate matching children eligible for adoption with parents seeking to adopt. Most states maintain web sites to facilitate adoption of children in the foster care system. Still other states provide information to private agencies who maintain web sites. In 2001, 50,000 children in the foster care system were adopted (Administration for Children and Families, 2003).

Finding the Birth Parent

Because they seek to determine their complete history or because they are curious or have some other reason, many adults who were adopted seek to identify their birth parents. There is a good deal of disagreement as to whether and how this process should be facilitated. Some experts believe that contacting the birth parents might make them feel guilty about the adoption. Also, the birth parents might reject the adopted person, who might then have an unhealthy reaction to that rejection.

Before World War II, it was common practice for adoption records to be open. However, after the war, the combination of an increase in out-of-wedlock pregnancies and a conservative mood in the country resulted in adoption's going "into the closet." Adoption records became sealed so that secrecy could be maintained. Since then, only two states, Alaska and Tennessee, have passed legislation to open these records.

More recently, residents of the state of Oregon decided this issue for themselves (Sanchez, 1998). In November 1998 Oregon voters approved a ballot initiative requiring the state to unseal confidential birth records. On request, adoptees would be given all the information about their past—in spite of the wishes of their birth parents. As you can imagine, this precipitated an outcry from opponents and supporters alike. The American Civil Liberties Union opposed the initiative, arguing that it was an invasion of the privacy earlier promised to birth parents who placed their children for adoption. Supporters argued that the question was, Who should have more rights? A parent who gives up a child or the child who was adopted? Clearly they came down on the side of the child. Since Oregon's decision, two other states have adopted an unqualified right to view adoption records—Tennessee and Alabama—and two other states make records available if birth parents have not filed an objection—Delaware and Nebraska.

Discussion Questions

1. What are the methods of abortion, and in what situations are they used?
2. Create a personal chart showing your own dimensions of human sexuality that relate to the abortion issue. After seeing all the issues involved, have you altered your position on abortion?
3. Explain the types of adoption available and the way each works.

Application Questions

Reread the chapter-opening story and answer the following questions.

1. The author Anna Quindlen appears to take a situational view of abortion: She thought abortion was OK for a bright college student but had second thoughts about an older and financially secure adult (herself). Does situation matter? In which situations is it acceptable to get an abortion? In which situations is it unacceptable?
2. The chapter also mentions the possibility of adoption. Should Quindlen have counseled her freshman with information about adoption? Explain why or why not.

Critical Thinking Questions

1. When the issue of abortion versus adoption is discussed, the father rarely enters into the discussion. Should the father have control over whether or not a woman can have an abortion or give a child up for adoption?
2. When do you believe that life begins? At conception? At a certain point in fetal development? At about 24 weeks, when the fetus can survive outside the womb (albeit with neonatal intensive care)? At about 35 weeks, when most babies can sustain life without medical intervention? Explain your decision.
3. Because many infertile couples want to adopt a child, why are there not more incentives for women to place children of unexpected pregnancies up for adoption? What could be done to motivate such a practice? Should the federal government be involved in such an effort?

Critical Thinking Case

In the late 1970s, Dr. Milfred Jefferson, an African-American surgeon and chairperson of the national Right to Life organization, stated that abortion was genocide. She believed that a federally funded abortion program was aimed at eliminating the poor, African-American population of the United States. Dr. Jefferson cited statistics showing that 30% of all abortions funded by Medicaid were performed on African Americans (while African Americans made up about 11% of the population). She said that "abortion is accomplishing what 200 years of slavery and 300 years of lynching didn't."

Opponents argue that the disproportionate number of Medicaid-funded abortions performed on African-American women resulted from higher representation of African Americans among the poor in the United States; hence, they would have more need of financial support for abortions. Along these lines, people of lower socioeconomic status have less access to sex education, birth control information, and prescription birth control.

Abortion rates are still disproportionately high for African Americans (National Center for Health Statistics, 2000). In 1997, the abortion rate for whites was 19.3 per 100 live births; the abortion rate for Hispanics was 26.8 per 100; the abortion rate for African Americans was 54.3 per 100—2.8 times the rate for whites!

Exploring Personal Dimensions

What is your feeling about abortion? Place an A, B, C, D, or E in the blank to the left of each of the thirty items below, using the provided scale:

A. I *strongly agree* with the statement.

B. I *tend to agree* with the statement (some reservation).

C. I am *undecided* (uncertain about my feelings or have no feelings one way or the other).

D. I *tend to disagree* with the statement (some reservation).

E. I *strongly disagree* with the statement.

_______ 1. Abortion penalizes the unborn for the mother's mistake.

_______ 2. Abortion places human life at a very low point on a scale of values.

_______ 3. A woman's desire to have an abortion should be considered sufficient reason to do so.

_______ 4. I approve of the legalization of abortion so that a woman can obtain one with proper medical attention.

_______ 5. Abortion ought to be prohibited because it is an unnatural act.

_______ 6. Having an abortion is not something to be ashamed of.

_______ 7. Abortion is a threat to our society.

_______ 8. Abortion is the destruction of one life to serve the convenience of another.

_______ 9. A woman should have no regrets if she eliminates the burden of an unwanted child with an abortion.

_______ 10. The unborn [child] should be legally protected against abortion because it cannot protect itself.

_______ 11. Abortion should be an alternative when there is contraceptive failure.

_______ 12. Abortions should be allowed because the unborn [child] is only a potential human being, and not an actual human being.

_______ 13. Any person who has an abortion is probably selfish and unconcerned about others.

_______ 14. Abortion should be available as a method of improving community socioeconomic conditions.

_______ 15. Many more people would favor abortion if they knew more about it.

_______ 16. A woman should have an illegitimate child rather than an abortion.

_______ 17. Liberalization of abortion laws should be viewed positively.

_______ 18. Abortion should be illegal, for the Fourteenth Amendment in the Constitution holds that no state shall "deprive any person of life, liberty, or property without due process of law."

_______ 19. The unborn child should never be aborted no matter how detrimental the possible effects on the family.

_______ 20. The social evils involved in forcing a pregnant woman to have a child are worse than any evils in destroying the unborn child.

_______ 21. Decency forbids having an abortion.

_______ 22. A pregnancy that is not wanted and not planned for should not be considered a pregnancy, but merely a condition for which there is a medical cure, abortion.

_______ 23. Abortion is the equivalent of murder.

_______ 24. Easily accessible abortions will probably cause people to become unconcerned and careless with their contraceptive practices.

_______ 25. Abortion ought to be considered a legitimate health measure.

_______ 26. The unborn child ought to have the same rights as the potential mother.

_______ 27. Any outlawing of abortion is oppressive to women.

_______ 28. Abortion should be accepted as a method of population control.

_______ 29. Abortion violates the fundamental right to life.

_______ 30. If a woman feels that a child might ruin her life she should have an abortion.

Source: Snegroff, S. *Abortion attitude scale.* Saluda, NC: Copyright Family Life Publications. Reprinted by permission.

To score this instrument, use the following point values for items 3, 4, 6, 9, 11, 12, 14, 15, 17, 20, 22, 25, 27, 28, and 30 only: A = 5, B = 4, C = 3, D = 2, E = 1.

For items 1, 2, 5, 7, 8, 10, 13, 16, 18, 19, 21, 23, 24, 26, and 29 use the following scale: A = 1, B = 2, C = 3, D = 4, E = 5.

Now add your points; the score should fall between 30 and 150. A score of 30 represents an unfavorable attitude, a score of 90 represents a neutral attitude, and a score of 150 represents a favorable attitude toward abortion.

Sexuality Online

Go to the web component for *Exploring the Dimensions of Human Sexuality* at sexuality.jbpub.com for web exercises, additional resources related to this chapter, and student review tools.

Suggested Readings

Gorney, C. *Articles of faith: A frontline history of the abortion wars.* New York: Simon & Schuster, 1998.

Henshaw, S. K. Factors hindering access to abortion services, *Family Planning Perspectives, 27* (1995), 54–59, 87.

Henshaw, S. K. Unintended pregnancy in the United States, *Family Planning Perspectives, 30* (1998), 24–29, 46.

Kincaid, J. *Adopting for good: A guide for people considering adoption.* Grove, IL: Intervarsity Press, 1997.

Saul, R. Abortion reporting in the United States: An examination of the federal-state partnership, *Family Planning Perspectives, 30* (1998), 204–211.

Sifferman, K. A. & Strohm, R. L., eds. *Adoption: A legal guide for birth and adoptive parents (layman's law guide).* Edgemont, PA: Chelsea House, 1997.

CHAPTER 10

Sexual Techniques and Behavior

FEATURES

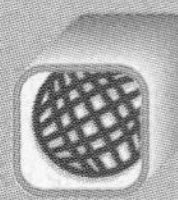

Global Dimensions
Global Religious Views on Sexuality

Gender Dimensions
Differences Between Male and Female Sexual Fantasies

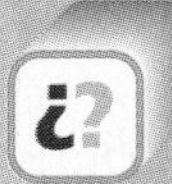

Ethical Dimensions
Should People Who Do Not Feel Comfortable with Oral or Anal Sexual Activity Learn to Enjoy These Activities?

Multicultural Dimensions
Does Level of Education Influence Sexuality?

Communication Dimensions
Word Choice Affects Study Results

CHAPTER OBJECTIVES

1 Identify the historical basis for present-day societal, religious, and/or cultural attitudes toward masturbation.

2 Cite the prevalence of sexual fantasy, describe its content and function, and note differences in male and female sexual fantasies.

3 Describe the role of touch, sight, smell, sound, and taste in sexual foreplay. Then list and describe various positions of sexual intercourse, including their advantages and disadvantages.

sexuality.jbpub.com

The Importance of the Senses
Global Dimensions: Global Religious Views on Sexuality

INTRODUCTION

One often hears that the 20th century's sexual revolution has led to more promiscuity and sexual freedom. The following excerpt, written before a different sort of revolution, the American Revolution, shows that many sexual techniques have not changed in a long time:

> *As I kept hesitating and disconcerted under this soft distraction, Charles, with a fond impatience, took the pains to undress me; and all I can remember amidst the flutter and discomposure of my senses was some flattering exclamations of joy and admiration, more specially at the feel of my breasts now set at liberty from my stays, and which panting and rising in tumultuous throbs, swell'd upon his dear touch, and gave it the welcome pleasure of finding them well form'd, and unfail'd in firmness.*
>
> *I was soon laid in bed, and scarce languish'd an instant for the darling partner of it, before he was undress'd and got between the sheets, with his arms clasp'd round me, giving and taking, with gust inexpressible, a kiss of welcome, that my heart rising to my lips stamp'd with its warmest impression, concurring to my bliss, with that delicate and voluptuous emotion which Charles alone had the secret to excite, and which constitutes the very life, the essence of pleasure. . . .*
>
> *But as action was now a necessity to desires so much on edge as ours, Charles, after a very short prelusive dalliance, lifting up my linen and his own, laid the broad treasures of his manly chest close to my bosom, both beating with the tenderest alarms: when now, the sense of his glowing body, in naked touch with mine, took all power over my thoughts out of my own disposal, and deliver'd up every faculty of the soul to the sensiblest of joys, that affecting me infinitely more with my distinction of the person than of the sex, now brought my conscious heart deliciously into play: my heart, which eternally constant to Charles, had never taken any part in my occasional sacrifices to the calls of constitution, complaisance, or interest.*

The preceding excerpt, from John Cleland's 1749 novel Fanny Hill, or Letters of a Woman of Pleasure, *shows that erotic literature has detailed sexual liaisons for centuries.*

Relatively few people actually set out to learn effective sexual arousal techniques. What learning takes place often occurs through trial and error (with plenty of both). The results may be total pleasure, or they may be shame and embarrassment, confusion, and perhaps sexual dysfunction. Furthermore, such naivete and ignorance too often result in unwanted pregnancies. We believe that a strong foundation of sexual knowledge includes not only anatomical and physiological facts but also specific information about what people find sexually stimulating. Therefore, this chapter covers nonphysical means of arousal, as well as techniques in beginning play (foreplay), sexual intercourse, and oral–genital sexual activity.

Solitary Sexual Behaviors

The two solitary sexual behaviors we discuss in this section are masturbation and fantasy. We should note, however, that although these are usually solitary behaviors, they can also be engaged in with a partner in the form of mutual masturbation or shared sexual fantasizing.

Masturbation

masturbation
Self-stimulation of the genitals.

One need not have a partner to be sexually stimulated. **Masturbation** is the stimulation of one's own genitals for sexual pleasure. As Woody Allen said in the movie *Annie Hall,* masturbation is sex with the person you love most.

Negative Attitudes: A Matter of History

Many of our attitudes regarding sexual activity are part of our cultural past. Masturbation is a good example of this. Ancient Hebrews believed they were partners of God in replenishing the Earth. In addition, they needed male

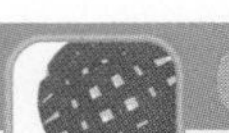

Global DIMENSIONS

Global Religious Views on Sexuality Different religions confront sexual behaviors and sexual mores differently. For example, in Judaism, a *mikva* (ritual bath) is prescribed for women who have just finished menstruating to cleanse her physically and spiritually. Muslims and Jews perform circumcisions as part of their religious rituals, although they perform them at different times and for different reasons. Muslim circumcision of men is a rite of passage into manhood and of women is a means to prevent them from being easily sexually aroused and, therefore, potentially unfaithful to their husbands. In Jewish practice, circumcision is performed only on young male infants 8 days old and represents a covenant with God. In Catholicism, abortion is a sin, because the religion teaches that life begins when fertilization occurs; the mother has no more status than does the unborn. In several other religions, abortion is allowed to remain a decision between the pregnant woman and her physician.

If you have a religion, what does it teach about sexuality? Perhaps you will want to interview a member of the clergy to understand better the rules, regulations, rituals, and rationale behind these teachings.

sexuality.jbpub.com

offspring to maintain the patriarchal system and to supply needed labor. Consequently, laws were enacted to discourage nonprocreative sexual behavior. Any sexual activity that did not potentially lead to conception was devalued.

Many believe this attitude is best represented by the story of Onan in Genesis in the Old Testament. Onan was the brother of Er, whom God slayed because he was "wicked." However, Er had not yet conceived any children with his wife, Tamar. It was Judaic law that the next of kin of the husband must impregnate the widow so that the dead man had an heir. God, therefore, ordered Onan to impregnate Tamar, but Onan, not wanting to sire a child who would not be his, "wasted his seed" on the ground by withdrawing his penis just before ejaculation. The Lord killed Onan for this indiscretion, and, erroneously, masturbation came to be nicknamed *onanism*. Christian mores were influenced greatly by Jewish codes of behavior, and, consequently, masturbation was condemned by Christian law as well.

To this day our attitudes toward masturbation are colored by these ancient proscriptions. For example, although Freud believed masturbation to be a normal childhood practice, he feared that if carried into adulthood it would interfere with the formation of healthy sexual relationships. As recently as 1976 the Vatican stated in a *Declaration on Sexual Ethics* that masturbation was an "intrinsically and seriously disordered act." In 1993, Pope John Paul II reaffirmed that masturbation is an immoral act.

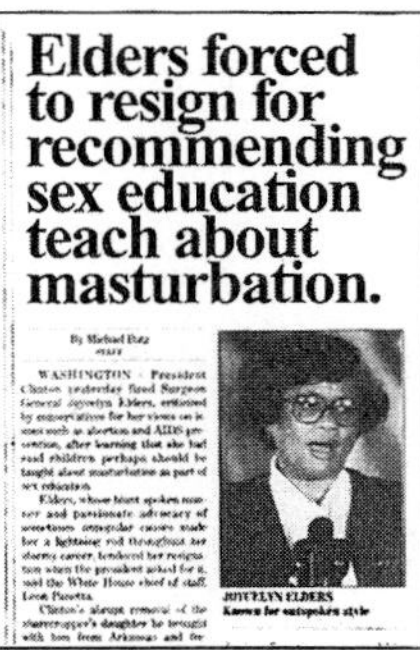

Elders forced to resign for recommending sex education teach about masturbation.

IT APPEARS MASTURBATION IS CAUSING OUR GOVERNMENT TO GO BLIND.

The President can deny Joycelyn Elders her job as Surgeon General. Unfortunately, he cannot deny the fact that today's generation of teenagers is more sexually active than any of its predecessors. A fact that makes an intelligent approach to sex education, even when it includes subjects like masturbation, more important than ever. After all, we live in the age of AIDS. And that's something we should never lose sight of. For information call 1-800-235-2331.

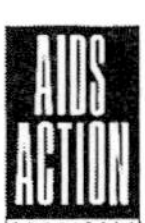

The Danger

No physiological harm can be attributed to masturbation. It will not cause insanity, sterility, sexual dysfunction, or any other physical affliction. Nor is there evidence that masturbation leads to an inability to establish meaningful sexual relationships. The primary danger associated with masturbation is within the individual's own mind—the guilt or shame he or she may feel about masturbating. Masturbation is so common that human sexuality experts now consider it a normal sexual act. It is normal to masturbate, and it is normal not to. As all sexual behaviors are, masturbation is a matter of personal choice. Awareness of this current thinking should go a long way toward alleviating a good deal of the guilt and shame people feel about engaging in this behavior.

Prevalence

As was discussed in Chapter 2, sexual research is fraught with limitations. Consequently we can only present data from several different studies and present a composite view about the prevalence of masturbatory behavior. The majority of studies have found that approximately 90% of adult males and slightly more than 60% of adult females report having masturbated (Arafat & Cotton, 1974; Downey, 1980; Hunt, 1974; Kinsey, Pomeroy, & Martin, 1948, 1953). These figures have remained remarkably consistent through the years (Clement, 1990). In fact, studies in the 1990s found that 60% of American men and 40% of American women had masturbated in the past year. Among couples living together, 85% of the men and 45% of the women had masturbated within the past year (Laumann, et al., 1994; Michael, et al., 1995).

Techniques

Males masturbate by stroking the shaft of the penis, often stimulated by erotic literature, films, or videos. Some men use gadgets to assist them. Artificial vaginas, furlike clothes, inflatable dolls, and other devices have been reported as masturbatory aids by some men.

Women masturbate by rubbing the vulva—in particular, the clitoris—or inserting an object (a finger, a dildo, a banana, or a similarly shaped object) into the vagina. There are, of course, many variations on this theme, and the use of a vibrator to stimulate the vulva, cream to decrease friction on the area rubbed, pillows or other soft objects to rub the genitals against, and squeezing together of the thighs are all common adjuncts to the standard masturbatory techniques (see Figure 10.1).

Masturbation is a pleasurable, common, and varied sexual behavior; it is devoid of physical harm; it is more prevalent in men than women; and it continues even after marriage. The appropriateness of this and other sexual behaviors, however, relates to one's acceptance of them without guilt or shame and one's religious and moral points of view. As with other sexual behaviors, whether to masturbate is a personal choice.

Fantasy

Fantasies are thoughts and images, daydreams, and scenarios. In a sexual context, we call these **sexual fantasies.**

sexual fantasies
Thoughts, images, and daydreams of a sexual nature.

Prevalence of Sexual Fantasies

Sexual fantasies are quite commonplace. One researcher surveyed middle-class women and found that only 7% had never experienced sexual daydreams or fantasies (Hariton, 1973). Earlier, Kinsey had found that 84% of men and 67% of women had sexual fantasies. Other researchers have also found sexual fantasies prevalent; for example, when studying college students, Sue (1979) found that 60% of men and women fantasized during sexual intercourse; Crepault and associates (1977) reported that 94% of their sample of women engaged in sexual fantasies; Zimmer and colleagues (1983) found that 71% of men and 72% of women fantasized about sex in order to become more sexually aroused; and Masters, Johnson, and Kolodny (1985)

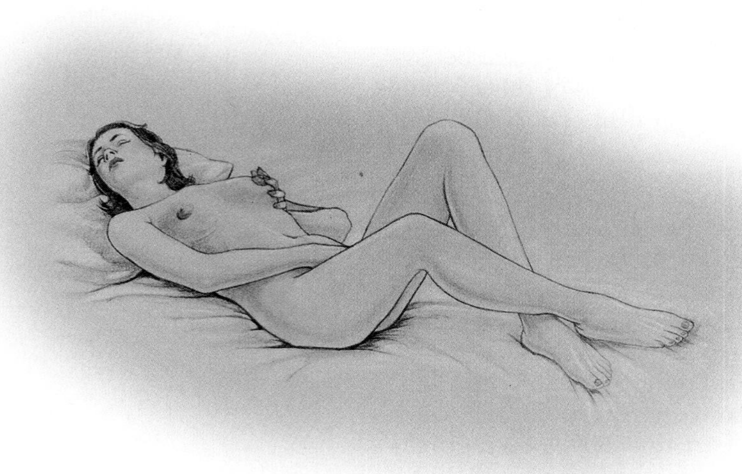

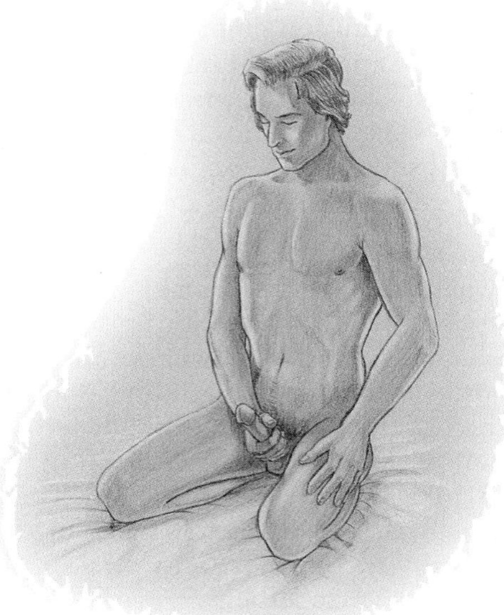

FIGURE 10.1 Masturbatory techniques.

reported that 86% of the women they studied fantasized abut sex. In addition, sexual experience appears related to sexual fantasies. For example, in two studies, women with more coital experience reported more sexual fantasies than women who were virgins or had less sexual experience (Brown & Hart, 1977; Knafo & Jaffe, 1984).

Content of Sexual Fantasies

The content of sexual fantasies is both similar and dissimilar when gender is the variable. Interestingly, when males and females are by themselves they tend to fantasize about engaging in sexual activities with their usual partners; however, when they are engaged in sex with their usual partners, they fantasize about sex with someone else (for example, a movie star or a model)

♂♀ Gender DIMENSIONS

Differences Between Male and Female Sexual Fantasies

In one of the author's college classes, students are asked to write their most erotic fantasy on one side of a sheet of paper. They are then instructed to write the letter *M* or *F* on the back to indicate male or female. Of course, students can opt out of this exercise regarding what males and females find erotic, but they seldom do. The papers are collected and placed face up on a long table. Students read the fantasies, one at a time, and try to determine whether a male or a female wrote each. When all the fantasies are read, the males meet in one room and the females in another and generalize about what the opposite sex seems to find erotic. The following are typical observations:

1. In both male and female fantasies, the males were active and the females passive. In other words, males were doing "it" (whatever "it" happened to be) to the females.
2. The female fantasies involved more of a relationship between the sexual partners than did the male fantasies. For example, many females described sexual activity after a walk on the beach, dinner, or long conversation. Many female fantasies involved people with whom the writer actually had had a long-term relationship, whereas the male fantasies included more quick sex. For instance, some male fantasies involved picking up a hitchhiker and doing "it" in the back seat of the car. Others described encounters with strangers in elevators, shopping malls, or locker rooms.
3. The male fantasies were more likely to include more than one opposite-sex partner; for example, "I walked into my apartment and there were the Dallas Cowboy Cheerleaders. Boy did we get it on!" The female fantasies seldom included more than one sexual partner, but when they did, they were more likely to include both opposite-sex and same-sex partners.
4. Female fantasies included a more detailed description of the setting than did male fantasies. Females described the colors in the room, the music in the background, the candles flickering, or the bright sun-filled, leafy knoll of grass. If males described anything, it was the sexy clothing the objects of their fantasies were in the process of shedding.

The findings from our sexuality class are similar to those reported by other sexuality experts. For example, Barclay (1973) reported male sexual fantasies were more explicit and included less emotional content than did female sexual fantasies, whereas female fantasies included more romantic elements. In a review of the differences between male and female sexual fantasies, Masters, Johnson, and Kolodny (1985, 350) conclude, "Several studies have shown that the sex fantasies of women tend to be more passive than those of men (women tend to visualize their role in the fantasy as having something done to them by someone else, rather than being the active 'doer')." Obviously, there are many exceptions to these findings. Some men include romantic elements in their fantasies and some women do not. Some women include explicit, active sexual behavior by them and some men do not. However, as a generalization, it appears the findings of our students are valid.

TABLE 10.1 Male and Female Sexual Fantasies During Intercourse

Fantasy Content	% Males	% Females
Sex with a former lover	43	41
Sex with an imaginary lover	44	24
Oral–genital sex	61	51
Group sex	19	14
Being forced into a sexual relationship	21	36
Being observed engaging in sexual intercourse	15	20
Being found sexually irresistible by others	55	53
Being rejected or sexually abused	11	13
Forcing others to have sexual relations with you	24	16
Having others give in to you after resisting	37	24
Observing others engaging in sex	18	13
Sex with a member of the same sex	3	9
Sex with animals	1	4

Source: Sue, D. Erotic fantasies of college students during coitus, *The Journal of Sex Research, vol. 15* (1979). Reprinted with permission from The Society for the Scientific Study of Sexuality.

(Leitenberg & Henning, 1995). Although quite a diversity in the content of sexual fantasies exists, other prevalent fantasies are having oral–genital sex, being found sexually irresistible by others, and having sex forced upon oneself. Table 10.1 presents the frequencies of various sexual fantasies by gender. Sexual fantasies may also include group sex, sex with celebrities, voyeuristic activities (peeping or watching others engaged in sex), sadomasochism, or experimentation with other partners or other activities. In a 1995 study that reviewed more than 200 other studies of sexual fantasies, the researchers concluded that women's fantasies tended to include sex with a new male partner, sex with a celebrity, seduction of a younger man or boy, and sex with an older man. Men's favorite fantasies included seeing women nude and having sex with a new female partner, multiple sex partners, and the power to drive women wild (Leitenberg & Henning, 1995).

foreplay
Physical contact preceding sexual intercourse.

Functions of Sexual Fantasies

Sexual fantasies serve several purposes. They are a source of pleasure, and, as such, they enhance sexual arousal. Furthermore, sexual fantasies allow people to test and rehearse various sexual activities if they are concerned about being judged by their partners. In this way the activity is tested in a nonthreatening setting and no one knows whether it works out. And sexual fantasies allow people to acknowledge sexual feelings without acting on them.

There is also research to indicate that sexual fantasies may be helpful in overcoming sexual anxiety (Coen, 1978). Consequently, many sexual therapists encourage fantasies in counseling clients with sexual dysfunctions. In fact, low sexual desire in women has been found to be associated with a lack of sexual fantasizing (Nutter & Condron, 1983).

In addition, sexual fantasies allow us to be "better" than we really are; that is, better lovers, more confident, more experienced, more risky, and more desirable. They also provide us with a safe means of engaging in sexual activities in which we may never wish to participate. For example, though some women fantasize about being forced to have sex, few would actually want that fantasy to come true. It is hypothesized that the frequency with which a woman reports this forced-sex fantasy is a function of her desire to be risqué in her sexual behavior but not accountable for it, because our society generally frowns on sexually adventurous women. Another interpretation of this forced-sex fantasy is that women seek greater power rather than less, so they fantasize that they are so desirable that the man cannot resist (Leitenberg & Henning, 1995). Although Hunt (1974) found twice as many women had this fantasy as men, he did find 10% of men also had submission fantasies.

Sexual fantasies also provide us with a means of fulfilling our every desire while not hurting ourselves or those we love. It is a private and safe way of doing anything we want. It is a means of acting out our wildest dreams while never acting improperly. For example, we may wonder what sex with an animal would be like, or what the experience of sex with our lover's friend would feel like. By fantasizing about these situations we do not harm ourselves, our lovers, or our pets, yet we can experience the situation vicariously. Fantasies of this kind are safe as long as they do not become obsessive. If they do, therapy may be indicated.

There are those who argue that sexual fantasies are unhealthy. For example, Apfelbaum (1980) believes fantasizing during sex with a partner can decrease the degree of trust and intimacy in the relationship. Others have taken a similar point of view (Hollender, 1970; Shainess & Greenwald, 1971). However, the predominant view is that sexual fantasizing can enhance sexual relationships as long as it does not become obsessive and as long as there is no compulsion to act out the fantasy. Some fantasies may be acted out with the consent of the sexual partner, but if one person feels uncomfortable, problems may arise. Guilt or shame may lead to other psychological and/or sexual problems. With the willing consent of both partners, however, acting out sexual fantasies can actually enhance sexual satisfaction and improve the relationship. It appears, though, that most sexual fantasizers do not intend to act out their fantasies, and, if they do, they may be disappointed. Nancy Friday (1975) reports that most individuals who have acted out their sexual fantasies were disappointed. It seems that reality seldom matches fantasy.

Sexual Behavior with Others

Foreplay is the physical contact that usually precedes coitus or oral–genital sexual activity. Generally foreplay includes touching, kissing, biting, and genital fondling. The word *foreplay* is really a misnomer, because this behavior can be enjoyed for itself and need not be a prelude *(fore-)* to anything. All such activity is meant to express love, sensuousness, desire, or all these feelings. We might more appropriately term this activity *pleasuring each other.* However, foreplay does also serve to prepare the participants, both psychologically and physically, for coitus.

The importance of foreplay to sexual enjoyment has been widely acknowledged. Data (Hunt, 1974) shows that unmarried people less than 25 years of age spend an average of 15 minutes in foreplay and another 15 minutes in intercourse, whereas Kinsey's 1948 data showed that a majority of males reached orgasm just 2 minutes after penile insertion. Michael and colleagues (1994) found that for 69% of men and 71% of women, intercourse took from 15 minutes to one hour. Because women need more time to be vaginally lubricated sufficiently for intercourse than men do to achieve erection and be ready (Masters & Johnson, 1966), perhaps this acknowledgment represents an increased understanding of women's needs to be sexually stimulated for a longer period than men before coitus.

Myth vs Fact

Myth: Sexual fantasies mean a person is fixating on sex and needs either to get professional help or to work hard to stop fantasizing.
Fact: Sexual fantasizing is prevalent and is not indicative of a sexual problem. Many males and females fantasize both before and during sexual intercourse, even if engaged in sexual intercourse with their usual partner.

Myth: Women who fantasize about being raped are "sick" and, if raped, get what they deserve.
Fact: First of all, no one "deserves" to be forced to engage in any sexual activity against his or her will. Second, having a fantasy does not indicate that someone actually wants the fantasy to come true. Rape fantasies may even indicate a woman's wish to be so desirable that men cannot resist her rather than a desire to give up control to a male.

Myth: Masturbation is normal for young people but can interfere with the healthy sexual relationship of older people, especially if they are married.
Fact: There is no evidence that masturbation is harmful either physically or psychologically. In fact, there are some times when a sexual partner is unavailable and masturbation can serve as a healthy sexual outlet. Furthermore, many married people with regular sexual intercourse still enjoy masturbating.

Myth: It is unfortunate, but people with disabilities cannot have a meaningful sex life because of the restrictions placed on them by their disabilities.
Fact: Certainly some disabilities place restrictions on sexual positions or sexual stamina. Still, there are many accommodations that can be made so that people who have heart disease, who are physically disabled, or who are ill can achieve and maintain meaningful sexual lives.

The Importance of the Senses

Sexual stimulation in foreplay, intercourse, or any other activity involves the imagination and all of the senses: touch, sight, smell, hearing, and taste.

Touch

Sensual touching is central to sexual stimulation. Although the skin is not a sexual organ as such, stroking the skin on any part of the body can contribute to and even initiate sexual arousal. The gentle stroking of a partner's face, ear, or neck can be both exciting and effective at communicating affection. Furthermore, each manner and intensity of body contact carries its own kind of stimulation. Gentle touching, where the fingers barely make contact with the skin and perhaps focus on one part of the body, can be tantalizing. Caressing—gentle stroking or rubbing—is firmer than gentle touching and communicates affection or appreciation. Firmer touches, too, can be sexually arousing. Hugs, embraces, and squeezes are all expressions of caring. Some might consider a full-body massage the ultimate expression of the sensual touch.

So sensual touching is not necessarily focused on the genitals. But once the body and emotions are primed for sexual activity, touching in and around specific areas of the body is intensely stimulating. The breast (especially the nipple), the inner thighs, the clitoris, the penis, the neck, the ears, and the navel are particularly receptive to sensual touching because of an abundance of nerve endings. However, touching of some of the sensitive genital areas (for example, the vulva or the glans) can result in irritation unless some kind of lubricant is used. Of course, the best lubricant is that produced vaginally by the woman herself. However, any lotion, such as hydroxyethyl cellulose (K-Y) jelly, that does not contain alcohol is also safe and useful for this purpose (unless you are using a condom, in which case Vaseline should not be used). Touching on all parts of the body can be of a teasing nature: moving here, then there, but not there (though almost), then back here. Genital touching should be done in a gentle manner, because rough handling (for example, of a testicle) could result in injury.

We should not overlook the use of touching for sexual self-stimulation. Masturbation is often the method by which people learn which body areas and which types of touching are most stimulating for them. Vibrators have become popular both for masturbating and for sexually stimulating partners. Many couples masturbate each other to orgasm and find this form of sexual activity very exciting and a safe alternative to intercourse.

As with other sexual behaviors, good communication is important for guiding partners in touching each other effectively. Such phrases as "I like that," "That hurts," and "Keep doing that, but just a little more gently (or more firmly)" will help your partner use touching on the specific areas and in the particular ways most stimulating to you. If you are the toucher and do not get this feedback, ask for it.

Sight

The power of visual images is clear everywhere in modern society—for example, in advertising, in films, and in television. These images sometimes work on us without our notice, but it is possible to use sexual imagery consciously for sexual stimulation. Sexual partners sometimes use sexual imagery in books, magazines, films, and photographs to become aroused together. Clothing can also serve this purpose. Men and women often dress in a manner termed sexy, not only to attract others but to add to their partners' or their own sexual excitement. Some people are excited by the sight of hair, eyes, legs, or other body parts. Partners can learn to make use of each other's particular visual stimulants to initiate or enhance sexual arousal.

Smell

The popularity of perfumes and colognes is probably attributable to their potential for arousing sexual interest. It is no small wonder that the old-time bordello is associated with highly perfumed and painted women (even though these ladies might have been a far sight raunchier than their counterparts in the modern media). Animal studies have identified smell as being more important in many species than sight or sound in attracting a mate. Substances called **pheromones** are secreted by some female animals to attract male sexual partners. Conversely, unpleasant smells such as bad breath can interfere with sexual arousal. Attention to normal body hygiene can prevent these problems.

pheromones
Substances that when secreted have a specific scent found to be sexually arousing.

Although it has long been suspected that humans produce pheromones, it is only recently that scientists have verified this. Human pheromones do not actually serve as sexual attractants, but they do alter the timing of women's menstrual cycles. The Monell Chemical Studies Center and the University of Pennsylvania Medical School (Cutler, et al., 1986) studied this issue for several years and found that women who experience coitus weekly are more likely to have normal menstrual cycles, fewer infertility problems, and milder menopauses than women who either are celibate or have sexual intercourse only sporadically (Rensberger, 1986). It seems that male aromatic chemicals secreted from sweat glands in the armpits, nipples, and genitalia are transmitted to their sexual partners by smell and skin absorption. Once transmitted, these chemicals affect the woman's reproductive system.

Women also produce a pheromone that affects other women's menstrual cycles. For years anecdotal reports indicated that women who live together or who work together seem to have synchronous menstrual cycles. These reports now have evidence both to support and to explain them (Preti, et al., 1986).

The manner in which human pheromones work is not fully understood. The suspicion is that molecules of the substances reach receptors of the nervous and endocrine systems and act on them to stimulate signals transmitted in the brain. These brain signals influence the endocrine system's secretion of hormones, and these hormones influence the woman's reproductive system.

There are several potential practical applications of this knowledge regarding human pheromones. For example, nasal sprays might be developed to alleviate certain kinds of infertility problems, to regulate the menstrual cycle (for instance, to make the rhythm method of birth control more effective), or to effect the onset of menopause or minimize its effects.

Hearing

Have you ever heard the expression "Whisper sweet nothings in my ear"? Well, those murmurings are not just nothings! Words and sounds before and during coitus can be sexually stimulating, as can music that contributes to an erotic atmosphere. Sexual talk can take many forms. Some people are aroused by "dirty words," and others are completely turned off by them. Similarly, some people find moaning during sexual activity to be exciting, whereas others are unimpressed with such guttural goings-on. Furthermore, some people report that saying or hearing "I love you" after orgasm can be one of the most exciting and romantic experiences in the world (Haffner and Schwartz, 1998). Once again, communication between sexual partners is the key.

Taste

The use of the mouth can be quite sexually arousing. Kissing, when both partners attend to it, can be intensely stimulating, whatever the variation: open mouth, closed mouth, a nibble here, a nibble there, a tongue darting

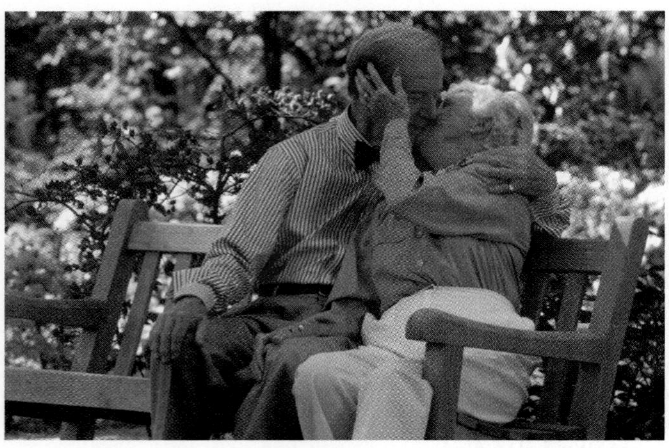

Kissing can be a very erotic, sensual activity in and of itself.

from spot to spot, and lips or teeth closing gently on a sensitive body part. Kissing with tongues touching (soul kissing, French kissing, deep kissing) can also take various forms. More on the use of the mouth, tongue, and teeth is discussed in the section on oral–genital sexual behavior. As with the other senses, taste can also be a turnoff. Obviously French kissing someone who has bad breath or licking a smelly body can be anything but arousing. Proper body hygiene and communication on such simple matters between sexual partners can go a long way toward improving sexual relations.

In the following sections, we discuss specific sexual behaviors and provide guidance for enhancing sexual satisfaction through the use of these activities.

Oral–Genital Sexual Behavior

cunnilingus
The stimulation of the female genitalia by the mouth, lips, and/or tongue of the sexual partner.

fellatio
Oral contact with a male's penis.

69
Two partners' simultaneous stimulation of each other's genitalia orally. The numerals 6 and 9 visually describe the body positions.

Oral–genital sexual behavior involves contact between the mouth, lips, and tongue of one partner and the genitals of another. When a female's genitals are orally stimulated, the act is called **cunnilingus** (meaning in Latin "one who licks the vulva"). When the penis is taken into the partner's mouth, the act is called **fellatio** (from the Latin *fellare,* meaning "to suck"). As with most sexual acts, some find oral–genital sexual contact sexually arousing; others are indifferent to it or find it repulsive. It is generally agreed, however, that oral–genital activity is quite common. Hunt's (1974) study, for example, indicated that 90% of married couples below age 25 years had experienced oral–genital sexual stimulation. More recently, Michael and associates (1994) found that 77% of men and 68% of women reported having given oral sex *to* a partner, and 79% of men and 73% of women had received oral sex *from* a partner.

Many of the techniques described as foreplay are applicable to oral–genital sexual activity. Thus a teasing approach, gentle in nature and varied in form, involving the mouth, lips, and tongue is particularly stimulating. Some women report especially enjoying the licking or sucking of the clitoris and labia minora or a thrusting of the tongue into the vagina. Men are often aroused when their partners lick the underside of the penile shaft and the glans or lick or lightly hold a testicle in the mouth. Again the testicles and clitoris are very sensitive and should be treated gently. And, of course, attention to personal hygiene is important to maximal—and even—minimal—pleasure.

Sexual partners need to discuss whether ejaculation should occur in the mouth during fellatio. Contrary to rumor, the ejaculate is not fattening when swallowed; however, it does have a unique taste. Some like or are indifferent to the taste; others dislike it. One word of caution here, though: Because the ejaculate can contain HIV if the male is infected, unless the relationship has been monogamous for some time and both partners are known to be HIV-free, the ejaculate should not be swallowed. In any case, whether the ejaculate is swallowed or not does not need to diminish the pleasure of either partner.

When couples orally stimulate one another simultaneously, the act is referred to as **69** (because their bodies in position resemble the numbers 6 and 9 (Figure 10.2). Couples can perform 69 side by side or with one partner on top of the other, depending on which position they consider more comfortable and stimulating. Some couples prefer to stimulate one another simultaneously, whereas others find they cannot concentrate on their own pleasurable sensations while concentrating on pleasuring someone else.

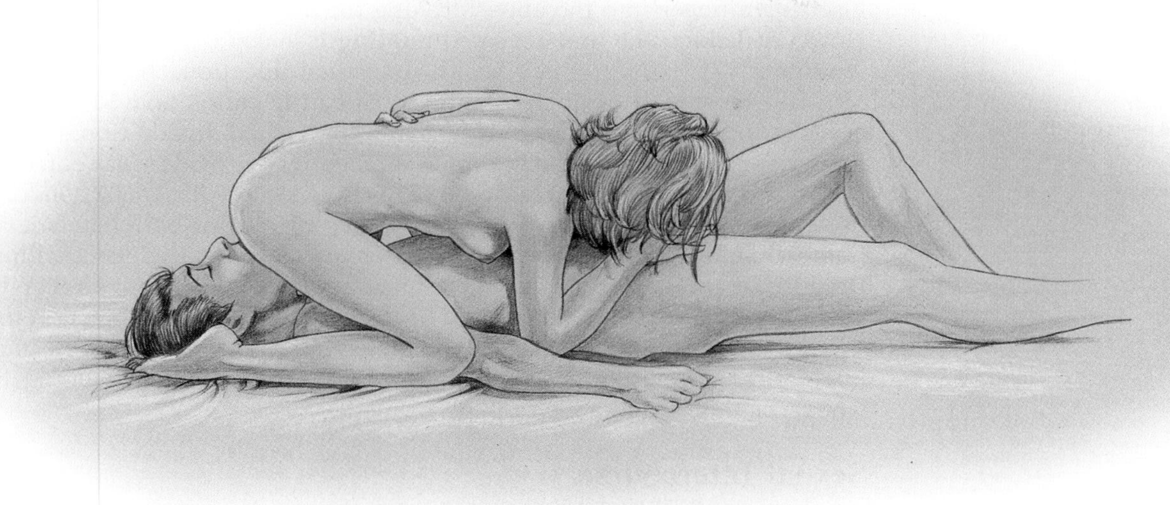

FIGURE 10.2 Simultaneous oral–genital stimulation.

Partners also need to discuss the need for a male to wear a condom and a female a dental dam during oral–genital contact. These behaviors decrease, although they do not eliminate, the possibility of contracting an HIV infection, as well as other sexually transmitted infections. That is why they are called "safer sex" behaviors. To be "safer," partners should consider agreeing to engage in these behaviors.

Ethical DIMENSIONS

Should People Who Do Not Feel Comfortable with Oral or Anal Sexual Activity Learn to Enjoy These Activities?

Some people believe that the more sexual acts one experiences, the more sexually satisfied one will be, and that to enhance our sexual lives, we need a variety of sexual expressions and sexual excitation. They feel that those who are not comfortable with oral–genital sexual activity or anal intercourse ought to be instructed in how to engage in these activities and given counseling to relieve any shame, guilt, or anxiety associated with them. People with this viewpoint argue that to ignore this discomfort is to forever accept a less satisfying sexual life than is possible; and when sexual partners have different desires related to oral and anal sexual activity, there is a threat to the relationship itself.

Others believe that sexual expression can occur in many forms and that no one person need accept all forms for himself or herself. If some sexual activities are uncomfortable, these people argue, choose other activities to include in your sexual repertoire. People should not be coerced into behaviors that they find repulsive; that is not fair. Furthermore, if one partner desires oral or anal sexual activity and the other does not, a good relationship will result if the one who does want these activities understands and accepts the other's feelings. Anything short of that and the relationship is probably not worthwhile anyhow.

What do you believe a couple who disagrees on this issue should do?

Anal Stimulation

analingus
Licking of the anus.

anal intercourse
Insertion of the penis into the anus.

dildos
Artificial penises.

Some people enjoy becoming sexually aroused anally, because there are numerous nerve endings in that area. Partners can stimulate each other by inserting a finger into the anus, stroking the anal opening, or licking the area. However, licking the anus, termed **analingus**—also commonly referred to as "rimming"—is risky to one's health. Intestinal infections, such as *Escherichia coli,* can be spread through analingus, as can hepatitis and STIs. This threat exists even though the anus may be carefully washed. In addition, minute tears that occur in the anus during **anal intercourse** provide easy entry into the body for organisms that cause STIs. This is especially likely if a condom is not used. Penile penetration of the anus is also possible, for both heterosexual and homosexual couples. **Dildos** (fake penises) can also be used for anal insertion. Because of the nature of the anus, one should take care not to tear the surrounding tissue (a lubricant should be used), and to prevent infection the penis should be thoroughly cleansed immediately after anal insertion. Because anal intercourse is one of the risk behaviors for HIV, a condom should be used whenever this sexual activity is performed.

Sexual Intercourse

Variety may truly be the spice of life, at least relative to coital (penile–vaginal intercourse) positions. Although most authorities recognize four basic positions of sexual intercourse, the variations on these themes are infinite. A leg thrown over here, an arm positioned there, a hand fondling this, lips doing that can all slightly alter the sexual experience so that it differs from past experiences. Consequently this section can serve only as a guide, not the last word, on coital positions.

In addition to the desire for variety, other situations—such as pregnancy, obesity, or poor health—may dictate certain modifications. For example, it is more comfortable for a pregnant or obese woman to be on top rather than have her partner press down on her abdomen. Similarly, a man with arthritic knees may not be comfortable with his knees bent in the on-top position. In addition, some coital positions may influence the effectiveness of a condom—male or female. As an example, when the man lies on his back with the woman on top, there may be some seepage of semen from the condom, especially if it is not placed on the penis correctly. When the man is on top, this is not as likely.

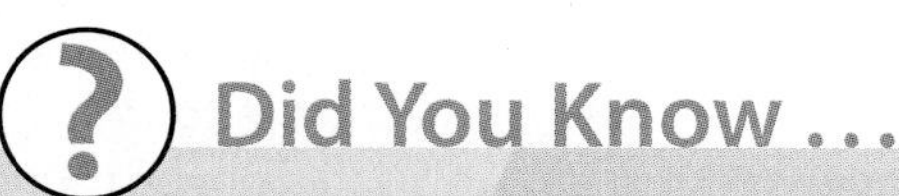

In a study of more than 100 white men and women aged 80 to 102 years who were living in retirement homes, there was more sex than you might imagine. Here are some of the findings:

1. The most common sexual activity was touching and caressing (82% of men and 64% of women). Masturbation was second (72% of men and 40% of women). Sexual intercourse was third (63% of men and 30% of women).
2. Seventy percent of men and 50% of women said they often or very often fantasized or daydreamed about intimate relations with the opposite sex.
3. Only about 25% of men but almost 50% of women said they had no interest in sex.

Source: Ageless sex, *Psychology Today* (March 1989), 62.

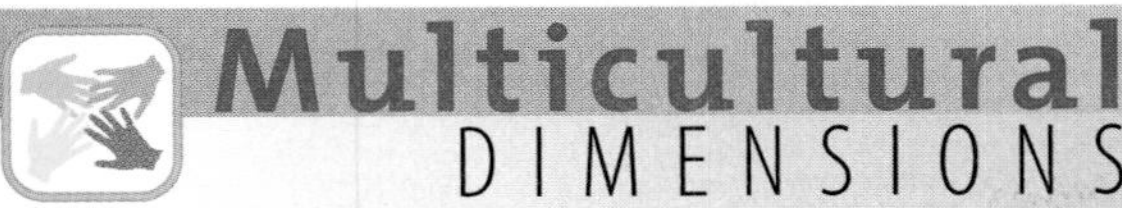

Multicultural DIMENSIONS

Does Level of Education Influence Sexuality?

Sexual practices vary greatly from person to person and from couple to couple. Yet, these practices seem to be influenced by education. Lauman and colleagues (1994) found that sex and education were related in the following ways.

1. Whereas 72% of men with any college education reported their last sexual encounter took between 15 minutes and 1 hour, only 61% of men with less than a high school education reported it took that long. With women, the results were comparable. Seventy-four percent of women with any college education reported their last sexual encounter took between 15 minutes and 1 hour, whereas only 60% of women with less than a high school education reported it took that long.
2. Although 81% of men and 78% of women with some college education reported having ever performed oral sex on a partner, only 59% of men and 41% of women with less than a high school education reported having ever performed oral sex on a partner. And although 84% of men and 82% of women with some college education reported ever having oral sex performed on them, only 61% of men and 50% of women with less than a high school education reported ever having oral sex performed on them.
3. In terms of anal intercourse, 28% of college-educated men and 24% of college-educated women reported ever having that experience, whereas only 21% of men and 13% of women with less than a high school education reported experiencing anal intercourse.

It appears that being educated results in being less conservative sexually. Why do you think that is the case?

1. *Man on top.* The man-on-top position (Figure 10.3) is sometimes called the "missionary position" or the male superior position. The position has a lot going for it: It allows full frontal body contact, which is usually pleasurable; because the couple is lying down, their hands are free to roam; and because they are facing each other, partners can kiss, talk, and watch each other's expressions. This position is also considered the most effective for increasing the chances of pregnancy, but whether or not you call that an advantage depends on your circumstances. On the negative side, sexuality therapists do not recommend this position for men who have difficulty controlling ejaculation.

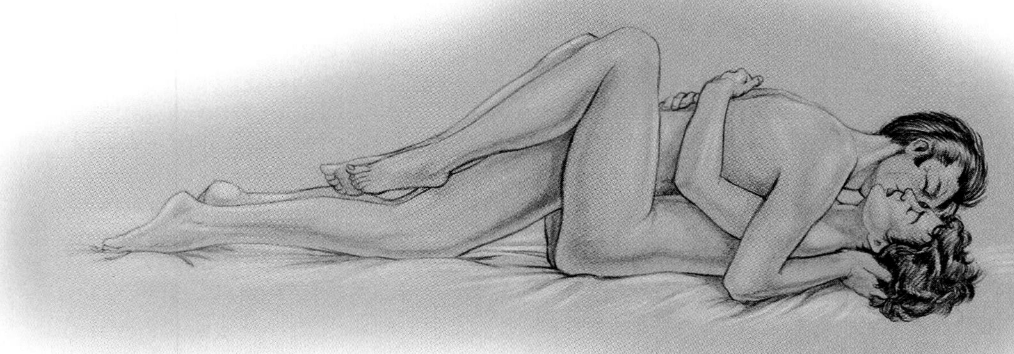

FIGURE 10.3 Man-on-top position.

FIGURE 10.4 Woman-on-top position.

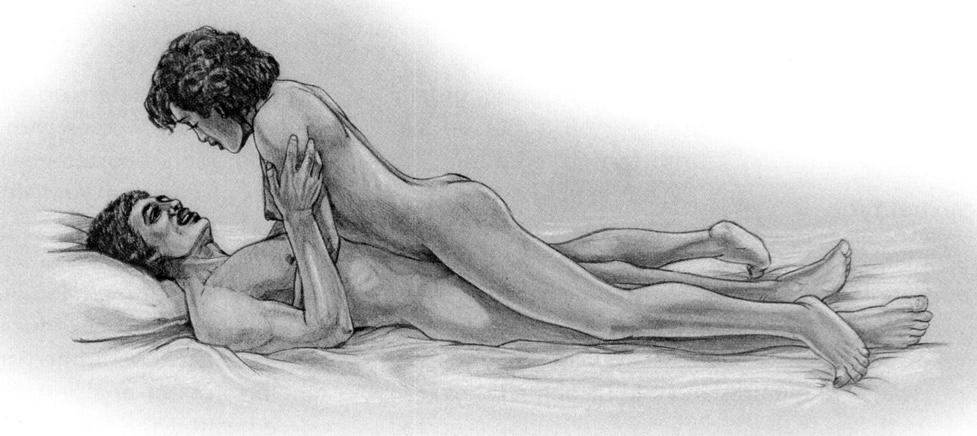

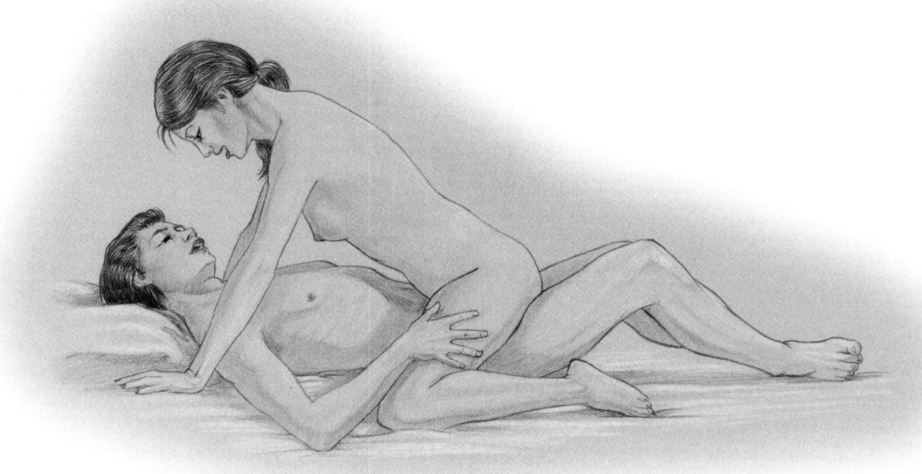

2. *Woman on top.* In the woman-on-top position, also called the female superior position (Figure 10.4), the woman can be either prone or on her knees. In either case this position permits more clitoral stimulation by either partner than the man-on-top position. Thus a woman who does not receive sufficient clitoral stimulation to achieve orgasm through coitus alone can reach orgasm through manual stimulation in this position while her partner's penis is inside her vagina. In this way she can experience the pleasure of orgasm around an erect

Did You Know . . .

A study of more than 3,400 Americans (Michael, 1994) found that

1. The mean age of first intercourse has increased by about 6 months since the 1970s.
2. Whereas males report curiosity as the reason for having their first intercourse, females report affection for their partner as the primary reason.
3. Thirty-two percent of 18- to 24-year-olds report ever having only 1 sexual partner. However, 34% report having had 2 to 4 sexual partners, 15% 5 to 10 partners, 8% 10 to 20 partners, and 3% more than 21 partners. Males consistently have more sexual partners than do females. In fact, 17% of all males report having had more than 21 sexual partners.

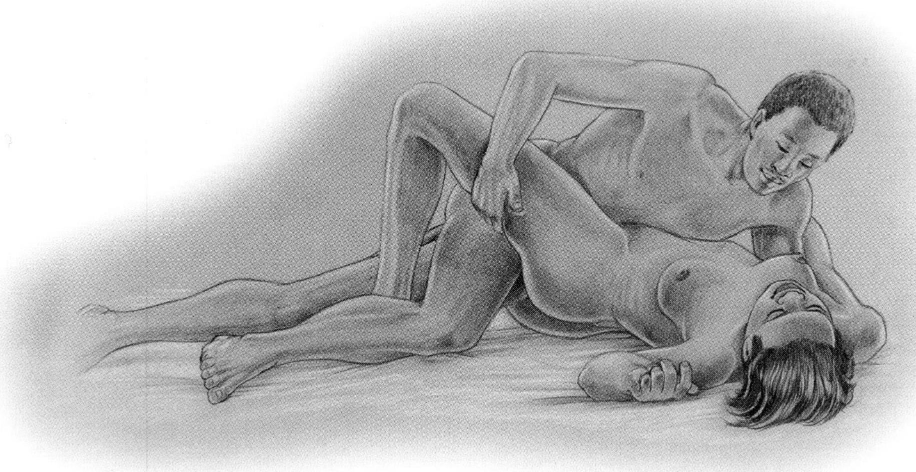

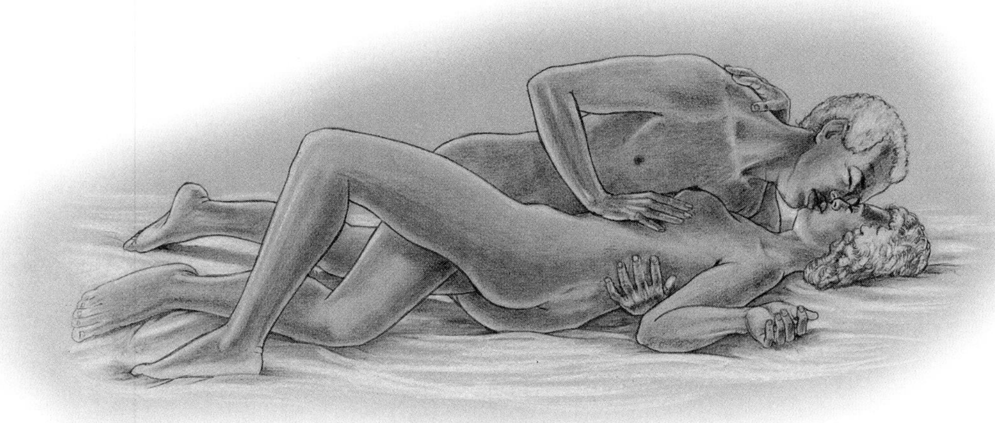

FIGURE 10.5 The side-by-side position. Note the subtle variations that are possible.

penis while the man has the pleasure of feeling her orgasmic contractions on his penis. In addition, the woman is free to move rather than being pinned under her partner. This is a good position for men who are attempting to control their orgasms; the squeeze technique (described in Chapter 15) is easy to use because the penis is relatively accessible. Another advantage is that both partners' hands are free, allowing them to caress each other. The one disadvantage of this position is that the effort by the man necessary for thrusting his penis can be tiring because the woman's weight is bearing down on his pelvis. Consequently women might do more of the movement in this position than in some others.

3. *Side-by-side.* In the side-by-side position (Figure 10.5), neither person is bearing the weight of the other. This is a relaxing position, because pelvic thrusts do not meet as much resistance as with the woman or man on top. However, because arms and legs may be pinned under other arms and legs, blood circulation can be temporarily cut off, making periodic switching or adjustment necessary for comfort. The side-by-side position also allows for kissing and face watching, and it

FIGURE 10.6 The rear-entry position.

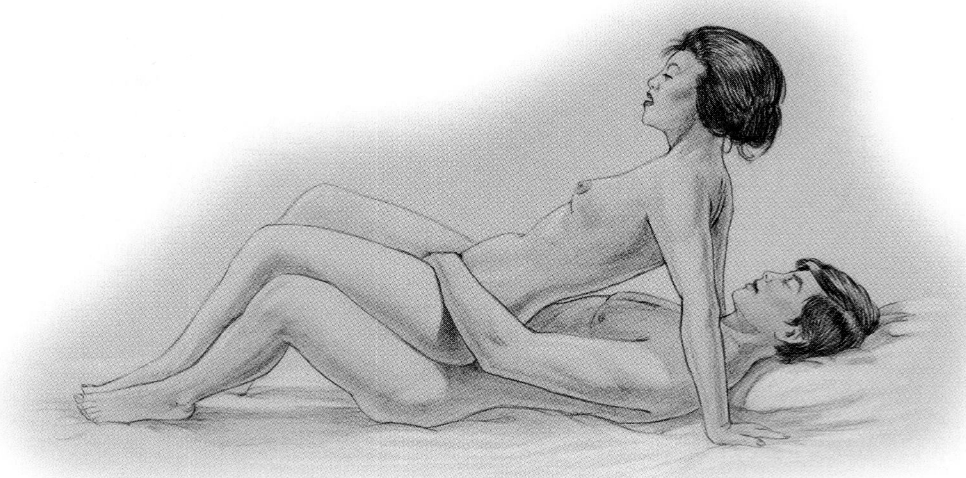

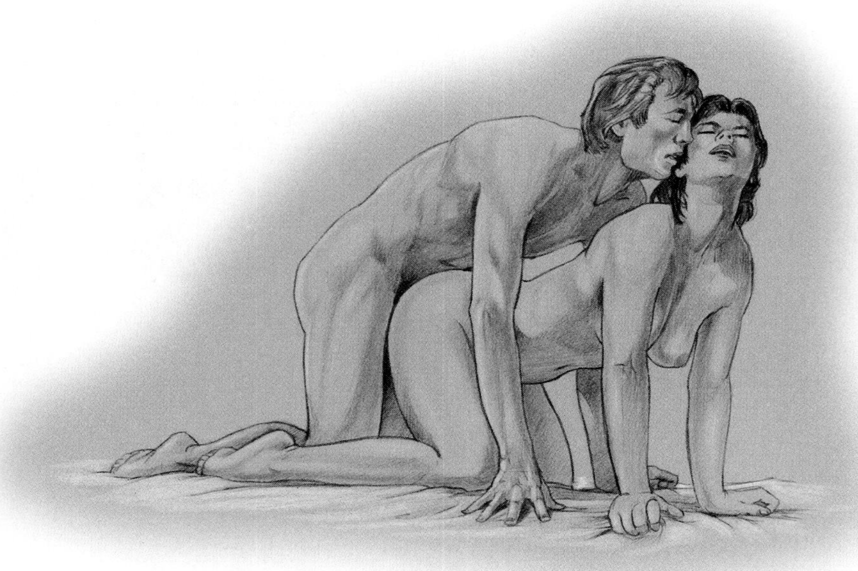

too frees the hands for stroking and caressing. However, it is sometimes difficult to keep the penis in the vagina in this position, and even vigorous thrusting can result in little or no clitoral contact. Still, hands work well here too, as in the woman-on-top position.

4. *Rear entry.* The rear-entry position (Figure 10.6) can be performed in two ways: with both people lying down, either side-by-side or with the woman atop the man, or with the partners kneeling (called the "dog position" for reasons clear to anyone who has seen dogs copulating). In either case the male's hands are free to fondle his partner's breasts and stimulate her clitoris. The disadvantages of this position include the lack of face-to-face contact and the feeling of

some people that they are being animal-like (others find this position sexually stimulating for this very reason). People who try the rear-entry position for the first time may be surprised by the sound effects: air may enter the vagina and produce noises when it leaves (some sexologists have termed this sound a "vart").

Once again we should say that the variety of coital positions is limited only by your imagination. Coitus, or any other sexual activity, can be pleasurable and exciting when the technique is pleasurable and exciting and when partners follow their inclinations. However, sexual techniques alone may not always be satisfying. The bond between sex makers that sometimes turns them into lovemakers can be as important as technique. A loving relationship of responsible people can add much to the pleasure obtained from sexual activity. Still, the very nature of sexual expression is pleasing, and it is obvious that sexual behavior can be enjoyed by people who are not in love but still care for each other. Whether such sexual behavior is moral or legal, however, is another issue, which depends on your ethics and society's—an issue discussed in Chapter 18.

Sexual Behavior of Homosexuals

With regard to the sexual activity of homosexuals, they enjoy most of the same activities as heterosexuals (Figures 10.7 and 10.8). One difference that has been noted, however (Tripp, 1976), is that intimacy and closeness seem to be more important than what is specifically done by the partners. People seem to have stereotyped ideas of specific sexual acts in which homosexuals participate. In contrast to these myths, both male and female homosexuals appear to take their time and make sexual activity last longer. They seem to prolong the pleasure rather than rush to orgasm (Masters & Johnson, 1979). Perhaps this is due to the fact that a person stimulating another person of the same sex can better understand what that person enjoys. Contrary to pop-

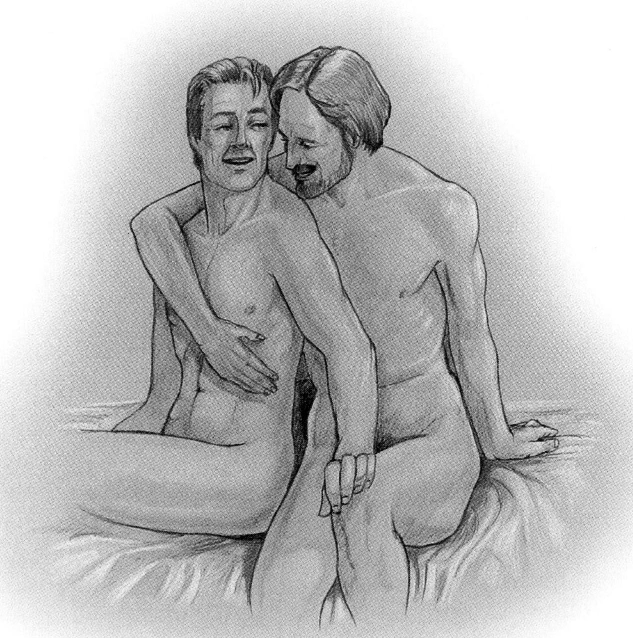

FIGURE 10.7 Gay men engage in varied sexual activities.

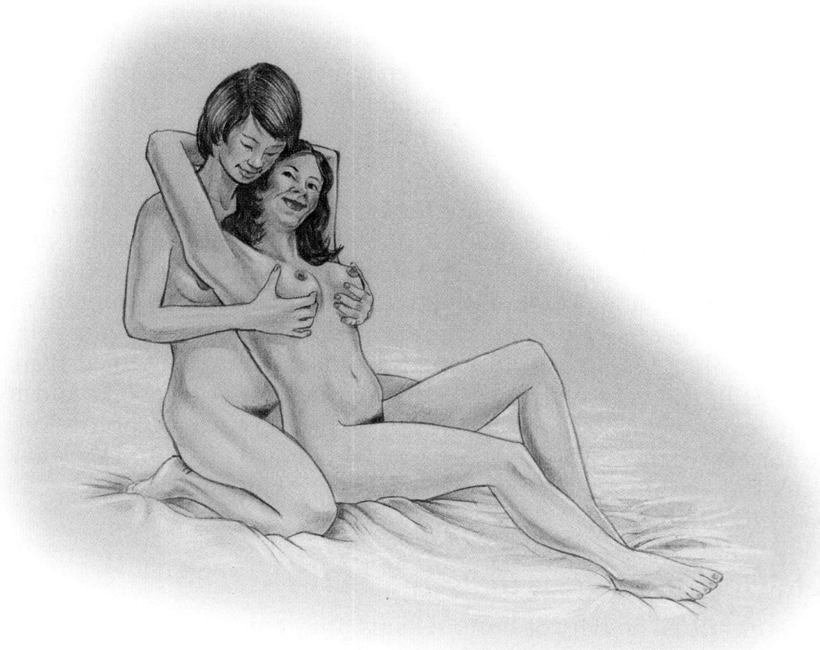

FIGURE 10.8 Oral and manual stimulation, and touching, are some of the sexual activities enjoyed by lesbians.

ular belief, male homosexuals do not generally have a preference to receive or insert the penis (Greenberg, 1973). Some people are under the misconception that one man plays the male and the other plays the female. This is not the case.

Masters and Johnson (1979), on the basis of their study of homosexuality, have reported a number of findings about the specific sexual behavior of homosexual men and women.

1. There are no major differences between the fantasy patterns of homosexuals and heterosexuals.
2. Homosexuality is learned and is definable only by overt behavior.
3. Homosexuality is a pattern of sexual interaction that a person can move into or out of at any time in life.
4. Physiologically homosexuals respond exactly as heterosexuals do to the same sexual stimuli—no sexual stimulus is unique to homosexuals.
5. Homosexuals are as amenable to treatment (with partners of their own choice) for sexual inadequacy as are heterosexuals.
6. Among established couples, homosexuals get more pleasure from lovemaking, even without intercourse, than do heterosexuals.

From a developmental standpoint, it is common for male and female homosexuals and bisexuals to have a history of sexual activity with the same and opposite genders, and to become sexually active during their early teens. No significant gender differences are found in lifetime prevalence rates or ages at initiating homosexual practices, but females tend to become sexually active at an older age than males and engage in more heterosexual activity. Sexual practices follow an initiation sequence beginning with manual sexual activity during their early teens and leading to further sexual activities during the middle and late teens (Rosario, 1996).

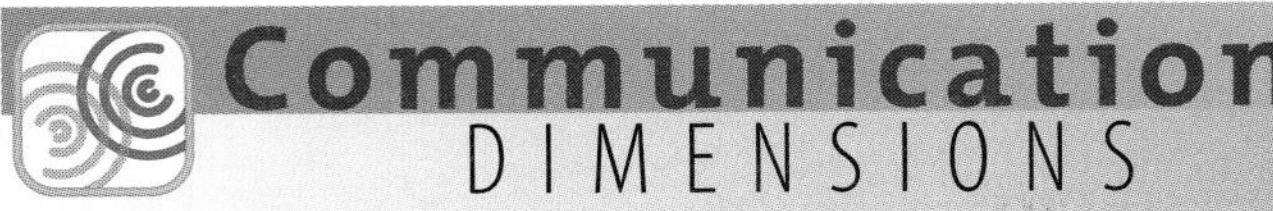

Word Choice Affects Study Results

Some years ago Blumstein and Schwartz (1983) conducted a study of couples and how often they "have sex." Lesbian, male homosexual, heterosexual nonmarried couples, and heterosexual married couples participated. They reported that lesbian couples "have sex" far less frequently than any other type of couple and that lesbian couples are less "sexual" as couples and as individuals than anyone else. In their sample only about one-third of the lesbians in relationships of 2 years or longer "had sex" once a week or more; 47% of lesbians in long-term relationships "had sex" once a month or less, and among heterosexual married couples only 15% "had sex" once a month or less. They also reported that lesbians seemed to be more limited in the range of their "sexual" techniques than did other couples.

In commenting on the Blumstein and Schwartz study, Frye (1997) points out that what 85% of heterosexual married couples are doing more than once a month and what 47% of lesbian couples are doing less than once a month is not the same thing. She indicates that the comparison is not accurate because the focus has been on sexual activity whereby a penis is inserted. When the only activity that counts as "doing it" involves interactions that include some sort of penile activity, she says, it is "no wonder [lesbians] discover [themselves] to 'do it' rather less often than do pairs with one or more penises present."

Frye feels that we would get a clearer picture if we start with a wide field of passions and bodily pleasures and create meanings that weave a web across it. She says:

> *I suggest that we begin the creation of a vocabulary that can encode and expand our meanings by adopting a very wide and general concept of "doing it." Let it be an open, generous, commodious concept encompassing all the acts and activities by which we generate with each other pleasure and thrills, tenderness, and ecstasy, passages of passionate carnality of whatever duration or profundity. . . . Our vocabulary will arise among us as we explain and explore and define the pleasures and our preferences across this field, teaching each other what the possibilities are and how to make them real.*

Lesbian Sexual Activities

In lesbian lovemaking, oral sexual activities are common, as are manual stimulation and tribadism. **Tribadism** is the rubbing of genitals against someone's body or genital area. Touching, caressing, and hugging—the emotional components of lovemaking—play a large role in lesbian lovemaking. Vaginal penetration with dildos is rare. In fact, lesbians tend to do more overall genital stimulation, rather than direct clitoral stimulation; as is often the case in heterosexual relationships (Masters & Johnson, 1979).

> **tribadism**
> Rubbing genitals against someone's body or genital area.

Gay Sexual Activities

Homosexual men engage in foreplay activities similar to those of heterosexuals, such as hugging, kissing, petting, and nipple stimulation. Anal intercourse is actually the least frequent male homosexual activity. More often, gay men participate in mutual masturbation or fellatio (oral sex). Laboratory studies by Masters and Johnson (1979) showed that gay men were likely to pay more attention to the area of the penis on the lower side than heterosexual couples.

Exploring the DIMENSIONS of Human Sexuality

Our feelings, attitudes, and beliefs regarding sexuality are influenced by our internal and external environments. Go to sexuality.jbpub.com to learn more about the biological, psychological, and sociological factors that affect your sexuality.

Biological Factors

- Sexual stimulation involves all five senses—touching, seeing, hearing, smelling, and tasting.
- Physical characteristics can enhance or inhibit sexual activities. For example, varying positions of intercourse offer varying degrees of comfort, depending on weight, physical stamina, or physical limitations.
- Foreplay allows for vaginal lubrication and erection before penile insertion.
- Physical disabilities may limit some sexual activities.
- Safer sexual activities decrease the risk of STI or HIV transmission.

Sociocultural Factors

- Sexual experience plays a role in what you find arousing.
- Sodomy laws prohibit certain sexual activities; however, these laws are rarely enforced.
- People who have more education tend to be less conservative sexually.
- Many religions prohibit certain sexual activities, such as premarital sex and masturbation. Pope John Paul II reaffirmed masturbation as an immoral act in 1993.
- School sexuality education programs often reflect community standards about what is perceived to be acceptable sexual behaviors. Parent and peer reactions to sexual information affect your perception of sexual activities.

Psychological Factors

- Emotional involvement with a partner plays a role in sexual pleasuring.
- Sexual fantasies are common among males and females.

CASE STUDY

Many factors influence what we find sexually arousing. Biologically, a physical disability may limit some sexual activities; on the other hand, it may also lead to other activities that are equally stimulating for a partner.

Psychologically, emotional attachment lends itself to sexual pleasuring. The greater the emotional attachment to someone we feel, often the greater the sexual pleasuring.

Schools play a broad role in developing our sense of what is acceptable or unacceptable. Community standards have an influence on what is taught, and that in turn influences student perceptions. Some fundamentalist religions ask young people to sign a public pledge to abstain from premarital sexual activity.

Communication is an important dimension. You and your partner need to be able to communicate what techniques you find sexually arousing. In addition, you must be able to communicate your love.

Family and friends influence sexual opinions as well. For example, comments by family and friends about the Clinton–Lewinsky affair may have influenced your perception of both extramarital activity and oral sexual activities.

Discussion Questions

1. Discuss the many dimensions that shape current attitudes toward masturbation and fantasies. How do male and female fantasies differ?
2. Explore the role of the senses, oral–genital contact, and various intercourse positions and sexual stimulation. Describe how sexual contact with another person can be made safer.

Application Questions

Reread the chapter-opening story and answer the following questions.

1. Many people are surprised to find that such an erotic novel dates back to the mid-18th century. Given that your ancestors reproduced (if they had not, you would not be reading this text), why is it widely believed that sexuality in the 1700s was inferior to today's sexuality?
2. One major change in sexual techniques since the novel was written is the more common prevalence of oral–genital sex. What might have prompted such a change?
3. This novel, as well as *Lady Chatterly's Lover* and many others, was banned in Boston, meaning that the book was not allowed to be sold in the city. The ban was finally rendered legally useless by the mid-20th century. How do current efforts to ban or limit the distribution of sexually explicit materials differ from the efforts of our ancestors?

Critical Thinking Questions

1. Explain why the former president, Bill Clinton, fired Joycelyn Elders, then surgeon general, for advocating the teaching of masturbation during school sexuality education. Although she may be correct in her thinking, should Elders have considered the diversity of the country, including those who would adamantly oppose the idea?
2. Is it better to do what is natural during sexual activity with a partner or to act according to what is learned in books such as this one?

Critical Thinking Case

The author Susan Minot, in her short story "*Lust*," mentions sexual technique: "I lay back with my eyes closed, luxuriating because he knew all sorts of expert angles, his hands never fumbling, going over my whole body, pressing the hair up and off the back of my head, giving an extra hip shove, as if to say *There*" (p. 15). But Minot continues the description as though the "expert" was very cold and unloving in his sexual activities.

Critics of sexuality education argue that knowing of the existence of the Grafenberg spot, erogenous zones, and the like, makes sexual relationships too mechanistic. Each partner is trying so hard to recall what is stimulating and how to stimulate it that the spontaneity that makes sexual relationships so enjoyable is lost. People would be better off just "flying by the seat of their pants." Is that not the way sex has been conducted for eons? Have we not done all right with that system for generation after generation? Why add science to a nonscientific experience? Just lie back and enjoy yourself.

Others agree that sexual relationships have been adequate in the face of little knowledge of sexual arousal and response. However, they argue, adequate is not good enough. With knowledge of how the body is organized—for example, where nerve endings are accumulated—and how to achieve increased sexual excitement, sexual relationships could be enhanced. Further, there is nothing wrong with consciously, even during a highly emotional sexual encounter, thinking of how best to please your partner, because that means that your partner will be thinking of how best to please you. The result will be a more sexually satisfying relationship.

What do you think? Spontaneous sexual experiences or mechanistic ones? Thoughtless sexual experiences or thoughtful ones?

Exploring Personal Dimensions

Assessing Your Techniques of Sexual Arousal

Are the techniques of sexual arousal you use effective? Do you know what other techniques of sexual arousal are available to you? To find out, answer the following questions. A discussion follows.

1. Do you fantasize about sex? How often?
2. What do you fantasize about when you fantasize about sex?
3. Do your sexual fantasies when you are with your partner differ from those when you are alone? If so, describe the difference.
4. Do you discuss your sexual fantasies with anyone else? If so, why? If not, why not?

Discussion

In a summary of research on sexual fantasies that reviewed more than 200 studies, the *Washington Post* reports the following information. Compare your responses to the typical responses of other adults.

1. Men average seven sexual fantasies a day, five of these triggered by outside stimuli such as watching a beautiful woman and two by inner thoughts. Women average five sexual fantasies a day, three from outside stimuli and two from their internal selves.
2. Women's favorite sexual fantasies involve a new sexual partner, sex with a celebrity, and sex with either a younger man or boy or an older "gent." Men's sexual fantasies include observing women nude and having sex with a new partner, sex with multiple partners at the same time, and having the sexual prowess to "drive women wild."
3. When men and women are alone, their sexual fantasies tend to be of their usual sexual partner, if they have one. Ironically, though, when they are actually engaged in sexual activity with their usual sexual partner, they tend to fantasize about sex with someone else. Often, this fantasy involves a celebrity.
4. Because many men and women feel guilty about fantasizing about someone else while being engaged in sexual activity with their usual partner they do not discuss their sexual fantasies with their partner. A mere 26% of men and only 32% of women tell their sexual partner about their fantasies.

Well, how do you compare with the average adult female or male? Is there anything about your sexual fantasies that you will work to change?

Source: Tasker, F. X marks the fantasy, *The Washington Post* (July 27, 1995), D5.

Sexuality Online

Go to the web component for *Exploring the Dimensions of Human Sexuality* at sexuality.jbpub.com for web exercises, additional resources related to this chapter, and student review tools.

Suggested Readings

Caster, W. *The lesbian sex book.* Boston: Alyson Publications, 1993.

Comfort, A. *The joy of sex.* New York: Crown, 1972.

Comfort, A. *The new joy of sex.* Westminster, MD: Random House, 1995.

Cooper, P. The art of sex: 20 ways to perfect your style, *Men's Health* (April 1990), 38–40.

DeAngelis, B. Sexual secrets men are afraid to share, *Redbook* (February 1990), 96–97, 136.

Ellenberg, D. & Bell, J. *Lovers for life: Creating lasting passion, trust and true partnership.* Santa Rosa, CA: Aslan Publishing, 1995.

Friday, N. *Men in love.* New York: Delacorte Press, 1980.

Friday, N. *Women on top: How real life has changed women's sexual fantasies.* New York: Simon & Schuster, 1991.

Haffner, D. & Schwartz, P. *What I've learned about sex.* New York: Perigee Books, 1998.

Hertford, J. *A pocket guide to loving sex.* New York: Carroll and Graf Publishers, 1995.

Kroll, K. & Klein, E. *Enabling romance: A guide to love, sex, and relationships for the disabled (and people who love them).* Kensington, MD: Woodbine House, 1995.

Lever, J. & Schwartz, P. *The great sex weekend.* New York: Perigee Books, 1998.

Love, P. & Robinson, J. *Hot monogamy.* New York: Dutton, 1994.

Plaud, J. J., et al. A multivariate analysis of the sexual fantasy themes of college men, *Journal of Marital and Family Therapy, 23* (1997), 221–230.

Sipski, M. & Alexander, C. *Sexual functioning in people with disability and chronic disease.* Frederick, MD: Aspen Publishers, 1997.

Strassberg, D. S., et al. Forces in women's sexual fantasies, *Archives of Sexual Behavior, 27* (1998), 403–414.

Winks, C. & Semans, A. *The good vibrations guide to sex.* Pittsburgh: Cleis Press, 1995.

CHAPTER 11

Sexual Orientation

FEATURES

Multicultural Dimensions
Race and Ethnicity and Same-Sex Sexual Behavior

Gender Dimensions
Male and Female Same-Sex Sexual Behavior

Ethical Dimensions
Research on Causes of Homosexuality

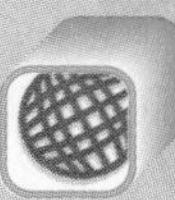

Global Dimensions
Attitudes About Gay Males in Mexico and the United States

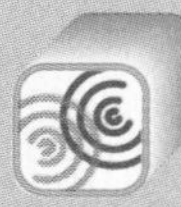

Communication Dimensions
Comunication About Gay and Lesbian Athletes

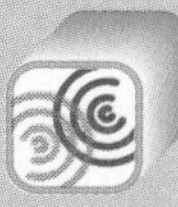

Communication Dimensions
Coming Out

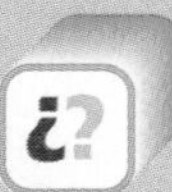

Ethical Dimensions
Should Gay Marriages Be Legal?

CHAPTER OBJECTIVES

1. Define sexual orientation, including heterosexuality, homosexuality, situational homosexuality, and bisexuality. Discuss the validity of the Kinsey continuum.
2. Compare and contrast the theories of sexual orientation, including biological, psychological, and sociocultural theories.
3. Discuss homosexual life, including the challenges specific to homosexuality.
4. Discuss social issues that affect homosexuals.

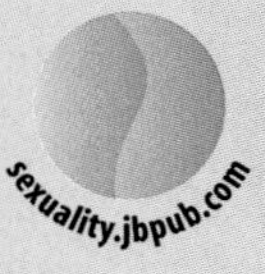

sexuality.jbpub.com

Theories of Sexual Orientation
Homophobia
Coming Out
The Gay Rights Movement

INTRODUCTION

By all appearances, Brad was an archetypal early-1970s high school male: a "good" student, a "really nice" guy with a willingness to help out with school projects and panache in fixing cars. He dated several girls. But his relationship with Peggy was extra special. They were best friends, hanging out together and attending high school parties and dances as a couple. They also engaged in a variety of sexual activities.

At first Brad could not quite understand why the idea of sexual intercourse with Peggy did not appeal to him as much as it should. Eventually Brad realized that he was gay. Peggy was hurt at first about the abrupt end of their relationship, but she cared about Brad enough to remain a close friend.

After high school, Brad attended a local college and continued to hang out with his high school friends who had accepted his sexual orientation, rather than venturing out to meet people who might not have been so accepting. Gay bashing was common, and Brad had a legitimate fear for his safety. During this time, the early 1980s, he met Brian, whom he has been with ever since.

Brad felt comfortable "coming out" to his friends, but he did not tell his elderly parents for fear of their reaction. This silence caused a bit of a problem, because his parents (and relatives) were forever introducing him to "nice girls" and wondering why nothing ever came of the dates Brad claimed he had. About the time Brad turned 30 years old, over dinner one evening, his father said to him, "You're gay, aren't you?" Although Brad's parents may have initially been hurt or confused, or may have questioned their own parenting, they continued to love and support Brad.

For Brad, as for many gays and lesbians, the AIDS crisis took a terrible toll. Many friends became sick and died. Many of Brad's friends learned about and began practicing safer sexual activities, no longer going to bathhouses or having quick, anonymous encounters. Brad attended rallies to promote governmental funding for AIDS research.

Brad was lucky: Both he and Brian tested negative for HIV. One thing that HIV did teach Brad, however, was that although he and Brian had been together for many years in a committed relationship, their situation was quite different from that of a legally married couple. When one of Brad's close friends died of AIDS, Brad's friend's parents, who did not want to believe their child was gay, demanded all his assets—which the deceased had intended to leave for his partner. Because the parents had the legal standing in the state in which the death occurred, the grieving partner lost everything. Even while his friend was dying, the parents were allowed to make all medical decisions and legally barred the partner from hospital visits.

In marriages, spouses automatically have each other's power of attorney, which means that if one spouse is incapacitated, the other has control over his or her affairs. A gay couple must go through lawyers in order to ensure that each partner has power of attorney for the other. Because Brian and Brad had purchased a home together and had made various other investments together, they realized it was imperative for them to complete the proper documentation to protect each other.

Brad's story illustrates many of the dimensions of sexual orientation. Sexual orientation takes time to develop and has an impact on many aspects of a person's life. In this chapter, we look at the ways that the many dimensions of human sexuality interact to determine sexual orientation.

Sexual Orientation

People have various feelings about sexual orientation—and even the topic of sexual orientation. The Sexuality Information and Education Council of the United States (SIECUS) position statement on sexual orientation (1995) is as follows:

> *Sexual orientation is an essential human quality. Individuals have the right to accept, acknowledge, and live in accordance with their sexual orientation, be they bisexual, heterosexual, gay, or lesbian. The legal system should guarantee the civil rights and protection of all people, regardless of sexual orientation. Prejudice and discrimination based on sexual orientation is unconscionable.*

A person's **sexual orientation** is one's erotic, romantic, and affectional attraction to the same sex, to the opposite sex, or to both. **Sexual identity** refers to an inner sense of oneself as a sexual being, including one's identification in terms of gender and sexual orientation. **Sexual preference** is a term once used to describe sexual orientation—**bisexuality** (attracted to both sexes), **heterosexuality** (attracted to members of the opposite sex), and **homosexuality** (attracted to members of the same sex). This term is now outdated because sexual orientation is no longer commonly considered to be one's conscious individual preference or choice; instead it is thought to be formed by a complicated network of social, cultural, biological, economic, and political factors (Sexual orientation and identity, 1998).

For our purposes, the terms *homosexual* and **gay** are used interchangeably to apply to either males or females. The term **lesbian,** however, applies only to a female homosexual.

The Kinsey Continuum

No clear-cut line separates homosexuality and heterosexuality; in fact, it is more accurate to think of these orientations as being on a continuum. Figure 11.1 shows a seven-point continuum of sexual orientation originally devised by Kinsey. Most of us probably experience varying degrees of sexual orientation; that is, most of us are attracted to both sexes, even though we may act in only one way sexually.

The notion of a continuum of sexual orientation helps explain not only differences among people but also a phenomenon known as **situational homosexuality**—that is, sexual behavior limited to specific circumstances in which members of the same sex are generally deprived of contact with the other sex. Homosexual activity in a single-sex school or in a prison, for example, does not necessarily indicate that the individuals involved are primarily homosexual. They may never participate in homosexual activity in other situations, and their orientation may prefer sexual activity with the other sex. However, because people of the other sex are not available to them, and because they prefer sexual activity with another person to masturbation exclusively, they engage in sexual behavior with people of the same sex. You may have participated in sexual activity with someone of the same sex sometime in your life; however, unless you are sexually attracted to people of the same sex, fall in love with people of the same sex, have sexual behaviors with people of the same sex, and identify yourself as a homosexual, you are not classified as a homosexual.

The distinction we wish to make is between specific behavior and one's sexual orientation. A person's engaging in sexual activity with someone of

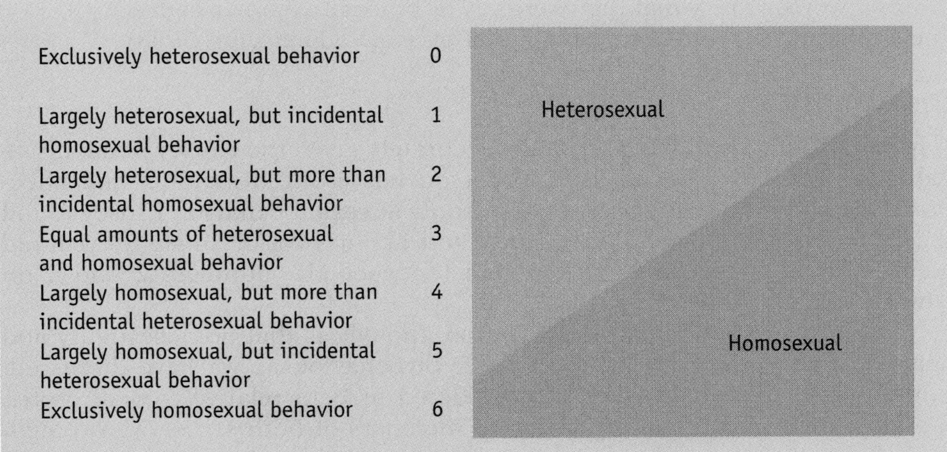

FIGURE 11.1 Kinsey Sexual Orientation Continuum The Kinsey continuum refers only to homosexual or heterosexual *behavior;* remember that it was developed in the 1950s. If such a continuum were developed today, it would likely refer to erotic, romantic, and affectional attraction, as do our definitions of sexual orientation. It would also probably recognize that a person's behavior and sexual orientation might differ. For example, a person can be heterosexually married, have sexual intercourse with a spouse, and still be a homosexual or a bisexual.

sexual orientation
One's erotic, romantic, and affectional attraction to the same sex, to the opposite sex, or to both.

sexual identity
Inner sense of oneself as a sexual being, including one's identification in terms of gender and sexual orientation.

sexual preference
Term formerly used to describe sexual orientation that is now outdated, because sexual orientation is no longer commonly considered to be a conscious individual preference or choice, but to be formed by a complicated network of factors.

bisexual
One whose erotic, romantic, and affectional attraction is toward both sexes.

heterosexual
One whose primary erotic, romantic, and affectional attraction is toward members of the other sex.

homosexual
One whose primary erotic, romantic, and affectional attraction is toward members of one's own sex.

gay
Male or female homosexual. (*Gay* used alone probably refers to a male, though it is acceptable to refer to a *gay female.*)

lesbian
Female homosexual.

situational homosexuality
Homosexual behavior limited to circumstances in which members of the same sex are deprived of contact with the other sex.

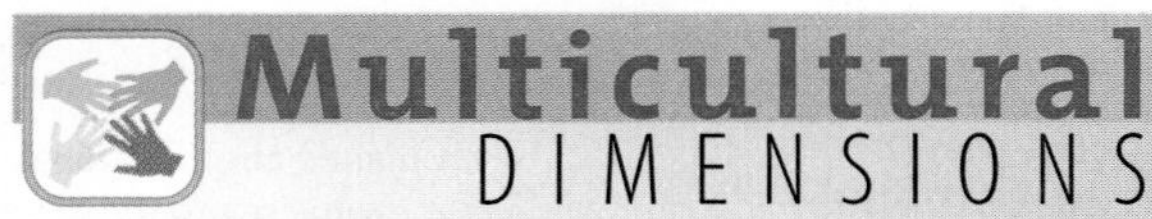

Race and Ethnicity and Same-Sex Sexual Behavior Laumann and associates (1994) reported some differences in the rates of same-sex sexual behavior for people with different racial and ethnic backgrounds in the United States. For example, the proportion of people reporting same-sex sexual behavior since puberty was as follows.

White = 7.6% of males and 4% of females
African American = 5.8% of males and 3.5% of females
Hispanic = 8.8% of males and 3.8% of females
Asian = no males and 3.3% of females

The same researchers also asked people which sexual behaviors they found "very appealing." The following proportions found sexual activity with a same-sex partner "very appealing."

White = 3.3% of males and 2.7% of females
African American = 2.9% of males and 3.5% of females
Hispanic = 2.9% of males and 4.4% of females
(Sample sizes for other groups were too small to be meaningful.)

Interestingly, in most cases the proportion of people who find same-sex sexual behavior to be "very appealing" is lower than the proportion who have participated in it. We are not certain of the reason(s) for this, but perhaps some of those who participated were experimenting and learned that the behavior did not appeal to them after all.

the same sex does not indicate that person is a homosexual; someone's not engaging in sexual activity with the same sex does not indicate that person is not a homosexual. Sexual orientation is not the same as sexual behavior.

Many of us take our sexual orientation for granted; however, about 11% of junior and senior high school students may not be sure of theirs. Uncertainty about sexual orientation declines with age, from about 26% of 12-year-old students to 5% of 17-year-old students. About 20% of gay and bisexual men surveyed on college campuses knew that they were gay or bisexual in junior high school, and 17% said they knew in grade school. Six percent of gay or bisexual women knew that they were gay or bisexual in junior high school; 11% knew in grade school (Gay, lesbian, and bisexual adolescents, 1998).

Bisexuality

If homosexuality is difficult to define accurately given the Kinsey scale, bisexuality is even more so. A bisexual person has erotic, romantic, and affectional attraction to both sexes. Looking only at sexual behavior, Kinsey found that 9% of single 30-year-old women and about 16% of single 30-year-old men could be categorized as bisexual (between the numbers 2 and 4 on Kinsey's scale).

The problem with this categorization, though, is that homosexuality and heterosexuality are more than a matter of behavior, as we have discussed. Consequently, bisexuality can be considered to be a relatively equal erotic, romantic, and affectional attraction to members of both sexes, even though an individual may have a favorite attraction or behavior.

MacDonald (1981) defines *bisexuality* as enjoying and engaging in sexual activity with members of both sexes or recognizing the desire to do so. Because bisexual behavior usually involves only one other person at any one time, some sexuality experts prefer terming it **ambisexual** behavior; that is, sexual behavior and attraction that fluctuates from a relationship with a same-sex partner to one with an other-sex partner.

ambisexual
A person whose sexual relationships fluctuate, from relationships with same-sex partners to relationships with opposite-sex partners.

As with homosexuality, our definition of bisexuality allows that someone who at one time engaged in bisexual behavior may not be a bisexual, and, someone who has never participated in bisexual behavior could be a bisexual. For example, someone may fantasize about sexual relations with members of both sexes and find himself or herself attracted to people of both sexes but may never have engaged in sexual relations with a same-sex partner. This person may nevertheless be bisexual. In fact, one study found that bisexuals fantasize a great deal about sexual activity with both males and females (Storms, 1980).

Another way of looking at this is to realize that sexual identity (orientation) and sexual behavior are two distinct measures, and one is not necessarily consistently predictive of the other. For example, women who self-identify as "lesbian" may have male sexual partners because of economic necessity, societal or cultural expectation, or erotic desire. Similarly, women who identify themselves as "bisexual" or "heterosexual" may have either or both male and female partners (Rankow, 1996).

For people who are really homosexual but are unwilling to acknowledge their sexual orientation even to themselves, bisexuality may be a means of coping. Many of these people eventually accept their homosexuality without the need to mask it with bisexual behavior. Others remain bisexual throughout their lives because their sexual attraction is truly to both sexes. Still others engage in bisexual behavior for a time but sooner or later revert to heterosexuality.

Bisexuals point to the variety that characterizes their sexual relationships. They are able to enjoy fully the sexual pleasures of both males and females and are open to the most erotic of activities. One of the disadvantages of bisexuality, though, is the suspicion it provokes in both the heterosexual and the homosexual community. In one sense, bisexuals are both like and unlike these groups; however, it is often the "unlikeness" that is the focus. Homosexuals view bisexuals as homosexuals who are afraid to admit to their preference. Some homosexuals reject sexual relations with bisexuals for this reason. It seems that lesbians are even more rejecting of bisexual women than are male homosexuals of bisexual men. Some lesbians want bisexual women to declare openly their lesbianism and insist there is no such thing as a true bisexual.

On some college campuses, new student organizations for bisexuals who feel shunned by gay-student support groups are emerging (Morgan, 2002). Interestingly, supporters of the new groups say many of the previous groups established for gay, lesbian, and bisexual students have exhibited the very kinds of intolerance and discrimination they were designed to fight. The name for this behavior is *biphobia,* or antipathy toward those who identify as bisexual. Supposedly, some gay students belittle bisexuality as a "cop-out" to avoid identification as gay. Others say that bisexuals are confused about their real sexual orientation.

Bisexuals are referred to in many ways: as "switch hitters," "AC–DC," or "people who swing both ways." The way these individuals determine that they are bisexual varies. Some women bisexuals say that some of their needs can be met only by men, whereas other needs can be met only by women (Blumstein & Schwartz, 1976). Male bisexuals tend to express their bisexuality as a means of achieving variety and creativity in their sexual lives (Masters, Johnson, & Kolodny, 1985). Many bisexuals first experience sexual activity with a same-sex partner who is a close friend. Others find their way to bisexuality through group sex. In any case, the causes of bisexuality, as do the causes of heterosexuality and homosexuality, remain unknown.

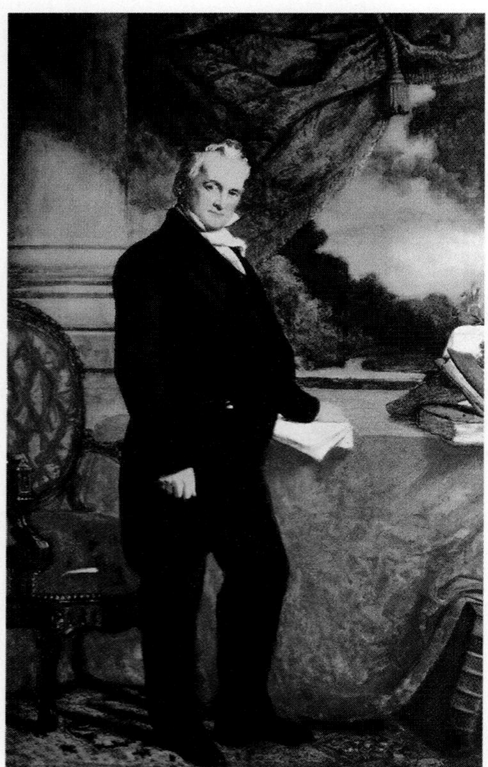

James Buchanan—the country's only unmarried president—was said to have been involved in a homosexual relationship with William Rufus De Vane King—the country's only unmarried vice president (under Franklin Pierce). During their 23-year friendship, they were longtime roommates in Washington, DC.

Homosexuality in the Population

It is hard to know exactly how many homosexuals live in U.S. society; most still choose to keep their sexual orientation hidden. Consensus among authorities is that male homosexuals outnumber lesbians by two or three to one, although this ratio is frequently debated. A conservative estimate is that there are about 6.2 million gays in the United States (or about 2.5% of the population), whereas gay activists say that 25 million is a more accurate figure, which would be about 10% of the population (Gay and lesbian issues, 1991). Various researchers have come up with various numbers for the prevalence of homosexuality in the United States. In summarizing data on the prevalence of homosexuality, the Kinsey Institute (2003) indicated that anywhere from 2% of women and 4% of men to 7.5% of women and 7.7% of men consider themselves to be homosexual. Although these figures appear to apply to people at the extreme right-hand side of the Kinsey continuum (numbers 5–6), it is not known for sure exactly which people are included in the estimates. It does indicate, however, that, statistically speaking, a number of your friends and classmates have homosexual orientations, as do a number of your teachers. A similar proportion of any group, whether they be laborers, musicians, or professional athletes, probably have homosexual orientations as well. For instance, a more recent study than Kinsey's (Fay, et al., 1989) found that approximately 20% of men had a homosexual experience at least once in their lives.

As might be expected, it is not easy to conduct research related to sexual orientation. For example, a content analysis of 144 studies suggested that women and bisexuals were underrepresented, and, in about one-third of the studies, participants' sexual orientations were assumed rather than assessed (Chung, 1996). In another study, involving 3,054 students in grades 9–12, 6.4% reported same-sex contact (Faulkner, 1998).

In Chapter 2 we discussed the National Health and Social Life Survey (NHSLS). It has often been stated that about 10% of our population is homosexual; however, "all of the recent population-based surveys of sexual behavior, including this one, have found rates that are much lower than 10%" (Laumann, et al., 1994). In the NHSLS it was found that 4.9% of men and 4.1% of women had had same-sex sex partners since age 18 years; 4.1% of males and 2.2% of females had same-sex sex partners in the last 5 years; and 2.7% of men and 1.3% of women had had same-sex sex partners in the last year. Only 2% of males and 0.9% of females had a homosexual sexual identity, and 0.8% of males and 0.5% of females had a bisexual sexual identity (Laumann, et al., 1994).

In addition to the number of homosexuals who hide their orientation and the difficulty of defining exactly who is included on Kinsey's continuum, another reason for the disparity in the estimated number of homosexuals relates to political implications. For example, those lobbying for greater gay rights need to show that large numbers of people are affected by this issue. If they can demonstrate political clout—that is, a large voting bloc—they can convince politicians to support their causes. That support can translate into legislation that assures gays the rights and privileges they feel have long been denied to them. However, it is in the interest of those opposed to gay rights for these estimates to be lower, because such lower numbers would marginalize gay people. That is one reason why some gay rights organizations estimate that 10% of the population is homosexual and others use a much lower figure.

Same-sex couples head nearly 600,000 homes in the United States, according to census data considered the federal government's most thorough count

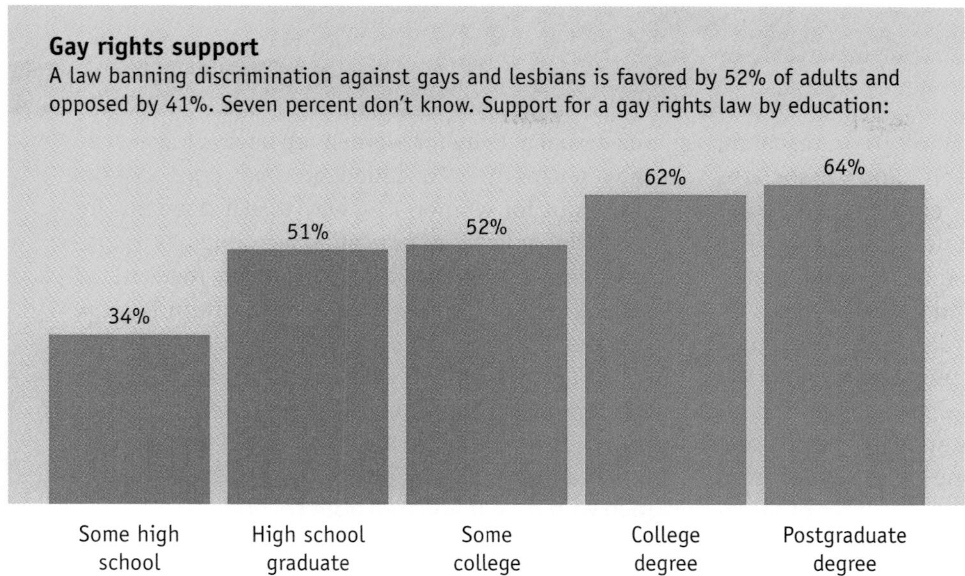

FIGURE 11.2 Gay rights support.
Source: Harris Poll by A. R. Carey and S. Ward. *USA Today* (Oct. 26, 1998), 1.

yet of homosexuals (Census shows nearly 600,000 same-sex couple homes, 2001). A gay or lesbian couple heads a household in nearly every county in America. Sixteen percent of the same-sex couple homes are in California, 8% in New York, and 7% in Texas. However, such living arrangements still make up a tiny share of the nation's households—just over 0.005% of the 105.5 million U.S. homes. The results also dispel stereotypes that homosexuality is limited to large urban areas and college towns.

Heterosexuality in the Population

Regardless of the exact numbers of homosexuals and bisexuals in U.S. society, it is safe to assume that the sexual orientation of most people is heterosexual. Because of this, some heterosexuals may have a difficult time understanding and supporting the need for equal rights and opportunities for people with different sexual orientations. Some heterosexuals may even be guilty of heterosexism, which means they think about human experience only in heterosexual terms and ignore or put down homosexual behaviors. They also may stereotype homosexuals in a negative manner and view them as dangerous to others.

It is interesting to note that gay rights support increases by level of education, as seen in Figure 11.2 (Carey & Ward, 1998).

Theories of Sexual Orientation

Although many studies have been done on the subject, no one knows exactly what factors shape sexual orientation. Some argue that biological factors account for a homosexual, heterosexual, or bisexual orientation. Others claim that psychological factors or learned behavior is responsible. Determining an accurate method for defining and identifying sexual orientation for the purpose of constructing representative samples of homosexuals, bisexuals, and heterosexuals is a goal of researchers. Different definitions and measures have been used to develop samples since the 1860s, when the topic of sexual orientation first attracted widespread research interest. If advances

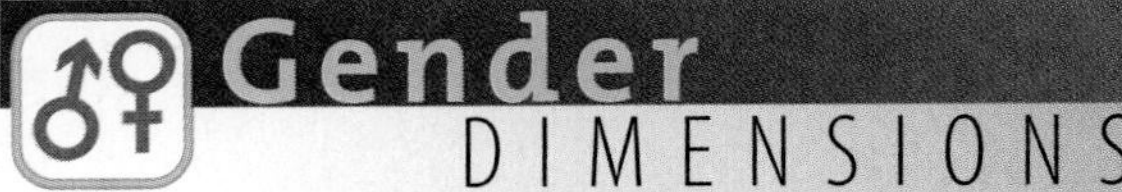

Male and Female Same-Sex Sexual Behavior As part of their research, Laumann and associates (1994) consistently found higher levels of same-sex sexual behavior among males than among females. For example, 2.1% of females and 4.1% of males reported having same-sex sex partners in the past 5 years; 4.1% of females and 4.9% of males reported having same-sex sex partners since age 18 years.

Except for one variable, the appeal of having sexual activity with someone of one's own sex (which is higher for females than for males), the rates of same-sex sexual activity for women are always lower than the rates for men. Education, however, does seem to stand out for women in a way that it does not for men. Higher levels of education are generally associated with higher rates on any given measure of same-sex sexual behavior. But this pattern is more pronounced for women than it is for men. For example, in general women with a high school degree or less report very low rates of same-sex sexual activity. However, women who have graduated from college report a higher level of same-sex sexual activity than men who have graduated from college.

in the understanding of sexual orientations are to be made, it is critical that definitions and measures of sexual orientation be standardized (Sell, 1997).

Because the vast majority of people are heterosexuals, most theories about sexual orientation relate to homosexuality or bisexuality. It is as though heterosexuality is the "norm" and homosexuality and bisexuality are indications that something went wrong. These theories are described in the following paragraphs.

Biological Theories

Biological theories of the development of homosexuality include genetic factors and hormonal factors.

The Genetic Theory

The genetic theory of the cause of homosexuality states that something in a person's genes causes that person to be sexually attracted to members of the same sex. The most frequently cited evidence for this view is the study by Kallman (1952). Kallman studied twins (both fraternal and identical) who grew up in the same home. Fraternal twins do not share an exact genetic inheritance, whereas identical twins do share the same genetic material (they occupied the same ovum). Consequently, the environments are the same for both sets of twins, but the difference is in the genetic makeup. Kallman found identical twins had a 95% concordance rate (both twins were homosexual) compared to a 12% concordance rate for fraternal twins. He concluded that homosexuality is a function of genetic predisposition. Whitam and Diamond (1986) reported a concordance rate of 75% for identical twins and a 19% rate for fraternal twins, thereby supporting the genetic theory. However, numerous other studies over the years (Heston & Shields, 1968; Zuger, 1976) have not been able to verify Kallman's findings. Furthermore, Kallman's selection of twins for his studies was criticized. He chose twins from prisons, psychiatric settings, and charitable organizations, thereby restricting the ability to generalize his results to twins living in more typical situations.

Several studies have supported the idea of a genetic connection to homosexuality. For example, Hamer and associates (1993) studied genetic material from 40 pairs of gay brothers and found identical pieces of the end tip of the

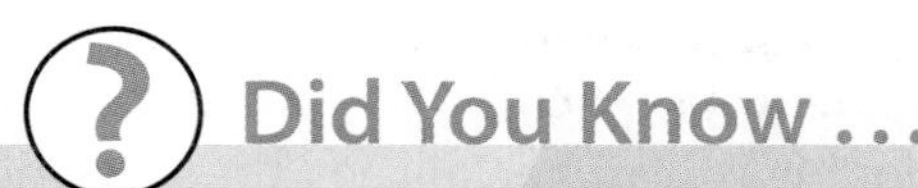

In *Biological Exuberance* (St. Martin's Press, 1990), the linguist and cognitive scientist Bruce Bagemihl attempts to dispel the myth that humans are the only species who practice homosexuality. In fact, he found that homosexual activity has been documented in more than 20% of the 2,000 species whose sexual activity has been observed. The following are a few examples discussed in his book:

- Male giraffes wrap their necks together until both are sexually aroused.
- Homosexual activities account for 50% of sexual activity among bonobos (chimplike apes).
- A male greylag goose may pair with another male goose for 15 years.

Source: Kluger, J. The gay side of nature, *Time, 153, no. 16* (April 26, 1999), 70.

X chromosome to a much greater degree than would have been anticipated. They concluded that there may be one or more genes that play a role in predisposing some men to homosexuality.

Many researchers feel that the most promising support for a biological reason for sexual orientation comes from genetic studies. There is a great deal of evidence that gay male and lesbian sexual orientations run in families (Bailey, et al., 2000; Dawood, et al., 2000; Kendler, et al., 2000).

Sexuality experts do caution that a specific gene linked to homosexuality has not been identified. Also, because of the complexity of sexual orientation, it is likely that a possible genetic link is only part of the picture.

McGuire (1995) indicates that genetic analysis of behavioral differences among humans requires both careful experimental design and appropriate genetic models. He believes that all studies of the genetic basis of sexual orientation of men and women have failed to meet one or more of the criteria for such a research study—valid and precise measures, appropriate methods, randomly selected subjects, appropriate sample sizes, and appropriate genetic models.

The Hormonal Theory

The hormonal theory of the cause of homosexuality states that homosexuality is a result of hormonal imbalances that occur before or after birth. Because it is known that prenatal hormonal treatment in animals can lead to different male and female behavior patterns (Dorner, 1968; Hutchinson, 1978; Money & Ehrhardt, 1972), some theorists have concluded that these same conditions might cause homosexuality. Evidence for this view can be found in the work of several researchers. For instance, Dorner and associates (1975) studied the responses of homosexuals and heterosexuals to injections of the hormone estrogen and found these responses to differ. Furthermore, Gladue and colleagues (1983) found that when homosexual men were administered estrogen, their patterns of secretion of luteinizing hormone (LH) changed to be more like those of heterosexual women; in addition, their testosterone levels remained lower for a longer time than did heterosexual men's when both groups were administered estrogen. Studies have also found that a prenatal excess of androgen in females is associated with a greater incidence of lesbianism (Ehrhardt, Evers, & Money, 1968; Money & Schwartz, 1977) and that a prenatal deficiency in androgen production in males is associated with an increased incidence of male homosexuality.

One research project tentatively identifies prenatal exposure to the synthetic estrogen diethylstilbestrol (DES) as predisposing female offspring to lesbianism (Ehrhardt, et al., 1985). Another researcher alleges the existence of anatomical differences in the size of parts of the brains of homosexual and heterosexual men (LeVay, 1991). Yet another researcher has pointed out that there is little evidence supporting the hormonal theories and that sexual orientation is more likely determined by other personal and cultural factors (Doell, 1995).

As is the case with the genetic theories, there are problems in research on the hormonal causation of sexual orientation. There is no convincing evidence that sexual orientation is the result of either prenatal or postnatal hormonal imbalances, or that homosexuality causes these imbalances. However, research continues in this area.

Psychological Theories

Psychological theories of the development of sexual orientation consider psychoanalytical factors and the influence of learned behavior. Although these theories were historically believed, they have not been proved valid. Today many experts do not support these theories.

The Psychoanalytical Theory

Psychoanalytical theories of the cause of sexual orientation relate to parental and family characteristics. Sigmund Freud postulated that everyone is born with the potential to be bisexual. Whether or not someone becomes heterosexual or homosexual is, Freud believed, a result of circumstances that affect the child's psychosexual development. For example, if a young boy is unable to resolve the Oedipal complex (an attraction for his mother) satisfactorily and becomes "fixated" at this phase of psychosexual development, he may become homosexual; or if the boy continues to fear castration ("castration complex"), he may grow up to be homosexual.

Irving Bieber and colleagues (1962) fueled this view of the influence of family background when he compared the family backgrounds of 106 homosexual men and 100 heterosexual men and found differences. Specifically, Bieber found that homosexual men more often had overprotective and dominant mothers and weak, passive, and detached fathers than did heterosexual men. Bieber hypothesized that this family upbringing made men homosexual because they were fearful of interacting with women and unable to identify with their father. The problem with Bieber's study was the manner in which he acquired his sample of homosexual men. Because there is a social stigma associated with homosexuality, thereby making many homosexuals unwilling to admit to their preference, it has often been difficult to find gay men and women to study. Consequently, homosexual samples have in the past too frequently been obtained from either psychiatric settings (patient populations), prisons, or the military. The ability, therefore, to generalize these results to socially functional homosexuals is suspect. Bieber's sample was obtained from patients undergoing psychoanalysis. As Clark and Epstein (1969, 575) state:

> *One does not go into prisons and mental hospitals or clinics to study normal heterosexuality and then generalize to the population at large; therefore, to do so with homosexuals, as has been done so often in past research dealing with this area, is to study a sample already selectively loaded with psychopathology which may not be truly representative of the whole homosexual population.*

On the one hand, evidence supporting Bieber's theory exists in the larger-than-usual population of homosexuals who have such family characteristics. On the other hand, there are many heterosexuals who grew up in similar households but never became homosexual. Clearly this theory remains just that—a theory.

The Learned Behavior Theory

Behaviorists believe that homosexuality is the result of situations experienced usually early in childhood and reinforced throughout one's life. For example, someone may experience an unsuccessful and unsatisfying heterosexual relationship that leads him or her to experiment with homosexuality, with which they find satisfaction. The attitude of many people is that "if they only had an effective lover, they'd never be homosexual." Others believe homosexuals are physically unattractive to the opposite sex, so their only sexual outlet is someone of the same sex. Dew (1985) found that many college students had this view. Others believe that an early childhood homosexual experience "recruits" people to homosexuality.

Studies are not supportive of these viewpoints. Homosexuals do not differ from heterosexuals in terms of their frequency of dating in high school (Bell, Weinberg, & Hammersmith, 1981), they often report having had sexual experience with people of the opposite sex (Klach, 1974; Martin & Lyon, 1972), and they are not seduced into homosexuality as children (Bell, Weinberg, & Hammersmith, 1981). As with the other theories, the learned behavior theory demands further investigation before it can be supported.

Recently some researchers have argued that we have no business trying to determine the cause of homosexuality until we are able to determine what causes any form of sexual orientation. In other words, we are what we are, and why we have certain sexual orientations might be scientifically interesting; however, it has very little practical significance. Whether or not you accept this type of reasoning, the fact is that we still do not know why some people are homosexual and others heterosexual.

Integrated Theories

The integrated theory of the development of sexuality—homosexuality is just one form—argues that physical, psychological, and learned factors are involved. A good explanation of this view has been offered by the renowned endocrinologist John Money (1987). Money describes societies in which homosexuality is a precursor of heterosexuality. For example, in the large area in the Pacific between Sumatra through Papua New Guinea and Melanesia, homosexuality is institutionalized. Males between the ages of 9 and 19 years move out of their families' homes into the long-houses in the center of the village. There they engage regularly in homosexual activity until they reach marriage age (19 years). After marriage, homosexual activity stops or is kept to a minimum. Likewise, the Sambian people in the eastern part of New Guinea require a boy just before puberty to give up his mother's milk for the "milk" (semen) of men. That is the only way the boy can grow and mature into a man. In fact, omission of this phase would stigmatize the man as deviant, rather than stigmatizing him as deviant for participating, as it might in American culture.

In the examples cited, homosexuality is a part of society and is learned behavior. Still, there is evidence presented by integrated theorists of the biological aspects of homosexuality. Experiments on certain animals have shown that the brain can develop in contrast to the body's form and structure. In one such study, pregnant lambs were injected with testosterone at a critical point in the pregnancy, and the resulting ewe was homosexual. That is, its brain was masculinized and it acted exactly as a ram acts in its mating and urinating behaviors. However, it possessed ovaries that secreted estrogen.

Integrationists, then, conclude that the prenatal influence on sexuality is important but that it plays out in a social context. Therefore, sexuality (heterosexuality, bisexuality, and homosexuality) is a function of the interaction of all of these factors: biology, hormones, cultural expectations, learned behavior, and psychological variables.

Two Landmark Studies

Two 1991 studies concerning gay men renewed enthusiasm for research into the causes of sexual orientation. In one investigation, Simon LeVay, a neuroscientist at the Salk Institute in San Diego, California, studied the brain tissue of men who had died of AIDS (LeVay, 1991). In particular, LeVay analyzed a part of the hypothalamus known to be involved in the development of typical male sexual behavior. When monkeys have lesions in this part of the brain, they exhibit fewer male sexual behaviors, although their sexual drive remains intact. Under extreme magnification, LeVay found that the size of one of the nuclei (INAH-3) in this area was twice as large in heterosexual men as in homosexual men. In fact, the size of these nuclei in homosexual men was similar to that in heterosexual women. This was not the first time that a difference in the brain tissue of homosexual and heterosexual men was found. Earlier, Swaab and Hofman (1990) reported a difference in the size of another part of the brain. However, LeVay's work was the first to identify a difference in an area of the brain known to be related to sexual orientation.

Some have concluded that this provides evidence for the causes of homosexuality, if not for sexual orientation in general. However, LeVay is the first to point out that whether the smaller nuclei caused or are the result of homosexuality is still left unanswered. In addition, the possibility exists that a third factor, one that influences both sexual orientation and the size of this part of the brain, may not have been identified yet. Several studies have been planned to answer these questions and to improve understanding of the relationship between biology and sexual orientation.

The second notable study was conducted by J. Michael Bailey and Richard C. Pillard, one from Northwestern University and the other from Boston University. Bailey and Pillard (1991) studied identical twins, fraternal twins, and adopted brothers, among whom one of each pair had declared himself to be homosexual. They found that the more genetically similar each was to his gay brother, the more likely he was to be gay, also. Homosexuality was found in the remaining number of each pair in 52% of the identical twins (who developed from the same ovum), 22% of the fraternal twins (who developed from different ova), and only 11% of the adopted brothers (who

Ethical DIMENSIONS

Research on Causes of Homosexuality

As can be seen from information presented in this chapter, many researchers are interested in what determines sexual orientation or, perhaps for some, what causes homosexuality. They would argue that it is important to know what factors determine sexual orientation because if causes are known, then sexual orientation could be influenced in whatever way might be desired.

Others argue that research into the cause(s) of homosexuality is unethical and should not be undertaken because it assumes more often than not that homosexuality is a form of mental illness or an undesirable deviance from the heterosexual norm, which should be cured (Schuklenk & Ristow, 1996).

Do you think research about the causes of sexual orientation (or homosexuality) is ethical or unethical?

share no common genetic material). The researchers estimated that between 30% and 70% of the determining factors of homosexuality are genetic. However, questions remain: Even if 70% is genetic, what accounts for the other 30%? What role do prenatal hormonal secretions play? What role does environment play once the child is born?

No single scientific theory about what causes sexual orientation has been substantiated. Studies to associate orientation exclusively with genetic, hormonal, or environmental factors have so far been inconclusive.

Effect of School Environment

Something not often considered related to sexual orientation is the environment found in educational institutions. For example, how do teachers deal with the topic of sexual orientation or with students with various sexual orientations? How do heterosexual peers treat gays, lesbians, and bisexuals?

Telljohann and associates (1995) reported that less than half of a random sample of 211 high school health teachers taught about homosexuality. When taught, it was most commonly taught for less than one class period. Only one in four teachers perceived himself or herself as competent in teaching about homosexuality. One in five teachers said students often used abusive language when describing homosexuals. One-third of health teachers indicated that gay and lesbian rights are a threat to the American family and its values. More than half of the health teachers indicated that gay and lesbian support groups would not be supported by their school administrators. Interestingly, only 10 states require educators to include information about sexual orientation in their sexuality education programs (Haffner & Gambrell, 1993).

Harris (1997) claimed that schools, especially junior high schools and high schools, are failing to accept gay, lesbian, and bisexual youths equally and teach acceptance to fellow students and faculty. She indicated a need for better role models in the career development of lesbian and gay youth, the importance of incorporation of the topic of homosexuality in the curriculum, and the need for open discussions about gay and lesbian issues at school.

Two men, Benjie Nycum and Mike Glatze, began traveling the country in 2001 to help promote positive self-image and a sense of belonging for gay youth. They have a web site called "Young Gay America" that they support with earnings from their day jobs. They provide safe sex information on the web site, post poems and essays from readers, and spend hours each night answering e-mails asking for advice. In addition, there are more than 2,000 gay–straight alliances in schools in the United States that can help create the integration that is so crucial for gay kids "feeling a sense of belonging" (Lotozo, 2003).

Although not all sexual minority youth experience difficulties, a number of issues frequently confront students who begin to perceive themselves as gay or lesbian. These include identity conflict, feelings of isolation and stigmatization, peer relationship problems, and family disruptions (Marinoble, 1998). Because awareness of a homosexual sexual orientation sometimes occurs quite early in life, it is vital that school personnel at all levels be active and informed in addressing this topic.

Fontaine (1998) pointed out that gay adolescents face the same developmental challenges as their heterosexual counterparts, with the added burden of attempting to incorporate a stigmatized sexual identity with little support from school personnel. Teachers either avoid the topic of homosexuality or, when discussing it, frequently present it in a negative manner.

Ryan and Futterman (2001) pointed out that although the vast majority of lesbian and gay youth become well-adjusted adults who lead satisfying, productive lives, their additional developmental challenges require a range of coping skills and adaptation. Unfortunately, unlike most of their heterosexual

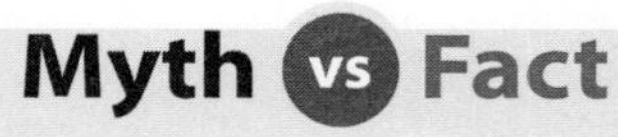

Myth: A homosexual can be easily recognized as being different from heterosexuals.
Fact: Only a small proportion of homosexuals are what can be termed "visible homosexuals." The vast majority look and act just as everyone else does and differ only in their sexual orientation.

Myth: Gay men really want to be women and lesbians really desire to be men.
Fact: Most homosexuals are perfectly happy with their sex; they just prefer relationships with someone of the same sex.

Myth: Homosexual males are effeminate and weak, and homosexual females are masculine and physically strong.
Fact: Sexual orientation has nothing to do with one's body type or style of movement, nor does body type dictate sexual orientation.

peers, they have no built-in support system. They must learn to identify, explore, and ultimately integrate a positive adult identity despite persistent negative stereotypes of lesbian and gay people. They also must learn to protect themselves from ridicule, verbal and physical abuse, and exposure. The social and emotional isolation experienced by gay and lesbian youth is a unique stressor that increases risk for a range of health problems.

Russell (2001) added support to this idea by indicating that gay and lesbian youth have more threats of violence as well as experiences of violence, have substance use and abuse rates well above the national average, and have a higher risk of thinking about and attempting suicide. In addition, Sadowski (2001) indicates that verbal, physical, and sexual harassment of gay and lesbian students is widespread in U.S. schools and that many teachers and administrators do not deal effectively with such incidents.

Staley and coworkers (2001) indicated that the individual consequences of living as an openly gay person can be profound—rejection by family and friends, physical violence and verbal abuse, insensitive health and social services, loss of jobs or housing, and lack of protection under the law. Homosexual boys are more likely than heterosexual boys to report poor body image, binge eating, and suicide attempts.

Black and Underwood (1998) mentioned that schools are the one location through which all youth pass, and school personnel have a major effect on their healthy development. There must be a healthy school setting for all students. This means allowing students to learn, grow, develop, and reflect their diversity without fear of violence, harassment, and prejudice. Such an environment would enable all students to develop accurate perceptions of homosexuality, dispelling feelings of hatred and contempt, which when left unchallenged lead to discrimination, gay bashing, and the perpetuation of homophobia.

Many school personnel have been reluctant to include sexual orientation in their antidiscrimination policies. Some researchers feel that schools' hostile environment forces 28% of gay and lesbian students to drop out. Sixty-five percent of teachers in one Colorado survey had never taken a course that included information on homosexuality (Reese, 1997).

The climate at the college and university level is also important. Eliason (1996) surveyed 1,287 university employees about attitudes toward lesbian, gay, and bisexual employees and students. Twenty-five percent of the subjects had negative attitudes, and 47% did not favor granting health benefits to partners of lesbian, gay, and bisexual employees. She concluded that the overall campus climate remained hostile because of a large number of negative attitudes.

More and more universities are signaling to prospective students that they have gay-friendly campuses. For example, in 2003 Stanford University gave every freshman a CD highlighting the campus's gay and lesbian resources, including its community center. San Jose State University regularly features gay and lesbian people in its brochures. Several forces are driving the growing momentum to make gay students feel welcome. Students are coming out earlier and are searching for colleges where they will find social acceptance. As the gay population increases its visibility, students and scholars are demanding the same outreach efforts that ethnic groups and women fought for years ago. Also, school admissions staff are realizing that homosexual students comprise an important demographic that should be reached in some way (Vo, 2003).

Lesbian, gay, and bisexual educators sometimes choose to "come out" or publicly reveal their sexual orientation. Waldo and Kemp (1997) investigated the effect of a gay instructor's coming out on his students' attitudes toward lesbians and gay men. A survey was administered to students at the beginning and the end of a semester. Midway through the semester, the gay instructor disclosed his sexual orientation to his students as part of a lesson on sexual orientation. Students in his section demonstrated improved attitudes, while students in a heterosexual professor's class showed no change in attitudes. It appears that a gay instructor's coming out may positively affect his students' attitudes toward lesbian, gay, and bisexual people. However, these efforts by individual instructors are only a small part of the more comprehensive institutional efforts needed to create a healthier climate for the appreciation of sexual diversity.

In one study of gay and lesbian adolescents aged 14 to 21 years, half of the students said that homosexuality had been discussed in their classes, and 50% of the females and 37% of the males said it was handled negatively (Gay, lesbian, and bisexual adolescents, 1998). Clearly there is much progress to be made here.

Research indicates that supportive programs in schools can make a difference (Sadowski, 2001). For example, schools that had gay–straight alliances and school-based support groups for gay and lesbian students and their "straight allies" were much more likely to be welcoming places for sexual minority students. Teacher training about gay and lesbian issues can also improve school climate.

Homosexual Life

As we grow and develop, many challenges confront us regardless of our sexual orientation. Typically homosexuals are happy, well-balanced people just like anyone else. They basically enjoy the same activities as other people, have similar goals in life, and in recent years have been able to enjoy parenthood through adoption or, for some lesbians, through artificial insemination. This is not often the picture that heterosexuals get, however, because it is more commonly problematic behavior that is seen. For example, happy, healthy homosexuals do not seek psychotherapy more often than happy, healthy heterosexuals do; but we often tend to generalize about all homosexuals from those few who do seek help. If we did the same thing with heterosexuals, we would have a very skewed picture of what heterosexuals are really like.

Many homosexuals, however, are more likely to experience certain kinds of challenges than are heterosexuals. For example, we know that many gay, lesbian, and bisexual students experience harassment and are the victims of hate crimes in high school. Although many report that they received support regarding sexual orientation issues from someone at school, in one study more than 35% reported a previous suicide attempt (Jordan, 1997).

Gay, lesbian, and bisexual youth must cope with prejudiced, discriminatory, and violent behavior and messages in their families, schools, and communities. These often result in isolation, fear of stigmatization, and lack of peer or familial support (Just the facts about sexual orientation and youth, 2000).

In May 1999, James Hormel, a San Francisco businessman and Democratic Party contributor, became the U.S. ambassador to Luxembourg. The appointment followed a 3-year delay in the Senate, threats by a senator to block all other Clinton appointees, and a constitutional maneuver by Clinton during the congressional Memorial Day recess. Although no doubts were raised as to Hormel's abilities to serve his country, senators wanted to block his appointment because he was the first openly gay U.S. ambassador nominee.

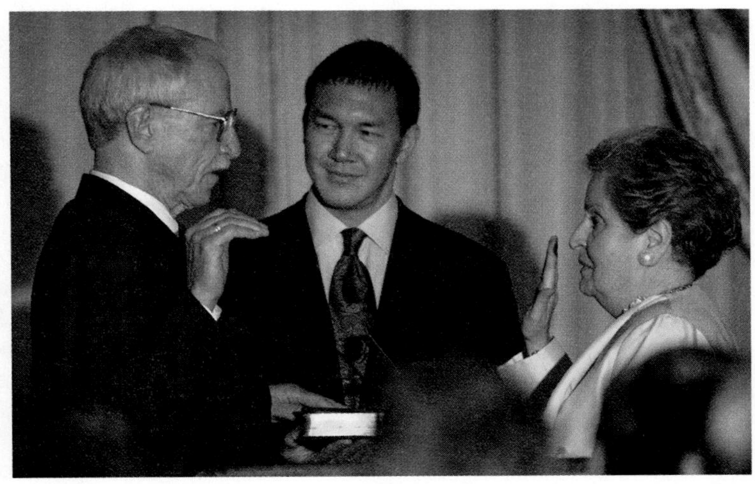

Myth vs Fact

Myth: Homosexuals want to seduce children into a life of homosexuality.
Fact: Although some homosexuals seduce children, most sexual abuse of children is committed by heterosexuals. Both situations are intolerable, but to blame homosexuals alone for the sexual abuse of children is wrong.

Myth: Homosexuals should not be teachers.
Fact: It would be clearly wrong for a teacher of any sexual orientation to seduce students or to encourage them to adopt a particular sexual lifestyle, but there is no reason to expect such behavior to be more or less prevalent among homosexuals.

Myth: Homosexuals are suffering from a mental illness.
Fact: When homosexuals and heterosexuals are matched by age, IQ, and education, mental health experts cannot find differences in adjustment between the two groups.

Myth: Homosexuals are poor security risks.
Fact: There may have been some foundation for this belief in the past because homosexuals were easy targets for blackmail; however, as society grows less homophobic and as many homosexuals identify themselves publicly, the supposed risk should evaporate.

An interesting case of discrimination was reported by Young (2002). A Christian group at Central College, in Iowa, forced one of its student leaders to give up his position as president of the InterVarsity Christian Fellowship because he would not disavow his homosexuality. The same person was also president of the student government at the college. Leaders of InterVarsity asked him to resign his leadership position because he would not agree to a statement that the only acceptable form of sexual activity is that of a man and a woman who are married. This led to a debate at the college about whether the InterVarsity Christian Fellowship should continue to be recognized on the campus.

Lesbian, gay, and bisexual youth have higher than average rates of depression, suicide attempts, substance abuse, sexually transmitted infections, school failure, family rejection, and homelessness (Kreiss & Patterson, 1997). In addition, students reporting same-gender contact are more likely to report fighting and victimization resulting in elevated risk of injury, disease, and death resulting from violence, substance abuse, and suicidal behaviors (Faulkner, 1998).

Living in an environment in which many people do not accept differences in sexual orientation can also be a challenge. Malaney (1997) reported that 60% of college students heard derogatory comments directed at their gay, lesbian, and bisexual friends. A review of the research also indicates that discrimination against gay and lesbian workers occurs in the workplace (Badgett, 1996).

One relatively recent development on some college campuses has been the establishment of fraternities for gay students. As of 2003 there were perhaps two dozen gay fraternities around the country; about half of them have sprung up since 1998. The University of South Alabama, Kent State University, and Florida International University (FIU) are among the universities that have them. At FIU the Gamma Lambda Mu men took great pains to spell out the precise limits of their bonding. Their bylaws state that brothers may not date one another. They want to prove to their classmates that gay men can join together in the spirit of service and camaraderie and not for sexual activity. Gay and lesbian groups have gained acceptance on most college campuses, but entry into the Greek system has been much more slow (DeQuine, 2003).

As discussed in Chapter 2, Alan Bell and Martin Weinberg (1978) studied the lifestyle of homosexuals and concluded that a more appropriate term than *homosexuality* would be *homosexualities*. They found that homosexual relationships could be categorized as (1) *closed couples* living together in committed, stable relationships; (2) *open couples* living together with less emotional involvement and having intercourse outside the relationship; (3) *functionals,* sexually active people uncommitted to any partner; (4) *dysfunctionals,* sexually active people with sexual problems who are dissatisfied with their sexual orientation; and (5) *asexuals,* those unhappy about being homosexual and less active sexually.

An increasing number of gays seek marriage, even though these marriages are not usually legally recognized. Some lawmakers simply ignore the issue, and others have gone out of their way to institute laws prohibiting gay marriages. Sometimes homosexuals decide to have a marriage ceremony even though it may not be legally recognized. This can lead to other interesting issues. For example, the topic of same-sex marriage ceremonies in campus churches has sparked controversy at several universities (Same-sex weddings on campuses, 1997).

Reform Jewish rabbis have the option of presiding at gay commitment ceremonies. In approving this option, Jewish leaders said, "It is not sinful to be a gay and lesbian," and "Gay and lesbian Jews, and the committed relationships they form with their partners, deserve the recognition and respect due to people created in the image of God" (Thompson, 2000).

Except that both people are of the same sex, the marriages usually resemble heterosexual ones in every way. It is interesting to note that at least in Denmark the divorce rate for homosexuals is only 17%, compared to 46% among heterosexuals. Reasons given for this difference include that newly married homosexuals are older on average than newly married heterosexuals, that many have been in their relationships for years beforehand, and that because of society's objection to overt homosexuality only those who are strongly motivated to marry do so (Jones, 1997).

The Social Scene

In the United States the homosexual subculture is centered on private clubs, homosexual bars, and homophile organizations. These organizations are designed to help protect homosexuals, promote their rights, promote a positive image of the gay lifestyle, and help the general public better understand homosexuality. Clubs, bars, and organizations give homosexuals opportunities to fraternize with other gays and perhaps develop social and/or intimate relationships.

Gay bars are most often cocktail lounges that cater to either male or female homosexuals, but usually not to both. They are places where dancing and socializing occur. Other than their clientele, gay bars are not very different from typical heterosexual bars.

Since the AIDS scare, gay baths attended by gay men are less popular, and many localities have actually passed legislation defining them as health hazards and outlawing them. This is because sexual activity with a stranger has been identified as a high-risk activity for HIV transmission. However, where they are legal, many gays still attend these facilities. The baths usually are dimly lit, with many rooms for dancing and socializing. The typical bath visit involves checking one's clothes on entering, being issued a towel, and finding a partner who is willing to have sexual activity in one of the private

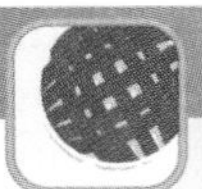

DIMENSIONS

Attitudes About Gay Males in Mexico and the United States

Significant differences exist between the homosexual behaviors of Mexican males in Mexico and those of middle-class Anglo males in the United States. Most Mexican homosexual males appear to have strong preferences for playing either the anal insertive or the anal receptive sexual role, but not both. Although they may engage in fellatio, anal intercourse provides the ultimate sexual satisfaction.

In Mexico there is a widely held belief that feminine males prefer to play the female (receptive) role. The link between effeminacy and homosexuality also results in a belief that as a result of this role preference feminine males are sexually interested only in masculine males with whom they play the passive sexual role.

One effect of homosexual role playing in Mexico is that only the feminine male is labeled as a "homosexual." The masculine self-image of Mexican males is not threatened by their homosexual behavior as long as they play the anal insertive role and also have a reputation for having sexual relations with women.

Compared to Mexican males, Anglo males are generally believed not to have a strongly developed preference for playing one sexual role over the other, and not necessarily to look on anal intercourse as the preferred or ultimate technique in homosexual sexual encounters. It seems unusual for Anglo males to adhere in the United States to a particular role, and fellatio is the most frequently practiced sexual technique.

Source: Zinn, M. B., Hondagneu-Sotelo, P., & Messner, A. *Through the prism of difference.* Boston: Allyn & Bacon, 1997.

rooms or in the "orgy" room. Homosexuals seeking impersonal sexual activity can find it at the baths.

Another place where some homosexual men meet to find a sexual partner is in public restrooms. Sexual activity in public toilets, known as "tearooms," has long been a significant and controversial part of gay culture. Concern increased on many college campuses when a web site that listed popular places for sexual activity between men, including bathrooms at dozens of colleges nationwide, was discovered (Hoover, 2003). Some college police conducted undercover stings and routinely questioned men who appeared to be loitering around bathrooms. In a twist of technology, the same web site that allowed users to post messages about their "cruising" experiences helped police determine where the activity was happening, and to gauge the success of their operations to discourage it. The tearooms have a distinct culture. Men use signals to approach each other. The sexual activity, usually fellatio, is quick. Words are rarely spoken between partners. Some people argue that colleges should not intrude upon activities that take place behind closed doors, even if the doors are those of bathroom stalls. Others feel that using a public bathroom is different from doing something in the privacy of one's own home. They consider it an issue of public decency and assert that people do not want to be solicited for sexual activity or to witness it.

The impersonal nature of the sexual activity that takes place in the stalls of the restroom is often the attraction; for others it is the only place they feel comfortable meeting sexual partners. The public has on numerous occasions been shocked to learn that a well-known figure—usually not known to be homosexual—frequents a particular public restroom to engage in homosexual acts. The restroom affords the anonymity desired while still providing a sexual outlet. These restrooms are known to harbor the tearoom trade and are subject to periodic police raids. As with the baths, however, the anonymity of the public restroom has the disadvantage of increasing the chances of contracting HIV. As such, they have become less frequently employed as a place for casual sexual activity.

Although clubs, bars, and organizations are often safe places for homosexuals, there is a fear of police harassment and of possible discovery. In addition, some homosexuals desire to have more open and intimate relationships.

In a permanent relationship, living together seems to be more important to lesbians than to male homosexuals. Many gays of both sexes believe that steady love relationships are quite meaningful and enjoy the warmth and understanding of such relationships.

Social Issues and Homosexuals

Additional issues related to homosexual life are being considered all the time. For example, Burdon (1996) found that within intimate relationships heterosexuals engage in deceptive behavior more than homosexuals or bisexuals. The degree of openness about their homosexuality is unrelated to deceptive behavior among homosexuals and bisexuals.

The issue of homosexuals becoming parents has been controversial. Some people feel homosexuals and bisexuals should have the same rights to be parents as heterosexuals; others are fearful of the potential influence homosexuals may have on the sexual identities of their children. Interestingly, Costello (1997) found that homosexual and bisexual parents are willing to be active in fostering a sexual identity different from their own in their children.

Crawford and Solliday (1996) assessed the reactions of 97 college students to vignettes describing situations in which diverse couples were trying to adopt a young boy. The subjects were more likely to see homosexual couples as creating a dangerous environment for the child, being more emotionally unstable, and being less likely to be awarded custody of the child than heterosexual couples.

A majority of respondents to a large telephone survey found divorce, sexual intercourse before marriage, interracial relationships, and single motherhood acceptable. However, 57% considered homosexuality unacceptable. Respondents were willing to grant homosexuals basic rights, such as freedom from harassment or the right to earn a living. But they stopped short of sanctioning anything that might imply they considered homosexuality the moral equivalent of their own behavior (Rosin & Morin, 1998).

Since 1994 the military has had a "Don't ask; don't tell" policy. This means that military officials are not supposed to ask about the sexual orientation of members of the military, but that they are supposed to discharge openly gay troops. Because the military is struggling to recruit and retain good people, leaders look the other way to retain an experienced service member. At the same time, cases of antigay harassment have more than doubled (to almost 1,000 cases per year). Incidents ranged from verbal taunts and death threats to assaults and one murder (Stone, 2000).

As we have mentioned, learning more about sexual orientations can result in a more positive attitude about various behaviors. For example, viewing a documentary film (*The times of Harvey Milk,* 1983) about the events surrounding the life and death of a prominent gay politician had a significant and positive effect on attitudes toward homosexuals of 115 college students (Riggle, Ellis, & Crawford, 1996).

However, even in professional journals there may be biases related to sexual orientation. A content analysis of 13,217 articles published in marriage and family therapy journals showed that only 77 (0.006%) focused on gay, lesbian, and/or bisexual issues or used sexual orientation as a variable (Clark & Serovich, 1997).

In 1993 the American Medical Association (AMA) banned discrimination against gay, lesbian, and bisexual doctors by adding the words *sexual orientation* to the AMA nondiscrimination bylaws. Despite progress such as increasing support services for gay medical students, two-thirds of medical students reported hearing antigay comments from a classroom instructor, 42% said that clinical faculty had made negative remarks about homosexuality, and 7% indicated that their homosexuality had been criticized personally by an instructor. Gay and lesbian patient care needs to be integrated throughout the medical school curriculum (Wallick, 1997).

Evidence is accumulating that lesbians experience certain elevated health risks when compared to heterosexual women. These include increased risk of breast cancer, untreated sexually transmitted infections, and barriers to health care (Ellingson, 2002). The reasons for these risks are not totally clear. Reasons for increased breast cancer may include childlessness (associated with a 36% increase in the risk of development of breast cancer), higher rates of obesity and alcohol use, and less likelihood to practice breast self-examination and receive clinical breast exams. Although the prevalence of sexually transmitted infections is generally lower among lesbians than among heterosexual women, risk reduction behaviors also seem to be lower. Reasons given for relatively low frequency of early detection behaviors include low perceived need, fears of and experience of homophobic care providers, and lack of insurance.

In spite of some positive changes, it is interesting to note the influence of a patient's sexual orientation on the therapist's perception of the patient's mental health. Four hundred and seventeen therapists reviewed hypothetical case histories in which the patient was either heterosexual or homosexual. Patients labeled as homosexual received diagnoses of more severe mental illness than did those labeled as heterosexual (Rubinstein, 1995).

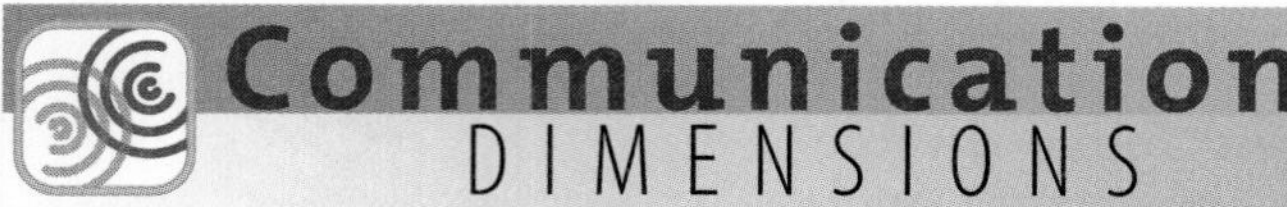

Communication About Gay and Lesbian Athletes

Being accepted and being accepting can be issues for college athletes. Traditionally there is an assumption that male athletes are heterosexually virile and desirable. Female athletes can face a very different perception—that they are all lesbians or bisexual. Straight women can go to great lengths to avoid that stereotype, leaving their homosexual teammates out in the cold. The highly visible men's sports of football, basketball, hockey, and baseball remain the most unaccepting of homosexual athletes. Athletes who perform individually, rather than on teams, may have an easier time being accepted (Jacobson, 2002 [1]).

In 2002 the Rice University football coach was quoted as saying that "while he would not necessarily kick a player off the team for being gay, he probably would think hard about doing so." Immediately, the president of Rice University indicated the need for the coach to affirm his commitment to the university's nondiscrimination policy and to apologize for "the damage done by his comments." The coach did so (Jacobson, 2002 [2]).

There are examples of communication difficulties related to homosexuality in pro sports, also. For example, in 2002 it was rumored that Mike Piazza, All-Star catcher for the New York Mets, was gay. Responding to the rumors, Piazza said that the Major Leagues are ready for gay players, but he is not one of them.

Also in 2002, Esera Tuaolo, who had played defensive tackle in the National Football League for 9 years, revealed that he was gay. He said that he retired from pro football in 1999 because of failing knees and shoulders, but also because of the discomfort he experienced hearing players make disparaging remarks about gays. One of his former teammates said, "Had other players known Tuaolo was gay, he would have been eaten alive" (Airing it out, 2002).

Communication related to homosexual athletes remains an important social issue.

Although approval of gays and lesbians has increased in recent years, disapproval remains formidible. In a May 2001 Gallup Poll, 43% of Americans surveyed said that homosexuality should not be considered "an acceptable alternative lifestyle" (O'Keefe, 2001). Between 1998 and 2001, supporters of gay and lesbian rights lost 13 of 18 initiatives at the state and local levels and many anti-gay-rights referendums are under way across the country. Gay and lesbian advocates tend to blame ignorance, bigotry, and fear based on misinformation, inflexible mores, and myths for this lack of support.

Obviously, many social issues influence our feelings and reactions toward people of different sexual orientations. A humanistic outlook on homosexuality assumes that people freely choose sexual behaviors on the basis of their sexual desires, needs, and ways of seeking closeness and intimacy. The humanist is less concerned with the choice of sexual partner or the preference for certain sexual acts than with the creation of mutual intimacy and closeness and mutual acceptance in a climate of enhancing each person's personal satisfaction. In other words, whatever two partners decide to do in the privacy of their sexual encounters by expressed mutual consent and joint planning is morally right and ethically responsible (Garai, 1996).

Do you think we need to make changes in society's views, or do you feel conditions are fine the way they are?

Can You Tell Who Is Gay?

One of us recently invited a gay male to speak in his class and was amused by the students' reactions to the guest. The guest speaker's visit was announced a week in advance, to allow the students time to envision what this person might look like. Why not close your eyes for a moment and imagine for yourself how this person looked?

Well, the next week in walked this "hunk." The women in the class, in particular, were stunned. How could such a gorgeous male specimen be wasted? All he needs is a sexy woman who really knows what she is doing! This guy does not even speak with a lisp or walk funny! Many of these attitudes were actually expressed during the discussion that ensued.

These students' attitude was that any man who was attractive and could have any woman he wanted would surely have no reason to be gay. Only those who were unattractive, who walked with a "swish," or who spoke with a lisp—and therefore could not "make it" with someone of the opposite sex—"resorted" to homosexuality. The data just do not support this view. The great majority—some estimate 90%—of homosexuals are not visibly identifiable. Homosexuality is not just a choice made because no other choice is available. And attractiveness is unrelated to homosexual orientation.

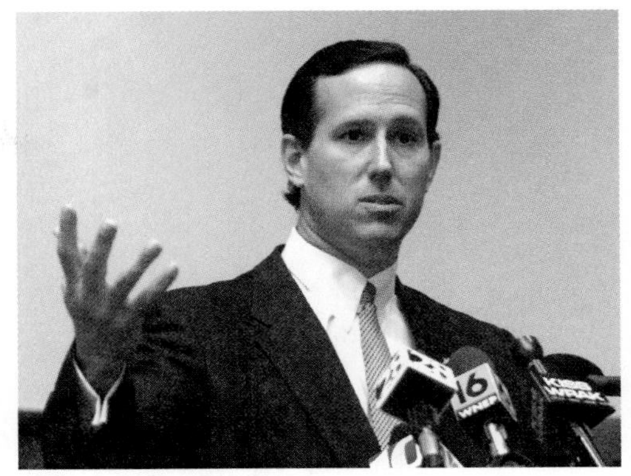

On April 7, 2003, in an interview with the Associated Press, Senator Rick Santorum is quoted as comparing consensual homosexual sexual activity to bigamy, polygamy, adultery, and even incest. Sen. Santorum later admits to having a problem "with homosexual acts" and "acts outside of traditional heterosexual relationships." While the senator's remarks sparked quite an uproar in the media, the White House did not immediately denounce the senator's comments. What message regarding the government's view of homosexuality does this send to the American public?

Homophobia

Although society's attitudes are gradually becoming more accepting, there are still many people who have strong negative feelings about homosexuals. **Homophobia** is an irrational fear of homosexuality in others, a fear of homosexual feelings within oneself, or an unhappiness with one's own homosexuality. Homophobia probably results from ignorance, a belief in the common myths about homosexuality, or even the tendency to judge homosexuals as immoral. People with strong negative feelings often reveal their homophobia by openly insulting homosexuals and even subjecting people suspected of being homosexual to verbal or physical assault. Also homophobics are often careful to avoid behaving in ways that could be interpreted as homosexual, for example, by shunning certain kinds of clothing or physical activities.

According to FBI statistics, the number of hate crimes based on sexual orientation increased from 767 in 1992 to 1,317 in 1999. These numbers represent 11.6% of all reported hate crimes in 1992 and 16.7% in 1999 (Gays, lesbians and bisexuals rank third in reported hate crimes, 2001). It is clear that hate crimes based on sexual orientation are increasing.

homophobia
An irrational fear of homosexuality.

heterosexist
An attitude that reinforces heterosexuality as the privileged and powerful norm.

We talked about school settings earlier; here it is appropriate again to mention teachers. Butler and Byrne (1992) found a group of 97 undergraduate elementary education majors to be slightly homophobic. They pointed out that even slightly homophobic attitudes among elementary educators is a concern because they are in a unique position to significantly affect the attitudes of many students. They suggested that reducing homophobia must begin at the personal level. In addition, a teacher can ask the following questions to create a more accepting classroom environment: (1) Do I make **heterosexist** (characterized by the belief that heterosexuality is the privileged and powerful norm) assumptions? (2) Do I ignore homophobic remarks? (3) Do I blame my audience for their own misinformation? (4) Do I use educational materials that assume that all my students are heterosexual?

Logan (1996) made a couple of interesting observations related to homophobia. She found that males were more likely to rate themselves as homophobic than females. She also argued that broadly applying the term *homophobic* to describe antihomosexual responses is inaccurate and inappropriate and that most antihomosexual responses are more prejudicial than phobic.

Matchinsky and Iverson (1996) studied 108 heterosexual college students and found more positive attitudes toward homosexuality in those working toward a psychology degree than in those with only one course in psychology.

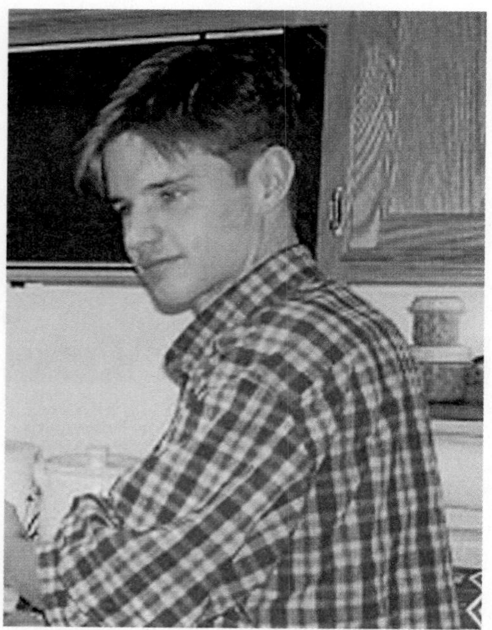

In October 1998, Matthew Shepard, a gay University of Wyoming student, made a pass at Aaron McKinney in a bar. Hours later, McKinney and an associate set out to avenge McKinney's embarrassment. They tied Shepard to a fence post, pistol-whipped him, and left him to die. The attack was denounced nationwide as a hate crime and drew media attention to the horrors that homophobia could unleash.

They also found that those who believed in a psychological cause of homosexuality were more homophobic than those who believed in a biological cause.

Adams and coworkers (1996) explored the susceptibility of homophobic and nonhomophobic men to homosexual imagery. They found that 80% of the homophobic participants experienced moderate to definite erections while viewing a male homosexual video, compared with only one-third of the nonhomophobic men. Strangely, the homophobes' own assessments of their arousal were low; they did not think, or at least did not admit, that they were aroused. Adams indicated that the findings support thinking that homophobia is the result of repressed homosexual urges or a type of latent homosexuality.

Black and Underwood (1998) reported that more than 40% of the clients of the Institute for the Protection of Lesbian and Gay Youth in New York City had suffered from homophobic violence. When this violence happens at school, dropping out seems to be the only choice for many victims.

Walters and Hayes (1998) commented on the prevalence and cultural influences on homophobia in the United States. They suggested that, as social institutions reflecting cultural values, schools, colleges, and universities sanction an environment that ignores the value of gay students, staff, and faculty. Institutional homophobia dismisses the legitimacy of these individuals by refusing to establish a homosexually affirmative environment and by refusing to deal with prejudice, discrimination, and abuse against homosexuals in the same way they protect other oppressed groups. People who work with students should be trained to recognize, address, and challenge homophobia.

Coming Out

The lifestyle of a gay person is greatly influenced by the extent to which he or she decides to remain in the closet—to keep his or her sexual orientation a secret—or to **come out**—accepting that orientation and making it public. Each choice can be made in varying degrees.

> **come out**
> Accept and make homosexual orientation public.

The decision to come out involves several stages: (1) acknowledging, (2) accepting, and (3) openly expressing one's homosexuality. Some homosexuals never acknowledge their sexual orientation even to themselves. The first step in coming out is usually to realize that one does not fit the heterosexual model. The second step is acceptance, a step that sometimes requires that the individual overcome a learned negative view of homosexuality that becomes a negative view of himself or herself.

Even when a homosexual or bisexual reaches the acceptance stage, he or she can still decide to remain in the closet. It is generally easier to pass as a heterosexual than to take the final step toward openness. However, a person who can live publicly within his or her true sexual orientation generally has a better chance of living a happier life than one who remains secretive. In some situations, however, such as being a parent, the pain of coming out may far outweigh that of staying in the closet.

Telling the family—whether parents, siblings, spouses, or children—can also be extremely difficult, and many people who would prefer an open homosexual life choose not to face this ordeal.

For most people, the process of deciding to come out begins during school years. As students, few homosexuals choose to disclose their sexual orientation to principals, teachers, counselors, or friends. Reasons cited for nondisclosure include fear of the consequences and not wanting others to know. Most of those who did disclose their sexual orientation received positive feed-

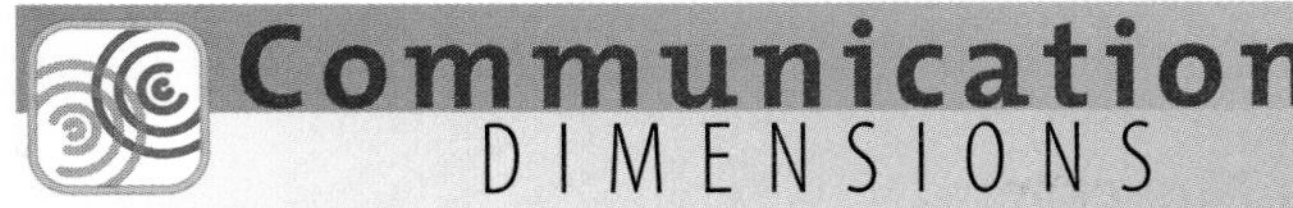

Communication DIMENSIONS

Coming Out Each of us may be in a position to communicate with someone who is thinking about coming out. A few facts and a few communication suggestions may be helpful. First, the facts:

1. Coming out can be important as an affirmation of one's sexual orientation.
2. Coming out can jeopardize some relationships.
3. Coming out can promote a sense of pride in one's sexual orientation and, in the long run, actually improve relationships with both gay and straight people.
4. Coming out is usually a two-part process—first, coming out to oneself; second, coming out to others.
5. Coming out to oneself may involve gradually dealing with denial, putting matters into focus, and even dealing with personal homophobia.
6. Coming out to others probably involves stages—first involving a few very close friends or relatives, later more relatives, and then a larger public, such as employers, fellow students, and coworkers.
7. Some gays may be out only to a certain degree. For example, only families and very close friends know about their sexual orientation.

Here are a few communication suggestions from professional counselors (Black & Underwood, 1998) that can be helpful to all of us:

1. Coming out should be postponed until the person has a reasonably high sense of self-worth and a support network.
2. The person should be secure in his or her identity before coming out to others.
3. The person should be helped to weigh the pros and cons of coming out and to examine why he or she wants to come out.
4. People who are planning to come out, or who are coming out, usually need a great deal of support and encouragement from others.
5. It is not our responsibility to "make" the person straight or gay. It is our responsibility to help provide a supportive environment.
6. It is important to be ourselves and be sincere.
7. Confidentiality must be respected.
8. Communication should be done in a helpful way but not in a forceful way.
9. Use words that do not assume that everyone is or should be heterosexual. For example, substitute terms such as *partner* or *significant other* for *boyfriend* or *girlfriend.*
10. Role playing can be used to help someone who is going to come out to be prepared to handle a variety of situations.

back for doing so, but both positive and negative consequences of coming out have been reported. Gay men were aware of their sexual orientation at an earlier age than lesbians and were more likely to recommend disclosure to principals and teachers. Females were more likely to disclose only to females, whereas males were likely to come out to both males and females. Both groups were cautious about coming out in the school setting (Harris, 1997).

It is not possible to predict others' response to disclosure. This move can result in a student's experiencing everything from lack of support, isolation, rejection, and ostracism to unfair discipline, taunting, harassment, verbal slurs, persistent random acts of violence, and outright vicious beatings. Students must carefully consider the pros and cons of coming out and examine *why* they want to come out. In any case, coming out should be postponed until the student achieves a reasonable degree of self-esteem and a support network (Black & Underwood, 1998).

Earlier we indicated that gay instructors who come out often positively influence their students' attitudes toward lesbian, gay, and bisexual people (Waldo & Kemp, 1997). Unfortunately, it is difficult if not impossible to know what the reactions of people will be. For many reasons, the decision to come out remains difficult for most homosexuals.

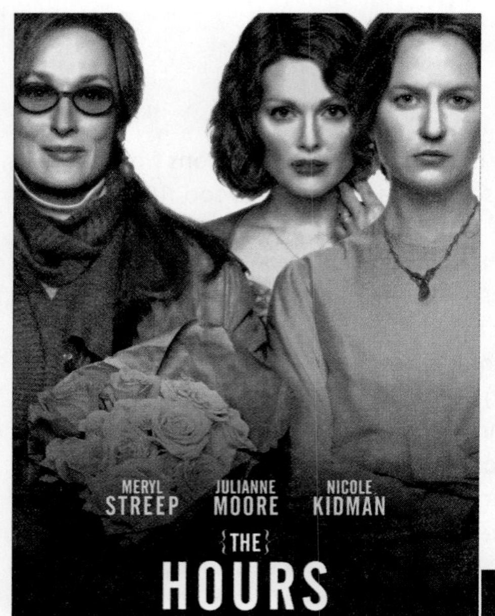

As society grows increasingly comfortable with the topic of homosexuality, more and more films have emerged that treat the issue of homosexuality as the backdrop to the story, not the main story line. The Academy Award–winning film, *The Hours,* depicts three women living different lives at different points in history. While homosexuality does touch upon their lives, the primary message is that of their individual quests for love, individuality, and fulfillment.

Just a few years ago, featuring a homosexual character on a television sitcom would most likely result in a show's cancellation. Today, one of television's most popular comedies proudly and overtly addresses the topic of homosexuality. *Will & Grace,* which focuses on the unique relationship between Will, who is gay, and his best friend, Grace, who is straight, won three Emmys in 2000. Through the experiences of Will and Grace and their friends Jack and Karen, the show frankly and hilariously explores the universal subjects of friendship, sex, relationships, and love, whether heterosexual or homosexual.

The Gay Rights Movement

Gay and lesbian organizations can help gays deal with the stresses experienced as a result of their sexual preference. There are many different organizations that can provide the social support needed to manage such stressful life situations as coming out or staying in the closet. The support of people who understand what you are experiencing and who can offer advice can be invaluable. One of the authors has studied the effects of homophile organizations on several aspects of their members' health. During the first study (Greenberg, 1973), it was found that homosexual members felt more alienated than heterosexual nonmembers but did not differ in their self-esteem. The question then became whether the organization helped people to become less alienated and to feel better about themselves, or whether people had joined the organization that way. A subsequent study (Greenberg, 1976) looked at this question and found that self-esteem remained constant from the time a person joined the organization throughout his or her membership. However, alienation did change as a result of membership. New members soon became less alienated, probably because now they had compatriots with whom they had a common interest and goal. After 1 year in the organization, however, members' alienation levels rose again, probably because they realized the difficulty of achieving desired societal changes and the slowness of any progress. Even then, though, it is helpful to have others with whom to share these frustrations.

The gay rights movement has progressed, largely because of these homophile organizations and their ability to mobilize their membership to march, to vote, and to boycott when necessary. The movement began in earnest after a raid by the New York City police on the Stonewall gay bar in June 1969. That raid led to a 2-day riot that forever changed the tolerance level of the gay community toward societal prejudice based on sexual orientation. As a result, gays have presented a united front in voting for political candidates who are willing to sponsor their causes. In cities such as San Francisco and Washington, DC, where there are significant numbers of homosexual citizens (voters), politicians are particularly sensitive to gay rights issues. In these cities, gays have made a difference in those elected to public office.

There is no way to know whether social activities, such as the gay rights movement, have influenced other aspects of society or whether aspects of society have influenced gay rights. There is no question that there is more openness about homosexuality in today's society. A prime example of this was Ellen DeGeneres's decision to come out on her TV show in 1998. Another example is the way that homosexual films have moved into the mainstream. In movies, homosexuals were first ignored, then scorned. By the early 1990s, with the AIDS epidemic, homosexuals began to be pitied in films. Films about them tended to be about their homosexuality and not about their overall lives. There are now more movies about homosexuals than ever, but these movies deal with overall issues and not just people's homosexuality and generally appeal to viewers of all sexual orientations (Corliss, 1998).

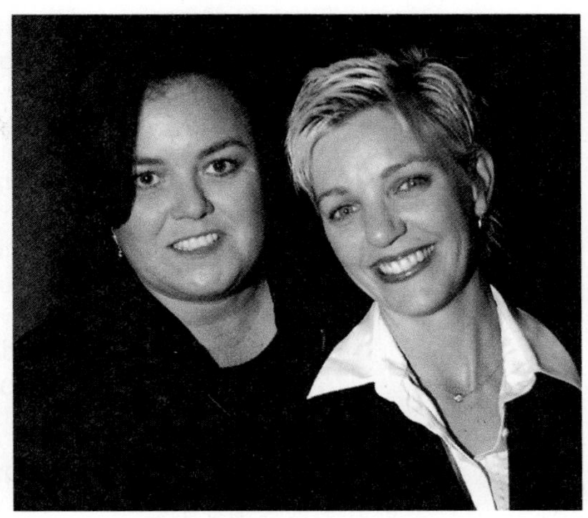

Increasingly, gay men and lesbians are choosing in vitro fertilization or adoption in order to start their own families. The issue of gay and lesbian adoption has recently been in the media after former talk-show host Rosie O'Donnell publicly criticized President Bush's opposition to gay adoption. O'Donnell, who is openly gay, has three adopted children and says that her own experiences as a mother make her certain that gay people should have the right to be parents.

Legal Rights

Marriage in the United States is more than a public recognition of love. It is also a legally binding contract, providing the married couple with myriad tax and legal support benefits, from which gay relationships are usually excluded.

Gays have long argued that marriage is not a requirement for a strong family unit. In 1989, Mayor Ed Koch of New York City agreed (Koch grants benefits for domestic partners, 1989). He issued an order recognizing domestic partnerships of gays. Not merely symbolic, Koch's declaration meant that gay city employees who had live-in companions could be eligible for death benefits. It also allowed labor unions to negotiate for health benefits for such families.

Not all of New York City's politicians agreed with Koch. One argued, "I think that Koch's executive order undermines one of society's most essential institutions: marriage." Koch responded, "Over time, society changes. So must the government that serves it. Practices or policies that might have seemed unacceptable to our grandparents or unusual to our parents seem equitable, indeed necessary, to our generation. We honor the past, but we cannot be held captive to it."

Following are some of the legal benefits for married couples.

- *Income taxes*—In many instances, married couples receive a lower tax rate than would two individuals filing separately. (An exception to this, known as the "marriage penalty," occurs when both spouses earn relatively equal high incomes and consequently pay a higher rate than they would as individuals. This is currently being addressed by Congress.) At any rate, any income tax benefits for married couples do not include gay couples.
- *Adoption*—Many states do not allow gay couples to adopt children. Even states that do allow it generally put married couples first in line.
- *Estate taxes*—Married couples do not have to pay any federal estate taxes (and usually only a limited amount of state estate tax) on the death of a first spouse. State laws provide (for people without wills)

Ethical DIMENSIONS

Should Gay Marriages Be Legal? Given the many legal benefits for married couples, there seems to be increasing pressure to legalize gay marriages. Those who feel gay marriages are not proper, for whatever reasons, would argue that we should not make gay marriages legal. Those who feel we have an ethical responsibility to treat all people equally, and to recognize the rights of various groups, would argue that gay marriages should be legal.

In recent years there have been measures considered in some states to recognize the legal rights of people involved in same-sex partnerships. The question of whether it is ethical to provide or not to provide legal sanction to these partnerships fosters interesting debates.

that property moves directly to the spouse (or spouse and children, depending on the state). Unless a gay couple has an updated will (and most people in the United States do not), the biological family of the deceased can claim all possessions.

- *Employment benefits*—Married couples share a variety of benefits from work (health, dental, life insurance, to name some) that gay partners do not. Many Fortune 500 companies have instituted policies in recent years to allow gay partners such rights, but there is no law requiring this. Companies like Disney and Apple offer these benefits to recruit and retain high-quality talent. Whereas many large companies can afford to do this, many smaller companies are not so inclined.
- *Social Security survivorship benefits and pensions*—At death, the law provides that the surviving spouse receive continued benefits. Not so for gays.
- *Disability decision making*—If a married person becomes seriously injured and needs medical care decisions made for him or her, the law provides that spouses can make those decisions. But in cases in which parents or siblings of a disabled gay person do not approve of his or her relationship, they can—and often do—challenge the domestic partner's decisions in court.

You can see from this list that there are many problems related to legal rights of gay couples. There is much to be done to ensure equal rights for all married couples.

In 2000, Vermont became the first state to approve same-sex unions. Although the term *marriage* was not used, this bill provided homosexual couples with essentially the same rights as heterosexual couples (Drummond, 2000).

Should same-sex couples be allowed to marry legally? Some people feel that same-sex couples should have the same human rights as others. They argue that when people work, pay taxes, enter into lifetime commitments, and raise children, there is no reason they should not be afforded the same social and legal benefits and status as heterosexual couples—including legal marriage. In opposition to this idea, however, an alliance of conservative groups campaigned for a 28th amendment to the U.S. Constitution that would prevent same-sex couples from getting married legally. The proposed Federal Marriage Amendment reads in part: "Marriage in the United States shall consist only of the union of a man and a woman. Neither this Constitution or the constitution of any state, nor state or federal law, shall be construed to require that marital status or the legal incidents thereof be conferred upon unmarried couples or groups" (Should same-sex couples be allowed to marry legally? 2003).

In 2001 the Belgian government approved a bill to legalize same-sex weddings. It made Belgium the second country in the world to recognize gay marriages, after its northern neighbor, the Netherlands (Ames, 2001). In 2003, the Canadian government also decided to recognize gay marriages.

In 2003 the U.S. Supreme Court struck down state sodomy laws as demeaning to homosexuals, and said the government has no authority to regulate the sexual behavior of "consenting adults acting in private" (Murphy, 2003). Many people felt that this decision would have far-reaching implications for the popular discussion about gay rights. For example, some said that by essentially acknowledging gay relationships as legitimate, the Supreme Court justices gave the gay rights movement a new credibility in debates about marriage, partner benefits, adoption, and parental rights.

Should lesbian and gay couples be allowed to adopt children? Some people start with the premise that homosexuality is wrong and believe that such a relationship is an inappropriate context in which to raise children. Because they fear that sexual orientation and behaviors can be learned, they fear that a child raised by a lesbian or gay couple would be more likely to become a lesbian or gay man. Others do not believe that sexual orientation determines one's ability to parent. They feel the most important requirements are the abilities to love, support, and care for a child. Most lesbians and gays were raised by heterosexual parents. Therefore, they believe being raised by a lesbian or gay couple will not create lesbian or gay children any more than being raised by a heterosexual, married couple would guarantee heterosexuality (Should lesbian and gay couples be allowed to adopt? 2003).

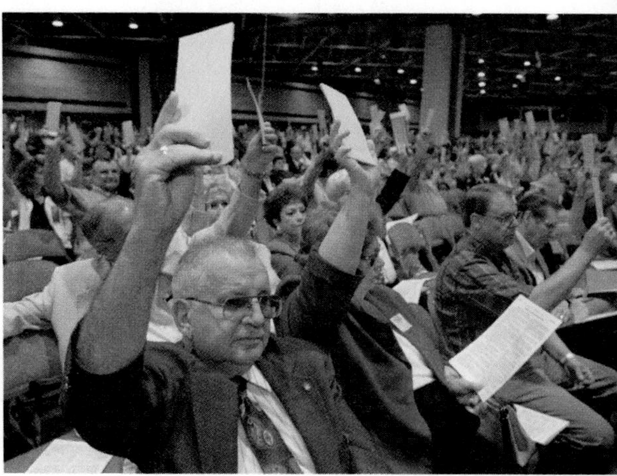

The Southern Baptists voted to boycott Disney for extending employee benefits to domestic partners and for allowing unofficial "Gay Week" at its Florida theme park. Disney's terse official response questioned why anyone would wish to deprive anyone else of basic benefits.

Finally, freshmen entering college have their own ideas about legality and homosexuality. Thirty-six percent of men and 20% of women think it is important to have laws prohibiting homosexual relationships. Forty-seven percent of men and 63% of women think same-sex couples should have the right to legal marital status (Characteristics of freshmen, 2001).

Homosexuality and HIV and AIDS

Acquired immune deficiency syndrome (AIDS) is of particular concern to male homosexuals. AIDS is discussed in detail in In Focus: HIV and AIDS, so we will limit our discussion here to the effect of HIV and AIDS on the homosexual community.

AIDS was first discovered in homosexual men who had a rare cancer called Kaposi's sarcoma. Since then we have learned that AIDS can affect anyone. It is not the group one belongs to that puts one at risk; it is the behavior in which one engages. One of those high-risk behaviors is anal intercourse. Regardless of the sexual orientation of those engaging in anal intercourse, they are placing themselves at risk of contracting the human immunodeficiency virus (HIV), which causes AIDS, for several reasons. Anal intercourse can tear the tissue of the rectum and thus provides a route of entry for HIV. Blood vessels are located close to the skin's surface in the rectum, and it is thought that this, too, may play a part in HIV transmission. Because anal intercourse is a sexual activity in which some homosexual men participate, they are at high risk.

In addition, the more sexual partners one has, the greater the risk of contracting HIV. Again, this is true regardless of sexual orientation. However, because homosexual relationships do not have the same social acceptance or legality as do heterosexual relationships—for example, homosexual lovers cannot legally marry—these relationships tend to be less stable. Thus, some gays are likely to have more sexual partners than do heterosexuals.

Furthermore, because pregnancy is not an issue for homosexual men, the need to use a condom was previously dismissed. Now, however, gay men use condoms more effectively and more frequently than do straight men.

Recognizing their high-risk status, the gay community has organized a massive educational campaign to inform people how to engage in sexual activity in the healthiest way possible. As a result, homosexual men have begun altering their sexual behavior; they engage in anal intercourse less frequently and they are more likely to use a condom when participating in high-risk sexual behavior (Coates & Stall, 1990). The result has been a decrease in the number of infected homosexuals (Winkelstein, et al., 1987).

Exploring the DIMENSIONS of Human Sexuality

Our feelings, attitudes, and beliefs regarding sexuality are influenced by our internal and external environments. Go to sexuality.jbpub.com to learn more about the biological, psychological, and sociological factors that affect your sexuality.

Biological Factors

- Research into genetic factors for homosexuality has been inconclusive. No specific gene has been identified. Any genetic link would be only part of the picture for determining sexual orientation.
- Research into hormonal imbalances (either prenatal or postnatal) has proved inconclusive. No specific hormonal factors have been identified. Any hormonal link would be only one aspect of determining sexual orientation.

Sociocultural Factors

- Homosexual students often feel isolated and stigmatized.
- Family life can be disrupted by disclosure of homosexuality.
- Different cultures view homosexuality in different terms.
- Some states have laws making homosexual sexual activities illegal. Further, gay marriages do not have legal standing for state or federal benefits. Many large corporations have begun to offer employee benefits for domestic partners.

Psychological Factors

- Most theories that the influence of mothers or early sexual experiences lead to changes in sexual orientation have been discounted.
- Most homosexuals lead lives as fulfilling and satisfying as those of most heterosexuals.

CASE STUDY

No single scientific theory about the biological causes of sexual orientation has been substantiated; neither have any psychological theories. It is likely that the biological, psychological, and sociocultural factors interact to influence our sexual orientation. Because the dimensions change over time, an individual's sexual orientation may change over time as well.

Culturally, not all societies view homosexuality in the same manner. In areas of the Pacific such as Papua New Guinea, boys regularly participate in homosexual activities until they reach the age of marriage (19 years). In Mexico, only a male who plays the receptive role in anal intercourse is considered homosexual.

Socially, gays and lesbians in the United States can feel stigmatized and socially isolated as a result of fear of disclosure. Those who disclose their orientation ("come out") face discrimination and possibly even violence. Further, family and friends may reject them.

Discussion Questions

1. What defines a person's sexual orientation? Is sexual orientation constant throughout life, or can it change over time?
2. Describe the theories of the causes of sexual orientation, and whether or not research supports theoretical claims.
3. Compare and contrast the homosexual lifestyle with the heterosexual lifestyle.
4. What are the social issues surrounding homosexuality? How do such issues adversely affect homosexuals?

Application Questions

Reread the chapter-opening story and answer the following questions.

1. Explain why Brad was dating and engaging in sexual activities with Peggy if he thought he was gay.
2. Discuss the social and psychological effects on people who are unable to disclose their sexual orientation and introduce a lifetime partner to friends and family.

Critical Thinking Questions

1. If a genetic link were found for homosexuality, how might that affect those found to have the gene? Would society accept homosexuality as an inherited "defect"? Or would homosexuals encounter more discrimination in the workplace, in the military, and so on?
2. Assuming that studies claiming that only a small percentage of the population is gay are correct, why should efforts be made to accommodate such a small minority?
3. Consider the current "Don't ask; don't tell" policy of the U.S. military. Should sexual orientation make a difference on the battlefield?
4. Given that many states ban same-sex sexual activity, is it ethical to vote admitted homosexuals into public office?
5. If homosexuality had no social stigma, would there be more or fewer people living as homosexuals? Explain your answer.

Critical Thinking Case

When the filmmaker Debra Chasnoff's son started kindergarten, she had more to worry about than the other parents. Her son thought that having two moms was great—but what would the other kids tell him?

From her own experience with school systems, Chasnoff started a film project, *It's Elementary,* which was completed in 1996. She and Helen Cohen, the film's coproducer, toured the country and filmed teachers in classrooms as they described gay and lesbian lifestyles to children. Their goal was to show that the classroom could be a place where children are taught tolerance and acceptance of lifestyles different from those of their own families.

Originally, the film was used in school systems and colleges to educate teachers about the prejudice that exists among young children regarding homosexuality. But more recently, the film has caused quite a stir on the airwaves. After PBS turned it down for national distribution, San Francisco's KQED agreed to sponsor the film.

During the early summer of 1999, 89 of 347 public stations scheduled it, 17 more were on board, and 53 were considering it. This caused some anger among the Christian Right and other conservative groups who do not believe the film should be broadcast where children might watch it without supervision, although the stations had scheduled it for nighttime airing. They also argued that the film does not take parents' rights into consideration (Ness, 1999).

What do you think? Should teachers be encouraged to educate elementary school children about the topic of homosexuality, or should this responsibility be left to parents? Should films like *It's Elementary* be broadcast on national TV if the goal is to get people talking and thinking about educational issues?

Exploring Personal Dimensions

Take a few moments to measure the strength of your feelings about homosexuality and gender identity by using this values grid.

Place in the appropriate square of the grid the *italicized* key term in the questions following that shows how you feel about the question. Note that you will be identifying the *degree* of your feelings, not whether they are positive or negative. Fill in all 16 squares, placing only one key term in any one square. (You may change your mind as you go along if you discover other key words about which you feel more or less strongly.) After you complete the grid, look it over to see how strong your feelings are. If you can find a willing partner, compare your grids and discuss your responses.

	Very Strongly	**Strongly**	**Mildly**	**No Reaction**
1. How would you feel if your closest *friend* told you he or she was a homosexual?	❑	❑	❑	❑
2. How do you feel about *two girls* who greet each other with a kiss after a long summer vacation?	❑	❑	❑	❑
3. How do you feel about *two boys* greeting each other with a kiss after a long summer vacation?	❑	❑	❑	❑
4. How do you feel about a person who would *beat up* a homosexual for fun?	❑	❑	❑	❑

5. How do you feel about two *girls holding hands* on the way to class?	❑	❑	❑	❑
6. How do you feel about girls wearing *boys' clothes?*	❑	❑	❑	❑
7. How do you feel about boys wearing *girls' clothes?*	❑	❑	❑	❑
8. How do you feel about two *boys holding hands* on the way to class?	❑	❑	❑	❑
9. How do you feel about *boys* who do not like sports?	❑	❑	❑	❑
10. How do you feel about *girls* who do like sports?	❑	❑	❑	❑
11. How do you feel about taking *group showers?*	❑	❑	❑	❑
12. How do you feel about a man taking over the household *chores?*	❑	❑	❑	❑
13. How do you feel about a male *hairdresser?*	❑	❑	❑	❑
14. How do you feel about a woman who becomes a *construction worker?*	❑	❑	❑	❑
15. How do you feel about going out only with persons of the *opposite sex?*	❑	❑	❑	❑
16. How do you feel about going out only with persons of the *same sex?*	❑	❑	❑	❑

How did you feel about these questions? Did any of them bother you for any reason? Why or why not? Do you have strong feelings about homosexuality?

Source: Bruess, C. E. & Greenberg, J. S. *Sexuality education: Theory and practice.* Sudbury, MA: Jones and Bartlett Publishers, 2004.

Sexuality Online

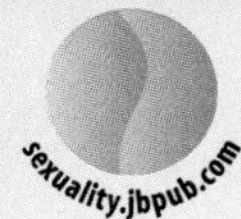

Go to the web component for *Exploring the Dimensions of Human Sexuality* at sexuality.jbpub.com for web exercises, additional resources related to this chapter, and student review tools.

Suggested Readings

Bohan, J. S. Teaching on the edge: The psychology of sexual orientation, *Teaching of Psychology, 24, no. 1* (1997), 27–32.

Cahill, S., Mitra, E., & Tobias, S. *Family policy: Issues affecting gay, lesbian, and transgender families.* Washington, DC: Gay and Lesbian Task Force, 2003.

D'Augelli, A. R. Lesbian, gay, and bisexual development during adolescence and young adulthood, in *Textbook of homosexuality and mental health,* Cabaj, R. P. & Stein, T. S., eds. Washington, DC, American Psychiatric Press, 1996.

D'Emilio, J., Turner, W. B., & Vaid, U., eds., *Creating change: Sexuality, public policy, and civil rights.* Gordonsville, VA: V.H.P.S., 2000.

Esterberg, K. Gay cultures, gay communities: The social organization of lesbians, gay men, and bisexuals, in *The lives of lesbians, gays, and bisexuals: Children to adults,* Savin-Williams, R. C. & Cohen, K. M., eds. Fort Worth, TX: Harcourt Brace College Publishers, 1996.

Golombok, S. Adoption by lesbian couples, *British Medical Journal, 324* (June 15, 2002), 1407–1408.

Gottlieb, A. R. *Out of the twilight: Fathers of gay men speak.* Binghamton, NY: Haworth Press, 2000.

Haumann, G. Homosexuality, biology, and ideology, *Journal of Homosexuality, 28, no. 1–2* (1995), 57–77.

Howard, K. & Stevens, A., eds. *Out and about campus: Personal accounts by lesbian, gay, bisexual, and transgendered students.* Los Angeles, CA: Alyson Publications, 2000.

Marcus, E. *What if someone I know is gay? Answers to questions about Gay and lesbian people.* Newark, NJ: Penguin Putnam, 2000.

Rothblum, E. D. *Preventing heterosexism and homophobia.* Thousand Oaks, CA: Sage Publications, 1996.

Swan, W. K. *Gay/lesbian/bisexual/transgender public policy issues: A citizen's and administrator's guide to the new cultural struggle.* New York: Harrington Park Press, 1997.

Weinrich, J. D. Biological research on sexual orientation: A critique of the critics, *Journal of Homosexuality, 28, no. 1–2* (1995), 197–213.

CHAPTER 12

Sexuality in Childhood and Adolescence

FEATURES

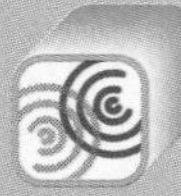
Communication Dimensions
Ten Tips for Discussing Sexuality Scandals with Children

Ethical Dimensions
Is It Ethical to Ignore Your Child's Developing Sexuality?

Gender Dimensions
How Gender Stereotypes Affect Sexuality

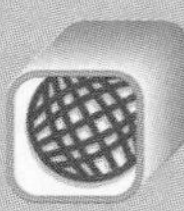
Global Dimensions
Teenagers and Sexuality Around the World

CHAPTER OBJECTIVES

1. Explain why an infant is a sexual being; include the role that touch plays in development.
2. Explain the sexual development of children from preschool through the early elementary years.
3. Describe the differences in puberty for boys and girls.
4. Identify the three developmental stages of adolescence.
5. Discuss the prevalence of sexual abuse and sexual harassment of children and adolescents.

sexuality.jbpub.com

Sexual Development During Preschool and Early Elementary Years
The Media as Sexuality Educator of Children
Late Adolescence

INTRODUCTION

As you have learned earlier in this textbook, we are sexual beings from birth to death. But people often have difficulty understanding what we mean when we say children are sexual beings. As you will read in this chapter, parents need to think about helping their children grow up into sexually healthy adults from the very first months after birth.

It is not always easy. Even though one of us has been a sexuality educator for more than 20 years, she has often faced situations with her own children that she did not know how to deal with at first. Here are two true stories.

> *When my daughter was a toddler, we had taught her the names of all the parts of her body: "This is your nose, this is your stomach, this is your vulva, these are your knees." One day, we were visiting a Georgia O'Keeffe exhibit at a prestigious museum. She was in a backpack on my husband's back. After we had walked through several rooms of large paintings of flowers, she exclaimed, quite loudly, "Look, Mama! Vulvas!" My husband, who was quite shaken, replied in an equally loud voice, "The car. The car. She wants to know where the car is." I, however, was quite pleased at her insight!*
>
> *Many years later, when our son, Gregory, was 4 years old, we were on a car trip playing "Twenty Questions." We had determined that the person to be guessed was alive, a woman, and in the news. It was Gregory's turn: "Is it Monica Lewinsky?" I almost stopped the car! We had never talked with Gregory about the presidential scandal, except to use it to talk about lying. I asked quietly, "Greg, who's Monica Lewinsky?" holding my breath for the answer. He said, "You know, Mom. She's the teenage figure skater." "No," I replied, trying not to laugh, "That's Tara Lipinsky."*

Of course, at 4 years old, Gregory did not understand much about the sexual aspects of the Clinton–Lewinsky crisis. We talked to him about how President Clinton had lied and added that in our home, we believed that it was bad to lie. His questions were pretty simple to answer.

The eighth-graders in my Sunday school class had many more questions, and they were decidedly related to the sexual details. Why was there semen on the dress? Did many women keep these kinds of souvenirs? How many

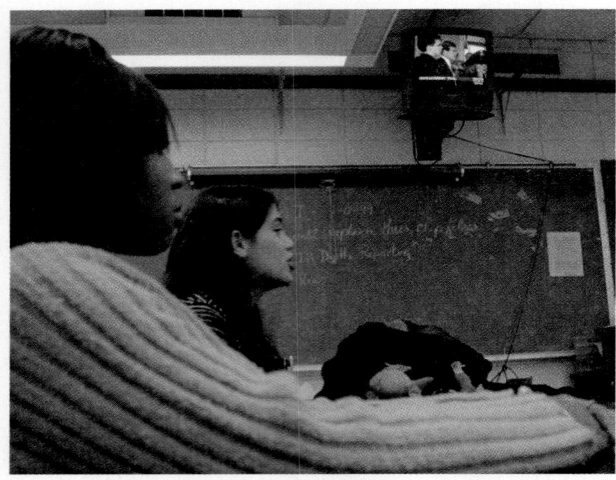

Many parents found it hard to discuss former president Bill Clinton's sexual relationship with Monica Lewinsky. However, it is important to realize that parents teach their children about sexuality with what they say—as well as by what they do not say. By not saying anything about the presidential affair—or similar incidents in the news—parents may be inadvertently telling their children not to ask questions about sexuality.

married adults have affairs? Why did they not have intercourse? It was indeed a "teachable moment."

During the year when the story of Bill Clinton and Monica Lewinsky unfolded, I received many calls from parents who were confused about how to answer their children's questions about the crisis in the White House. How much should they tell their children? Should they answer their children's questions directly? Should they try to shield their children from the news?

Sexual Development of Infants and Toddlers

Sexuality education begins in the delivery room. Of course, we are not talking about giving newborn babies facts about reproduction or sexual behaviors. But think for a minute: What is the first or second question parents ask after the birth of a child? They ask, "Is it a boy or a girl?" And sexuality education about gender roles begins.

Newborn babies develop sexually. In some ways, the first 18 months of life is one of the most important times for learning about love and touch and developing a sense of trust in the world. It is during their infancy that babies learn they are loved and learn how to love when parents kiss them, hug them, and talk to them. Babies also learn whether care providers will meet their needs or whether they will have to tough it out. They learn quickly whether they can count on their care providers to respond to their basic needs.

Actually, biological sexual development begins during pregnancy. Prenatal ultrasound technology has verified that the sexual response system begins to develop in males during the middle stages of gestation. Erectile response begins to appear at around 16 weeks; respiratory function does not begin until almost 12 weeks later. And, although sexual response in female fetuses is not readily observable, it is assumed that the capacity for lubrication begins at this time as well.

infants
Babies from birth to 1 year old.

During the first few months of life, **infants,** babies from birth to 1 year, begin to discover their bodies. By 7 or 8 months, they discover their hands and toes. About the same time, boys discover their penis. Girls, on average, seem to discover their vulva about 2 months later. Infants love to put their fingers and toes into their mouths, and they love to touch their genitals. Baby boys have erections regularly throughout the day and during sleep, as many as three or more times a night. Infant boys may become erect simply by crying, coughing, stretching, or urinating. Baby girls' vaginas are believed to lubricate about just as often, although this is not easily observable, and studies on this topic have not been done.

The Importance of Touch

Cuddling and stroking babies help them learn that their bodies feel good when they are touched and also helps cement the parent–child bond. In fact, research shows that parents should hold their babies as much as possible. A loving touch helps babies grow and develop. And when touch is violated, as in the horrifying cases of child abuse and parental neglect, the child may

Communication DIMENSIONS

Ten Tips for Discussing Sexuality Scandals with Children

If a sexuality scandal of a high public official or a popular entertainer makes headlines, most likely any child in elementary school will hear about it. If a child is in middle or high school, one can be certain he or she has heard a great deal.

Many parents wonder whether they need to discuss these scandals at all. Certainly, everyone would prefer not to talk about well-known government officials or celebrities and sex in the same breath.

The question parents need to ask is, Whom do I want to tell my children about this sad situation? Another child on the playground? An acquaintance on the school bus? They are unlikely to tell other children the facts in a clear way. And only parents can give their children the values they wish to impart to them.

Here are some tips for discussing scandals with your children:

1. Think about values as they relate to the current situation. What are your family values about sex outside marriage, fidelity, telling the truth? If parents believe that individuals involved in the scandal behaved wrongly, then they should explain this to their children.
2. Find out what the children already know. Do not wait for them to ask questions. That may never happen. You can start by saying, "Tell me what you've heard about. . . ." You may be surprised how much they know.
3. Ask them to tell you what certain words mean to them. For example, a child may say that a celebrity had "oral sex" and think that means kissing.
4. Clarify the facts. Give short, age-appropriate answers. A short answer on "oral sex" for a child below the age of 10 years is, "Adults kiss, hug, or touch each other in special ways to show caring and share sexual pleasure. Oral sex is one way." Ask preteens or teenagers for their definition. Then correct any misinformation.
5. Use these talks to encourage good decision making. Even the smallest child understands that decisions have consequences. You can talk to preteens and teens about the importance of making good decisions about sexuality. Young people (and adults) need to understand that they do not have to act on sexual feelings and that they need to differentiate between life-enhancing and harmful sexual behaviors.
6. Use television news as a springboard for discussion. Do not let children younger than 13 years old watch this coverage alone. Talk during the commercials about what you think. Ask children what they think.
7. Help your children understand the larger issues surrounding sexuality scandals. These issues will affect the families of those involved, careers, and possibly the welfare of the nation.
8. Keep the lines of communication open. Talk. Do not lecture. Continue your conversation over the next few weeks. Remember that this is not a one-time discussion. Your children need your ongoing support in dealing with this issue.
9. If you have not talked about sexuality to your children before, start now.
10. You do not have to answer questions about your personal life. The answer to "Do you and Daddy do that?" is "Daddy's and my sex life is personal. When you are an adult, you will decide what sexual behaviors are comfortable for you."

grow into an adult who may be incapable of having healthy adult sexual and intimate relationships.

Touch is one of the first ways that a baby learns he or she is loved. Some psychologists theorize that a loving touch helps set the stage for adult intimacy. Touching and holding infants teach them how parents feel about them. When I am crying, will I be picked up? Can I count on you to show me that you love me? Responding to infants' needs teaches them that the world is a predictable, safe place. It boosts their self-confidence and their ability to believe that when they need help and support, they will get it. When parents and caregivers convey love and delight when they hold their infants, the infants learn they are loved. Conversely, if the adults are scared or tentative or uncomfortable, the infant seems to learn that he or she is not quite all right. In fact, babies who are not touched enough may be at risk for the disorder called **failure to thrive** and may die. (Not all cases of failure to thrive are related to a lack of touching; some babies have an inability to take nourishment.) We should remember that early messages conveyed by touching or the lack of touching may persist throughout life.

failure to thrive
Syndrome whereby babies do not gain weight or achieve developmental milestones.

Developing a sense of trust in the world is an important foundation for adult mental health, including sexual health. The developmental psychologist Erik H. Erikson wrote that the first psychosocial crisis in life is to resolve "basic trust versus basic mistrust." According to Erikson, between birth and 18 months of age, children learn whether their needs will be met and whether they can trust the people and the world around them. If their needs are met, they develop the ability for intimacy and a sense of hope. Erikson wrote that feeding is the primary way that an infant resolves these issues: Can I trust that they will feed me when I am hungry (Erikson, 1950)?

In the early 1960s, two researchers did an important experiment with rhesus monkeys. They separated some monkeys from their mothers at birth and offered them surrogate wire mothers to hold. Some of the surrogates were only wire frames; others were covered with soft fabric. The monkeys would cling to a dummy covered with soft fabric but rejected one made up just of wire, even when it had a bottle of milk attached. In other words, the baby monkeys preferred a soft touch to being fed when that comfort was not there. The baby monkeys denied touch grew up to be troubled adult monkeys. They were more likely to bite and scratch; the males did not approach females sexually; and the females were mostly infertile (Bullough & Bullough, 1994). Some psychologists believe that such studies show that a lack of touch in infancy can affect future adult sexual and intimate relationships.

Teaching Body Parts

Bath time and diaper changes are wonderful times to start teaching a child about body parts—*all* the parts of his or her body. Many parents play this game to teach body parts with their 5- or 6-month-old children: "Here is your nose, here's your tummy, here are your knees, here are your toes." In addition to teaching the names of these body parts, these parents may be inadvertently conveying an early message about their willingness to address sexual issues. These parents may be communicating to their child that many (one-third) of the body's parts have no names and that they are different from all the other parts of the body. How much more sex-positive it would be if parents could learn to say, calmly and without flinching, "Here's your nose, here's your tummy, here's your penis (or vulva), here are your knees, here are your toes." Thus all the parts of the body that the baby is exploring have names, and parents can speak about all of them.

Parents should treat all body parts equally. When parents use euphemisms only for the genitals, they give their child a message that these parts of the body are shameful or different. They may, without meaning to or realizing it, even introduce a sense of guilt about certain parts of the body. These feelings sometimes persist into adulthood, making it difficult for grown men and women to be comfortable with their bodies and sexual feelings. They may also affect a child's ability to tell about sexually abusive incidents accurately.

Infant Genital Touching

Babies begin to explore their genitals during diaper changes. This usually happens at about 7 to 10 months, a little after they discover that they have fingers and toes. And they experience for themselves that it feels good to touch all the parts of their bodies.

Many parents are uncomfortable when they see their babies touch their genitals. They wonder what, if anything, they should do. They wonder whether their child is masturbating or is becoming obsessed with this behavior. This type of genital exploration is not the same as masturbation; it is generally not purposeful and not directed at orgasm. It is about exploring and learning more about the body.

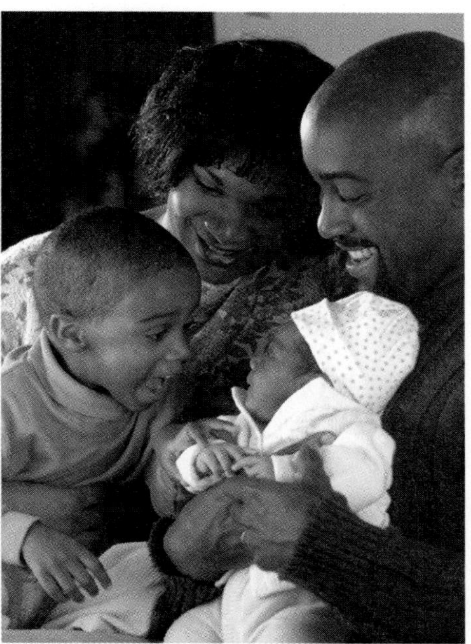

The affection displayed by parents sets an example for their children. Parents who are violent or abusive to each other around a child also set an example for the child to follow.

Gender During the First Three Years

There are some innate differences between boy babies and girl babies. Studies indicate that boy babies may be more active and irritable than girl babies. On average, girl babies seem to reach such developmental milestones as sitting up, reaching for objects, and talking earlier than do boy babies (Beal, 1994).

Boys and girls are also socialized differently from their earliest moments of life. In fact, parents' expectations for their children as males and females may start before birth. Mothers who know the sex of their fetus in utero even describe fetal movement differently. Pregnant mothers of boys say that the fetus's movements are strong and vigorous, whereas pregnant mothers of girls describe them as lively or moderate. When pregnant women do not know the sex of the fetus, they use words that are more gender neutral. Although studies show that male fetuses are not really more active than female fetuses, gender stereotypes affect perception even before a baby is born (Beal, 1994).

Many people prepare differently for their new baby when they know whether the child is a boy or a girl. Parents-to-be often select different wallpaper and accessories for the nursery, different-colored infant clothes, and different announcement cards. Even new-baby congratulations cards are rigidly divided into pink or blue. Pastel yellow and green are available for those who do not know the sex and want to buy clothes or paper the nursery before the child's birth; in fact, often that is all that is available. Today, even newborn disposable diapers are coded blue and pink and feature different characters, although throughout history, genderless diapers did just fine.

With today's frequent use of amniocentesis and ultrasound, many parents *do* know the biological sex of their child months before his or her birth. And for some parents, it is during the middle trimester of the pregnancy that they begin to think about how they want to raise that boy or girl child. Although it may be politically incorrect to say so, most parents secretly hope for a child of one sex or the other. In fact, surveys of people about to become parents in the United States have found that for many the ideal birth order is first a son, then a daughter (Haffner, 1999).

Studies of parents with newborn babies show that parents often speak differently to boy infants and girl infants. In fact, many parents hold, play with, and even touch their baby girls differently than they do their baby boys. Some studies have even found that parents' views of their new babies differ by sex during the first 24 hours of life. Parents rate their new girl babies as more delicate, finer, and softer than they do their boy babies; newborn sons are rated as stronger, firmer, and hardier than newborn daughters (Beal, 1994).

During the first year of life, parents continue to treat their sons and daughters differently. Studies show that mothers look at their daughters more than they do their sons, hold them more, touch them more, and cuddle them more. Mothers are more emotionally expressive to daughters: They smile at them more, talk to them more, and respond to their needs more quickly. Even in the first few months of life, these behaviors encourage girls to be more social and more emotional than boys. Mothers wait longer to tend to their sons' needs, and those extra few unattended minutes perhaps give them a greater beginning sense of autonomy and independence. Fathers play with and talk to their infant sons more than they do their infant daughters, and many fathers adopt a rougher kind of horseplay with their sons than they do with their daughters (Beal, 1994).

During the first 18 months of life, children themselves are also beginning to learn the differences between males and females. Babies pick out male and female voices as early as 6 months of age. Between 1 year and 18 months, babies look longer at photographs of people of their own sex than they do of people of the other sex. Studies show that most children by the age of 3 years can identify both photographs and dolls as male or female and can tell an adult whether they are a boy or a girl (Beal, 1994).

During the first 3 years of life, children are learning the difference between boys and girls and beginning to identify themselves as male or female. By 3 years old, they know that they will grow up to be a man or a woman, and they are absorbing a remarkable number of gender stereotypes.

Children learn to divide the world into "male" and "female" before they reach the age of 2 years. Depending on the behaviors they see in their homes and preschools, they identify certain behaviors as male or female. For example, in some studies, children as young as 2 years have told researchers that girls like to play with dolls and boys like to play with trucks. They say that girls like to cry and boys like to hit. They divide adult jobs into male jobs and female jobs. They even assign genders to colors: pink and purple stuffed animals are deemed girls; black and brown stuffed animals are deemed boys. And they may even change their behaviors to fit these gender stereotypes. For example, girls and boys in the first 18 months have basically identical levels of aggressive behavior, but by the age of 2 or 3 years, girls act less aggressive than boys. Both boys and girls seem to have learned that aggression is acceptable behavior for boys but not for girls. And there is some evidence that there are indeed differences in male and female brains that account for some of the differences in behaviors by children of different sexes.

It is almost a cliché to say that children learn from what they observe around them. But research clearly shows that children from traditional homes are much more likely to learn these gender stereotypes. Parents often provide very different types of toys to girl and boy infants and toddlers. Girls get dolls, stuffed animals, kitchen appliances, jewelry, and dress-up clothes. Boys are given cars, trucks, balls, and sports equipment. In a study of toy catalogs, almost every catalog rigidly divided the pages into toys that were played with only by boys and toys that were played with only by girls. Girls were sometimes pictured playing "boys' games" such as ball or science projects, but no boys were pictured with dolls, kitchens, or other "playing house" toys. In every catalog, the erector set was accompanied by a picture of a boy (Haffner & Casselman, 1995). Many psychologists believe that these toy selections actually affect skills in later life: Girls learn more about nurturing and boys have more of an opportunity to develop reasoning and spatial relation skills.

Sexual Development During Preschool and Early Elementary Years

During the years from age 3 years to age 5 years, children begin to develop a strong sense of gender and what that means to them and the people around them. They are finishing with toilet training, and if they are in school or a day care center, they have probably observed other children and learned for themselves that boys and girls have different body parts. They are very curious about their own and other people's bodies. This is the age when a child is first likely to ask, "Where did I come from?"

Preschool Genital Touching

Three- and 4-year-olds delight in their own bodies. And just as they learn it feels good when they run, jump, and cuddle, they are also discovering that it feels good when they touch their own genitals. Most professionals believe that preschool children touch their genitals as a natural part of child development. In a 1998 study of mothers of 2- to 5-year-olds, about 25% of mothers reported that their sons and 15% reported that their daughters touched their genitals in public. Sixteen percent of both preschool boys and girls had been observed masturbating with their hands (Friedrich, et al., 1998).

Toddlers and preschoolers touch their genitals in a much less purposeful way than older children and adolescents, and many do so without embarrassment or anxiety. In fact, it is not unusual in a preschool to have several of the boys touching their penis unconsciously throughout the day. Little girls find it pleasurable to touch their vulva and clitoris as well.

Many children appear not even to be aware that they are touching their genitals in this way. Some children do discover that this activity helps them calm down. Many children touch their genitals right before naps or bedtimes to help them fall asleep. (Just as for adults, some children never touch their genitals at all. It is normal for a preschooler to touch the genitals and it is normal for him or her not to.)

Attraction to Parents

Sigmund Freud felt that 3- to 5-year-old boys develop fantasies of possessing their mother sexually and become jealous of their father. He named it the **Oedipus complex** after the Greek tragedy in which Oedipus unknowingly kills his father and then marries his mother. According to Freud's theory, this period is accompanied by castration anxiety; boys fear that their father will retaliate against their interest in their mother by cutting off their penis. Freud also theorized that girls develop an **Electra complex;** they develop "penis envy" and want to take their father away from their mother. Girls, he said, reject their mother because they blame her for their lack of a penis. Freud named this "complex" the Electra complex after the Greek tragedy in which a princess helps kill her mother.

Oedipus complex
Libidinal feelings of a child toward the parent of the opposite sex and hostile or jealous feelings toward the parent of the same sex.

Electra complex
Freud's theory that 3- to 5-year-old girls want to take their father away from their mother.

Most modern psychologists debunk these ideas. Feminist psychologists critique Freud's views as extremely sexist, and anthropologists point out that these "complexes" are not found in all cultures. Still, it is not uncommon for preschool children to prefer the parent of the opposite gender at this time.

Preschool children love their parents intensely and may be confused about whether all love is expressed romantically. Many children try to kiss their parents romantically. Some even try to imitate adults they have seen in person or on TV or in the movies by putting their tongue into their parents' mouths.

Preschool children sometimes may even seem jealous when their parents show affection to each other. In one study, 13% of mothers of 2- to 5-year-olds reported that their children became upset when they saw adults kiss (Friedrich, et al., 1998).

Questions About Reproduction

Some time between the ages of 2½ and 5 years, children ask, "Where did I come from?" Children at this age are often very curious about pregnancy and birth. According to psychologists, at around the age of 4 years, children understand that babies do not just spontaneously appear and that something must have happened for this process to begin.

Little children are known to be concrete thinkers, and they are very literal. One study found that children who are told that "a seed is planted in the mommy" actually picture plants growing inside their mothers (Bernstein, 1994). Being told that a baby grows in the mother's stomach may frighten a child who associates stomachs with food and eating and may cause her or him to wonder then why fathers, who also have a stomach, do not have babies.

The psychologist Anne C. Bernstein did research with small children about how they understand reproduction (Bernstein, 1994). She labels the preschooler asking about reproduction a "geographer." The emphasis really is on the *where:* They want to know *where* the baby comes from and *where* it was before it was born. Preschoolers can be offered a very simple answer: "You grew in a special place inside Mom called a uterus. You began from a tiny egg (the size of a pencil dot) from Mom and an even tinier sperm from Dad." This will satisfy most preschoolers. If they ask, "But how did I get into the uterus?" they can be given a very simple definition of sexual intercourse:

> *When two grown-ups love each other, they like to kiss and hug and touch each other in ways that feel good. Sometimes, the man and woman place the man's penis into the woman's vagina. The man's penis releases sperm into the woman and sometimes a baby begins.*

Preschoolers and Sex Play

Many adults remember playing "doctor" or "house" with other children. Playing doctor, including undressing each other and examining each other's genitals, is quite common. As many as half of adults remember engaging in childhood sexual play (Leitenberg, et al., 1989). (It is interesting to note that throughout the years, playing doctor seems to be the usual scenario for most of this sex play. Without an adult sexual context, children know that doctors look at patients' genitals: further evidence that this behavior usually indicates curiosity, not a desire for erotic fulfillment.) Most child development experts see this type of sex play as expected and natural childhood sexual curiosity. If the children are of the same age and stage of development, experts do not believe that it is harmful. And studies of adults show that engaging in childhood sexual play does not seem to have any effect, either positive or negative, on adult sexuality (Leitenberg, et al., 1989).

What is going on here? Preschool-age children are curious about their bodies and about other people's bodies. They may especially be curious about the bodies of the other gender. At this age, they are also mimicking adult behavior as they play house, firefighter, and doctor. They are trying on roles and behaviors. Combining curiosity and role playing often leads to what some experts have labeled "childhood sex play." This curiosity leads to touching, and children may discover that this type of touching feels good.

In fact, some sexologists even believe that early childhood sex play teaches children some important skills. They point to studies of monkeys: In monkeys, early (preadult) sex play lays the foundation for successful male–female reproduction in adulthood. Monkeys who are raised in isolation

TABLE 12.1 A Quick Way to Assess Whether Childhood Sex Play Is Likely to Be Harmless or Whether Parents Should Be Concerned

	EXPECTED	PROBLEMATIC
Age of children	Similar	More than 3 years apart
Children seem	Giggly, curious, happy	Aggressive, angry, fearful, withdrawn
Activities	Undressing, playing doctor ("You show me yours, I'll show you mine")	Oral, anal, or vaginal intercourse; penetration with fingers, objects
After parental intervention	Behavior stops	Behavior continues

and do not have this opportunity never copulate or reproduce, even when paired with an experienced mate (Bullough & Bullough, 1994).

There is a big difference between normally harmless child sexual play and play that is exploitative or abusive. Children do not normally engage in painful sexual behavior, oral–genital contact, or simulated or real intercourse or penetration with fingers or objects with another child, and they do not engage in normal sexual play with children more than a few years older than they are. These behaviors may indicate a child who *may* have been sexually abused. (They could also indicate exposure to inappropriate TV or videos.) Table 12.1 provides some guidelines on distinguishing between harmless play and exploitative, inappropriate behaviors.

latency period
Outdated Freudian theory that children aged 6–12 years old have no sexual feelings or interest.

Elementary School Years

The early elementary school years (kindergarten to grade 3) are years of tremendous growth and change. Naps and playtime give way to homework and tests. Preschool teacher hugs may be replaced by neutral hellos. The class of 12 now has 20 children, and individual attention is no longer the rule. Children begin to learn about sexuality issues from other children on the bus or the playground.

Freud wrote that the period from 6 years old to puberty was a sexual **latency period,** meaning that children this age are not interested in sex; they are too busy growing socially and intellectually. Unfortunately, this out-of-date theory continues to be used to fight sexuality education for elementary school children.

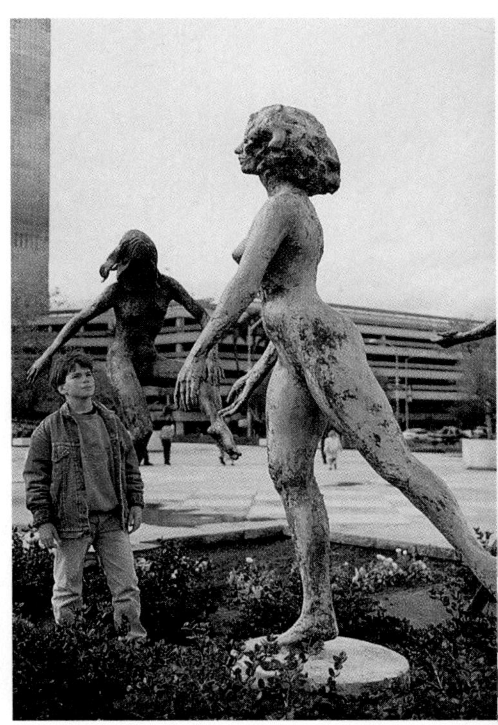

Children are naturally curious about sexuality.

Nothing could be less realistic than this concept of latency. Five- to 8-year-olds continue to be very interested in sexual issues; it is just that their interest is no longer as apparent to the adults in their lives as it used to be. Some professionals believe that the concept of latency is mostly the product of a sexually repressive culture; in cultures in which sexuality is openly expressed, children continue to show these interests throughout childhood. In a 1998 study of more than 11,000 children aged 2 to 12 years, mothers reported that they had observed sexual behaviors in children at all of these ages. For example, 14% of 6- to 9-year-old boys were still touching their genitals in public, 40% did so at home, 20% tried to look at people nude, 8% wanted to watch nudity on TV, and 14% were very interested in girls. Girls this age also exhibited sexual behaviors that were observed by their mothers: 20% had been observed touching their genitals, 20% tried to look at people nude, 8% wanted to watch nudity on TV, and 14% were very interested in boys. And that is just the behavior that the mothers were able to observe (Friedrich, et al., 1998)!

As mentioned, 5- to 8-year-olds continue to develop as sexual persons, and they are very curious about pregnancy and birth. They develop strong friendships, and most boys and girls show a strong preference for playing with children of the same gender. They become even more aware of socially defined gender roles; they have a clearer idea about what is expected of boys and what is expected of girls. They may continue to engage in sex play with children of both genders, although they are much more likely to do it where they will not be discovered by adults. And in private, their exploration of their genitals may become more purposeful.

Some sexologists believe that the period from age 5 years to age 8 years is critical in sexual development. According to Dr. John Money, each person develops a love map during the first years of life, similarly to the way we develop a native language, and, he says, love maps are completed by around the age of 8 years. Dr. Money (1997) defines **love maps** this way:

> *A developmental representation synchronously existent in the mind and the brain, depicting the idealized lover, the idealized love and sexual affair, and the idealized solo or partnered program of sexuerotic activity projected in private imagery and ideation or in observable performance.*

love maps
Fixed ideas in our brains of idealized romantic and sexual partners.

secondary sexual characteristics
Changes occurring during adolescence—such as growth of pubic hair, breast development, and testes and penile development.

breast budding
First stage of breast development in females, whereby breast tissue elevates as a small mound.

In other words, our love maps develop in our brains and help us develop a picture of our idealized romantic and sexual partner including preferred build, race, color, temperament, and look as well as our preferred sexual behaviors in adulthood. According to Dr. Money, by the age of 8 years, these love maps are pretty well established.

And many professionals believe that the elementary school years are the most important time for people to develop as moral thinkers, and that development is important to adult sexual health. While they are preschoolers, children believe that their way of thinking is the only way possible. But in early elementary school, children begin to understand that there may be other points of view and ways to consider a situation. They can begin to understand the "golden rule": Do unto others as you would have them do unto you.

Developing an ability to empathize and make good decisions is part of the foundation for adult sexual health. A sexually healthy adult is able, for example, to make decisions about his or her sexuality that are consistent with his or her own values and to discriminate between behaviors that are life-enhancing and those that may be harmful to oneself or others.

The Media as Sexuality Educator of Children

The media—television, movies, magazines, even the news—are among many children's most prominent sexuality educators. As the Reverend Jesse Jackson once said: Television is now children's third parent. Television and movies teach children about what it is to be a man or a woman, how men and women relate to one another, what is attractive, and what is "sexy." And most parents do not like the messages that many television programs and movies give children about these issues. Too often, television and movies are sexist, violent, exploitative, and degrading. Few programs model honest, equitable relationships between men and women, and almost none shows people practicing responsible sexual behaviors.

Television shows contain an amazing amount of sexual content. In fact, there are on average more than *eight sexual interactions per hour on network television,* two-thirds of which involve physical behaviors. And unbelievably, less than 10% of these scenes with sexual content mention sexual risks, consequences, or responsibilities—such as contraception, condoms, unintended pregnancy, abortion, or sexually transmitted infections (Rideout & Hoff, 1996).

After sleeping and attending school, children aged 6 to 8 years spend more time each week watching television than they do playing, eating, doing chores, participating in sports, or attending church or synagogue. American children watch an average of 24 hours of television a week. By the time an American child graduates from high school, he or she will have spent 18,000 hours in front of a TV set, compared to only 13,000 hours in a classroom. And a child will view a staggering 20,000 commercials a year as part of that television time (Rideout & Hoff, 1996).

And few media are completely "safe." Even programs rated "G" or "family viewing" may have messages that are not consistent with your values about sexuality. Three out of four "family hour" programs on network TV contain some sexual content, up from 43% in 1976. Thirty percent featured scenes with a primary emphasis on sex, up from 9% in 1976 (Rideout & Hoff, 1996).

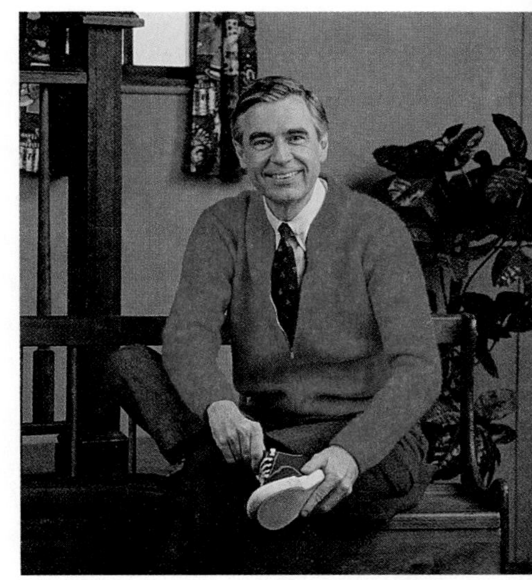

Although it was clearly intended for preschoolers, the second largest audience for *Mister Rogers' Neighborhood* was preadolescents, who want to hear that they are special and that they are OK just as they are. What other media programs offer positive self-esteem messages to preadolescents?

Sexual Development During Puberty

Puberty, teenager, and *adolescence* are not interchangeable words. *Puberty* is the stage of maturation when a human being becomes capable of sexual reproduction. *Teenager* is defined chronologically: a teenager is a young person between the ages of 13 and 19 years. *Adolescence* is actually a relatively new concept: It is the period of development that extends from puberty (or the end of childhood) through the attainment of full adult status. Before 1900, and still today in many developing societies, children marry shortly after puberty and begin their adult responsibilities. Today, as more and more American young people stretch their college and graduate school education through their 20s and even 30s—and then return to live in their parents' homes—some have wondered when contemporary U.S. adolescence ends: At 30 years? When you buy your own home? Have your own children? Before your midlife crisis?

Preparing for Puberty

Young people, at some time between the ages of 8 and 16 years, go through a predictable process of biological development called *puberty.* Normal pubertal changes, indicated by the development of **secondary sexual characteristics** such as breast buds and pubic hair, may begin as early as age 8 years for girls and as early as age 9 years for boys, but some teens may not begin these changes until they are 15 or 16 years old. The median age for puberty to begin for boys is between 11 and 12 years; for girls, it is between 10 and 11 years. Still, average means that half of young people begin this process earlier, and half begin it later. The process of puberty from the first physical changes to obtaining a fully adult body and full reproductive potential may last 4 or 5 years. On average, boys begin and end puberty about 1 year to 2 years later than girls do.

The first noticeable sign of puberty in girls is generally the development of **breast buds;** the breast begins to elevate as a small mound. Later, the breast and the nipple get bigger. A 1997 study of more than 17,000 girls found that on average African-American girls start developing breasts just before age 9 years, and white girls start at about the age of 10 years. Light, sparse pubic and underarm hair begins to appear about 6 months later. Girls begin to experience a growth spurt, often growing as much as several inches in a year. Their genital and underarm areas begin to produce sweat glands, and body odor may result. Most girls begin menstrual periods about 2 years after breast budding begins, but some girls have completed breast development before their first period, and some girls' breasts continue to develop for many years after.

Boys experience many of the same changes. During puberty, they too develop light, sparse pubic and underarm hair, and their sweat glands become activated. Between the ages of 12 and 14 years, their penis and scrotum begin to enlarge. At first, the testes become larger, and the skin on the scrotum reddens and coarsens. As boys mature, their penis starts to grow longer. Pubic hair slowly becomes darker, and it starts to curl.

Girls today are experiencing first menstruation at earlier ages than girls growing up three or four decades ago. The average age for first menstruation, **menarche** (pronounced "men-ar-key"), in the United States is now 12½ years. That means that many girls have their first period before the end of seventh grade, and many begin as early as fourth or fifth grade. It also means that many girls will at least be in the eighth grade before their first period, and some may be seniors in high school before they get a period. All of these situations are normal.

menarche
First menstruation.

Tanner scale
Scale developed by Dr. John Tanner for measuring pubertal development in boys and girls.

gynecomastia
Glandular tissue development in the breasts of boys.

Puberty for Girls

As we mentioned, puberty begins with the development of secondary sexual characteristics. In most girls, breast budding occurs at around age 9 or 10 years but can begin as early as 7 and as late as 13½ years. During puberty, the breasts develop, and the internal (ovaries, uterus, vagina) and external (labia, clitoris) sexual organs increase in size. The uterus increases in size by five to seven times. On average, the process of puberty in girls takes 4 years, but it can be as quick as 1½ years to as long as 8 years.

In 1997, a study appeared in the medical journal *Pediatrics* that surprised many professionals and parents. It found that at least one-quarter of girls began puberty, as marked by the appearance of breast buds, by the third grade (Herman-Giddens, 1997). And yet, many parents wait until fifth or sixth grade to prepare their daughters for the first period. The age of menarche depends on numerous factors: race, genes, nutrition, and culture. And for unknown reasons, it occurs later in rural communities and in big families. The onset of menarche may be dependent on the proportion of body fat. The mean percentage of body fat at menarche is 24%. This may explain why female athletes and ballet dancers, who generally have a lower percentage of body fat, often have delayed puberty (Neinstein, 1991).

Too many young women say they are not being prepared adequately for pubertal changes. Some girls receive only minimal education in school or at a youth group meeting. In a focus group (Louis Harris and Associates, 1997) on adolescent female health, one 12-year-old girl said:

> *That was a big thing in the fifth grade. We had boys' education and girls' education. There was this little pamphlet we got. My friends and I were upset for the whole week.*

Other girls report that they received only scant information from their mother or older siblings or friends. In the same focus group, one girl reported, "On my tenth birthday, they gave us this little package, and it was like a pad and a little booklet." Another girl reports that she really did not get the information she needed: "I think that if I knew what it was, that all girls get it, and I was told that this is going to happen to everyone, that it doesn't hurt, and that it's fine, I think it would have been all right. But in a sense, you feel such shame."

Many pediatricians use a measurement called a **Tanner scale** to rate physical sexual development in both boys and girls (see Table 12.2).

TABLE 12.2 **Tanner Scale for Girls**

Tanner Stage	Pubic Hair	Breasts
1	None	None
2	Sparse	Small breast buds
3	Darker, begins to curl	Breasts and nipples enlarged
4	Coarse, less curly than adult	Continued breast development
5	Adult triangle	Mature; nipple projects

TABLE 12.3 **Tanner Scale for Boys**

Tanner Stage	Pubic Hair	Penis/Scrotum
1	None	Childlike
2	Sparse	Scrotum: reddened, thinner, larger
		Penis childlike
3	Darker, begins to curl	Penis length increases
		Scrotum continues to enlarge and darken
4	Coarse, less curly than adult	Penis increases in length and circumference
5	Adult	Adult

Puberty for Boys

Puberty in boys begins on average during the sixth or seventh grade, but in some boys it begins at 9 years, and in others puberty does not begin until they are almost 14 years old. The first physical sign is usually an increase in the size of the testes; unlike breast budding in girls, this is unlikely to be observed by parents. During puberty, the penis doubles in size. By Tanner stage 3 (see Table 12.3), ejaculation has usually occurred, and there may be some production of sperm. In fact, some sexologists call this "spermenarche," to correspond to the first period of girls (menarche). Most often, a boy experiences this as nocturnal emissions, or wet dreams. By Tanner stage 4, males are fertile and able to cause a pregnancy. The average length of time for a boy to go through puberty is 3 years, but it can vary from 2 to 5 years.

A 2001 study of teenage boys found that today's boys are beginning puberty sooner than their fathers, perhaps as much as 6 months sooner. African-American boys begin pubic hair and genital maturation earlier than whites and Mexican Americans. There is, however, no evidence that teens are completing puberty earlier (U.S. boys may be hitting puberty sooner, 2001).

Significant numbers of boys are troubled by a condition called **gynecomastia.** During puberty, they begin to develop an increase in the glandular tissue around their breasts; in fact, these boys sometimes are very worried and fearful that they are growing breasts or turning into a girl. Nearly one in five 10-year-olds will have this kind of tissue development. In rare cases, gynecomastia may be the result of diseases that are rare in young people: liver

hypogonadism
Decreased activity of the gonads that may result in retardation of growth and sexual development.

hyperthyroidism
Excessive functional activity of the thyroid gland.

hypothyroidism
A deficiency of thyroid activity.

precocious puberty
Pubertal development before the age of 7 years.

imaginary audience
Belief in early adolescence that other people are looking at you as if you are onstage.

conformity with peers
Desire to be like everyone else.

disease, **hypogonadism, hyperthyroidism,** or **hypothyroidism.** It could also be a sign of drug use. However, most of the time it is just a variation of male pubertal development, and it usually resolves itself within 1 year to 1½ years. It continues longer than 2 years in fewer than 1 in 10 boys.

Early and Late Developers

Although the majority of young people finish puberty a few years after the start of their teen years, some begin puberty much earlier and some go through it much later. Both early and late developers face special challenges.

Some children begin puberty much earlier than age 9 or 10 years. Some children even enter what is called **precocious puberty** in the first year of life. Some girls begin pubertal development as early as age 3 years, and although it may not be an indicator of a medical problem, it should be discussed with a physician. Interestingly, this seems to be largely the result of genetic coding in girls, and most often there is no underlying disease. Conversely, precocious puberty in boys is much more likely to be an indication that something is wrong. If parents observe pubertal changes in a boy younger than 7 years old, they should see a health practitioner for a medical evaluation and possible interventions.

As we mentioned, some children enter puberty at around the age of 8 years—in third grade! In fact, a study found that this is actually much more common than many parents and practitioners had thought. As many as one-quarter of African-American girls and about 10% of white girls begin puberty by the age of 7 years (Herman-Giddens, 1997).

Early-developing girls have special problems. Because they look more mature, adults often expect them to act more mature. A third- or fourth-grade girl with developing breasts may feel awkward and want to hide her body. She may be relentlessly teased by her male and female classmates. She may indeed feel that she is not normal. Conversely, late development in boys may be more of a problem than early development. A 15- or 16-year-old boy who is still short, has no facial hair, and has a high voice may be relentlessly teased.

What Is Normal?

Early, late, and average developers *all* share a common concern: *Am I normal?* Rapid body changes can be very confusing. Nine- to 12-year-olds can become obsessed with their appearance. In fact, psychologists say preteens have an **imaginary audience:** They think that everyone is looking at them. Getting dressed and preparing their hair and faces can take hours. They need adult reassurance that they are attractive, and they need to understand that it is not true that everyone is looking at them.

They are concerned about their height and breast size or penis size, and they wonder whether they are too developed or too underdeveloped. They wonder whether their feelings, which sometimes fluctuate immensely, are normal. It is important to reassure preadolescents that they are developing according to their own personal genetically predetermined clock. When they ask questions like "How come I don't have my period yet?" or "Why am I the shortest boy in the class?" the question behind the question is almost always "Am I normal?"

Physical development does not occur separately from emotional or social development. The physical changes in children are often much easier to accept than the emotional and social ones. Parents of 9- to 12-year-olds often wonder, "What happened to my nice, sweet, obedient child? How come she never seems to want to do anything with us anymore? How come he doesn't want to be seen with me?"

Dr. Bob Corwin, a New York state pediatrician, has said to parents, "During childhood you are the hammer; during adolescence, you are the anvil." What he meant was, that until adolescence, it is the parents' job to teach, teach, and teach, and during adolescence, sometimes parents just need to be there. Dr. Bob Selverstone has written: "It is fine for the child to walk away from the parent—you are preparing them for a life on their own. You must assure them that you won't walk away from them" (Selverstone, 1989).

The reality is that during preadolescence and the years following it, conflicts with parents peak. Yet, it is important to know that only about one in six teenagers and parents experience a severe disruption in their parent–child relationship (Haffner, 1995). Preadolescents are just beginning to separate from their parents, but they are also still looking to their parents for guidance and support.

Emotional Changes in Preadolescence

The rapid physical changes of puberty we have described initiate many psychosocial changes. Preadolescents are beginning to move toward independence and are often very self-conscious of their bodies. Their fluctuating hormones often lead to extreme moodiness and unexplainable feelings. One minute, they desperately want parents to help them; another moment, they are yelling, "You just don't understand" and slamming the door to their room. Children at this age become very sensitive to what they perceive as adult criticism or advice, although they can be relentless in their criticism of parents ("Mom, you're not really going to wear that to the school concert?"). They may even be embarrassed by parents.

Children at this age also need to test parental authority and sometimes the authority of teachers and other adult figures in their lives. This may include trying out values that are different from their parents'. The research literature demonstrates that most teenagers go through a period of seeming to reject their parents' values; yet, by the time they reach adulthood, almost all of them adopt values similar to their parents'.

Friends become very important during the preadolescent years. Being popular is of utmost importance. The good news is that needing to be just like friends, known by psychologists as **conformity with peers,** peaks in early adolescence and then starts to decline. The bad news for parents is that peer pressure can be intense during this period and usually dictates the type of sneakers that are acceptable, the length of one's skirt and pants, and even the coolness of being seen with one's parents. It also can lead to experimentation with cigarettes, alcohol, and sex.

Cliques often emerge during this period. Depending on where one lives, there are the jocks, the nerds, the skaters, the preppies, the hippies, the populars, the burnouts, and the freaks. Preadolescents may for the first time feel pressure to engage in certain activities to be part of a group, and, for some young people, that means experimenting with smoking, shoplifting, or cheating on tests. Among eighth graders, a surprising 30% have a cigarette at least once a day, 13% have used marijuana, two-thirds say they have tried alcohol, a quarter say they are current drinkers, and 28% say they have been drunk at least once (Carnegie Corporation of New York, 1992).

Preadolescents are also beginning to develop a sense of identity. Their ability to think abstractly has just begun. They frequently daydream and turn inward and imagine acting out different roles. Daydreaming is normal and actually quite healthy. Giving a child a diary or journal and then respecting his or her right to keep it private can be an effective way to encourage a new adolescent to think about and explore his or her feelings. Many parents worry that their preadolescent child is spending hours alone in his or her room; this time alone can be an important part of growing up. Of course, if a child

Myth vs Fact

Myth: People become sexual at puberty.
Fact: People are sexual from birth to death. Although people sexually mature at puberty and become capable of reproduction, infants and children experience sensual feelings and identify themselves as boys and girls.

Myth: Dressing boys in blue and girls in pink teaches them about their gender.
Fact: By the time they are 3 years old, almost all boys and girls identify themselves by the correct gender and know that they will have that gender throughout their lifetime. Clothes colors do not make a difference.

Myth: Children in elementary school go through a latency period about sexual issues.
Fact: Elementary school children remain very interested in sexuality-related issues, and many continue to be involved in sex play with friends or genital self-pleasuring. They have just learned to hide this behavior from adults.

Myth: The average age of first intercourse has plummeted in the past 5 years.
Fact: The biggest change in adolescent sexual behavior occurred in the 1970s. The average age of first intercourse has decreased by 1 year since 1971.

Myth: Most teenagers have had sexual intercourse.
Fact: Only about half of teenagers aged 15–19 years have had sexual intercourse.

Myth: Masturbating more than once a week is harmful.
Fact: There is no "standard" for frequency of masturbation. Once is too often if you do not like it. Frequency is highly individual, and it is not harmful as long as it does not interfere with school, work, or relationships.

has no interest in family or friends, a lack of interpersonal connections may indicate a more serious problem.

Children at this age can seem very dramatic. They often feel that they are continuously onstage. They may become convinced that their problems are unique and no one understands them.

Masturbation

During puberty, many boys and girls begin to masturbate for sexual pleasure. Research shows that as many as three-quarters of boys and about half of girls below the age of 15 years masturbate (Coles & Stokes, 1985). And unlike when they engaged in more casual genital touching as children, many of these young people are seeking orgasm and pleasure. Masturbation is often the first way that young people—and sometimes adults—experience orgasm or ejaculation.

Boys, in particular, seem to "take up" masturbation at puberty. Parents of adolescent boys are often concerned about the amount of time their sons seem to be spending locked in the bathroom or bedroom. In our experience, boys are often worried that they are masturbating too often and wonder whether their desire to masturbate is normal. And some girls have these same types of questions too.

How much is too much? The sexuality educator Sol Gordon says, "Once is enough, if you don't like it." If masturbation is interfering with a child's school, homework, friends, or family life, it is being done too often. Otherwise, frequency is highly individual. Some adults masturbate every day; some, once a year. And some people never masturbate. In fact, teenagers need to know that although many preteens, teens, and adults masturbate, some never do.

Sexuality in Adolescence

There is public and professional consensus about what is sexually unhealthy for teenagers. Professionals, politicians, and parents across the political spectrum share a deep concern about unplanned adolescent pregnancy; out-of-wedlock childbearing; STIs, including AIDS; sexual abuse; date rape; and the potential negative emotional consequences of premature sexual behaviors.

However, there is little public, professional, or political consensus about what is sexually healthy for teenagers. The public debate about adolescent sexuality has often focused on which sexual behaviors are appropriate for adolescents and ignored the complex dimensions of sexuality.

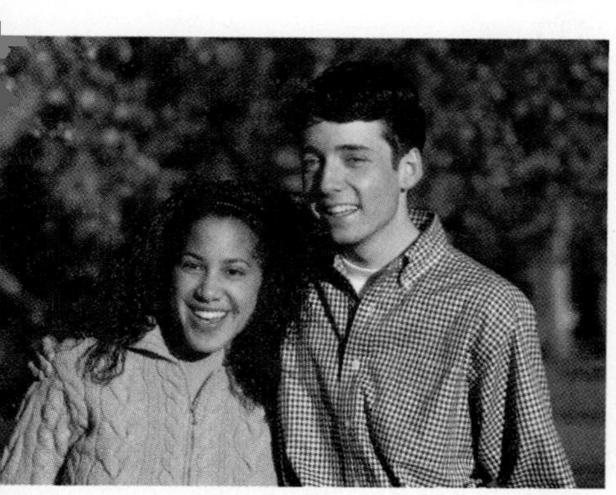

Many adults become concerned when their adolescent children begin to explore their emerging sexuality. But honest communication between an adult and a child can help him or her develop into a sexually healthy adult.

Some groups support the "Just say no" approach to adolescent sexuality. They believe that the only healthy adolescent sexuality is abstinence from all sexual behaviors until marriage and that adults should work to eliminate teen sexual experimentation. Another approach could be described as "Just say not now." This philosophy encourages young people to abstain until they are more mature but, given the high rates of teenage sexual involvement in intercourse, recommends that it is important to provide young people with access to contraception and condoms regardless of whether adults approve of their behavior. This approach might also be labeled "If you can't say no, protect yourself!" Other adults adopt a "Don't ask; don't tell" posture and simply pretend that adolescent sexuality and sexual behavior do not exist.

In 1994, the Sexuality Information and Education Council of the United States (SIECUS) convened the National Commission on Adolescent Sexual Health. The following sections are adapted with permission from the commission's report, "Facing Facts: Sexual Health for America's Adolescents."

The commission report called for a new approach to adolescent sexual health. They said that society has a responsibility to help adolescents understand and accept their evolving sexuality and to help them make responsible sexual choices, now and in their future adult roles. Adults must focus on helping young people avoid unprotected and unwanted sexual behaviors. Individual adults and society in general must help adolescents develop the values, attitudes, maturity, and skills to become sexually healthy adults.

The following statement reflects the consensus of the National Commission on Adolescent Sexual Health (1994):

> *Becoming a sexually healthy adult is a key developmental task of adolescence. Achieving sexual health requires the integration of psychological, physical, societal, cultural, educational, economic, and spiritual factors.*
>
> *Sexual health encompasses sexual development and reproductive health, as well as such characteristics as the ability to develop and maintain meaningful interpersonal relationships; appreciate one's own body; interact with both genders in respectful and appropriate ways; and express affection, love, and intimacy in ways consistent with one's own values.*
>
> *Adults can encourage adolescent sexual health by:*
>
> - *Providing accurate information and education about sexuality;*
> - *Fostering responsible decision-making skills;*
> - *Offering young people support and guidance to explore and affirm their own values; and*
> - *Modeling healthy sexual attitudes and behaviors.*

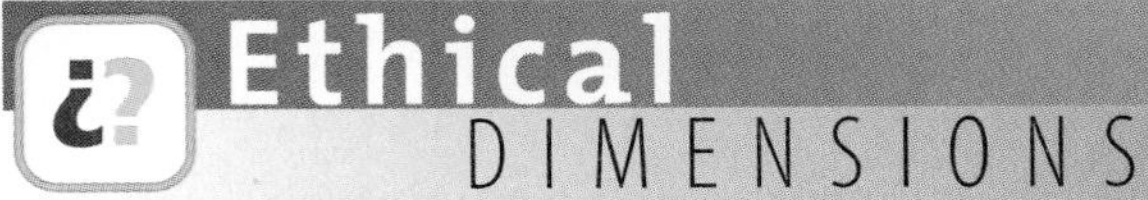

Is It Ethical to Ignore Your Child's Developing Sexuality?

One of us once attended a presentation with a group of Swedish sexuality educators who were talking about the difference in sexual mores between Sweden and the United States. One of the Swedish women told us a story about her first sexual experience. She was 17 years old and very much in love. She and her boyfriend told her parents that they were ready to have sexual intercourse, and they asked to make love in her bedroom at home. The next morning, her parents served them breakfast in bed to celebrate this passage! The American educators were stunned.

Many parents vehemently oppose the idea that their teenagers might have sexual intercourse. They teach "Just say no." Other parents ignore their teenager's growing involvement with another teen, adopting a "Don't ask; don't tell" policy. Other parents talk openly and honestly to their children and encourage them to talk to them if they are thinking about intercourse so they can help them get contraception.

But even these parents usually stop at inviting their teen children to have sex in their home, and we cannot imagine even among the most progressive parents we know serving their child and lover breakfast in bed!

The boundaries between parents and their teen children about sexuality are often difficult to negotiate and raise many moral and ethical issues. Is it ethical to ignore a teen's developing sexuality? Is it ethical to withhold information about contraception and condoms? Does talking about condoms and contraception encourage teens to experiment with sexual behaviors? Should parents help a teen obtain contraception, or is a teen who is old enough to be having intercourse old enough to go to a clinic or a drug store unassisted? And if you know your teen child is having intercourse, should you allow him or her to do so in your home? While you are out? Overnight? And what is your responsibility to the other child's parent?

How did your parents handle these issues? How do you think you will handle them when you are a parent? What issues do you need to think about in answering these questions?

Society can enhance adolescent sexual health if it provides access to comprehensive sexuality education and affordable, sensitive, and confidential reproductive health care services, as well as education and employment opportunities. Families, schools, community agencies, religious institutions, media, businesses, health care providers, and government at all levels have important roles to play.

Society should encourage adolescents to delay sexual behaviors until they are ready physically, cognitively, and emotionally for mature sexual relationships and their consequences. This support should include education about:

- *Intimacy;*
- *Sexual limit setting;*
- *Resisting social, media, peer, and partner pressure;*
- *Benefits of abstinence from intercourse; and*
- *Pregnancy and sexually transmitted disease prevention.*

Society must also recognize that a majority of adolescents will become involved in sexual relationships during their teenage years. Adolescents should receive support and education for developing the skills to evaluate their readiness for mature sexual relationships. Responsible adolescent intimate relationships, like those of adults, should be based on shared personal values, and should be:

- *Consensual;*
- *Non-exploitative;*
- *Honest;*
- *Pleasurable; and*
- *Protected against unintended pregnancies and sexually transmitted diseases, if any type of intercourse occurs.*

Adolescent Development

Discussions about adolescent sexuality often are predicated on an adult perception of how "things should be" rather than on an appreciation of the dynamics and goals of adolescent development and maturation.

Adolescence is the time when young people develop the knowledge, attitudes, and skills that become the foundation for psychologically healthy adulthood. Adolescence is a period characterized by rapid changes and the need to achieve many significant developmental tasks. Nevertheless, although adolescence can be a time of great conflict and distress, the majority pass through it successfully. Children who enter adolescence with the most social or psychological disadvantages are likely to experience the greatest difficulties. Indeed, it may be that the greatest barrier to healthy development is a lack of education and economic opportunities (Peterson & Leffert, 1994).

The Three Stages of Adolescence

Developmental psychologists and health professionals have categorized adolescence into three developmental stages: early adolescence, middle adolescence, and late adolescence. These stages are key to understanding adolescents' behavioral decisions and adolescent sexuality. Table 12.4 summarizes these stages.

While reading this section, it is important to remember that there is no such thing as an "average adolescent." Individual adolescents vary widely in the pace of their development. For example, in any group of 13-year-olds, some might function as 9-year-olds, and some as 16-year-olds. There is also a high degree of variation within each adolescent: For example, a physically mature 15-year-old might function emotionally as a 12-year-old in dealing with parents and yet cognitively as a late adolescent in dealing with math problems.

TABLE 12.4 Highlights of Adolescent Developmental Stages

Early Adolescence

Females ages 9–13; males ages 11–15

- Puberty as hallmark
- Adjusting to pubertal changes such as secondary sexual characteristics
- Concern with body image
- Beginning of separation from family, increased parent-child conflict
- Presence of social-group cliques
- Identification in reputation-based groups
- Concentration on relationships with peers
- Concrete thinking but beginning of exploration of new ability to think abstractly

Middle Adolescence

Females ages 13–16; males ages 14–17

- Increased independence from family
- Increased importance of peer group
- Experimentation with relationships and sexual behaviors
- Increased abstract thinking ability

Late Adolescence

Females ages 16 and older; males ages 17 and older

- Autonomy nearly secured
- Body image and gender-role definition nearly secured
- Empathetic relationships
- Attainment of abstract thinking
- Defining of adult roles
- Transition to adult roles
- Greater intimacy skills
- Sexual orientation nearly secured

Source: Reprinted with permission from Haffner, D. *Facing facts: Sexual health for America's adolescents.* New York: SIECUS, 1995.

Adolescent growth and development—and adolescent sexuality—are not singular or stable. They are plural and dynamic. For most young people, adolescence does not entail an absolutely predictable, consistent set of developmental tasks; nor does it unfold in a singular, universal fashion. Adolescent sexuality emerges from cultural identities mediated by ethnicity, gender, sexual orientation, class, and physical and emotional capacity. Adolescent development is affected by parents, other family members, and other adults, as well as schools and the peer group.

Early Adolescence

The **early adolescent** (females aged 9–13 years, males aged 11–15 years) experiences body changes more rapidly than at any time since infancy—secondary sexual characteristics begin to appear; growth accelerates; and physical changes require psychological and social adjustments of the adolescent, family, and other adults. These young people are often concrete thinkers and therefore have difficulty projecting themselves into the future. This phenomenon creates problems when young people are asked to modify their behaviors and delay gratification to achieve a distant future goal. The young adolescent is

early adolescence
First stage of adolescence, defined by pubertal changes—usually ages 9–13 years for females and ages 11–15 years for males.

beginning to separate from the family but usually values parental guidance on important issues. Conflicts with parents usually peak at the height of these pubertal changes, yet only 15% of teenagers and their parents experience a severe disruption in the parent–child relationship (Peterson & Leffert, 1994). Peer norms, especially identification with a particular group or set of groups, assume increasing importance.

Experimenting with some sexual behaviors is common, but sexual intercourse of any kind is usually limited. Males may initiate intercourse during this stage but most often delay regular sexual activity until middle or late adolescence. Adolescent girls are much less likely to begin having sexual intercourse at this age. Of those who do, many are in relationships with much older males.

Young adolescents seek to develop a sense of identity, connection, power, and joy. For many adolescents in communities that do not support the development of personal identity in other ways, drugs and sexual experimentation may provide a way to achieve it. Early sexual involvement is one way that disadvantaged youth may meet developmental needs for power, identity, connection, and pleasure (Selverstone, 1989). Involvement in sexual behaviors may not be motivated by sexual pleasure but rather may reflect peer norms, boredom, conflicts with adults, low self-esteem, and poor ability to control impulsivity (Durban, DiClemente, & Seigel, 1993).

Middle Adolescence

Middle adolescence (females aged 13–16 years, males aged 14–17 years) is the stage that most typifies the stereotype of "teenager." The transitions in this stage are so dramatic that they seem to occur overnight. The secondary sexual characteristics become fully established, and, for girls, the growth rate decelerates. Abstract thought patterns begin to develop in significant proportions of middle adolescents.

middle adolescence
The typical "teenage years," usually ages 13–16 years for females and ages 14–17 years for males.

late adolescence
Period of transition to adulthood, beginning usually at age 16 years for females and age 17 years for males.

conceptual identity
Who am I in my world?

functional identity
What adult roles will I play in the world?

cognitive development
Explains the ability to think concretely or abstractly.

sexual self-concept
Who am I as a sexual being?

Middle adolescents are sometimes described as feeling omniscient, omnipotent, and invincible. These feelings provide young people with the support to develop increased autonomy but may also put them at risk. Although studies suggest that adolescents feel no more invincible than adults who are risk takers (Quadrel, et al., 1993), a sense of invincibility, coupled with a developing ability to predict consequences, allows some adolescents to participate in risk-taking behaviors and believe that they cannot be harmed—for example, "I can drive a car even though I have never taken a driving lesson," "I can stop a bullet and not die," "I can have unprotected sexual intercourse and not become pregnant or get HIV."

As adolescents continue the process of separation from the family, they cling more tightly to the peer group that they defined for themselves in early adolescence. The peer group begins to define the rules of behavior. Parents generally place more value on long-term issues such as the importance of education and career preparation than peers do. The desire to be accepted by the peer group often influences such issues as experimentation with drugs or sexual behaviors. By its acceptance or rejection, the peer group influences the adolescent's self-image.

Sexuality and sexual expression are of major importance in the life of many middle adolescents. As they move through rapid developmental changes, adolescents at this stage often focus on themselves and assume others will too. Many middle adolescents choose to show off their new bodies with revealing clothes such as miniskirts and muscle shirts. Although adults may define these styles as sexually provocative, that may not be the intent of the middle adolescent.

Middle adolescents often fall in love for the first time. Again, because they are self-centered, their love object may serve as a mirror and reflect characteristics that they admire; that is, they may not love an individual for him- or herself. Sexual experimentation is common, and many adolescents first have intercourse in middle adolescence.

Late Adolescence
Teenagers in **late adolescence** (females aged 16 years and older; males aged 17 years and older) are explicitly moving toward adult roles and responsibilities. Some are beginning full-time jobs; others are beginning families. Many are preparing for these adult roles. The late adolescent completes the process of physical maturation. Many young people at this stage achieve the ability to understand abstract concepts, and they become more aware of their limitations and how their past will affect their future. They understand the consequences of their actions and behaviors, and they grapple with the complexities of identity, values, and ethical principles. Within the family, they move to a more adult relationship with their parents. The peer group recedes in importance as a determinant of behavior, and sexuality may become closely tied to commitment and planning for the future.

Adolescent Developmental Tasks

Developmental psychologists have identified six key developmental tasks for adolescents. Becoming a sexually healthy adult depends on the completion of these key developmental tasks (Haffner, 1995). The six key tasks are as follows:

1. ***Physical and sexual maturation:*** Adolescents mature biologically into adults, a process that occurs at an earlier chronological age than it did in the past.
2. ***Independence:*** Adolescents develop autonomy within the structure that gave them nurture and support during their childhood. This is usually the family but may include some similar surrogate structure. The parent–child relationship is transformed during adolescence, as the young person develops autonomy while obtaining the skills to maintain satisfying relationships within the home and with others.
3. ***Conceptual identity:*** Adolescents establish and place themselves within the religious, cultural, ethnic, moral, and political constructs of their environments.
4. ***Functional identity:*** Adolescents begin to prepare themselves for adult roles in society. By identifying their competencies, they discover how they will support themselves and contribute to their own families and society.
5. ***Cognitive development:*** Children and young adolescents are concrete thinkers and focus on real objects, present actions, and immediate benefits. They have difficulty projecting themselves into the future. During adolescence, young people develop a greater ability to think abstractly, plan for their future, and understand the effect of their current actions on their future lives and other people.
6. ***Sexual self-concept:*** During adolescence, young people tend to experience their first adultlike erotic feelings, experiment with sexual behaviors, and develop a strong sense of their own gender identity and sexual orientation.

The pursuit of these developmental tasks answers three psychosocial questions that adolescents ask themselves: Am I normal? Am I competent? Am I lovable and loving (Scales, 1991)? Many adolescent behaviors can be attributed to the search for affirmative answers to these questions.

social cognition
Ability to see a situation from another person's point of view.

Physical and Sexual Maturation

As noted in the section on puberty, sexual maturation differs significantly among young men and young women. On average, young girls begin pubertal events 1 to 2 years before boys. The adolescent female completes the process of puberty in 3 to 5 years, whereas for males, the process lasts 4 to 6 years.

- *Young people today are reaching sexual maturity at a much younger age than in the past.* Today, most girls experience menarche (first menstruation) at 12–12½ years of age. Records from family bibles around the time of the American Revolution indicate an age of menarche of approximately 17 years. In 1860, the average age of menarche was somewhat older than 15 years in Europe and Northern America. During the 20th century, the age at menarche declined an average of 3 months per decade until 1960. Since 1960, the average age of menarche appears to have remained constant at 12–12½ years, with slight ethnic and urban–rural differences in the United States (Neinstein, 1991).
- *Early pubertal development is associated with an increased likelihood for early experimentation with sexual behaviors, in particular intercourse.* Girls and boys who mature early are more likely than others to have sexual intercourse as teenagers (Chilman, 1990; Paikoff & Brooks-Gunn, 1991).
- *The discrepancy between maturation among young women and young men is one factor that may contribute to some young women's seeking partners older than they are.* This difference in age places young women at considerable risk for sexual exploitation.
- *Adjusting to the biological changes of puberty is a major task of early adolescence, and society does not adequately prepare or support young people during these changes.* A significant minority of young women do not receive education about menstruation before menarche, and few adult men can recall receiving information on pubertal maturation before their first ejaculation or nocturnal emission. Many adolescents are embarrassed by or ashamed of normal pubertal events. Sexual health for adolescents includes an ability to appreciate one's own body and to view pubertal changes as normal. Achievement of these goals is dependent on parents' and other trusted adults' preparing young people in advance of pubertal events, as well as supporting them during this important transition.

Cognitive Development

During adolescence, young people develop a range of intellectual characteristics that increase the probability that they will be able to become sexually healthy adults. Ideally, this includes developing the ability to reason abstractly, to foresee consequences of actions, and to understand the social context of behaviors. Adolescents develop an increased ability to control impulsivity, to identify the future implications of their actions, and to obtain control of their future plans.

Decision-making abilities increase during adolescence. Conformity with one's peers peaks in early adolescence. In middle adolescence, people develop the skills to strengthen the capacity for autonomous decision making. They begin to develop a better understanding of personal risks, possible consequences, and the need to obtain more information (Peterson & Leffert, 1994).

Developmental age and general level of cognitive and emotional development may influence adolescent sexual decisions, contraceptive use, and safer sex practices. An adolescent's degree of cognitive maturity may place limits on his or her ability to plan for sexual relationships, clearly articulate personal values, negotiate with a partner, and obtain contraception and condoms. Further, the adolescent's ability to form empathetic relationships is dependent on **social cognition:** the capacity to see a situation from another person's perspective. Social cognition is one aspect of cognitive development. Understanding one's feelings and the feelings of others is central to emotional growth.

THEY SAY WALL STREET
IS A MAN'S WORLD.
THEY'RE ONLY HALF RIGHT.
THE $TREET
A new series from the creator of Sex and the City
FOX FALL

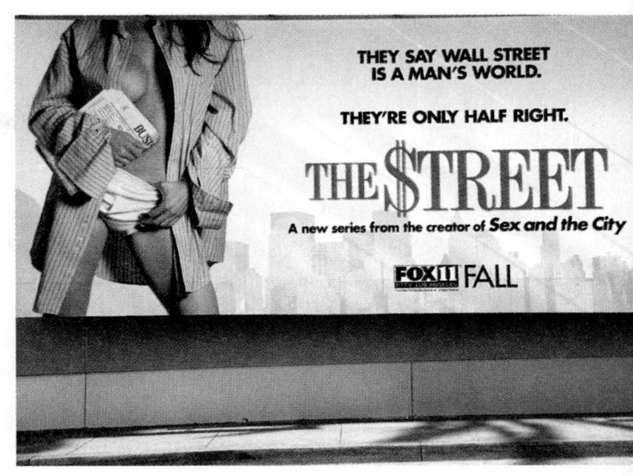

What is the message of this billboard? What messages do you think this gives women regarding their worth in a professional setting? What is the message to young women who might see this depiction of a half-clad woman?

Sexual Self-Concept

Sexual self-concept, an individual's evaluation of his or her sexual feelings and actions, develops during adolescence. Young people develop an increasing sense of gender identity as men and women. An understanding of one's sexual orientation also develops during adolescence: Young people become more aware of their sexual attractions and love interests, and adultlike erotic feelings emerge. Sexual experimentation is common among all groups of adolescents.

During adolescence, young people solidify their gender identification by observing the gender roles of their parents and other adults. Gender identification includes understanding that one is male or female, as well as understanding the roles, values, duties, and responsibilities of being a man or a woman. Most young people have a firm sense of their maleness or femaleness before adolescence, but in adolescence, clear identification with adult masculine and feminine models emerges. It is essential that adolescents have men and women in their environment who convey the values, behaviors, and attitudes of appropriate gender role models. By interacting with psychologically healthy adult men and women, adolescents learn who they are and how to behave in appropriate ways.

Sexual Orientation

One's sexual orientation often emerges in adolescence. In one study of students in grades 7–12, 88% of teenagers described themselves as predominantly heterosexual, 1% described themselves as bisexual or predominantly homosexual, and 11% were "unsure" of their sexual orientation. Uncertainty about sexual orientation diminished with chronological age; 26% of the 12-year-olds were "unsure" compared with only 5% of the 18-year-olds (Remafedi, et al., 1992).

In retrospective studies, many gay and lesbian adults identify adolescence as a period of confusion about their sexual identity. Although a majority of adult gay men recall feeling different as children (Bell, Weinberg, & Hammersmith, 1981), most did not self-identify as gay until their late teenage years. Gay males begin to believe that they might be homosexual at an average age of 17 years (Bell, Weinberg, & Hammersmith, 1981); lesbians, at an average of 18 years. Gay males act on their homosexual feelings at a mean age of 15 years, whereas lesbians report an average age at first genital sexual experience at 20 years (Bell, Weinberg, & Hammersmith, 1981). "Coming out," or disclosing one's sexual orientation to others, generally does not occur until adulthood.

Adolescent Sexual Behavior

Almost all American adolescents engage in some type of sexual behavior. Although policy debates have tended to focus on sexual intercourse and its negative consequences, young people explore dating, relationships, and intimacy from a much wider framework. *Sexual behavior is almost universal among American adolescents.*

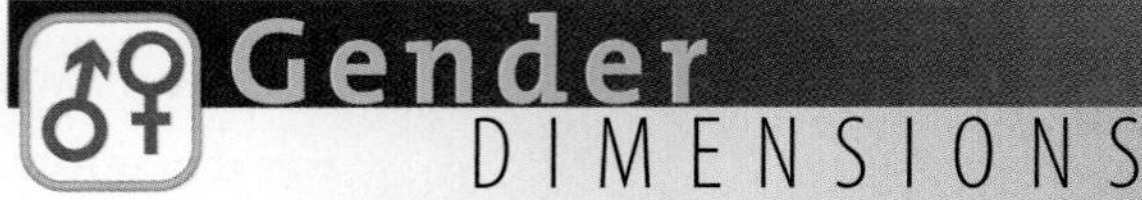

How Gender Stereotypes Affect Sexuality

Gender-role stereotypes impede both young men and young women in attaining sexual health. Young women may learn that "It is better to be cute and popular than smart," "Girls have few sexual feelings," and "Girls who carry condoms are bad." Boys may learn that "Real men are always ready for sex" and that "Guys should never act like girls." One study found that teenage males who agree with traditional cultural messages about masculinity are more likely than other young men to use condoms less consistently (or not at all) and to say that if they made a partner pregnant, they would feel like a "real man"; they are also less likely to think men share the responsibility for preventing pregnancy (Pleck, 1991).

Although patterns of sexual involvement are increasingly similar for boys and girls, persistent gender stereotypes mean that young women still experience their sexual behaviors quite differently (Thompson, 1990) than young men do. In a 1994 poll, young women reported that they were more likely to regret their sexual experiences, more likely to label the relationship "love," less likely to report their sexual experiences as pleasurable, and more likely to bear the brunt of negative outcomes than their male counterparts (Roper, 1994).

Why do these different standards continue to exist? Will they ever change?

Consider these statistics:

- A majority of American teenagers date.
- Of American teenagers, 85% have had a boyfriend or girlfriend.
- Of American teenagers, 85–90% have kissed someone romantically.
- Of American teenagers, 79% have engaged in "deep kissing" (Coles & Stokes, 1985; Roper, 1994).

The majority of adolescents move from kissing to other more intimate sexual behaviors during their teenage years.

- More than half of all teenagers have engaged in "petting behaviors." By the age of 14 years, more than half of all boys have touched a girl's breasts, and one-quarter have touched a girl's vulva (Coles & Stokes, 1985).
- By the age of 18 years, more than three-quarters have engaged in heavy petting (Roper, 1994).
- One-quarter to one-half of young people report experience with fellatio and/or cunnilingus (Coles & Stokes, 1985; Newcomer & Udry, 1985). Almost half of boys aged 15–19 have received oral sex and 4 in 10 have performed oral sex on a girl (Gates & Sonenstein, 2000).
- 2–5% of teenagers report some type of same-gender sexual experience (Coles & Stokes, 1985; Remafedi, 1992; Roper, 1994).

Some data suggest that the progression from kissing to noncoital behaviors to intercourse differs among different groups of adolescents. Many teenagers move through a progression of intimate behaviors; lower-income teenagers are less likely to follow this progression, moving more rapidly from kissing directly to sexual intercourse (Brooks-Gunn & Furstenberg, 1990).

Teenagers Who Have Intercourse

More than 80% of Americans first have intercourse as teenagers (Alan Guttmacher Institute, 1994). More than half of women and almost three-quarters of men aged 15–19 years have had sexual intercourse. However, despite the large numbers of young people who experiment with a variety of sexual behaviors, intercourse is generally less widespread and certainly less frequent than many teenagers and adults believe. The majority of teenagers use contraceptives as consistently and effectively as most adults.

Teenagers have always engaged in sexual behaviors. However, in the past, at least for teenage women, intercourse was reserved for engaged or married couples, and marriage often took place in the teen years. When an out-of-wedlock pregnancy occurred, "shotgun" marriages were frequently the answer, or girls were sent away to stay with relatives until the baby was born and adopted. It may surprise readers to note that the birthrate for adolescents peaked in 1957 (Alan Guttmacher Institute, 1994). In fact, the adolescent birthrate is significantly lower than it was 40 years ago. In 1955, 90 of every 1,000 15- to 19-year-old women gave birth; by 1999, that number had dropped to 50 of every 1,000 (The National Campaign to Prevent Teenage Pregnancy, 2001). Nevertheless, in the last two decades, there has been a significant change in the numbers of young people who have had intercourse at young ages. At each age of adolescence, higher proportions of teenage men and women have had sexual intercourse today than had done so 20 years ago. Nevertheless, teenage pregnancy rates are falling; they had reached a level of 90.7 in 1997. Both abortion rates and birth rates have declined (Morbidity and Mortality Weekly Report, 2000).

Contraceptive use has also increased substantially during this time. In 1979, fewer than half of adolescents used a contraceptive at first intercourse (Forrest & Singh, 1990); in 1988, two-thirds did so. By 1990, that proportion had increased to more than 70% (National Center for Health Statistics, 1995). Surveys suggest that as many as 60% of teenagers now use condoms; these proportions are two to three times higher than those reported in the 1970s (Centers for Disease Control and Prevention, 2000). However, in every survey, fewer than half of the teenagers who recently used condoms did so all of the time (Cates, 1991). Condom use is especially critical for teens and college students; one-half of all new cases of STIs occurred in people under the age of 25 (American Social Health Association, 1998).

Consider these additional facts:

- The majority of teenagers wait until middle and late adolescence to have intercourse (AGI, 1994; Centers for Disease Control and Prevention, 2000). Table 12.5 shows data on high school students who have ever had sexual intercourse, by gender, race, and grade level.
- In the United States, the average age at first intercourse is 16 for males and 17 for females (AGI, 1994; Centers for Disease Control and Prevention, 1994).
- The majority of teenagers report they do not feel peer or partner pressure to have intercourse (Roper, 1994; Smith, 1988).
- The majority of teenagers who have intercourse do so with someone whom they love or seriously date (Roper, 1994).

TABLE 12.5 **High School Students Who Have Ever Had Sexual Intercourse by Gender, Race, and Grade**

	Female	Male	TOTAL
White	44%	44%	44%
African-American	66%	80%	73%
Hispanic	46%	52%	52%
Grade 9	34%	42%	38%
Grade 10	44%	42%	43%
Grade 11	50%	49%	50%
Grade 12	62%	60%	61%
TOTAL	47%	49%	48%

Source: Morbidity and Mortality Weekly Report, 47, no. SS-3 (August 14, 1998).

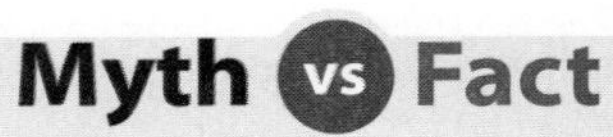

The Percentage of Teens Who Have Dangerously Incorrect Opinions

Here are the percentages of teens who believe the following myths:

Having sex every now and then without a condom is "not that big of a deal." 11%

Oral sex is "safe sex." 21%

Birth control pills are effective in preventing HIV/AIDS. 21%

Birth control pills are effective in preventing other STIs. 22%

Condoms break so often they are not worth using. 22%

Teens need a parent's permission to get condoms. 24%

It's unhealthy for girls to use birth control pills. 38%

Teens need a parent's permission to get birth control pills. 50%

Source: Teens still believe myths that can kill, *Family Life Matters, 43* (Spring 2001), 1, 6.

- Typically, teenage men and women who have sexual intercourse do so less than once a month (AGI, 1994; Sonenstein, Pleck, & Lu, 1991). Nevertheless, parents often have a difficult time dealing with an adolescent child who is having sexual intercourse. One-third of teens who have had intercourse did so in the past three months (Centers for Disease Control, 2000).
- The majority of teenagers who have intercourse use contraception. Two-thirds of adolescents use a contraceptive the first time they have intercourse (AGI, 1994), and more than three-quarters do so on an ongoing basis (AGI, 1994). Almost 60% used a condom at last intercourse (Centers for Disease Control and Prevention, 2000).

Table 12.6 shows data on condom and birth control pill use by teenagers.

For some adolescents, particularly the youngest, intercourse is developmentally disadvantageous. For many adolescents, sexual involvement is pleasurable, safe, and normative. However, for a significant minority of young people, these behaviors can be quite risky and dangerous. In particular, young adolescents who become involved in sexual behaviors are more likely to become pregnant, more likely to get an STI, and more likely to be in an exploitative relationship.

Although intercourse is relatively rare for young adolescents, in some population groups, it is quite common. According to a national youth poll, in 1990, 20% of females and 34% of males have intercourse before they are 15 years old (Centers for Disease Control and Prevention, 1992). Intercourse is developmentally disadvantageous for young adolescents because they do not have the cognitive or emotional maturity for involvement in intimate sexual behaviors, especially intercourse.

Teenage sexual behavior, particularly among the youngest teenagers, is often not voluntary, and young people who have been sexually abused often experience delays in cognitive, social, emotional, and psychological development. In fact, 12.5% of teen girls and 5.2% of teen boys report a history of forced sexual violence (Centers for Disease Control and Prevention, 2000). In addition, compared with other adolescents, they have first voluntary intercourse at younger ages, a larger number of partners, and a greater likelihood of adolescent pregnancy and childbearing (Boyer & Fine, 1992).

TABLE 12.6 Percentage of High School Students Using Condoms and Birth Control Pills at Last Sexual Intercourse, by Gender, Race, and Grade Level

	Condom Use			Pill Use		
	Female	Male	TOTAL	Female	Male	TOTAL
White	49%	62%	56%	25%	17%	21%
African-American	59%	68%	64%	15%	9%	12%
Hispanic	40%	55%	48%	13%	7%	10%
Grade 9	58%	59%	59%	8%	8%	8%
Grade 10	53%	65%	59%	17%	8%	12%
Grade 11	55%	65%	60%	19%	12%	16%
Grade 12	43%	61%	52%	30%	19%	24%
TOTAL	51%	63%	57%	21%	13%	17%

Source: Morbidity and Mortality Weekly Report, 47, no. SS-3 (August 14, 1998).

Teenage women have male sexual partners who are on average 3 years older than they are. The National Center for Health Statistics reports that in almost 70% of births to teenage girls, the fathers were age 20 years or older (National Center for Health Statistics, 1995). A California study found that the younger the mother, the greater the partner age gap. Among mothers ages 11 and 12 years old, the fathers' age averaged nearly 10 years older (California Vital Statistics Section, 1992).

The earlier a teenager begins having intercourse, the more partners she or he is likely to have. Eight percent of teens have had sexual intercourse before the age of 13 years (Centers for Disease Control and Prevention, 2000). Young people whose first intercourse occurred before age 13 years are nine times more likely to report three or more partners than those adolescents whose first sexual intercourse was at age 15 or 16 years (Centers for Disease Control and Prevention, 1992). Among 15- to 24-year-olds who had initiated intercourse before age 18 years, 75% report having had two or more partners, and 45% report having had four or more partners (MMWR, 1992).

The self-assessment exercise at the end of this chapter raises many of the questions that a young person—indeed, an adult—needs to consider to determine his or her readiness for a sexual relationship.

Sexual Abuse of Children and Adolescents

Sexual abuse occurs in all types of homes. It happens hundreds of times a day in the United States. Indeed, as many as 200,000 children are reported to be sexually abused in the United States each year. Seven percent of girls younger than 12 years old say that they have been sexually abused, and 4% of boys that age say that they have been sexually abused (Louis Harris and Associates, 1997). Girls are more likely to be sexually abused than boys, and men are more likely to be the assailants than women. However, boys are also victims of sexual abuse, and some abusers are women. And sexual abuse is every parent's nightmare.

sexual abuse
The psychological exploitation or infliction of unwanted sexual contact on one person.

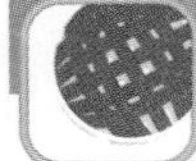

Global DIMENSIONS

Teenagers and Sexuality Around the World

Young people around the world experiment with sexual behaviors. Young people in northern European countries and the United States have first intercourse at similar ages, but northern European teenagers have much lower pregnancy and STI rates. European countries tend to be more open about sexuality, and their official governmental policies focus on reducing unprotected intercourse rather than on eliminating sexual behaviors. There is a greater availability of sexual information and reproductive health services for teenagers.

The United States has one of the highest adolescent birth rates in the world. Teenagers in Sweden, the Netherlands, Canada, Great Britain, France, and the United States have similar levels of sexual intercourse, but teenagers in other countries are much more successful than U.S. adolescents at preventing pregnancy and disease. For example, Sweden has one-third and the Netherlands has one-sixth the U.S. rate of teenage pregnancies, despite similar levels of teenage sexual intercourse. A 1985 study of 37 industrialized countries found that a major reason for the difference is that European teenagers use contraception effectively (Jones, et al., 1988).

According to the study's authors:

- Teenagers in these countries are not too immature to use contraceptives consistently and effectively.
- Teenage pregnancy rates are lower in countries where there is greater availability of confidential contraceptive services and comprehensive sexuality education (Jones, et al., 1988).

Sexual Abuse of Children

Most parents teach their children not to talk to strangers, accept candy from people they do not know, or ever get into a car with a stranger. Indeed, many preschools and kindergartens offer "stranger danger programs." However, the reality is that, in 90% of the cases, the assailant was someone in the child's family or someone close to the family.

Children can also be sexually abused by other children. This is different from the sex play described earlier in this chapter. In sex play, children are usually of the same age, they are engaging in light-hearted exploration, and they appear to be enjoying themselves—at least until they realize they have been "discovered" by an adult. And, in general, once they are told by an adult that they should stop, they do.

Some children, however, engage in inappropriate behaviors and become sexually abusive to other, usually younger, children. This may include engaging in oral or genital sex with other children, with or without their consent. Many of these children have been sexually abused themselves, and many of them have inappropriately been exposed to sexually explicit materials or adult erotic behavior. In one study, all the girls who had sexually abused other children (about 25% of childhood abusers are girls) and most of the boys had been molested themselves, often years before they committed these crimes against other children (Finkelhor, 1986). In a case reported widely in the news, three boys in Dallas aged 11, 8, and 7 years were charged with abducting, beating with a brick, and sexually assaulting a 3-year-old girl whose mother went into the house to make a phone call.

Here are some possible signs of child sexual abuse:

- The child has an unusual discharge from his penis or her vagina. A doctor should be called immediately. It is most likely just an allergic reaction to new soap or bubble bath or wearing of a wet bathing suit too long, but it could also be a sign of a sexually transmitted infection. A pediatrician can tell the difference.
- The child compulsively masturbates in public, after the parent has repeatedly told him or her that this is private behavior.
- The child tries to get other children or adults to touch his or her genitals or repeatedly tries to touch adults' genitals after being told to stop.
- The child begins to be more interested in sex or engaging in sexual behaviors than playing with friends, going to school, or engaging in other activities.
- The child engages in sex play with children who are several years older than he or she is.
- The child manually stimulates or has oral or genital contact with pets.
- The child repeatedly draws pictures with the genitals as the primary focus.
- The child begins to exhibit disturbing new toilet behaviors.
- The child engages in oral–genital sex with another child.

Sexual Abuse of Adolescents

Sexual assault is not uncommon among adolescents. Six percent of boys and 15% of girls are sexually assaulted before their 16th birthday. In a study of teenage girls in foster care, 43% reported experiencing some type of sexual abuse. The most prevalent type of abuse was being touched or fondled by an adult against her wishes. One in six reported that she had been forced to have intercourse with an adult. One-third of the young women had been sexually abused before their 10th birthday (Polit, Cozette, & Thomas, 1990). Ten thousand women younger than 18 years old were raped in 1992 (Child Welfare League, 1994). In fact, one-quarter of rape victims are women 11 to 17 years of age (National Victims Center and Crime Victims Research and Treatment Center, 1992). Nearly three-quarters of young women who had intercourse before age 14 years reported having had intercourse involuntarily (AGI, 1994; Child Welfare League of America, 1994).

A disproportionate number of young women who become pregnant during adolescence are victims of childhood sexual abuse. In one study of teenagers who were pregnant or were parents, 70% of whites, 42% of African Americans, and 37% of Hispanics had been sexually abused as children (Boyer & Fine, 1992). In another study, 64% of parenting and pregnant teens reported that they had had at least one unwanted sexual experience (Child Welfare League of America, 1994).

Gay, lesbian, and bisexual teenagers face an additional form of abuse related to their sexuality. A study in New York City found that of lesbian, gay, and bisexual teenagers reporting an assault, almost half reported that the assault was related to their sexual orientation, and for almost two-thirds, the assault happened within their families (Hunter, 1990).

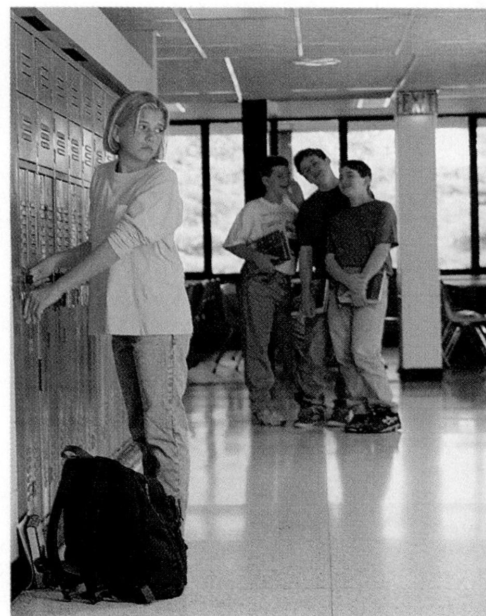

Sexual harassment in schools is common. What type of program could be instituted to help stop such harassment?

Sexual Harassment

Sexual harassment is a fact of life in most middle and high schools. *Sexual harassment in school* is defined as "unwanted and unwelcome sexual behavior that interferes with the student's life." Sexual harassment includes unwanted sexual comments, jokes, and gestures; receiving from another student sexual pictures, photographs, and notes; sexual graffiti about a specific student in the bathroom or locker room; spreading of sexual rumors; flashing or mooning; touching, grabbing, or pinching in a sexual way; brushing against another student in a sexual way; pulling clothes off; blocking another student in a sexual way; and forcing kissing and other sexual behaviors. In a study conducted by the American Association of University Women in 1993, 85% of girls and 76% of boys in grades 8 through 11 reported that they had been victims of one of these behaviors (Bryant, 1993). One-third had been harassed by the time they reached sixth grade. And almost 6 in 10 of these students report that they have engaged in these offensive behaviors themselves!

sexual harassment
Unwanted sexual behavior that interferes with the student's life.

Most sexual harassment in schools occurs openly in classrooms and hallways, rather than in secluded areas. Students are usually harassed by other students, but in one in five cases, they are harassed by adult employees. And students report that this type of sexual harassment affects their lives. Girls in particular report that they feel less confident and more afraid to go to school after incidents of sexual harassment. This same study found that students are not likely to tell adults about these incidents. Only 7% told a teacher, and only one-quarter told a parent (Bryant, 1993).

Schools are supposed to protect students against sexual harassment. Schools need to have sexual harassment policies, with clear penalties for perpetrators, which should be communicated to students and parents. A clear procedure for handling complaints of sexual harassment should be established. A May 1999 U.S. Supreme Court decision found a school financially liable for harassment that occurred between two students (Haffner, 2001).

Exploring the DIMENSIONS of Human Sexuality

Our feelings, attitudes, and beliefs regarding sexuality are influenced by our internal and external environments. Go to sexuality.jbpub.com to learn more about the biological, psychological, and sociological factors that affect your sexuality.

Biological Factors

- Puberty changes boys and girls into men and women.
- Genetic coding affects the onset of puberty and general overall appearance.
- Reproduction becomes possible after menarche and spermenarche.
- Sexual arousal and response become important issues in an adolescent's life.
- Physical appearance changes dramatically during puberty, affecting body image.
- Growth and development, in terms of physical and mental maturity, greatly affect a person's self-concept.

Sociocultural Factors

- Socioeconomic status affects sexual behaviors. Lower-economic status youths have sexual intercourse earlier than teens who are more well off, and they experience a higher rate of STIs and births.
- Religion and ethnic heritage affect beliefs about sexuality and permissiveness.
- Many cultures' double standard expects boys to be sexually aggressive and girls to remain sexually passive.
- Media and ad information often convey information to adolescents about sexuality and sexual behavior.
- Friends often convey false information about sexual behaviors to adolescents.

CASE STUDY

Sexual maturation is a time of constant physical and psychological changes. At the same time, deeply rooted sociocultural influences, once able to provide a sense of comfort, now may cause confusion.

Many adolescents feel they have almost no control over physiological changes and the accompanying mood swings. In an attempt to preserve the child's body they once had, some girls attempt to control their food intake. But a girl with a bad self-image may develop an obsession with food intake that leads to an eating disorder.

Boys also feel out of control, experiencing erections and hormonal surges at almost any stimulus.

A cultural double standard does not help. Boys who do not want to be permissive feel out of place, as do girls who want to experience sexual behaviors. Such confusion can lead to sexual experimentation—usually in the form of unsafe sexual practices.

Psychological Factors

- Emotions are dramatically affected by hormones, which cause dramatic mood swings for adolescents.
- Early or late developers may have issues with securing their body image.
- Sexual experience used to be gained slowly, starting with kissing games, moving to petting, then intercourse. Today's teens often move directly from kissing to intercourse.
- Self-concept is influenced by social status and peers.
- Learned attitudes and behaviors are put to the test as the body goes through constant physical changes.

Discussion Questions

1. Discuss how touch, including genital touching, differs for infants and toddlers versus adolescents.
2. Describe the roles that parents, peers, and the media play in teaching preschoolers and early elementary students about sexuality.
3. Compare and contrast puberty in boys and girls, both physiologically and emotionally.
4. Identify and describe the three stages of adolescence, including the development of sexual self-concept.
5. Distinguish between expected childhood sex play and behaviors that could be abusive.

Application Questions

Reread the chapter-opening story and answer the following questions.

1. On *Mister Rogers' Neighborhood,* Fred Rogers sings a song that says, "Boys are special on the outside/Girls are special on the inside." Is there any reason to tell a young child more than that?
2. Some parents choose to teach their young children about sexual intercourse and reproduction; many other parents do not want their children learning such information. Given that children repeat what they know, is it important to respect the rights of those who—for religious or cultural reasons—want such information withheld from their children?
3. Given that children do hear national news at some point, did the mass media handle the Monica Lewinsky affair with adequate discretion? If you were a reporter *and* a parent, how would you balance the responsibility to report the news but protect young children?

Critical Thinking Questions

1. You are the parent of a 4-year-old and have just received a phone call from a parent who has a child the same age. It seems the two children were in the garage "examining" each other. The other parent is furious, accusing your child of initiating the "perversities." What do you say to the parent? What do you say to your child?

   You have 10 minutes before your child arrives home, time enough to check out the SIECUS web site. What information helps you talk to your child?
2. Some pressures of adolescence are the result of society's double standard—that it is OK for men but wrong for women to be interested in engaging in sexual behaviors. Given what the chapter says about normal sexual feelings, what pressures does a double standard place on women? On men?

   Is it possible for society to eliminate the double standard and emphasize equality? If so, would society choose that both men and women have an equal right to say yes or no to sexual experiences? Explain your answer.
3. Refer to Table 12.6 when answering these questions. What is the influence of race and ethnicity on condom and birth control use? What might account for these differences? What is the influence of age on condom and birth control use? Why might condom use be higher in the 9th grade than in the 12th grade? How might pill use influence condom use? How can young people who choose to engage in sexual intercourse be encouraged to use both birth control pills and condoms?

Critical Thinking Case

Adolescents have a hard enough time coming to grips with their sexuality even if they receive proper information and support. But few do. In addition, some school-based sexuality education programs have a "fear-based" component. The aim of many fear-based programs is abstinence outside marriage. There is nothing wrong with teaching abstinence; however, many fear-based programs tend to distort information and use incorrect information to make their point.

The SIECUS web site features a large section on fear-based programs, with general information and critiques of seven fear-based programs.

Choose one fear-based program and prepare a critique. What are the strong points and weak points of the program? How could it be improved? Would the fear techniques used in the program have prevented you from engaging in sexual activity?

Exploring Personal Dimensions

Readiness for a Sexual Relationship

Teenagers and young adults often wonder, "How do I know if I am ready for sex?" The following checklist may help them assess their readiness for mature sexual relationships (Winship, 1983).

This checklist may help adolescents *and* adults evaluate whether they are ready for a mature sexual relationship with a partner. Ideally, these criteria would be met *before* a young person or an adult engaged in intimate sexual behaviors, including any type of intercourse. Think about your own decisions or the decisions of people you know. Do they meet these criteria?

Are you and your partner

_____ Physically mature?
_____ Patient and understanding?
_____ Knowledgeable about sexuality and sexual response?
_____ Empathetic and able to be vulnerable?
_____ Committed to preventing unintended pregnancies?
_____ Able to handle responsibility for positive consequences?
_____ Able to handle responsibility for potential negative consequences?
_____ Honestly approving of your behavior?

Is your relationship

_____ Committed, mutually kind, and understanding?
_____ Do you trust and admire each other?
_____ Have you experimented with and found pleasure in nonpenetrative behaviors?
_____ Have you talked about sexual behaviors before they occur?
_____ Is your motivation for a sexual relationship pleasure and intimacy?
_____ Do you have a place for the sexual relationship that is safe and comfortable?

Source: Haffner, 1995.

Sexuality Online

Go to the web component for *Exploring the Dimensions of Human Sexuality* at sexuality.jbpub.com for web exercises, additional resources related to this chapter, and student review tools.

Suggested Readings

Adolescent health: State of the nation. Atlanta: Centers for Disease Control, 1995.

AIDS sexual behavior and intravenous drug use. Washington, DC: National Academy Press, 1989.

Bernstein, A. *Flight of the stork.* Indiana: Perspectives Press, 1994.

Brindis, C. D. *Adolescent pregnancy prevention: A guidebook for communities.* Palo Alto, CA: Health Promotion Resource Center, Stanford Center for Research in Disease Prevention, 1991.

Dryfoos, J. *Adolescents at risk.* New York: Oxford University Press, 1990.

Greydanus, D. E., ed. *Caring for your adolescent: Ages 12–21.* New York: Bantam Books, 1992.

Guidelines for comprehensive sexuality education. New York: SIECUS, 1991.

Haffner, D. *Facing facts: Sexual health for America's adolescents.* New York: SIECUS, 1995.

Haffner, D. *From diapers to dating.* New York: Newmarket Press, 1999.

Haffner, D. *Beyond the Big Talk,* New York: Newmarket Press, 2001.

Hayes, C. D. *Risking the future: Adolescent sexuality, pregnancy and childbearing.* Washington, DC: National Academy Press, 1987.

Herdt, G., ed. *Gay and lesbian youth.* New York: The Haworth Press, 1989.

Jones, E. F., Forrest, J. D., Goldman, N., Henshaw, S., Lincoln, R., Rosoff, J. I., Westoff, C. F., & Wulf, D. *Teenage pregnancy in industrialized countries.* New Haven, CT: Yale University Press, 1986.

Lawson, A. & Rhode, D. L., eds. *The politics of pregnancy: Adolescent sexuality and public policy.* New Haven: Yale University Press, 1993.

A matter of time: Risk and opportunity in the out-of-school hours. New York: Carnegie Corporation of New York, 1992.

Millstein, S., Petersen, A., & Nightingale, E. *Promoting the health of adolescents.* New York: Oxford University Press, 1993.

National Campaign to Prevent Teengage Pregnancy. *No easy answers.* Washington, DC: National Campaign, 1999.

Savin-Williams, Ritch. *And Then I Became Gay.* New York: Routledge, 1998.

Sex and America's teenagers. New York: The Alan Guttmacher Institute, 1994.

Wilson, P. *When sex is the subject.* Santa Cruz, CA: Network Publications, 1991.

Web Sites About Teenage Sexuality

www.sxetc.org

www.teenpregnancy.org

www.teenwire.com

CHAPTER 13
Sexuality in Adulthood

FEATURES

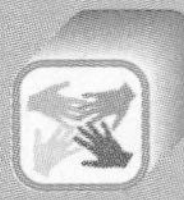
Multicultural Dimensions
The Jefferson–Hemings Affair

Communication Dimensions
Tempted by Digital Dalliances

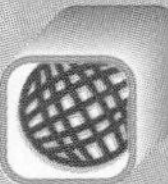
Global Dimensions
Divorce in China

Multicultural Dimensions
The Boomer Sandwich

Ethical Dimensions
Should Donor Eggs Be Used to Let Women Older Than 50 Years Produce Viable Babies?

Gender Dimensions
Coming to Terms: Masculinity and Physical Challenges

CHAPTER OBJECTIVES

1. Discuss the major theories of love and sexuality.
2. Describe the typical college relationship, including sexual activities.
3. Cite the factors that have led to the increase in the number of single people and the postponement of marriage.
4. Evaluate the advantages and disadvantages of cohabitation.
5. Describe the characteristics of a happy marriage.
6. Discuss the reasons for the high number of divorces.
7. Describe changes that occur during the aging process.
8. Discuss the sexuality challenges for the disabled and ill, as well as how to overcome them.

sexuality.jbpub.com

Cohabitation
Multicultural Dimensions: The Jefferson–Hemings Affair
Types of Marriage
Divorce

INTRODUCTION

Lynn and Chris first met in a small town's only junior high when they were 12 years old. By high school, they had become friends and had their first date at the homecoming dance their sophomore year. After a couple of years of dating, they lost their virginity together at age 16 years. Throughout high school, they stayed together and began planning for college and a life together.

They applied to the same colleges and entered the college where they were both accepted. The struggles of college produced many changes, but they made a conscious effort to change together. As they grew up together, they did things they perceived to be more grown up: traveling, saving up for an apartment, and the like. During their junior year, they got an off-campus apartment in the heart of the local city.

Although they had been together for more than 5 years and were engaged, they were surprised at their parents' reactions—shock and dismay—to their living together. After all, it was the late 1970s, and both families had had other relatives who had lived together. Lynn and Chris saw living together as a "next step" toward marriage. Why, they thought, was society so backward?

Surviving college made them more determined to pursue their dream of life together, with children and good jobs. At age 24 years, they married. Four years later, a first child was born; 3 years later, a second child. With each change, they managed to adapt. But slowly—almost imperceptibly—they realized that they were not always changing in the same ways.

As they hit full stride in their careers in their mid-30s, and their children reached school age, decisions had to be made. Holding a high-level management position that requires long hours and travel also requires support at home—with children and housework. The old saying "Behind every great man, there's a great woman" today would be phrased as "A successful person has family support."

Lynn supported the family by working from a home office and taking care of the children—schools, homework, sick days, vacation days, doctor and dentist appointments, play dates, sports, and extracurricular activities. Chris rarely returned home from work before 7:30 P.M., worked many weekends, and traveled around the world. Conflicts developed over what was important in their lives, and, because Chris made more money than Lynn, issues concerning how to spend also arose. Chris's lack of time at home increased tensions. Eventually, Lynn discovered that Chris was having an affair with a business associate.

After considering the possibility of divorce for several years, Lynn and Chris finally proceeded—after 14 years of marriage and almost 25 years together. The children stayed with Lynn, and Chris was ordered to pay child support and alimony. Both Lynn and Chris expressed a feeling of relief after the divorce was finalized.

Lynn and Chris had a great deal of positive support from friends, many of whom had been divorced themselves. It seemed that society had begun to accept divorce. But once again, they were surprised by the reaction of their parents, who felt that they should stay together and try to work out their problems. Some things never change!

In this chapter we continue our exploration of the life cycle, picking up in young adulthood. We first explore how people fall in love, then we follow the life cycle from singlehood, through cohabitation, marriage, and divorce. Finally, we take a look at sexuality and the elderly.

Love and Sexuality

What is love? How do you know when and whether you are in love, whether you are loved, or whether you love another person? These questions have been asked through the ages by young people just beginning to long for and seek intimacy outside their parental families. And through the ages love has never grown any easier to define. There are many types of love—love of one's parents, of a friend, of a pet. Perhaps the most difficult sort of love to describe is love of a person with whom one could potentially share a sexual relationship.

Theories About Love

Love may take a variety of forms, as Greek philosophers long ago demonstrated: *eros,* passionate and/or erotic love; *agape,* a selfless, giving love; *storge,* affectionate love, usually of the type parents have for their children; *ludus,* playful love (partners keep the relationship at a distance by keeping love at a game level); and *mania,* a love consumed by emotional extremes such as misery, possessiveness, and jealousy.

Erich Fromm presented his ideas about love in *The Art of Loving* (1956). He distinguishes brotherly love, motherly love, erotic love, and self-love. He believes that loving is an art—something that must be learned and practiced. Fromm indicated that immature love is characterized by a dependent relationship between two people, and mature love is characterized by care, responsibility, respect, and knowledge of the loved person. He defines erotic love as a craving for total union with another person that is exclusive and enduring.

Abraham Maslow distinguished between B-love and D-love (1968). Those who experience B-love (short for *Being* love) are unselfish in their love for another; those who experience D-love (short for *Deficiency* love) are selfish and have a strong need for love.

Types of Love

Love takes many forms and can be distinguished as romantic love or conscious love. Romantic love, also known as passionate love, is characterized by almost total absorption in another, with strong feelings of elation, sexual desire, anxiety, and arousal. This form of love is often accompanied by physiological reactions—perspiration, stomach churning, blushing, and increased pulse rate.

People have very different ideas of what is romantic, as shown by a readers' survey in *Psychology Today* (Rubenstein, 1983). Common romantic themes include walking on a moonlit beach, having a quiet dinner at home, kissing in public, or making love all weekend. Some saw romance typified by heightened emotions while others thought of intense and painful emotions.

Intense, passionate love is most likely to occur early in a relationship. At this point people often overlook faults, avoid conflicts, and ignore logic and reasoned consideration. Conscious love, on the other hand, is a more realistic view of another person. We see both the strengths and weaknesses of the loved one and do not depend completely on him or her to fulfill our needs and give us what we ourselves lack. The sexual activity in conscious love may be more rewarding than in romantic love because the sexual behavior communicates and expresses loving feelings. People who have an honest view of each other can enjoy giving as well as receiving. People who feel romantic (passionate) love are often intent on receiving pleasure and fulfilling their desires, rather than on giving and taking equally.

In addition to being romantic or conscious, love can take various forms—erotic, friendship, devotional, parental, or altruistic. In erotic love there is a type of biological "chemistry" that binds lovers together and leads them to form a binding relationship (Lee, 1988). Individuals experiencing erotic love are preoccupied with their love and constantly think about their partner. Erotic love becomes less intense as time goes on, but even at a lower level it can be a positive part of a relationship.

Friendship involves deep and intimate feelings, but these are not physical. The Greek term for this type of friendship or liking is *philia*. Although there are many similar attitudes and feelings among lovers as well as friends, lovers tend to differ from friends in sexual intimacy, exclusiveness, and fascination (Davis, 1985). Men and women can be friends without becoming sexually involved.

Devotional love does not involve physical contact and is a very specific kind of love. This type of love is most likely to be directed to a god, a country, an ethnic group, or other significant groups or institutions.

Parental love can be intense, but the feelings are different from other forms of love. Infants and children learn this type of love through holding and touching—even very early in life. For some people, parental love represents the most intense form of love they will ever feel.

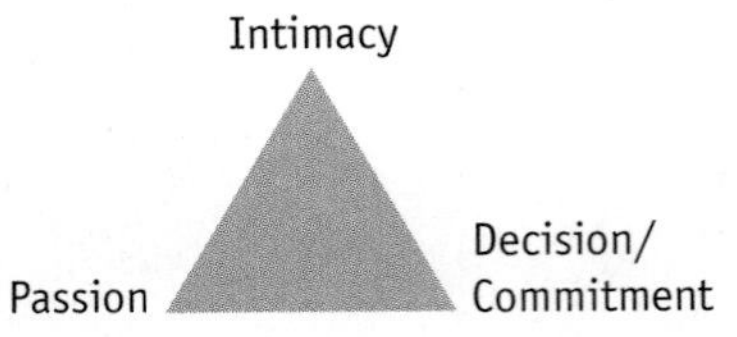

FIGURE 13.1 Sternberg's triangular theory of love.

Altruistic love is a generous giving of the self. Some say this is a special form of parental love; it is seen in people who spend great amounts of time doing church work, volunteering in hospitals, and assisting others in a variety of ways. Some people who work in helping professions, for example, as therapists or teachers, might find they have a great capacity for altruistic love.

Sternberg (1986) has proposed a triangular theory of love suggesting that there are three components of love: intimacy, passion, and decision/commitment. These components can be visualized as points on a triangle (Figure 13.1); the triangle metaphor is used to show how a couple can be matched or mismatched in the love they have for each other. The top of the triangle is intimacy, which is the emotional component of love, according to Sternberg. Here are feelings of mutual understanding, bondedness, willingness to share, giving of emotional support, and valuing of the other person as part of your life. Passion is the motivational drive of love that includes physical attraction, sexual relations, and romance. Passion can usually differentiate romantic love from love in a friendship or of a family member. This component is usually first in a relationship but is also the first to fade. Passion and intimacy are interwoven and one may precede the other, depending on how the relationship begins. Decision/commitment is the cognitive component of the triangle, as one makes the decision to love the other person and then makes the long-term commitment to maintain the relationship.

Perfectly matched involvements of partners exist when the vertexes of the triangles are equally matched and are at the same level. Closely matched couples may be slightly off on one of the components, and this is usually not a perilous situation. Moderately mismatched partners exhibit mismatching at one or two of the vertexes and the partners are at different levels within those components. For example, they may be equally matched on the passion vertex, but one partner is slightly more committed and has greater feelings of intimacy than the other. A severely mismatched couple is one whose partners may be equally committed but are very disparate in the passion and intimacy components.

This theory of love may help partners determine whether they are on the right track in their relationship and may help diagnose any problems.

Sternberg (1988) has outlined eight types, or phases, of love based on his triangular model. They are listed in Table 13.1.

TABLE 13.1 Sternberg's Types (Phases) of Love

1. **Nonlove:** All three components of love are absent. Most personal relationships are of this type.
2. **Liking:** Intimacy is present, but passion and commitment are not.
3. **Infatuation:** There are passionate desires, but intimacy and commitment are not present. This is a kind of "love at first sight."
4. **Empty love:** Commitment exists, but passion and intimacy are missing. Relationships that once had passion and intimacy can become stagnant.
5. **Romantic love:** There is no commitment, but there is passion and intimacy.
6. **Companionate love:** A combination of intimacy and commitment exists, but passionate attraction has died down. The relationship becomes a kind of committed friendship.
7. **Fatuous love:** Passion and commitment are present, but intimacy is not. This type is associated with whirlwind romances and "quickie marriages."
8. **Consummate love:** This is the complete measure of love involving passion, intimacy, and commitment. It can be very hard to achieve this type of love, and even harder to maintain it.

Source: Sternberg, 1988.

Characteristics of Romantic Love

Because we are focusing on human relationships and sexuality in this text, it is appropriate to consider briefly the characteristics of romantic love—companionship, intimacy, caring, commitment, sexual activity, and romance. Companionship involves sharing experiences and receiving emotional support from each other. At first this characteristic might not seem as exciting as some of the others, but over time it can be enduring and very necessary.

Intimacy involves sharing thoughts and feelings with a person who is considered very special. Whereas traditionally women and not men revealed their innermost thoughts, in recent years there is a tendency for both genders to disclose highly personal feelings within a relationship (Hatfield, 1988; Pearson, 1985).

Caring is the desire to do things for another person without expecting anything in return. As in most other aspects of a relationship, balance is important. For example, it is possible to think of situations in which there is so much caring that the relationship is completely one-sided.

Commitment means pressing on with a relationship even during difficult times. When conflict or problems exist, commitment is needed to give other aspects of love a chance to grow.

Sexual activity sometimes seems to be the major part of romantic love; however, there are many couples who love each other but have a minimal amount of sexual activity. Sexual activity alone, even when highly pleasurable, is not enough to maintain a poor relationship (Blumstein & Schwartz, 1983). There does seem to be a connection between sexual activity and positive relationships, but a good relationship probably has a positive influence on sexual activity, rather than the converse.

The decision to participate in sexual activity can be very simple for some people, and very complicated for others. Sexual activity can have different meanings for different people. It can be a validation of deep intimacy in a relationship, it can be a way to help get to know another person, it can be done to promote reproduction, it can reduce sexual tension, it can produce excitement and risk, and for some it can be a form of recreation.

For many college students it is helpful to base decisions about sexual activity on their values. Some students may have clear guidelines based upon what they have learned from their family, their religion, or their peers; others may not have such guidelines. In either case it may be wise to consider personal values in life and relationships before getting sexually involved. This can mean thinking about the role of relationships and sexual activity in life at that time, what norms are most highly valued and why, and what should be done for protection against unwanted pregnancy and sexually transmitted infections if a decision is made to participate in intimate sexual activity. Communication about these decisions with a potential partner is especially important. Suggestions for such communication were provided in Chapter 3.

Love as a Relationship Develops

The nature of love typically changes as a relationship develops. For example, the passionate or romantic love of an early stage might evolve into a companionship type of love. This does not mean that passion and romance have evaporated; nor does it mean that the relationship is not as good as before. It simply means that there are common stages of relationships, and they can all be of high quality. Relationships can be thought of as having different phases of growth. At any stage there are ways to promote better relationships.

Hormonal and Chemical Aspects of Love

The characteristics and types of love presented so far have been mainly based upon emotional, psychological, and spiritual kinds of feelings. Some experts argue that hormonal and chemical factors are also involved in love. One reason may be related to brain chemistry. Another relates to **pheromones,** which are chemical substances secreted by some animals that supposedly affect the reproductive behavior of another same-species animal.

Related to brain chemistry, during the intense passion of a developing love relationship some people report a natural high, almost as though they were on drugs. Researchers (Liebowitz, 1983; Walsh, 1991) reported that this "high" results from surging levels of three brain chemicals that allow brain cells to communicate with each other. They are similar to amphetamine drugs and cause effects such as giddiness, euphoria, and elation. As with use of amphetamines, the "high" typically does not last—perhaps because the body develops a tolerance for the chemicals just as it does for amphetamines, or perhaps because the intensity of the relationship decreases.

The same researchers also point out that there are brain chemicals that help explain why some relationships develop into long-term loving relationships. These substances, called **endorphins,** are morphine-like chemicals that help cause a sense of security, tranquility, and peace. The researchers feel that these chemicals help explain why abandoned lovers may feel such a loss. They are not getting their doses of feel-good chemicals.

The topic of pheromones has received greater attention in recent years. For over a hundred years scientists have documented the effects of pheromones on mating behavior in insects and animals. The big question has been, Do pheromones have the same effects on humans?

In 1986 Dr. Winnifred Cutler began to document the effects of human pheromones (Link & Copeland, 2001). Those who believe in human pheromones claim they send signals that are picked up by organs inside the nose. We cannot smell them, but they supposedly can have a major impact on sex drive, increase in fertility, and regulation of women's menstrual cycles. Behaviors that are reported to increase as a result of pheromones include making conversation, expressing an interest in another person, being responsive to another person, paying unsolicited compliments, overtly flirting, brushing up against another person, and becoming sexually excited.

On the basis of the concept that there are natural human pheromones, entrepreneurs developed numerous products designed to mimic the alleged effects of pheromones. These include towelettes with pheromones as well as creams and oils that are supposed to help with sexual attraction. It is too early to tell whether or not such products are effective—and even the basic effects of pheromones are not agreed upon by experts.

Love Problems

With all its positive aspects, love can also create problems. Perhaps the most obvious ones are rejection, jealousy, and falling out of love. Being turned down by another person (rejection) can be difficult to experience. This can happen at various stages of a relationship, and fear of rejection is natural. Of course, as with so many other aspects of life, obtaining the many positive benefits of a relationship always entails a gamble (such as the possibility of rejection). Dealing with rejection can be difficult for some, but often it simply involves trying again. If a strong relationship already exists, it might be wise to use good communication skills and talk about the rejection with the other person. Couples counseling can help single and married couples. At any rate, rejection can also be used as a learning experience to help in future relationships.

In their *Psychology Today* readers' survey, Salovey and Rodin (1985) defined *jealousy* as the "thoughts and feelings that arise when an actual or desired relationship is threatened." People were more likely to experience jealousy if they had a low opinion of themselves, saw a large difference between what they were and what they wanted to be, and valued highly visible traits such as wealth, fame, popularity, and physical attractiveness. Few differences in men's and women's jealous feelings were found in the survey, except that women showed certain behaviors more than men, such as searching through a lover's belongings or using extensive questioning.

Some jealous feelings are probably natural, but jealousy is also a bothersome feeling that can get in the way of good love relationships. It can be helpful to understand why jealous feelings occur, to use good communication skills to talk about jealousy within a relationship, and to avoid doing things that might contribute to a partner's jealous feelings. For some, effective means of coping with jealousy are thinking about one's positive qualities, selectively ignoring some activities that might be upsetting, and simply containing feelings of jealousy. It might be wise to recognize jealous feelings and accept and deal with them as part of an overall relationship.

What Causes Attraction?

Many factors contribute to attraction and falling in love. Unlike in the fairy tale in which the prince marries the commoner, in real life we are usually attracted to someone we consider attainable. This attraction differs from adolescent crushes on movie stars, sports stars, politicians, or teachers. In adulthood, we seek intimate relationships with someone who can love us in return.

Most North Americans marry someone who has the same sociocultural dimensions, someone whose race and ethnicity, religion, age, and social class are similar to their own (Henslin, 1995). A 1994 study showed that most Americans met their spouses at school, church, or work or through friends (Laumann, et al., 1994). Why do we like people who are like us? One explanation is that doing so provides us with validation for our personality characteristics and beliefs (Baron, 1998). Similarity is a very powerful determinant of attraction.

Gender also plays a role in mate selection. Researchers interviewed more than 9,000 young adults (males and females), all in their 20s, who lived in 33 countries. Subjects were given a list of 18 traits and asked to rank them in terms of most (1) to least (18) desirable in a potential mate (Buss, et al., 1990). The results are listed in Table 13.2.

Buss and associates found a gender difference as well: Males in all cultures in the study placed an emphasis on youthfulness and attractiveness. Data showed that at the time of marriage, the average male was 2 to 5 years older than his partner. Women, however, placed an emphasis on mates who were somewhat older, had better prospects for financial security, and were industrious. Buss explains the difference in terms of evolutionary needs: Males select younger, physically attractive women because such characteristics are viewed as good indicators of reproductive success. Women select older, more

TABLE 13.2 **Ranking of Desirable Traits in a Partner (Male and Female Combined)**

1. Mutual attraction (love)
2. Dependable character
3. Emotional stability and maturity
4. Pleasing disposition
5. Good health
6. Education and intelligence
7. Sociability
8. Desire for home and children
9. Refinement, neatness
10. Good looks (ranked higher by males)
11. Ambitious and industrious
12. Good cook and housekeeper
13. Good financial prospects (ranked higher by females)
14. Similar education
15. Favorable social status or rating
16. Chastity (ranked higher by males)
17. Similar religious background
18. Similar political background

established males because such characteristics are viewed as good indicators of security for their offspring (Buss, 1994).

Sexuality During the College Years

A national survey of more than 269,000 freshman college students revealed information about sexual attitudes (Kellogg, 2001). About 54% thought abortion should be legal, 42% (55% of males and 33% of females) thought that if two people really like each other it is all right to have sexual intercourse even if they have known each other only a very short time, 27% thought there should be laws prohibiting homosexual relationships, 56% thought same-sex couples should have the right to legal marriage status, and 22% thought the activities of married women are best confined to the home and family.

Before the late 1960s, there were strict rules on campuses about men's and women's socializing. Older readers may remember the "one foot on the floor" rule: Women were allowed to have men in their college dorm room only with the door open and only with each person's having one foot on the floor. Curfews were common. Coed dorms were nonexistent.

Today, most campuses have long given up these types of rules. Intercourse on college campuses has increased dramatically: 12% among college men and 35% among college women during the period from 1965 to 1980 (Rubinson & Rupertis, 1991). The prevailing sexual norm on most campuses is "permissiveness with affection."

In one study comparing students in 1973 and 1988, definite trends emerged. The percentage of women having casual sexual relations with more than one person increased, as did the percentage of women having intercourse within a meaningful relationship. Men, too, were more likely to have casual sexual intercourse in 1988 as compared to 1973 (Dunn, et al., 1992). Most studies done during the 1980s and 1990s report that between 75% and 85% of students have had sexual intercourse (Reinisch, et al., 1995; Wiley, et al., 1996). Most college students report that they are heterosexual; only 1% identify as homosexual and 2% as bisexual (Reinisch, et al., 1995).

While not necessarily pertaining only to students attending college, here are some interesting statistics about males and females of college age. By their late teenage years, at least 75% of all men and women have had intercourse, and more than two-thirds of all sexually experienced teens have had two or more partners. Among sexually experienced people in their 20s, 31% of men and 20% of women had more than one sexual partner in the past year (Sexual and reproductive health, 2002).

Late high school and early college years are a time of transition to sexual activity for males. Fewer than 25% are sexually experienced by age 15, but more than 90% have intercourse before their 20th birthday. Slightly more than 20% of sexually experienced men have had only one partner by their late teens, and about 30% have had six or more (In their own right, 2002).

It is important to point out, however, that one in six college students is a virgin. Among virgins, 40% report that they have not met the right person yet and 38% have religious beliefs that support chastity until marriage (Survey USA, 1998).

Types of Relationships

Most college students are involved in a steady relationship. In one study, almost three-quarters of undergraduate students said that they were in a monogamous relationship (Stebleton & Rothenberger, 1993). Most college students appear to be serially monogamous; that is, they are sexually exclusive with one partner at a time. In one study, 53% of the sexually experienced college men and 60% of the sexually experienced college women were involved in an exclusive love relationship. Still, significant percentages of college students have casual sexual activity. Fourteen percent of young women and 38% of young men report that they have had casual intercourse with more than one partner during their college years (Dunn, et al., 1992).

Significant proportions of college students have had several sexual partners. In one study, 38% of men and 36% of women had had vaginal intercourse with more than five partners. Although on average, these young people had been having sexual intercourse for less than 4 years, males reported an average of eight female partners and females reported an average of six male partners (Reinisch, et al., 1995). In a national phone survey of college students, 36% of males and 21% of females reported that they had had nine or more partners (Survey USA, 1998).

The Institute for American Values (Mulhauser, 2001) interviewed 1,000 college women and reported that dating among college students is all but dead. Apparently, college students either participate in random hookups or are in a very serious relationship. For many, there is nothing in between. Hooking up does not have to mean having sexual intercourse. In fact, 39% of the respondents were virgins. Dating, however, was not reported to be very common. One-third of the women said they had been asked on two or fewer dates. Of the seniors interviewed, only 50% said they had been asked on six or more dates since college started. Because few people are asking for dates, what is left is an informal hookup.

Previously, noncollege singles in their 20s were almost entirely overlooked in research about sexual behavior and attitudes. Popenoe and Whitehead (2001) found that this group aspire to marriage and expect their marriage to last a lifetime. However, many are first looking to get ahead on their own. Both men and women are committed to making it on their own and getting a place of their own before marriage. The mating culture is described as "sex without strings and relationships without rings." Sexual activity is viewed as being for fun. Casual sexual activity is an expected part of the dating scene. The threat of HIV and AIDS looms large over the dating scene. However, although both men and women fear AIDS, it is mainly the women who take the initiative and responsibility for protection. Both men and women see the club scene as a place for drinking, fun, and casual sexual hookups. In seeking a high-quality relationship, these men and women say you should look for a partner through church, friends, or school. Entering a relationship usually means postponing sexual activity until you get to know each other. Before becoming seriously involved, couples often are tested for HIV and AIDS. Once a couple can prove to each other that they have recently tested negative, they are less vigilant about using condoms.

Overall there has been an increase in "casual" sexual relationships among high school and college students (Surveys show change in attitudes toward sex among high school and college students, higher incidence of "casual" and "oral sex," 2003). Thirteen hundred Ohio 7th- to 11th-grade students were interviewed about dating, relationships, and sexual activity. About 55% had engaged in intercourse and one-third of those had engaged in intercourse with "someone whose attachment went no further than friendship." The study also reported a significant shift in attitudes toward oral sexual activity, noting that respondents consider it "an acceptable alternative" to intercourse and different from sexual intercourse. The proportion of young adults who have engaged in oral sexual activity has risen; one-third of 15- to 17-year-olds and two-thirds of 18- to 24-year-olds have engaged in oral sexual activity.

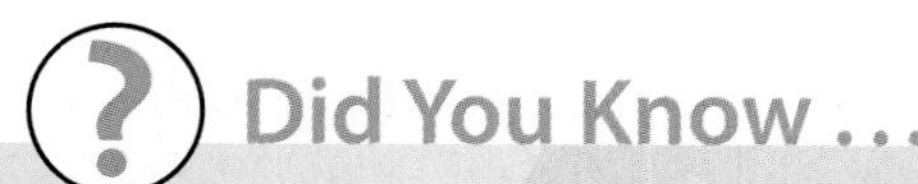

During the early 1970s, college couples' living together was making the news for the first time. At an informal press gathering, President Richard Nixon was asked, "When you were at Whittier College, was there much sex on campus?" The startled Nixon is said to have given a smirk and replied, "No . . . most of it took place in the dorms!"

Safer Sexual Activities and College Students

Most studies of condom use among college students date from the early 1990s; the results then indicated that condom use was relatively rare. Studies found that between 15% and 41% of students reported that they always used condoms, and the more partners a person had, the lower the rate of condom use (Lewis, et al., 1997). A 1998 telephone survey of college students was much more encouraging; 54% reported that they always or almost always use condoms, and 24% said that they sometimes did. Still, one in five reported that he or she almost never used condoms (Survey USA, 1998). As a result, one in five males and nearly one in three college age females have been infected with an STI (Reinisch, et al., 1995).

Relatedly, it is interesting to note that 6 in 10 pregnancies involving teenage fathers end in a birth; 4 in 10 end in an abortion. Thirteen percent of abortions each year involve teenage men. Also, most males use a condom the first time they have intercourse, but condom use subsequently declines and reliance on female methods increases. Condom use is more common among males who are not in a union than among those who are cohabiting or married (In their own right, 2002).

One of the early pieces of advice in HIV prevention was "Know your partner well." The belief was that partners should be able to trust each other to be honest. However, one study showed that more than one-third of the college men and one-fifth of the college women who were involved in a self-described monogamous relationship had been sexually unfaithful to their partner (Stebleton & Rothenberger, 1993). In another study of young people at several colleges in California, 60% of the women and 47% of the men believed that they had been lied to for the purposes of sexual activity (Mays & Cochran, 1993). Men are five to seven times more likely to lie than women in order to have sexual relations; 33% of men admit to lying, as compared to 7% of women (Stebleton & Rothenberger, 1993).

Communication is the key to an honest and protected sexual relationship. Yet, most studies indicate that college students do not talk before they have sexual activity. In one study, three-quarters of college-age men and one-third of women never asked partners about their past sexual history (Stebleton & Rothenberger, 1993). Several researchers have found low levels of communication about condoms, safer sex, HIV, and STIs between college students before their first sexual encounter (Lewis, et al., 1997). However, in almost all cases, sexually experienced college students said that they would use condoms if their partners insisted (Lewis, et al., 1997).

Singlehood

For most heterosexual young adults—male and female—singlehood is a temporary status. The vast majority of people eventually marry, but they are delaying marriage longer than in the past. In 1970, the median age for first marriage was 20.6 years for women and 22.5 years for men (Renzetti & Curran, 1998); by 1997, it had reached 25 years for women and 26.8 years for men (Schmid, 1998). Still, the number of young singles and people who never marry has increased dramatically since the 1960s. (The role of elderly singles is discussed later in this chapter.)

Singles delay or avoid marriage for several reasons, including improved social attitudes toward being single, increased caution inspired by high divorce rates, and increased availability of effective contraceptives (Renzetti & Curran, 1998). In addition, some singles enjoy the freedom from unnecessary commitments, opportunities to meet new people and develop new relationships, room for personal growth, and the ability to have a varied sex life that is free of guilt (Sullivan, 1998). Further, there is less societal pressure than there used to be to marry at an early age.

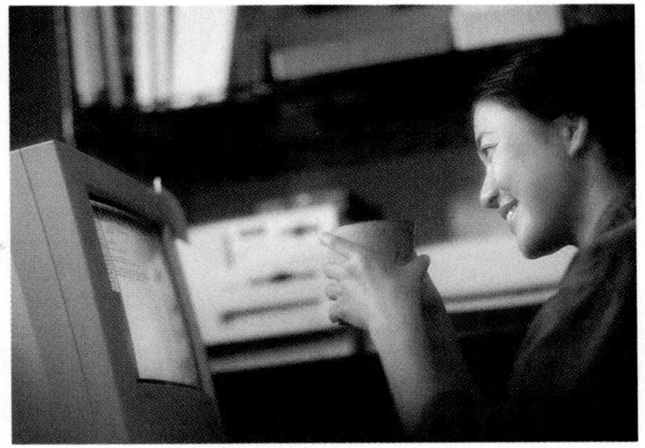

Add the Internet to the places to meet singles. On singles bulletin boards, singles can read extended personal ads, complete with photos. In chat rooms, singles have the opportunity to "meet" and "talk" to prospective dates in a safe environment. But be wary—experts warn that a first encounter with someone met on the Internet should be in a public place, perhaps among other friends.

But probably the most important reason why young people delay marriage are economic constraints (Bedard, 1992). In the last 30 years, housing prices have increased significantly, while the number of jobs that pay a wage adequate for establishing an independent household has declined. Consequently, 53% of people aged 18–24 years and 12% of people aged 25–34 years live at home with their parents (Renzetti & Curran, 1998).

The sociologists Bumpass, Sweet, and Cherlin found that although young people have postponed the age at which they first marry, they have not postponed the age at which they set up housekeeping together. If cohabiting couples were counted as married, the rate of family formation and age at first marriage would show little change since 1970 (Bumpass, Sweet, & Cherlin, 1991). Whether this situation, derived from 1980s data, still prevails is unclear.

The number of people who never marry has increased in the past three decades. In 1970, never-marrieds accounted for 18.9% of males and 13.7% of females. By 1997, 27% of males and 20.2% of females older than 18 years had not married (U.S. Bureau of the Census, 1998). Nearly 14 million people (34.5% of people between the ages of 25 and 34 years) had never married (see Table 13.3). More than half (54.2%) of African Americans in this age group had never married (Schmid, 1998). The number of cohabiting people is not high enough to account for this increase.

Of course, some people who are single would like to get married. Online dating, once viewed as a refuge for the socially inept and as a faintly disrespectable way to meet other people, is quickly becoming a fixture of single life for adults of all ages, backgrounds, and interests. More than 45 million Americans visited online dating sites in just one month in 2003, up from about 35 million in one month in 2002. Spending by subscribers on web dating sites has soared, rising to about $100 million or more per quarter in 2003, up from under $10 million per quarter in 2001. Some people feel that the traditional means for getting people together are not working as well as they did previously, and that there is a need for something new. As more people choose to marry later in life, few social institutions have arisen to replace the role that local communities, families, and schools once played. The Internet is

TABLE 13.3 Never-Married Persons as a Percentage of Total Population by Gender and Age, 2001

Age	Male	Female
All ages 15 years old and over	31.3	25.1
15–19	98.5	95.9
20–24	83.7	72.8
25–29	51.7	38.9
30–34	30.1	21.9
35–44	18.0	13.0
45–54	9.5	8.6
55–64	5.5	4.9
65 and over	4.2	3.6

Source: U.S. Bureau of the Census, *America's families and living arrangements.* Washington, DC: U.S. Department of Commerce, 2001.

filling that need. For many, there is a disconnect between who people say they are online and what they really are like. However, many people have found success through Internet dating and feel that online dating may be making it more acceptable to openly signal what they want. But gender rules still seem to apply. Men say women rarely send the first e-mail note. As word spreads of successful matches, the stigma of advertising for a romantic partner online rather than waiting for friends or fate to conjure one is fading (Harmon, 2003).

Cohabitation

cohabitation
Situation in which people who live together and share a sexual relationship are not married.

Cohabitation is the situation in which people who live together and share a sexual relationship are not married. Just a generation or two ago people who lived together were said to be "living in sin"—a remark meant as religious scorn, not humor. In fact, until around 1970, cohabitation was illegal in all 50 states (*Economist,* 1999). Today cohabitation is not regarded as negatively as it used to be.

One reason for the increased acceptance of cohabitation is the vast increase in the number who cohabitate—from 439,000 in 1960 to more than 4.2 million in 1998 (Popenoe & Whitehead, 2001; U.S. Bureau of the Census, 1998); an additional 1.5 million same-sex partners cohabit (Miller & Solot, 1999). Further, half of all women aged 25 to 39 years have cohabited at some point; roughly 30% of these women cohabited before their first marriage. Of unwed couples in 1997, 1.47 million had a child younger than age 15 years (U.S. Bureau of the Census, 1998).

Looking at the numbers in another way, there was a 71% increase in the number of unmarried partners living together between 1990 and 2000 (Census: Unmarried couples increase, 2001). Census 2000 showed that the number of unmarried-partner households increased to 5.5 million, of which 4.9 million were made up of heterosexual partners. In 1990 unmarried-partner households accounted for 3.5% of all households, whereas in Census 2000 they accounted for 5.2% of all households.

Another reason for the increased acceptance of cohabitation is that major corporations, in an effort to hire and keep high-quality employees, have extended "domestic partner benefits" to both homosexual and heterosexual cohabitors (Miller & Solot, 1999). More than half of Fortune 500 companies have extended such benefits. A further reason is the availability of effective contraceptives that reduce the fear of pregnancy among couples who wish to live together but not to start families.

Cohabitation is not new. The 1933 opera *Porgy and Bess,* which takes place in an African-American ghetto in Charleston, South Carolina, features a comical scene in which a huckster lawyer preys on the deprived citizens, offering divorces for people who once lived together. The lawyer convinces Porgy to buy a divorce, so that he can legally cohabit with Bess!

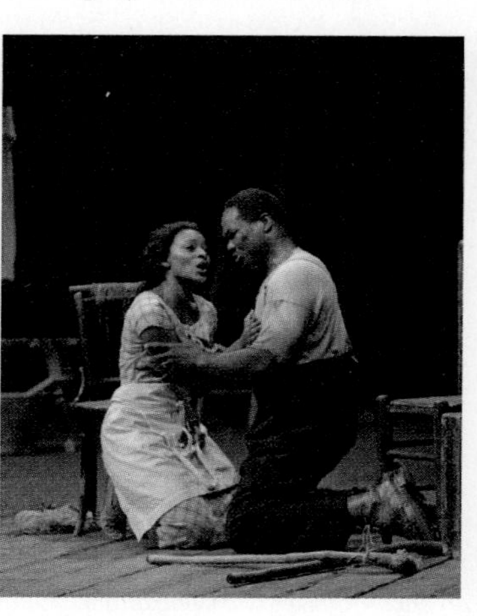

Advantages to Cohabitation

Many reasons are given for living together. They include finding out more about the habits and character of a partner, wanting to test compatibility, avoiding the risks of being "trapped in an unhappy marriage," working on personal "issues" before deciding to marry, and saving money (Poponoe & Whitehead, 2001).

Disadvantages to Cohabitation

Unmarried couples may experience discrimination in housing, insurance, taxes, child custody, and other areas. (These are some of the same issues that homosexuals face; see Chapter 11.) They may also face pressure to marry from parents and friends—who may have social and religious backgrounds different from the cohabitors'.

Some people, especially divorced people, become cohabitors because they do not want the legal and economic "entanglements" of another marriage should the relationship end. In reality, though, the legal "entanglements" of marriage can also prove to be legal "entitlements." When cohabitors break up, one partner may lose financially because of inability to prove that assets were jointly purchased. Also, if one partner dies without a will, property would pass to surviving family members—not to the intended surviving partner. For example, in Massachusetts, the property would go half to parents, half to siblings, and none to partner. Further, if a partner is disabled or hospitalized, the cohabitor has no rights to make medical decisions and can even be legally barred from hospital visits.

Are Cohabitations Successful?

Do cohabiting couples have a higher rate of success if they marry later than do married couples who did not live together first? A critical look at the body of research fails to prove whether prior cohabitors have better marriages or not.

Researchers have found that most cohabitations are not "till death do us part." Most cohabitations last 2 years or less (Bumpass & Sweet, 1991), and the longest cohabitations occur between marriages (Come live with me, 1999).

A controversial 1999 report, from Rutgers University's National Marriage Project, illustrates why critical thinking is important when we are reviewing studies. The report, "Should We Live Together? What Young Adults Need to Know About Cohabitation Before Marriage," contains no new research—it is simply a review of previous research studies. However, because the report was sponsored by "conservative, traditional family foundations" (Boorstein, 1999), the contents deserve a critical review.

The report alleged that cohabiting weakens potential future marriages by increasing the likelihood of divorce and domestic violence. Among the studies cited was a 1992 study of 3,300 adults (from the National Survey of Families and Households) that found that couples who live together before marriage are 46% more likely to divorce than those who did not. "The longer you cohabit, the more tolerant you are of divorce," says David Popenoe, a sociologist who cowrote the study. "You're used to living in a low-commitment relationship, and it's hard to shift that kind of mental pattern" (Labi, 1999).

However, the report does not differentiate among the many dimensions of human sexuality. According to the Alternatives to Marriage Project (which supports cohabitation), religion plays a key role. Couples who cohabit are less religious and more likely to believe that divorce is an acceptable choice for a marriage gone bad. In contrast, people who marry without living together first tend to be more religious and more strongly opposed to divorce (Miller & Solot, 1999). Thus, religion is a stronger indicator of divorce than simple cohabitation.

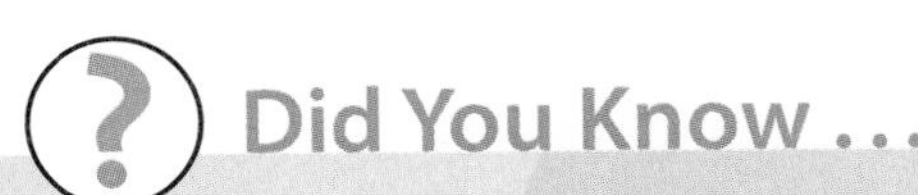

The United States' cohabitation rate of about 5% is low compared to the rate in other countries, such as Sweden and Norway, where 12% of heterosexual couples cohabit (Renzetti & Curren, 1998).

A further criticism of the National Marriage Project report is that it does not control for the socioeconomic dimension. On average, married couples have higher income than unmarried couples. Dorian Solot, cofounder of the Alternatives to Marriage Project, suggests that "studies that purport to compare happiness or domestic violence rates between married and unmarried couples are actually seeing the effects of wealth. Wealthier people have better health care, better neighborhoods, better access to education, and more choices in their lives" (Miller & Solot, 1999).

Further, statistics from earlier studies were manipulated to fit the conservative values of the sponsor. For example, Larry Bumpass, a sociologist at the University of Wisconsin and the director of the study previously cited that claims that cohabitation increases the divorce rate by 46%, notes that the divorce rate has stabilized—even gone down—while the rate of cohabiting has skyrocketed. According to Bumpass, "If cohabitation was causing an increase in divorce, you would have expected the divorce rate to accelerate, but it's not. . . . To lay everything on the doorstep of cohabitation is to fail to recognize the dramatic change that is occurring in the way marriage is viewed" (Boorstein, 1999; Labi, 1999).

Manning (2001) reported on racial and ethnic differences in childbearing in cohabiting unions. She found that Hispanic women were 77% more likely than white women to conceive a child in cohabitation. Black women were 69% more likely than white women to do so. Among women who became pregnant while cohabiting, Hispanic women were almost twice as likely and black women were three times as likely as white women to remain cohabiting with their partner when the child was born. In addition, children born to Hispanic women in cohabiting unions were 70% more likely to have been planned than were those born to cohabiting white women.

There are also a growing number of older Americans living together (Census: more elderly live together, 2002). The reasons vary, but for many it is a combination of bad experiences in previous marriages, the desire to keep their finances separate, and for some, loss of benefits if they remarry. There are at least 112,000 households headed by someone 65 years or older with an unmarried partner.

So, is cohabitation a positive or a negative thing? There are different opinions among different people. For example, some reports indicate that marriages of people who have cohabited and later marry are significantly more likely to end in divorce (Living together before marriage may hurt—not help—chances of successful match, 2002). Some people feel this is partly because people who choose to live together tend to be younger, to be less religious, or to have other qualities that put them at risk for divorce. Seventy percent of those who lived together for at least 5 years did eventually marry, but after 10 years 40% had broken up, as compared to 32% who did not live together first. Others argue that marriage is too great a commitment and prefer cohabitation (Should people not cohabit before getting married? 2003). They feel that the emphasis should be on the commitment between two people and that the quality of the relationship is the most important consideration. They indicate that society discriminates against people who wish to commit themselves to another person and remain unmarried.

Marriage

Marriage has changed over the years, but in many respects it has remained the same. June is still the most popular time to marry, more adults marry than never marry, and marriage is still a legal entity. It involves a fee to the

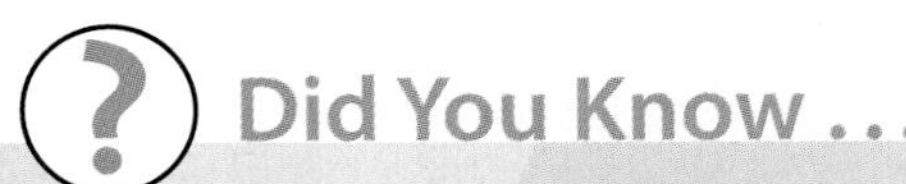

Facts About Unmarried-Partner Households from Census 2000

1. Five and-a-half million couples were living together but not married, up from 3.2 million in 1990.
2. Most of the unmarried-partner households had partners of the opposite gender (4.9 million); about one in nine (594,000) had a partner of the same gender.
3. Of the same-gender unmarried-partner households, 301,000 had male partners and 293,000 had female partners.
4. Unmarried partners are more likely than married couples to live in metropolitan areas.
5. California contained one of every eight unmarried-partner U.S. households.
6. Opposite-gender unmarried partners tend to share household activities more equally than married couples.
7. Four of 10 opposite-gender unmarried-partner households have children present.
8. One-third of female partner households and one-fifth of male partner households contain children.
9. Partners in opposite-gender unmarried-partner households are 12 years younger, on average, than partners in married-couple households.

Source: Simmons, T. & O'Connell, M. Married-couple and unmarried-partner households: 2000, in *Census 2000 special reports.* Washington, DC: U.S. Department of Commerce, 2003.

county, a marriage license, and a marriage ceremony—either civil or religious. Although there is no legal requirement that a wife take the husband's last name, she usually does. In most marriages the woman is still more likely to be the one who uses a contraceptive (Mosher & Pratt, 1990). Most Americans spend most of their lives within a marital relationship.

Although most people marry, the marriage rate has fluctuated and so have the ages at which people marry. The highest marriage rate (marriages per 1,000 population) in the past few decades was 10.9 in 1972. In 1982 it was 10.8, and it steadily declined until it was 8.8 in 1996. In 1999 it was 8.6, in 2000 it was 8.5, and in 2001 it was 8.4. In 2001 there were 2,327 marriages (Births, marriages, divorces, and deaths: 2001, 2002). The age at first marriage steadily increased from a median age of 22.5 years for the male and 20.3 years for the female in 1963, to 23.6 years for the male and 21.8 years for the female in 1980, to 25.9 years for the male and 24 years for the female in 1990. In 1998 it was 27 years for men and 25 years for women (U.S. Bureau of the Census, 1998b.) In 2000 it was 26.8 years for men and 25.1 years for women (America's families and living arrangements, 2001).

Popenoe and Whitehead (2001) reported that although older age at first marriage seems detrimental to marriage as an institution, it may have a strongly positive effect. This is because it appears to be by far the most important factor for a leveling off of divorce rates. On the other hand, there can be disadvantages to the trend for postponing marriage to much older ages. For example, it can result in increased exposure to the hazards of nonmarital sexual activity and childbearing, sexual exploitation, loneliness, and lack of social integration. The question of the optimal age at which to marry, then, is still open. It seems best to wait until the early 20s, but how much beyond that cannot be answered definitively.

The age at remarriage after a divorce has also steadily increased. It was 36.3 years for males and 31.8 years for females in 1963, 37.1 years for males and 32.8 years for females in 1985, and 37.4 years for males and 34.2 years for females in 1990 (U.S. Bureau of the Census, 1998b).

The number of interracial married couples has also increased. For example, in 1980 there were 651,000 interracial married couples, and in 1997 there were 1,264,000 (U.S. Bureau of the Census, 1998c). Interracial marriages between younger people increased most, and both African Americans and whites who marry interracially tend to have higher status than those who do not marry interracially (Heaton & Albrecht, 1996).

Pugh (2001) reported on a continued rise in mixed-race marriages, which totaled about 1.5 million in 2000. Adding Hispanics who marry outside their ethnic group raised the total of mixed marriages to 3 million. Even though ethnic barriers are softening as the population becomes more diverse, this figure still represents only 5% of all U.S. marriages. Within racial and ethnic groups, mixed marriage rates vary widely. Hispanics and Asians, the nation's fastest growing minority groups, marry partners of different races at about three times the rate of blacks and five times the rate of whites. Asian women and black men are more than twice as likely to marry outside their groups as Asian men and black women.

Although about 10% of the adult population (19.3 million adults) were divorced as of 1997, about 109.2 million adults (55.9% of the adult population) were married and living with their spouse in 1997 (U.S. Bureau of the Census, 1998c). Because it is clear that a majority of people choose to be married, it is appropriate to consider the attraction of marriage and marriage partners.

The Attraction of Marriage

The attraction to marriage is the result of several factors:

1. *Marriage provides companionship.* It is nice to have someone committed to spending time with you and sharing important occasions in your life.
2. *Marriage provides for emotional security.* The intimate nature of the marital relationship can help alleviate the anxieties, fears, and insecurities you experience in today's society.
3. *Marriage provides for a sexual outlet.* The knowledge that your sexual needs will be satisfied in a loving, caring relationship can be quite appealing.
4. *Marriage can improve your self-esteem.* Just knowing that you are worthy enough for someone else to marry can make you believe you are an attractive, appealing, valuable person.
5. *Marriage can provide financial security.* The addition of another wage earner, or someone who can earn money while you contribute to the partnership by doing chores that would cost money to pay someone else to do, can make you more financially able to live the life you desire.
6. *Marriage can legitimize reproduction.* If you want children and believe they will do best in a socially sanctioned family—a marriage—you may want to be married.

Obviously, marriage has numerous attractions that have made it the predominant family lifestyle. However, not all these attractions are present in all marriages, and, depending on the expectations before the marriage and

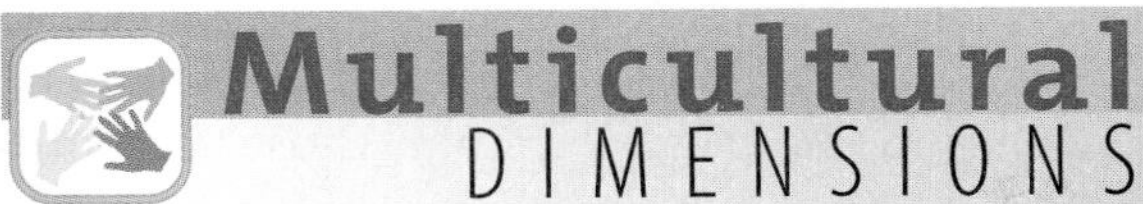

Multicultural DIMENSIONS

The Jefferson–Hemings Affair

If you think the presidential sex scandal surrounding Monica Lewinsky went on for a long time, consider the case of Thomas Jefferson. In 1801, the newly elected Jefferson was first accused of having children with a young black slave named Sally Hemings. But it was not until the fall of 1998 that DNA tests proved that descendants of the Hemings family were indeed related to Jefferson. Sally Hemings's youngest son, Eston, was fathered by either Thomas Jefferson or his brother.

The DNA findings do more than put to rest a question of paternity; they also lay the foundation for all the Jefferson descendants—African American and white—to join together as one openly biracial family. For the first time, descendants of Jefferson's slave were welcomed at the annual gathering of the Monticello Association (the organization of descendants of Jefferson's white daughters) at Monticello on May 15, 1999.

"It's not just our story—it resonates for the whole country," said Dr. Michelle Cooley-Quille, a Hemings descendant and a clinical psychologist at John Hopkins University, who attended the event. Her father was denied entry into the Monticello Association and denied burial at Monticello, a privilege accorded to all members, when he died in 1997. "It's symbolic of what we've been denied but where we belong."

Indeed, the Jefferson clan has followed the multicultural path of many Americans. The number of official interracial marriages was 1,264,000 in 1997, almost double the 651,000 in 1980. However, as the Jefferson story suggests, there have been many unrecorded interracial relationships during the history of the United States. The growing acceptance of contemporary interracial marriages—as well as the acceptance of our past—is a positive step in the direction of racial harmony.

Sources: Reed, D. Jefferson reunion adds slave's kin, AP/AOL (May 6, 1999); Edwards, T. M. Family reunion, *Time, 125, 21* (November 23, 1998); Cawthorne, N. *Sex lives of the presidents.* New York: St. Martin's, 1998; U.S. Bureau of the Census. *Statistical abstract of the United States 1998.* Washington, DC: U.S. Government Printing Office, 1998.

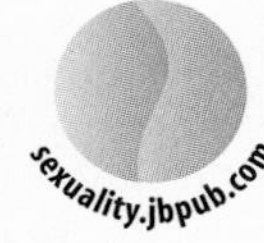

on other important considerations—such as the personality traits of the partners and their love for each other—the resultant disappointments either are overlooked or are deemed important enough to cause divorce.

It is interesting that, in general, American women are waiting to begin families. The average American woman was almost 25 years old when she had her first child in the year 2000. That is compared to an average age of 21.4 years for a first birth in 1970. The average age of mothers for all births rose from 24.6 years to 27.2 years over three decades (American women waiting to begin families, 2002).

Choosing a Life Partner

Interestingly, when and if you choose another person with whom to form a lifelong commitment, that person will most likely be similar to you in many ways. Most people choose others of similar religion, age, social class, race, and education (Baron, 1998). When two people join together after 20 or 30 or more years of living independently of each other, they have all the problems of adjustment you can imagine. They may have to learn to eat the same foods, wake and go to sleep at the same times, and put up with each other's myriad idiosyncrasies. In other words, they have enough problems without adding still others that occur when they have different religions, social classes, educational backgrounds, and so on. It would be unfair, however, to overlook the relationships that work in spite of the partners' dissimilarities. That elusive concept, love, can do wonders with problems. However, the odds against partners of dissimilar backgrounds are greater than those for similar partners.

A "premarital inventory" developed at the University of Minnesota could be helpful for those contemplating marriage (Zaslow, 2003). It is an example of how researchers have studied divorced couples to see which questions they wish they had asked before taking the leap. Sample items include the following: We have some important disagreements that never seem to get resolved, and I am satisfied with the way we have decided to share household duties. It is available at www.lifeinnovations.com.

Promoting a Happy Lifelong Commitment

Advice from many sources tells you how to be happy in a relationship. For example, Wallerstein (1996) lists nine "psychological tasks" that are the pillars on which good lifelong relationships rest:

1. To separate emotionally from the family of one's childhood so as to invest fully in the relationship.
2. To build togetherness based on mutual identification, shared intimacy, and an expanded conscience that includes both partners and protects each partner's autonomy.
3. To establish a rich and pleasurable sexual relationship.
4. For couples with children, while protecting their own privacy, to embrace the roles of parenthood and to absorb the effect of a baby's entrance into the marriage.
5. To confront and master the inevitable crises of life.
6. To maintain the strength of the relationship in the face of adversity. It should be a safe haven in which partners are able to express their differences, anger, and conflict.
7. To use humor and laughter to keep things in perspective.
8. To nurture and comfort each other, satisfying each partner's needs for dependency and offering continuing encouragement and support.
9. To keep alive the early romantic, idealized images of falling in love while facing the sober realities of the changes wrought by time.

The extent to which a husband is tied to his parents can make or break a new marriage. Both spouses report higher levels of satisfaction in marriage when the husbands are free of excessive guilt, anxiety, mistrust, responsibility, inhibition, resentment, and anger in relation to their mother. Couples are also better adjusted when husbands possess a good ability to manage and direct practical affairs without help from their father. In addition, as stated earlier, people are more likely to be attracted to and marry someone of the same personality type (Latest research on marital adjustment and satisfaction, 1998).

Silberman and Robinson-Kurpius (1998) indicate that previous research showed that a satisfying relationship includes three aspects of love—intimacy, passion, and commitment. In their research they found that intimacy (intensity of liking [love], depth and breadth of exchange, sharing of resources and feelings) followed by passion are the strongest predictors of marital satisfaction.

While studying the influence of religion on marital stability, Call and Heaton (1997) found that the frequency of church attendance has the greatest positive effect on relationship stability. When both partners attend church regularly they have a much lower risk of divorce than partners who do not.

There are many lists of characteristics that promote a happy relationship. Hales (1986) indicates that in relationships that endure, the partners are best friends who communicate well, both verbally and emotionally. They can handle negative emotions and develop ways to deal with conflict. They are diplomatic, trust each other, and are committed to their union. They have some shared interests and are adaptable to change. They are willing to learn the skills to make their marriage last.

Rice (1997) lists eight secrets of happy couples. They use pet names that help them to feel close to each other. They work closely together on some projects. When the going gets tough, they do not call their parents—but they do stay connected to their parents. They do not keep debit–credit accounts of who does what around the house. They learn the art of constructive arguing, and they listen to each other. They give each other gifts and often write little notes. They never mock each other. They also take "for better or worse" seriously.

A controversial way to promote a good-quality commitment advocates that the wife become a "surrendered wife" (Edwards, 2001). This approach advocates that she should not control, criticize, or interrupt her husband. If she does, she should apologize for being "disrespectful." She should tell him what she wants, but if he does not agree, she should stay mum and do what he wants. She should never ask about his feelings. Critics argue that this idea is a throwback, is destructive, and does not protect women. Supporters indicate this can promote "an empowering" experience and a good relationship.

There is even a video game designed to help promote relationships. It is called *Sims* (short for simulation) and the idea is simple (Grossman, 2002). You control an ordinary suburban family. You make them dinner at night and send them to work in the morning. You turn on the TV when they are bored and put them to bed when they are tired. The family wrestles with the everyday demands of job, family, housework, and personal care. The object is to keep your Sims well fed, solvent, healthy, entertained, and happy. The video game is designed to re-create real-life interpersonal relationships; to date, 20 million copies have been sold in 17 languages.

Types of Marriage

In some states heterosexual couples who have lived together for a specified period and who have represented themselves as married are recognized as legally married. These associations are called **common-law marriages.**

About 56% of children live in a **nuclear family**—a couple and their children. This is up from 51% in 1991. The portion of children living in any sort of two-parent family, including nuclear families, those living with stepparents, and those in other arrangements, is about 71% (down from 73% in 1991) (Meckler, 2001).

Peer marriages are relationships in which couples have worked out at least a 60–40 split on child rearing, housework, and control of discretionary funds and consider themselves equal (Schwartz, 1994). Most partners in peer marriages work outside the home. Partners in peer marriages require lots of honesty, a dedication to fair play, flexibility, generosity, and maturity.

In some families the fathers stay at home and the mothers work outside the home. Stay-at-home dads do the same household activities as stay-at-home moms, but they also mow the lawn, fix the dishwasher, and clean the gutters. There is not a complete role reversal when the father stays at home. Working mothers also only partially give up their traditional role. When they go home, they tend to be the "traditional mom." In a stay-at-home father

common-law marriage
The recognition by some states that heterosexual couples who have lived together for a specified period and have represented themselves as married are in fact legally married.

nuclear family
A married couple and their children.

peer marriage
Relationship in which partners have equal status.

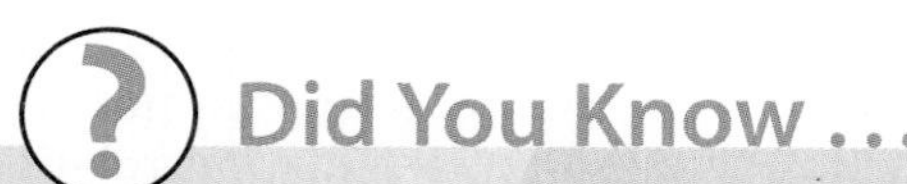

A middle-income couple will spend $156,690 (in 1999 dollars) to raise a child born in 1998 to age 17 years—$240,000 when factoring in inflation. Here is where it went:

1. Housing = 33%.
2. Food = 18%.
3. Transportation = 15%.
4. Child care/education = 9%.
5. Clothing = 7%.
6. Health care = 7%.
7. Other (entertainment, books, and so on) = 11%.

Sources: Carey, A. R. & Tian, Q. Cost of raising kids, *USA Today* (Oct. 27, 1998), 1; Cost of raising child to 17 rises to $156,690, study says, *Boston Globe* (April 22, 1999).

family, if a child gets hurt or wakes up at night and both parents are available, the child will go to either the mother or the father. In a traditional family the child will go to the mother 80% of the time and the father 20% of the time (Working moms turn traditional when they're home, 1998).

stepfamily
A family with children that is formed as a result of remarriage.

About 16.5% of children live in a **stepfamily**, also called a *blended family*, compared to about 15% in 1991 (Meckler, 2001). Stepfamilies can be more complex than the families of first marriages, but, contrary to myth, stepfamilies have a high rate of success in raising healthy children. Stepkids seem to be very resilient. Their major source of problems is parental conflict left over from a first marriage. Stepfamilies experience most of their troubles in the first 2 years; after 5 years, stepfamilies are more stable than first-marriage families, because second marriages are generally happier than first marriages. Stepfamilies are not just make-do households limping along after loss. All members experience real gains, notably the opportunity to thrive in a happier relationship (Rutter, 1994).

One researcher indicates that there are seven basic types of relationships—three of them happy and four of them unhappy (An arrangement of marriages, 1993). The four unhappy ones make up about 75% of marriages and are labeled *devitalized, financially focused, conflicted,* and *traditional.* These relationships hinge on external elements, leisure activities, religious attitudes, financial management, children, family and friends—and distress dominates. The three happy ones make up 25% of relationships and are labeled *balanced, harmonious,* and *vitalized.* In these relationships the partners are held together by smooth working of most or all factors intrinsic to relationships—personality compatibility, communication, conflict resolution, and sexuality.

With about 50% of the annual 2.3 million new marriages in the United States destined to end in divorce, an increasing number of couples are turning to prenuptial agreements to protect their assets in the event of a marital breakup. Most such agreements simply state how assets will be divided in case of divorce or death (A binding agreement before you tie the knot? 1997). Some people argue that prenuptial agreements contribute to marital happiness; others believe they contribute to distrust and overemphasize personal assets.

In Louisiana and Arizona, it is legal to back up marriage laws with tougher, individually designed and legally mandated divorce standards. This is called a *covenant marriage.* In this marriage style, the option of walking out is eliminated. For example, Louisiana's covenant marriage requires premarital counseling and, for divorce, 2 years of living apart plus mandated marital counseling. The goal is to make marriage more committed (Russo, 2000).

Building a good relationship obviously takes a lot of effort. There are sources of help for couples desiring to use them. For example, the Association for Couples in Marriage Enrichment is an organization designed to preserve and strengthen relationships.

Sexual Behavior in Marriage

Nonmarital sexual behavior has received more attention from researchers and reformers alike than sexual behavior in marriage. Nevertheless, it is possible to make important observations and generalizations about marital sexual activity. Bell and Gordon (1972) observed that two major changes have occurred in marital sexual relations, both of which have had a greater effect on women. First, because more reliable contraceptives are available, the relationship between intercourse and conception is no longer beyond the control of the couple. This eliminates the fear of pregnancy and thereby increases sexual satisfaction. Second, there is relatively new emphasis on the wife's right to expect as much sexual satisfaction as the husband, with the result that communication regarding sexual matters in marriage is even more important than before.

Today's married couples have sexual intercourse more often, experience more sexual pleasure, and engage in a greater variety of sexual activities and techniques than the people surveyed in the 1950s. There is now more precoital activity and it tends to last longer than in earlier years. Oral stimulation of the breasts and manual stimulation of the genitals have increased, as has oral–genital contact (Clements, 1994; Laumann, et al., 1994).

The National Opinion Research Center (NORC) study found that frequency of sexual interactions is a factor of age, relationship duration, and marital status. In general, married couples engage in sexual activities more frequently than singles; cohabiting couples engage in sexual activities more often than married couples (Laumann, et al., 1994). Nearly 40% of married couples engage in sexual activities twice a week, compared with 25% of singles (Elmer-Dewitt, 1994).

The frequency of sexual intercourse in marriage tends to decrease the longer a couple is married. For example, for newly married couples the average rate of sexual intercourse is about three times per week. In early middle age, the average rate is about one-and-a-half to two times a week. After age 50 years the rate is about once a week or less. This does not mean that sexual activity is not important or that the marriage is no longer satisfactory. The decrease may be the result of biological aging, fatigue, and a decrease in sex drive (Call, Sprecher, & Schwartz, 1995). Higher levels of sexual satisfaction and pleasure are found in marriage than in extramarital relationships or in singlehood (Laumann, et al., 1994).

We can ascribe these changes to a loosening up of society in general and to the fact that even heterosexual sexual activity has come out of the closet. It is now permissible to talk about sexual behavior freely with one's partner and with others and to read books such as Alex Comfort's *Joy of Sex* without guilt or shame. Thus, communication between partners has become more open and honest and certainly has had an effect on their lovemaking. We can also cite the positive effects of the women's movement, which has been growing in strength since the late 1960s. As was noted earlier, women have become more aware of their capacity for and their right to sexual satisfaction through orgasm. As a result they have been assuming an active role in lovemaking and in communicating what turns them on. When their partners have responded positively, one result has been that partners spend more time exploring each other sexually, attending to each other's bodies, and experimenting with various coital positions that may better satisfy women's needs.

Many married people also masturbate. Hunt's survey (1974) found that 72% of young married males and 68% of young married females masturbated. The frequency rates were higher for husbands (once or twice a month) than for wives (less than once a month). The reasons married people cite for masturbating vary. Some people masturbate when they are separated from their partner. Some do so as a variation on their sexual experience. Also some couples like to watch each other masturbate as part of their mutual sexual activity. Others masturbate because they do not achieve satisfaction with their partner and are unwilling to forgo it altogether.

Do married couples have as much sexual activity as they would like? The majority of wives and husbands in Hunt's study reported that the frequency was about right (Hunt, 1974), but almost 49% of the women and 30% of the men reported that they wanted intercourse more often. Certainly some couples participate in sexual activity much more and others much less than the average. It is possible that, on the whole, people tend to overemphasize sexual activity in marriage.

Gagnon and Simon (1973) suggest that we can gain perspective by comparing rates of sexual activity with the frequency of other things we do. First, we might think of nonsexual activities that people perform in the course of a year and their frequency. We eat regular meals about 1,000 times per year, and go to and from work twice a day. Many homemakers in the suburbs, it is said, run 10 errands with the car each weekday. By comparison marital sexual activity does not occur with very great frequency.

Second, we can consider the time involved. People report that marital intercourse commonly takes about 10 to 20 minutes. If couples engage in intercourse 150 times per year, taking 20 minutes per act to be the average, the total is about 50 hours per year. We spend 2,000 hours working (40 hours times 50 weeks), 1,000 hours watching television (about 3 hours per day), and perhaps 250 hours commuting (1 hour per day). Marital sexual activity does not consume a great deal of our time.

Are married couples generally satisfied with their sex life? According to Hunt's data, a majority of married people—60% to 66%—are satisfied. Two-thirds of the men in the sample rated their marital coitus as very pleasurable, whereas about 60% of the women said the same. Most women who said they found coitus very pleasurable were 35 to 44 years old; the men so reporting were younger. It appears, then, that as women mature and gain sexual experience, they enjoy their experiences more than at a younger age, and men experience more of their pleasure when they are young.

Though their information is sparse and not based on long-term investigation, some studies suggest that there are changes in sexual satisfaction throughout a marriage. Two researchers (Frank & Anderson, 1979) who surveyed married couples found three distinctive sexual stages of marriage: (1) *Early marriage*—years of satisfaction. Almost all couples found sexual activity pleasurable and satisfying in the beginning. Of the couples married fewer than 5 years, 91% of the women and 95% of the men indicated that their sex life was either satisfying or very satisfying. About 18% of the couples in this group had sexual intercourse four or five times a week, and more than 33% reported a frequency of two to three times a week. (2) *The middle years*—the era of distractions. During the middle years—from about 5 to 20 years—the stresses and crises of adult life apparently had a negative impact on the couples' sex life. Husbands and wives reported that they were distracted from their sexual relationships with each other,

Myth vs Fact

Myth: Single adults have more sexual activity than married adults.
Fact: The 1994 national survey of adults 18 to 59 years old found that married adults had more sexual activity than single adults.

Myth: Liberals enjoy sex more than conservatives.
Fact: In the same study, marriage was a great equalizer. Married couples, regardless of religious or political background or past sexual history, have roughly the same amount of sexual activity. And conservative women report more frequent orgasm than liberal women.

Myth: Almost all married couples have affairs.
Fact: Only 25% of men and 15% of women report that they have had an extramarital affair.

Myth: People lose interest in sexual activity as they get older, and, by their 60s, few people are having sexual relationships.
Fact: People can have a satisfying sexual life as they age. Sexual relationships may change as a couple ages, but many couples in their 60s, 70s, and 80s report pleasurable, exciting sexual relationships.

though they tended to express this distraction in different ways. Men maintained their interest in sexual activity but were troubled by attractions to women other than their wives. Wives seemed to lose interest in sexual activity itself and reported that it was more difficult to relax before intercourse. More couples reported satisfaction than dissatisfaction, yet more than 30% of the husbands and 40% of the wives reported too little foreplay in their sex life. (3) *The later years*—a time for tenderness. Couples married more than 20 years rated their marriage high in satisfaction and compatibility, although they had a less glowing view of their sex life. Sexual frequency was less than for younger couples, and the men reported increased difficulty in achieving and maintaining erections. The men seemed to accept this situation and rated their sex life as satisfactory, but the women reported more dissatisfaction, describing themselves as less excited, less confident, and more resigned. "In fact, over one-half of the women in their 40s used the word 'resignation' to describe their feelings about their sexual relationship." In analyzing their findings, Frank and Anderson concluded that it is not so much the quality of sexual performance that counts in a marriage as the quality of the feelings that acccompany the sexual activities.

One factor that can contribute to problems in marital sexual activities is timing—particularly in the years when couples are both raising children and working hard at their jobs. Married people often have sexual activities late in the evening after a long day and just before sleep. The presence of children in the family can make it hard for parents to find time to be alone. Because many people feel that a quiet and private time is necessary for sexual activities, there may be pressure to "work sex in" during the short evening.

Extramarital Relationships

Despite all the media hype over the past few years about extramarital sexual activity by government officials, the reality is that most people are faithful to their spouses. In the NORC study, a relatively large number of adults reported that they have been completely monogamous during the course of their marriage. Only 10% of women and 25% of men reported that they had had an extramarital sexual relationship (Laumann, et al., 1994)—far below the 50% of men and 25% of women reported by Kinsey back in 1948 and 1953.

Because husbands are more involved in extramarital sexual relations than wives are, presumably without their spouse's knowledge, more women may be at risk of STIs than has been thought. Research is not available on what proportion of husbands have same-gender relationships outside their marriage. However, married men and women who perceive themselves to be at no (or low) risk of STIs and HIV may in fact be at risk because of their partner's extramarital sexual activities (Laumann, et al., 1994).

Extramarital sexual activity can take place in two different contexts: one in which the partners have no agreement (nonconsensual context) and one in which the partners agree to have sexual relations with someone else (consensual context).

Nonconsensual Extramarital Sexual Activity

Married people engage in **nonconsensual**—and therefore usually secret—extramarital relationships for many and complex reasons. On a practical level one's spouse may be unable to have sexual intercourse because of illness, or a couple may be separated for a long period. Thus the person deciding on an extramarital relationship does so in order to have sexual relations at all. But in other situations an individual might search for someone outside the marriage simply to add excitement or variety to life. Another might

nonconsensual
In this context, a married person's engaging in sexual intercourse without the consent of the spouse.

feel dissatisfied sexually with his or her partner and look for a more satisfactory emotional and physical relationship while maintaining the marriage. Or a person might feel drawn to someone outside the marriage by sexual attraction alone and choose to act on that attraction.

Movies, television, and other popular media have given the impression that marital infidelity is on the upswing, but the NORC study (Laumann, et al., 1994) found that generally this was not true. Hunt (1974) also found that men tend to have their flings at an earlier age (younger than 25 years old), whereas women tend to engage in affairs at a later period of life, around 35 to 40 years.

A number of forces tend to restrain or increase extramarital sexual activity:

1. Because religiously devout people tend to have lower rates of extramarital sexual activity, rising rates can be predicted from the decline in traditional religious activity.
2. Those who participate in nonmarital sexual intercourse are more likely to participate in extramarital activity, too.
3. Because women are more aware of their right to sexual satisfaction than in years past, some females are more likely to now seek sexual pleasures outside marriage.
4. The more money a person has, the greater is the opportunity for extramarital sexual activity.
5. The changing role of women in the labor force is also a factor; women who work outside the home have a greater opportunity for extramarital activity than women who do not.

Although there are cultures in which it is expected that married people will have affairs, most people in the United States say they believe in monogamy and want it in their marriage. However, two of three married couples experience an affair during their marriage, and 17% of divorces are caused by infidelity. Traditionally, more men than women take part in affairs, but women are catching up. Affairs are a sign that the wandering spouse is dissatisfied in the marriage. It can be a way of expressing pain and confusion that the person cannot verbally articulate. However, this does not necessarily mean that he or she wants to end the marriage. An affair can be a way of expressing that there are problems that need to be resolved. (Stanton, 2001).

What are the effects of extramarital sexual relationships on a marriage? Initially, many people who learn their spouse has been having affairs feel both betrayed and emotionally devastated, especially if they believe their spouse to be honest, loyal, and loving. When they learn of the affair, there is a chance that the marriage will fall apart quickly. However, if the couple can talk about the situation, taking the opportunity to improve their communication and assess their own relationship, the marriage does not necessarily dissolve.

Sometimes the type of extramarital relationship has a great effect on the eventual outcome. When a spouse has engaged in a one-night stand, the other spouse might be likely to forgive and forget. If the extramarital affair was intimate, was long-lasting, and involved a strong emotional commitment, however, the other spouse may find it difficult to get over the unfaithfulness.

consensual
In this context, a married person's engaging in extramarital sexual activity with the knowledge and permission of the spouse.

open marriage
A marriage in which partners allow each other to have intimate and emotional relationships with others.

swinging
Swapping of mates for sexual activities.

Consensual Extramarital Sexual Activity

There are many types of **consensual** activities; we discuss the two major ones—open marriage and swinging. **Open marriage** became publicized with the appearance of George and Nena O'Neill's book, *Open Marriage,* in 1972.

The O'Neills believed that traditional marriage was too confining and limiting for the partners and that one partner could not fulfill all the intimate needs and expectations of the other. They described an open marriage as one in which the partners allow each other to have intimate and emotional relationships—sexual or nonsexual—with others. For instance, the married couple might decide that each partner is entitled to one night a week alone to engage in another intimate relationship. The idea is that this arrangement allows the married couple to grow and contribute more to the marriage. Another aspect of the open marriage is the renewable contract. The partners formally agree that extramarital relationships are permitted in the marriage and might even foster support, loyalty, and trust between partners but that the partners may change their contract regarding extramarital activity as they continue to grow. The idea here is that the agreement is flexible and renewable so that neither partner is forced to stand by a commitment that he or she no longer feels.

Swinging is the exchange of partners among married couples. (This phenomenon used to be called *wife-swapping,* but the term lost favor with the rise of the women's movement because of its suggestion that wives were property and that men made the decisions.) All those involved participate willingly, and both partners in a marriage usually engage in it simultaneously.

Swingers object to calling this type of activity extramarital, because they view it as part of the marriage relationship. One study has shown that most swingers do not want emotional involvements outside the marriage and that active swingers usually engage in this kind of sexual activity about once every

Communication DIMENSIONS

Tempted by Digital Dalliances A marriage these days can be short-circuited with nothing more than a computer and a modem. CBS News Correspondent Thalia Assuras takes a look at how sexual relationships online are forcing courts to consider where to draw the line between virtual sex and adultery.

More than 40 million home computers are connected to the Internet, and it's estimated that sexually oriented chat rooms number in the tens of thousands. Computer analyst Nancy Tamasaitis says digital dalliances are steaming up cyberspace and threatening marriages. Tamasaitis said, "I think it shows that there are a lot of people that are very bored and unhappy with their marriages."

Take the case of Tami, who asked not to be identified. She said her 10-year marriage was heading toward divorce court after she had cybersex and phone sex with a married man thousands of miles away. "It's something that makes you feel good, because somebody is giving you attention that maybe you're not getting in your relationship," Tami said.

In many cases, virtual sex can lead to real sexual activity. The question is, if the relationship is not consummated and remains online only, is that adultery? Most states define adultery as the physical act of having intercourse with someone who is not your spouse. But divorce attorney Harry Schaffner says, the Internet is forcing the law to change that definition. "It can be considered mental cruelty. It can lead to irreconcilable differences that cause an irretrievable breakdown of the marriage," Schaffner says of virtual sex.

But not always. Sex therapist Dr. Patti Britton contends Internet interplay is a way to spice up a stale marriage, from the safety of your home. "Cybersex or cyber-dating is a viable option for people who want to find ways to feel their juices flow again," says Dr. Britton.

Tami says her cyberaffair is over. But, she cautions, because computers are everywhere—and so easy to use—cybersex can be difficult to resist.

2 weeks (Gilmartin, 1975). Most often swingers find one another by advertising in tabloids or in special magazines devoted to swinging.

People who engage in swinging are apparently very ordinary outside their sexual life. Bartell (1970) found that even though swingers describe themselves in the ads as very exciting, they really are quite dull, and television watching and swinging are their main recreational activities. The same study found that most female swingers are homemakers, that most couples who engage in swinging are conservative in their thinking, and that although husbands usually initiate the idea of swinging, wives eventually become more interested in continuing it. Whitehurst (1985) also found that males are reluctant to continue the swinging, and females are reluctant to enter into the activity. With the AIDS epidemic and high rates of other STIs, however, swinging may be on a downward slide.

Divorce

Today, for every two marriages there is one divorce. For couples marrying today, the chance is less than one in three that they will remain together permanently (Baron, 1998). There are many reasons that marriages break up. Among these are greater economic independence of women, greater ease of getting a divorce, decreased stigma attached to divorce, unrealistic expectations for marriage, communication difficulties, infidelity, and feelings of incompatibility (Center for Families in Transition, 2003).

The divorce rate peaked in 1979 at 5.3 per thousand population; the highest number of divorces (1,213,000) occurred in 1981. Since that time, the rate of divorce and the number of divorces have declined. For example, in 1990 there were 1,175,000 divorces and a divorce rate of 4.8 per thousand population. In 1997 there were 920,000 divorces and a divorce rate of 4.2 per thousand population (Divorce, 1998; U.S. Bureau of the Census, 1998). In 1999 the divorce rate was 4.1 per thousand, followed by rates of 4.2 and 4.0 in 2000 and 2001, respectively (Births, marriages, divorces, and deaths, 2002). The slowing of the divorce rate may be due to the greatly increased number of cohabiting couples, whose breakups are not recorded in divorce statistics. In all, about 10% of the adult population—19.3 million adults—were divorced as of 1997 (Schmid, 1998).

In 2001 the National Center for Health Statistics reported new data on marriage, divorce, and remarriage (First marriage dissolution, divorce, and remarriage in the United States, 2001). The center reported that 43% of first marriages end in separation or divorce within 15 years. One in three first marriages ends within 10 years and one in five within 5 years. The study also showed that duration of marriage is linked to a woman's age at first marriage; the older a woman is at first marriage, the longer the marriage is likely to last. For example, 58% of marriages of brides younger than 18 years old end in separation or divorce within 15 years compared with 36% of those who married at age 20 years or older. Younger women who divorce are more likely to remarry: 82% of those divorced before age 25 years remarry within 10 years, compared with 68% of those divorced at age 25 or later.

At the same time, there has been little change in such traditionally high divorce rate differences between those who marry when they are teenagers compared to those who marry later, and the nonreligious compared to the religious. Both teenagers and the nonreligious who marry have considerably higher divorce rates (Popenoe & Whitehead, 2001).

The significant effect of divorce on family life cannot be exaggerated. The spouse who maintains custody of the children has to supervise their care,

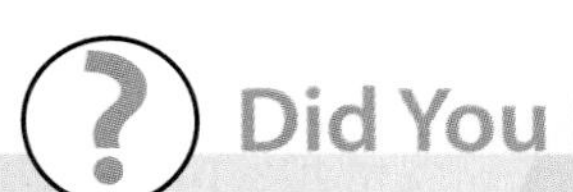

Did You Know . . .

The Top Ten Myths of Divorce

1. **Half of all marriages end in divorce.** If today's divorce rate continues, the chance that a marriage contracted this year will end in divorce is probably a little higher than 40%.
2. **Second marriages tend to be more successful than first marriages.** The divorce rate of remarriages is higher than that of first marriages.
3. **Living together before marriage is a good way to reduce the chance of divorce.** Those who live together before marriage have a considerably *higher* chance of divorce.
4. **Problems caused for children of divorce are not long-lasting.** Many such problems are long-lasting and become worse in adulthood.
5. **Having a child will improve a marriage and prevent divorce.** The decreased risk is far less than it used to be.
6. **After divorce, the woman's standard of living plummets while the man's greatly improves.** The difference is not as great as previously thought, but the gender gap is real. A woman's loss is about 27% and a man's gain is about 10%.
7. **When parents do not get along, children are better off if their parents divorce.** Only the children in very high-conflict homes benefited from the conflict removal that divorce can effect. In lower-conflict marriages that end in divorce, the situation of the children is often much worse.
8. **Children who grow up in a home broken by divorce have as much success in their own marriages as those from intact homes.** Children of divorce have a much higher rate of divorce than those from intact families.
9. **After divorce, children involved are better off in stepfamilies than in single-parent families.** There seems to be no difference between the two.
10. **Being very unhappy at certain points in a marriage is a good sign that the marriage will end in divorce.** Eighty-six percent of a large national sample who were unhappily married indicated 5 years later that they were happier. Three-fifths of them said they were "very happy" or "quite happy."

One additional myth: It is usually men who initiate divorce proceedings. Two-thirds of all divorces are initiated by women.

Source: Adapted from: Popenoe, D. The top ten myths of divorce. National Marriage Project, [Online]. Available: http://marriage.rutgers.edu/pubtoptenmyths.htm.

earn enough money to meet their needs, and provide, usually without help, the love and affection all children crave. In addition, the divorced parent must reestablish a social life at the same time the emotional scars from the failed marriage are healing. The children may blame themselves for the divorce and must manage without the constant contact with one parent.

Because divorce is rather common, there are many studies on the topic. Many have focused on the effects of divorce. DiIuilio (1997) found that divorce can be hazardous to people's health and that of those around them. Divorced men who smoke have a 71% greater risk of premature death from cancer than married men who smoke, and divorced women lose 50% more time to injury and illness annually than married women. Children of divorce have a greater likelihood of dropping out of school, suffering depression and other mental and emotional problems, engaging earlier in sexual activity, becoming addicted to alcohol or drugs, procreating outside wedlock, falling economically below the poverty line, committing suicide, and getting divorced (Kahn, 1998).

Every year, more than 1 million children in the United States experience the divorce of their parents. The most important factor in how divorce affects a child's life is how parents treat each other and their children during and after the divorce (Divorce and children, 2001).

The question of whether or not divorce creates long-term negative effects for children has long been debated (Does divorce create long-term negative effects for children?, 2003). Some studies indicate that about twice as many children of divorced parents have emotional problems. In addition, they have greater challenges negotiating relationships once they are older, have a greater chance of choosing the "wrong" partner, and are much more likely to divorce. Critics of this research question these findings. They point out that most of the studies do not involve interviews with the children, but instead are colored by caregivers' views of how a divorce affects children. Some researchers indicate that children of divorce often have a greater sense of responsibility, independence, and maturity than their counterparts whose parents have remained together. In addition, if there has been great discord and constant fighting in the household, a divorce can provide relief to the children who have been living in that highly stressful setting.

Long-term effects of divorce have also been studied. Thabes (1997) examined the long-term adjustment of women divorced for more than 5 years who had not remarried. She found that 26% of the women had a clinically significant problem with depression. Cherlin, Chase-Landsdale, and McRae (1998) examined the long-term effects of parental divorce on individuals' mental health after the transition to adulthood. They found that a parental divorce during a person's childhood continued to have a negative effect on his or her mental health in adulthood.

There have been some governmental attempts to help prevent divorce. For example, in 1997 the British government started a campaign to increase public awareness of and access to marriage-support programs. The project represented a clear stand by the government. By contrast, most divorce-related bills proposed in the United States have been innocuous and undemanding. In Michigan and Maryland, for example, proposed laws prescribed a delay in granting marriage licenses to couples who refused to take marriage-skills classes (Russo, 1997). Louisiana attempted to encourage people to take marriage more seriously by creating covenant marriages, whereby couples are required to undergo premarital counseling and seek additional counseling if needed during the marriage. Instead of a "no-fault" divorce, a covenant marriage allows either spouse to seek a divorce only on the grounds of adultery, felony, abandonment, spousal or child abuse, or living apart for 2 years (Wagner, 1998). Many states also require divorcing parents to take a state-mandated class aimed at reducing harm to children.

Single-Parent Families

single-parent family
For whatever reason, only one parent who is living with a child or children.

Families with a single parent **(single-parent families)** are becoming increasingly prevalent. According to the U.S. Census Bureau, the number of single-parent families increased greatly between 1970 and 2000, from 6% to about 32% of all families (America's families and living arrangements, 2001). Almost 30% of children younger than 18 years old live with a single parent. Among African Americans 62% of children younger than 18 years live with a single parent (U.S. Bureau of the Census, 1998). Single-mother families increased from 3 million in 1970 to 10 million in 2000, while the number of single-father families grew from 393,000 to more than 2 million. Reasons for this shift include occurrence of a larger proportion of births to unmarried women; the

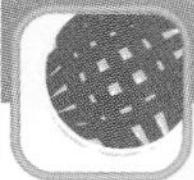

Global DIMENSIONS

Divorce in China Because of rapid increases in both extramarital affairs and divorces, in 1998 a "marriage and family law" was drafted in Beijing. This law resulted from 10 years of study and stipulates that husband and wife have an obligation to "mutual fidelity"; people who are unfaithful will be considered "guilty parties," and in the case of divorce the guilty party will be obliged to compensate the injured party. At the same time, living apart for 3 years will be considered grounds for divorce.

Over the last 20 years, the divorce rate in China has been steadily rising. It has risen more than 120% since 1986. In 1997 it reached one-quarter of the marriage rate.

In 1980 infidelity was the cause of divorce in only 14% of the cases, whereas by 1990 the figure reached 40%. With economic liberalization in China came a gradual increase in extramarital affairs and a corresponding increase in the number of divorces. Social change, the increasing mobility of the population, peasant migration to the cities, the arrival of foreign companies, and trends in foreign emigration have all contributed to the rising divorce rate. The divorce rate is highest in the big cities—32% in Beijing and 34% in Shanghai.

Source: Shuoming, J. For or against sexual liberation? *China Focus, 6, no. 10* (Oct. 1, 1998), 1+.

delay of marriage, which means that adults were single for more years; and the growth in divorce among couples with children (America's families and living arrangements, 2001).

Usually when we think of single-parent families, we think of them as being headed by women. Although this is generally true—about 80% of single-parent families are headed by women—the number of men heading such families is rising dramatically. For example, the number of single-father households rose 62% from 1990 to 2000. The portion of the country's total 105.5 million households that were headed by single fathers doubled in a decade, to 2% (Single-father homes on the rise, 2001).

Father-headed single-parent families often place the father in a new role. We say often because nowadays men in two-parent families more and more are helping with what were heretofore considered to be the wife's household chores and responsibilities. For these husbands the adjustment to heading a single-parent family will be less difficult. They are accustomed to cooking, cleaning, nurturing, and changing diapers. For the more traditional husband, the adoption of these necessary chores and responsibilities, added to the financial and emotional burdens of divorce, means that a more significant adjustment is required.

Life in a single-parent family can be stressful for the adult and the children. Members may unrealistically expect that the family can function as a two-parent family does and may feel that something is wrong if it cannot. The single parent may feel overwhelmed by the responsibility of caring for the children, maintaining a job, and keeping up with the bills and household chores. Typically, the family's finances and resources are drastically reduced by the parents' breakup.

Single-parent families deal with pressures and potential problem areas that the nuclear family does not have to face (Single parenting and today's family, 1998):

- Visitation and custody problems
- The negative effects of continuing conflict between the parents

- Fewer opportunities for parents and children to spend time together
- Negative effects of the breakup on children's school performance and peer relations
- Disruptions of extended family relationships
- Problems caused by parents' dating and entering new relationships

The demand for social services to meet the special needs of single-parent families is growing. Because single-parent families often have financial, psychological, custodial, and other needs that are more acute than those of conventional two-parent families, they need counseling and/or support groups. Many single parents have the added responsibility of providing role models for their other-sex children. Day care, a virtual necessity (as it also is for many two-parent households), solves some problems, yet it may also be a source of anxiety, or at least concern, for financial, educational, psychological, or other reasons.

Although some of these research findings might seem discouraging—or they might seem wrong to readers who come from single-parent families—it is important to remember that these findings refer to trends in groups and have no bearing on particular individuals. Children in single-parent families are often very successful. Our intention here is to suggest that single parenthood does require special care and consideration. Perhaps most of all, the special needs of single-parent families should be understood both by family members themselves and by teachers, employers, and others with whom they interact. To meet this need for understanding, a group called Parents without Partners serves as a sounding board and a source of counsel for single parents.

The need for good parenting skills remains constant regardless of the parent's marital status. However, the situation can be more demanding for both the parents and the children in single-parent households. The following are some suggested guidelines.

1. Be honest with your children about the situation that caused you to become a single parent.
2. In case of a separation or divorce, assure children that they are not responsible for the breakup of the relationship.
3. Try to maintain as much of the same routine as possible.
4. Do not try to be both mother and father to the children. Establish a family atmosphere of teamwork.
5. In the case of divorce, acknowledge that the relationship between you and your former partner is over, and do not encourage your children to hope for reconciliation.
6. Reassure children that they will continue to be loved and cared for (by both parents, if true).
7. Do not use children to gain bargaining power with a separated or divorced spouse.
8. Encourage relatives to help children maintain a sense of belonging to a continuing family.

Popenoe and Whitehead (2001) have provided helpful information to summarize this section. For example, they indicate that the percentage of children who grow up in fragile—typically fatherless—families has grown enormously from 1960 to 2000. This is mainly due to increases in divorce, out-of-wedlock births, and unmarried cohabitation. Children in such families have negative outcomes at two to three times the rate of children in married two-parent families. Also, in mother-headed single-parent families there was an enormous increase in the percentage of mothers who have never married, from 4% in 1960 to 40% in 1998. In earlier times, most single mothers were divorced or widowed. Today the number of never-married single mothers is higher than that of divorced mothers. A major reason for the increase in number of never-married single mothers is that single motherhood has become a permanent status for many women.

Sexuality and Aging

There was a time when it was believed that sexual desire and functioning became unimportant with age. Although a gradual decline in sexual activity occurs around age 50 years and accelerates after age 70 years, sexuality remains an important part of life into old age (Sanders, 1999).

Understanding the sexuality of elders is important because of the rapidly increasing elderly population. The population of U.S. citizens aged 65 years and older grew from 25.5 million in 1980 to 34.1 million in 1997, and 35 million in 2000. The population of those aged 85 years and older almost doubled from 2.2 million in 1980 to 4.2 million people in 2000 (12% of the older population) (U.S. Bureau of the Census, 1998; The 65 years and over population, 2001). As people live longer, it is important to understand how sexuality is affected in the later years.

The number of elderly Americans, especially women, living independently after losing their spouse has increased sharply. Some 70% of widows lived by themselves in 1997, up 56% from 1970. During the same time, the number of widowers increased from 53% to 60%. Overall, 46.3% of American women older than 65 years were widows. Just 7.4% of elderly women were divorced. The number of elderly women still living with their husband rose from 34% in 1970 to 40% in 1997 (Schmid, 1998).

Cultural expectations play an important role in sexuality for older people. In 70% of societies, the elderly are expected to remain sexually active—and they do. A study by Winn and Newton (1980) found that in 22% of societies, women are actually expected to become less sexually inhibited as they age.

Many studies have confirmed that people remain sexually active into their 70s and 80s. Bretschneider and McCoy (1988) found that 62% of the men and 30% of the women they studied engaged in intercourse. These people ranged in age from 80 to 102 years. DeBeauvoir (1973) revealed that 70% of those men older than 65 years of age who were listed in *Who's Who* had sexual intercourse on an average of four times a month. And Kaplan (1974) found that women tend to want more rather than less sexual activity as they approach their middle and older years.

In 1998, The National Council on the Aging conducted a telephone survey of 1,300 Americans above the age of 60 years. They found that nearly half engage in sexual activity at least once a month, and 4 in 10 said they would like to engage in sexual activities more frequently than they currently do. Three-quarters of the men and the women said that they are emotionally satisfied or even more satisfied with their sexual activities than they were in their 40s. Forty-three percent said that sexual relations were just as good as or better than they were in their youth, and 43% said they were less satisfying.

Older men were more than twice as likely to report wanting more sexual activity than women, and men were much more likely to be sexually active than women older than 60 years. Nearly two-thirds of senior men are currently sexually active, whereas only 37% of women are currently sexually

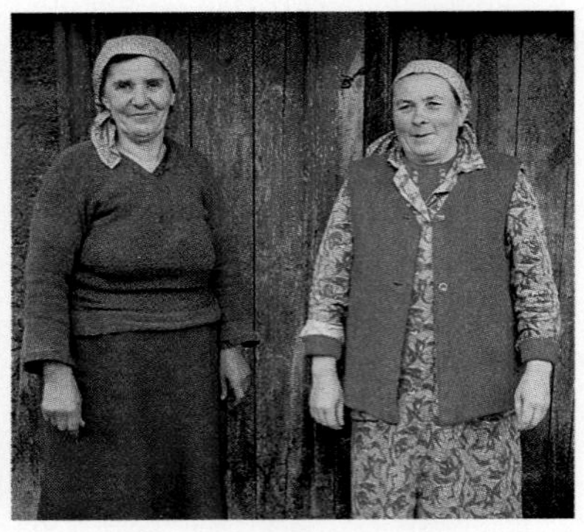

The Abkhasian people of Georgia (a republic of the former Soviet Union) often live to be more than 100 years old. One reason they believe they live so long are their sexual customs. The Abkhasian people believe that sexual energy should be conserved. They do not marry until about age 30 years and do not believe in premarital sexual activity. It is essential that a bride be a virgin. In marriage, sexual activity is considered a pleasure to enjoy, but for the sake of one's health it should not be overdone.
Source: Henslin, 1986

active. This gap exists partially because women live longer and thus are much more likely to be widowed than men. However, men were much more likely to say that a medical condition prevents them from engaging in sexual activities (51% of men, 12% of women) and that medications are reducing their sexual desire (44% of men, 16% of women).

Prevalent in our society is the performance ethic, which is concerned with the frequency of intercourse and orgasm. As we mature (age, if you will) it becomes apparent that other types of sexual activity become important (Foster, 1979). These include caressing, hugging, petting, kissing, and sharing of intimacies. As Masters and Johnson indicated, people who experience a satisfying sexual life in their early years will most likely continue this pursuit. However, those people who are today 65 years and older lived under very different mores. Your grandparents and possibly your parents led more restricted sexual lives, especially the women. Women were not taught about masturbation, nor were they taught to ask that they be sexually satisfied.

Older people cannot only be sexually satisfied by having relationships with others; they can also experience active sexual behaviors by themselves. Masturbation is a viable activity for older people (Wasow & Loeb, 1979), especially women. If the male loses the capacity to maintain erections, women can masturbate; or men can masturbate to orgasm even after they can no longer become erect. Mutual masturbation becomes popular, once again, as it may have been when they were younger.

Physiological changes are often attributed to changes in sexuality associated with aging. However, onset of menopause for women and declining levels of testosterone for men represent only one factor in sexuality changes. Psychological and sociocultural changes occur as well (Sanders, 1999).

Some sexual dysfunction (discussed in Chapter 15) associated with aging, such as erectile disorder, can now be overcome with pharmacology. The drug Viagra can restore the physical ability to have an erection; however, it does not rekindle the psychological or social aspects that make for a loving relationship. Viagra poses special problems to a relationship: A woman may wonder whether the erection is caused by the drug or by attraction to her. The couple needs to learn how to resume lovemaking after what may have been a 10-year or longer hiatus (Renshaw, 1999).

Psychological changes also occur across the aging process, such as changes in mood. For women, causes may include stress, health problems,

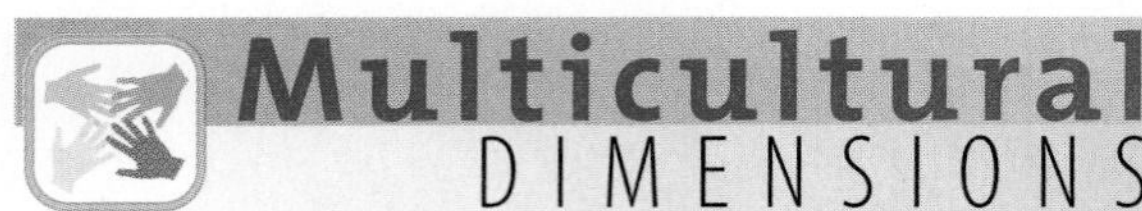

Multicultural DIMENSIONS

The Boomer Sandwich

A study done by the American Association of Retired People on 45- to 55-year-olds (the sandwich generation) showed how different cultures take care of their own (The Boomer sandwich, 2001). Compared with other generations, this one is better educated (38% are college graduates compared with 23% of the general population). More of them are married (67%, well above the national average). They are also more economically secure (almost a third earn more than $75,000 a year).

Who helps their aging relatives most? Forty-two percent of Asian Americans provide care for their aging relatives compared with 34% of Hispanics, 28% of African Americans, and 19% of whites. Those born outside the United States are much more likely to care for or support older family members (43%) compared with those who are born in the United States (20%). Overall 69% do not want their children to have to look after them when they get older.

menopause, hormone replacement therapy, and other lifestyle changes. For men, they may include a shift in focus from career to increased focus on family, challenge to the male role as leader and protector of the family, increased need for affirmation and acceptance, or irritation and anger with aging (especially the physical changes) (Sanders, 1999).

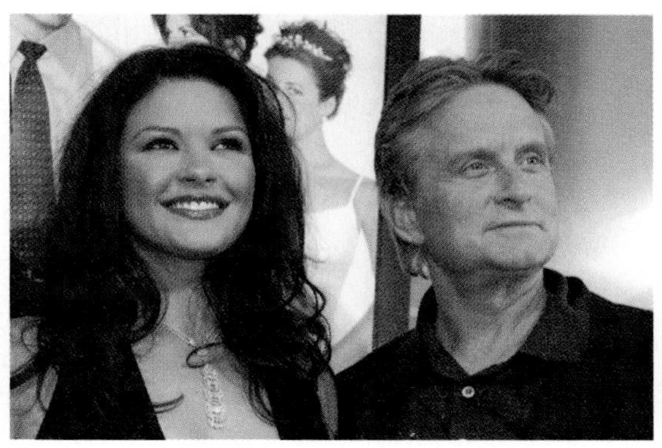

A common occurrence in Hollywood, both on- and off-screen, is that of a romantic involvement between an older man and a significantly younger woman. The marriage of Catherine Zeta Jones to Michael Douglas, 25 years her senior, hardly sets a precedent. Does this sort of relationship reinforce the view that images of attractiveness include older men, but not older women? Would the routine pairing of older women and younger men, such as occurred in 2003 with Demi Moore (40 years old) and Ashton Kutcher (25 years old) receive such widespread acceptance?

Social factors affecting psychological changes include the fact that socialization of people in their 70s, 80s, or 90s in regard to sexuality is substantially different from that of those in their 30s or 40s. For example, images of sexual attractiveness tend to be youth oriented and may affect the self-esteem of aging women (Sanders, 1999). Ironically, men are sometimes viewed as more attractive as they age. And Hollywood movies often capitalize on this double standard by pairing an older, experienced male actor with a young actress.

In addition, the acceptability of some sexual activities has changed over the past few decades. Thus, whereas younger people may engage in more oral sexual activities than their predecessors, older adults are less likely to engage in oral sex (Laumann, et al., 1994).

Interestingly, Pfeiffer (1975) found that some long-married couples actually experience more sexual satisfaction during their older years. Once their offspring are out of the house and they are retired from working, they can devote more time to each other and have more fulfilling and rewarding lovemaking.

The Physiology of Aging

As people age, they change physiologically. Physical, hormonal, neural, and vascular changes associated with aging can affect sexual functioning and behavior (Sanders, 1999). However, current research can help dispel some long-held myths about aging and sexuality.

Physiological changes in the female may result in some minor changes in sexual response. The vaginal lips do not swell as much during sexual excitement in older women, the vagina takes longer to become lubricated, and the length and width of the vagina decrease by the age of 60 years. However, older women still have the capacity to reach orgasm and enjoy sexual activity. In one community sample of 141 women, menopausal status and hormonal variations did not significantly predict sexuality variables such as frequency of sexual intercourse, frequency of sexual thoughts, or negative sexual feeling factor (Sanders, 1999).

The relationship between menopause and a woman's sexuality has often been misunderstood. Although menopause can produce uncomfortable symptoms (hot flashes, bloating, swelling of breasts, back problems, migraines), most women get through this stage quite well and function satisfactorily. They probably cope with menopause as well as they coped with other stressful events in their lives.

One important question for women going through menopause is whether or not to take hormones to help with their symptoms. Estrogen may be taken by itself or in combination with progesterone. These hormones have also been prescribed to help prevent osteoporosis (thinning of the bones) and possibly to prevent heart disease. Taking of such hormones has been a controversial issue since 2002, when studies raised questions about the safety of hormone replacement therapy (HRT). A huge federally funded study of HRT involving more than 16,000 women was abruptly stopped when researchers discovered that long-term use (more than 5 years) of HRT was not lowering the risk of heart disease and stroke, as had been thought, but raising it along with the risk of breast cancer and blood clots. HRT is still the best treatment available for relief of night sweats, hot flashes, and mood swings. Women and their physicians have to decide whether these benefits outweigh the potential risks of HRT (Hormone replacement therapy, 2003).

Some experts have replaced the term *hormone replacement therapy* with *menopausal hormone therapy* (MHT). In 2003 the Food and Drug Administration ordered that labels for all postmenopause drugs containing estrogen with or without progestin describe the risks of MHT and advise that women use the lowest dosage for the shortest time possible (Hormone labels will warn of risks, 2003).

The popular myth that women will cease to be sexually active with the estrogen decrease (or cessation) is simply not true. It would seem that women may enjoy sexual relations more after menopause, because they no longer menstruate and have no need for contraceptives. Some people incorrectly think that a **hysterectomy** ends a female's sexual activity. In general this is not true, because removing a woman's uterus has no effect on her sexual functioning. As long as the ovaries are left in place, there should be no change in sexual response. In fact, some women may find they respond better because the possibility of pregnancy has been eliminated.

hysterectomy
Surgical removal of the uterus.

Men also experience changes as they age. An older man requires more time to become erect and to ejaculate than a young man. However, the widely held belief that testosterone levels decline with age may not be accurate. The Massachusetts Male Aging Study, based on a random sample of 1,700 men aged 40 to 69 years, found that when sociodemographic, psychosocial, health, and lifestyle characteristics were taken into account, age was not related to testosterone levels. It is possible that any decline in testosterone levels may be related to illness rather than physiological processes. Further, androgen-receptor sensitivity may change with age, so that even normal plasma levels of testosterone may not be adequate to sustain former levels of sexual functioning (Sanders, 1999).

Direct physical changes do occur in men as they age: The testes become smaller, the scrotal skin becomes thinner and less elastic, seminal fluid may become thinner and be produced in lower quantities, and sperm become less lively. Erections occur more slowly and the plateau phase lasts longer. Another important occurrence is that older men do not feel imminent ejaculation—it is less forceful. It is common for the refractory period to become longer as men age. One possible advantage of slower response is the likelihood that middle-aged and older men can prolong sexual activity and actually be better sexual partners. It should be remembered, however, that even elderly men continue to produce sperm and can become fathers if appropriate precautions are not taken.

The capacity to enjoy sexual experiences is not lost in older men, as it is not lost in older women. Masters and Johnson (1966) maintain the importance of continued and frequent sexual experiences for aging males:

> *If elevated levels of sexual activity are maintained from earlier years and neither acute nor chronic physical incapacity intervenes, aging males usually are able to continue some form of active sexual expression into the 70- and even 80-year age groups.*

Masters and Johnson further indicate that women who do not regularly participate in sexual activity tend to have difficulty accommodating a penis when they do attempt sexual intercourse. Those who can accommodate a penis and have adequate lubrication are likely to have maintained regular sexual response (once or twice a week).

Ethical DIMENSIONS

Should Donor Eggs Be Used to Let Women Older Than 50 Years Produce Viable Babies?

Women older than 50 years are just as likely to conceive and deliver a baby with donor eggs as younger women are. Many people argue that there is no medical reason why healthy women in their 50s should not have babies with donor eggs. They say that people in their 60s and 70s are much more active than in past years, so they have enough stamina to raise a child. Also, knowing that they can reproduce after age 50 will take the pressure off some women to reproduce when they are younger. They can concentrate more on their marriage and their careers and not worry about child rearing until later in life.

Others feel that it is wrong for a woman older than 50 years to reproduce. They feel that there is a much higher possibility of their offspring's being orphaned at a young age. Even if people are healthy and active, statistics show that many people die in their 60s and 70s. If that happens, relatively young children will be without parents for more of their lives. Also, for healthy people, raising a child takes a lot of energy and it is more likely younger parents will have that energy.

Do you think donor eggs should be used to let women older than 50 years reproduce? At what ages should women be allowed to reproduce?

Source: Rubin, R. Donor eggs can let women over 50 produce viable babies, *USA Today* (November 11, 2002), 9D.

Barriers to Sexual Activity in Later Years

Although health problems can interfere with sexual activity for older people, they need not end all sexual activity. For example, arthritis or lower back pain might require understanding and a variety of sexual positions. Diabetes can result in diminished sexual response, but sexual pleasuring can still provide satisfaction. Stroke victims might lose some control of speech or movements but still be capable of sexual response under appropriate conditions.

Heart attacks are sometimes of particular concern in relation to sexual activity. Some people think that sexual activity may bring about a heart attack, and although in reality this is not a common problem, heart attack victims often hesitate to return to sexual activity. In general, those who have been sexually active before the heart attack will have little, if any, problem being sexually active again. Of course it makes sense to improve personal health as much as possible after a heart attack. Those who have a proper diet, exercise appropriately, and control stress responses are most likely to have satisfactory sexual activity as well.

The availability of partners for the older divorced or widowed person can present severe restrictions on intimacy. How can one have a successful relationship if there are no possible mates? Older women outnumber older men; they tend to live 7 years longer and they generally marry men a few years older than they are. Hence the older woman, who is supposed to have sexual relationships only with her spouse, is alone.

Another problem that exists for older men and women is that their sphere of friendships may be couples—that is, pairs. If one of only a few single people, the person may be omitted from social activities or may appear to be a fifth wheel, and so he or she is not very comfortable with other couples. This indeed limits sexual activity; even more importantly, it may limit intimacy and friendships in later life.

For older people living in nursing homes, there might be additional problems. For example, nursing home personnel sometimes resist sexuality programs (Starr & Weiner, 1981). People may be segregated to discourage sexual activities. Medications may be prescribed without considering their effects on sexual functioning; for example, some high blood pressure or arthritis medications can lessen sexual response. Fortunately, attitudes of the staff in nursing homes as well as the families of those in the homes are changing. This is an excellent example of the need to accept people of all ages as sexual beings.

It should be noted that there are times when couples may want to sleep apart, because medication may cause a person to snore loudly, shake violently, or talk loudly, making it uncomfortable for the other partner. As well as elderly adults, some younger couples choose to sleep in separate bedrooms for similar reasons. It should be remembered that sexual activity can occur in either bedroom and at any time during the day or evening.

Aging and Safer Sexual Activity

STI and HIV are generally thought of as diseases that the young must worry about. But the increasing number of sexually active elders has also been a factor in the increase in cases of STI and HIV. People 50 years and older account for about 13% of AIDS cases in the United States. They actually are more vulnerable to HIV infection because the linings of the vagina and anus become more fragile and more susceptible to tears during intercourse, providing a direct path into the bloodstream for the virus. The immune system also tends to grow weaker with advancing age. To make matters worse, older people are only one-fifth as likely as those in their 20s to be tested for HIV. So the infection is typically not diagnosed until a late stage. It is important that older adults take the same safer sexual precautions as younger people (AIDS risk rising in older people, 2003). As the older population continues to increase, the increase in STI and HIV is likely to continue at a corresponding rate.

One problem is that many people link pregnancy and STI risk. An elderly woman may not think to use a condom—after all, pregnancy is not possible (Broom, 1999). But condom use and safer sexual practices are still needed throughout life to prevent the transmission of STIs and HIV. And because an elderly man can impregnate a woman late into his life, safer sexual practices for men must include contraception.

Homosexuality Among the Aging

As with all sexual beings, homosexuals eventually become old and need to deal with problems caused by aging. The loss of partners and friends may be compounded for older gay men, who saw many of their friends die of AIDS during the 1980s and 1990s. For them, AIDS meant that the good-byes that would have been said as they approached old age were made not only to lifelong friends but also to younger and younger men (Swartz, 1998).

Because they grew up in such a sharply homophobic society, many gays are still cautious about coming out. Kehoe suggests that many elderly lesbians are still careful about coming out in today's somewhat more accepting society because they have become accustomed to hiding their identity (Kehoe, 1989). When older gay men or lesbians do not disclose their sexual identity, they prevent themselves and others from sharing in a comprehensive understanding of their lives (Altman, 1999).

Many gays may decide to keep their sexual identities secret because of fears of receiving biased or inferior services from doctors, attendants, or nursing homes. Help is available from Senior Action in a Gay Environment (SAGE), an organization concerned with senior lesbians and gays. They provide social services, individual and group therapy, and home visits for the homebound. They also act as advocates on behalf of older lesbians and gays.

Sexuality for the Physically and Mentally Challenged

Nearly 40 million Americans have illnesses or disabilities that limit physical activity, and about 38% of them are older than 65 years of age. Injuries from accidents are one source; less researched are the effects on sexuality of Alzheimer's disease, Parkinson's disease, diabetes, heart disease, multiple sclerosis, severe arthritis, and stroke. Invasive surgical procedures, antidepressants, blood pressure medicines, and other prescription drugs may also affect the sex drive (Pope, 1999).

Sexual challenges are especially prevalent as aging occurs. Although the average American lives to almost 74 years of age, he or she spends the final 11.7 years in poor health (Donatelle, 1998). For example, as discussed in detail in Chapter 15, about 30 million American men suffer from erectile disorder, which has many causes. The former senator and presidential candidate Bob Dole experienced erectile disorder caused by surgery for prostate cancer. Ten years later, he agreed to be a spokesperson for erectile disorder (in the ads paid for by Pfizer, maker of Viagra).

Although we think of physical or mental challenges and illness as physical (biological) dimensions of sexuality, psychological and sociocultural dimensions also come into play. Mild depression is common among not only those with a chronic illness but also their caregivers and spouses, and it affects the couple's sexual activities (Pope, 1999). Further, an illness or disability may force a person to withdraw from normal social activities, thereby removing him- or herself from social support. Those who suffer from a disability also may suffer from body-image or gender-identity problems (Gerschick & Miller, 1998).

As with any sexual problem, it is not just the ill or disabled spouse who suffers. Both partners have to come to terms with changes in sexuality. Communication becomes a critical tool for acceptance of a new sexuality.

Physical Challenges

Physical challenge can result in any number of specific problems—for example, low energy levels, blindness or limited vision, movement problems, sensory loss, and the need to manage bags or tubes. Nevertheless, the challenged can generally find, or be helped to find, creative ways of overcoming such impediments to physical intimacy. For example, although most of us tend to focus on stimulating the genital area, in fact, the whole body can be stimulated and aroused. We can achieve sexual satisfaction—and possibly orgasm—without an erect penis or a well-lubricated vagina. With conscious intention and learning, anyone can use any part of the body in an infinite number of ways to achieve sexual satisfaction. For the challenged—as well as for the able-bodied—such learning can lead to a rich sexual life.

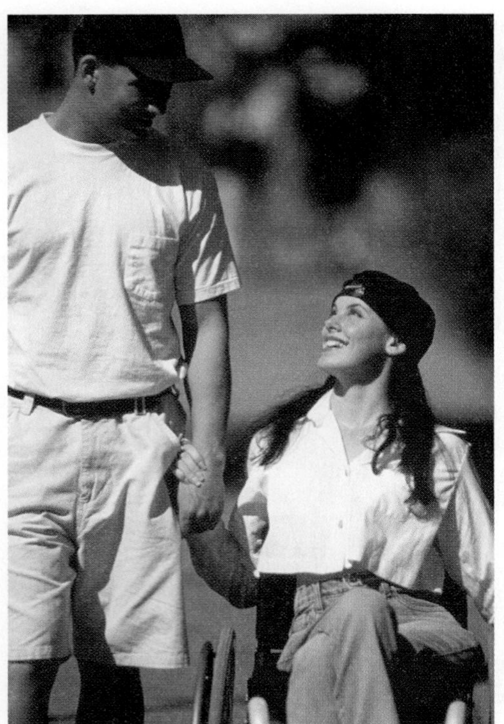

Disabilities do not have to prevent individuals from experiencing all the dimensions of human sexuality.

Even though sensory challenges, such as blindness and deafness, do not directly influence overall sexual responsiveness, they may affect sexuality. For example, people who have been blind for most or all of their life may have difficulty in understanding a partner's anatomy. Fortunately, educational programs, including learning about sexual anatomy and intercourse positions through the use of models, can be very helpful.

Deaf people may also have special challenges related to sexuality. For example, some of the usual communication routes may be blocked. Deaf people may miss words in lipreading or may be misunderstood when using sign language if others are not familiar with it. As people without such challenges do, those with sensory challenges may feel afraid or embarrassed when attempting to communicate about sexuality. Educational programs are needed for the sensory challenged just as they are needed for people without such challenges.

Cerebral palsy usually does not preclude interest in sexual activity, fertility, or ability to experience orgasm. Depending upon the nature and extent of problems with muscle control, those with cerebral palsy may have difficulty with certain sexual activities or positions. In addition, social rejection or feelings of inadequacy may become problems. Fortunately, education and counseling to help those with cerebral palsy understand their sexuality and learn appropriate social skills can help improve body image and ability to have intimate relationships.

Sometimes challenged people have to adapt their behavior to meet new conditions. For example, a woman with severe arthritis of the hip joints may find she cannot spread her legs wide enough for intercourse in the standard frontal position or that the weight of a partner's body may produce pain. She can employ rear entry or side-by-side coital positions that reduce or eliminate discomfort.

It is important to recognize certain aspects of sexual functioning in paralyzed individuals (Woods, 1979):

1. Some components of the human sexual response cycle (such as erection) are mediated by spinal-cord reflexes. Therefore, it is not necessary to have pathways from the brain to the sex organs. For example, stimuli resulting from pressure or tension in the pelvic organs or from touch excite impulses that can cause erection.
2. The level of the spinal-cord lesion and the degree of interruption of nerve impulses influence the nature of sexual functioning. For example, the local reflexes important in female orgasm are thought to be integrated into the lumbar and sacral regions of the cord.
3. Gratification can be obtained from sexual responses other than those from the sex organs during sexual stimulation. Many physically challenged people develop other areas of stimulation to high levels.
4. Adaptation of previous sexual practices may be needed after spinal-cord injury. Sexual activity may need to take place in different positions, and sexual aids may be helpful.
5. Fertility and the ability to bear children are usually not lost by women with spinal-cord injuries.

Gender DIMENSIONS

Coming to Terms: Masculinity and Physical Challenges

Men with physical challenges are marginalized and stigmatized in American society. The image and reality of men with challenges undermine cultural beliefs about men's bodies and physicality. The body is a central foundation of how men define themselves and how they are defined by others. Bodies are vehicles for determining value, which in turn translates into status and prestige. Men's bodies allow them to demonstrate the socially valuable characteristics of toughness, competitiveness, and ability.... Thus, one's body and relationship to it provide a way to comprehend the world and one's place in it. The bodies of men with challenges serve as a continual reminder that they are at odds with the expectations of the dominant culture. As anthropologist Robert Murphy writes of his own experiences with disability:

> *Paralytic disability constitutes emasculation of a more direct and total nature. For the male, the weakening and atrophy of the body threaten all the cultural values of masculinity: strength, activeness, speed, virility, stamina, and fortitude.*

This article seeks to sharpen our understanding of the creation, maintenance, and re-creation of gender identities by men who, by birth, accident, or illness, find themselves dealing with a physical challenge. We examine two sets of social dynamics that converge and clash in the lives of men with physical challenges. On the one side, these men must deal with the presence and pressures of hegemonic masculinity, which demands strength. On the other side, societal members perceive people with disabilities to be weak....

Recently, the literature has shifted toward understanding gender as an interactive process. Thus, it is presumed to be not only an aspect of what one *is*, but more fundamentally it is something that one *does* in interaction with others.... Whereas previously gender was thought to be strictly an individual phenomenon, this new understanding directs our attention to the interpersonal and institutional levels as well. The lives of men with challenges provide an instructive arena in which to study the interactional nature of gender and its effect on individual gender identities.

In *The Body Silent*, Murphy (1990) observes that men with physical challenges experience "embattled identities" because of the conflicting expectations placed on them as men and as people with disabilities. On the one side, contemporary masculinity privileges men who are strong, courageous, aggressive, independent, and self-reliant.... On the other side, people with challenges are perceived to be, and treated as, weak, pitiful, passive, and dependent.... Thus, for men with physical challenges, masculine gender identity and practice are created and maintained at the crossroads of the demands of contemporary masculinity and the stigmatization associated with disability. As such, for men with physical disabilities, being recognized as masculine by others is especially difficult, if not impossible, to accomplish. Yet not being recognized as masculine is untenable because, in our culture, everyone is expected to display an appropriate gender identity.

Source: Kimmel, M. S. & Messner, M. A. *Men's lives.* Needham MA: Allyn & Bacon, 1998.

Sexuality and Illness

The ill are another group whose sexuality has mainly been ignored. In the past both patients and medical personnel avoided any mention of sexual topics, no doubt because both were too embarrassed to discuss them. Now questions about sexual history are often asked in addition to standard questions about medical history. And physicians, patients, and partners are encouraged to discuss, when relevant, the effects of illness or other medical problems on sexual functioning.

Diabetes, neurological disorders, gynecological disorders, inflammation of the male's prostate gland, castration, rectal surgery, and heart attacks usually have a direct (or assumed) effect on sexual functioning. But people with other nonrelated physical medical problems often experience sexual problems caused by psychological factors. Some of us, for example, feel guilty when we get sick and try to determine where the fault lies. Because the topic of sexuality is a leading producer of guilt, we may consciously or unconsciously avoid sexual activity. We may even allow illness to restrict our sexual life, not because restriction is necessary but because we failed to ask medical personnel whether restriction was actually required.

To reduce sexual problems associated with illness, we need to feel that sexuality is appropriate to discuss, and we need to be aware of guilt feelings. And, in all cases of illness, we need to take responsibility for finding out the earliest and safest time to resume normal sexual activity to prevent other detrimental effects on interpersonal relationships, as well as on self-concept. For example, after a heart attack it would be helpful to know the following (Cambre, 1978):

1. More than 80% of heart attack patients can resume normal sexual activity.
2. These patients should be cleared for sexual activity by a doctor, but this can usually be done about 4 to 8 weeks after an attack.
3. As with other forms of physical activity, it is wise to get the body in shape gradually. Thus, masturbation or mutual foreplay might be helpful activities.
4. During sexual activity, maximal stress on the heart lasts about only 4 to 6 minutes. This is far less than that experienced in many other activities.
5. It is important to relax and avoid other stress factors. Contributing factors such as marijuana, other drugs, heavy drinking, a heavy meal, or an extramarital affair would put additional strain on the heart.
6. A practical physiological test of readiness is 10 minutes of rapid walking (120 paces per minute), followed by climbing two flights of stairs in 10 seconds (two steps per second). When a heart attack victim can do that, it should be safe to return to normal sexual activity.

The American Heart Association (1998) recommends that when people who have heart disease engage in sexual activities they

- Choose a time when they are rested, relaxed, and free of the stressful feelings produced by the day's schedules and responsibilities
- Wait 1 to 3 hours after eating a full meal, so that digestion can take place
- Select a familiar, peaceful setting that is free of interruptions
- Take medicine before sexual relations if prescribed by a physician

Alzheimer's disease also affects sexuality. Some Alzheimer's sufferers develop a loss of libido, whereas others develop hypersexuality—a constant desire to engage in sexual activities. However, an affected spouse may demand sexual activity but not even recognize his or her own spouse. Caregivers say that the sexual encounter may be emotionless, mechanical, or marred by inappropriate behavior, such as giggling (Pope, 1999).

Did You Know . . .

Persons with physical, cognitive, or emotional challenges have a right to sexuality education, sexual health care, and opportunities for socializing and for sexual expression. Family, health care workers, and other caregivers should receive training in understanding and supporting sexual development and behavior, comprehensive sexuality education, and related health care for individuals who have these challenges. The policies and procedures of social agencies and health care delivery systems should ensure that services and benefits are provided to all persons without discrimination and their caregivers have information and education about ways to minimize the risk of sexual abuse and exploitation.

Source: Position statement of Sexuality Information and Education Council of the United States, 1995.

We also need to realize that sexual problems can be expressed through physical symptoms; a person who asks for an examination of the genital area because of a supposed concern about cancer may actually be seeking an acceptable way to talk about a sexual difficulty. The relationship between illness and sexuality needs to be understood in order to help reduce the incidence of problems in medical settings and to increase our acceptance of both ourselves and others when illness is present—either in or out of the hospital.

Emotional Challenges

Throughout this text we have emphasized a comprehensive concept of human sexuality. One excellent example of this concept is the influence of emotional states upon sexual responsiveness. Many life problems, such as stress, problems at work, death of a friend or relative, or work overload, may interfere with sexual interest or response. Apprehension about intimacy, fear of pregnancy, or possibly fear of contracting of an STI may influence relationships with others. Depression or poor self-esteem can also create problems related to intimate relationships.

Whatever the reason, emotional well-being has a strong influence on overall sexuality and on sexual response. It can be helpful to understand that, at times, lack of interest in sexual activity or even inability to respond can be natural and common. Fortunately, these situations are usually temporary and can be effectively handled through personal understanding or professional counseling if needed.

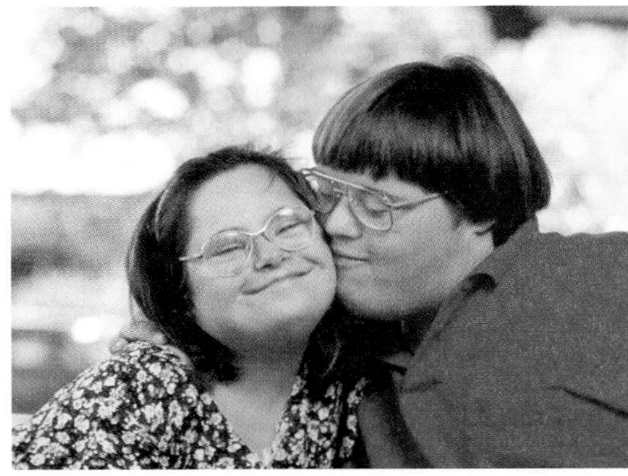

Despite many factors that must be considered, including safe sex and the ability to make proper decisions regarding sexuality, the mentally challenged are certainly capable of participating in sexual relationships. With the support of education and counseling, the mentally challenged can often greatly benefit from the affection and intimacy encountered through a sexual relationship.

Sexuality of the Mentally Challenged

For many years, the sexuality of the mentally challenged was dealt with by restricting or preventing sexual behavior; indeed, the mentally challenged were sterilized to prevent any chance of pregnancy. The societal fear was that the mentally challenged would have mentally challenged children and that they would not be able to care for their children properly—thus, costly medical care would be needed. A turning point in the rights of the mentally challenged occurred with the election of President John F. Kennedy in 1960. His mentally challenged sister, Rosemary, had a profound effect on him and was a major factor in his proposing of legislation to educate and help the mentally challenged (Wilson, et al., 1996).

There are more than 2.5 million mentally challenged individuals in the United States. Approximately 85% are considered to have "mild mental retardation" (American Psychiatric Association, 1994); they experience few or no obvious impairments in perceptual functions (seeing or hearing), and their retardation is not recognized until they take intelligence tests at school. Most reach an academic level of about sixth grade and are able to live and function individually (Wilson, et al., 1996). Most of these people live and work among us. The 1999 movie *The Other Sister,* with Juliette Lewis and Giovanni Ribisi, portrays a mentally challenged couple who desperately want to have as complete a life as possible.

Mentally challenged people who are allowed to have sexual relationships can and do build feelings of affection and tenderness that appear to contribute to their happiness and tranquility. In 1970, the United Nations passed a resolution supporting the right of mentally challenged individuals to sexuality education, cohabitation, and marriage. Although the rights of the mentally challenged are indisputable, their ability to make proper decisions regarding sexuality is often disputed.

As everyone else can, the mentally challenged can benefit from sexuality education and counseling. Because being challenged is just one more dimension of human sexuality, it needs to be factored into the decision-making process. For example, Depo-Provera or a long-term contraceptive might be selected instead of oral contraceptive pills, because contraceptive effectiveness would not depend on remembering to take a pill every day. Through factual knowledge, role playing, and personal experience, the mentally challenged are able to have fulfilling sexual lives.

Personal and Social Support

Society in general continues to deny the sexuality of the ill and the challenged. If this situation is to change, we need to remember that these people are sexual beings in the same way as everyone else. We also need to prevent public service personnel from denying the sexuality of their clientele. Attention must be paid to policy decisions influencing human services; to approaches used to serve the ill and the challenged; and to attitudes of those working with these people, as well as of society in general. Organizations that provide services to the ill and challenged need to teach classes in sexuality, not only for their patients but also for their patients' relatives and those who work with them.

Exploring the DIMENSIONS of Human Sexuality

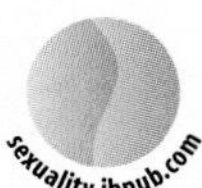

Our feelings, attitudes, and beliefs regarding sexuality are influenced by our internal and external environments. Go to sexuality.jbpub.com to learn more about the biological, psychological, and sociological factors that affect your sexuality.

Biological Factors

- Physiological changes, such as the onset of menopause for women and androgen-receptor sensitivity for men, affect sexuality for the aging. However, elderly couples can still engage in a sexually satisfying relationship.
- Nearly 40 million Americans have illnesses or challenges that limit physical activity. Many of these conditions affect sexuality.
- Nearly 30 million American men suffer from erectile disorder, which is usually pharmacologically treatable.

Sociocultural Factors

- Most Americans are attracted to people who have the same sociocultural dimensions—race and ethnicity, religion, age, and social class.
- Singlehood, cohabitation, and divorce have become more acceptable to society in general; however, some social stigma and discrimination still exist. The common societal expectation is still that people eventually marry.
- More people are postponing the age of first marriage. Reasons include economic constraints, greater caution due to high divorce rates, and greater availability of contraception.
- People who attend church regularly are less likely to cohabit and less likely to divorce.
- Louisiana passed a covenant marriage law in which couples must undergo premarital counseling. Instead of having a "no-fault" divorce, the couple can only seek divorce for cause—adultery, felony, abandonment, abuse, or living apart for 2 years.

Psychological Factors

- Romantic love is characterized by strong feelings of elation, sexual desire, anxiety, and arousal.
- Happy relationships help people to handle negative emotions and deal with conflict.
- Divorces result in emotional scars for both partners and their children. A parental divorce during childhood continues to have a negative effect on adult mental health.

CASE STUDY

The life cycle of sexuality, from high school graduation through aging, offers many opportunities to see the interaction of the dimensions of human sexuality.

Consider the aging process: Biological changes, especially in levels of hormones, can bring about psychological changes, such as in mood. In addition, a psychological shift occurs in men as they shift their attention from career to family. Cultural expectations affect elderly adults' perceptions and expectations of their sexuality.

New advances in pharmacology such as the introduction of Viagra may solve a biological problem, but the couple must then solve the psychological and social problems related to reintegrating the ability to have an erection in the relationship. Although medication can solve most erectile disorder issues, an erection is also a function of psychosocial sexual attraction—something that cannot yet be purchased.

Discussion Questions

1. Compare and contrast the different theories about love. Which do you agree with? Explain why.
2. Summarize the studies about college relationships and sexual activities.
3. Discuss why increased numbers of people are remaining single.
4. Compare the advantages and disadvantages of cohabitation versus marriage.
5. Discuss why marriage is popular.
6. Discuss the reasons for divorce. What can be done to help protect children?
7. Discuss how and why the aging process affects sexuality.

Application Questions

Reread the chapter-opening story and answer the following questions.

1. The names Lynn and Chris were deliberately used as pseudonyms because they are names used by both genders. When you read the story, who did you think was the male? the female? Explain your answer. Then switch the genders of Lynn and Chris and reread the story. Does it strike you differently now? Why?
2. What advice from the chapter might have helped Lynn and Chris have a better marriage?

Critical Thinking Questions

1. Should mildly mentally challenged people be allowed to have children? Would they be any better or worse than typical parents (who have to learn from the start as well)? If mentally challenged parents are denied reproduction rights, what about those who have diagnosed psychiatric illness (such as depression)?
2. An increasing percentage of the population is remaining permanently single. Discuss whether this trend appears to be long term or just temporary. What are its implications for population growth? The future of social security?
3. Because of all the problems that divorce causes, should it be outlawed? What effects would such a law have on families?
4. Write a prenuptial agreement, indicating your expectations and responsibilities in marriage. Be sure to include how financial decisions, household tasks, child rearing responsibilities, and so on, will be handled. Would such a document help or hinder a marriage?

Critical Thinking Case

Although dual-income families have become the norm, equal sharing of housework is not. In one survey of dual-income families (Galinsky, Bond, & Friedman, 1993), women claimed greater responsibility for shopping (87%), cooking (81%), cleaning (78%), and paying bills (63%); men were more often responsible for repairs (91%).

The concept of the woman's having a greater share of the housework after working all day is known to sociologists as the "second shift" (the first shift is work; the second shift is home) (Henslin, 1995). Combining the time spent working at work and at home, each year women put in an extra month of 24-hour days compared to their spouses (Hochschild, 1989). Further, most of women's tasks with children involve "maintenance"—feeding and bathing, taking them to the doctor, helping with homework. Men, in contrast, "help out" with fun activities—going to the movies or the park.

Consider which dimensions of human sexuality influence the continuation of this phenomenon. What could be done to break out of stereotyped roles and create a more equal home environment?

Exploring Personal Dimensions

Are You Ready for Marriage?

The following quiz, developed by three clinical psychologists and marriage therapists, can help you decide whether marriage is right for you at this point in your life. Respond as honestly as you can to the following statements. Indicate which of the two choices more closely reflects your personal opinions and priorities by placing a check before line a or b. (If you have a mate, you might each fill out the quiz separately, and then compare your answers.)

1. _____ a I wouldn't feel alive unless I were married.
   _____ b Give me liberty or give me death.
2. _____ a My "favorite things to do" are typical of married people.
   _____ b My hobbies and interests are those of a single person.
3. _____ a Being married can give me more of the security I want.
   _____ b Being single can probably give me more of the career opportunities I want.
4. _____ a I'd love to vacation alone somewhere with my spouse.
   _____ b I'd love to vacation with different people at different times.
5. _____ a Married means being sexually content.
   _____ b Single means being sexually content.
6. _____ a I prefer the stability and security of married life.
   _____ b I prefer the self-reliance and adventure of single life.
7. _____ a I want sex and affection from one reliable person.
   _____ b I want a variety of lovers.
8. _____ a Marriage is underrated.
   _____ b Marriage is overrated.
9. _____ a I'm willing to work to make my spouse happy.
   _____ b I don't want to be responsible for my mate's happiness.

10. _____ a It's morally more correct to live a married life.
_____ b I'd like to do things when I want, without family constraints.
11. _____ a I'm ready to share my life and my credit cards.
_____ b I'm ready to share good times, but let's not get too serious.
12. _____ a I believe that people should be married.
_____ b I think people are happier if they are single.
13. _____ a Sex is best with one's spouse.
_____ b Sex is too delicious to limit it to one person.
14. _____ a My career plans can tolerate or maybe even benefit from my being married.
_____ b My career plans benefit from my being single.
15. _____ a I prefer the majority of my friends to be married.
_____ b I prefer the majority of my friends to be single.
16. _____ a A marriage can be a beautiful experience.
_____ b A marriage can be a trap.
17. _____ a I'd like to know whom I'll be sleeping with for the rest of my life.
_____ b I don't want to know whom I'll be sleeping with for the rest of my life.
18. _____ a Today's smart people are getting married.
_____ b Today's smart people are single and enjoying it.
19. _____ a The pleasures of marriage are wonderful.
_____ b The risk of a bad marriage more than offsets any pleasure.
20. _____ a "Love" and "marriage" go together.
_____ b "Love" and "independence" go together.
21. _____ a I don't mind sharing bank accounts and expenses.
_____ b I'm too independent to enjoy sharing my money with a spouse.
22. _____ a I want to pour all my love into a permanent relationship.
_____ b I'm not happy with an exclusive love relationship.
23. _____ a The economic advantages of being married are important to me.
_____ b I like the idea of being single so I can spend my money as I wish.
24. _____ a Being married is important from a moral/religious standpoint.
_____ b Morality and religion have little to do with marital status.
25. _____ a Lovemaking with one's spouse is certainly best.
_____ b The many sexual opportunities of being single are a great advantage.
26. _____ a My greatest chance for personal growth is through marriage.
_____ b My greatest chance for personal growth is through independence.
27. _____ a I'd prefer to share the risks of life with a spouse.
_____ b My privacy is too important for me to enjoy being married.
28. _____ a I want a reliable lifetime relationship in marriage.
_____ b I'd rather live free and easy and singly.
29. _____ a I'd be willing to make major changes, such as moving to another state, to help a spouse.
_____ b I'm not ready to move, or make other major changes, to help a spouse.

30. _____ a Marriages are made in heaven.
_____ b Marriages are too often made in hell.
31. _____ a My recreational interests are family oriented.
_____ b My recreational interests are for singles.
32. _____ a I'd enjoy the security involved in being married.
_____ b I prefer the freedom of being single.
33. _____ a I would love to have children.
_____ b I don't want the responsibility of a family.
34. _____ a Being married offers joint tax returns and other financial benefits.
_____ b I prefer to spend my money the way I want to.
35. _____ a I prefer sex and affection with my spouse for life.
_____ b I prefer love affairs with many people.
36. _____ a I prefer the steady companionship of being married.
_____ b I prefer the excitement of companionship with many lovers.
37. _____ a I'd enjoy spending leisure time with my spouse.
_____ b I like spending my leisure time as I please.
38. _____ a If I have to choose between career advancement and marriage, I choose marriage.
_____ b If I have to choose between career advancement and marriage, I'll take career.
39. _____ a Married people can count on sexual satisfaction from a trusted partner.
_____ b Single people can find lovers from an endless pool of possibilities.
40. _____ a Marriage requires major compromises, and I'm willing to make them.
_____ b Marriage requires major compromises, and I'm not yet ready to make them.

Scoring the Quiz

1. Count the number of your "a" responses and write the total here: _____
2. Compare your number of "a" responses with the following scale to determine your level.

0–20 = Low readiness
21–30 = Medium readiness
31–40 = High readiness

Interpreting Your Score

Low marriage readiness If you scored here, your values are heavily weighted toward a single lifestyle. Even if you've found a partner who shares your interests and values, the importance you attach to marriage at this time isn't enough to ensure success. Don't marry on the assumption that your values will change. They may not. And you shouldn't marry on the basis of other people's expectations or views about being married. *Yours* are the only ones that really count when it comes to marriage.

Though you may not value married life now, marriage readiness can develop rapidly. You may grow tired of the freedom and lifestyle that characterize being single, or come to appreciate more those elements associated with being married. Continue to review your marriage readiness from time to time, but do NOT marry until your values will support it.

Medium marriage readiness Your values blend support for both single and married lifestyles, which means there's a certain level of risk if you choose to get married at this time. Probably the most important issue for you to consider is your potential mate's marriage readiness. Someone with a high readiness level can add stability to the relationship, increasing the likelihood of its success. On the other hand, someone without it would dramatically reduce your already uncertain potential for a good marriage.

If he/she is less ready for marriage than you, be wary of demands for concessions. For example, he/she may say, in effect, "Do what I want or I'm getting out. I don't really want to be married as much as you do anyway." This is a destructive gambit; don't be pushed into a decision you're not ready to make.

A second major issue for you is the parity "fit" between you and your potential mate—your approximate equality in terms of personality, status, and appearance. Medium marriage readiness provides little cushion against the costs of an unequal match. High parity may lead to a successful marriage even if one or both partners possess only medium marriage readiness. But as the parity levels decrease, the greater the need for both partners to have a strong commitment to their marriage.

High marriage readiness Your values strongly support married life, and your only challenge will be to find the right match. Be on guard, however, against projecting your own high level of marriage readiness onto a potential mate. The key for you is to realize that although you may be ready, you still need to choose your partner wisely.

Sexuality Online

Go to the web component for *Exploring the Dimensions of Human Sexuality* at sexuality.jbpub.com for web exercises, additional resources related to this chapter, and student review tools.

Suggested Readings

Dornbusch, S. M., Herman, M. R., & Lin, I-C. Single parenthood, *Society, 33, no. 5* (1996), 30–32.

Howell, S. H., Portes, P. R., & Brown, J. H. Gender and age differences in child adjustment to parental separation, *Journal of Divorce and Remarriage, 27, no. 3–4* (1997), 141–158.

Hoyt, C. 22 minutes to a better marriage, *McCalls, 124* (Apr. 1997), 124+.

Johnson, D. R. & Booth, A. Marital quality: A product of the dyadic environment or individual factors? *Social Forces, 76, no. 3* (1998), 883–904.

Morrow-Kondos, D., Weber, J. A., Cooper, K., & Hesser, J. L. Becoming parents again: Grandparents raising children, *Journal of Gerontological Social Work, 28, no. 1–2* (1997), 35–46.

Pierce, A. R. Who's raising baby: Challenges to modern day parenting, *The World and I* (February 2002), 306–317.

Pontisso, D. A call for reform: The U.S. Commission on Child and Family Welfare report, *Children Today, 24, no. 2* (1997), 26–27.

Popenoe, D. & Whitehead, B. D. The state of our unions 2000: The social health of marriage in America, The National Marriage Project. Rutgers, The State University of New Jersey (2001). Available: http://marriage.rutgers.edu/state_of_our_unions%202000%20text%20only.htm

Schwartz, P. Love is not all you need, *Psychology Today* (May/June 2002), 56–58, 60–62.

CHAPTER

14 Sexually Transmitted Infections

FEATURES

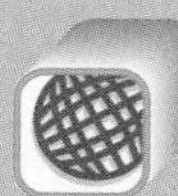

Global Dimensions
STIs Around the World

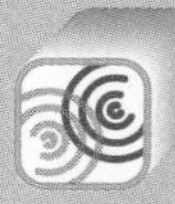

Communication Dimensions
Talking with a Partner About STI Prevention

Multicultural Dimensions
STIs and Minorities

Ethical Dimensions
Notifying Partners About STIs

CHAPTER OBJECTIVES

1. Define STIs and SRDs, describe how are they transmitted, and discuss the reasons for their prevalence.
2. Discuss the bacterially based STIs, including incidence, transmission, symptoms and complications, and diagnosis and treatment.
3. Discuss the virally based STIs, including incidence, transmission, symptoms and complications, and diagnosis and treatment.
4. Discuss the ectoparasitic infestations, including transmission, symptoms and complications, and diagnosis and treatment.
5. Describe ways that STIs and SRDs can be prevented.

sexuality.jbpub.com

Prevalence of Sexually Transmitted Infections
Bacterial Infections
Viral Infections

INTRODUCTION

Jessica was enrolled in one of our human sexuality classes. One day after class, she asked whether she could stop in during office hours to discuss something "private." Over the years, we have learned that "private" can mean many things: a student just found out she is pregnant, is being abused by a romantic partner, or is concerned about a sexual disorder. In Jessica's case, though, it was a concern that she might have an STI.

Jessica went on to describe a sexual encounter with Rodney that culminated in sexual intercourse. Shortly afterward, Jessica noticed a rash on her inner thighs and became alarmed. As soon as she described her concern about having contracted an STI, I knew I would have to refer Jessica to a physician at the campus health center for testing and diagnosis. I am an educator, not a medical doctor, and I know my limitations. Still, I could not refer her immediately for fear that she would think I was uninterested and be disinclined to discuss with me other concerns she might have in the future. Consequently, we discussed the reasons for her concern—the rash appeared, Rodney had not used a condom, they had not employed any other method of birth control, she met Rodney only the week before at a party and she did not really know him well—and we explored any other symptoms she described. Although I did not feel qualified to discuss whether Jessica had an STI, I did take advantage of our private time together to talk about the wisdom of coitus without the use of a condom and/or any other method of birth control and explored with her the decision to engage in coitus with someone she had only recently met.

It turned out that all Jessica had was a rash caused by nylon underpants she wore during her weekly jog. The relief on her face said it all, and I doubt that Jessica forgot that scare the next time she was faced with a decision regarding whether to engage in sex. That is not to say that she will refrain or become abstinent, although those are certainly possibilities and decisions others have made, but rather that she would understand better that any choice to engage in sexual activity is accompanied by both potentially pleasurable and potentially disturbing consequences—contracting an STI, one of those disturbing consequences, is always a possibility.

Although Jessica did not have an STI, we have encountered other students who did. Fortunately, most of those students were diagnosed early enough and treated successfully. This chapter describes the more common STIs, ways they can be prevented, and ways they are treated when they are not.

What Are Sexually Transmitted Infections?

sexually transmitted infections (STIs)
Infections that are primarily contracted through sexual contact.

sexually related diseases (SRDs)
Diseases of the reproductive system that can occur in either sexually active or sexually inactive individuals.

The term **sexually transmitted infections (STIs)** describes infections that can be contracted through sexual intimacy. Sexual intimacy includes oral–genital and anal sex, as well as vaginal intercourse. At least 20 STIs have been identified. There are also diseases of the sexual organs referred to as **sexually related diseases (SRDs),** which are disorders of the reproductive tract that occur in both sexually active and sexually abstinent individuals. These can be caused by organisms that live in the healthy body but under certain conditions, such as stress, diabetes, drug use, and other health-related problems, affect the delicate chemical balance of the body and cause disease conditions of the sexual organs. Some cancers are also considered to be SRDs. A sexually related infection can sometimes be transmitted to a sexual partner, and the conditions under which this occurs are discussed in this chapter.

Whatever the sexual disease, whether contracted during sexual activity or occurring in an abstinent individual, it affects the individual's feelings about his or her sexuality. Some people feel that anyone with a disease of the sexual organs is unclean, evil, and immoral; that a sexual disease is a punishment for sexual intimacy; and that only those of low socioeconomic and low educational status contract these diseases.

There is no truth to these beliefs. Organisms live in our bodies and can multiply when our resistance is low or, as mentioned earlier, when other conditions exist. Pathogenic organisms can sometimes adjust to their habitat, proliferate, and even change in ways that cause symptoms of disease. Not only can they affect the body of an infected individual, but they are sometimes transferred to another individual through sexual activity.

Prevalence of Sexually Transmitted Infections

Sexually transmitted infections have become quite common, even though we have seen a decline in the rates of some particular STIs. There are many reasons for the prevalence of STIs. For example, whereas most states require physicians to report to health departments HIV and AIDS, gonorrhea, and syphilis cases, this was not always the case. Therefore, to compare current STI rates with periods in which reporting was not required would certainly make it appear that there are more cases, in fact, there may not be. In addition, since the 1960s there has been a change in attitudes about sexual behav-

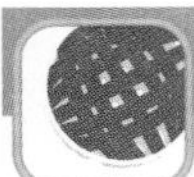

DIMENSIONS

STIs Around the World

There are wide variations in STIs around the world. Some countries have a high incidence; others have a lower one. The reasons for these differences may at first appear obvious but on further inspection are extremely complex. For example, it is assumed that lack of education is related to STIs, and, in fact, in some countries that is the case. Better educated people have access to information about STIs, their transmission, and their prevention. Furthermore, better educated people are more likely to have better paying jobs, allowing them to act on their STI knowledge (purchase condoms, for example). Yet, this is not always the case. For example, the World Health Organization (1998) cites Sub-Saharan Africa as the region of the world most affected by HIV. In the 44 countries of this region, the majority of the infections occur among the most literate men and women.

There are several possible explanations for this surprising finding. First, more schooling may be associated with a cultural change that is also associated with behaviors that increase the risk of disease. The World Health Organization states that this may be especially true for women, who without education may be less socially mobile and be exposed to a narrow spectrum of social and sexual relations. More education also means more money to support high-risk behaviors, such as paying for prostitutes or supporting a number of sexual partners.

The reason people contract STIs varies from country to country and even within subpopulations in any one country. The keys to preventing STIs at a policy level are understanding these differences and responding to them systematically.

ior. More frequent sex and earlier sex have meant an increase in the number of people subjected to STIs. Other variables include the following:

1. There is considerable social pressure for social and sexual contact, along with widespread ignorance about sexual health and disease transmission.
2. The traditional restraints on sexual behavior are weakening as families and society in general become more loosely knit. Families are more mobile; relocation can threaten the stability of family members as they move away from the support system offered by the extended family and community. Adolescents and young adults are now reared in an atmosphere favoring more personal freedom and less adult supervision. More and more families have two parents in the workforce; adolescent and young adult family members are frequently employed while attending school; and many more adolescents than in the past are unattended during certain times of the day.
3. Adolescence is a time of physical, psychological, and biochemical change and development. There is a wide range in the speed of adolescent development. Physiological maturing occurs at a faster rate than do intellectual, social, and emotional maturing. This places young people in a position of biological readiness for activities that have physical and emotional consequences for which they are not prepared. Often they face sexual decisions that affect their interests and they are not able to judge.
4. Current social values have led to widespread expectations of instant gratification. Learning, growing, and achieving goals require persistence; there seems to be a strong sense of urgency to act now, accompanied by a need for immediate satisfaction.

5. An "everybody-does-it" attitude undermines convictions about individual responsibility. Thus adolescents who feel stifled by external controls and are eager for independence often take actions, frequently sexual in nature, for which they are unprepared.
6. New modes of contraception have not eliminated unwanted pregnancy, but they have all but eliminated the fear of it. In the past this fear effectively inhibited sexual activity among many people of childbearing age.

One result of the combination of these factors has been an increase in sexual activity among most people—not just the young. This increase, in turn, has led to a rise in the incidence of STIs. There is no doubt that the risk of exposure is greater in people who are sexually active, especially with more than one person, because the chance of contracting an STI increases with the number of sexual contacts.

In spite of these social factors, and because of several other variables such as the fear of HIV infection, the rates of several STIs have decreased dramatically. However, accompanying this decrease in rates for some STIs is an increase in rates for others. The rates, signs, symptoms, potential complications, and means of diagnosing and treating the more prevalent STIs are presented in the following sections.

Bacterial Infections

Some STIs are caused by bacteria. Among these are gonorrhea, nongonococcal urethritis, chlamydia, and syphilis. It is not uncommon for these bacterial infections to be transmitted from one partner to the other, and treatment therefore often requires refraining from sexual activity until the bacteria have been eliminated.

Gonorrhea

Incidence

Gonorrhea ranks high on the list of reportable communicable diseases. Only chlamydia is more prevalent. The incidence of gonorrhea decreased from 1970 to 1996. However, it increased to 132 per 100,000 population in 1999 (Centers for Disease Control and Prevention, 2001) (Figure 14.1). The aver-

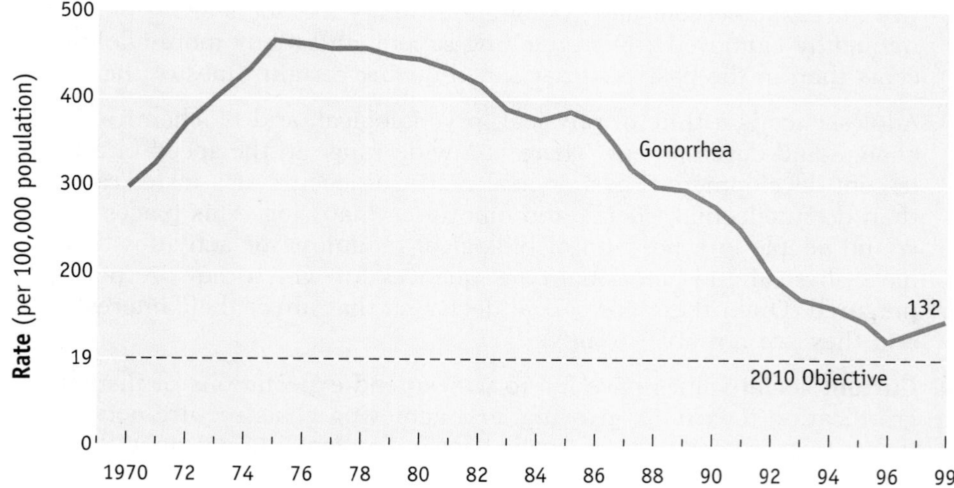

FIGURE 14.1 Gonorrhea—reported rates: United States, 1970–1999, and the Healthy People Year 2010 objective. *Source:* Division of STI Prevention. *Sexually transmitted disease surveillance, 1999.* U.S. Department of Health and Human Services, Public Health Service. Atlanta: Centers for Disease Control and Prevention (September 2000), 15.

age annual decrease in gonorrhea between 1986 and 1996 was about 25 cases per 100,000 persons. This decrease was consistent across gender and age (see Figure 14.2). In 1999 there were 360,076 cases of gonorrhea reported in the United States. Gonorrhea rates remain higher than the Healthy People 2010 national health objective of 19 new cases per 100,000 persons.

When gonorrhea rates are examined by race and ethnicity, wide variations are evident. In 1997, African Americans accounted for approximately 77% of reported cases of gonorrhea. The gonorrhea rates in 1999 were 803 cases per 100,000 for African Americans, 67 for Hispanics, and 27 for non-Hispanic whites. The gonorrhea rate for African-American adolescents 15 to 19 years of age was almost 25 times greater than the rate for white adolescents. African-American females aged 15 to 19 had a gonorrhea rate of 3,691, whereas African-American adolescents between 15 and 19 had a gonorrhea rate of 2,831 (Division of STI Prevention, 2000). Among 20- to 24-year-olds, the rate for African Americans was 30 times greater than for whites of the same age (3,426 versus 116, respectively).

To put these figures into perspective, it is expected that many other cases of gonorrhea are not reported because of the social stigma still associated with STIs and the reluctance of Americans to address sexual health in an open manner. Because gonorrhea can result in pelvic inflammatory disease, sterility, ectopic pregnancy, and other serious health conditions, the number of Americans subjected to these risks, in spite of the declining rate of gonorrhea, is still disturbing.

Transmission

Gonorrhea is caused by a bacterium known as ***Neisseria gonorrhoeae,*** also called *gonococcus*. This bacterium grows in the mucous membrane, the moist protective coat that lines all orifices (openings) of the body. The mucous membranes lining the mouth, throat, vagina, cervix, urethra, and anal canal are all very receptive to gonococcus. When contact occurs between the site of gonococcus in one person and the moist membrane of another—as in all forms of sexual activity—bacteria are transferred. Thus oral–vaginal, oral–anal, penile–anal, oral–penile, oral–oral, and genital–genital contact can result in the transmission of the disease from an infected person to the other partner. Out-

gonorrhea
A sexually transmitted infection that commonly starts with inflammation of the mucous membrane lining of the openings of the body (mouth, vagina, etc.).

Neisseria gonorrhoeae
The bacterium that causes gonorrhea; also known as *gonococcus*. Street names include "clap" and "drip."

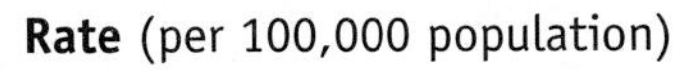

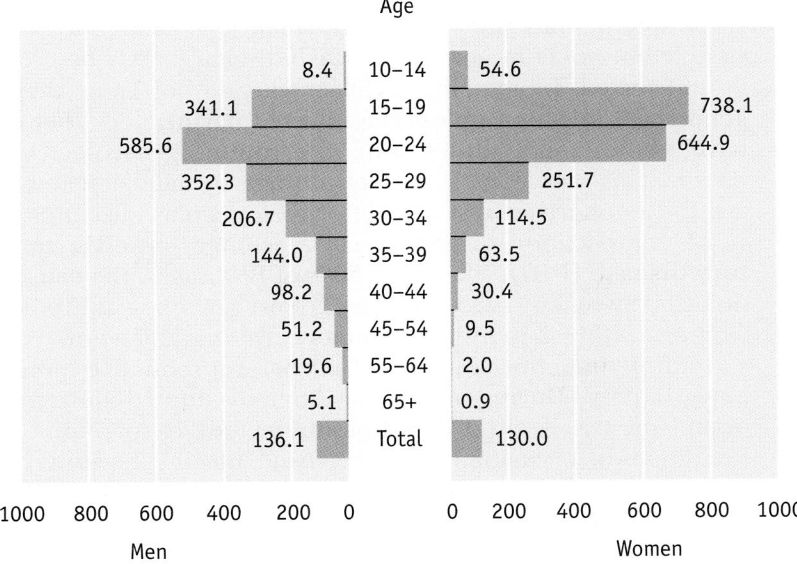

FIGURE 14.2 Gonorrhea—age- and gender-specific rates: United States, 1996. *Source:* Division of STI Prevention. *Sexually transmitted disease surveillance, 1999.* U.S. Department of Health and Human Services, Public Health Service. Atlanta: Centers for Disease Control and Prevention (September 2000), 21.

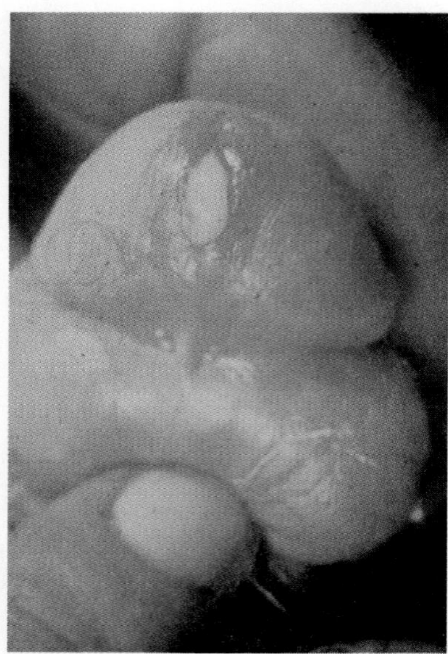

Although 90–95% of males with gonorrhea experience some symptoms, almost 80% of women are asymptomatic. For males, the gonorrhea "drip" is a common symptom.

side the body, however, the gonococcus dies in a few seconds, making it next to impossible to transmit the disease via toilet seats, cups, towels, or other articles used by an infected person. Interestingly enough, although bacteria travel from the mucous membrane of the infected partner to that of the uninfected partner, they sometimes die during transfer. Thus, exposure does not always result in infection. It is thought that a man has about a 10% chance of contracting gonorrhea from a single exposure to a partner with the infection. A woman, however, has a greater than 40% chance of contracting the disease from a single exposure, because the mucous membrane lining of the vagina, having a large surface area, is particularly receptive to gonococcus invasion. Any small irritations in the mucous lining can allow the organism rapid entry into the woman's system. For men and women, after multiple exposures to an infected individual the attack (infection) rate increases to 80% to 90% (Fiumara, 1987). Oral–genital sexual activity can result in *gonococcal pharyngitis* (gonorrhea of the throat) in either gender.

Symptoms and Complications

Males are more likely than females to exhibit symptoms of gonorrhea. It is estimated that 90% to 95% of men infected with gonorrhea have symptoms (Schwebke, 1991a; Smith, Schoonover, Lauver, & Allen, 1990). The males who exhibit symptoms do so within 2 to 10 days after contact; 3 to 5 days is the most likely interval. The primary sites in males are the urethra and the rectum. Symptoms include the sudden onset of frequent, painful urination (dysuria) and a discharge of pus from the urethra. Some males have tenderness in the groin area and noticeable swelling of lymph nodes. In anal gonorrhea, symptoms include membrane irritation, discharge, and painful defecation.

Complications in the male are seen within 2 to 3 weeks without treatment. Infection spreads up the *genitourinary tract,* the posterior urethra, the prostate, the seminal vesicles, and the epididymis. Sometimes acute inflammation of the prostate occurs, accompanied by pelvic tenderness and pain, fever, and urinary retention. Inflammation of the epididymis may occur; it can be recognized by a feeling of heaviness in the affected testicle, inflammation of the scrotal skin, and sometimes swelling in the lower part of the testicles. If the gonococcal infection spreads to the other testicle, infertility is a possible complication.

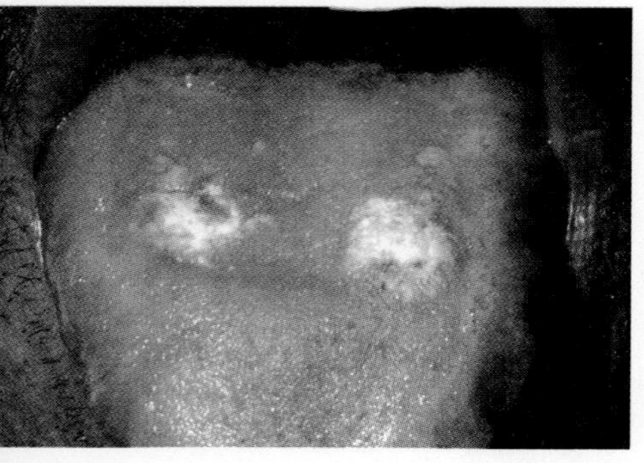

Gonorrhea lesions on the tongue.

As many as 80% of the females who contract gonorrhea have no symptoms. The cervix is the primary infection site in females, and although it may be inflamed, symptoms may not be evident. Inflammation of the Bartholin's glands is possible but not common. A yellowish discharge may be present but may remain undetected. In actuality most females do not know they have a gonorrheal infection unless the infected partner tells them or they have a smear and culture done in a routine gynecological examination. This fact alone should encourage sexually active women to ask for a gonorrhea test as part of their regular checkups.

A complication of gonorrhea in women is **pelvic inflammatory disease (PID).** In 33% to 50% of PID cases, the cause is gonorrhea (Swinker, 1985). If the gonorrhea goes untreated in a woman, within 2 months the gonococcal organisms may cause an ascending infection into the internal reproductive organs and pelvic cavity. During menstruation and immediately after, the organisms travel rapidly. Symptoms include dyspareunia (painful intercourse), occasional nonmenstrual uterine bleeding, inflammation of the fallopian tubes with subsequent tubal infection, vaginal discharge, general abdominal pain, and fever up to 102°F. PID is a common complication in women. As the body defenses try to

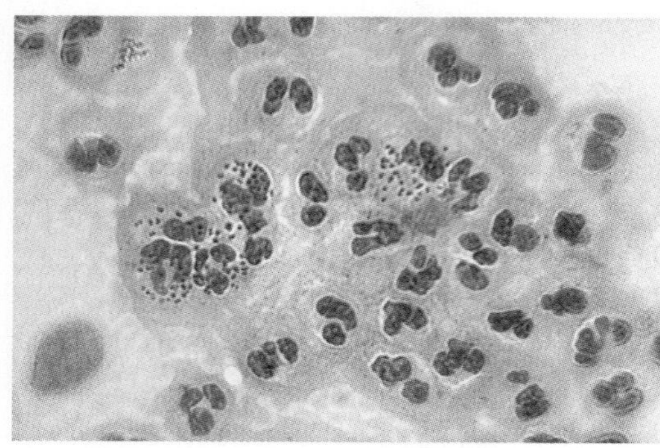

Neisseria gonorrhoeae is the cause of gonorrhea.

wall off the infection, scarring of the fallopian tubes can occur and infertility can result.

Extragenital complications of gonorrhea (those that occur in areas other than the genitals) include *gonococcal arthritis* and *gonococcal dermatitis.* These are sometimes referred to as *disseminated gonococcal infection.* Gonococcal arthritis affects the hands, wrists, ankles, knees, and elbows. Gonorrhea is the primary cause of arthritis in pregnant women and the most common cause of infectious arthritis in the United States. Gonococcal dermatitis, a rash, is most frequently seen on the hands and lower extremities. White blisters appear and eventually darken, leaving the body without scars. *Gonococcal endocarditis,* inflammation of the heart valves, is a serious but rare gonorrheal complication. Finally, *gonococcal ophthalmic infection* can occur in the newborn; that complication has been reduced by treating the eyes of all babies with silver nitrate tetracycline, or penicillin, at birth.

Diagnosis and Treatment

The most accurate method of diagnosing gonorrhea is by means of a culture of discharges taken from various body sites. In the male the urethra is the most common site of infection, and a sample of the discharge should be taken there. Throat and rectal cultures are taken if the patient's sexual activity with an infected person involves these body areas. In the female the discharge sample is taken with a cotton-tipped applicator inserted into the cervical opening, because the environment in this area is optimal for gonococcus. Other sites from which cultures can be developed are the throat, rectum, and vagina. When gonococci are present, approximately 96% of the organism is isolated in these areas.

For many years the treatment of choice for gonorrhea was penicillin. In 1976, however, a strain of gonococcus resistant to all forms of penicillin appeared (Antibiotic-resistant strains, 1987). Called **penicillinase-producing *N. gonorrhoeae* (PPNG),** this organism produces a substance that inactivates penicillin. PPNG was originally linked to foreign travel, but this is no longer the case. Today the number of reported cases of PPNG in the United States continues to rise, as infections are reported in a vast majority of the states.

Three additional resistant strains of gonorrhea have also appeared. The first is known as **chromosomally mediated–resistant *N. gonorrhoeae* (CMRNG),** an organism that contains intranuclear DNA capable of rendering its cell membrane impermeable to penicillin (Fiumara, 1987). The second strain is **tetracycline-resistant *N. gonorrhoeae* (TRNG).** This strain of gonorrhea, similar to PPNG, produces a substance that inactivates tetracycline. The third resistant strain is **ciprofloxacin-resistant *N. gonorrhoeae.*** This strain, discovered in 1991, is resistant to the new drug ciprofloxacin. Approximately 6% of gonorrhea bacteria were found to be PPNG-resistant, 9% were CMRGN-resistant, 14% were TRNG-resistant, and 0.04% were resistant to ciprofloxacin. That amounts to approximately 29% of gonorrhea cases resistant to some antimicrobial treatment.

The current treatment of choice for gonorrhea consists of an intramuscular injection of the drug ceftriaxone or 500 mg of ciprofloxacin administered orally. Other drugs have also been used, such as cefixime, ofloxacin, and doxycycline, all of which are administered orally. Because it is suspected that over half of those infected with gonorrhea have a coexisting chlamydial infection, a dual-therapy regimen that includes a drug for the gonorrheal infection as well as doxycycline or azithromycin for the chlamydial infection has been recommended. As with all drug regimens, special populations, for example, pregnant women, require special precautions and alterations.

pelvic inflammatory disease (PID)
Infection of the reproductive organs, particularly the uterus and fallopian tubes, and the pelvic cavity.

penicillinase-producing *N. gonorrhoeae* (PPNG)
Strain of gonococcus resistant to all forms of penicillin.

chromosomally mediated–resistant *N. gonorrhoeae* (CMRNG)
Strain of gonorrhea resistant to penicillin because its DNA makes its cell membrane impermeable to penicillin.

tetracycline-resistant *N. gonorrhoeae* (TRNG)
Strain of gonorrhea that produces a substance that inactivates tetracycline.

ciprofloxacin-resistant *N. gonorrhoeae*
Strain of gonorrhea resistant to the drug ciprofloxacin.

Nongonococcal Urethritis

nongonococcal urethritis (NGU) Inflammation of the urethra caused by *Chlamydia trachomatis,* and *Ureaplasma urealyticum, Mycoplasma hominis, Trichomonas vaginalis,* herpes simplex virus, and unknown organisms.

Chlamydia trachomatis An intracellular parasite that causes chlamydial infections.

chlamydia A term that encompasses several major diseases caused by *Chlamydia trachomatis,* including genitourinary tract infection, a type of conjunctivitis in newborns, a type of pneumonia in infants, lymphogranuloma venereum, and trachoma.

Incidence

Nongonococcal urethritis (NGU) and its potential companion, *nongonococcal cervicitis* (in females), are STIs characterized by inflammation of the urethra and cervix, respectively. The signs and symptoms of NGU are similar to those of gonorrhea. If there are indications of urethritis and a laboratory test rules out gonorrhea, NGU is diagnosed.

Before the 1990s this condition was called *nonspecific urethritis* because its causes were unknown. Today researchers have been able to identify several organisms that are believed to cause NGU. Approximately 30% to 40% of NGU cases are caused by *Chlamydia trachomatis. Ureaplasma urealyticum, Mycoplasma hominis, Trichomonas vaginalis,* and herpes simplex virus are thought to be the causative agents in another 30% to 40% of cases. The cause of the remaining cases is still unknown (Sexually transmitted disease summary, 1990).

Symptoms

NGU symptoms in males include discharge from the penis and a burning sensation during urination. Women who have NGU-related infection sometimes report a mild vaginal irritation, burning, or discharge. At least 70% of infected women, however, are believed to be asymptomatic. Additionally, it is estimated that 10% of infected men may be asymptomatic (Fiumara, 1986a). NGU is not a reportable communicable disease so we have no official count of cases in the United States. It is estimated that cases of NGU equal or surpass those of gonorrhea, ranging from 2 to 5 million cases annually (Cancila, 1986; Problems arise with the "other STIs," 1987).

Treatment

Treatment consists of either 100 mg of doxycycline taken twice a day for 7 days or a single dosage of 1 g of azithromycin, both administered orally. Alternatively, erythromycin or ofloxacin may be used.

Chlamydia

Incidence

Chlamydial infections, caused by the intracellular parasite ***Chlamydia trachomatis,*** are the most common STIs in the United States today. The Centers for Disease Control and Prevention (CDC) of the Department of Health and Human Services states that because case reporting remains incomplete, estimating the total number of **chlamydia** cases is extremely difficult. However, in 1999 there were 659,441 chlamydial infections reported (Division of STI Prevention, 2000). From 1987 through 1999 reported cases of chlamydia increased from 51 cases per 100,000 persons to 254 cases per 100,000 (see Figure 14.3). This increase reflects increased screening, recognition of the nature of asymptomatic infection (especially in women), as well as actual increases in the disease. In 1991 treatment for chlamydial infections cost more than $1 billion in health care costs (Stein, 1991).

Reported cases of chlamydia in women far exceed reported cases in men (405 cases per 100,000 to 95 per 100,000, respectively). Rates for women are highest in the 15- to 19-year-old age group (2,484 per 100,000 persons) and for 20- to 24-year-olds (2,187 per 100,000) (see Figure 14.4).

Chlamydial infection is an umbrella term that encompasses four major diseases caused by *C. trachomatis:* (1) a genitourinary tract infection in adults, (2) inclusion conjunctivitis (an acute eye infection) in newborns and chlamydial pneumonia in infants, (3) trachoma (a chronic eye infection), and (4) lymphogranuloma venereum. The two diseases of most concern in the

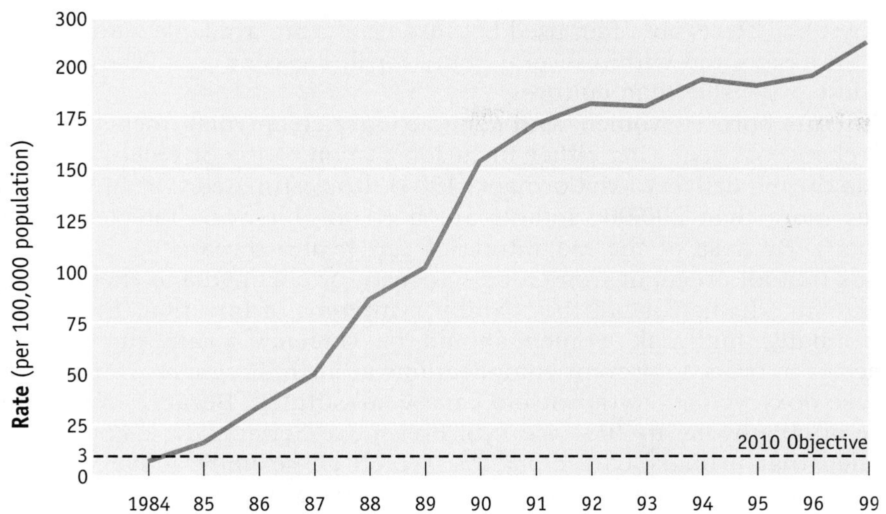

FIGURE 14.3 Chlamydia—reported rates: United States, 1984–1999. *Source:* Division of STI Prevention. *Sexually transmitted disease surveillance, 1999.* U.S. Department of Health and Human Services, Public Health Service. Atlanta: Centers for Disease Control and Prevention (September 2000), 10.

United States are adult genitourinary tract infection and infant conjunctivitis and pneumonia (Hopkins, 1983).

Symptoms and Complications

Genitourinary tract chlamydial infection has been called "the silent STI." Early symptoms of this infection are often mild and therefore unrecognized. Approximately 75% of infected people are asymptomatic. Symptoms, in those who exhibit them, occur 1 to 3 weeks after exposure. In men the most common symptoms include pain or burning on urination and a white, watery discharge from the penis. Women may note painful urination, a vaginal discharge, and abdominal pain.

Diagnoses and Treatment

To diagnose chlamydia, a layer of cells is scraped from the affected area. One of three tests is then used. A culture test for chlamydia is preferred by the CDC because of its sensitivity and specificity. Rapid assay tests and fluores-

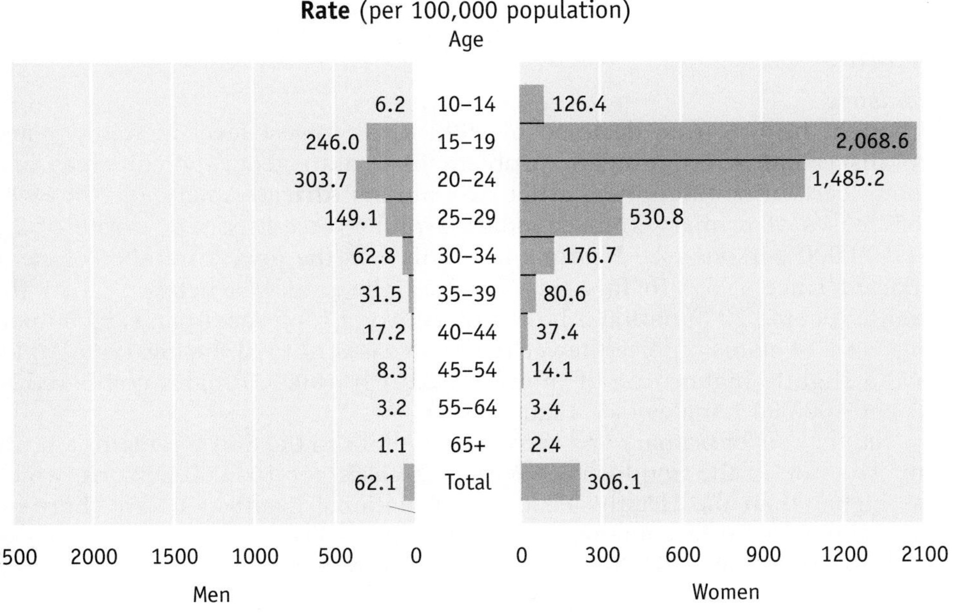

FIGURE 14.4 Chlamydia—age- and gender-specific rates: United States, 1999. *Source:* Division of STI Prevention. *Sexually transmitted disease surveillance, 1999.* U.S. Department of Health and Human Services, Public Health Service. Atlanta: Centers for Disease Control and Prevention (September 2000), 13.

cent antibody tests are often used because results are available within 15 minutes for assays and within several hours for fluorescent tests. These tests are also less expensive than cultures.

Infants born to women with genitourinary chlamydial infections have a 70% chance of acquiring either inclusion conjunctivitis or chlamydial pneumonia during delivery (McCormack, 1984). It is estimated that in the United States more than 200,000 infants are born to chlamydia-infected mothers annually. Because of the magnitude of this health threat, the CDC recommends that all pregnant women be screened for chlamydia at their first prenatal visit, whether or not they exhibit symptoms of infection (Stein, 1991). Additionally, high-risk women should be screened again in their third trimester in order to prevent complications at birth. Pregnant women should not use doxycycline; erythromycin can be substituted. Because of the prevalence of chlamydia, in 2001 the U.S. Preventive Services Task Force recommended that primary care clinicians screen all sexually active women 25 years of age and younger for chlamydia as part of regular health care visits (Agency for Healthcare Research and Quality, 2001).

Treatment

Chlamydial infections are easily treated in their early stages. The treatment of choice is a single 1-g dosage of azithromycin administered orally or 100 mg of doxycycline administered orally twice a day for 7 days. Alternatively, either erythromycin or ofloxacin may be used. To minimize the risk of reinfection, patients are asked to refer their sexual partners for evaluation, testing, and treatment and to refrain from sexual intercourse with any partners who have not been treated. Reinfection is of prime importance. Researchers have found that nearly 20% of teenage women who have had a chlamydial infection are reinfected within 2 years (Xu, et al., 2000). In fact, women aged 15 to 19 years old are four times as likely as 30- to 44-year-old women to have one repeat infection and five times as likely to be reinfected at least twice.

Unfortunately, because of the asymptomatic nature of the infection and the similarity of symptoms for chlamydia and gonorrhea, many cases of chlamydia are either improperly treated or untreated. Untreated chlamydia can lead to PID in women and to epididymitis in men. In both genders the possibility of sterility exists. Screening is therefore recommended for persons with more than one sex partner, and especially for women younger than 35 years old (NIAID, 1987a).

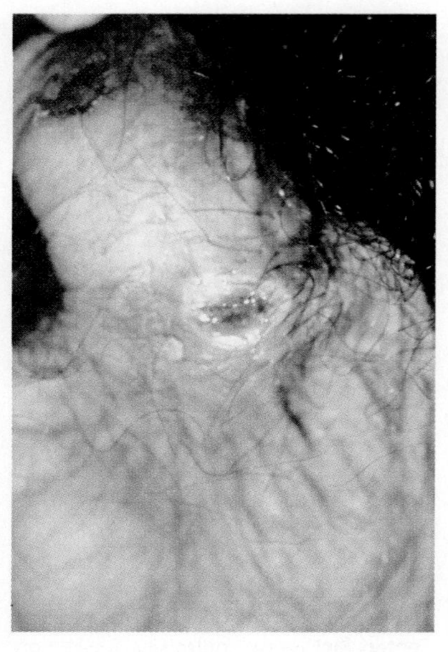
Chancres of primary syphilis on penis.

Syphilis

Incidence

Although the U.S. rate declined in 1999 to its lowest level in many years, syphilis remains a significant problem in certain geographical areas and among certain populations, particularly among African-Americans. In 1999, 6,657 cases of primary and secondary syphilis were reported, a rate of 2.5 per 100,000 persons (see Figure 14.5). This was the lowest number of cases reported since 1959. In fact, in 39 states, the rate was below that of the Healthy People 2000 national health objective of four cases per 100,000 persons, and 14 states reported fewer than five cases in total during 1999. Males have a slightly higher rate of infection: 2.9 per 100,000 males compared to 2.0 per 100,000 females (see Figure 14.6).

Yet, the rate of primary and secondary syphilis in the South remains a problem. The rate in the South in 1999 was 4.5 cases per 100,000 persons, which was higher than the Healthy People 2000 national health objective. Furthermore, the national rate among African-Americans was a disturbing 15.2 cases per 100,000 persons: 30 times greater than the rate for non-Hispanic whites.

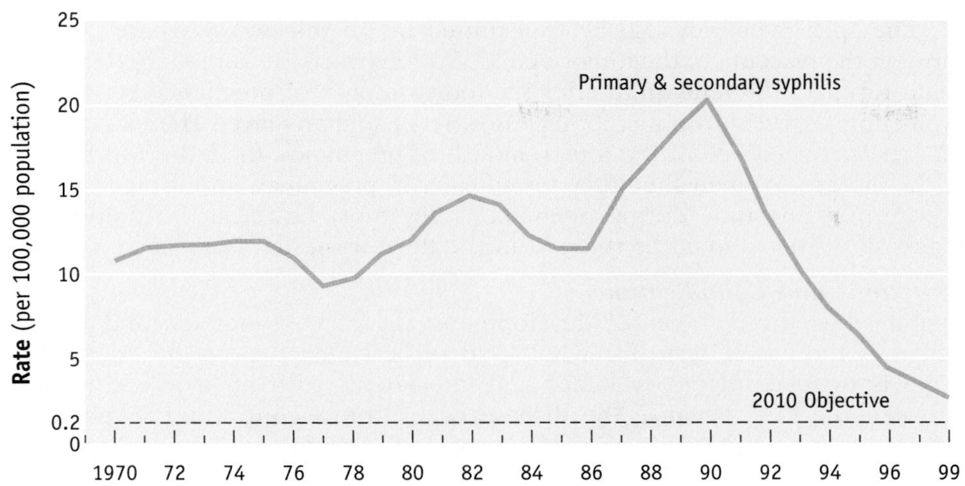

FIGURE 14.5 Primary and secondary syphilis—reported rates: United States, 1970–1999, and the Healthy People Year 2010 objective. *Source:* Division of STI Prevention. *Sexually transmitted disease surveillance, 1999.* U.S. Department of Health and Human Services, Public Health Service. Atlanta: Centers for Disease Control and Prevention (September 2000), 29.

Also of concern is congenital syphilis (that acquired prenatally or at birth). Although rates of congenital syphilis have also declined, in 1999 the rate was 14.3 cases per 100,000 live births. This was lower than the 1998 rate of 21.6. Yet, eight states reported increases in their congenital syphilis rates between 1998 and 1999, and 22 states reported a rate of more than five cases in 1999. In 1999, 28 states had congenital syphilis rates that exceeded the Healthy People 2010 national health objective of 1 case per 100,000 live births (Division of STI Prevention, 2000).

Transmission

The cause of **syphilis** is *Treponema pallidum,* a spirochete organism that requires a warm, moist area to survive. The **spirochete** is thin and corkscrew-shaped and is transmitted from the open lesions of the infected person to the mucous membranes or cuts in the skin of the other person. The organism can be transmitted by vaginal, anal, or oral–genital contact. Only a few hours after the time of contact, the spirochete reaches the bloodstream of the newly infected person.

syphilis
An STI caused by the spirochete *Treponema pallidum.*

spirochete
A spiral-shaped bacterium, one of which, *Treponema pallidum,* causes syphilis.

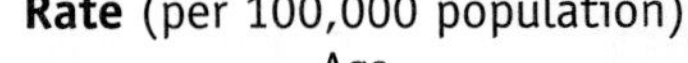

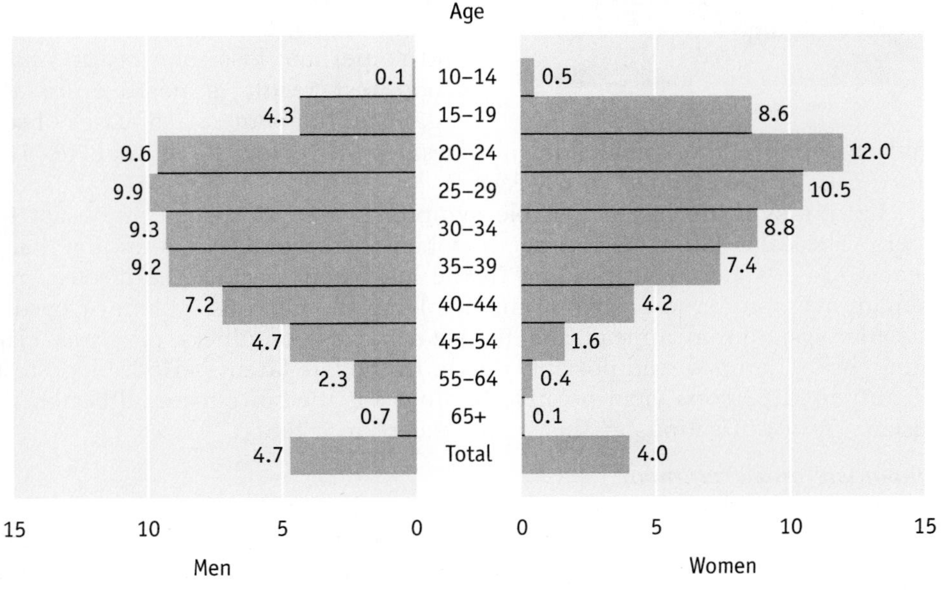

FIGURE 14.6 Primary and secondary syphilis—age- and gender-specific rates: United States, 1999. *Source:* Division of STI Prevention. *Sexually transmitted disease surveillance, 1996.* U.S. Department of Health and Human Services, Public Health Service. Atlanta: Centers for Disease Control and Prevention (September 2000), 33.

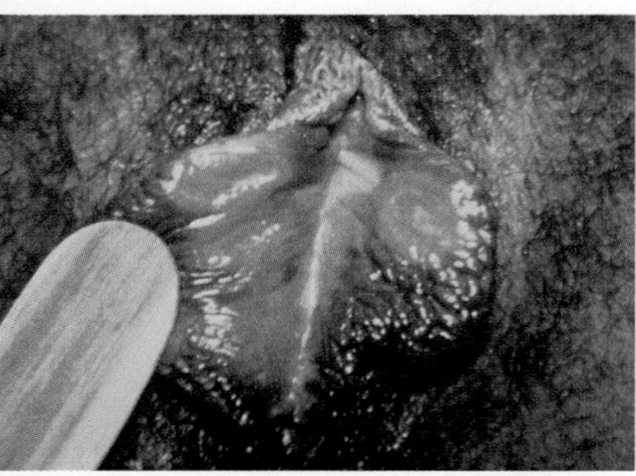

A chancre is symptomatic of the primary stage of syphilis. Often, though, the chancre can appear on hidden parts of the female genital areas, making the disease asymptomatic by appearance. A woman who suspects that her partner has syphilis should therefore request a medical exam or test.

The spirochete can also be transmitted by an infected pregnant woman through the placenta to the unborn child. Syphilis bacteria cannot cross the placenta to infect the fetus until after the fourth month of pregnancy because of protection provided by a membrane known as Langhan's layer. Therefore, if the mother is treated before the fourth month of pregnancy, the baby will be free of the disease. Women should be tested early in pregnancy, and if they suspect exposure at any time during pregnancy, they must be retested. Additionally, high-risk women should be retested in the third trimester (Schwebke, 1991b).

Symptoms and Complications

Syphilis has three stages of development: primary, secondary, and latent. *Latent* is the newer term for what used to be called the *tertiary* stage; this stage is divided into early latent and late latent, with no true delineation between the two, because the disease occurs on a continuum. Syphilis is infectious during the primary, secondary, and early latent stages.

Primary syphilis manifests itself by the appearance of a painless lesion, called a ***chancre.*** The chancre can appear from 10 to 90 days after exposure; on an average it appears in 21 days. Usually one lesion forms, generally on the glans penis in the male and the cervix in the female; however, the walls of the vagina and the tissues of the labia can also be sites of chancres. Because the lesions occur most frequently on hidden genital areas, they often remain undetected. Lesions can also appear on the nipples, anus, scrotum, or mouth.

Unfortunately the chancre disappears with or without treatment within 2 to 6 weeks. A person who suspects that he or she has been exposed to syphilis should have a blood test and not assume that the disappearance of the lesion means absence of the disease. During the primary stage, however, a blood test result may be negative; thus the test should be repeated. If possible, material exuding from a lesion suspected of being syphilitic should be examined under a microscope in what is called the *darkfield technique.* Sometimes this procedure, too, is repeated.

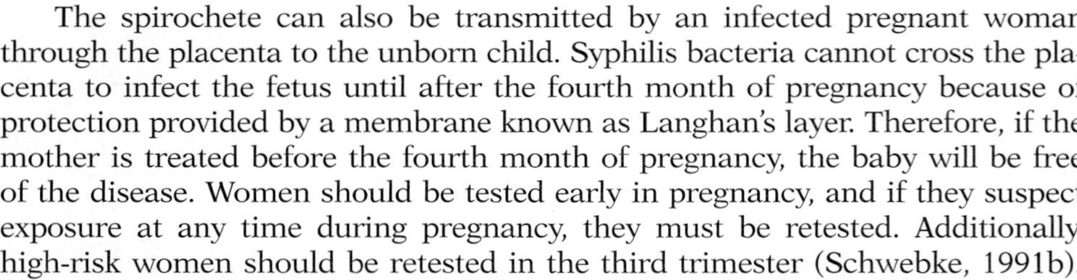

In the secondary stage of syphilis, a generalized rash can appear on the body 6 weeks to several months after initial exposure. Although the rash disappears within a few weeks, medical treatment should be sought for the underlying syphilis bacteria, *Treponema pallidum.*

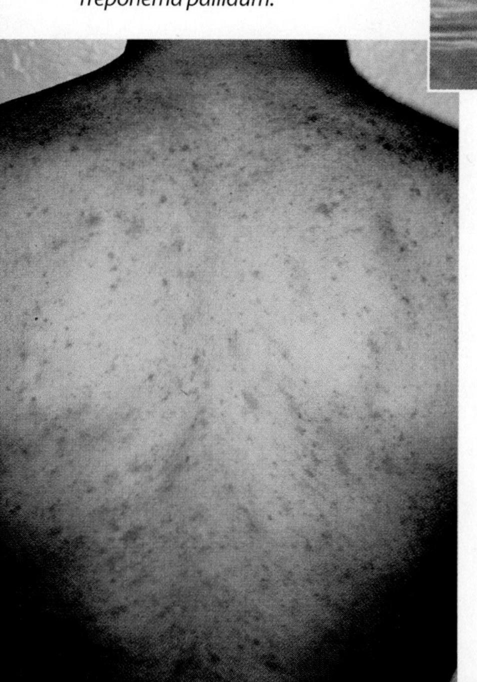

Secondary syphilis is usually characterized by a generalized rash that appears on the body 6 weeks to several months after initial exposure. The rash does not itch, and it too subsides without treatment. Sometimes in this stage mucous patches are found in the mouth. A dull, depressed feeling; fever; and some hair loss may occur, and a blood test result is positive for the organism. In about 25% of cases of secondary syphilis, the spinal fluid also tests positive for the spirochete. This stage usually lasts from 2 to 6 weeks.

Latent syphilis has no visible symptoms, and this stage may last for years. The early latent period begins when the secondary symptoms disappear and ends 1 to 4 years later. In the late latent period, the disease may remain asymptomatic or symptoms involving the nervous system or cardiovascular system may appear. The disease can cause blindness, paralysis, crippling, brain damage, and possibly death. In the late latent period, blood tests of untreated persons yield positive findings for the spirochete, although the disease is not infectious at this stage (except to a fetus).

Diagnosis and Treatment

As noted, early diagnosis is made through a darkfield microscope examination of the material exuding from the chancre or rash, if possible, and through blood testing. The current treatment of choice is 2.4 million units of benzathine penicillin G, usually in one megadose, injected into the buttocks muscles. Because this penicillin is excreted from the body slowly, a constant level of the drug is maintained in the blood for a number of days.

Viral Infections

Some STIs are caused by viruses. Among these are herpes genitalis, hepatitis B, and genital warts. These STIs are among the most difficult to eradicate because the viruses that cause them remain in the body even after symptoms subside. However, as we discuss, there are effective treatments for viral STIs.

Herpes Genitalis

Incidence

The cause of **genital herpes** is a virus called ***herpes simplex virus (HSV)***, which belongs to a family of more than 70 herpesviruses. Humans play host to four herpesviruses:

1. Herpes simplex virus, the agent for fever blisters and genital herpes
2. Cytomegalovirus, a virus that can cause death or retardation if acquired by a fetus
3. Varicella-zoster virus, the agent that causes chickenpox and shingles
4. Epstein-Barr virus, the agent of Burkitt's lymphoma in humans

primary syphilis
The first stage of syphilis most generally manifested by the appearance of a painless lesion called a *chancre*.

chancre
A painless lesion that is symptomatic of the primary stage of syphilis and appears at the site of contact.

secondary syphilis
The second stage of syphilis, characterized by a rash.

latent syphilis
A stage of syphilis that may last for years: early latent (about 1 to 4 years in duration) and late latent (may last for years), may be symptom-free or cause degenerative complications.

genital herpes
An STI characterized by tiny fluid-filled blisters that appear on the genitals and in the genital tract.

herpes simplex virus (HSV)
The virus that causes oral and genital herpes infections.

Communication DIMENSIONS

Talking with a Partner About STI Prevention

Many of our students react incredulously when we suggest they speak with a potential partner about STIs before engaging in sex. "It would ruin the moment," they argue. In frustration, we sometimes respond, "Contract an STI and then let us know about ruining the moment!" If that were all we offer our students, they would be right to be angry. Instead, we also provide them with suggestions to communicate with a potential sexual partner about preventing STIs:

- Begin the conversation before matters are "hot and heavy." Once people are sexually excited, it is more difficult for them to make sensible decisions or to participate in meaningful conversation.
- Make inspecting genitalia part of sexual play. Laughter, soft touch, and expressions of admiration can make the moment enjoyable rather than clinical.
- Suggest that your partner examine you for signs of disease first. This will make it less threatening when it is your partner's turn to be examined.
- Discuss your prior sexual history, as it relates to STI risk, with your partner before asking your partner to share his or her history. Engage in this discussion by disclosing as much detail as you feel comfortable discussing. If expressed in an erotic manner, this discussion can be sexually stimulating as it concurrently accomplishes the purpose of preventing exposure to disease-causing organisms.
- Demonstrate effective communication skills. Lean forward, nod your head, and look your partner in the eyes to communicate interest. Periodically paraphrase what your partner has said and what you guess he or she is feeling to demonstrate you have been listening. Do not interrupt, raise your voice, or frown in a way that interferes with your partner's communication.

There are ways to make communicating about STIs less embarrassing, less confrontational, and more effective. Discussing STIs with sexual partners is important. Your very health, maybe even your life, may depend on it!

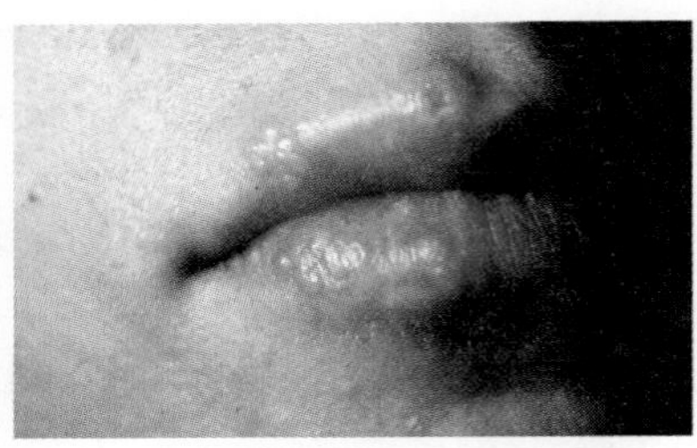

Herpes simplex virus 1 can manifest itself as a cold sore.

In 1961, it was found that two types of HSV exist; type 1 (HSV-1) is seen more frequently in areas of the body above the waist; type 2 (HSV-2) is seen more frequently below the waist. Although most cases of recurrent genital herpes (70%) are caused by type 2, 5% to 30% are caused by type 1. In addition, genital herpes can also appear above the waist. For example, when HSV is transmitted through oral–genital sex, a sore may appear on the mouth.

Most patients who experience a first episode of HSV-2 infection experience recurrent episodes of genital lesions. However, clinical recurrences are much less frequent for HSV-1 infection than for HSV-2 infection. Therefore, identifying the causative agent has implications for treatment and counseling. For patients who have frequent recurrences of lesions (six or more recurrences a year), daily oral administration of acyclovir (400 mg twice a day) can decrease the rate of recurrence by 75% or greater.

Genital herpes has been diagnosed in 45 million Americans (Division of STI Prevention, 2000); many other cases remain undiagnosed (Figure 14.7). The Year 2010 national health objectives set a goal of reducing the incidence of genital herpes from 17% of the population to 14%. It is believed that 50% of pregnant women have antibodies to herpes that have developed as a result of a past contact with a herpesvirus and pass the antibodies to their unborn child through the placenta. Possibly as many as 70% of children 10 to 14 years of age have herpes antibodies, and by 50 years of age about 90% of people have such antibodies, which indicate that they have had some contact with a herpesvirus.

Symptoms and Complications

A herpes infection may be categorized into four stages (Fiumara, 1986b). **Primary herpes genitalis** corresponds with the time of actual infection by the herpesvirus and the formation of antibodies. A primary (first occurrence) herpes infection can be very painful but can also be completely symptom free. Less than 40% of those infected experience noticeable signs and symptoms. The other infected individuals become carriers of the herpesvirus and are unaware of their infection (Johnson, et al., 1989). The time between exposure and development of the primary infection is 2 to 20 days, with an average of 6 days (Smith, Lauver, & Allen, 1990). In women the cervix is the main site of infection, although the vagina and vulva may also be involved. Symptoms include painful lesions, a sluggish feeling, and fever, along with possible lymph-node enlargement. Tiny blisters form, filled with a clear fluid in which the virus thrives. The area may become reddened and infected, and when blisters appear the site is in its most infectious state. The open lesions

primary herpes genitalis
The first stage of a genital herpes infection; it begins with infection by the herpesvirus and the formation of antibodies. Common symptoms include painful lesions in or around the genital area, a sluggish feeling, fever, and possibly swollen lymph nodes. Up to 75% of infected persons may be asymptomatic in the primary stage.

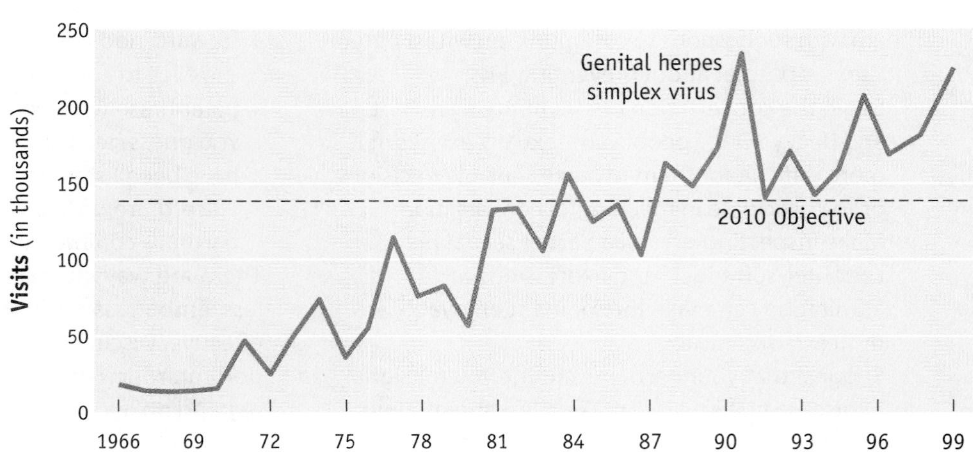

FIGURE 14.7 Genital herpes simplex virus infections—initial visits to physicians' offices: United States, 1966–1999, and the Healthy People Year 2010 objective. *Source:* Division of STI Prevention. *Sexually transmitted disease surveillance, 1999.* U.S. Department of Health and Human Services, Public Health Service. Atlanta: Centers for Disease Control and Prevention (September 2000), 36.

crust over as healing begins. In men, blisters and ulcers appear on the glans penis and the shaft, and urethritis may also develop. In both genders blisters sometimes appear on the thighs and buttocks. Some people experience itching, tingling, or burning sensations where a lesion will appear, known as the **prodrome.**

Once antibodies are formed the virus enters the **latent herpes genitalis** stage. Antibodies do not protect against reinfection, but they do tend to make any recurrent infection less severe. During the latent stage the herpesvirus travels up the afferent nerve to the sacral ganglion, where it remains inactive (Figure 14.8). At this point in the infection there are no signs and symptoms and transmission of the virus is believed to be rare.

prodrome
Itching, tingling, or burning sensations occur where a herpes lesion will appear.

latent herpes genitalis
In the stage of genital herpes characterized by inactivity of the herpesvirus an infected individual is asymptomatic and transmission of the virus is rare.

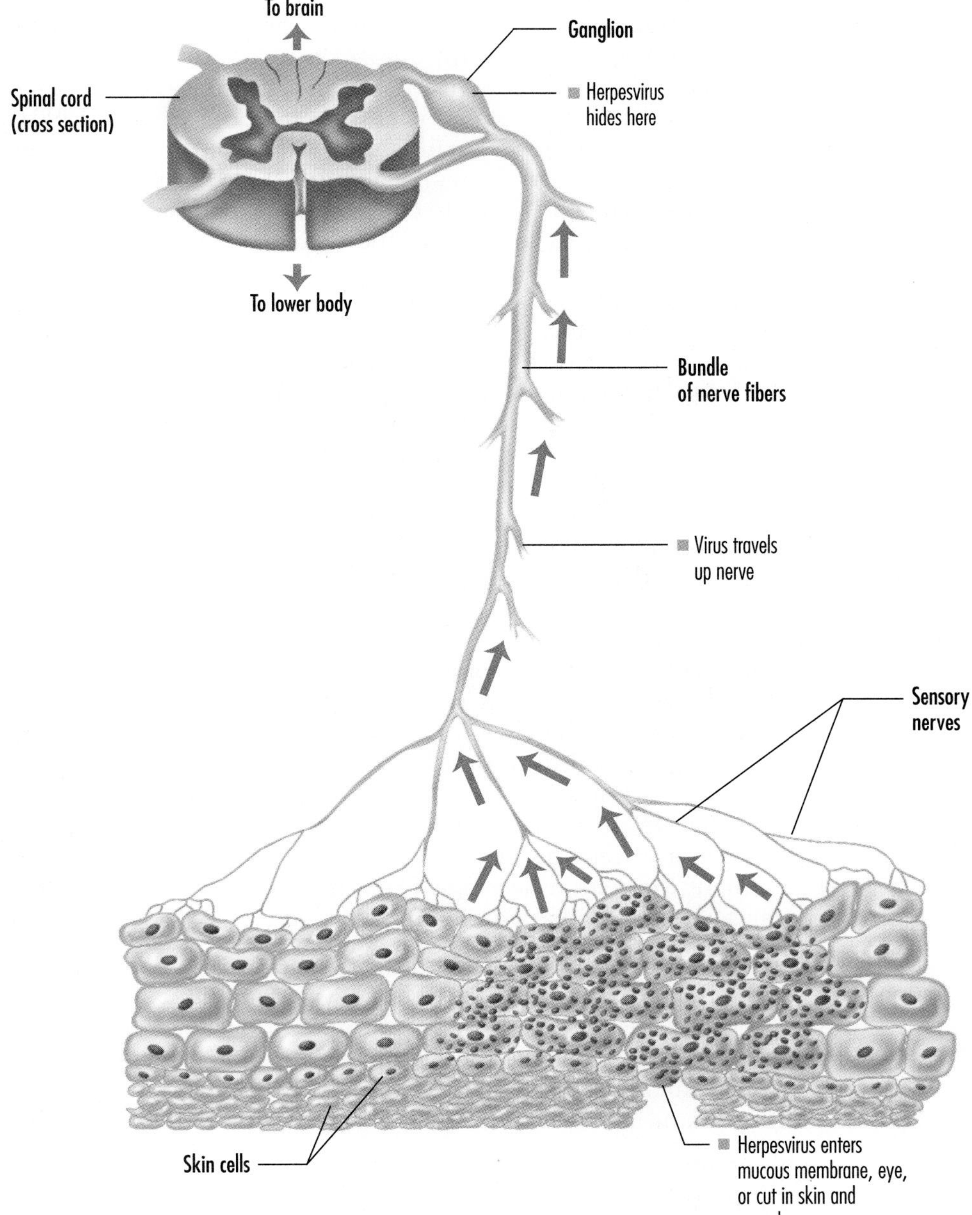

FIGURE 14.8 An initial herpes infection takes place when the virus (dots) enters cells of the mucous membranes, eyes, or skin. It reproduces and travels up (arrows) the sensory nerves until it reaches a ganglion (cluster of nerve cell bodies). There it hides, protected from attack by the body's immune system, which overcomes the infection at the place of entry. Though the entry wound soon heals, when conditions allow, the virus may later travel back down the nerve pathway to reinfect skin cells.

shedding herpes genitalis
During the third stage of a genital herpes infection virus is excreted from the body even though an infected individual experiences no signs or symptoms. This stage is believed to occur infrequently.

recurrent herpes genitalis
The fourth stage of a genital herpes infection is characterized by a reactivation of the virus and the appearance of blisters on the skin. Not all people with herpes have recurrences.

According to Dr. Nicholas Fiumara (1986b), the virus can become reactivated in the sacral ganglion without producing clinical signs. This occurrence is termed **shedding herpes genitalis.** During this stage, the virus is excreted from the body even though the infected individual is experiencing no symptoms. Yet it is possible for the virus to be transmitted to another person via sexual contact during this stage. It is believed that asymptomatic shedding occurs less than 1% of the time or about 1 day a year (Herpes without symptoms, 1986).

The fourth stage of a herpes infection is termed **recurrent herpes genitalis,** characterized by reactivation of the virus with clinical manifestations. During this stage the virus travels down the nerve root to the skin, often causing new herpes blisters to erupt. Many individuals experience prodrome symptoms before a recurrence. Symptoms of recurrent infections are usually milder than those of the primary herpes infection and are of shorter duration, lasting from 2 to 10 days. The lesions are infectious for about 5 days (Fiumara, 1986b). The frequency of outbreaks also varies, ranging from one or two recurrences in a lifetime to several outbreaks a month. Not all individuals who have genital herpes experience recurrences; it is estimated that about 40% of herpes cases are recurrence free (Smith, et al., 1990). Researchers have not been able to determine who experiences recurrences or which factors trigger recurrence. It has been suggested that stress, menstruation, or illness may bring on a recurrence; however, more research is needed to clarify the mechanisms at work in the recurrence stage of genital herpes (NIAID, 1987b).

The recurrence stage of herpes causes special problems for those infected. Recurrences are not always apparent as blisters may appear inside the genital tract where they cannot be seen, or symptoms may be so mild they are unnoticed. Psychological stress increases for many herpes sufferers because they are constantly in fear that symptoms will reappear. They are faced with the difficult decision of whether to tell new partners that they have had herpes. They feel vulnerable to rejection and therefore unwilling to share the information; but they feel guilty if they are not honest. A variety of local groups across the country help herpes sufferers express their feelings about the disease and work through emotional problems.

Diagnosis and Treatment

Most diagnoses of herpes are made from the clinical signs: The patient has the vesicle-type lesions and the herpesvirus is isolated by tissue culture (the current preferred diagnostic procedure) or by blood test or Pap test (which is less accurate than a tissue culture). Cultures are taken from saliva, semen, and the cervix. The virus is known to grow slowly at times, so a culture result is not concluded to be negative for 2 weeks. Even with this procedure, conclusive diagnosis cannot always be made.

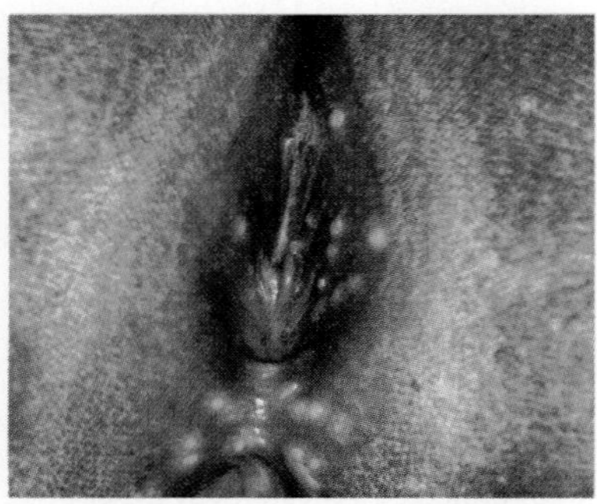

Symptoms of primary herpes genitalis include painful lesions, a sluggish feeling, and fever, along with lymph-node enlargement.

The best treatment for genital herpes is prevention. Some recommended preventive treatment procedures are as follows:

1. Many cases of genital herpes are transmitted by persons who are unaware that they have the infection or are asymptomatic when transmission occurs. In light of this realization, and because of the possibility of asymptomatic shedding of the virus between recurrences, it is recommended that condoms and spermicides always be used during sexual intercourse.
2. Persons with genital herpes should refrain from sexual activity when lesions or symptoms (prodrome) are present and inform their sexual partners that they have herpes. Prodromal symptoms precede herpes

recurrences and include itching and burning and a "pins and needles" sensation at the site of infection.

3. Because there is a risk of transmitting herpes to a fetus neonatally, childbearing-aged women who have genital herpes should inform their health care providers, especially those who care for them during a pregnancy, about the infection.
4. Those experiencing a first episode of genital herpes should be advised to seek episodic therapy with antiviral medications and to minimize or prevent recurring symptoms with suppressive antiviral therapy.
5. Sexual partners should be evaluated for genital herpes and counseled regarding the disease regardless of the results of that evaluation.
6. Patients should be informed that the presence of lesions makes them more susceptible to HIV infection. Therefore, special precautions to refrain from HIV high-risk behaviors should be taken.
7. Because stress can induce recurrences, it is advisable for persons with genital herpes to learn stress management techniques and employ them on a regular basis. These include relaxation techniques, such as yoga, meditation autogenics, and progressive relaxation, as means of perceiving events as less stressful (Greenberg, 2002).
8. To help prevent secondary infections and thereby prolong the recurrent episode, persons with genital herpes should be advised to wash the affected area with warm water and soap several times a day. Dry the area by patting it with a soft towel, sprinkle cornstarch or baby powder on the area to keep it dry, and wear loose-fitting cotton underwear to allow moisture to evaporate from the area (nylon traps moisture).

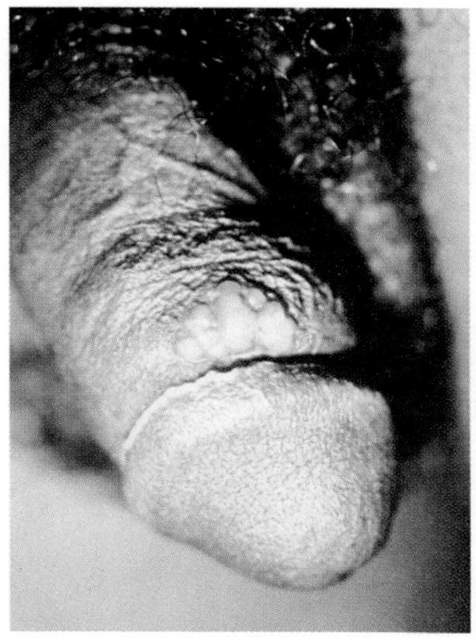

Herpes simplex on penis.

Although there is no cure for genital herpes, there is effective treatment that can manage the symptoms and minimize or prevent recurrences. For the first episode of genital herpes, 400 mg of acyclovir (trade name Zovirax) taken orally three times a day for 7 to 10 days is the recommended treatment. Alternative treatments are 200 mg of acyclovir taken orally five times a day for 7 to 10 days, or 250 mg of famciclovir taken orally three times a day for 7 to 10 days, or 1 g of valacyclovir taken orally twice a day for 7 to 10 days.

During recurrent episodes, treatment includes either 400 mg of acyclovir taken orally three times a day for 5 days, 200 mg of acyclovir taken orally five times a day for 5 days, 800 mg of acyclovir taken orally twice a day for 5 days, 125 mg of famiciclovir taken orally twice a day for 5 days, or 500 mg

Did You Know . . .

Individuals infected with an STI are at a higher risk for becoming infected with HIV, the virus that causes AIDS. Researchers believe that the genital lesions characteristic of STIs provide HIV with an easy entry point to the body. Thus, individuals who engage in unsafe sexual practices while an open lesion exists on the genitals lose an important line of defense against infection—unbroken skin.

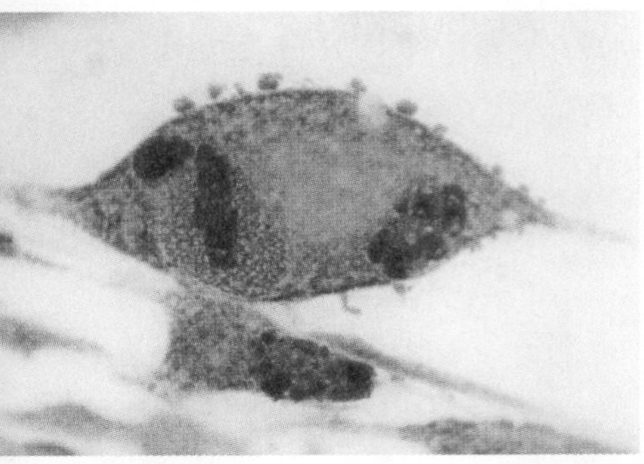

The herpes simplex virus magnified 360 times.

of valacyclovir taken orally twice a day for 5 days. Treatment also may be a daily regimen to reduce the frequency of genital herpes recurrences. These treatments, called *suppressive therapy,* can reduce recurrence by as much as 75% among patients who have frequent recurrences (six or more a year). Suppressive therapy consists of 400 mg of acyclovir taken orally twice a day, 250 mg of famiciclovir taken orally twice a day, 500 mg of valacyclovir taken orally once a day, or 1,000 mg of valacyclovir taken orally once a day (for patients who have more than 10 recurrences per year).

The most important adverse effects of genital herpes are the long-term problems; everyone—infected or not—needs to be aware of these. One serious implication is the association between the virus and cervical cancer, although this relationship is neither absolute nor conclusive. Epidemiological studies have suggested a fivefold increase in risk for cervical cancer in women with herpes virus type 2 infection (Sexuality update, 1987). Therefore it is generally recommended that women with genital herpes have a Pap smear every 6 to 12 months (Smith, Schoonover, Lauver, & Allen, 1990).

The other serious and more certain effect is the relationship between herpes and childbearing. Primary genital herpes during pregnancy poses the greatest risk to the fetus. If the initial infection occurs early in the pregnancy, the risk of spontaneous abortion (miscarriage) increases threefold (Johnson, 1986). Active genital herpes in pregnant women can have an adverse effect on the infant at the time of delivery. As already noted, the contagious virus is contained within the lesions. If vaginal lesions leak fluid during childbirth, the virus is transmitted to the infant and can result in encephalitis, brain damage, or both. Though less common, HSV can also be transmitted to a fetus through the placenta, thus causing infection before birth. The risk of infection to the infant during childbirth appears to be lower during recurrent infections (about 5%) than primary infections (as high as 50%) (Smith, Schoonover, Lauver, & Allen, 1990).

At this time it not considered practical or feasible to test all women for herpes during their pregnancies, but women with a history of herpes definitely should be examined weekly from 32 weeks of gestation until delivery to see whether lesions recur. Any primary genital herpes lesions are likely to be detected in the frequent routine prenatal visits. If genital herpes is present at the time of delivery the infant should be delivered by cesarean section. If laboratory examinations for active herpesvirus yield negative findings at delivery, the infant can be delivered vaginally with little risk of infection.

Hepatitis B

Incidence

Approximately 80,000 people in the United States are infected with a virus that attacks the liver and causes hepatitis B. In fact, it is estimated that 1 in 20 people in the United States is infected by hepatitis B virus (HBV) at some time in life. HBV is transmitted through blood or blood products, semen, vaginal secretions, and saliva. The risk of acquiring hepatitis B is greater if you (Centers for Disease Control, Frequently asked questions, 2002)

- engage in sexual activity with someone infected with HBV
- engage in sexual activity with more than one partner
- are a gay male and engage in sexual activities
- live in the same house with someone who has lifelong HBV infection
- have a job that involves contact with human blood

- use intravenous drugs
- have hemophilia
- travel to areas where hepatitis B is prevalent

Consequently, high-risk groups include those with multiple sex partners, gay men, sexual contacts of infected persons, intravenous drug users, infants born to infected mothers, health care and public safety workers, and persons who are on hemodialysis (Centers for Disease Control, Fact sheet, 2002).

Symptoms and Complications
Approximately 30% of those infected with HBV are asymptomatic. In those cases, only a blood test can reveal the disease. In other instances, in those infected the eyes or the skin turns yellow (jaundice); the appetite suffers; nausea, vomiting, fever, or stomach or joint pain may occur; and the person may feel extremely tired and unable to work for weeks or months. Although the mortality rate is lower than that of other forms of hepatitis, approximately 5,000 people die each year of untreated hepatitis B.

Diagnosis and Treatment
Hepatitis B is diagnosed by a blood test for hepatitis antibodies or antigens. At the time of this writing, there is no cure for hepatitis B. That is why prevention is so important. Once hepatitis B is diagnosed, treatment consists of bed rest and ingestion of adequate amounts of fluid to prevent dehydration. Usually feelings of fatigue subside in a few weeks, although they may not subside for several months in severe cases. For patients in whom liver disease develops, alpha interferon and lamivudine are two drugs that have proved to be effective in approximately 40% of patients.

As with all of the STIs, prevention is the first avenue of protection from infection by HBV. Of course, limiting the number of sexual partners and having no sexual activity with someone who is infected is good advice. In addition, refraining from handling blood or blood products, semen, vaginal secretions, and saliva is an effective preventive measure. And, of course, injecting no drugs, being tattooed or having body piercing from an artist who practices good health practices, and sharing no personal care items such as razors or toothbrushes are also good preventive practices. There is a vaccination to prevent HBV infection that has been available since 1982 (Centers for Disease Control, Hepatitis B vaccine: Fact sheet, 2002). The Centers for Disease Control and Prevention recommends that all newborns and children less than 19 years of age be vaccinated, as well as those who might be subjected to risk of infection (such as health care workers whose jobs expose them to human blood). The vaccination consists of three doses administered over several months.

Genital Warts

Incidence
Genital warts (condyloma acuminata), the result of a group of viruses called **human papillomaviruses (HPVs),** occur in most areas of the genitals and anus. In females the warts appear on the labia, in the lower area of the vagina, on the cervix, or around the anus; in males they appear on the glans, foreskin, and shaft of the penis; on the scrotum; and in the anal area as well. It is estimated that there are more than 20 million women with genital warts in the United States, and three-fourths of their sexual partners are infected (see Figure 14.9). The incubation period ranges from 3 weeks to 3 months after contact with an infected person. Some lesions are moist and some are dry; the moist lesions respond well to treatment. Most genital wart

genital warts
A virally caused STI characterized by wart-like lesions on the genitals.

condyloma acuminata
The technical name for the STI commonly known as genital warts.

human papillomavirus (HPV)
A virus that causes genital warts.

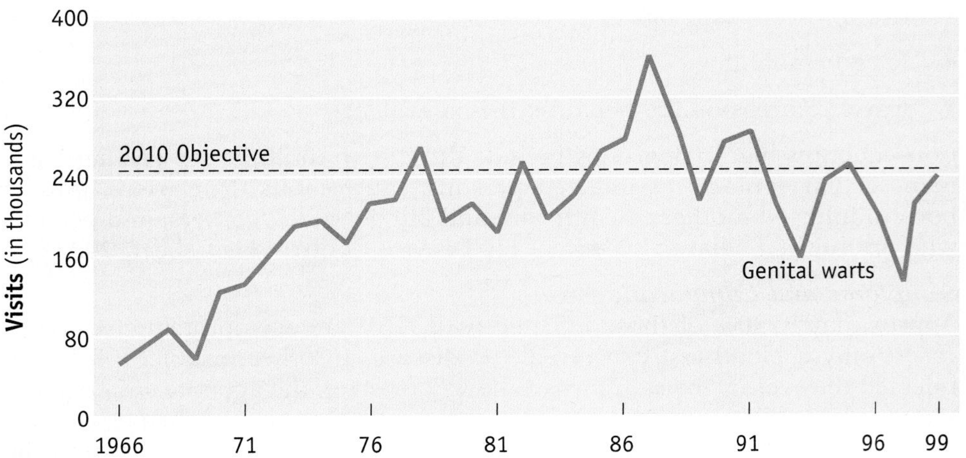

FIGURE 14.9 Human papillomavirus (genital warts)—initial visits to physicians' offices: United States, 1966–1999, and the Healthy People Year 2010 objective. *Source:* Division of STI Prevention. *Sexually transmitted disease surveillance, 1999.* U.S. Department of Health and Human Services, Public Health Service. Atlanta: Centers for Disease Control and Prevention (September 2000), 32.

infections are subclinical, meaning that they are not readily apparent to the infected individual and may often be overlooked by a physician during an examination. A study at the University of California at Berkeley found that almost half of the 467 young women who consulted the university health service for a routine gynecological exam were infected with HPV (Bauer, et al., 1991). Of the women examined, only 1% had genital warts visible at the time of examination, and only 9% had a history of genital warts. The rest of the women who had a positive test result for HPV had subclinical infection that would generally be undetected. Bauer and her colleagues believe that their results are applicable to other young college women.

Diagnosis and Treatment

Because it is difficult to diagnose subclinical cases of HPV infection, many cases are undetected. Several tissue biopsy tests are used by HPV researchers. The dot blot hybridization test is limited in the number of strains of HPV it can detect. Another test, the polymerase chain reaction (PCR) test, detects a more broad spectrum of HPV types (Nearly half of sexually active college women, 1991). Neither of these tests is routinely used by health practitioners to diagnose or detect cases of HPV infection. Most often a diagnosis of HPV infection is made by noting the appearance of warts. In moist areas of the body, they tend to be white, pink, or white to gray; in dry areas they are hard and yellow-gray.

The usual treatment for genital warts uses either cryotherapy or drug podophyllin. In cryotherapy the warts are frozen with liquid nitrogen. The tissue then dies and is replaced with healthy normal tissue. The drug podophyllin is an irritant that causes the outer skin containing the virus to be sloughed off. Neither of these techniques kills the virus; both remove the infected tissue. Podophyllin should not be used during pregnancy because it may cause birth defects (NIAID, 1987c). Surgery may be necessary to remove especially large warts (Krilov, 1991). Regardless of the method used to treat genital warts, the recurrence rate is high.

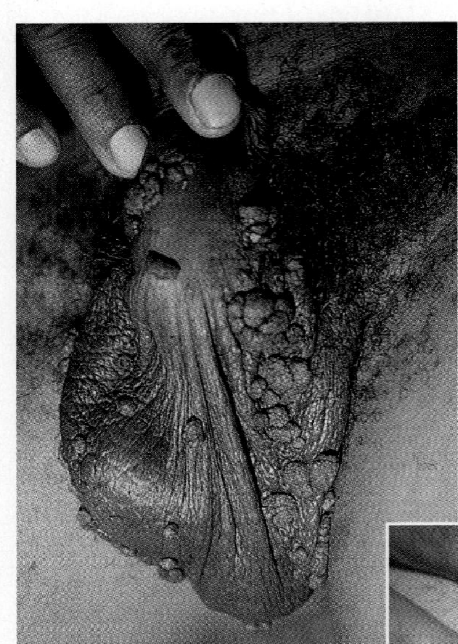

It is estimated that more than 20 million women and 15 million men have genital warts. Most people have a subclinical condition, which is to say, that the warts are not readily visible. Although the condition is treatable, it is not curable.

Patient-applied treatments are also available. These include podofilox solution or gel that is applied with a cotton swab or the finger to the infected area twice a day for 3 days, followed by 4 days of no treatment. This cycle can be repeated for up to 4 weeks. Imiquimod cream may also be applied at bedtime three times a week for as long as 16 weeks.

Vaginal Infections

One category of infection, vaginitises or vaginal infections, occurs in response to changes in an individual's own body and has, therefore, been referred to as a *sexually related disease* (SRD). Two of these vaginitises, trichomoniasis and candidiasis, can also be transmitted from partner to partner and are considered relatively common in women (see Figure 14.10).

trichomoniasis (trick)
A type of vaginitis that can be an STI or an SRD. Symptoms include a foul-smelling, foamy white or yellow-green discharge that irritates the vagina and vulva. Urethritis may also be present.

Trichomoniasis

Trichomonas vaginalis is a one-celled organism that burrows under the vaginal mucosa to cause **trichomoniasis,** or **trick.** According to the National Institute for Allergy and Infectious Diseases, the estimated annual incidence is approximately 3 million cases. The common mode of transmission is through sexual intercourse, but trichomoniasis can be contracted by prolonged exposure to moisture (for example, wet bathing suits, towels, or other clothing). Women who are pregnant or who use an oral contraceptive may be more prone to trichomoniasis infections. These women have high levels of progesterone, which increase the alkalinity in the vagina, creating a hospitable environment for the trichomonas organism. The main symptom of trichomoniasis is an odorous, foamy, white or yellow-green discharge that irritates the vagina and vulva. Frequently trichomoniasis is accompanied by urethritis. A microscopic examination of a sample of the discharge can reveal what caused the condition.

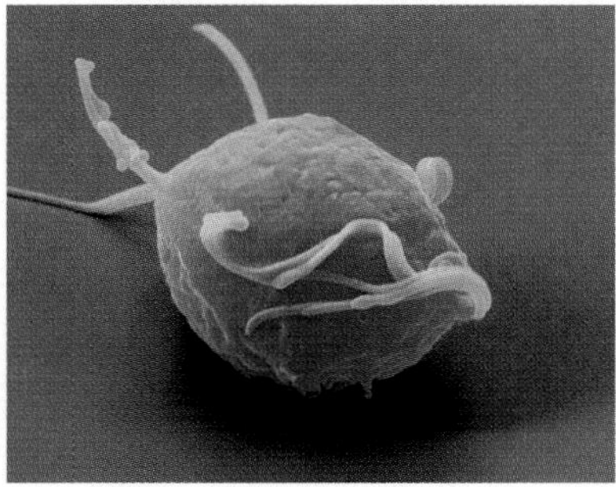

Trichomoniasis vaginalis is a common vaginal infection. Prolonged, untreated, or inadequately treated trichomoniasis can result in an increased risk of cancer.

Because the infection can be passed back and forth between partners (the Ping-Pong effect), both partners should be treated when trichomoniasis is confirmed in a woman. The man may harbor the disease organism but be asymptomatic. Metronidazole (trade name Flagyl) is the only effective systemic drug used. Some topical agents are sometimes also prescribed. Both partners follow the regimen, which is one megadose administered in 1 day. Consumer advocates have suggested, however, that metronidazole is linked with cancer, because cancer appeared in laboratory animals given

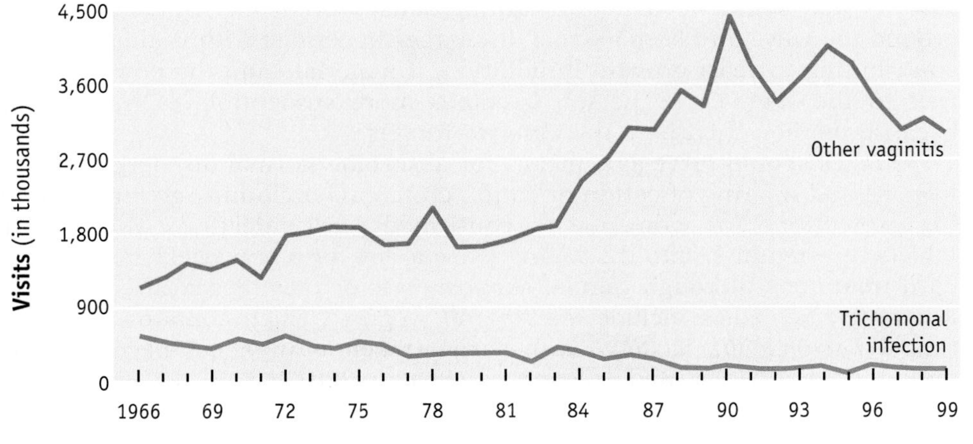

FIGURE 14.10 Trichomonal and other vaginal infections—initial visits to physicians' offices: United States, 1966–1996. *Source:* Division of STI Prevention. *Sexually transmitted disease surveillance, 1996.* U.S. Department of Health and Human Services, Public Health Service. Atlanta: Centers for Disease Control and Prevention (September 1997), 32.

massive doses of the drug. Others argue that much greater doses than those used in treating trichomoniasis were administered to these laboratory animals and that it poses no danger to humans. Nevertheless, an increased risk of cancer of the cervix does exist in women with a history of trichomoniasis infections. The white blood cell count lowers with the intake of Flagyl, but it returns to normal in a short time. If a second round of the drug is necessary, a white blood cell test is recommended. Prolonged, untreated, or inadequately treated trichomoniasis may result in a greater risk of cancer than does use of the recommended dosage of Flagyl, the only effective drug at this writing.

Flagyl should not be taken during the first 3 months of pregnancy; a pregnancy test should always precede prescription of this drug (Mead, Miller, & Thomason, 1987). Also, both partners taking metronidazole are advised against drinking alcoholic beverages because of undesirable side effects, such as headache and nausea.

candidiasis
A common form of vaginitis, sometimes called a yeast infection, which is caused by the fungus *Candida albicans.*

lactobacilli
Bacteria in the vagina that aid in keeping it healthy; also called *Doderlein bacilli.*

pubic lice
A parasite, commonly referred to as crabs, a louse that grips the pubic hair and feeds on tiny blood vessels of the skin.

pediculosis lice
Also known as crabs, of three common types: *Pediculus corporis,* a body louse; *Pediculus capitis,* a head louse; and *Pediculus pubis,* a pubic louse.

Candidiasis

The second most common form of vaginitis, **candidiasis,** also called *moniliasis, Monilia,* or *yeast infection,* is caused by the fungus *Candida albicans.* This fungus normally lives in the vagina, where it grows well in the alkaline environment. It is also known to be present in the mouth and intestine of many men and women. On occasion when the **lactobacilli,** or *Doderlein bacilli,* that are necessary for a healthy vaginal condition are reduced in number, the yeast multiply and outgrow other vaginal organisms. Women normally have these lactobacilli in the vagina, where they are necessary to maintain a healthy environment. They protect against a variety of infections, particularly those caused by bacteria in the urinary tract and the colon. The protective lactobacilli can be reduced by general poor health or lowered resistance, by too frequent douching, and by use of antibiotics (which can kill the lactobacilli as well as the bacteria causing the disease for which the antibiotic is prescribed). When the normally acid environment is changed, the yeast multiply and outgrow other vaginal organisms, resulting in a white and curdy discharge. Examination reveals a whitish plaque around the vagina and on its walls. Itching, frequently associated with a rash or redness of the vulva, is common. In advanced cases intercourse is painful, and burning and discomfort occur during urination.

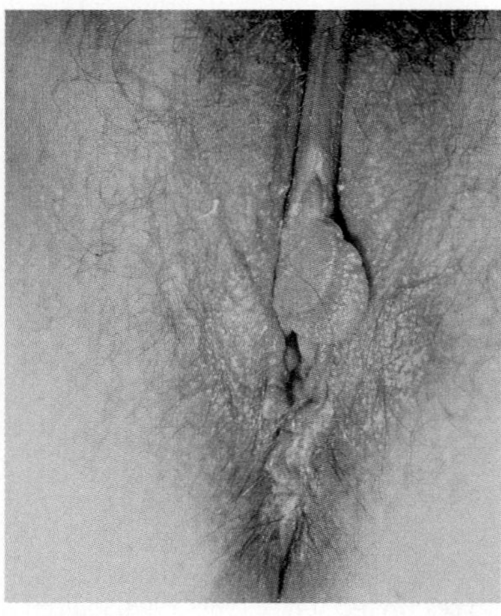

The second most common form of vaginitis is candidiasis, or yeast infection. It can result in white and curdy discharge, as shown here.

Oral contraceptives and deodorant sprays also alter the vaginal environment, making it more susceptible to fungus growth. Wearing of tight jeans and nonabsorbent nylon underwear and outer clothing and prolonged exposure to wet, synthetic material bathing suits prevent air from circulating around the vulva and keep normal discharges in contact with vaginal tissues, contributing to yeast growth. In addition, if material from the bowel is carried to the vagina, the person becomes more susceptible to moniliasis, because the bowel harbors the *Candida* fungus.

Clothes should serve as a means for absorbing normal discharges. Good hygiene and wearing of cotton or cotton-crotch underclothing go far in offering protection. For women with confirmed yeast infections, mycostatin tablets inserted high into the vagina twice a day for a few weeks is the standard treatment, although vaginal suppositories or creams can also be used. Alternative remedies include tea tree oil, yogurt (which contains the antifungal *Lactobacillus acidophilus*), garlic (taken orally), echinacea (taken orally), gentian violet, and oregano oil (Phalen, 2001).

Ectoparasitic Infestations

There are two common STIs that are not diseases, as such, but are infestations of parasites. These are pubic lice and scabies. Parasites are found among all socioeconomic classes and are spread by close physical contact.

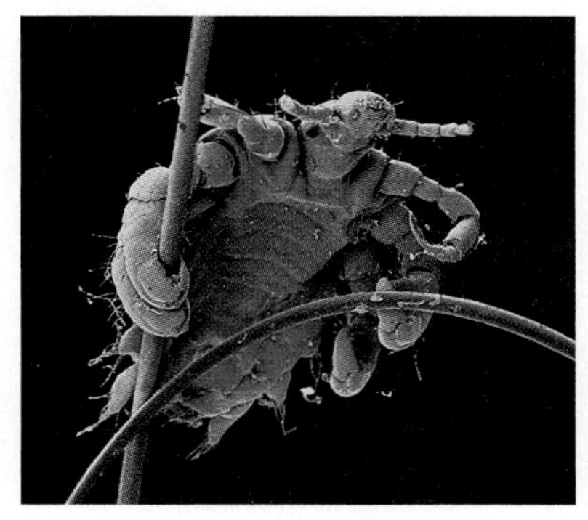

Pubic lice, commonly called "crabs," are usually transmitted from person to person by sexual contact. Direct treatment, plus cleaning of clothes and bedding, eliminate the lice.

Pubic Lice

Pubic lice, commonly referred to as crabs, are parasites. Actually there are three different kinds of lice, known as **pediculosis lice,** and each seems to prefer its own habitat. *Pediculus corporis* is a body louse; *Pediculus capitus* is a head louse; and *Pediculus pubis* is the louse of the pubic area. Pubic lice are usually transmitted from person to person by sexual contact. The organism grips the pubic hair and feeds on tiny blood vessels of the skin.

Female crabs live 1 to 2 months and lay up to 10 eggs a day. As they feed on the human skin and blood, they irritate the skin, causing itching and occasionally swelling of glands in the groin. The nits, or eggs, stick to the

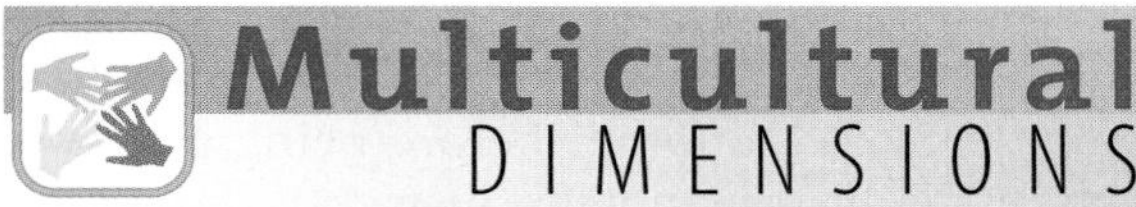

STIs and Minorities Surveillance data show high rates of STIs for some minority racial or ethnic groups compared with rates for whites. Race and ethnicity in the United States are risk markers that correlate with other more fundamental determinants of health status such as poverty, access to high-quality health care, health-care-seeking behavior, illicit drug use, and residence in communities with high prevalence of STIs.

- Chlamydia trends show consistently higher rates among women.
- In 2001, African-Americans accounted for 75% of total cases of gonorrhea. The overall gonorrhea rates were 782.3 cases per 100,000 for African-Americans and 74.2 for Hispanics compared to 29.4 for non-Hispanic whites.
- In 2001, African-American females 15 to 19 years old had a gonorrhea rate of 3,495.2 cases per 100,000 population. African-American men in this age group had a gonorrhea rate of 1,794.1 per 100,000. These rates were on average 46 times higher than those of 15- to 19-year-old white adolescents. Among 20- to 24-year-olds, the gonorrhea rate among African-Americans was almost 24 times that of whites.
- Since 1990, rates of primary and secondary syphilis have declined among all racial and ethnic groups. However, rates for African-Americans and Hispanics continue to be higher than for non-Hispanic whites. In 2001, African-Americans accounted for 62.5% of all cases of primary and secondary syphilis. Although the rate for African-Americans declined from 12.2 cases per 100,000 population in 2000 to 11.0 per 100,000 in 2001, the rate was 15.7 times the non-Hispanic white rate of 0.7 per 100,000.
- In 2001, the rate of congenital syphilis in African-Americans was 37.8 per 100,000 live births and 20.1 in Hispanics compared to 1.8 in whites.

Reducing the prevalence of many of these STIs in minority populations will require a combination of strategies. Of course, education about prevention is important. Still, education will not have a significant effect in minority populations if not combined with strategies to reduce poverty, increase access to good-quality health care, decrease drug abuse and the sharing of drug "works," and create comprehensive sexuality education programs that start in schools at early ages and continue through community agencies into the adult years.

Source: Division of STI Prevention. *Sexually transmitted disease surveillance, 2001.* U.S. Department of Health and Human Services, Public Health Service. Atlanta: Centers for Disease Control and Prevention (September 2002).

pubic hair with a thick substance. Aided by body warmth, the eggs hatch and the new lice perpetuate the cycle of feeding on the human before dropping off. They can live for about 1 day off the body and are visible to the naked eye on clothing and bedsheets. Two different preparations are effective: A-200 Pyrinate, an over-the-counter preparation, and gamma benzene (Kwell), available only by prescription. Either one is applied to the pubic hair. Directions should be carefully followed. One dose is usually curative, but sometimes the nits, though inactive, adhere to the pubic hair for weeks after treatment unless removed. A fine-toothed comb dipped first into vinegar, then into water, and combed through the pubic hair dissolves them. And, of course, clothing and bed linen used before treatment should be washed.

scabies
Skin irritation caused by a tiny mite that is transferred from one person to another by close contact, sexual or otherwise.

Scabies

Scabies is caused by a tiny mite that can barely be seen. The organism generally lives for up to 2 months. The female burrows under the skin at night, probably for the warmth of the human host, and the results are intense itching and the formation of pus. There is a characteristic distribution pattern of scabies. It is seen most commonly on the wrists, in the spaces between the fingers, under the breasts, and on the buttocks. Nodular scabies (raised lesions) can last up to 1 year. The mites lay two to three eggs a day, and in 2 or 3 weeks a new cycle begins. Because the incubation period is 4 to 8 weeks, one individual can transmit scabies to another before being aware of its existence. Close contact that is usually (but not exclusively) sexual can transmit the mites. Scabies is rarely contracted from clothing, bedding, or toilet seats.

To diagnose scabies, a physician scrapes a burrow and puts the scraping on a slide, often with mineral oil to make the swimming mite more readily visible. Kwell is the medication used to treat scabies, as well as crabs. It must be applied very judiciously, because it can be toxic to some people. In particular there is concern about the safety of pregnant women's using Kwell (NIAID, 1987d).

Prevention

On the one hand, STIs are often like other diseases in that, for many, there are effective treatments that result in elimination of the disease. On the other hand, for some STIs, even though there are effective treatments, there are no cures (for example, herpes genitalis). Still other STIs have only recently had potentially effective treatments developed to treat them and, until then, inevitably led to incapacity and death (for example, syphilis). Even when cured, people who have contracted some STIs can be affected for their entire lives, for example, when the disease results in infertility. Sexually transmitted infections, therefore, are serious conditions that we would be best advised to prevent. Fortunately, there are actions we can take to prevent contracting an STI or at least minimize the likelihood of contracting one.

Abstinence

The most certain way to avoid contracting an STI is to abstain from sexual activity, meaning not just coitus. As we have learned, STIs can be contracted through oral sex and anal sex as well.

For some people, abstinence is a viable choice. However, it is clear that for many others, abstinence is not acceptable. This may be for many rea-

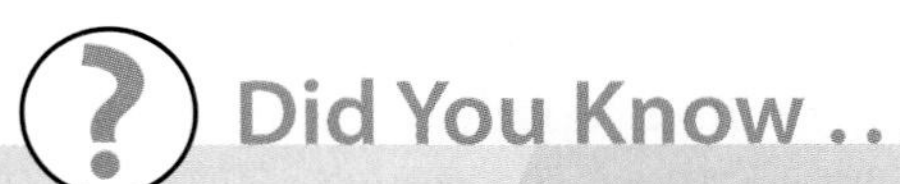

Did You Know . . .

Although it is impossible to determine the exact number of STIs each year, it is agreed that the cost of these diseases is extensive. One estimate is that STI expenditures on direct medical care and related services, as well as the indirect costs associated with the loss of productivity, totaled $10 billion in 1994 (Donovan, 1997), and this estimate excludes costs attributed to HIV and AIDS.

sons. They may have an interest in sex and find it so pleasurable that they are not willing to forgo it. They may be older and not married and intend never to marry. They may be homosexual with legal marriage unavailable to them. For those not willing to remain abstinent, other strategies for preventing contraction of an STI are available.

Monogamy

If a sexual partner is STI-free, and he or she is the only person with whom you engage in sexual activity, then you will not contract an STI. Monogamy with an uninfected partner, though, can be problematic. How are you to be sure your partner is uninfected? If the relationship is a long-term one, there probably is a greater reason to assume your partner is uninfected if he or she tells you so. However, unless you see the results of medical tests for STIs, you can never really be sure. Furthermore, even if the results are negative for HIV, for instance, sufficient antibodies may not have been formed to allow the test to detect them. This usually takes months. Last, even if you assume a partner is monogamous, some seemingly trustworthy sexual partners have been shown to be anything but. For these reasons, relying on monogamy with an uninfected partner as protection against contracting an STI can be risky.

¿? Ethical DIMENSIONS

Notifying Partners About STIs There are many reasons why people with STIs choose not to notify their sexual partner(s) about their infection. They may be embarrassed to do so, they may be married and have contracted the STI during extramarital sex or homosexual contact, or they may not want anyone to know about their infection for fear they will not be able to get dates or other sexual partners.

In spite of these concerns, some people believe that all sexual partners, past and present, should be notified of a sexual partner's STI status. In this way, they can get tested and retested if they are infected. And they can prevent the spread of the infection by refraining from sex with other people until they are disease-free.

Yet, some people argue that *absent any signs or symptoms,* notifying a sexual partner might do more harm than good. For example, if the disease was contracted during an extramarital affair, notification might result in divorce. If contracted during homosexual activity, notification might mean the loss of a job or other discriminatory actions. Furthermore, notification might unduly frighten the unsuspecting partner, causing potentially unhealthy consequences associated with stress.

What do you think is the ethical thing to do?

Reduce the Number of Sexual Partners

If a person is unwilling or unable to maintain a monogamous relationship, decreasing the number of sexual partners lessens his or her odds of contracting an STI. The greater number of sexual partners, the greater the likelihood that one of them will be infected.

Refrain from the Use of Alcohol and Other Drugs

Decisions regarding important aspects of your life deserve thoughtful consideration. What more important decision is there than that concerning whether you will engage in an activity that has the potential of causing serious, sometimes life-threatening illness? Alcohol and other drugs can interfere with decision making by decreasing inhibitions and affecting judgment. Therefore, protection against STIs should include abstention from the use of mind-altering drugs.

Myth vs Fact

Myth: If you get syphilis, you will know it because a rash will break out.
Fact: A rash may not appear until secondary syphilis has occurred. Furthermore, although a chancre (a sore) may develop early in the course of the disease, it may not be visible or may be dismissed as inconsequential. Also, in women, the early signs of syphilis may not be readily visible on the genitalia.

Myth: Gonorrhea is no more serious than the common cold and can be cured easily.
Fact: Gonorrhea can cause infertility, arthritis, or endocarditis (inflammation of the heart valves). In addition, certain antibiotic-resistant strains of gonorrhea raise concern about the ability to continue to treat this STI with present medications.

Myth: If you get an STI once, you acquire an immunity to it and cannot contract it a second time.
Fact: You do not have immunity to STIs and can therefore contract them anew each time you have contact with the disease-causing organisms.

Myth: Sexually transmitted infections occur only in or on the genital organs.
Fact: You can acquire an STI through oral–genital contact, in which case the signs of the disease would occur in the mouth and on the face. Or, you can have contact with an STI-causing organism by touching an infected area with your fingers, in which case the signs of the disease would appear on your fingers and hands.

Discuss STI Concerns with Potential Sexual Partners

Any new sexual partners should discuss concern about STIs before engaging in sexual activity. Whether they know they are infected, the high-risk behaviors they have engaged in and the results of any medical screenings they have had should be shared. This kind of a conversation can lead to concern about a potential sexual partner and a decision to refrain from sex altogether—or at least until a new medical screening can be obtained. Such a conversation will also make it easier to engage in the inspection of external signs of STIs described in the following section.

Examine Yourself and Your Partner

Although it may be embarrassing for some people, inspecting yourself and your sexual partner for signs of STIs can help prevent their spread. However, if this activity is done as sexual play, the embarrassment can be minimized.

Examine the skin of the genitals for lesions, blisters, and infected sores. Genital warts, chancres, and signs of herpes can be detected in this way. Note any foul-smelling odors. For males, the penis should be checked for any discharge by "milking" the urethra. This can be done by holding the penis and squeezing it gently but firmly. For females, the vulva should be examined for any external signs of infection. In addition, evidence of any vaginal discharge should be sought by inserting a finger into the vagina.

Because you are not a medical expert, do not rely on your own inclinations or interpretations of any unusual signs you notice. If any doubt is raised by your inspection, refrain from sexual activity until a medical screening has been arranged. That does not mean you have to abandon your relationship with a partner who has signs of an STI or that you have to be abandoned if you have these signs. All it means is that you need to protect yourself and a sexual partner from a disease that can be prevented with a little caution and patience. Recognizing an STI is disturbing and sometimes scary. However, until the results of medical screening are obtained, and afterward if the results indicate an STI, partners should express caring and concern.

Use Latex Condoms

The pores of a latex condom are too small for some organisms that cause STIs to penetrate. Therefore, the use of a latex condom during coitus and fellatio is effective in reducing the risk of contracting an STI. The National Institutes for Health formed a panel of experts to study the effectiveness of condoms in preventing STIs and HIV and AIDS. The panel concluded that condoms are effective in preventing HIV and AIDS and gonorrhea acquired by men from women (American Public Health Association, 2001). They also concluded that there was not conclusive epidemiological evidence that condoms prevented the transmission of chlamydia, syphilis, chancroid, trichomoniasis, genital herpes, and human papillomavirus infection. These findings have, unfortunately, been misinterpreted in too many media reports. The panel did not state that condoms did not prevent these STIs. Rather, they only stated that there was no convincing epidemiological evidence that they do. They stated that more studies were needed to warrant such a statement. Experts still recommend the use of condoms to reduce the risk of HIV and AIDS and STIs, awaiting the supportive evidence they expect to have soon.

It should be noted that condoms can only decrease the risk of contracting an STI, not eliminate it. Condoms will not offer protection against STIs that are transmitted by contact with other parts of the body—diseases such as herpes, warts, or ectoparasitic infections.

Avoid High-Risk Behaviors

Because organisms that cause STIs are present in semen and vaginal secretions, the goal is to prevent them from being transmitted from an infected person to a person not infected. Coitus without the use of a condom can result in the depositing of semen that includes disease-causing organisms within a partner's body. So can fellatio without a condom and cunnilingus without a dental dam. Anal sex is a particularly high-risk behavior because the friction creates fissures (tears in the lining) in the anus, allowing easy entrance to disease-causing organisms into the bloodstream. Furthermore, because organisms that cause STIs reside in the blood, using needles or other products that may contain drops of blood from another person puts one at high risk for disease. Sharing needles is one of the more common ways of contracting HIV in the United States.

Other Protective Measures

Still other behaviors can lessen the likelihood of contracting an STI or increase the likelihood of detecting one at an early stage:

- Wash the genitals before and after sex.
- Obtain regular medical checkups.
- Inspect the genitalia regularly.
- Do not share razors, hypodermic needles, or scissors.
- Do not handle towels, wet bedding, or undergarments immediately after these have been in contact with another person.
- For women, using a diaphragm, spermicide, or other barrier method of contraception may offer protection against some STIs.

If you suspect you have been exposed to an STI, see a physician or visit a health clinic in your community or on your campus. It is unwise to try to diagnose and treat the condition yourself. It is also extremely important to comply with the treatment regimen, which includes taking all the medication prescribed at the appropriate times and returning for any follow-up visits. Also, if you have an STI, notify your partner(s). Failing to tell a partner

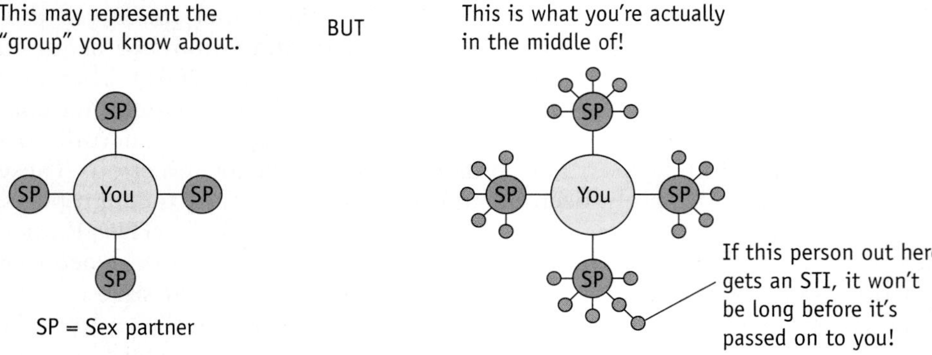

FIGURE 14.11 STIs: a fact of life for the sexually active. By sexually active, we do not mean having a lot of sex. Instead we are using the term to mean having sex with different people. In general, the fact of life is that, sooner or later, sexually active people will either be exposed to an STI or contract one.

of the possibility of infection could result in the spread of the disease, not just to a single individual but possibly to many (see Figure 14.11).

Sexuality Education and STIs

Alarmed at what they called the "hidden epidemic," the Institute of Medicine (IOM) convened a 15-member expert panel in 1994 to strategize ways to address the STI problem. The IOM concluded that society's unwillingness to confront sexual issues is the main barrier to responding to STIs (Eng & Butler, 1996). The IOM report went on to explain that this attitude hinders the dissemination of accurate, straightforward information about STIs in educational programs for adolescents and interferes with communication between parents and their children and between sexual partners. Furthermore, this attitude compromises health care professionals' ability to counsel patients, impedes research on sexual behavior, and leads to unbalanced messages being sent via the media. The members of the expert panel noted several studies that found that almost two-thirds of respondents knew little or nothing about STIs other than HIV and AIDS and that most people seriously underestimate their risk of acquiring an STI, as well as its consequences.

The need for education about STIs is evident, has long been overlooked, and requires the involvement of many different segments of our society, working together to prevent their occurrence and to develop more effective treatments if and when they do occur.

Exploring the DIMENSIONS of Human Sexuality

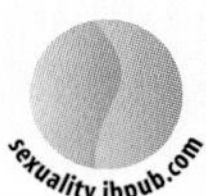

Our feelings, attitudes, and beliefs regarding sexuality are influenced by our internal and external environments. Go to sexuality.jbpub.com to learn more about the biological, psychological, and sociological factors that affect your sexuality.

Biological Factors

- STIs are contracted primarily through sexual contact.
- SRDs are diseases of the reproductive system that can occur in either sexually active or sexually inactive individuals. For example, cervical cancer has been linked to herpes type 2.
- Individuals with an STI have a higher risk of becoming infected with HIV, possibly because the genital lesions characteristic of STIs give HIV access to the body.
- STIs can be passed to a baby both before and during birth.

Sociocultural Factors

- Society's unwillingness to confront sexual issues is a major barrier in responding to STIs.
- Some ethnic groups have higher rates of STIs than others. Southern states have higher rates of syphilis than the national average.
- Economically, the cost of treating STIs—and the associated lost productivity—probably exceeds $10 billion per year.

Psychological Factors

- Having an STI affects an individual's feelings about his or her sexuality.
- Learning later in life that you became sterile because of an undiagnosed STI can have a devastating psychological effect.
- Psychological stress increases for genital herpes sufferers because they constantly fear that symptoms will reappear. They must decide whether to tell new partners of their condition and face potential rejection.

CASE STUDY

Sexually transmitted infections are quite prevalent, especially among young people. Some STIs and SRDs are curable; some are treatable but chronic. Because many cases are asymptomatic or early symptoms are ignored, treatment does not occur. The STI can then be transmitted further.

Having a curable STI is at a minimum embarrassing. Yet having a chronic STI like genital herpes or genital warts can have a profound psychological impact on a person's life. The STI will affect the individual's sexual activities for an entire lifetime. The fear of rejection after informing a potential sexual partner might cause the individual to say nothing. Self-esteem can diminish.

Socially, race and ethnicity correlate with fundamental determinants of health status such as poverty, access to health care, health-care-seeking behavior, and residence in areas with a high prevalence of STIs. Thus, a higher prevalence of gonorrhea or syphilis among African-Americans has social—not biological—underpinnings.

Prevent STIs through abstinence, monogamy, reduction in the number of sexual partners, abstinence from alcohol or other drugs, communication with partners, examination of yourself and your partner, use of latex or polyurethane condoms, and avoidance of high-risk behaviors.

Discussion Questions

1. What are STIs, how are they transmitted, and what are the reasons for their prevalence?
2. What are the bacterially based STIs? Include their incidence, transmission, symptoms and complications, and diagnosis and treatment in your answer.
3. What are the virally based STIs? Include their incidence, transmission, symptoms and complications, and diagnosis and treatment in your answer.
4. What are the ectoparasitic infestations? Include their incidence, transmission, symptoms and complications, and diagnosis and treatment in your answer.
5. List the key ways to prevent STIs, evaluating the theoretical and user effectiveness of each in the real world.

Application Questions

Reread the chapter-opening story and answer the following questions.

1. Jessica chose to ask her human sexuality professor about her potential STI. Why didn't she go to the student health clinic or her primary care physician?
2. The author describes several of the "private" conversations students wish to have with human sexuality professors, concerning pregnancy, abuse, sexual disorders, and STIs. Where on your campus (or in your community) could you go for help for each of these problems? Be specific, creating a list with phone numbers.
3. Should professors discuss personal sexuality issues with students? Explain why or why not.

Critical Thinking Questions

1. Applications for marriage licenses in many states require a blood test for syphilis but not for the other STIs. Because many STIs are asymptomatic, should marriage tests require testing for all the major STIs? What difficulties would implementing such a program involve? (Hint: Consider how each disease is diagnosed.)
2. How can undetected STIs affect fetuses and newborns?
3. Criminal laws generally provide that someone who deliberately inflicts harm on another person should be punished. Civil laws allow the victim to seek compensation for harm done. Should people who know they are infected with STIs but who have unprotected sex with others and infect them be prosecuted? Should the people they infect be able to sue for physical and psychological damages?

Critical Thinking Case

Most of us believe that STIs afflict young people. But STIs strike people of all ages—including senior citizens. People who are widowed or divorced do not become asexual; rather, they usually begin dating new people. In fact, 90% of postmenopausal women remain sexually active.

Dr. Peter Leone, medical director of the Wake County, North Carolina, STI Clinic, says: "Women who are past menopause often think they can't get an STI. People link pregnancy and STI risk. But methods to prevent pregnancy aren't the best ones for preventing STIs. On the other hand, some people think, 'Why should I use a condom? I can't get pregnant.' "

Although the STI incidence rates per 100,000 people has remained low for senior citizens, the number of seniors is growing dramatically. So, even if rates remain low, the number will continue to increase. Consequently, people 50 years old and older have 10% of the total AIDS cases in the United States.

Consider your parents or your parents' friends who are divorced or widowed. How could you, as a student in this class, give them information about taking responsibility for their sexual behavior?

Ironically, it seems that senior citizens share the attitude of young people regarding sexual behavior: It cannot happen to me. Explain this attitude. Do young people and seniors have different reasons for their beliefs?

Exploring Personal Dimensions

Can You Be Assertive When You Need to Be?

To take the necessary actions to prevent contracting an STI, you will have to be assertive: That is, you will need to resist pressure to engage in sexual activity if you choose not to, and you will need to insist on the use of a condom and other safer sex precautions if you decide to engage in sex. Do you have assertiveness skills? To find out, write an assertive response to each of the situations described.

1. You are on a date and your partner insists on engaging in a sexual activity that you decide is not for you at that time. You say:

   ____

   ____

   ____

2. Your partner argues that condoms diminish the sensation. You respond by saying:

   ____

   ____

   ____

3. Your partner states that she or he has been tested for STIs and the test result was negative. Therefore, there are no reasons for using safer sex techniques. You respond by saying:

____

____

____

To be assertive, you need to:

1. Specify the behavior or situation to which the statement refers.
2. Relate your feelings about that situation.
3. Suggest a remedy or what your preference is.
4. Identify the consequences of the change: What will happen if it occurs and what will happen if it does not occur.

Now check your responses and revise them to be consistent with these assertiveness principles.

Sexuality Online

Go to the web component for *Exploring the Dimensions of Human Sexuality* at sexuality.jbpub.com for web exercises, additional resources related to this chapter, and student review tools.

Suggested Readings

Hansfield, H. H. *Color atlas and synopsis of sexually transmitted diseases.* New York: McGraw-Hill, 1992.

Holmes, K. K., Mardh, P. A., Stamm, W. E., Sparling, F., & Wasserheit, J. *Sexually transmitted diseases.* New York: McGraw-Hill, 1998.

Monif, G. R. *Understanding genital herpes (women's health care series).* New York: Parthenon Publishing Group, 1996.

Morse, S. A. *Atlas of sexually transmitted diseases and AIDS.* St. Louis: Mosby-Year Book, 1996.

Nevid, J. A. & Nevid, J. S. *Choices: Sex in the age of STIs.* Boston: Allyn & Bacon, 1997.

Sonnex, C. *A general practitioner's guide to genitourinary medicine and sexual health.* Port Chester, NY: Cambridge University Press, 1996.

Wisdom, A. & Hawkins, D. A. *Diagnosis in color: Sexually transmitted diseases.* St. Louis: Mosby-Year Book, 1997.

I»N»T»E»R chapter FOCUS

HIV and AIDS

FEATURES

Multicultural Dimensions
AIDS Among Asian Americans

Ethical Dimensions
Should HIV Testing Be Mandatory for Pregnant Women?

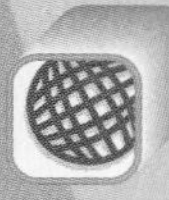
Global Dimensions
AIDS in Africa

Gender Dimensions
Women and AIDS

CHAPTER OBJECTIVES

1. Describe acquired immunodeficiency syndrome (AIDS), the opportunistic diseases associated with it, and how the human immunodeficiency virus (HIV) invades the body and causes AIDS.
2. Discuss different treatments for HIV and AIDS, including how the mortality rate has declined as a result of these treatments.
3. Cite ways in which HIV infection can be prevented.

sexuality.jbpub.com

Prevention of HIV Infection and AIDS
Global Dimensions: AIDS in Africa
HIV and College Students
Gender Dimensions: Women and AIDS

INTRODUCTION

Tom applied for a graduate assistantship in our department and, because of his impressive academic record and the nature of his experiences, was awarded one. He was a pleasure to have around, always smiling and willing to help in whatever way he could. Because of his personality and his conscientiousness Tom's graduate assistantship was extended into the next year and several years thereafter.

It was during his fourth year with us that Tom began losing weight and missing some days at school. Attributing it to the flu or a similar condition, no one seemed to take much notice—that is, until Tom started missing even more days and looking emaciated. Before long, the rumor spread that Tom had AIDS and did not have long to live. Unfortunately, the rumor was true and before many more months, Tom died.

With today's new medications and combination of medications, Tom might be alive today. Or at least he would have lived longer with HIV than he did. Of course, that troubles those of us who knew and cared for Tom. However, other issues are also troubling. Until he told us, we did not even know Tom was gay. He contracted HIV through unprotected sex. Why did he feel the need to hide his identity, and how much torment did that hiding create? More to the point, what did we (the department, the faculty, the university, and the society at large) convey to Tom that led him to conclude we would reject him if we knew his secrets? And how many others are in a situation similar to Tom's and are in torment as he was?

We hope that this chapter, by presenting information about HIV and AIDS, will help us all become more understanding of those who are wrestling with not only the physical and psychological effects of HIV infection but the social consequences as well.

Acquired Immune Deficiency Syndrome (AIDS)

Acquired Immune Deficiency Syndrome (AIDS)
A syndrome caused by the human immunodeficiency virus (HIV), characterized by a depressed immune system and the presence of one or more opportunistic diseases.

opportunistic diseases
A major manifestation of AIDS, diseases that occur in the presence of a suppressed immune system.

human immunodeficiency virus (HIV)
A retrovirus that causes AIDS.

retroviruses
A group of viruses consisting of ribonucleic acid (RNA) surrounded by a protein coat that can convert their RNA into deoxyribonucleic acid (DNA) once they have invaded a living cell, allowing them to take over the cell and reproduce themselves.

Acquired Immune Deficiency Syndrome (AIDS), so named because it attacks and slowly destroys the body's immune system, was first identified by American physicians in mid-1981. At that time, physicians noted the unusual occurrence of five cases of *Pneumocystis carinii* pneumonia among previously healthy homosexual men in Los Angeles. Soon thereafter, reports surfaced of a rare form of cancer, Kaposi's sarcoma, also among young homosexual men in New York and California. These observations led to the recognition of AIDS, a disease characterized by **opportunistic diseases** in an immune-compromised individual. Diseases such as *Pneumocystis carinii* pneumonia and Kaposi's sarcoma are labeled opportunistic because they rarely occur in young healthy individuals, instead relying on the opportunity presented by a depressed immune system. AIDS is considered a syndrome because it is characterized by a range of opportunistic diseases, rather than one particular disease (Table IF3.1).

Research conducted by Robert Gallo at the National Institutes of Health and by Luc Montagnier and colleagues at the Pasteur Institute in Paris led to the discovery of a new virus believed to cause AIDS. Gallo named the virus human T-lymphotropic virus type III (HTLV-III); Montagnier identified it by the name lymphadenopathy-associated virus (LAV). In May 1986 the International Committee on Taxonomy of Viruses announced its recommendation that the virus be consistently identified by the name **human immu-**

TABLE IF3.1 **Common Opportunistic Diseases**

Cancers
Kaposi's sarcoma
Primary lymphoma of the brain
Protozoal and Helminthic
Cryptosporidiosis, intestinal (causing diarrhea for over one month)
Pneumocystis carinii pneumonia
Strongyloidiasis (pneumonia, central nervous system [CNS] infection, or disseminated infection)
Toxoplasmosis (pneumonia or CNS infection)
Fungal Infections
Aspergillosis (CNS or disseminated infection)
Candidiasis (esophagitis)
Cryptococcosis (pulmonary, CNS, or disseminated infection)
Histoplasmosis (disseminated)
Bacterial Infection
Atypical *Mycobacterium* species other than *M. tuberculosis* or *M. leprae* (disseminated infection)
Viral Infection
Cytomegalovirus (pulmonary, gastrointestinal tract, or CNS infection)
Herpes simplex virus
Chronic mucocutaneous ulcers persisting longer than one month
Pulmonary, gastrointestinal tract, or disseminated infection
Progressive multifocal leukoencephalopathy (presumed papovavirus)

Source: Allen, J. R. Definitions: Surveillance definition of AIDS, in *AIDS: A basic guide for clinicians,* Ebbeson, P., et al., eds. Philadelphia: W. B. Saunders, 233–234.

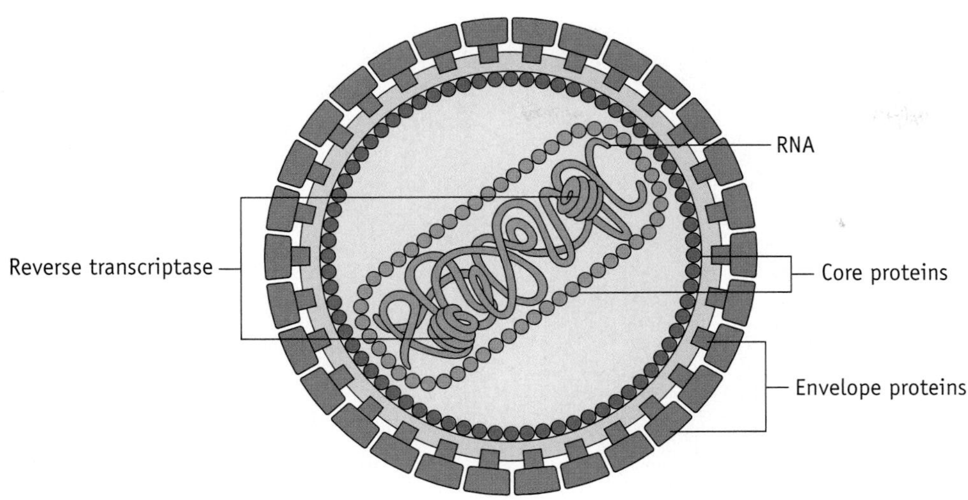

FIGURE IF3.1 HIV consists of an outer shell, or protein envelope, that surrounds a protein core that protects the ribonucleic acid (RNA) and the enzyme reverse transcriptase. *Source: FDA Consumer* (October 1987), 10.

nodeficiency virus (HIV) (AIDS virus gets new name amid feuding, 1986). Today we know that HIV is the cause of AIDS.

HIV belongs to a special class of viruses called **retroviruses.** Retroviruses consist of a protein shell surrounding the genetic material ribonucleic acid (RNA) (Figure IF3.1). For HIV to attack a human cell it must first attach itself to a special receptor on the cell's surface. In humans HIV attaches to T4 lymphocytes, a type of white blood cell that plays an important role in the immune response to disease. Once attached to the T4 cell, HIV enters the cell and releases its RNA. The RNA is then converted into DNA by an enzyme (reverse transcriptase) also carried by HIV. This HIV DNA then combines with the cell's DNA, causing the cell to reproduce HIV (Figure IF3.2). In essence, HIV converts the cells it attacks into factories producing HIV, which then go on to infect other T4 cells. As this process progresses, T4 cells are destroyed and the body becomes unable to defend itself against organisms that would normally be no threat to health. Thus the opportunistic diseases that characterize AIDS infect the individual, usually leading to death.

Incidence of HIV and AIDS

As noted in Table IF3.2, through December 2001, more than 807,000 adults and adolescents and more than 9,000 children had acquired AIDS. HIV infection is the eighth leading cause of death in the United States. Between 1985

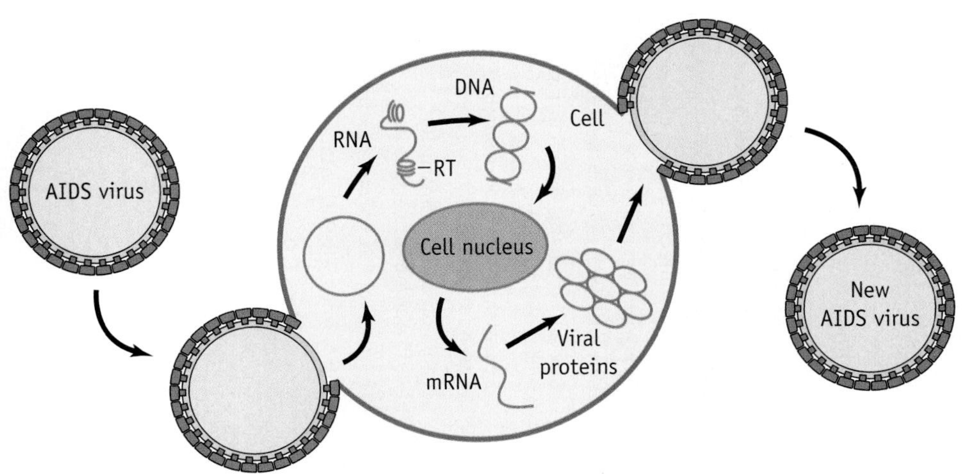

FIGURE IF3.2 HIV infection and replication in a human cell. The virus enters the cell and releases RNA, its genetic material. Using the enzyme reverse transcriptase (RT), the virus converts its RNA into deoxyribonucleic acid (DNA), which enters the cell nucleus and combines with the cell DNA. The cell's altered genetic material then produces messenger RNA (mRNA), which codes for new virus. *Source: FDA Consumer* (October 1987), 10.

TABLE IF3.2 **AIDS Cases by Age Group, Exposure Category, and Sex, Reported Through December 2001, United States**

Adult/adolescent exposure category	Males				Females				Totals[1]			
	2001		Cumulative total		2001		Cumulative total		2001		Cumulative total[2]	
	No.	(%)	No.	(%)	No.	(%)	No.	(%)	No.	(%)	No.	(%)
Men who have sex with men	13,265	(42)	368,971	(55)	—	—	—	—	13,265	(31)	368,971	(46)
Injecting drug use	5,261	(16)	145,750	(22)	2,212	(20)	55,576	(39)	7,473	(17)	201,326	(25)
Men who have sex with men and inject drugs	1,502	(5)	51,293	(8)	—	—	—	—	1,502	(3)	51,293	(6)
Hemophilia/coagulation disorder	97	(0)	5,000	(1)	9	(0)	292	(0)	106	(0)	5,292	(1)
Heterosexual contact:	2,762	(9)	32,735	(5)	4,142	(37)	57,396	(41)	6,904	(16)	90,131	(11)
Sex with injecting drug user	549		9,821		937		21,736		1,486		31,557	
Sex with bisexual male	—		—		192		3,801		192		3,801	
Sex with person with hemophilia	5		69		8		425		13		494	
Sex with transfusion recipient with HIV infection	19		446		13		619		32		1,065	
Sex with HIV-infected person, risk not specified	2,189		22,399		2,992		30,815		5,181		53,214	
Receipt of blood transfusion, blood components, or tissue[3]	105	(0)	5,057	(1)	113	(1)	3,914	(3)	218	(1)	8,971	(1)
Other/risk not reported or identified[4]	8,909	(28)	57,220	(9)	4,606	(42)	23,870	(17)	13,515	(31)	81,091	(10)
Adult/adolescent subtotal	31,901	(100)	666,026	(100)	11,082	(100)	141,048	(100)	42,983	(100)	807,075	(100)

TABLE IF3.2 AIDS Cases by Age Group, Exposure Category, and Sex, Reported Through December 2001, United States (Continued)

Pediatric (<13 years old) exposure category	Males				Females				Totals[1]			
	2001		Cumulative total		2001		Cumulative total		2001		Cumulative total[2]	
	No.	(%)	No.	(%)	No.	(%)	No.	(%)	No.	(%)	No.	(%)
Hemophilia/coagulation disorder	0	(0)	229	(5)	0	(0)	7	(0)	0	(0)	236	(3)
Mother with/at risk for HIV infection:[4]	79	(85)	4,113	(88)	71	(87)	4,171	(95)	150	(86)	8,284	(91)
Injecting drug use	17		1,626		16		1,612		33		3,238	
Sex with injecting drug user	8		763		7		728		15		1,491	
Sex with bisexual male	2		91		3		95		5		186	
Sex with person with hemophilia	1		18		0		15		1		33	
Sex with transfusion recipient with HIV infection	0		11		0		14		0		25	
Sex with HIV-infected person, risk not specified	22		656		16		683		38		1,339	
Receipt of blood transfusion, blood components, or tissue	1		74		1		80		2		154	
Has HIV infection, risk not specified	28		874		28		944		56		1,818	
Receipt of blood transfusion, blood components, or tissue[3]	2	(2)	241	(5)	0	(0)	140	(3)	2	(1)	381	(4)
Other/risk not reported or identified[5]	12	(13)	78	(2)	11	(13)	95	(2)	23	(13)	173	(2)
Pediatric subtotal	93	(100)	4,661	(100)	82	(100)	4,413	(100)	175	(100)	9,074	(100)
Total	**31,994**		**670,687**		**11,164**		**145,461**		**43,158**		**816,149**	

[1]Includes one person whose sex is unknown.

[2]Includes persons known to be infected with human immunodeficiency virus type 2 (HIV-2). See *MMWR, 44* (1995), 603–606.

[3]In 41 adults/adolescents and 2 children AIDS developed after they received blood screened negative for HIV antibody. Thirteen additional adults acquired AIDS after receiving tissue, organs, or artificial insemination from HIV-infected donors. Four of the 13 received tissue, organs, or artificial insemination from a donor who tested negative for HIV antibody at the time of donation. See *N Engl J Med* 1992;326:726–732.

[4]Thirty-four adults/adolescents are included in the "other" exposure category who were exposed to HIV-infected blood, body fluids, or concentrated virus in health care, laboratory, or household settings, as supported by seroconversion, epidemiological, and/or laboratory evidence. See *MMWR, 42* (1993), 329–331, 948–951; and XI International Conference on AIDS; Vancouver, Canada: July 7–12, 1996;1:179 [abstract Mo.D.1728]. One person was infected after intentional inoculation with HIV-infected blood. Additionally, 221 persons acquired HIV infection perinatally and were diagnosed with AIDS after age 13 years. These 221 persons are tabulated under the adult/adolescent, not pediatric, exposure category.

[5]Includes five children who were exposed to HIV-infected blood as supported by seroconversion, epidemiological, and/or laboratory evidence: one child was infected after intentional inoculation with HIV-infected blood and four children were exposed to HIV-infected blood in a household setting (see *MMWR, 41* (1992), 228–231, and *N Engl J Med, 329* (1993), 1,835–1,841). Twelve of the children had sexual contact with an adult with or at a high risk for HIV infection (see *Pediatrics* 1998;102:e46).

Source: Centers for Disease Control and Prevention. *HIV/AIDS Surveillance Report, 13, no. 2* (2001), 14.

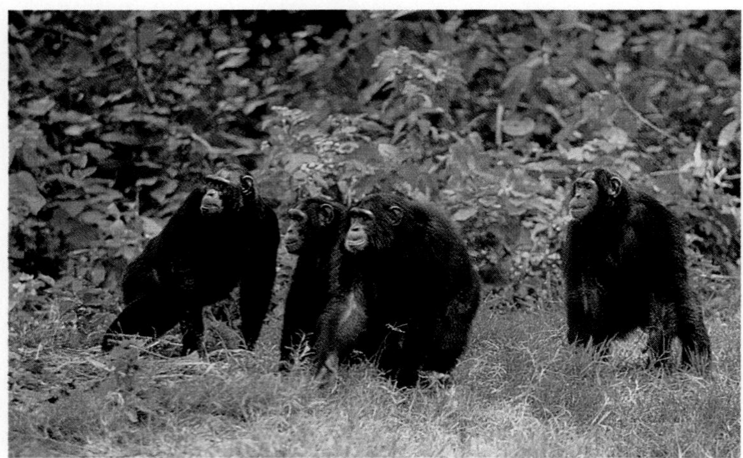

In February 1999, Dr. Beatrice Hahn of the University of Alabama at Birmingham announced that she had tracked HIV's ancestor to a virus that has long infected *Pan troglodytes*, a subspecies of African chimpanzees. In an effort to help human HIV patients, researchers are looking into why the monkeys do not appear to become sick from the virus.

and 2000, almost 325,000 white Americans, 283,000 African-Americans, and 138,000 Hispanics contracted AIDS. Almost five times as many American males as females contracted AIDS between those years. HIV infection is the fourth leading cause of death among African-Americans and the fifth leading cause of death among Hispanics (Centers for Disease Control and Prevention, 2000).

HIV affects different age groups at different rates. Whereas HIV infection is the sixth leading cause of death among 15- to 24-year-olds, it ranks third among 25- to 44-year-olds. What these rankings indicate is that HIV is contracted when people are teenagers and in their early 20s and is manifested after several years when they are older.

Although the death rate from HIV infection increased steadily from 5.5 per 100,000 in 1987 to 15.6 per 100,000 in 1995, it dropped for the first time to 11.1 per 100,000 in 1996. This drop was primarily a result of new treatments, although education campaigns may have played a part. This drop is in no small part related to the increased funding for HIV and AIDS research, which increased dramatically over the years. In 1985, $205 million was spent by the federal government on HIV and AIDS. By 2001 that number had increased to $14.2 billion (National Center for Health Statistics, 2002).

The World Health Organization reports that there were some 31 million HIV infections in 1997. Most of these appeared in Sub-Saharan Africa (almost 21 million), another 6 million in South and Southeast Asia, and slightly more than 1.5 million in Latin America and the Caribbean. In North America, there were 860,000 infections in 1997. In contrast to the incidence

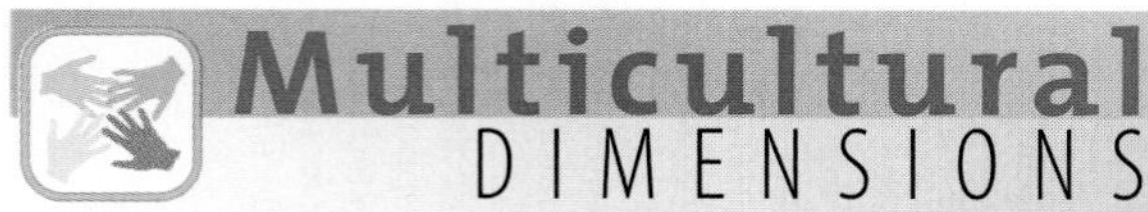

Multicultural DIMENSIONS

AIDS Among Asian Americans

The incidence of AIDS in the Asian-American community is assumed to be small. However, there are problems with this assumption. For example, when Asian-Americans are grouped together, diverse ethnic and racial subgroups are ignored. There are 28 Asian subgroups and 20 Pacific Islander subgroups. Chinese and Filipinos make up the two largest Asian subgroups, followed by Japanese, Asian-Indians, and Koreans. The result is that certain subgroups may actually have a high incidence of HIV infection and others a low incidence. One study (Jew, 1991) did find such a wide difference: 66.5 cases per 100,000 among Thai-Americans and 2.7 per 100,000 among Korean-Americans. Grouping Asian-American subgroups together conceals the need for intervention in particular subgroups. In addition, shame often prevents Asian-Americans who are infected from revealing that fact to their families and friends, thereby falsely lowering the apparent incidence rate. Furthermore, language barriers sometimes prevent Asian-Americans from communicating their HIV status to health providers and authorities who maintain health data.

It is estimated that by the year 2050, the Asian-American population will have increased by 356% (Lin-Fu, 1993), constituting 11% of the population. If this projection is accurate, there will be 41 million Asian-Americans in the United States by the year 2050. It is time that HIV and AIDS in the Asian-American community be studied more systematically and interventions adopted as necessary.

Did You Know . . .

Do mosquitoes transmit HIV? Scientific experiments have shown that HIV does not multiply in insects such as biting flies, mosquitoes, and bedbugs (Miike, 1987). Additionally, it has been noted that the mouths of such insects cannot hold enough blood of one person to be capable of infecting another person (Booth, 1987). Epidemiological evidence also supports the hypothesis that transmission by insects does not occur.

in the United States, where most cases of HIV are the result of homosexual contact, the majority of HIV infections in those other regions of the world are transmitted by heterosexual contact.

Transmission

HIV is found in large concentrations in two human body fluids: semen and blood. This is related to the large number of white blood cells present in these body fluids. It appears that a concentration of HIV is probably necessary for the transmission of HIV from one individual to another. Thus the most common modes of transmission are those that involve the exchange of semen or blood between individuals. Unprotected sexual intercourse with an infected individual is the most common way that infected semen is transmitted; however, cases of AIDS related to artificial insemination have been reported (Confirmation of transmission, 1986). The majority of AIDS cases in the United States, 49%, have involved men who had sex with men (Table IF3.2). The prevalence of anal intercourse among homosexual and bisexual men and their often large number of sexual partners have been cited as reasons for this large percentage of cases.

Of the total reported adult/adolescent AIDS cases, approximately 11% appear to be related to heterosexual transmission (Centers for Disease Control, 2000). In the United States, this transmission category includes individuals who reported heterosexual contact with a person considered to be at risk for AIDS and of individuals born in a country where heterosexual transmission is believed to be the major mode of transmission. Heterosexual transmission is of particular concern to women—for them 38% of reported cases are thought to have been transmitted by heterosexual contact, compared to only 5% of male reported cases. Many women who become infected with HIV through heterosexual contact have partners who are injecting drug users. Women in this category are not necessarily injecting drug users themselves; they become infected through sexual intercourse with partners who are.

The transmission of HIV related to injecting drug use is growing rapidly. Through December 2000, injecting drug use was associated with HIV transmission in 25% of all reported AIDS cases. Infection occurs through the sharing of needles contaminated with HIV. Additionally, these injecting drug users can transmit the virus to their sexual partners through intercourse, and, in the case of female injecting drug users, to their infants pre- or postnatally. Injecting drug use is currently thought to constitute the major threat of HIV transmission to the heterosexual population. This mode of transmission disproportionately affects the urban poor and minority populations, especially African-Americans and Hispanics. It is estimated that 38% of African-Americans and Hispanic men with AIDS are injecting drug users. The number of injecting drug users among minority women with AIDS is 43% of the reported cases of AIDS in African-American women and 47% of

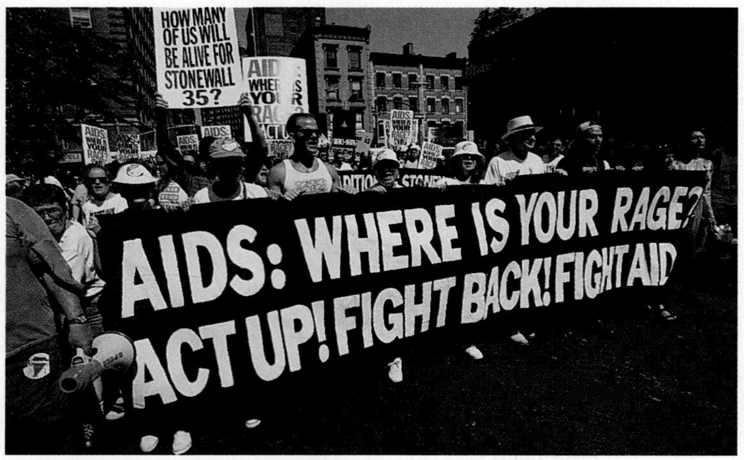

The efforts of the gay community to garner media attention for the HIV and AIDS crisis brought it to the forefront of the nation's medical agenda during the 1980s. Because of these efforts, HIV and AIDS research and medical funding garnered a far greater percentage of government spending than it would otherwise have, which resulted in a significant reduction of HIV incidence in the mainstream gay community. Unfortunately, within the gay community, gay men are currently experiencing a resurgence of the HIV and AIDS epidemic. In actuality, we have little more today in the way of prevention than we had two decades ago. Despite the efforts of both the gay and mainstream communities and tremendous scientific advances in treatments for the virus, this crisis is far from averted.

reported AIDS cases in Hispanic women (Centers for Disease Control, 2000).

Between 1979 and mid-1985 HIV transmission through blood transfusions was of great concern to health professionals and the public. In the spring of 1985 an HIV antibody test was approved by the FDA for the purpose of screening blood donations. **Antibody** tests do an excellent job of protecting the nation's blood supply from contamination with HIV. There is, however, still a slight risk that the test will miss HIV antibodies (resulting in a false negative test result). Additionally, the test may not detect HIV-infected blood because a person who is infected with HIV may not produce a detectable level of antibodies for up to 3 months after infection. It must be emphasized that this risk is very small. The CDC and the American Red Cross reported that the risk of contracting AIDS through blood transfusions was about 1 in 28,000 in 1987 (Blood supply grows safer, 1990). Additionally, they reported that the chance that HIV-infected blood will not be detected through the blood screening process was decreasing by more than 30% a year. There is no risk of becoming infected with HIV through donation of blood.

AIDS and the Gay Community

Originally, AIDS was discovered in gay men. Of course, it was soon realized that risky behavior is associated with HIV infection, not one's sexual identity or one's country of origin. (Haitians were targeted with discriminatory immigration regulations because of the relatively high incidence of AIDS in Haiti.) However, given the high incidence of HIV infection in the gay community, much effort has been made to educate gays about safer sex practices. This effort has been quite successful: Gay men have been engaging in sex with fewer partners (Seigel & Raveis, 1993), using condoms more frequently during sex (although rates among gay men have since risen again), and somewhat decreasing anal sexual intercourse behavior. Further, gay men who are infected tend to discontinue their sexual activities, for many reasons: They may not feel up to it physically, they may not be able to acquire a willing sexual partner, they may perceive themselves as less attractive as the disease progresses, they may become depressed, and they may be concerned about infecting another person. It is for these reasons that many gay men choose a sexual partner who is also HIV-positive (Hoff, et al., 1992).

Not to be overlooked is the effect of the lobbying efforts by the gay community—males and females—for increased funding for AIDS research and more rapid approval of drugs with the potential for treating HIV infection and AIDS. As more and more people, including celebrities (for example, Rock Hudson, Keith Haring, and Greg Louganis) contracted HIV, the alarm was sounded throughout the gay community. That alarm led the way to successful local and national lobbying efforts. When compared to that for other diseases, funding for AIDS research far exceeds its ranking in terms of deaths or incidence, a direct result of the gay community's involvement. Imagine what the status of treatment for HIV and AIDS would be today, not

antibodies
A class of proteins secreted by the immune system that bonds with antigens. Antibodies fight off disease-causing organisms.

silent infection
A stage of HIV infection characterized by no symptoms other than the presence of HIV antibodies.

symptomatic infection
The second stage of HIV infection, characterized by HIV antibodies as well as general signs and symptoms such as swollen lymph glands, fatigue, unexplained weight loss, night sweats, persistent fever, and diarrhea.

to mention the advancements on the horizon, without the gay community's efforts.

Stages of HIV Infection

Once an individual is infected with HIV, the natural course of the infection progresses in three stages. The first stage is **silent infection.** This stage is an asymptomatic period during which the only evidence of infection is the presence of HIV antibodies. However the development of antibodies takes at least 2 weeks, and it is often 6 to 8 weeks before antibody levels are high enough to be detected by current tests.

Some infected individuals (it is not known how many) progress to the second stage of infection—**symptomatic infection.** This stage consists of several general signs and symptoms, the most prominent of which is persistent swelling of the lymph glands, especially in the neck, armpits, and back of the mouth. Other common signs include fatigue, unexplained weight loss, night sweats, persistent fever, and diarrhea. It is currently believed that most, if not all, individuals who have symptomatic HIV infection will progress to the third and final stage—AIDS.

In the latest reporting period at the time of this writing, in the year 2001 there were 42,983 cases of AIDS reported in the United States and its territories (Figures IF3.3 and IF3.4). People who have AIDS have all the general signs and symptoms of infection described, but they also have one or more of the opportunistic diseases such as *Pneumocystis carinii* pneumonia or Kaposi's sarcoma. HIV can cross the blood–brain barrier and cause personality changes, deterioration of memory and judgment, dementia, and brain tumors (Redfield & Burke, 1989).

Although AIDS is classified as a terminal disease, people now live with AIDS for a long time. Newer medication regimens, accompanied by an enthusiastic research agenda, lead some to conclude that eventually AIDS will be considered a chronic disease (like hypertension and diabetes) that can be controlled, if not eradicated.

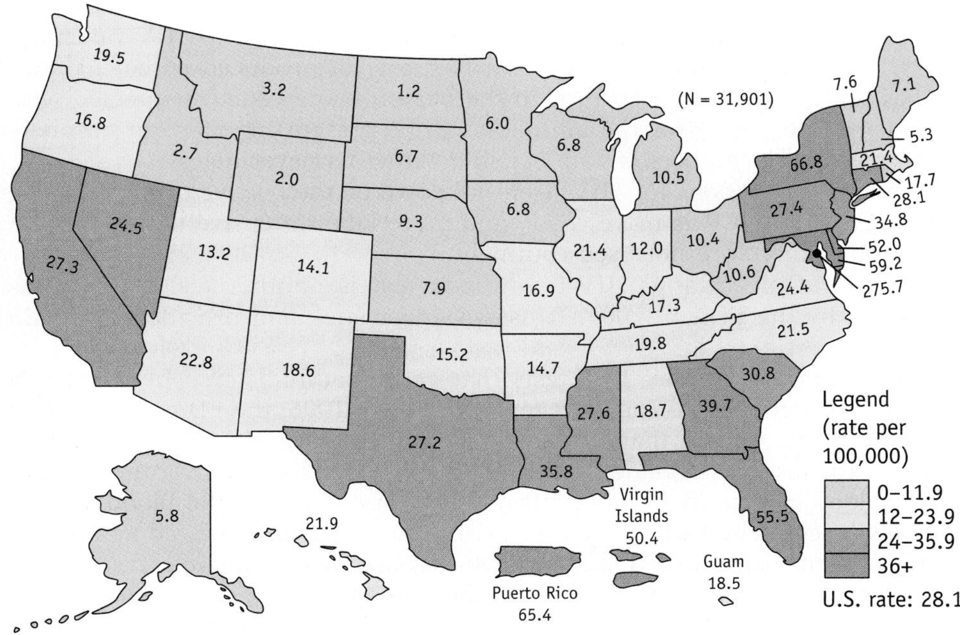

FIGURE IF3.3 Male adult/adolescent annual AIDS rates per 100,000 population, for cases reported in 2001, United States. *Source:* Centers for Disease Control and Prevention. *HIV/AIDS Surveillance Report, 13, no. 2* (2001), 12.

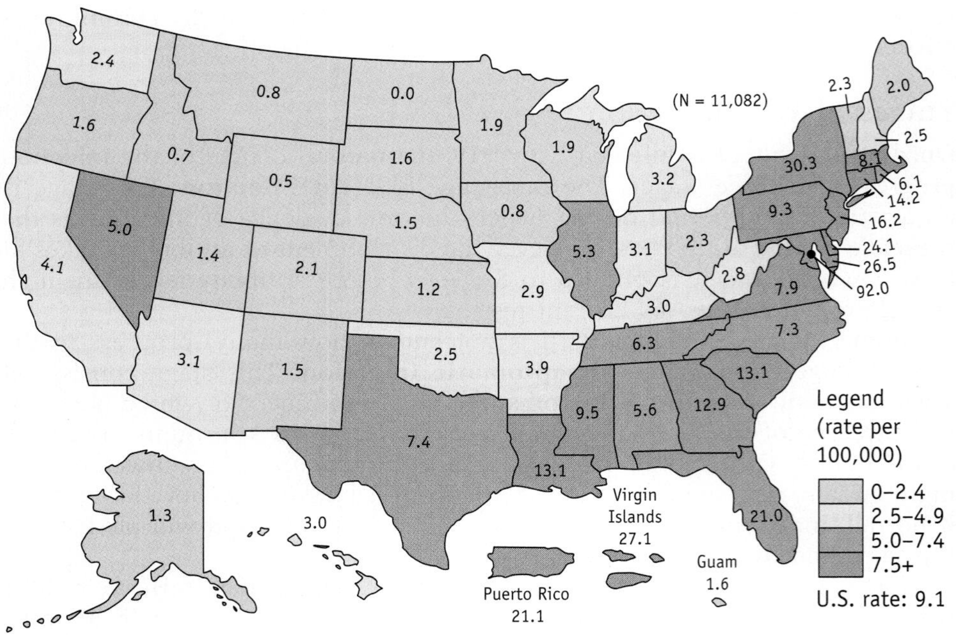

FIGURE IF3.4 Female adult/adolescent annual AIDS rates per 100,000 population, for cases reported in 2001, United States. *Source:* Centers for Disease Control and Prevention. *HIV/AIDS surveillance report, 13, no. 2* (2001), 12.

Testing for HIV

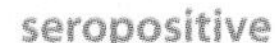

seropositive
The result of a blood test for antibodies to HIV that indicates that such antibodies have been found in the blood.

seronegative
The result of a blood test for antibodies to HIV that indicates no presence of such antibodies.

There are several HIV tests. The initial one performed is called the *enzyme-linked immunosorbent assay (ELISA)* test. The ELISA test identifies the presence of HIV antibodies. If antibodies are present, the person is said to be **seropositive.** If no antibodies are present, the person is said to be **seronegative.** However, even though the test results show that HIV antibodies are present, they may be "false positive." Therefore, once the ELISA finding is positive, a more sensitive, and more expensive, test is administered, the Western blot. If the Western blot result confirms the presence of HIV antibodies, the person can be assured that he or she is infected. It should be noted that both of these tests do not directly test for the presence of HIV. Rather, they test for the presence of antibodies produced in response to HIV infection. Thus, it is possible that the infection has not yet produced sufficient antibodies to be measured even though the person being tested is infected with HIV. If it is too early for the antibodies to be present in sufficient numbers to be measured, the person can transmit the virus nevertheless.

One test that looks for HIV itself is known as the *polymerase chain reaction (PCR)*. The PCR is more costly and more labor-intensive than the other tests and is therefore not used routinely.

The OraQuick Rapid HIV-1 antibody test is another test, which was approved by the FDA in 2003. It uses a finger stick and provides results in 20 minutes.

In addition, there are HIV tests that can be administered by oneself in one's home, similarly to early pregnancy tests. In 1996, the FDA approved an HIV home-test system that uses blood samples collected at home. Components of the test, the Confide HIV Testing Service, include an over-the-counter home blood collection kit, a certified laboratory to whom the blood sample is mailed, counseling when the results are presented, and assured anonymity of the person being tested. Negative results are made available through an automated message, although the person can speak to a counselor if he or she chooses. Positive results are communicated by a professional who provides counseling.

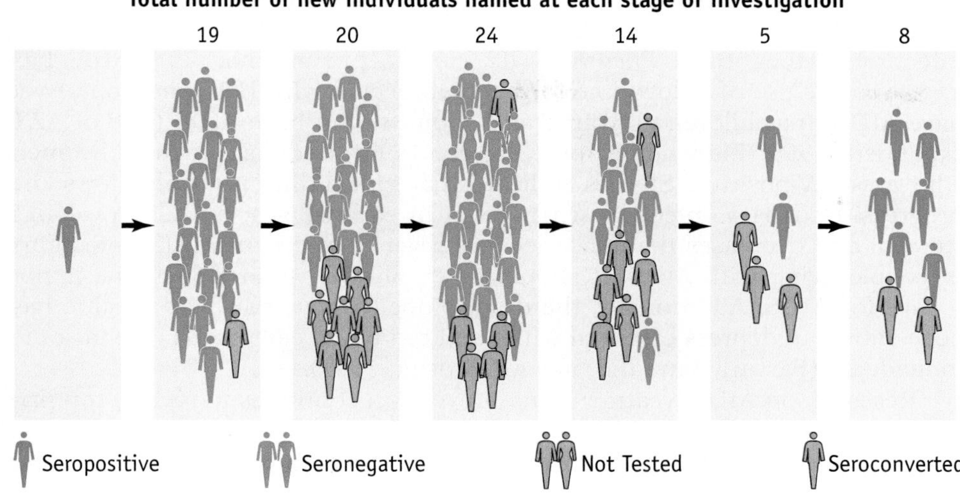

FIGURE IF3.5 Partner notification programs can be highly productive, as illustrated by results of a South Carolina investigation that began with one HIV-positive man. Of the 19 sexual contacts he named, all but one were tested, and three were seropositive. Those three then named 20 sexual contacts not already identified, leading to the discovery of two more HIV-positive men, who in turn named 24 other previously unidentified contacts, and so forth. When the investigation reached its end point of no new HIV-positive contacts, it had identified a total of 90 persons at risk, tested 68 of them, and found 12 who either were seropositive or seroconverted 6 months after initial testing.

An oral HIV test is now available. In 1997, the Whitman-Walker Clinic in Washington, DC, was the first major AIDS clinic in the United States to administer this oral test. The oral test, OraSure, requires a person to place a flat inch-long cotton swab, attached to a stick, between the gum and cheek for 2 minutes. The swab draws fluid from the mucous membrane, which contains HIV antibodies if the person is infected. This test is ideal for persons who are afraid of needles.

An individual who receives a positive HIV test finding should be given medical and psychological counseling as well as education intended to prevent HIV transmission to others. Additionally, it is important at this time to initiate the process of *partner notification*. The CDC recommends that "persons who are HIV-antibody positive should be instructed in how to notify their partners and to refer them for counseling and testing. If they are unwilling to notify their partners, or if it cannot be assured that their partners will seek counseling, physicians or health department personnel should use confidential procedures to assure that the partners are notified" (Partner notification, 1988).

The notification of partners is an important step in stopping the spread of HIV (Figure IF3.5). However, an HIV-positive person may not feel capable of contacting sexual or needle-sharing partners for a variety of reasons, including fear of discrimination or legal action (Judson, 1990). In one study, Marks and associates (1991) found that 52% of sexually active HIV-positive persons did not inform their partners of their HIV antibody status. In such instances, when an HIV-infected person does not feel able to disclose HIV antibody test results, a representative from the health department should notify and counsel the partner(s) of that person. The name of the HIV-positive individual is not revealed; nor is the alleged HIV exposure date. Thus confidentiality is maintained for HIV-infected individuals while knowledge of exposure to HIV is provided to partners.

Treatment of HIV and AIDS

In 1987 the FDA approved **zidovudine** (brand name Retrovir; formerly azidothymidine [AZT]) as the first drug licensed in the United States for the treatment of AIDS patients. Zidovudine is an antiviral drug that slows the

zidovudine
The first drug (brand name Retrovir) (also known as AZT) approved by the FDA for the treatment of AIDS. This antiviral drug slows the replication of the AIDS virus, thus slowing the course of the syndrome.

replication of HIV in human cells. Originally, zidovudine was approved for use by AIDS patients who had not had Kaposi's sarcoma or opportunistic infections other than *Pneumocystis carinii* pneumonia. The FDA has approved the use of zidovudine for people infected with HIV who do not yet have AIDS, for children as young as 6 months who have AIDS (Use of AZT expanded, 1990; Zidovudine for children, 1990), and for pregnant women who are HIV-positive. Studies indicate that zidovudine not only slows the progression of HIV infection when given in early stages, but also prolongs survival and decreases the incidence and severity of opportunistic infections in people living with AIDS. It should be emphasized that zidovudine is not a cure for AIDS. Additionally, the drug is not without risks; zidovudine has been shown to depress essential white and red blood cell production in some individuals (Fast-tracking the first AIDS drug, 1987).

Research on AIDS treatment and prevention continues to receive top priority. The results of this research have been the development of several possible vaccines now being tested and of a new generation of drugs to treat HIV infection.

¿? Ethical DIMENSIONS

Should HIV Testing Be Mandatory for Pregnant Women? If pregnant women are infected with HIV, they can pass on that infection to their babies in utero. Yet, there is a simple way to prevent many of these babies from being born infected—that is, by administering to pregnant women a regimen of the AIDS drug AZT. In fact, the likelihood of HIV transmission to babies of HIV-positive pregnant women drops from approximately 26% to 8% when AZT is administered. For this reason, many physicians and legislators advocate that pregnant women be required to be tested for HIV as part of their routine prenatal care. In that way, the danger to the fetus is identified, and AZT can be administered to the women whose fetuses are at risk.

However, this issue is more complicated than it appears at first glance. For example, if women are required to be HIV tested during prenatal care, many will forgo prenatal care in order to avoid the test and its possible repercussions. These repercussions may include losing one's job, one's housing, or one's partner. In addition, a woman who lives in a rural area may not be able to find a physician willing to manage her pregnancy and help in the delivery of her child. Avoiding prenatal care, though, places the fetus at risk of being born at low birth weight and/or with a variety of birth defects. Still, opponents of mandatory testing point out that no other segment of society is required to be HIV tested. Therefore, to require this of pregnant women is to discriminate against these women. There is no disagreement that pregnant women ought to be counseled about the risks and benefits of being tested and that there is a treatment to help prevent their babies from being born infected with HIV even if they are infected. But, the choice to be tested for HIV should be the woman's.

Proponents of mandatory HIV testing for pregnant women argue that counseling alone will not persuade enough women to be tested. Too many would choose to avoid testing, and the result would be that too many babies would be born with HIV. To protect the babies, they maintain, women should be required to be tested and their HIV status determined. Only then can pregnant women infected with HIV be administered AZT, thereby indirectly treating their fetuses. In addition, women who test positive for HIV can be educated about the risk of breastfeeding, another means through which HIV can be transmitted to their babies.

Should the privacy of the mother be protected, or is her privacy less important than the benefits to the fetus? This is not only a policy issue, it is also an ethical issue. On which side of this argument do you find yourself?

The Vaccine

In 1998, after an experimental AIDS vaccine had been tested on animals, 5,000 volunteers began receiving injections. The volunteers consisted of people at high risk for HIV infection, such as gay men and women whose sexual partners were infected. Manufactured by VaxGen, Inc., the vaccine AIDSvax, is made of dead virus and therefore cannot cause HIV infection. However, it is hoped that it will produce antibodies in sufficient number to provide protection against HIV.

Triple-Drug Therapy

The new generation of drugs has produced the most dramatic advancement in the fight against AIDS to date. There are now three classes of antiretroviral drug therapies (Elion, 1997):

1. *Nucleoside reverse transcriptase inhibitors* (zidovudine, didanosine, stavudine, and so on): These drugs block the action of reverse transcriptase, thereby preventing HIV RNA from reproducing.
2. *Protease inhibitors* (such as indinavir, nelfinavir, ritonavir, and saquinavir mesylate): These drugs shut down HIV replication by preventing the viral enzyme protease from cutting other viral protein into shorter pieces needed by HIV to make new viral copies for infecting new T4 cells.
3. *Nonnucleoside reverse-transcriptase inhibitors* (such as delavirdine and nevirapine): These drugs block the reverse transcriptase directly.

These medications are administered together in what is called *combination therapy,* or the *AIDS cocktail.* Combination therapy makes sense because it attacks the virus at different steps in the life cycle rather than at one step. Studies have reported that combination therapy delays the progression of HIV infection to AIDS and reduces mortality rate (Hammer, et al., 1996; Katzenstein, et al., 1996). However, combination therapy is expensive. It is estimated that the annual cost of treating patients at the HIV stage is approximately $4,000, and the annual cost for treating a patient at the AIDS stage is $25,239—and these figures are in 1995 dollars (Gable, et al., 1996). In 2003, it is estimated that the average annual cost of treating someone with HIV is between $10,000 and $15,000; for AIDS the annual cost is between $15,000 and $22,000. The effect of these astronomical costs is that some people with AIDS, such as the poor or unemployed, cannot afford the most effective treatments available to them; the government has to decide how much financial support to provide for the treatment of AIDS (an economic issue with tax implications); and the most effective treatments are withheld from Third World countries where HIV

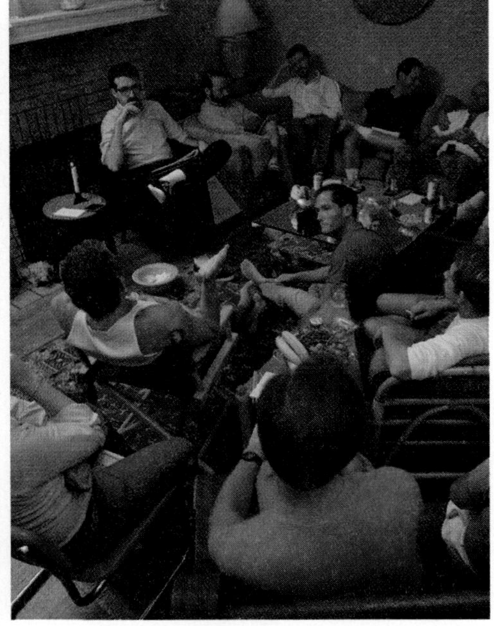

People with HIV must cope not only with the knowledge of their illness but also with society's fear of HIV. Support groups offer emotional support and firsthand advice on coping with the illness.

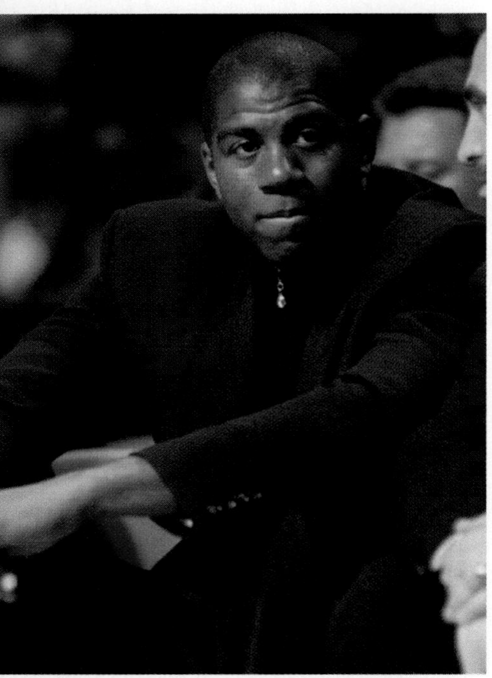

In November 1991, the basketball star Magic Johnson announced that he had acquired HIV virus through unprotected sexual intercourse with an unknown infected woman. Magic provides living proof of the effectiveness of the AIDS cocktail: The level of HIV in his body has been reduced to an undetectable level.

and AIDS are prevalent (both a financial and an ethical issue). In 2000, though, drug companies started discounting drugs to Third World countries so more people with HIV and AIDS could be treated. And recognition of the financial costs, not to mention all the other costs of contracting HIV to the person and the person's friends and family, leads many experts to conclude that the best way to prevent HIV and AIDS is by educational campaigns.

Prevention of HIV Infection and AIDS

Until a cure for AIDS is discovered, efforts to prevent HIV infection and AIDS will be critical to controlling this epidemic. Currently there are two major emphases: (1) preventing the initiation of behaviors or conditions that will put an individual at risk of infection and (2) changing behaviors to reduce the chances that an individual will become infected if exposed to HIV (Ibrahim, 1991).

The best method available to prevent infection with HIV is abstinence: abstaining from sexual activity with an HIV-infected partner and abstaining from injecting drug use. This is an important message of HIV and AIDS education efforts—especially for adolescents and young adults who are in a developmental stage at which sexual and drug experimentation is common. Today such experimentation carries a deadly risk of HIV and AIDS.

Abstaining from sexual activity throughout one's life is impractical and undesirable for most people. For those who are uninfected and sexually active, maintaining a mutually faithful monogamous relationship with an uninfected partner also prevents the sexual transmission of HIV. And each partner would also need to abstain from injecting drug use, another high-risk behavior for HIV transmission.

Many people have previously engaged in behaviors that put them "at high risk" of being infected with HIV. People should be considered at risk if they have shared needles or syringes to inject drugs or steroids; are male and have had anal sex (even once) with another male; have had sex with someone they believe may have been infected with HIV; have had another STI; received blood transfusions or blood products between 1978 and 1985; or have had sex with someone who has any of these risk characteristics. In addition, the more sexual partners a person has had, the greater the chances that person will have had contact with an HIV-infected person. Magic Johnson brought this point home to many people when he announced to the world that he was infected with HIV from unprotected sexual intercourse with a woman he could not identify because of his numerous sexual partners over the years. It is important to remember, however, that unprotected sexual intercourse with just one person is risky if that person is infected with HIV.

If an individual decides to engage in sexual activity with a person who is at risk for or is infected with HIV, public health authorities recommend

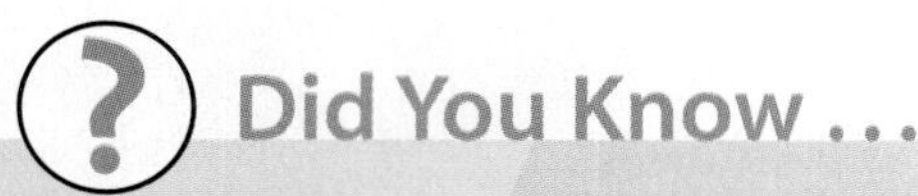

The World Health Organization, in collaboration with UNAIDS, released the *AIDS Epidemic Update* in December 2002, which estimated that five million new infections with HIV occurred in 2002.

that a condom be used during sexual intercourse (vaginal or anal). Latex condoms have been shown to be an effective barrier to HIV (Tests confirm condoms block AIDS virus, 1986). Although condoms are not 100% effective in preventing HIV transmission, they are considered to be among the most important components of safer sex.

Yet, even with all the educational efforts and mass attention directed at the issue of condoms and safer sex, studies indicate that most people do not consistently use condoms. Joseph Catania and colleagues (1992) examined a random sample of 1,770 unmarried multiethnic San Franciscans and found that only 9% of heterosexual men and women reported "always" using a condom during sexual intercourse. Even more disturbing is the finding that 46% of the heterosexual men and 61% of the heterosexual women reported "never" using condoms. The gay and bisexual men in this study reported significantly higher rates of condom use: 48% reported "always" using condoms. Yet even in this high-risk group (homosexual and bisexual males living in San Francisco), 10% reported that they "never" used condoms and 41% reported that they "sometimes" used condoms. In an analysis of the National Survey of Family Growth (Piccinio & Mosher, 1998), researchers investigated the contraceptive method used by women aged 15–44 years. They found that 23% used condoms. When broken down into various categories, younger women, African-American women, more highly educated women, higher-income women, and never married women were the most likely to have employed condoms. Yet, condom use in none of these groups even approached 50%.

In 1990, the CDC surveyed a representative sample of 11,631 U.S. high school students about their sexual behavior (Sexual behavior among high school students, 1992). A majority of the students surveyed (54.2%) reported that they had engaged in sexual intercourse; 39.4% reported having had sexual intercourse within the past 3 months. Of those latter students, only 44.9% indicated that they had used a condom during their last act of intercourse. In a study of adolescent use of condoms (Ford, Sohn, & Lepkowski, 2001), researchers found that condoms were used in 59% of relationships, although not necessarily during every sexual intercourse encounter. White adolescents were more likely to use condoms than either African-American or Hispanic adolescents; adolescents whose partners were of a different race or ethnicity were more likely to use condoms; and the longer the relationship, the more likely it was condoms were used. Further research is needed to identify educational programs that successfully increase condom use in people at risk for HIV infection.

Other safer sex strategies are also recommended. If an individual or a sexual partner is at risk for HIV infection, he or she should avoid mouth contact with the penis, vagina, or rectum. Sex with prostitutes should also be avoided, because both male and female prostitutes are often injecting drug users. The possibility of prostitutes' having sexual intercourse with high-risk individuals is also great.

Because the current antibody tests for HIV are not 100% accurate, those who are at high risk of HIV infection and those who are known to be infected are asked not to donate blood. Women infected with HIV should prevent pregnancy, as HIV can be transmitted to the unborn child (see the Ethical Dimensions box on page 552).

Screening tests for HIV are an important preventive tool. It is currently recommended that those who have engaged in any of the risk behaviors described take an HIV antibody test. There are many public and private testing sites that provide confidential or anonymous HIV testing. HIV testing should always be accompanied by counseling and education as well. Even

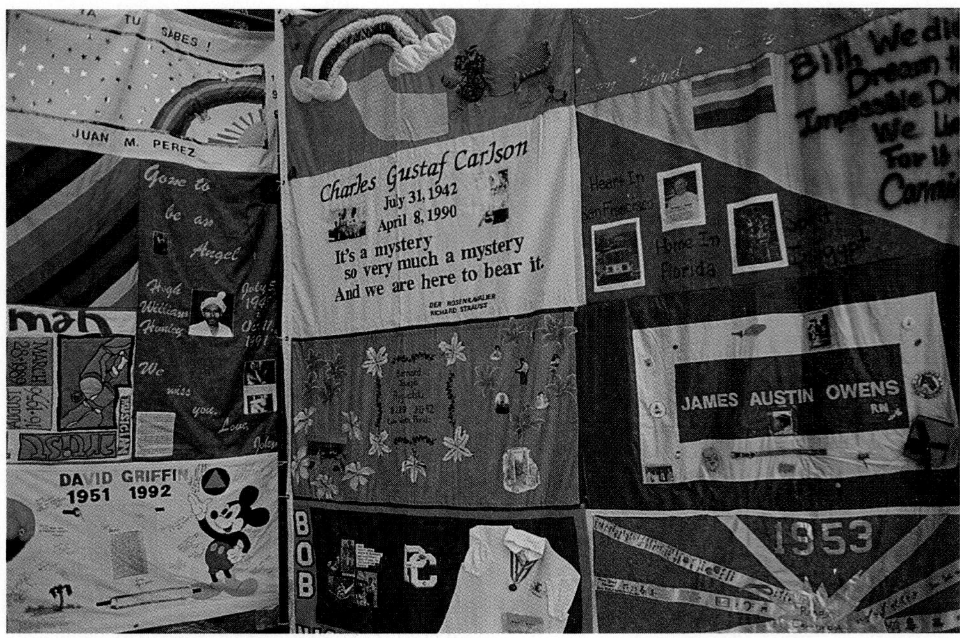

The remarkable AIDS quilt is made up of 44,000 panels, each representing a life lost to AIDS. It was created both as a living memorial for those who died and as a brilliant way to help the public visualize the growing toll that AIDS was taking.

for those who test negative, the time of finding out their results can be an important "teachable moment."

Of course, among the ways to prevent the spread of HIV are for those who are infected to let their sexual partners know of their HIV status and to take all the necessary precautions to prevent its transmission. Many people do disclose their HIV status to their partners. Still, in a review of several studies of this issue, the American Public Health Association found that only 60% of those who knew they were infected with HIV disclosed this information to all their partners (Many people, 1998). Of the 40% who did not share this information, half of those did not tell their primary partner. To make matters worse, only 42% used condoms all of the time during sexual intercourse. Given that disclosure can lead to stigmatization and other consequences that have been described previously in this chapter, it is understandable, though not acceptable, that some people who are HIV-positive refrain from informing others. In the end, however, this is selfish and dangerous.

HIV and AIDS and Young Adults

HIV and AIDS are of particular concern for young adults who have a lot of years left to live. Unfortunately, the HIV and AIDS rate for young adults is a growing problem. In 2001, 42,983 adolescents and adults below age 25 years had contracted HIV. The reasons for the large number of AIDS among young adults include the following.

- Young adults tend to have more sexual partners, thereby increasing their risk of encountering one who is HIV-positive.
- Young people tend to consider themselves invulnerable and are therefore more likely to engage in sexual intercourse without using a condom.
- Young people may feel self-conscious about purchasing condoms and therefore not have them available when they decide to engage in coitus.

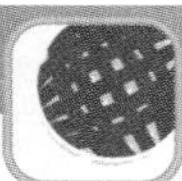

Global DIMENSIONS

AIDS in Africa Imagine! In some areas of Africa, 25% of the population is infected with HIV. The United Nations reported that in 1997, throughout the world, more than 30 million people were infected with HIV (Parts of Africa, 1998). The highest rates of infection for 15- to 49-year-olds are in 21 countries south of the Sahara. In Botswana and Zimbabwe, 25% of adults are infected, and in 13 other African countries at least 10% of adults are infected. In some African cities, more than one-third of adults are infected. Further, when pregnant women who attend prenatal clinics in some major African cities are tested for HIV, 70% are determined to be seropositive. The concern is not only for these women but also for their babies, many of whom will be born infected. From 1981 through the beginning of 1998, 8.2 million African children had seen their mother die of AIDS. In East Africa, 40% of children younger than 16 years of age had lost one or both parents to AIDS.

The African situation is even more perilous when one considers these countries' inability to afford costly drugs shown to be effective in treating HIV infection and AIDS. Triple-drug treatment, becoming routine in the United States, for example, is unheard of in many parts of Africa and other developing countries. In a humanitarian gesture, drug companies have begun discounting these drugs to Third World countries.

Still, in countries that have organized effective prevention programs, such as Senegal, Tanzania, and Uganda, the rates of infection are slowing. In Uganda, HIV prevalence decreased from 13% in 1994 to 9.5% in 1997. In Senegal, the HIV infection rate had remained stable at 2%.

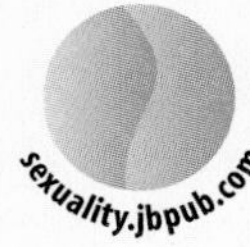

- For some of the reasons given, young people become infected with STIs more often than older people; that incidence in turn makes them more susceptible to contracting HIV.
- Young adults tend to use mood-altering drugs that diminish their capacity to make healthy decisions when they are sexually aroused.

However, in recent years young people have tended to change some high-risk behaviors. For instance, the proportion of 15-year-olds who engage in coitus declined between 1988 and 1995 (from 27% to 22% among women and from 33% to 27% among men) (Department of Health and Human Services, 1997). The Healthy People 2010 National Health Objectives goal is that 75% of males and females ages 15 to 17 years will have never engaged in sexual intercourse. In addition, the rate of condom use by African-American women has increased twofold (from 12% to 25%). However, the Healthy People 2010 objective is to increase further the number of sexually active African-American women who use condoms, recognizing that African-American women have a long way to go to decrease their risk of contracting HIV. In a study of the changes in sexual behavior between 1990 and 1992 of 18- to 49-year-olds, it was found that although there was little change in the number of multiple partners, in having a high-risk partner, or in obtaining an HIV test, there was a change in the use of condoms. Consistent condom use increased from 11% in 1990 to 20% in 1992 (Choi & Catania, 1996). These results were replicated by Piccinio and Mosher (1998), who reported condom use among 15- to 44-year-old Americans increased from 12% in 1992 to 20% in 1995. The researchers concluded that sexuality education has the potential to significantly affect the health of young Americans.

HIV and College Students

In the absence of a cure for AIDS and the prevalence of STIs, preventive measures will continue to be the primary method of responding to the threat of these diseases. Because young adults, such as college students, tend to have more sexual partners than those older or younger, they are particularly at risk for these diseases. That is why HIV and AIDS and STI educational campaigns have targeted this population. The results of these educational efforts have been heartening at times and disturbing at others.

In 1990, a survey of adult sexual behavior found that 13% had had sex with more than one partner in the year preceding the study, but only 8% of this group used condoms consistently (Leigh, Temple, & Trocki, 1993). In that same survey, the highest frequency of sex (daily) was among respondents who were younger than 30 years (14%). Shockingly in this day and age, of the 655 respondents who reported having had a sexual encounter with a new partner within the previous 5 years, only 25% said they had used a condom.

The good news is that young adults have adapted healthier behaviors in the years since. In a study of the changes from 1988 to 1995 in sexual behavior and condom use among teenage males, for instance, the proportion of 15- to 19-year-old males who reported ever having experienced sexual intercourse with a female declined from 60% to 55% (Sorenstein, et al., 1998). Furthermore, in 1995, 67% used a condom during their last sexual intercourse compared to only 57% in 1988. Overall, the proportion of males who had sexual intercourse without condoms declined from 37% in 1988 to 27%

Gender DIMENSIONS

Women and AIDS AIDS was originally identified as a disease affecting gay men. However, the face of AIDS has changed. Certainly, gay men are still the largest category of those infected with HIV in the United States. Yet, worldwide in 1993, 45% of new adult HIV infections occurred in women, and the number of female HIV infections was expected to equal the number of male infections in the year 2000. In the United States, new cases among women are increasing at a greater rate than among men, although men still have a greater number of cases.

Although HIV infection is affecting women to a greater extent than before, it is especially affecting women of color. Almost three-fourths of new infections are among African-American and Latino women. More alarming is that new infections occur more often in women aged 25 to 39 years than in other age groups. Given that these are the childbearing years, often these women's babies are born infected.

Poor women and women of color are more likely to contract HIV from a male sexual partner who is infected (most likely from intravenous drug use) than other women. They are also more likely to use drugs themselves, share needles, and/or engage in sex for drugs with other drug users who may be infected. Furthermore, poor women often lack access to education about AIDS and safer sex techniques, to medical care, and to economic and social support systems.

Instituting needle-exchange programs and community educational campaigns, putting health providers in the community through health clinics and walking of the neighborhoods, and using community health workers to encourage women to seek treatment are ways we can respond to the problem of women and AIDS.

in 1995. In another study concerning contraception methods used by American adults, it was found that, whereas the use of the birth control pill decreased between 1988 and 1995 from 31% to 27%, condom use increased from 15% to 20% (Piccinino & Mosher, 1998).

However, as evidenced by the preceding statistics, too many males and females still engage in unhealthy sexual practices that place them at risk of contracting an STI or becoming infected with HIV. Are college students, who are the most educated people in our society, ready to engage in safer sex? A study of 376 university students concluded that they are not (Dahl, Gorn, & Weinberg, 1997). With the rationale that carrying condoms is the one way to ensure that a condom is available when needed, researchers surveyed college students regarding their likelihood of carrying a condom in different situations (a bar, a concert, a party, and a first date). Part of the study involved the researchers' interviewing 346 students (137 females and 209 males) at a university bar known for "fun, cheap beer and . . . sex." They offered a five-dollar food coupon for every condom each student possessed. Only 16 students were carrying a condom (less than 5%). What do you think the results of this study would have been if it was conducted at a bar near your campus?

Why do college students not use condoms during sexual activities? A partial answer was provided by college students themselves in a study that asked them that very question (Bradford & Beck, 1991). Among the most frequently cited reasons for not using a condom were past failure or lack of experience with condoms, embarrassment in purchasing or using condoms, interference of the effects of alcohol with the use of condoms, hesitation to offend partners, belief that condom use decreases sexual pleasure, loss of spontaneity, loss of erection, lack of a condom when sexual intercourse was desired, low comfort level in communicating feelings about condom use with a partner, and fear of rejection if insisting on the use of a condom.

With so much at stake in terms of life and death, why do the factors cited seem so insurmountable to many college students and young adults?

Discussion Questions

1. Explain the ways HIV is transmitted, the stages of infection, the tests for infection, and how opportunistic diseases occur as a result of AIDS.
2. What treatments are available for HIV? What limits their worldwide availability?
3. List the safer-sex practices that reduce the risk of HIV transmission.

Application Questions

Reread the chapter-opening story and answer the following questions.

1. On June 25, 1998, the Supreme Court ruled that HIV-infected people are protected by a federal ban on discrimination against the disabled—even if they suffer no symptoms of AIDS. If that ruling had been made when Tim was diagnosed with HIV, do you think he might have been more willing to disclose his condition? Why or why not?
2. Regardless of the law, if you were a professor considering granting a graduate assistantship to a student (or an employer making a hiring decision), would the knowledge that the candidate was infected with HIV make a difference? How about if the person were being treated for cancer? Or heart disease? Why should such information make a difference?
3. How would you feel if you knew a fellow classmate or employee were HIV-infected?

Critical Thinking Questions

1. Is it fair that the federal government spends a disproportionate share of medical research money on HIV research? Put another way, should federal research money be spent in proportion to the number of people who contract an illness and die of it (such as cancer or heart disease)? Or should the potential threat of a disease's becoming more widespread take precedence?
2. You may remember this gender-related issue from another chapter: Men who carry condoms are considered to be "responsible." But women who carry condoms are considered "sluts." Given the need for more condom use to prevent the spread of STIs and HIV, how can this double standard be overcome?

Critical Thinking Case

Deciding whether or not to disclose HIV infection is clearly a troubling decision for anyone to make. But do people have an obligation to disclose that information to protect others?

Consider the case of the two-time double–Olympic diving gold medalist Greg Louganis, who was HIV-positive during his second Olympics. Louganis did not disclose his HIV status to Olympic officials. During one dive, Louganis hit the board with the back of his head and received a wound that bled. A doctor treated him without knowing of the HIV condition—and thus did not take extra precautions. Also, Olympic competitors are required to supply urine samples to test for illegal substances (such as steroids). Because urine would contain HIV, anyone handling Louganis's sample would have also been at risk unless proper precautions were taken.

Should Louganis have been required to disclose his status before the Olympics? What discrimination may result against an athlete who discloses his or her HIV-infected status? (You may reflect on the problems Magic Johnson faced when he disclosed his status.)

What about typical recreational athletes—people who work out in gyms, play basketball in leagues, fence (saber, epee, or foil), or participate in any recreational activity in which they can be injured accidentally? When do HIV-infected people need to disclose their status?

Exploring Personal Dimensions

Could You Negotiate Safer Sex?

The following items ask you to agree (A) or disagree (D) with the statements presented. Indicate the items about which you are unsure (U) of your response. Compare your responses to those of a friend. Discuss each item about which you said you were unsure of your response. Are there items about which you and a friend disagree? What changes or adaptations would you or your friend have to make in order to take on a safer orientation toward sex with a partner?

I believe that

_____ I could use a condom effectively.

_____ I could buy condoms without embarrassment.

_____ If my partner did not want to use a condom during sexual intercourse, I could convince him or her to do otherwise.

_____ Consumption of alcohol or use of other recreational drugs would in no way affect my determination to use a condom or to convince my partner to respect my wishes.

_____ Having to remember to buy, carry, and use condoms would interfere with sexual spontaneity.

_____ If I suggested using a condom, my partner would think that I must have had many previous sexual partners.

_____ I would feel comfortable insisting on using a condom with a new sexual partner.
_____ I would not feel self-conscious about putting a condom on myself (or on my partner).
_____ I would be able to discuss use of condoms with a partner even before we had any physical intimacy such as touching, caressing, or kissing.
_____ If I suggested using a condom, my partner would think I did not trust him or her.
_____ Using a condom during sexual intercourse would interfere with sexual pleasure or sexual functioning.
_____ Using condoms is an activity primarily for people who have many sexual partners.
_____ Having to use a condom might subsequently prove to be embarrassing to me or my partner if the mechanics of using one resulted in loss of erection.
_____ I could tactfully remove and dispose of a condom after sexual intercourse.
_____ I could convince my partner that use of a condom can be a stimulating part of sexual foreplay.

Sexuality Online

Go to the web component for *Exploring the Dimensions of Human Sexuality* at sexuality.jbpub.com for web exercises, additional resources related to this chapter, and student review tools.

Suggested Readings

Bartlett, J. G. & Finkbeiner, A. K. *The guide to living with HIV infection: Developed at the Johns Hopkins AIDS Clinic*. Baltimore, MD: Johns Hopkins University Press, 1998.

Branson, B. M. Home sample collection tests for HIV infection, *Journal of the American Medical Association, 280* (1998), 1699–1702.

Cohen, M. R. & Doner, K. *The HIV wellness sourcebook: An east/west guide to living well with HIV/AIDS and related conditions*. New York: Owl Books, 1998.

Fan, H., Conner, R. F., & Villarreal, L. P. *AIDS: Science and society,* 2nd ed. Sudbury, MA: Jones & Bartlett Publishers, 1998.

Gupta, G. R. (2001) Gender, sexuality, and HIV/AIDS: The what, the why, and the how, *SIECUS Report, 29* (2001), 6–12.

Hader, S. L., Smith, D. K., Moore, J. S., and Holmberg, S. D. HIV infection in Women in the United States: Status at the millennium. *Journal of the American Medical Association, 285* (2001), 1186–1192.

Huber, J. T. & Riddlesperger, K. *Eating positive: A nutrition guide and recipe book for people with HIV/AIDS*. Binghampton, NY: Harrington Park Press, 1998.

Ward, D. E. & Krim, M. *The Amfar AIDS handbook: The complete guide to understanding HIV and AIDS*. New York: W. W. Norton, 1998.

Watstein, S. B. & Chandler, K. *The AIDS dictionary*. New York: Facts on File, 1998.

CHAPTER 15

Sexual Dysfunction and Therapy

FEATURES

Gender Dimensions Characteristics of Dysfunction Between the Sexes

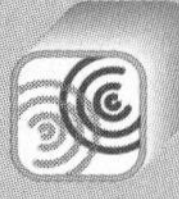

Communication Dimensions Discussing Sexual Dysfunction

Multicultural Dimensions Sexual Dysfunction and Latino Populations

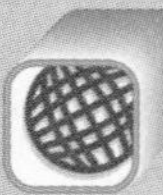

Global Dimensions Sexual Disorders Around the World

Ethical Dimensions Should Surrogates Be Used in Sexual Therapy?

CHAPTER OBJECTIVES

1. Describe the major male and female sexual dysfunctions, including the desire dysfunctions. Evaluate what makes the inability to perform sexually a clinical dysfunction.
2. Identify the multidimensional causes of sexual dysfunction, including the physical, psychological, and sociocultural aspects.
3. Compare and contrast the varied approaches to treating sexual dysfunctions. Explain why many different models of therapy exist.

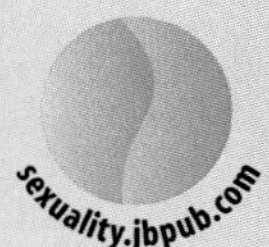

sexuality.jbpub.com

Gender Dimensions: Characteristics of Dysfunction Between Genders
Male Sexual Dysfunction
Female Sexual Dysfunction
Treating Sexual Dysfunction

INTRODUCTION

After he was diagnosed with prostate cancer in 1991, Senator Bob Dole underwent treatment, including surgery. He has since avidly promoted the importance of early detection and encouraged men to speak frankly with their doctors about prostate-related problems.

But it was in May 1998 that Dole made his biggest disclosure: He said on Larry King's talk show that he had been among the men who took part in the trials for the drug Viagra (sildenafil citrate). Viagra is a drug to treat men who have difficulty achieving an erection (erectile dysfunction). In effect, Bob Dole was admitting that he, as do millions of other men, had a sexual dysfunction—specifically, erectile disorder. The next day, Elizabeth Dole, his wife, was asked about the drug during a public appearance. She laughed and said with a beaming smile, "It's a great drug!"

Such public disclosures by celebrities and politicians make taboo topics—such as sexual dysfunctions—the subject of discussion among friends, colleagues, classmates, and even couples. Dole's 1998 public announcement, followed by commercials in March 1999, offered frank and genuine advice: If you have a problem, see a doctor. In the case of erectile disorder, about 80% of problems are physical and can be solved with a prescription or a medical procedure. Other disorders, though, have psychological or sociocultural dimensions at their root.

The Viagra story also touches on the socioeconomic and political dimensions of sexuality. As recently as the 1970s, insurers would not have covered treatments for erectile disorder, because the condition was believed to be psychological. Insurers began coverage as research proved there were physical causes as well. Coverage for Viagra is limited generally to 12 pills per month—the recommended dosage.

When the FDA approved Viagra on March 27, 1998, it was not covered under Medicaid. Thus, it was unavailable to those in lower economic brackets. But the political ramifications of denying this wonder drug to the poor caused an uproar. Politicians know that older citizens are more likely to vote. Thus, many states require Medicaid coverage for Viagra. Alabama pays for only 4 pills per month; Arkansas, Louisiana, and Maryland pay for 10; and Utah pays for 20 pills per month.

Sources: Why is Mrs. Dole smiling? *Washington Post* (May 9, 1998); Postmarketing safety of sildenafil citrate (Viagra), www.fda.gov/cder/consumerinfo/viagra/viagraupdate721.htm; Stark, K. Will insurers pay? Clamor for Viagra could cinch it, *Philadelphia Inquirer* (April 24, 1998).

Sexual Dysfunction

Are you perfect? What seems a silly question has great importance for sexual functioning. Of course none of us is perfect. And yet, the occasional inability to function sexually (for example, to achieve and maintain an erection or to secrete adequate vaginal lubrication) leads many of us to conclude that something is drastically wrong with us.

This lack of response may be caused by a number of factors that have no bearing at all on your sexual functioning. For example, the ingestion of alcoholic beverages can interfere with sexual response, as can use of a number of other drugs such as hypertension medication, narcotics, and barbiturates. In addition, some people have partners with whom it is difficult to respond sexually. For example, your partner may be unappealing, dirty, or smelly; he may know so little about sexual physiology that he attempts penile insertion before sufficient vaginal lubrication; or she may touch the scrotum and handle the testicles in a way that causes pain and discomfort. And yet, if the individuals with these sexual partners do not respond as one would expect under more conducive circumstances, they themselves are sometimes accused of having an "abnormality." It might be more accurate to suggest that those who are sexually responsive to dirty, smelly, clumsy sexual partners are the ones experiencing some abnormality.

The media also help to establish unrealistic sexual expectations that, when not met, may lead people to think of themselves as dysfunctional. For example, when movies portray gorgeous specimens of men and women in romantic settings, who seem to have nothing else on their minds but sex, and who are willing and able to engage in any sexual activity that comes to mind, we and our lovers may not measure up. We might conclude something is wrong with us or our love life, although in reality something is wrong with this portrayal. We will discuss the commercialism of sex in detail in Chapter 17. Suffice it to say here that soap operas, movies, plays, and advertisements sometimes lead people to decide they are not as sexually adequate as those they see "performing" on satin sheets with unblemished bodies glistening under flattering spotlights.

However, there are people who experience difficulty responding sexually and who wish their sexual responses could be healthier and more sexually satisfying. They may find it difficult to achieve and/or maintain an erection or to relax enough to allow penile penetration. They may ejaculate too soon, or they may experience disturbing pain during coitus. They may wonder why they do not feel sexually aroused enough or do not experience orgasm. Men and women, heterosexuals and homosexuals, experience these concerns.

They may be young or old, African-American or white, well educated or lacking in schooling, and from any socioeconomic group. The one characteristic they have in common, though, is dissatisfaction with their sexual life, and this dissatisfaction often affects other aspects of their relationships.

This chapter explores some of these matters. We discuss the kinds of sexual problems people experience, what causes these problems, and how they can be treated. Notice the difficulty in diagnosing particular sexual dysfunctions (even the experts do not always agree about whether a dysfunction exists) and the varied approaches to treating them once they are identified. This, too, is discussed and its implications explored. We begin with a definition of sexual dysfunction.

Sexual dysfunction is a chronic inability to respond sexually in a way that one finds satisfying. We do not use the term to describe those situations, common to many people, in which they are temporarily uninterested in sexual activity or unable to respond sexually because of exhaustion, excessive use of alcohol, anger, and so on. The key word in our definition is *chronic*—that is, a consistent long-term inability to respond. It applies both to people who have never had satisfactory sexual relations—primary dysfunctions—and to people who have had successful sexual relations at some time but are now having chronic difficulty—secondary dysfunction.

sexual dysfunction
A specific, chronic disorder involving sexual performance.

The amount of sexual dysfunction prevalent in society is difficult, if not impossible, to determine. But it has been estimated that at some time in their marriage, about half of all married couples experience sexual difficulties (Ende, Rockwell, & Glasgow, 1984; McCarthy, Ryan, & Johnson, 1975; Nathan, 1986) that can be classified as (chronic) sexual dysfunctions. Specialists in human behavior, such as psychiatrists, social workers, and psychologists, report that about 75% of their clients have sexual problems that may or may not be chronic (McCary, 1979). Obviously it is impossible to determine the number of people who do not satisfactorily respond sexually but who never seek treatment. But the number of people seeking treatment has increased in recent years.

There are several possible explanations for this increase. First, the increasing amount of information on the subject has made admitting sexual dysfunctions less embarrassing. Second, more effective therapy is now available and people are more willing to take advantage of it. Third, as the physiological features of sexual response are understood by more people, more nonorgasmic women and men with erectile problems realize they are not permanently unresponsive but have sexual dysfunctions that can be treated effectively. Fourth, the amount of sexual dysfunction might actually be increasing among men because as women become aware of their right to sexual satisfaction, more men may find themselves overanxious about meeting their partners' expectations.

The underlying cause of any sexual dysfunction may be either physical or psychological, but most experts agree that psychological causes, broadly defined, are much more prevalent, causing anywhere from 40% to 90% of sexual dysfunctions. Masters and Johnson's 1970 conclusion, which is probably still relevant, was that "sociocultural deprivation and ignorance of sexual physiology, rather than psychiatric or medical illness," were at the source of most sexual dysfunction. We would add that although poor communication about sex may not actually cause a dysfunction, it can certainly allow conditions to worsen rather than improve and can contribute to making otherwise temporary troubles chronic. Likewise, most problems are best solved through the cooperation of partners.

We now turn our attention to the types of dysfunctions people experience, and we begin with those experienced by men.

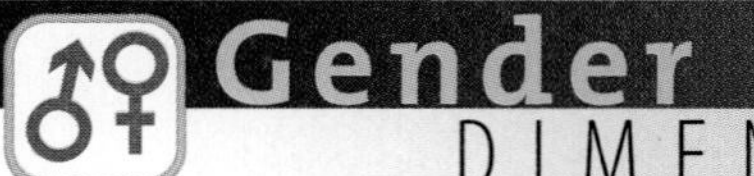

Characteristics of Dysfunction Between the Sexes

In the February 10, 1999, issue of the *Journal of the American Medical Association,* the results of a national study of the prevalence and predictors of sexual dysfunction in the United States were published. Here are the results by sex:

Females

1. The prevalence of sexual dysfunction in women decreases with increasing age, with the exception of problems with vaginal lubrication.
2. Nonmarried women are more than one and a half times as likely to have orgasmic dysfunction and sexual anxiety as married women.
3. Women who have graduated from college are half as likely to experience low sexual desire, orgasmic dysfunction, dyspareunia (pain in the genital area during sexual intercourse), and sexual anxiety as women who did not graduate from college. Overall, women with less education experience less pleasure with sex and more sexual anxiety.
4. African-American women have higher rates of low sexual desire and less sexual pleasure than white women. However, white women are more likely to experience dyspareunia.
5. Hispanic women experience lower rates of sexual dysfunction than other women.
6. Sexual arousal problems are more prevalent in women who have been sexually victimized through adult–child contact or forced sexual contact.
7. The total prevalence of sexual dysfunction in women is higher than in men (43% versus 31%).

Males

1. As men age, they experience more sexual dysfunction, in particular, erectile dysfunction and low sexual desire.
2. Nonmarried men experience more sexual dysfunctions than do married men.
3. Men who have graduated from college are only two-thirds as likely to experience premature ejaculation and half as likely to experience lack of pleasure from sex or sexual anxiety as men who have not graduated from high school.
4. Men with poor health experience a higher prevalence of sexual dysfunction, whereas poor health is associated only with dyspareunia in women.
5. Circumcised men experience the same prevalence of sexual dysfunction as noncircumcised men.
6. Men reporting same-sex activity are twice as likely to experience premature ejaculation and low sexual desire as men who have not experienced same-sex activity.
7. Male victims of sexual victimization are three times as likely to experience erectile dysfunction and two times as likely to experience premature ejaculation and low sexual desire as are other males.

Source: Laumann, E. O., Paik, A., & Rosen, R. C. Sexual dysfunction in the United States: Prevalence and predictors, *Journal of the American Medical Association, 281, no. 6* (1999), 537–544.

Male Sexual Dysfunctions

Sexual dysfunction in males can be traumatic. In our society, men are expected to be experienced and talented in matters of sex. They are supposed to be the leaders with their sexual partners, serving as a guide to sexual bliss. When men cannot perform in this manner, they may consider themselves less manly and, as a result, experience a range of other psychological problems.

In addition to the effect sexual dysfunctions can have on a man's psychological health, his relationships can be devastated. A man would most likely not want to initiate or participate in sexual activity when the results might be failure and a demonstration of ineptness. Only a masochist would allow himself to be placed in such a situation continually and, consequently, his sexual activity would become sporadic. The partner then might wonder why she was not good enough or appealing enough and the total relationship would be at risk.

Sexual dysfunctions need not be viewed as exclusively negative. There is a positive side to this situation. Researchers report that people who engage in sexual therapy often become less anxious, communicate better (Zilbergeld & Kilmann, 1984), become more assertive with their sexual partners (Tullman, et al., 1981), and feel more positive about their sexual selves (Cotten-Houston & Wheeler, 1983). You might not choose to have a sexual problem even if you could acquire these benefits of sexual therapy, but the fact that this potential exists is often a welcome surprise.

Men experience four main types of sexual dysfunctions: erectile dysfunction, premature ejaculation, ejaculatory incompetence, and dyspareunia.

Erectile Dysfunction

A man's difficulty in achieving and maintaining an erection is popularly known as **impotence.** This term is Latin and means "without power." The word *impotence* is used to connote that a man has lost power—is no longer "manly"—when he cannot achieve or maintain an erection. Furthermore, he has lost power as a lover and has lost his reproductive capacity. The more understanding, more professional, more sensitive, and more accurate term is **erectile dysfunction.** To imply that a man with a sexual dysfunction is generally without power is untrue and unfair and only exacerbates the situation. Men who are unable to achieve or maintain erections may be satisfying lovers nevertheless; they may be very effective at cunnilingus or manual masturbation. Furthermore, they may be in "powerful" positions (such as a corporate executive) or be adequate in all other aspects of their lives.

impotence
Difficulty in achieving and maintaining an erection.

erectile dysfunction
The inability of a man to maintain an erection long enough to have sexual intercourse; commonly known as *impotence.*

primary erectile dysfunction
A condition in which an adult male has never had an erection sufficient to engage in sexual intercourse.

secondary erectile dysfunction
A condition in which an adult male has previously had an erection sufficient to engage in sexual intercourse but no longer has.

There are an estimated 20 to 30 million American men who have an erectile dysfunction (Danoff & Katz, 1998). This includes 10% of men in their 60s, 25% in their 70s, 40% in their 80s, and more than half in their 90s (Endocrinology Society, 1998). Approximately 7% of younger men experience erectile dysfunction. Men who have never had an erection sufficient to have sexual intercourse are said to have **primary erectile dysfunction.** Men who have previously been able to maintain an erection long enough to have intercourse but subsequently have an erection problem are said to have **secondary erectile dysfunction.** Secondary erectile dysfunction is approximately 10 times more prevalent than primary erectile dysfunction (Kaplan, 1974; Kolodny, Masters & Johnson, 1979). Some men achieve an erection only to lose it on vaginal insertion. Others achieve and maintain an erection long enough during masturbation to have an orgasm but cannot be coitally connected and maintain that erection. These, too, are examples of erectile dysfunction.

Making a precise diagnosis of erectile dysfunction is not as easy as it might appear (Table 15.1). Many men are at times unable to have an erection or lose it before vaginal penetration. They may be uninterested in their partners, they may have ingested too much alcohol, or they may be using certain medications that interfere with the erectile reflex. How often does this have to occur before the condition is classified as erectile dysfunction? Masters and Johnson (1970) classified men

TABLE 15.1 DSM-IV: Diagnostic Criteria for Male Erectile Disorder

A. Persistent or recurrent inability to attain, or to maintain until completion of the sexual activity, an adequate erection.

B. The disturbance causes marked distress or interpersonal difficulty.

C. The erectile dysfunction is not better accounted for by another Axis I disorder (other than a Sexual Dysfunction) and is not due exclusively to the direct physiological effects of a substance (for example, a drug of abuse, a medication) or a general medical condition.

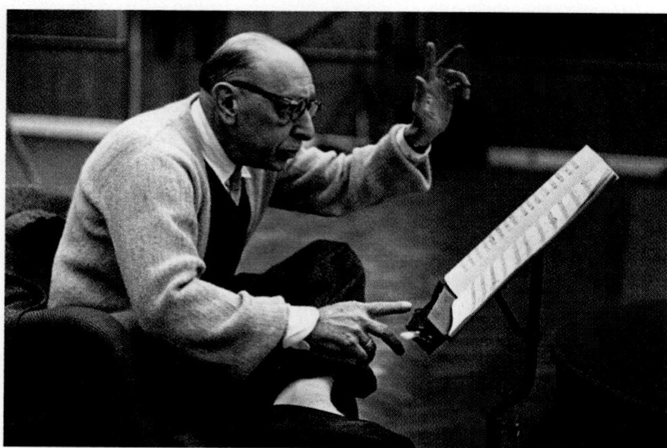

Up to the 1970s, before the advent of drug therapy, erectile dysfunction was believed to be mainly psychological in nature. Thus, most remedies focused on mind over matter. The legendary 20th-century composer Igor Stravinsky (1882–1971) once wrote to a friend that to overcome impotence you should eat a large meal and then visit a brothel! With today's knowledge, would a man who responded to a meal and a prostitute be considered to have erectile disorder?

who, in at least 25% of their sexual encounters, are unable to maintain an erection long enough for penile insertion as having secondary erectile dysfunction. Crooks and Baur (1990) believe it inappropriate to specify a cutoff point (for example, 25%). They prefer to ask the couple whether they believe a problem exists; if they say it does, then erectile dysfunction is diagnosed.

Erectile dysfunction is caused by myriad factors (Buvat, et al., 1990). Whereas it was previously believed that most erectile dysfunctions were caused by psychological factors, the latest thinking is that 70% are at least partially the result of physiological factors (Danoff & Katz, 1998). Among these factors are diabetes (Jensen, 1981; Maatman & Montague, 1985; Nidus Information Services, 1998); infections; the use of drugs or medications (Crenshaw, 1985); alcoholism; spinal-cord injury; injuries to the penis, testes, urethra, or prostate; and any condition that interferes with the flow of blood to the erectile tissue of the penis (Lewis, 1990; Wespes & Schulman, 1985). In addition, kidney disease, nerve damage (for example, from surgery), endocrine abnormalities, and neurological problems can cause erectile dysfunction. Even riding a bicycle more than 100 miles a week (obviously among serious bikers) can cause erection problems (Schroepfer, 1989).

Among the nonorganic causes are fear of sexual performance—"Will I be an adequate sexual partner or show my ineptitude?" This fear can result in a self-fulfilling prophecy; that is, the fear may make the man so anxious that he is unable to achieve and maintain an erection. The result could be lowered self-esteem, which itself feeds into the original fear. Thus, a cycle of erectile dysfunction develops. In addition, guilt or shame about sexual activity can interfere with an erection.

All men are capable of having difficulty in achieving an erection at one time or other, even college-age men. Perhaps they have just ingested alcohol, which is a central nervous system depressant; or they find their partner unappealing; or the surroundings are not conducive to sexual stimulation. In any case, infrequent erectile difficulties are not cause for alarm. However, if they persist, professional help should be sought.

Some novel ways to diagnose the causes of erectile dysfunction exist. For example, knowing men normally have erections during their sleep, physicians sometimes place electronic devices around the flaccid penises of men with erection problems while they sleep to determine the presence and frequency of erections (Parulkar, et al., 1988). If a problem exists during sleep, the cause is organic. A man who is concerned about an erection problem but who does not yet want to consult a physician or counselor can place a ring of postage stamps around his penis before going to sleep. If the stamps are placed snugly around the flaccid penis and an erection occurs, the ring of stamps will be broken in the morning. To determine further whether erectile dysfunction is a result of physiological causes, the man is questioned about how abruptly the problem presented itself. If it is a psychological problem it usually develops gradually; if it is physiological it usually develops abruptly (Stipp, 1987).

It is an unfortunate fact that erectile dysfunction can permeate an entire relationship. This is true not only because sexual activity is a significant part of a total relationship, and consequently has an effect on other aspects of the relationship, but also because the woman or man may blame him- or herself for the partner's erectile problems—"Am I not attractive enough?"

"Am I not skilled enough?" "What am I doing wrong?" Also, the sexual partner may assume that the problem stems from the man engaging in sexual activity with someone else. In any case, the effect may place such strain and pressure on the relationship that counseling should include these considerations among its foci.

Premature Ejaculation

premature ejaculation
The inability of a man to control ejaculation for a sufficient length of time during coitus.

Premature ejaculation, or rapid ejaculation, is the most common sexual dysfunction in men. However, as with some of the other dysfunctions, it is not easily defined. Years ago, *premature ejaculation* meant the man could not maintain penile insertion without ejaculating within a minimal amount of time (for example, 2 minutes) or could not perform a minimal number of penile thrusts before ejaculating. Masters and Johnson (1970) even proposed a definition that classified the ejaculate as premature if the man's partner was not satisfied in at least 50% of their coital episodes. Helen Singer Kaplan (1974) defined *premature ejaculation* as the man's inability to control his ejaculate voluntarily.

The problems with these definitions were several. The couples in these studies differed in their perception of what was premature. Some couples were perfectly happy for coitus to last a short period, whereas other couples were dissatisfied with only 2 minutes of insertion or a minimal number of penile thrusts. In addition, Masters and Johnson's definition overlooked the fact that some women do not experience orgasms during coitus and would not, regardless of the timing of their partner's ejaculation, achieve orgasm. Kaplan's definition neglected to recognize that men, as a rule, do not possess total voluntary control over ejaculation; this definition would classify most men as sexually dysfunctional.

Newer research considers the desires of the couple in the definition of premature ejaculation. For example, one definition divides premature ejaculation into a continuum ranging from ejaculation before penile insertion to ejaculation 7 minutes after insertion (Schover, et al., 1982). The ejaculate is not classified as premature, however, unless either the man or the woman considers it to be so. We define premature ejaculation as a condition in which the man cannot maintain vaginal insertion long enough—long enough as judged by the man himself and his partner—without ejaculating. This requires that either the man or his partner must be dissatisfied with the timing of the ejaculate for a problem to exist. This definition is consistent with that in the American Psychiatric Association's *Diagnostic and Statistical Manual (DSM-IV),* which states that premature ejaculation is "the persistent or recurrent ejaculation with minimal sexual stimulation, or, before, upon, or shortly after penetration and before the person wishes it." However, because this definition leaves open the questions of what is "minimal sexual stimulation" and what does "shortly" mean, we prefer our definition, which requires that either one or both partners perceive there to be a problem.

The effects of ejaculating prematurely can be harmful to the relationship and to the psychological health of the man. Men may feel less than manly and may have a lowered self-esteem (Perelman, 1980). Not wanting to disclose their problem, these men may refrain from sexual intercourse, thereby disappointing their partners and/or making them wonder about the viability of the relationship. Because premature ejaculation is estimated to affect 15% to 20% of all men at least moderately (Masters, Johnson, & Kolodny, 1985), the number of people affected—men and women—is significant.

Several self-help techniques for overcoming rapid ejaculation have been proposed (Trudel & Proulx, 1987). The use of a condom seems to help because the glans penis is not stimulated directly. Some men drink an alcoholic beverage to decrease the rapidity of their sexual response. Others allow themselves a rapid orgasm, or a small orgasm, knowing that the next one will take longer to arrive. Waiting for sufficient vaginal lubrication may also help prolong ejaculation. The glans penis may experience too much friction if the vagina is insufficiently lubricated, causing increased sensitivity and rapid ejaculation (Steege, 1981). Relaxing or switching positions to decrease muscle tension is another technique recommended, because rapid ejaculation is encouraged by too much muscular tension. Finally, creams designed to decrease sensitivity can be placed on the glans penis. Whether the benefit of controlling the ejaculate is worth the price of deadened sensations during coitus is a decision that only the man and his partner can make.

retarded ejaculation
A condition in which penile erection occurs during sexual intercourse but ejaculation does not; sometimes termed ejaculatory incompetence.

partial ejaculatory incompetence
A condition in which, during ejaculation, only a seepage of semen occurs, and orgasm lacks pleasurable sensations.

dyspareunia
Pain in the genital area during sexual intercourse.

Ejaculatory Incompetence
For some men, the problem is not ejaculating too soon but, rather, being unable to ejaculate in the vagina at all. This condition is known as **ejaculatory incompetence,** sometimes referred to as **retarded ejaculation.** When a man has never ejaculated in the vagina and is incapable of doing so, he is classified as having primary ejaculatory incompetence. When he has previously been able to ejaculate in the vagina but can no longer do so, he is classified as having secondary ejaculatory incompetence. These men may still be able to maintain an erection and/or stay sexually aroused. Or they may be

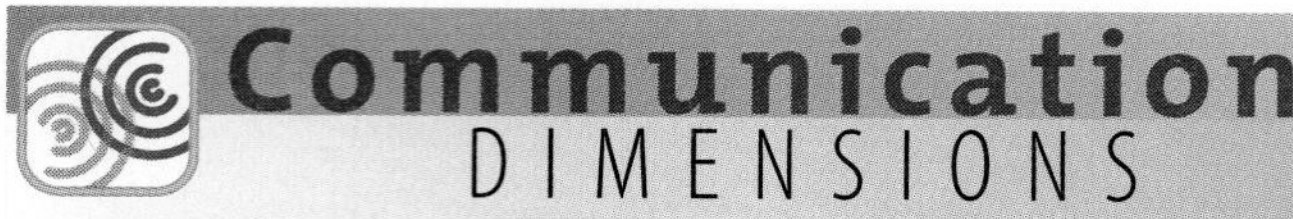

Discussing Sexual Dysfunction Two people who love and care for each other can deal with sexual dysfunction together. The key to the resolution of this situation, however, lies in the total relationship, not just the sexual part. Sexual communication is just one form of communication. If the relationship is characterized by ineffective communication in general, assuming that communicating about sex will be different is unrealistic. So, the first step in resolving sexual problems is to develop a relationship of caring, concern, mutual respect, and understanding. For this reason, some sex therapists work with clients to improve their interaction in general and concurrently help them respond to their sexual concerns.

Assuming that the relationship is minimally communicative, the first step is to provide support for each other and the promise of hope: "That's okay, honey; we'll get help and work it out." "It's not that I care any less for you, sweetheart, but something's interfering with my sex-making right now." This form of communication can reduce partners' anxieties that may be interfering with sexual function. Imagine the embarrassment of experiencing a sexual dysfunction and the resulting pressure during each subsequent sexual encounter. The fear of "failure" and the anticipation of disappointing one's partner can be so frustrating that they can feed on themselves, contributing to, and exacerbating, the sexual problem. Communicating that it is okay, that help can be obtained, that the problem will be faced together, and that there is a commitment to work to make matters better can go a long way in intervening between dysfunctional feelings and resulting dysfunctional sex.

Once counseling starts, the couple needs to continue communicating with each other but now must also begin communicating with the counselor. To be effective, communication with the counselor must be candid. Without candor, the source of the problems may never be uncovered, or at least it will take longer to discover. A commitment is then required to adhere conscientiously to the treatment regimen and remain with it until the problem is resolved.

Certainly, sexual dysfunction puts a strain on both people involved, but caring, supportive lovers can become even closer through facing this problem and overcoming it.

able to ejaculate through masturbation or oral–genital stimulation. Sometimes, though rarely, this condition can be specific to only one partner or to specific situations (Munjack & Kanno, 1979).

We use the term *ejaculatory incompetence* with some hesitation. It is unfair and inaccurate to suggest that men who have difficulty with ejaculating are incompetent. But because the professional literature refers to this condition as *ejaculatory incompetence,* we do so as well.

Another form of retarded ejaculation is called **partial ejaculatory incompetence.** This condition results in a "half" orgasm—that is, a seepage of semen without true orgasmic sensations. Kaplan (1974) writes of men who, when fatigued or in conflict, "come without realizing they have." Originally thought to be rare, this form of ejaculatory incompetence seems relatively common among men.

Ejaculatory incompetence is a disorder that may have interesting side effects. For example, the ability to maintain penile insertion for long periods without ejaculating may be valued by many men and appreciated by their sexual partners. However, the extreme of being unable to ejaculate in the vagina at all can result in the partner's questioning her own sexual abilities (Munjack & Oziel, 1980). In this case, the benefit of prolonged insertion quickly dissipates, and frustration and doubt set in. Another side effect is that when the man fakes orgasm to prevent his partner from feeling inadequate, not only does he remain sexually unsatisfied, but deceit, rather than trust and openness, can begin to characterize the relationship as a whole. As with many of the other sexual dysfunctions, treatment must be directed at the relationship as well as at the specific disorder.

Dyspareunia

Painful sexual intercourse is called **dyspareunia.** During sexual intercourse, men may feel pain in the penis, testes, or some other part of the body. Pain during coitus can be caused by both organic and nonorganic factors. For example, infections of the penis, foreskin, testes, urethra, or prostate can cause such pain, as can allergic reactions to a spermicidal cream or foam used as a contraceptive. Some men report irritation of the glans penis caused by an intrauterine device (IUD) string, which extends out of the uterus into the vagina.

Other causes of dyspareunia in men include a foreskin that is too tight and causes pain when an erection develops; smegma that has not been washed away from the glans penis and causes an infection and/or irritates the glans; and Peyronie's disease, in which fibrous tissue and calcium deposits develop in the area around the cavernous bodies of the penis and may cause pain.

Female Sexual Dysfunctions

Only relatively recently have females been allowed to express their sexual needs and to be viewed as entitled to sexual satisfaction at the same level as men's. However, a double standard is still alive and well. Some men consider women suspect if they initiate sexual activity or are vocal in appreciating it. They are still supposed to be coy, letting the man take the lead, for fear of what might be thought of them if they act too assertively. Given this situation, too many women have adopted a passive attitude toward sexual activity and sometimes have developed shame, guilt, or embarrassment about their sexual behavior. For some women, this has progressed into an inability to function in a sexually healthy and satisfying way. In particular, the sexual dysfunctions women sometimes experience are sexual unresponsiveness, orgasmic dysfunction, vaginismus, and dyspareunia.

TABLE 15.2 DSM-IV: Diagnostic Criteria for Female Sexual Arousal Disorder

A. Persistent or recurrent inability to attain, or to maintain until completion of the sexual activity, an adequate lubrication–swelling response of sexual excitement.

B. The disturbance causes marked distress or interpersonal difficulty.

C. The sexual dysfunction is not better accounted for by another Axis I disorder (except another Sexual Dysfunction) and is not due exclusively to the direct physiological effects of a substance (for example, a drug of abuse, a medication) or a general medical condition.

Sexual Unresponsiveness

Popularly known as **frigidity,** the condition in which a woman "is uninterested in sex" (Haas & Haas, 1990) or receives no erotic pleasure from sexually oriented stimulation is more appropriately termed **sexual unresponsiveness** or, technically speaking, female sexual arousal disorder (Table 15.2). The word *frigidity* connotes a cold feeling or a lack of emotion. On the contrary, the opposite might be true; that is, a woman may be a caring and sensitive person who is just unable to respond to sexual stimulation. The physiological manifestations of sexual unresponsiveness include lack of vaginal lubrication, lack of vasocongestion, and lack of change in the size of the vagina during sexual stimulation.

Sexual unresponsiveness can be caused by nonpsychogenic factors (such as low estrogen levels), shame, fear, guilt, or embarrassment about sexual activity or one's body. Before treatment can begin, the cause(s) must be identified. Obviously, if the causes are psychogenic in nature, treatment will differ from treatment for organic causes.

sexual unresponsiveness
Commonly referred to as **frigidity** or female sexual arousal disorder, a sexual dysfunction that causes a woman to experience little or no erotic pleasure through sexual stimulation.

orgasmic dysfunction
The consistent or frequent inability of a woman to achieve an orgasm.

vaginismus
The involuntary contraction of the muscles surrounding the vaginal entrance so that entry of the penis is prevented.

Orgasmic Dysfunction

Not all women can experience orgasm; this condition is known as **orgasmic dysfunction** (Table 15.3). Women who have never had an orgasm are said to have *primary orgasmic dysfunction,* or *primary anorgasmia* (some term this *inorgasmia*). Those who have at one time experienced orgasm but do not now are said to have *secondary orgasmic dysfunction,* or *secondary anorgasmia.* Some women have orgasms under certain circumstances but not others, for example, while masturbating but not when stimulated by a partner. This condition is referred to as *situational orgasmic dysfunction,* or *situational anorgasmia.* If the inability to experience an orgasm is limited to coital episodes, that is known as *coital sexual dysfunction,* or *coital anorgasmia.*

The data regarding the incidence of orgasmic dysfunction have been remarkably consistent over the years. Earlier studies that found that approximately 10% of women were coitally anorgasmic (Kinsey, Pomeroy, & Martin, 1953; Levin & Levin, 1975) have been supported by more recent research (Spector & Carey, 1990). Furthermore, only 30% to 44% of women report they usually experience orgasm through sexual intercourse without having the clitoris simultaneously stimulated (Ellison, 1980; Hite, 1976). These statistics have generated some controversy as to whether coital anorgasmia should be considered a problem. Remember our discussion of premature ejaculation, in which we stated the need for one or both of the sexual partners to feel a problem exists. Similarly, experts argue that if women achieve orgasm through direct clitoral stimulation or through oral–genital sex only, and they and their partners are satisfied with this, this should not be considered dysfunctional. It is further argued that coital orgasms are an inappropriate "goal" of sexual activity; a goal

TABLE 15.3 DSM-IV: Diagnostic Criteria for Female Orgasmic Disorder

A. Persistent or recurrent delay in, or absence of, orgasm following a normal sexual excitement phase. Women exhibit wide variability in the type or intensity of stimulation that triggers orgasm. The diagnosis of Female Orgasmic Disorder should be based on the clinician's judgment that the woman's orgasmic capacity is less than would be reasonable for her age, sexual experience, and the adequacy of sexual stimulation she receives.

B. The disturbance causes marked distress or interpersonal difficulty.

C. The orgasmic dysfunction is not better accounted for by another Axis I disorder (except another Sexual Dysfunction) and is not due exclusively to the direct physiological effects of a substance (for example, a drug of abuse, a medication) or a general medical condition.

imposed by men, who are only rarely anorgasmic, on women. The argument continues that because women's sexual response cycles have greater variability than men's, women are more content to enjoy sex—even coitus—without orgasm. Furthermore, most women can have regular orgasms, but not through intercourse alone. They require clitoral stimulation. If women do not experience orgasm through intercourse, they should not be considered dysfunctional.

An opposing view is presented by Masters, Johnson, and Kolodny (1985). They argue that accepting coital anorgasmia because it affects so many women is akin to accepting premature ejaculation as within normal limits, because both conditions affect approximately the same number of people. They continue that because many women who are coitally anorgasmic can be taught, through therapy, to achieve orgasms during coitus, why discourage these women from doing something about their coitally anorgasmic condition by describing it as normal? Finally, they argue there is no evidence that a large percentage of women are incapable of orgasm. Consequently, those who are incapable of orgasm should be offered help to rectify their situation.

Only about 5% of the cases of orgasmic dysfunction are the result of organic causes (Masters, Johnson, & Kolodny, 1985). Organic causes are usually such chronic illnesses as diabetes, alcoholism, hormone deficiencies, or pelvic infections. The other 95% are the result of psychogenic factors such as shame and guilt associated with sexual activity. These states of mind interfere with the woman's ability to relax and allow the natural body processes to occur. Each episode then feeds on the last, until coitus is anticipated with fear and embarrassment. It is no wonder that orgasms do not occur under these circumstances.

Vaginismus

Some women cannot relax the muscles around the entrance to the vagina enough to allow for penetration of the penis or even a narrower object, for example, a finger. The recurrent or persistent involuntary spasm of the outer third of the vagina that interferes with sexual intercourse is known as **vaginismus.** In less severe cases, spasms occur only when coitus is attempted. In even less severe cases, coitus is possible but is accompanied by discomfort. Figure 15.1 depicts the normal vagina opening as well as the contractions of the vaginal muscles during vaginismus.

Masters, Johnson, and Kolodny (1985) and Renshaw (1990) estimate that 2% to 3% of all postadolescent women have vaginismus. Interestingly, most

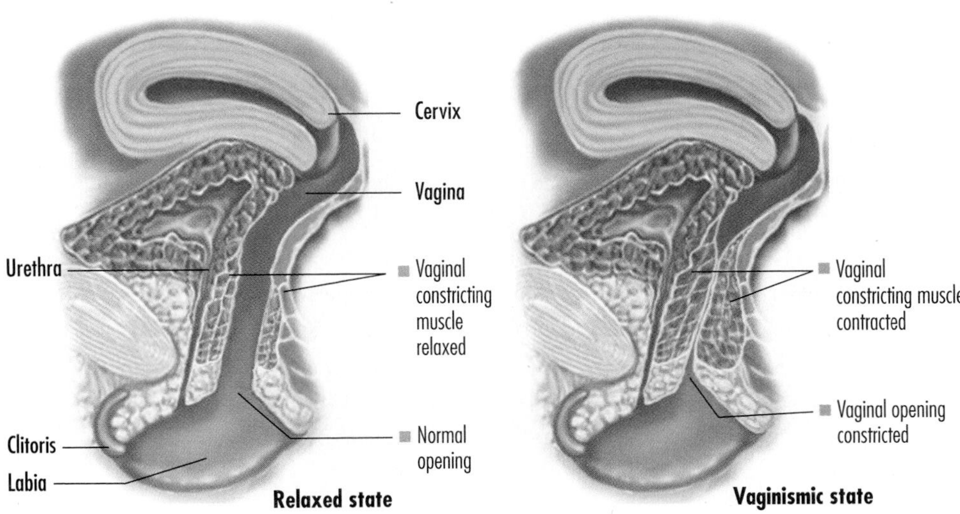

FIGURE 15.1 Vaginismus is the involuntary contraction of the muscles in the outer third of the vagina.

of them do not have a problem with sexual arousal. They experience vaginal lubrication normally, then enjoy foreplay, and they can be orgasmic (Kolodny, Masters, & Johnson, 1979). The causes of vaginismus are usually psychogenic: that is shame, fear, embarrassment, the most common cause of which is childhood sexual abuse (Perry, 1992). In addition, dyspareunia can lead to vaginismus. It is not difficult to imagine how a woman who experiences pain during sexual intercourse could tense up in fear of pain when penile insertion is imminent. In this case, when the dyspareunia is eliminated, the vaginismus usually disappears.

Vaginismus is also associated with erectile dysfunction in a woman's male partner, strong religious teachings about sexuality, homosexual feelings, and negative or hostile feelings about one's partner (Masters & Johnson, 1970).

Dyspareunia

Some women experience pain during sexual intercourse. Recurrent or persistent genital pain associated with sexual intercourse is known as *dyspareunia* (American Psychiatric Association, 1994). Although all women may experience some pain during some particular coital episode, dyspareunia is a chronic condition. Often this pain manifests itself as a burning feeling or cramping and may occur externally, in the vagina, or elsewhere in the pelvis. It is estimated that 1% to 2% of all women experience dyspareunia regularly (Masters, Johnson, & Kolodny, 1985).

Dyspareunia may be caused by disorders of the introitus, vagina, uterus, fallopian tubes, and/or ovaries. It may be a result of vaginal infections: yeast, bacterial, or trichomoniasis. Some contraceptive foams, creams, or gels or some condoms or diaphragms may irritate the vagina, resulting in pain during sexual intercourse. Even an intact hymen or scar tissue from a ruptured hymen can cause pain during penile insertion. More rarely, smegma—oily glandular secretions—accumulates under the clitoral hood and, when moved during coitus, may cause irritation and pain. Other pain may result when internal organs (such as the ovaries or uterus) are jarred during sexual intercourse (this may be remedied by the woman's being on top during coitus so she can control the depth of the penile thrusts).

One of the concerns regarding dyspareunia is its potential to lead to other sexual dysfunctions. For example, if a woman anticipates pain during coitus, she may tense her vaginal muscles, resulting in vaginismus; she may not be sexually responsive; or she may be anorgasmic. Treatment must identify any secondary dysfunctions and respond to those as well.

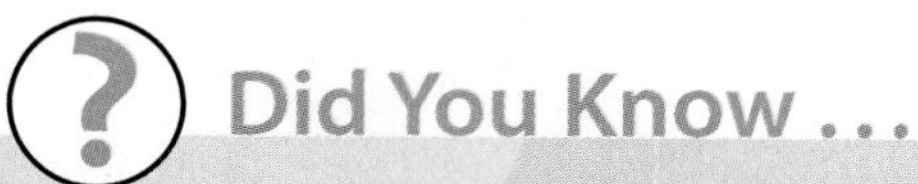

A testosterone-laced skin patch helped increase the sex drives of women who lost their libido after hysterectomies, according to a June 1999 study (Williams, 1999). The study followed only 57 women for only 9 months but laid the groundwork for further study. The study's primary author was Dr. Glenn Braunstein of the Cedars-Sinai Medical Center of Los Angeles. Critical thinkers will want to note, however, that the study's sponsor was Procter & Gamble, which makes a testosterone patch for men and wanted to find out whether it would be effective for women. Replicable results obtained in scientific studies with non-biased sponsors (e.g., the federal government) are needed to confirm—or dismiss—the results.

Sexual Desire Dysfunctions

In addition to the sexual dysfunctions described, both men and women sometimes experience problems with their interest in sexual activity. These dysfunctions include *inhibited sexual desire, dissatisfaction with sexual activity frequency,* and *sexual aversion.*

Inhibited Sexual Desire

Kaplan (1979, 1989) described **inhibited sexual desire (ISD),** sometimes referred to as *hypoactive sexual disorder (HSD),* as a lack of sexual appetite. It is characterized by a lack of interest in various types of sexual activity—for example, coitus, oral–genital sex, and even sexual fantasizing. People with ISD do not necessarily have some other sexual dysfunction as well. For instance, a man with ISD may not be interested in sexual activity initially but may be able to achieve an erection and have an orgasm once encouraged to participate; or a woman with a lack of interest in sexual activity may be orgasmic once convinced to participate.

inhibited sexual desire (ISD)
A lack of interest in sexual activity of various sorts; also called *hypoactive sexual disorder (HSD).*

primary ISD
A condition in which a person has always been uninterested in sexual activity.

secondary ISD
A condition in which a person was at one time interested in sexual activity but is no longer interested.

Primary ISD is a rare condition in which a person was not interested in sexual activity even as a child to the extent that he or she did not masturbate or fantasize about sexual matters. As adults, these people remain uninterested in sexual activity even if they are in a close relationship and/or married. More prevalent is **secondary ISD,** in which a lack of interest in sexual activity develops after a time of interest. With secondary ISD, lack of interest may be limited to a particular sexual partner or a specific situation. For example, the person may lack interest in sexual activity with the spouse but not with another lover, or in coitus but not in masturbation.

Defining ISD is as difficult as defining other sexual dysfunctions. Because each person's interest in sexual activity varies, when is too little interest really too little? When the lack of interest is specific to a sexual partner, is it the partner's fault? As we have stated, sexual interest in a smelly and dirty partner may be a dysfunction. One definition of ISD looks at the number of orgasms experienced in a certain period. Schover and associates (1982) diagnose ISD when the person experiences less than one orgasm every 2 weeks from masturbation or sexual activity with a partner. This definition ignores the fact that some women may be interested in sexual activity but are anorgasmic. In spite of this oversight, and as with several other dysfunctions discussed in this chapter, if the person or the couple does not perceive a sexual problem to exist, perhaps one does not. If the degree of interest between two people in a relationship is similar, and the relationship is otherwise healthy, should therapists advise the couple that they have a problem? Should they attempt to change the couple's degree of interest in sexual activity? Should one person accommodate his or her partner's lack of interest or adopt sexual behaviors to meet the interested person's needs? For example, should an uninterested person engage in oral–genital activity to satisfy the interest of the partner? Does this situation need correcting? These are not easy questions to answer.

The causes of ISD include organic and psychogenic factors. Approximately 10% to 20% of men with ISD have pituitary tumors that cause too much of the hormone prolactin to be produced. Excessive prolactin level reduces the level of testosterone produced and can lead to ISD or erectile dysfunction (Schwartz & Bauman, 1981). However, the majority of ISD cases are the result of such factors as poor self-esteem, a bad relationship, embarrassment regarding one's body, or a history of sexual abuse (Empower Health Corporation, 1998). ISD can also develop in response to another sexual dysfunction. For example, a man who has erectile dysfunction may develop ISD. When the thought of or opportunity for sexual activity is present, this man, rather than becoming excited, may envision only a threat to his self-image and, quite naturally, lack interest.

Dissatisfaction with Sexual Activity Frequency

Not everyone is as interested in sex as his or her partner. As we earlier described, a guest speaker in one of our classes characterized this disharmony as only a matter of the mind. To illustrate his point he referred to the way he responds to his spouse's occasional "Leave me alone, I've got a headache" when he is "ready and primed to go." Whereas some men would argue or pout, he usually says, "Where does your head ache?" and proceeds to massage her head and temples, cheeks and neck gently. After a while he moves to her shoulders and asks, "Does this feel good?" One full body massage later, his spouse's lack of interest has been transformed. Men and women alike can learn to tune into the temporary inhibition, exhaustion, anxiety, or preoccupation that may diminish a partner's sexual interest and learn how that person likes to be treated in such circumstances.

Regardless of the cause, study after study finds men more interested in sexual activity than women (Brecher, 1984; Mancini & Orthner, 1978; McCarthy, 1989; McCormick, 1979), but that should not lead us to assume that all men or all women are alike. This difference can have a negative effect on other aspects of a relationship. When this disparity in sexual interest is

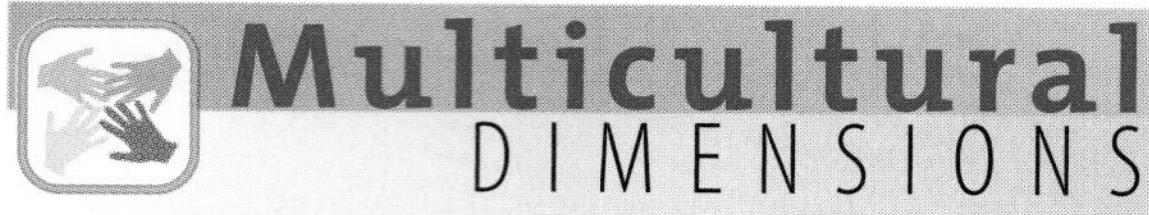

Sexual Dysfunction and Latino Populations

The Hispanic community, as do all subgroups within the United States, has some unique features that need to be considered regarding sexual dysfunction. Many of these features preclude Latinos from seeking professional help for sexual dysfunction. One of these is the language barrier. Not speaking English, or not speaking it well, means that if a sexual dysfunction arises, the person's ability to communicate the condition may prevent him or her from seeking help.

Hispanics also view the family as an extended one, not distinguishing between the nuclear family and the extended family. Cousins, aunts, uncles, and other family members are assumed to be part of the family, and advice is traditionally sought from family members as opposed to people outside the family, such as health professionals. However, matters of sexual function are considered inappropriate for a family discussion and, therefore, often are ignored.

Hispanics also maintain a sense of fatalism. Expressions such as *que sea lo que Dios quiera* ("it's in God's hands") and *esta enfermedad es una prueba de Dios* ("this illness is a test of God") are examples of this view of health-related problems. Therefore, a sexual dysfunction might be considered a matter for God, not for a sex therapist.

In addition, Latino communities tend to be male dominated, and that condition may interfere with admitting to a sexual dysfunction. In a project to enroll more children in government-sponsored health insurance programs, one of us found that what works for Anglo families does not work for Hispanic families. In Anglo families, it is the mother who is targeted for improving the health of the family's children. In Hispanic families we found it necessary to influence the fathers first. This is because of the concept of *machismo* (in which males are projected as strong, virile, powerful, and in control), which manifests itself in male-dominated families. Given the need to maintain this sense of machismo, Hispanic males are reluctant to admit a "weakness," especially a sexual dysfunction.

Culturally sensitive approaches are needed in all matters, particularly sexual ones. Sexual dysfunction is no exception.

Source: Perez, M. A., Pinzón, H. L., & Garza, R. D. Latino families: Partners for success in school settings, *Journal of School Health, 67* (1997), 182–184.

illuminated—that is, when one person feels he or she is pressuring the other or the other feels pressured—the potential for disagreement is evident. The result may be that both partners feel unloved and guilty (Zilbergeld & Kilmann, 1984). Accommodations are possible, however, as when a less interested partner helps his or her lover experience orgasm by oral–genital sexual activity or masturbation. To remedy this problem the couple must maintain effective communication rather than avoid it. In some cases, the assistance of a sex therapist may be warranted.

Sexual Aversion

Some people have an irrational fear—a phobia—of sexual activity that leads them to avoid it. That condition is termed **sexual aversion.** When sexual activity is even imagined, these people may experience a stress reaction: increased heart rate, muscle tension, perspiration, and nausea or diarrhea. Sexual aversion is usually caused by severe negative attitudes toward sexual activity expressed by parents, a history of sexual trauma such as rape or incest (LoPiccolo, 1985), the constant pressuring by a long-term partner, and/or gender identity confusion in men. Both men and women experience sexual aversion, and the therapy success rate is high for both (Kolodny, Masters, & Johnson, 1979; Schover, et al., 1982).

sexual aversion
An irrational fear of sexual activity.

Sexual Dysfunction and Self-Esteem

Some of us would like to think that sexual functioning is similar to other physical functioning—or that at least it ought to be considered so. If self-worth does not diminish when our digestive functioning goes haywire, why should we think less of ourselves if our sexual functioning is problematic? Well, no matter what we would like to think, sexual functioning is more closely connected to self-esteem than are other body processes. Men and women with sexual dysfunctions often feel less masculine or less feminine because they do not function sexually as they want to. Aside from their desire to function sexually for their own satisfaction, the sexually dysfunctional feel they are depriving their partners of satisfaction. Furthermore, they may fear that their partners will seek other sexual partners and/or leave them, fears that further diminish self-esteem. Not surprisingly, the partners of the sexually dysfunctional may also lose some self-esteem. They may feel that the dysfunction is due to their own lack of attractiveness, skill, or attention or that the partner no longer cares for them.

Therapists and counselors have become increasingly sensitive to the matter of self-esteem, of both the person experiencing sexual dysfunction and his or her partner.

Causes of Sexual Dysfunction

Sexual dysfunctions can have physical causes, psychological causes, and social causes. To prevent and treat sexual problems, these factors need to be understood.

Physical (Organic) Causes

It was previously believed that approximately 10% to 20% of male sexual dysfunctions were organic. Now we know that, at least for erectile dysfunction, 70% to 80% are the result of organic problems (Crenshaw, 1984; NIDUS Information Service, 1998; Stipp, 1987). Furthermore, many diseases and a number of drugs can alter sexual response. Erectile dysfunction can result from heart, kidney, and lung disease; from liver disease such as hepatitis, cirrhosis, and mononucleosis; from circulatory and blood vessel problems in which the penile veins allow blood to leak out of the erectile tissue (Rajfer, Rosciszewski, & Mehringer, 1988); and from a number of endocrine disorders such as hypothyroidism, Addison's disease, and diabetes. Erectile dysfunction can also result from infections of the urethra or prostate, tuberculosis, mumps, malnutrition, spina bifida, multiple sclerosis, leukemia, sickle-cell disorders, and thrombosis of the veins or arteries of the penis. Ejaculatory disturbances can result from some surgical procedures, such as those for cancer of the prostrate. Drugs known to decrease sexual responsiveness are alcohol and barbiturates, which, except in small amounts, are system depressants (Endocrinology Society, 1998). Certain antidepressants cause premature ejaculation. Medications that lower blood pressure also interfere with normal sexual functioning in males. However, frequent masturbation does not cause premature ejaculation, although premature ejaculation does seem to be related to a long history of withdrawal as a method of contraception (Pierson & D'Antonio, 1974).

Other than interviewing patients and obtaining a medical history, sex therapists have developed some unique ways to determine whether a sexual dysfunction is a result of physiological factors or is predominantly psychological. For example, a therapist who knows that a man with erectile dysfunction caused primarily by psychogenic factors has erections while he sleeps or when he arises in the morning may instruct the client to place a device (plethysmograph) around the penis that measures penile erection. This device graphs erections that occur during sleep (Tower Urology Group, 1998).

Although sexual dysfunctions in women are most likely the result of nonorganic factors, about 20% of them have physiological causes (Kaplan, 1983; Munjack & Oziel, 1980). For example, sexual unresponsiveness can result from disorders of major organs such as the heart or kidneys; orgasmic dysfunction may be caused by damage to the spine; vaginismus may be a consequence of anatomical or mechanical interference resulting from accident, surgery, or radiation for cervical cancer; and dyspareunia can result from infection of the vagina or allergic reactions. Given the many physical conditions that can cause sexual dysfunction, most sex therapists require that a client have a complete medical examination at the beginning of therapy.

Psychological Causes

Many sexual dysfunctions have no known physiological cause but, rather, a psychological basis. Anxiety related to meeting a partner's expectations, guilt about sexual relations or masturbatory behavior, shame about sexual behavior or about one's body, feelings of inferiority, and unconscious fear of castration or injury can all cause sexual dysfunctions. Decreased sexual desire, for example, can be caused by traumatic experiences, such as child sexual abuse, and by depression. Although erectile dysfunction is primarily caused by physiological factors, psychological causes are also at work. Among these are having a dominant, overcontrolling parent who may have caused low self-esteem; having conflicted homosexual feelings; and experiencing stress. Stress leads to an increase in the hormone epinephrine in the blood, which in turn can interfere with erection (of the penis or the clitoris). One researcher of sexual dysfunctions believes this could explain "the effects of performance anxiety" (Buvat, et al., 1990, 267).

Snegroff (1986) studied stressors associated with nonmarital sexual intercourse and found that males differed in some of these stressors and not in others. For males the following were of most concern.

1. Can I satisfy her?
2. Is my penis the right size?

3. Will I achieve and/or maintain an erection?
4. Will she want a commitment?
5. Will I perform well?

For females, the following were of most concern.

1. Can I satisfy him?
2. Will he like my body?
3. Will he respect me afterward?
4. Does he love/care for me?
5. Will I have an orgasm?
6. Are my breasts large enough?

A previous embarrassing sexual encounter in which the inability to be fully functional led to feelings of inadequacy can also lead to sexual dysfunction. Furthermore, orgasmic disorders also have psychological causes. Emotional reactions to one's partner can lead to resentment, shame, jealousy, boredom, or even disgust, which can cause an orgasmic disorder. These may be temporary feelings or, if the relationship experiences long-term disharmony, become permanent.

It is quite understandable that psychological factors can cause someone difficulty in functioning in an effective manner sexually. Is it any wonder that someone who is self-conscious about his or her body might not function well sexually? Imagine just waiting for a partner to laugh or cringe! Anxiety, guilt, and shame are hardly conducive to healthy sexual functioning.

Cultural Causes

Society also influences sexual functioning. For example, the double standard that judges women as less than moral if they actively seek sexual satisfaction can create shame and guilt that, in turn, interfere with normal

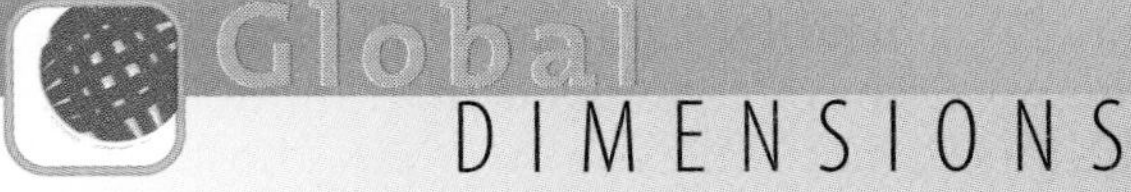

DIMENSIONS

Sexual Disorders Around the World The various perspectives and cultural mores of different countries may contribute to the development of sexual disorders, or at least to a diagnosis of a sexual dysfunction. For example, in China and other countries in which homosexuality is considered immoral, homosexuals, thinking every time they engage in sex they are doing something "dirty" and opposed by their society's expectations, might develop a sexual dysfunction. In Islamic countries in which female genital mutilation is customary, women may have hypoactive sexual disorder. On the island of Inis Beag, off the coast of Ireland, it is considered abnormal for women to experience orgasm. Therefore, women on the island engage in sex but prevent orgasm. Are they then experiencing orgasmic dysfunction? When men of Inis Beag attempt to ejaculate quickly so as to make sure their partners do not experience orgasm, are they then to be diagnosed with premature ejaculation?

In contrast, countries that have more relaxed sexual mores and accept a wider array of sexual behavior as "normal" tend to cultivate a sexually healthier population. For example, Sweden and Denmark have low rates of sexual dysfunction and teenage pregnancy. In Polynesian countries, known for encouraging sexual exploration at young ages, embarrassment and anxiety associated with sex are almost nonexistent.

Where you grew up and where you live now can have a tremendous effect on your sexual health. What influenced your sexual health? How?

sexual functioning. Furthermore, if the double standard is interpreted to mean that the male initiates sex and is more expert at it than a female partner, the pressure to behave in this manner can block the male's normal function. However, if females are taught to expect sexual satisfaction in their relationships comparable to that expected by their male partners, they might unintentionally put the onus for their fulfillment on their partners rather than assume that responsibility for themselves. With the onus placed on them, males may succumb to pressure and be unable to function as usual.

The way we perceive sex is also dependent on what our culture has taught us. Someone once said that sex is so "dirty" it should be saved for someone you love. Thinking of sex as dirty can create negative feelings such as embarrassment and guilt, which can result in sexual dysfunction.

Education, such as that to prevent HIV and AIDS, can also affect sexual function. For example, some people believe that premature ejaculation can be a function of men's not using condoms, because intercourse without a condom allows direct skin-to-skin stimulation, leading to premature ejaculation. Thus, with the advent of condom use as a means of preventing HIV and AIDS, it might be expected that fewer cases of premature ejaculation might occur, although some of the polyurethane condoms allow for more sensation than latex ones.

Others (Kaplan, 1989; University of Toronto Sexual Education and Peer Counseling Center, 1998) believe premature ejaculation results from boys' learning by their early teenage years to masturbate. Associated with their masturbatory behavior is guilt that causes them to speed up their orgasm. Having learned to ejaculate rapidly, they have difficulty controlling their ejaculation when they get older.

Religion is also related to sexual function. As one author states: "Rigid adherence to orthodox religious beliefs and practices is a common factor in the backgrounds of men and women with different forms of sexual dysfunction. Strict religious teaching—regardless of the particular religion—often results in negative attitudes toward sexuality. Individuals come to believe that sex is sinful" (Wilson, et al., 1996, 241). Of course, not all people who hold such religious beliefs develop a sexual problem, and these beliefs often influence behaviors in a healthy manner. Still, Masters and Johnson (1970) and other sex therapists have concluded that, in fact, strong religious beliefs increase the likelihood that a person who has those beliefs will experience sexual dysfunction.

Another significant cause of sexual dysfunction is related to a lack of information about sexual functioning—for example, not knowing or forgetting that foreplay is necessary to lubricate the vagina before penile entry. Other possible causes are nonsexual problems between sexual partners, ineffective communication (about sex and other matters), and traumatic past sexual experiences (for example, rape). Thus sexual unresponsiveness might, for instance, be caused by an inexperienced, inept, hasty, or insensitive lover; by situational factors, such as thoughts of a sick relative or deep-seated career concerns; or by sexual relations with impotent men.

Sexual Dysfunction and Aging

Elders have given up sex and have debilitating sexual dysfunctions. At least that is the prevailing myth. What is the truth?

In a survey commissioned by the National Council on the Aging (1998), 1,300 Americans 60 years of age and older were asked about their sex lives. The results go a long way toward eliminating the stereotype that elders have put sex aside in order to care for back pain, financial portfolios, or life in a nursing home. Here are the results:

- Nearly half of the elders surveyed reported engaging in sexual activity at least once a month.
- Of them 39% were satisfied with the amount of sex they have, whereas 39% wanted more sex.
- Men were twice as likely to report wanting more sex as women (56% to 25%, respectively).
- Only 4% stated they wanted sex less frequently.
- As people aged they engaged in sex less frequently; still, 57% of men and 30% of women in their 70s reported being sexually active.
- Of those questioned 74% of male respondents and 70% of female respondents said they were as satisfied or more satisfied with their sex life now than when they were in their 40s.
- For those who reported not having sex, the major reasons were a medical condition, decreased physical desire, and medications that reduce sexual desire.
- When asked what qualities elders sought in a "romantic partner," they identified high moral character, a pleasant personality, a good sense of humor, and intelligence; still 76% of men and 46% of women sought a partner interested in sex, and 67% of men and 48% of women wanted a partner to have an attractive body.

In summarizing the results of this survey, James Firman, president and chief executive officer of the National Council on the Aging, stated: "Our study debunks the prevailing myth about sexuality in older years. For many Americans, sex remains an important and vital part of their lives."

An alternative, and more humorous, way of looking at these results is the comment an elder made to a sexuality expert: "Look, everything we do may be slower, but we have more time."

Treating Sexual Dysfunction

In the past few decades many highly effective therapeutic approaches to sexual dysfunction have emerged (although love and concern between partners are still important). Masters and Johnson report an average cure rate for all sexual dysfunctions of 80%, with a 5-year relapse rate of only 5% (Masters, Johnson, & Kolodny, 1985). Helen Singer Kaplan (1974) reports that her treatment for vaginismus is almost 100% effective and that the great majority of women with orgasmic dysfunction are treatable.

Because the effectiveness of the various therapeutic approaches is well publicized, not only do more sufferers seek treatment—a positive step—but more and more people want to become sex therapists. As might be expected in a field that is emerging, charlatans and quacks, in addition to well-trained professionals, have set up practice. Therefore, anyone experiencing sexual problems would be well advised to investigate the training and experience of a sex therapist carefully before seeking that person's services. To help people select a professional therapist, the American Association of Sex Educators, Counselors, and Therapists (AASECT) has made public its requirements for certifying individuals as sex counselors or sex therapists. AASECT has also published a code of ethics. This code provides guidance for sex counselors and sex therapists, as well as for patients. Counselors and therapists whose behavior is inconsistent with this code may be incompetent and/or unethical.

Generally, sexual therapy for both men and women entails three components, regardless of the number and type of therapists involved: (1) an initial period of abstinence from coitus to reduce anxiety and facilitate communication; (2) the use of systematic tactile stimulation and exploration to focus on the giving and receiving of pleasure, rather than on the exclusive goal of orgasm; and (3) specific technical suggestions and direction, including sequences and variations on those techniques that facilitate and reinforce success.

Usually the couple is first seen together by the therapist or therapists. Then they are interviewed separately so they will feel free to discuss matters with the therapist that they might not yet feel comfortable discussing with their partner. Once the nature of the problem is identified, instruction and/or counseling can begin, following the sequence outlined earlier. Usually the couple is at first instructed to abstain from sexual intercourse and to learn how to experience pleasure in nongenital touching. Then genital fondling is allowed, and eventually coitus. The touching and coitus are private, away from the therapist's office, without the therapist present or in a room with one-way mirrors. Although it is rare, sometimes a *surrogate,* or substitute, partner is used to provide instruction, practice, and feedback for someone with a sexual problem. The use of sexual surrogates is highly controversial, both within the profession and among the public.

Approaches to Sexual Therapy

Several models of sexual therapy have been proposed. Perhaps a good place to begin a discussion of these models is first to consider a stepwise approach to sexual therapy.

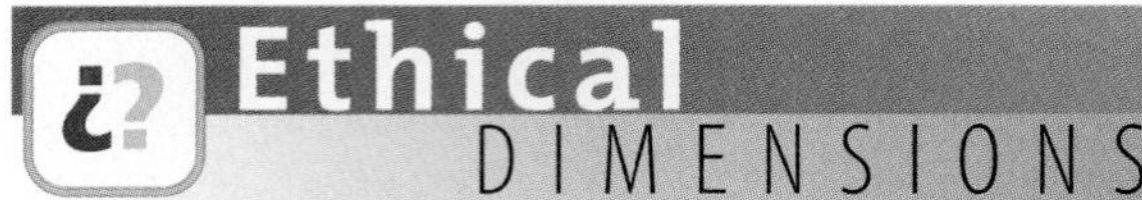

Should Surrogates Be Used in Sexual Therapy?

Early on, some therapists believed that the use of a substitute sexual partner was a vital and necessary component of sexual therapy. This substitute, or surrogate, was an experienced and trained sexual partner who could teach the sexually dysfunctional client effective sexual arousal techniques. Further, the surrogate let the client practice these techniques in a nonthreatening situation, because the surrogate was not a person with whom the client had a relationship or whom the client would ever see again. Advocates of the use of surrogates believed the therapy to be more effective if the client practiced on and received feedback from a real person.

Those opposed to surrogates usually based their arguments on one of two premises—either that sexual activity between people not married to each other is immoral or that the knowledge, skills, and attitudes learned with a surrogate are not readily transferred to one's usual sexual partner. A client's ability to function well with a surrogate does not ensure ability to function well with the usual sexual partner. Those arguing this position believed that sexual dysfunction is a problem between sexual partners and therefore needs to be worked out by both partners. Because the couple would have to practice sexually arousing techniques anyhow, why not practice them together from the outset of the therapy? And, finally, some people believed a surrogate was akin to a prostitute. Those employing such a method, therefore, should be subject to criminal prosecution.

Do you think surrogates should be used in sexual therapy? Why or why not?

The PLISSIT Model

Jack Annon (1976) suggested that relatively minor treatment may be effective for some sexual dysfunctions, whereas more intensive treatment may be required for others. Annon's model of sexual therapy is known as the **PLISSIT** model (an acronym of *P*ermission, *L*imited *I*nformation, *S*pecific *S*uggestion, and *I*ntensive *T*herapy). This model extends from the simplest to the more advanced levels of treatment.

PLISSIT
A model of sexual therapy that consists of moving through the stages of giving permission, limited information, specific suggestion, and, if that does not work, intensive therapy.

During the permission stage the therapist helps people accept their fantasies and desires and, where appropriate, even gives them permission *not* to engage in sexual intercourse until they are ready to do so. The therapist helps couples not to compare themselves with other couples or with an idealized sexual relationship.

During the limited information stage the therapist provides the factual information that may help the person become more functional sexually. For example, a person may not realize it is natural to fantasize about sexual activity or perceive it as a natural part of one's life. Information can give clients a more realistic perception, thereby removing an impediment to their sexual functioning. Other kinds of information, such as information about penis size and its limited effect on sexual satisfaction, clitoral sensitivity, or proper hygiene, may be all that is needed to help people overcome their sexual dysfunctions.

Specific suggestion is the level of therapy at which the therapist actually recommends activities for the clients. For example, self-stimulation, sensate focus, and the squeeze technique may be suggested. Many of these techniques were developed by Masters and Johnson (1970) but have since been modified by other sexual therapists. These techniques can help the person reduce sexual anxiety, improve communication between partners, or enhance arousal.

Intensive therapy may be required when permission, limited information, and specific suggestion are not successful in resolving a sexual problem. Intensive therapy entails a longer-term therapeutic treatment that identifies the deep-seated reasons that interfere with sexual functioning. This therapy has been called *psychosexual therapy* (Kaplan, 1974). Some therapists believe sexual dysfunction is caused by guilt or shame about sex, which leads to sexual anxiety, and the best treatment is intensive therapy to uncover the causes of these feelings.

The Masters and Johnson Model

William Masters and Virginia Johnson present a model of sexual therapy with several unique components. First, they believe that sexual problems are relationship problems, and, therefore, therapy works only with couples. Even seemingly healthy partners can learn how to respond and contribute better to their partner's response through sexual therapy. Second, they believe if couples are to be treated, the therapy team should be a couple—that is, a male and a female therapist. They believe that such a team can best appreciate the perspectives and best represent the couple in therapy. In addition, Masters and Johnson feel that clients can better identify with the therapist of the same gender, who may understand them better. Third, clients are medically screened for any potential organic causes of their dysfunction and given a complete psychological evaluation. Finally, treatment at the Masters and Johnson Institute is intensive; couples are seen every day for a 2-week period. This means that the couple must live near the institute, and there is significant expense. Masters and Johnson argue that this intensive interaction between the therapists and the clients is necessary initially to reduce anxiety and help the couple concentrate on overcoming the sexual problem.

Myth vs Fact

Myth: Sexual dysfunctions occur because someone either has been sexually abused or raped or has masturbated too often.
Fact: It is true that sexual abuse, such as rape and child abuse, can contribute to the development of a sexual dysfunction. Yet, there are many people who experience those traumatic events and never develop a sexual dysfunction. Regarding masturbation, there is no evidence that the frequency of masturbation is in any way related to the subsequent development of a sexual dysfunction.

Myth: Guys who "can't get it up" are not real men.
Fact: Most cases of erectile dysfunction are caused by physiological problems. To classify these men as less than real men is analogous to characterizing any man who has any physical illness as not a real man. The inability to achieve and maintain an erection is in no way related to manliness.

Myth: Women are not naturally interested in sex, so a woman who cannot be sexually aroused is quite normal.
Fact: Males and females have a natural interest in and capacity for sex. When they do not, they are exhibiting a sexual dysfunction termed *inhibited sexual desire* and should seek professional help to treat this condition.

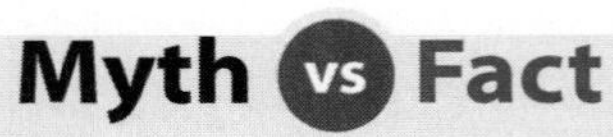

Myth: Treatment for sexual dysfunctions must entail counseling over the long term in order to be successful.
Fact: Treatments for sexual dysfunctions vary, depending on the nature of the particular dysfunction and the people involved. In many cases, the cause is a physical one, and medications can successfully treat it. In other cases, all that is needed is to educate the couple about effective techniques of sexual arousal. In relatively few cases is long-term counseling necessary.

Myth: Any couple who are not engaging in sexual activities frequently enough, with enough variety, and with orgasm have a sexual dysfunction for which they should seek sexual counseling.
Fact: Some experts believe that, for a sexual dysfunction to exist, one or both of the sexual partners must be dissatisfied with the sexual relationship. If both partners are satisfied, regardless of the nature of their sexual relationship, no sexual dysfunction exists.

Kaplan's Model

Kaplan (1974, 1979, 1983) employs many of the specific techniques of sexual therapy recommended by Masters and Johnson. However, Kaplan believes more intensive therapy is required to uncover the reasons for the sexual anxiety that interferes with normal sexual functioning. Kaplan's triphasic model consists of desire, arousal, and orgasm phases. Desire phase problems are the most difficult to treat because of their association with deep-seated psychological difficulties. Consequently, Kaplan recommends a longer period of sexual therapy to uncover the unconscious rationale for behavior and thought. Kaplan believes that sexual dysfunctions have their roots in multiple causes, some readily accessible and others requiring more intensive therapy to determine them. In addition, Kaplan treats premature ejaculation with the stop–start technique developed by James Semans (1956) rather than the squeeze technique developed by Masters and Johnson. Both the squeeze and the stop–start technique are described later in this chapter.

Other Approaches to Sexual Therapy

There are many other ways in which therapists treat sexual dysfunctions. For example, some behaviorists (LoPiccolo, 1977; Leiblum & Pervin, 1980) believe most sexual problems are learned and can be unlearned. Behaviorists use positive and negative reinforcement to encourage healthy behaviors and use gradual approaches to problematic sexual behavior. This latter approach is based on the early work of Joseph Wolpe (1958), who argued that one could not be anxious and relaxed at the same time. Consequently, Wolpe taught his clients deep muscle relaxation (for example, meditation) and gradually, over time, introduced more and more components of the anxiety-producing behavior. The sensate focus activity described later in this chapter is an example of Wolpe's desensitization technique.

Barbach (1975, 1980) organized groups of women to treat sexual dysfunction, in particular, orgasmic dysfunction and sexual unresponsiveness. Barbach's methods include exercises for the woman to do for herself. These exercises are also described later in the chapter.

Albert Ellis and Harper (1975, 1979) developed a therapy model he called *rational emotive therapy*. Ellis's model is based on the assumption that much of our behavior is a result of our thoughts and interpretations. Sexual problems arise from (irrational) thoughts and interpretations, and these problems can be treated by helping people recognize their irrationality and change these thoughts and interpretations into more rational ones.

Barry McCarthy believes that in the great majority of cases the sexual problem stems from a lack of knowledge, from communication problems, or from psychological difficulties. Consequently he views psychologists, social workers, marriage counselors, and ministers as better suited to working with such patients than physicians. In McCarthy's (1975) model of sexual therapy, a single therapist sees both sexual partners once a week, sometimes together, sometimes apart. This therapist is not a physician. Because a physical examination is a prerequisite to acceptance in the program, McCarthy considers a physician's skills unnecessary during therapy.

Treating Erectile Dysfunction

There are many effective ways to treat problems related to achieving and maintaining an erection. Because approximately 70% of cases of erectile dysfunction are caused by physical problems, medical scientists have successfully researched ways to counteract these physical limitations. These remedies include several different medications. A British researcher found a novel way to demonstrate the effectiveness of one of them. At a conference of urologists in Las Vegas in 1983, he presented a paper on the effectiveness of one of the medications and, in the middle of his presentation, stood up to show off his own erection, which he had induced with this drug. Urologists who began using the drug with their patients found it highly effective.

Many of these medications are injected into the penis and so are called *injection therapy* (men report only minimal pain). Until recently, the most commonly used injectable drugs were papaverine (brand name Pavabid or Cerespan) and phentolamine (brand name Regitine). Recently, however, another drug, alprostadil (brand name Caverject or Edex) has been used in injection therapy for erectile dysfunction and found to be even more effective (NIDUS Information Service, 1998). Alprostadil is usually sold in a six-dose kit that costs between $110 and $140. Erection occurs within 20 minutes of injection and lasts approximately an hour. An alternative way of administering alprostadil is by inserting a tube into the urethral opening and pressing a button that releases a pellet containing the drug.

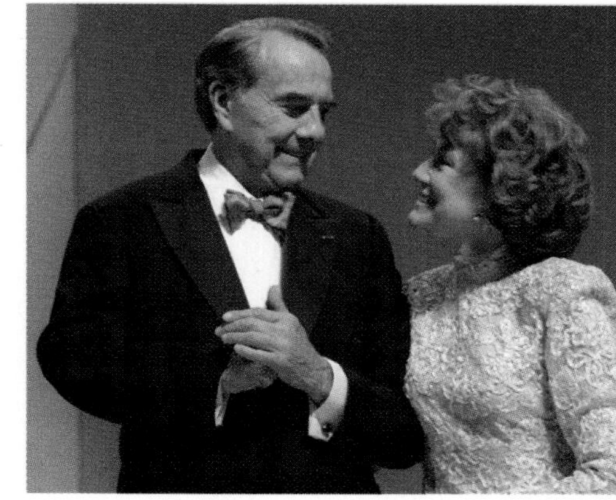

The former Senator Bob Dole decided in 1999 to do what he called a "public service announcement" sponsored by Pfizer, makers of Viagra. The ad addressed the subject of erectile disorder but did not directly endorse Viagra. Dole struggled with the decision to make the ad until he "thought about the 30 million men who live with this problem and are afraid to talk about it, and [then] it was easy for me to make up my mind."

Oral medications have also been found to be effective in treating erectile dysfunction. Although limited to men with hypogonadism (in which the testes do not produce sufficient amounts of testosterone), testosterone therapy has been used. More common has been the use of the drug yohimbine, which seems to improve blood flow to the penis.

Since 1997, excitement and a great deal of publicity have been focused on another drug, Viagra (sildenafil citrate). Viagra increases the level of cyclic guanosine monophosphate (GMP), a chemical that is produced in the penis during sexual activity whose function is to increase blood flow. Viagra is highly effective against erectile dysfunction, up to 70% to 97%, depending on the study (Goldstein, et al., 1998; Nidus, 1998; Reuters, 1998; Utiger, 1998), and when it is taken as prescribed, it is very safe. Although a few deaths of men who have used Viagra were reported, they were predominantly men who had cardiac disorders and used nitrate heart medications. Viagra is taken orally approximately an hour before sex but not more than once daily. It is not effective for men who experience inhibited sexual desire or no desire for their partners; desire must be present for Viagra to work.

An interesting "side effect" of Viagra may benefit women in an unforeseen way. Because Viagra is covered by some insurance companies and considered a medical treatment for a valid medical condition, health insurance companies are being lobbied to treat women in the same manner by including contraceptive services as a covered benefit. Such prestigious organizations as the American Medical Association and the American College of Gynecologists and Obstetricians have organized an effort to influence legislation that would require health insurance companies to include contraceptive pills as a covered benefit, as they do with other prescription drugs.

Another approach to organically caused erectile dysfunction is *bypass surgery*. When blood vessels that usually route blood to fill the cavernous bodies in the penis are blocked, surgeons can graft a blood vessel from another part of the body to bypass the blocked vessel, thereby allowing blood to flow into the cavernous bodies and make erection possible. However, very few men are candidates for this procedure, which is still considered experimental and has a high failure rate.

Sometimes the problem is not blood flowing into the cavernous bodies but blood leaking out (venous leakage). In this case, *venous ligation*, a surgical procedure that repairs the veins, can be employed. The problem with venous ligation, however, is that it is usually only a temporary remedy, and subsequent surgery is often required within a few years.

When erectile dysfunctions have irreversible physical causes, it is possible to treat them by implanting *penile prostheses,* commonly called *penile implants.* Approximately 200,000 of these devices were implanted in American men between 1982 and 1989 (Nidus Information Services, 1998), although this treatment has become the treatment of choice less frequently now that other effective and less traumatic treatments exist. There are three types of penile prostheses: semirigid rods, multicomponent inflatable implants, and self-contained inflatable implants. *Semirigid rods* contain stainless steel wires or plastic joints held together by a cable and coated with silicone. Two bendable rods are implanted in the corpus cavernosum, with the result that the penis is always erect (but it can be bent down).

Multicomponent inflatable implants involve placing an inflatable cylinder in the corpora, a fluid reservoir in the abdomen, and a pump in the scrotum. In preparation for intercourse, the male merely squeezes the pump, thereby moving fluid from the reservoir to the cylinders, causing the penis to become erect. When intercourse is completed, the male squeezes the pump release valve to move the fluid from the cylinder back to the reservoir.

Self-contained inflatable implants consist of two cylinders implanted in the penis, each containing a pump, fluid, and a release valve. When planning for intercourse, the male squeezes the penis glans, forcing fluid to move to the forward chamber, resulting in erection. At completion of coitus, the penis is slightly bent, causing the return of fluid to the storage area and a loss of erection.

Vacuum devices have also been successfully employed to treat erectile dysfunction. When the penis is placed in a plastic cylinder and a vacuum is created, causing blood to flow into the penis, an erection occurs. Once erection appears, a band is placed snuggly around the base of the penis to maintain the erection. Although this seems "unnatural," it is very effective when the psychological barriers are overcome. One note of caution: To prevent injury to the penis, only a medically approved device should be used, not one sold in sexual paraphernalia catalogues or magazines.

Many erectile dysfunctions do not have physical causes. These conditions are treated with counseling and several techniques described later in this section.

squeeze technique
A method of helping men control premature ejaculation whereby the penis is gently squeezed when the man senses ejaculation is imminent.

Semans stop–start
A method of controlling premature ejaculation (developed by James Semans) in which the man tells his partner to stop stimulating him when he feels ejaculation approaching.

Treating Premature Ejaculation

Two techniques are used to help men control premature ejaculation. The first is the **squeeze technique,** developed by Masters and Johnson (Figure 15.2), which entails a gentle squeezing of the penis while the man is experiencing full erection. When the man begins to feel the urge to ejaculate, the partner grasps the penis with the thumb on the underside where the shaft ends and the head begins and two fingers on the opposite side. The partner then squeezes for 3 to 4 seconds, after which the urge to ejaculate will have passed. After 15 to 30 seconds, stimulation is provided to full erection once more and the procedure is repeated as necessary. Eventually the man learns to control his ejaculation without his partner's help.

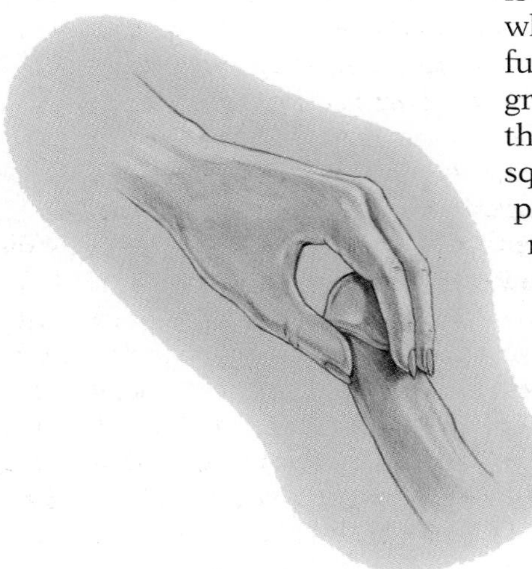

FIGURE 15.2 The squeeze technique. The man signals his partner to squeeze when ejaculation is approaching.

The second technique for learning ejaculatory control is called the **Semans stop–start method,** named for its developer, James Semans. The man lies on his back and concentrates on his feelings and sensations as his partner stimulates his penis manually (Figure 15.3). When he feels ejaculation approaching, he tells his partner to stop stimulating him. The couple repeats the procedure until the man learns ejaculatory control.

However, other remedies also exist. For example, changing the tempo of thrusting may result in decreased stimulation. Also, chang-

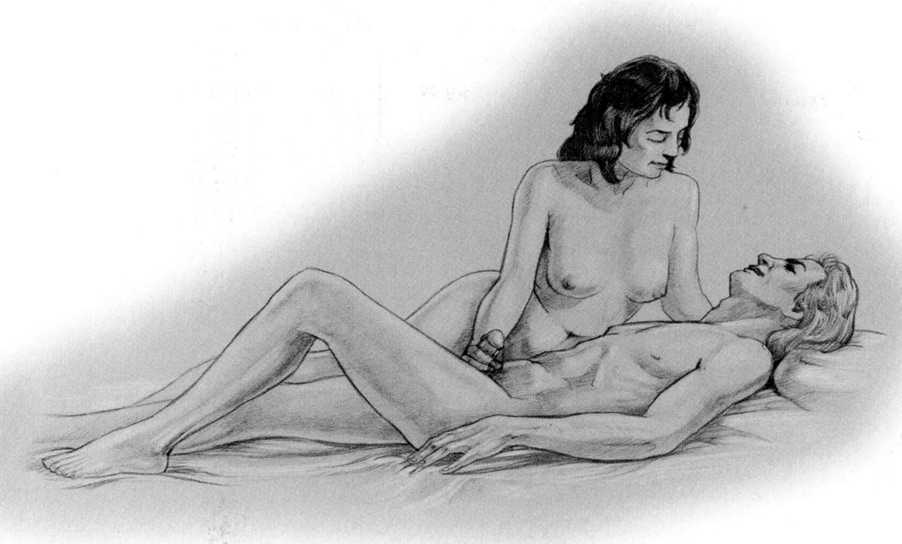

FIGURE 15.3 The Semans procedure. The man signals his partner to stop stimulation when he senses that ejaculation is close.

ing the angle or depth of penetration may help. Shifting one's thoughts to other events, talking to oneself ("self-talk"), and focusing on the nongenital aspects of the experience can all be of help in controlling ejaculation. Finally, some antidepressant medications, such as Prozac and Anafranil, have been found to control premature ejaculation (University of Toronto Sexual Education Centre, 1998).

Treating Retarded Ejaculation

The therapy for retarded ejaculation includes the technique known as sensate focus (described in the next paragraph), which helps the man focus on his sensual feelings and learn to derive pleasure from sexual behavior. Included in this treatment, in a stepwise fashion, is learning to ejaculate by masturbating alone, by masturbating with his sexual partner present, by asking the partner to masturbate him to ejaculation, and by asking the partner to masturbate him to the point just short of ejaculation and then inserting the penis into the vagina to ejaculate.

Sensate Focus

Sexual therapists treat sexual unresponsiveness in both men and women by teaching the couple a technique termed **sensate focus.** The idea behind this method is to encourage the man and woman to experience erotic feelings short of intercourse so that they will learn to accept sexual pleasuring (both giving and receiving) as part of their lives. The therapist gives the unresponsive partner permission and encouragement to feel nonthreatening sexual feelings, on the assumption that the client has withheld permission from him- or herself (for whatever individual subconscious reason). Eventually the therapy incorporates coitus into the sensate focus program. Figure 15.4 illustrates one of the sensate-focusing positions taught to couples.

sensate focus
A method of alleviating sexual unresponsiveness by procedures designed to encourage erotic feelings and sexual pleasuring.

Barbach's technique
A method of treating orgasmic dysfunction and sexual unresponsiveness developed by Lonnie Barbach that focuses on awareness of feelings and sensations through self-exploration and stimulation.

Barbach's Technique

Barbach's technique, effective in treating both sexual unresponsiveness and orgasmic dysfunction in women, has been widely disseminated to the general public through Lonnie Barbach's book *For Yourself: The Fulfillment*

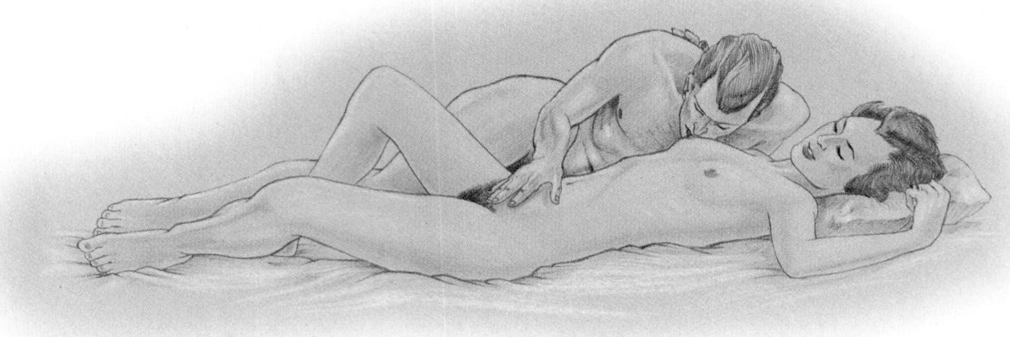

FIGURE 15.4 Sensate focus allows for nondemanding stimulation.

of Female Sexuality (1975). A woman begins the program by setting aside an hour a day for exploring her body visually (with a mirror) and manually (using body lotion or powder), all the time focusing upon feelings and sensations. Next she is led to do a vulva self-examination and vulva self-stimulation with a body lotion or oil. It is important at this stage that orgasm *not* be the goal of the self-stimulation. Rather the woman is encouraged to become aware of and focus on pleasurable sensations. Eventually the program leads the woman to seek orgasm by using the touching technique she found to be most pleasurable during the self-stimulation stage. The use of a vibrator is recommended for women who still find orgasm elusive after manual stimulation. However, after the woman experiences orgasm with a vibrator, she is encouraged to practice manual stimulation. This transfer is important in helping her to have orgasm with a sexual partner.

Combating Vaginismus and Dyspareunia

Vaginismus and dyspareunia are treated by a combination of education and practice. The education component entails instruction about the anatomy and physiology of the human sexual response and reproductive systems. Once it is understood that the problem stems from contraction of the muscles of the vagina that prevents penile penetration, training to control these muscles can begin. The best manner in which to carry out this training appears to be teaching the woman to contract and relax the muscles, becoming conscious of the sensations that accompany both contracted and relaxed vaginal muscles. Next slender rods—first a very narrow one and eventually wider ones—are inserted by the woman into the vagina with relaxed muscles. Once this is mastered (about 1 week), the next step is coitus, when the woman controls inserting the penis.

Dyspareunia, when not caused by physical problems, tends to stem from insufficient vaginal lubrication. In such cases the treatment is similar to that described for sexual unresponsiveness (that is, sensate focus).

Behavior Therapy Model

systematic desensitization
A means of overcoming anxiety by approaching the anxiety-provoking stimulus in small steps.

As stated previously, Joseph Wolpe developed a manner of treating anxiety as the cause of sexual dysfunction. Termed **systematic desensitization,** this model can be applied to people who are anxious about sex. Wolpe reasoned that if people were muscularly relaxed, they could not be anxious at the same time. Consequently, he taught people deep muscle relaxation techniques and then instructed them to think of the anxiety-provoking stimulus. For example, sexually dysfunctional patients might imagine their arms and legs are heavy, warm, and tingly (a relaxation technique called *autogenic training*). Once relaxed, they could imagine the sexual activity about which they feel anxious.

Systematic desensitization also assumes that the gradual introduction of anxiety-provoking stimuli will not produce anxious feelings. Thus, this technique involves a fear hierarchy: The initial stimuli are not anxiety provoking, but very gradually more anxiety-provoking stimuli are introduced. For example, the following might be the fear hierarchy of a married woman (Ted's wife) who experiences vaginismus:

1. I go out to a movie with Ted.
2. Ted and I return home and are alone.
3. Ted places his arm around me.
4. Ted nuzzles my neck.
5. Ted fondles my breast.
6. Ted takes my clothes off.
7. Ted removes his clothing.
8. Ted stimulates my clitoris and vagina.
9. Ted inserts his finger into my vagina.
10. Ted inserts his penis into my vagina.

The woman is then asked to imagine the first event in the fear hierarchy without feeling anxious—that is, without an increasing heart rate and rapid, shallow breathing. If she can imagine that event for 30 seconds without feeling anxious, she does deep muscle relaxation for 30 seconds. Then she moves to the next event of the hierarchy. The idea is to take very small steps from something that does not make her anxious to the point at which she is involved in the activity that was the problem (in the example, allowing penile insertion) (Greenberg, 1999).

Behaviorists are concerned with the behavior in question, not the underlying reasons for that behavior. They do not spend a great deal of time analyzing why someone feels or thinks as he or she does. Rather, they begin to manipulate the behavior so it is transformed into the desired behavior. To do this, therapists sometimes employ a technique called *shaping*. Shaping involves rewarding small behaviors along the way to developing the behavior that is the goal of the therapy. For example, if a person becomes anxious on dates and, therefore, refuses to accept a date, the therapist might have the person begin by just speaking to a love interest on the telephone. For doing that, he or she would receive a reward (for example, maybe a pass to a movie theater). To receive a reward the next week, however, the patient needs to spend a few minutes in face-to-face contact with that other person—and so on, until the patient goes out on a date without anxiety.

Self-Care Model

Several of the models and techniques of sexual therapy can be self-administered. For example, couples can employ the stop–start technique or the squeeze technique, and individuals can try systematic desensitization or shaping by themselves. They will thereby save some money and whatever inconvenience is associated with attending therapy. A good first step to solving problems associated with sexual functioning, given that any medical cause has been ruled out, is to employ these self-care techniques. If they are not successful, the person should consider seeking the help of a trained sex counselor or therapist. Often the trained eye can observe something that the untrained cannot.

Other Kinds of Therapy

There are other kinds of therapy that treat sexual dysfunction. However, forms of therapy and counseling that are not focused particularly on sexual response can also help people with sexual dysfunctions, especially when conditions are rooted in a more generalized lack of self-acceptance and self-esteem. Also beneficial in some cases is counseling or therapy directed toward improving communication in the nonsexual aspects of a relationship—for example, marriage counseling, family counseling, or crisis counseling for couples.

If you experience any of the sexual dysfunctions described in this chapter, you may want to ask your instructor or student-health service personnel for a referral to a qualified sex therapist. Paying attention to your sexual responsiveness is part of maintaining total well-being. A dysfunction in the sexual aspect of your life requires the same concern and treatment as any other chronic ailment. We are fortunate to live in a time when effective sexual therapy based on sound scientific research is generally available.

Choosing a Sex Therapist

For sex therapy to be effective, the therapist must be qualified. How can you determine this? Someone who claims to be a sex therapist is not necessarily competent in that particular area of expertise. To enhance your chances of choosing a qualified sex therapist, consider the following points:

1. *Does this person have a degree in a recognized profession related to counseling and therapy?* Psychology, marriage and family counseling, pastoral counseling, and social work are examples.
2. *Does this person hold a license or a certification related to counseling and therapy?* Some professions are licensed by the state (psychologists), whereas others are certified by professional organizations (for example, marriage counselors).
3. *Is this person certified by the American Association of Sex Educators, Counselors, and Therapists (AASECT)?* Certification by this professional organization attests to the training specific to sexuality issues the person has had.
4. *Do you know other people who have been helped by this therapist?* Sometimes the best referral is that of someone who has experienced therapy and benefited from it.

To begin choosing a sex therapist, consult local resources. A local hospital might be a good beginning. Perhaps the local medical association can make a referral. The psychology, counseling, social work, or health education department at your university might be able to help, as might your campus health center. Alternatively, you could contact AASECT for a referral in your area.

When first meeting the therapist, or talking with office personnel on the telephone, do not hesitate to inquire about the fee, the therapist's background and qualifications, the licenses and/or certifications the therapist holds, and the usual course of therapy provided for situations such as yours (length of treatment, type of treatment, and so on). Any therapist who objects to your asking these questions should be considered suspect. Reputable therapists should be glad that you are taking such an active interest in obtaining effective treatment. That sort of motivation is critical for a successful outcome.

Exploring the DIMENSIONS of Human Sexuality

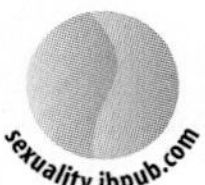

Our feelings, attitudes, and beliefs regarding sexuality are influenced by our internal and external environments. Go to sexuality.jbpub.com to learn more about the biological, psychological, and sociological factors that affect your sexuality.

Biological Factors

- Some sexual dysfunctions, including about 80% of erectile disorder cases, are of a physiological nature. Age is sometimes a factor, as normal changes in the human body affect sexual desire and arousal.
- Alcohol, drug abuse, and certain medications (e.g., for hypertension) can interfere with sexual response.

Sociocultural Factors

- The sexual double standard suggests that men be experienced and talented in sexual matters, leading their partners to sexual bliss. Failure to live up to such expectations can lead to psychological problems.
- Mass media create unrealistic sexual expectations that no real person can meet.
- Relationship problems can lead to some disorders.
- Rigid religious convictions that certain sexual activities are immoral may lead to negative attitudes toward sexuality.
- Masters and Johnson asserted in 1970 that "sociocultural deprivation and ignorance of sexual physiology, rather than psychiatric or medical illness" were the source of most sexual dysfunction.

Psychological Factors

- Sexual functioning is closely connected to self-esteem. Men and women with sexual dysfunctions often feel less masculine or feminine because they do not function as well sexually as they wish. Low self-esteem, guilt, or depression can lead to some sexual disorders.
- Gays seeking treatment for disorders must also confront society's negative attitudes about homosexuality.
- Failure to perform as expected can be devastating psychologically. In turn, such perceived failure would likely lead to isolation from sexual activities, which would cause further embarrassment. Fear of future sexual inadequacy can create a self-fulfilling prophecy that can result in lowered self-esteem.

CASE STUDY

Many of the sexual disorders are multidimensional. In fact, at different times, there can be different causes. Consider an otherwise healthy male who, after getting too little sleep during the week and ingesting too much alcohol, is unable to achieve and maintain an erection through intercourse. The dysfunction here is likely physiological. If he understands that alcohol and lack of sleep are to blame, he will probably be fine. However, if he perceives that he "failed" sexually, he may suffer from performance anxiety during his next sexual encounter.

Partners, too, may blame themselves for sexual dysfunction. When partners call into question their attractiveness or sexual ability, their self-esteem may suffer. Further, they may isolate themselves from sexual situations so as not to "cause" failure again.

Both sexuality education and communication can help couples avoid sexual anxiety. The former would help both partners realize why the initial dysfunction occurred. And communication could help both partners' self-esteem, by letting the other person know that he or she is desired.

Discussion Questions

1. Review the major male and female sexual dysfunctions, including features of diagnosis. What determines what a typical person might consider a sexual problem and what a sexual therapist diagnoses as a sexual dysfunction?
2. List the specific physical, psychological, and sociocultural dimensions that can affect sexual performance. Explain how each could have an effect. (Be specific: Religion is a factor, but state the specific religion. Would it affect all members of that religion or only specific people with a high degree of religious fervor?)
3. Examine the many types of sexual therapy available. Then evaluate which you think would work best for erectile disorder, vaginismus, and inhibited sexual desire dysfunction. Explain your answer.

Application Questions

Reread the chapter-opening story and answer the following questions.

1. Explain why when a celebrity or a politician discloses a personal problem, it seems easier for the general public to talk about the issue involved. Contrast that with how you might react if a classmate announced in class that he or she had a sexual dysfunction.
2. We know that Elizabeth Dole smiled when asked about Viagra. But if she had been asked about her sex life with Bob before his disclosure, how might she have reacted? Would she have revealed his "dysfunction" (related to prostate-cancer surgery)? If Viagra had not been developed, would either Bob or Elizabeth have realized that there was a dysfunction?

Critical Thinking Questions

1. Masters and Johnson claimed that male and female cotherapists were needed to treat a couple. They reasoned that only a person of the same gender as the client could really understand a sexual problem or dysfunction. Do you agree with Masters and Johnson, or could a couple be successfully treated by one therapist (of either gender)? Explain your answer.
2. The success of the drug Viagra was unprecedented: 36,000 prescriptions in the first week, 3.6 million in the first 4 months. Although it is clear that many of the patients had erectile disorders, there is strong anecdotal information to suggest that some men were experimenting with Viagra to improve their sex life. Consider the physical, psychological, and sociocultural dimensions of such experimentation (for example, belief you cannot perform without the pill, the ethics of getting a doctor to write a prescription). Would you take a drug that could possibly improve your sex life, even if it had associated risks?

Critical Thinking Case

Before the 1960s hardly anyone had heard of sexual dysfunction. However, soon after Masters and Johnson's book *Human Sexual Response* was published in 1966, the prevalence of sexual dysfunctions seemed to skyrocket. Some have argued that there are more sexual problems than in previous years because of the greater emphasis people place on sex today. We can now rent X-rated movies for home viewing or even order them into our homes via cable TV, we can purchase erotic print media at the local bookstore or listen to sexually charged music and lyrics on CDs and the radio, and we can even observe simulated sex during daytime hours on TV soap operas or on the Internet. This emphasis on sex, the argument continues, has created unrealistic expectations for people, and when they cannot "perform" as they observe others can, they become dysfunctional.

There is another view, however. Perhaps there was as much sexual dysfunction before 1966 as there is today; however, sex was not a topic for conversation, so problems remained undisclosed. The result was that people were unable to achieve sexual satisfaction.

What is your view? Is there more sexual dysfunction now, or has disclosure of sexual problems increased? Is the situation better today, or was it better before 1966? Is there too much pressure for people to "perform" sexually today?

Exploring Personal Dimensions

What Constitutes Sexual Dysfunction?

Perspectives on what constitutes a sexual dysfunction vary. One important consideration is that if you and your partner are satisfied with your sexual relationship, you probably do not have a disorder. If you do not participate in any sexual activity, skip this assessment. With that in mind, answer the following statements with one of the following responses:

a. Rarely or never b. Sometimes c. Often d. All or most of the time

1. I fantasize about sex.
2. I think about sex.
3. I am able to become aroused.
4. I remain aroused during sexual activities.
5. I enjoy having sex with my partner.
6. I engage in masturbation more than I feel is normal.
7. I worry about my sexual performance.
8. I feel worried about having sexual relations.

Male:

9. I experience pain when I have an erection or ejaculate.
10. I am able to achieve an erection.

Female:

9. I experience pain during intercourse.
10. I have difficulty reaching an orgasm.

This self assessment is not meant to be scored. Rather, it is intended as a tool to allow you to think critically about sexual performance and dysfunction.

After you have given initial responses to these questions, go back and review them two more times. The first time, consider whether you are satisfied with your initial response. In other words, think about whether you are happy with a particular aspect of your sexuality. Then consider whether your partner may be satisfied with your initial response.

For example, a man with a spinal-cord injury may not be able to achieve an erection. But that may be acceptable to both him and his partner, if they have found other satisfying sexual activities in which to engage.

Sexuality Online

Go to the web component for *Exploring the Dimensions of Human Sexuality* at sexuality.jbpub.com for web exercises, additional resources related to this chapter, and student review tools.

Suggested Readings

Altman, C. *You can be your own sex therapist: A systematized behavioral approach to enhancing your sensual pleasures, improving your sexual enjoyment.* Casper, WY: Casper Publishing, 1997.

Bartoi, A. G. & Kinder, B. N. Effects of child and adult sexual abuse on adult sexuality, *Journal of Sex and Marital Therapy, 24* (1998), 75–90.

Caverject: Injections for impotence, *Consumer Reports on Health* (March 1996).

Forman, R. & Forman, N. *Drug-induced infertility and sexual dysfunction.* Cambridge, England: Cambridge University Press, 1996.

Fowler, C. J. The neurology of male sexual dysfunction and its investigation by clinical neurophysiological methods, *British Journal of Urology, 81* (1998), 785–795.

Gentili, A. & Mulligan, T. Sexual dysfunction in older adults, *Clinical Geriatric Medicine, 14* (1998), 383–393.

Heiman, J. R., et al. Evaluating sexual dysfunction in women, *Clinical Obstetrics and Gynecology, 40* (1997), 616–629.

Hellstrom, W. J., ed. *Male infertility and sexual dysfunction.* New York: Springer-Verlag, 1997.

Kaplan, H. S. *The sexual desire disorders: Dysfunctional regulation of sexual motivation.* New York: Brunner/Mazel, 1995.

Murray, J. B. Physiological mechanisms of sexual dysfunction side effects associated with antidepressant medication, *Journal of Psychology, 132* (1998), 407–416.

INTER chapter FOCUS

Atypical Sexual Behavior

FEATURES

Communication Dimensions Communicating Accurately

Gender Dimensions Paraphilias and Gender Differences

Ethical Dimensions The Ethics of Chemical Treatment for Paraphilias

CHAPTER OBJECTIVES

1. Discuss how some atypical sexual behaviors exist on a continuum of sexual activity.
2. Describe the most common paraphilias.
3. Name and define paraphilias other than the most common ones.
4. Explain what can be done to treat paraphilias.
5. Summarize what is known about sexual addiction.

sexuality.jbpub.com

The Most Common Paraphilias
Sexual Addiction

INTRODUCTION

Varieties of sexual behaviors have been around a long time, as have many opinions about them. In February 1997, however, many people were surprised when a well-known NBC sportscaster, Marv Albert, known as the voice of the New York Knicks, was indicted on charges of assault and sodomy. His accuser, a 41-year-old female friend from Virginia whom he had known for 10 years, claimed that Albert viciously bit her several times on the back during an argument in his Washington hotel room.

The woman claimed that Albert became enraged when she refused to join in a "three-way" with him and another man and that he threw her on the bed and bit her on the back 10 to 15 times. Then, according to court documents, he forced her to perform oral sexual activity. After the woman sought treatment at a local hospital, the police were notified.

To many, the charges against Albert seemed very much out of character. For example, one of his producers said that on both a professional and a personal level he was a joy to be around. The executive producer of NBC sports said he was "in total shock" about the charges.

As the allegations were investigated, additional stories came out about Albert's sexual behavior, including his alleged fondness for wearing women's underwear and participating in threesomes. As a result, Albert was removed from sportscasting and taken off network shows. In July 1999 Albert returned to broadcasting as the radio voice of the New York Knicks.

Stories like the one about Marv Albert cause people to wonder about varieties of sexual behavior and talk more about them. Although many varieties of sexual behavior are relatively uncommon, it can be important to know more about them.

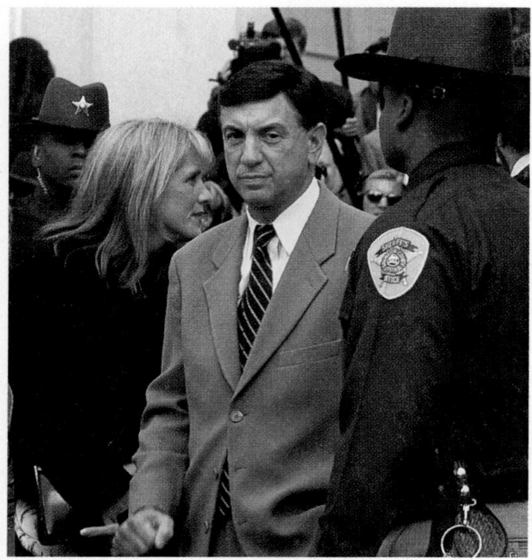

The sports broadcaster Marv Albert learned the negative consequences of participating in coercive sexual activities—arrest, embarrassment, punishment, loss of job and friends. Remember that if you ever consider taking part in such sexual activities, you too may suffer the same consequences.

Common Versus Atypical Sexual Behaviors

A few points about atypical sexual behavior in general should be noted before we consider specific behaviors. First, in many instances there are gradations of a sexual behavior existing on a continuum. For example, most people enjoy looking at other people. However, if someone spends many hours each day just looking at others, we would probably assume that person has a problem. There would be spots on the continuum between these two extremes that might be hard to judge. Is the behavior common or is it atypical? Is it acceptable or unacceptable? It is up to each individual, and society, to decide where on the continuum of sexual behavior activities become unacceptable. For instance, when is behavior obsessive (that is, the individual does not freely choose the behavior); when is it associated with emotional distress or with the inability to interact satisfactorily with other people; when is it forced on another person; when is it illegal?

Because many behaviors vary in degree, it is not surprising that many of us may recognize some degree of atypical behaviors or feelings in ourselves—perhaps only in private fantasies. In most instances, such behaviors or feelings should be accepted as natural—as long as they do not interfere with our optimal functioning or with the rights of others.

It is also common for us not to know a great deal about atypical sexual behaviors. Because in most cases such behavior is not common, and in most cases it is performed in private, it is difficult to study. Therefore, as we consider atypical sexual behaviors, many questions will be left unanswered.

It is also interesting that atypical sexual behaviors often occur in combination. For example, in the case of Marv Albert, he apparently did some cross-dressing along with participating in group sexual activity and violence.

Within this minichapter, we briefly discuss some of the most common atypical sexual behaviors. The more severe forms of sexual aggression (rape, incest, spousal abuse, sexual harassment, and child abuse) are discussed in Chapter 16.

The Most Common Paraphilias

Unusual or problematic sexual behaviors are scientifically known as paraphilias. **Paraphilia** means love *(philia)* beyond the usual *(para)*. There are about 30 different paraphilias, and each exists in fantasy and in reality. It is generally accepted that the prevalence and variety of paraphilias are greater in males than in females, but as indicated previously, in most instances little is known about them.

paraphilia
Literally meaning "love *(philia)* beyond the usual *(para)*," this term refers to various sexual behaviors previously referred to as deviant.

exhibitionism
Achievement of sexual gratification by exhibiting the genitals to observers.

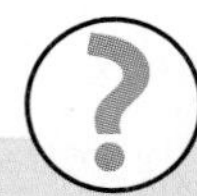

Did You Know . . .

Less than 2 years after he was fired by NBC after his guilty plea in his sexual behavior case, Marv Albert was rehired by NBC on June 29, 1999. Do you think that NBC was right to fire Marv Albert?

A paraphilia is distinguished by a preoccupation with an object or behavior to the point of being dependent on that object or behavior for sexual gratification. In most cases, types of sexual activity outside the boundaries of the paraphilia lack arousal or satisfaction unless the person fantasizes about the paraphilia at the same time (Paraphilia, 2001).

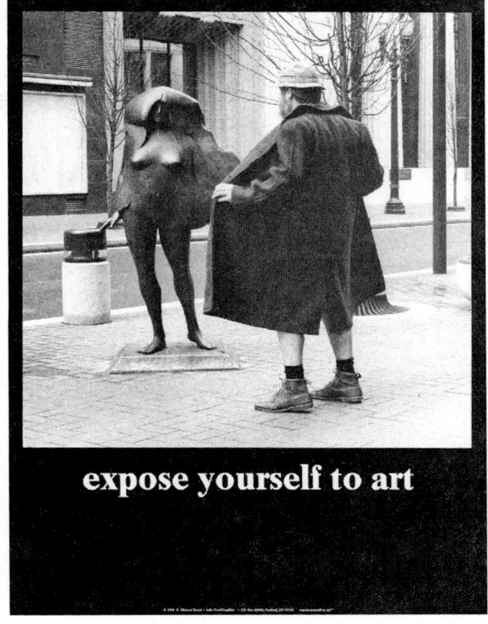

Although exhibitionists are often portrayed comically, in real life the phenomenon is quite different. Exhibitionists gain sexual pleasure from eliciting a harsh reaction to their unprovoked actions. It is best to ignore one if you are ever flashed.

Exhibitionism

Exhibitionism (commonly called *flashing* or *indecent exposure*) occurs when an individual achieves sexual gratification by exhibiting the genitals to observers. The American Psychiatric Association (1998) has officially defined exhibitionism as "over a period of at least six months, recurrent, intense sexually arousing fantasies, sexual urges, or behaviors involving the exposure of one's genitals to an unsuspecting stranger." Though exhibitionism is a good example of a sexual behavior that is difficult to classify as one that causes problems, we would probably agree that if someone's primary motivation in life is exhibitionism, that person has a problem. At what point does the behavior become abnormal?

The paraphilia of exhibitionism has its origins in the primate courtship or the allurement ritual of displaying the genitalia as an invitation to copulation. The male exhibitionist is compulsively driven to display his erect penis to elicit, from a stranger, a startle response ranging from curiosity to alarm or panic. A neutral response—for example, telling him that his penis should be covered in public—will bring the episode to a docile end (Money, 1984).

There is no definite support for any particular theory that explains the cause of exhibitionism. Descriptive studies of exhibitionists have tended to characterize them as having poor social skills, poor marital adjustment, poor heterosexual skills and less heterosexual activity, more difficulty in handling hostility and aggression, and more timid and unassertive behaviors (Blair & Lanyon, 1981).

Marshall (1991) suggested that exhibitionists have an important deficit in the capacity for intimacy and stated that this feature must be addressed in treatment. Silverstein (1996) pointed out that genital exhibitionism is motivated by a need for attention and admiration as well as a wish to overcome shame and feelings of inadequacy. Exhibiting oneself is done to create feelings of pride and power leading to sexual arousal.

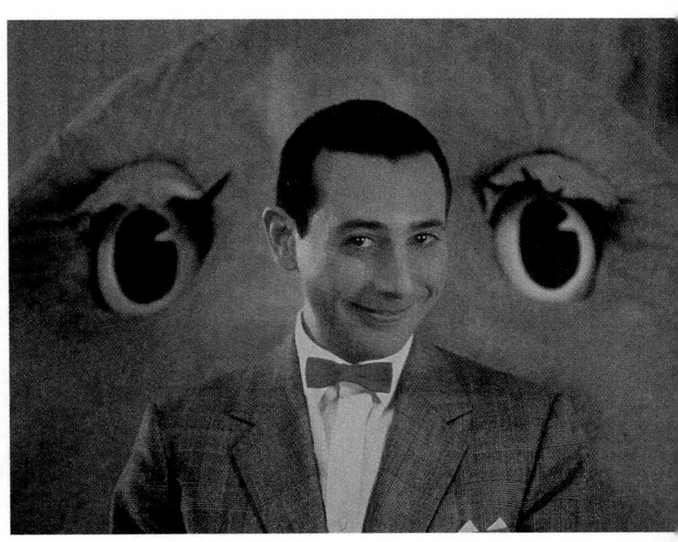

In 1991 Paul Reubens, the actor who created and played Pee-Wee Herman, was arrested by police and charged with "exposure of sexual organs" (masturbating) in an otherwise empty adult movie theater in Sarasota, Florida. Reubens immediately lost his TV job and was subjected to ridicule. Society was horrified that a children's television star would be involved in such activities. Years later, just when he seemed to be forgiven and had made a comeback, Reubens was involved in yet another scandal in which the police searched his home and, in 2002, charged him with "possession of material depicting children under the age of 18 engaging in sexual conduct." Regardless of an accomplished acting career, which includes one of the most popular children's television shows of all time, Paul Reubens may be best remembered in reference to the charges surrounding his atypical sexual behavior.

A few facts about exhibitionists might help to put this behavior into perspective. The exhibitionist receives sexual gratification through the victim's (observer's) response. Exhibitionists might achieve orgasm by the very act of exposure, but more likely they will masturbate either while exhibiting or later. Exhibitionists feel inadequate, they are afraid of rejection, they are shy, and commonly they have had unsatisfactory sexual relationships. They may be looking for attention or affirmation of their masculinity (most exhibitionists are male) or attempting to frighten others.

Although people often think exhibitionists are violent and aggressive, they usually are not. It is extremely rare for exhibitionists to do more than display the genitals. They do not want contact with a person. Punishment and imprisonment do not seem to prevent the recurrence of exhibitionism. Although it may be difficult, generally the best response is to ignore an exhibitionist and continue usual activities. In this way the exhibitionistic behavior is not reinforced.

voyeurism (scopophilia)
Obtaining of pleasure from watching people who are undressing or engaging in sexual behavior.

sexual masochism
Sexual gratification that results from experiencing pain.

sexual sadism
Sexual gratification that results from inflicting pain on another person.

Voyeurism

In a very general sense, the term **voyeurism** (or **scopophilia,** "love of viewing") means obtaining sexual pleasure from watching unsuspecting people undress or engage in sexual behavior. The American Psychiatric Association's (1998) official definition is "over a period of at least six months, recurrent, intense sexually arousing fantasies, sexual urges, or behaviors involving the act of observing an unsuspecting person who is naked, in the process of disrobing, or engaging in sexual activity." A "peeping Tom" is a voyeur. The voyeur learns from experience where to find people to watch. His erotic excitement lies in the forbidden act of looking at the person.

Voyeurs, who are often shy and lonely and lack social skills, commonly fantasize about having sexual relations with the people they are watching and often masturbate while fantasizing. Voyeurs derive satisfaction from the fear of being caught, the anonymity of the person being watched, and the fact that the person does not know he or she is being watched. Generally voyeurs are not violent and in fact are fearful of any contact with the people they observe.

Some degree of voyeurism probably exists in everyone. Society even condones some forms of voyeurism; for example, some magazines are designed to satisfy peoples' voyeuristic tendencies, and the popularity of sexually explicit movies and web sites is due to voyeurism.

Obscene Communication

The most common and traditional form of obscene communication has been obscene telephone calls; through the years there have also been many examples of obscene letter writing. In more recent years obscene e-mails have appeared as well.

Erotic telephone calling is a form of erotic distancing. As do the exhibitionist and the voyeur, the obscene caller or writer obtains sexual pleasure from a distance and not from direct contact with another person (Money, 1984). Telephone callers receive sexual gratification from making obscene remarks over the telephone, usually suggesting that the person meet them to have sexual relations (even though they would probably never go through with this). The recipient may be a stranger or a consenting listener. Professional consenting listeners, trained to take part in erotic telephone fantasies, charge for playing this role.

In a national survey in Canada, Smith and Morra (1994) found that 83.2% of females had received obscene or threatening telephone calls at some time in their life. Divorced and separated females, young females, and females living in major metropolitan areas were most likely to have been victims of this harassment. The typical caller was an adult male unknown to the victim. The majority of the respondents said that the calls affected them emotionally, and the most prevalent response was fear. Katz (1994) found that in the 6 months preceding a national survey in the United States, 16% of women had received at least one call. Women younger than 65 years old and those who were neither married nor widowed were more likely to receive such a call. It appears that obscene calls occur in a pattern.

Obscene telephone callers have counterparts in those whose primary turn-on is not genital sexual activity with a partner but erotic narrations or readings. The obscene letter writer or the obscene computer message sender is hoping for sexual gratification as well.

According to the U.S. Department of Justice, "Any comment, request, suggestion, proposal, image, or other communication which is obscene or indecent, knowing that the recipient of the communication is under 18 years of age" is illegal. In addition, "any indecent communication for commercial purposes which is available to any person under 18 years of age or to any other person without that person's consent" is illegal. These offenses are punishable by a fine up to $50,000 for each violation or imprisonment of up to 6 months or both (United States Code Annotated Title 47, 2003). Note that this covers any telecommunication device, including computers.

What should someone who receives an obscene communication do? Above all, people are advised to remain calm and not reveal shock or fright: These reactions can reinforce the message sender and increase the likelihood of repeated contact. The recommended response is to say nothing and end the communication. Most people who send obscene messages are not dangerous, and most do not make repeat contacts with the same person. In the case of obscene phone calls, it might be helpful to get an unlisted phone number, obtain caller ID, and/or contact the police about threatening or repeated calls.

Masochism and Sadism

Sacrificial paraphilias are those in which one or both partners atone for wicked acts by undergoing an act of penance or sacrifice. The penalty ranges from humiliation and hurt to a blood sacrifice and death. Self-sacrifice is masochism, and partner sacrifice is sadism. Either may be voluntary or forced (Money, 1984).

The American Psychiatric Association (1998) defines sexual masochism as "over a period of at least six months, recurrent, intense sexually arousing fantasies, sexual urges, or behaviors involving the act (real, not simulated) of being humiliated, beaten, bound, or otherwise made to suffer." It defines sexual sadism as "over a period of at least six months, recurrent, intense sexually arousing fantasies, sexual urges, or behaviors involving acts (real, not simulated) in which the psychological or physical suffering (including humiliation) of the victim is sexually exciting to the person."

Sexual masochism, therefore, is sexual gratification that results from experiencing pain. This might include scratching, biting, beating, and the use of various devices. The pain involved must be planned as a part of an overall experience; accidentally hitting a finger with a hammer is not the kind of experience the masochist wants. **Sexual sadism** occurs when an individual gets sexual gratification from inflicting pain on another person—the hallmark of sadism is intentional torture of the victim to sexually arouse the offender (Dietz, Hazelwood, & Warren, 1990). Sadists obviously make good

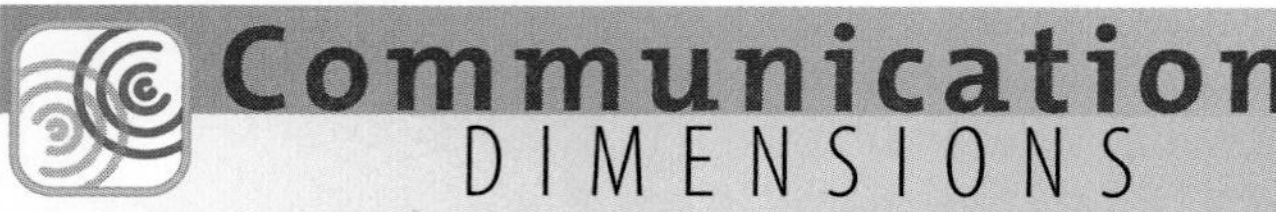

Communicating Accurately

With any sexual behavior, the concept of consent is crucial. For example, if a partner wants to be tied up, that might be fine; however, prior communication about the goal is important. A student once confessed (under the influence of alcohol) to a group of people that she wanted to be tied up. Another time, though, she said that her fantasy really involved being tied down with silk ribbons to a luxurious four-poster bed. Still later she said that what she really wanted was a partner who would initiate sexual activity with her. Thus, she did not always like being the aggressor, and her fantasy was really about having her lover "take charge." But in respect to her original assertions, that underlying desire would not have been known to a partner; nor would her desire for an initiating partner be fulfilled when she engaged in nonbondage activities. As always, effective communication is a must.

First, it is crucial to explain desires and intentions clearly in such situations. The student in our example was not clear, and this could have led to behavior or attempts at behavior that were not desired. This, in turn, could have caused overall relationship problems. Second, as with any form of sexual behavior, it is important to obtain consent. It is not enough to assume that you know what your partner meant or that consent is implicit because you have a good relationship. Without consent, sexual behavior is forcible. With consent, it can be enjoyable for everyone and contribute to a positive relationship.

partners for masochists, but sadomasochistic partner matching is difficult to achieve because it requires that the fantasies of the two people match completely. There is one sadistic scenario, however, that requires an unsuspecting partner or a stranger to be subjected to abuse. Sadism does not seem to be as common as masochism.

Domination and degradation are important to both the sadist and the masochist. Some psychiatrists feel that sadism is an expression of anger and hostility. Masochism, on the other hand, is sometimes thought to result from a belief that sexual activity is dirty and evil; therefore, the activity could be viewed as just punishment for sexual sins. It is difficult to understand the true psychology of these behaviors.

Sadomasochism is a paraphilia that combines both sadistic and masochistic sexual behavior. The main characteristic is the eroticizing of pain. What appears to the outsider to be painful is experienced as somewhat painful but mostly pleasurable and very sexually arousing to the sadomasochist. Sadomasochistic sexual encounters usually occur in the context of scripted scenes that simulate interactions between master and slave, employer and servant, and parent and child. Sadomasochists tend to alternate between masochistic and sadistic roles. In milder forms, dominance and submissive behaviors may be found in many relationships or may be an element of fantasy life (Sadomasochism, 2001).

There is more information available on masochism and sadism than on most other paraphilias, and a brief chronological review of a few studies will help to shed some light on these two behaviors. Weinberg, Williams, and Moser (1984) reported that although some persons engage in nonconsensual sexual violence such as rape or lust murders, for most participants sadomasochism is simply a form of sexual enhancement that they voluntarily and mutually choose to explore.

Glickauf-Hughes (1991) pointed out that masochists' relationships are characterized by masochists' loving objects who give nonlove in return. They tend to choose idealized but unloving partners with whom they behave as caretakers. Nakakuki (1994) proposed a concept of "normal masochism," seeming to imply that it does not have to be viewed as a negative behavior or psychological problem.

Shainess (1997) indicated that noticeable symptoms of masochism include low self-esteem, chameleonlike behavior, and, most important, the prevalence of linguistic forms, such as self-abasement and apology. All these ploys represent attempts to avoid contact with another person and maintain superiority while feeling worthless. It could be called a "system of self-destruction" aimed at proving superiority over others but inevitably failing.

Baumeister (1997) pointed out that masochism fosters temporary escape from the stressful awareness of one's ordinary identity. Litman (1997) suggested that sexual masochism is more widespread and can be more dangerous than current literature indicates. Danger can arise from being humiliated, endangered, and enslaved and being physically bound, restrained, and rendered helpless to the degree that life is threatened. He indicates that **bondage perversion** (deriving pleasure from being bound, tied up, or otherwise restricted) can be fatal—a mix of suicide and accident.

bondage perversion
Getting sexual pleasure from being bound, tied up, or otherwise restricted.

transvestite
A person who achieves sexual satisfaction from wearing clothes usually worn by the other gender.

Sexual masochism is more common in males, but the incidence in females is on the rise. Masochists often seek partners to tie up, humiliate, blindfold, or hurt. They may enjoy being whipped, beaten, shocked, or cut. Verbal abuse is common. Some masochists require pain or humiliation to function sexually (Masochism, 2001). Some sadists also require the pain or humiliation of a partner to function sexually. As long as it occurs with a consenting partner, sadism is not considered a psychological disorder. It is considered a disorder when it causes the person unhappiness or causes problems with work, social setting, or family. If the other person is not willing, sadism can be a severe and even criminal disorder. Sadism is much more common in males (Sadism, 2001). People who engage in masochism and sadism must be especially careful about diseases transmitted by body fluids, such as hepatitis and HIV.

Sadism and masochism are good examples of sexual behaviors in which we need to differentiate between fantasy and behavior. For example, many more people have reported sexual fantasies involving masochism and sadism than have actually participated in such behavior. It is possible to enjoy a sexual fantasy without needing to act it out in real life.

Transvestism

Transvestism is sometimes confused with transsexualism and homosexuality. A **transvestite** takes pleasure in wearing clothing of the other sex and is likely to achieve sexual gratification from doing so but may have no interest in having a sex-change operation or in relating sexually to members of the same sex.

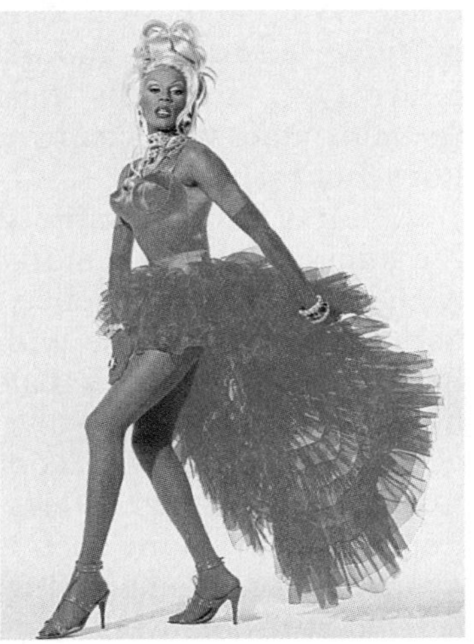

The cross-dresser RuPaul took cross-dressing to mainstream pop culture. He became a fashion model (both in magazines and on runways), a singer, and a talk show host. In case you are wondering, RuPaul takes almost 3 hours to get into his corset! However, the millions of dollars he has garnered has been worth the effort.

Some transvestites cross-dress only periodically, and the use of female clothes (most transvestites are males) may approximate a fetish. Others may wear female clothing under their male clothes. No one knows for sure why some people are transvestites, and it is interesting to note that most transvestites have quite normal heterosexual relationships.

One thousand and thirty-two periodic cross-dressers (transvestites) responded to an anonymous survey. Eight-seven percent described themselves as heterosexual. All except 17% had married. These transvestites strongly approved of both their masculine and feminine selves equally (Doctor & Prince, 1997). Although a majority of transvestites are heterosexual, a significant portion are bisexual, homosexual, or not sexually active with another person (Bullough & Bullough, 1997).

Most transvestites begin to experiment with cross-dressing when they are children or adolescents. Some feel guilty and uncomfortable about this preference; others do not. Many are happily married to people who understand their behaviors. Others have had relationships ruined by cross-dressing. There are numerous support groups for transvestites and their partners (Transvestism, 2001).

Fetishism

Fetishism is a paraphilia in which an inanimate object elicits sexual arousal. Articles of clothing and materials made of rubber, silk, fur, or leather are common fetishistic objects. The American Psychiatric Association (2000) defines the symptoms of fetishism as "over a period of at least six months, recurrent, intense sexually arousing fantasies, sexual urges, or behaviors involving the use of nonliving objects. The fantasies, sexual urges, or behaviors cause clinically significant distress or impairment in social, occupational, or other important areas of functioning."

The fetishist may masturbate while engaging in fetishistic behavior or may just enjoy stimulation from the objects. In a related paraphilia, **partialism,** people are aroused by a particular body part (breasts, muscular chests, feet, and so on). Most fetishes are practiced in private or with a willing partner.

Generally, a person who has fetishism must have the fetish present to become sexually excited. It usually begins in childhood or adolescence and is most common among males. Although many people are aroused by undergarments or other items, this is not considered fetishism except when a person cannot perform sexually unless the partner is wearing the items (Fetishism, 2001).

Most fetishes and partialisms are harmless. However, occasionally someone may commit burglary to obtain the fetish object.

Other Paraphilias

Bestiality

Bestiality (or **zoophilia**) is sexual contact with animals. In Kinsey's research (1948, 1953) about 8% of males and 4% of females reported having had sexual experiences with animals at some time. The frequency of bestiality was higher (17% for males) for those raised in rural areas. Men most often had sexual contact with farm animals; women most often had sexual contact with household pets.

Human sexual relationships with animals have been an interesting topic for some people for hundreds of years. Stories of human–animal contact are found throughout ancient folklore. For example, Zeus, in the form of a swan, had sexual intercourse with Leda, the queen of Sparta. Greek and Roman mythology portrayed females' having sexual relationships with bears, apes, bulls, goats, horses, wolves, snakes, and crocodiles. Historically, taboos against human–animal contact have been severe. The laws in many states treated bestiality as a felony. In eight states, the maximal penalty was life imprisonment. Many such laws remain on the books today (Bestiality, 2003).

Sexual experience with animals is usually only a transitory experience for young people who do not have acceptable sexual partners. It most likely occurs during adolescence, and most people move on to more common adult sexual relations with humans. True zoophilia exists only when sexual contacts with animals are preferred even when other forms of sexual contact are readily available (American Psychiatric Association, 2000).

Frottage

Frottage is the act of obtaining sexual pleasure from rubbing or pressing against a nonconsenting person. The American Psychiatric Association's official definition (2000) is "over a period of at least six months, recurrent, intense sexually arousing fantasies, sexual urges, or behaviors involving touching and rubbing against a nonconsenting person." It is likely to occur in crowds, on elevators, and in buses and subways. It is even possible that the frotteur will achieve orgasm. Women and girls, the usual recipients, generally find this behavior offensive. Normally no additional contact or other form of behavior follows.

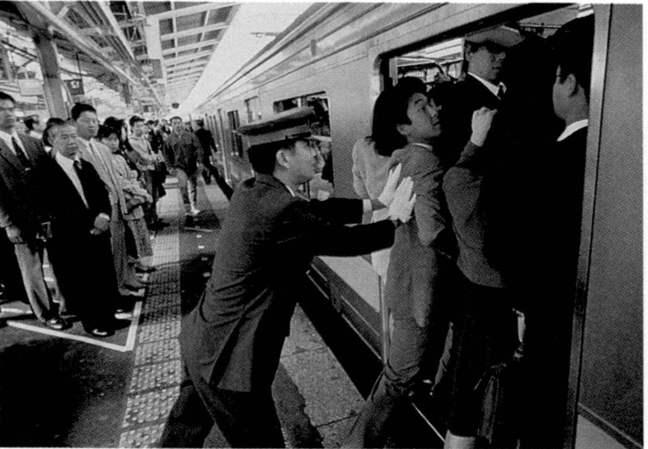

The overcrowding of subways in Tokyo and other Japanese cities lends itself to frottage, or deriving sexual pleasure from rubbing up against a nonconsenting person. The situation is exacerbated by the male-dominated Japanese culture, which prevents police from dealing with the problem.

Necrophilia

Necrophilia is a rather rare behavior in which a person receives sexual pleasure from viewing or having sexual relations with a dead person. Sometimes necrophiliacs (almost all of whom are men) pay women to pretend to be dead in order to provide sexual pleasure. This might even include dressing in a certain way, using white powder to look very pale, and lying very still. In this way the participants are simulated corpses.

Necrophiliacs are usually severely emotionally disturbed and sexually and socially inept and hate and fear women. Although local newspapers do not report instances, law enforcement officers indicate that bodies are sometimes stolen for this purpose.

fetishism
Paraphilia in which an inanimate object elicits sexual arousal.

partialism
Paraphilia in which sexual arousal is associated with a particular body part.

bestiality
Sexual contact with animals—also called *zoophilia.*

zoophilia
Sexual contact with animals—also called *bestiality.*

frottage
Obtaining of sexual pleasure from rubbing or pressing against another person.

necrophilia
Sexual relations with a dead person.

troilism
Having sexual relations with another person while a third person watches.

asphyxiophilia
Desire for a state of oxygen deficiency to enhance sexual excitement.

Troilism

Troilism is having sexual relations with another person while a third person watches. In one respect, troilism combines elements of exhibitionism and voyeurism. In another respect, it represents an illusion of prostitution (Money, 1984) because there are elaborate ruses and pretenses of prostitution. An example might be a husband's inviting another man to have intercourse with his wife. The husband watches and is able to get an erection. He then achieves penetration and orgasm, which are not possible unless his wife plays the role of a prostitute.

Troilism clearly does not qualify as a safe sexual activity. Because multiple partners are involved, this is a high-risk activity.

Asphyxiophilia

Asphyxiophilia is the desire for a state of oxygen deficiency in order to enhance sexual excitement and orgasm. It has also been called *erotic* or *autorerotic suicide, sexual suicide, autoerotic strangulation, autoerotic asphyxiation, hypoxophilia,* and *autoerotic accident.* Most information about asphyxiophilia is found in reports from police or doctors of forensic medicine who examine people who have died during this behavior (Innala & Ernulf, 1989).

Self-induced oxygen deficiency is used to produce sexual euphoria, increased excitement, or heightened orgasm during masturbatory activities. Reduced supply of oxygen to the brain results in giddiness, lightheadedness, or exhilaration that is reported to enhance sexual climax (Burg, 1987).

Oxygen deficiency can be induced in many ways. Because the circumstances and features of autoerotic deaths are not commonly known, they are often misinterpreted as suicides or homicides. And death can easily result, because cutting off the flow of blood to the brain can produce unconsciousness in as little as 5 to 10 seconds. Although the person probably did not intend to die, death results when an escape mechanism fails or the person cannot recover from self-induced oxygen deprivation.

Conservative estimates indicate that 500 to 1,000 autoerotic fatalities occur each year in the United States and that such deaths are steadily increasing. The majority of the victims are adolescents and young adults, almost all are male (96%) and white (94%), and most (73%) are not married (Bechtel, Westerfield, & Eddy, 1990).

There are several theories to account for life-threatening autoerotic behaviors: guilt associated with masturbation, risk-taking/thrill-seeking behavior, and psychological connections (such as castration anxiety or oral conflicts). Unfortunately, very little is known about intervention strategies to prevent or treat life-threatening autoerotic behavior (Saunders, 1989).

klismaphilia
Sexual arousal produced by the use of enemas.

coprophilia
Sexual pleasure associated with feces.

urophilia
Sexual pleasure associated with urine.

behavior therapy
Applying learning principles to help people change behavior.

Klismaphilia

In **klismaphilia** sexual arousal is obtained from enema use. Klismaphiles most often prefer the receiving role, but less commonly erotic arousal may be associated with administering an enema. The background of many individuals who show klismaphilia often indicates that as infants or young children they were frequently given enemas by concerned and loving mothers. This association with loving attention, or perhaps even sexual pleasure, learned early in life may eroticize the experience for some people, so they show a need to receive an enema for sexual satisfaction as adults. Because klismaphilia involves anal contact, it is not a safe sexual activity unless latex gloves are used, and there is great attention to cleanliness.

Coprophilia

In **coprophilia,** sexual pleasure is associated with feces. People who show coprophilia reach high levels of sexual excitement by watching someone defecate or by defecating on someone. The connection of feces with sexual arousal may also go back to childhood. Some children seem to enjoy holding back on a bowel movement and then carefully expelling the feces. It could also be that the connection between changing of soiled diapers and sexual stimulation during infancy eroticizes feces. Because it appears that HIV can be present in any body tissue or fluids, coprophilia is not a safe sexual activity.

Urophilia

In **urophilia,** sexual pleasure is associated with urine. Similarly to coprophilia, the person may want to urinate on someone or be urinated on. Again, as with coprophilia, there may be childhood beginnings for urophilia. For example, stimulation of the urethra during urination may become associated with pleasure, or there may have been stimulation from the changing of wet diapers. Urophilia has been referred to as "golden showers" or "water sports." Urophilia is not a safe sexual activity because HIV and other STIs can be transmitted through urine.

Treatment for Paraphilias

A number of issues surface when one considers treatment for paraphilias. For example, people with paraphilias often do not want treatment. Also, they often feel they cannot control their urges, so they cannot accept personal responsibility for their actions. However, personal responsibility is usually a prerequisite for successful behavior change. In addition, some helping professionals think it is not their responsibility to provide treatment for paraphilias—they believe it is the responsibility of the criminal justice system. In spite of these issues, it is appropriate to consider what might be done to help those with paraphilias. Possible treatments fall into three categories: (1) psychotherapy, (2) behavior therapy, and (3) pharmacological approaches (drug therapy).

Psychotherapy

Not much information is available about successful treatment of paraphilias by psychotherapy. The purpose of psychoanalysis is to discover unconscious conflicts that are believed to originate in childhood. If conflicts can be drawn to the surface and resolved, the hope is that the particular behavior can be changed.

Behavior Therapy

Behavior therapy applies learning principles to help people change their behavior. Many techniques have been used to help change paraphiliac behavior. For example, in systematic desensitization the therapist tries to break the link between a sexual stimulus (such as leather for a fetishist) and the inappropriate response (sexual stimulation). The client is taught to relax muscle groups so that relaxation replaces sexual arousal in response to the stimulus.

Gender DIMENSIONS

Paraphilias and Gender Differences Because it is hard to find accurate statistics about the incidence of paraphilias, it is also difficult to find a great deal of information about paraphilias and gender differences. Although we know that the majority of paraphilias occur among men, here is a brief summary of what is found in the literature on this topic.

1. Janus and Janus (1993) reported that
   a. Eleven percent of both men and women have had experience with bondage
   b. Six percent of men and 4% of women have participated in urophilia
   c. Eleven percent of men and 6% of women have engaged in fetishistic behaviors
   d. Six percent of men and 3% of women report cross-dressing
2. Kinsey, Pomeroy, & Martin (1948 and 1953) reported that
   a. Eight percent of men and 3% of women had experienced at least one sexual contact with animals
   b. Twenty-two percent of males and 12% of females in their sample responded erotically to stories with sadomasochistic (SM) themes
3. Regarding voyeurism, Person and associates (1989) reported that
   a. Among college students, 23% of women and 38% of men have watched their partners masturbate
   b. Eleven percent of women and 18% of men have performed sexual acts in front of mirrors
   c. Five percent of women and 4% of men have watched others engage in sexual intercourse

Ethical DIMENSIONS

The Ethics of Chemical Treatment for Paraphilias

Is it ethical to force paraphilic sex offenders to take hormones or tranquilizers to reduce their drives for paraphilic behaviors? Although in some cases Depo-Provera reduces the paraphilic sex drive to a level that allows the person to have a more normal sex drive, in others it causes a complete elimination of the sex drive—meaning that the individual has almost no interest in any sexual behavior (Levine, et al., 1990).

One difficulty is that some paraphilics enjoy their behavior. Therefore, they do not want treatment because they do not view their behavior as a problem.

Some experts would argue that chemical treatment for paraphiliacs should be required to protect other people from them. Others feel that such treatments should be required only for people who have paraphilias that violate the rights of others or harm them (Gijs & Gooren, 1996).

When faced with the possibility of arrest or imprisonment, paraphilic sex offenders could waive their right of informed consent and sign up for treatment just to avoid legal action. It can be difficult to balance the right of society to be protected from harm against the right of a person to avoid being given chemicals that may have undesired side effects.

Sources: Gijs, L. & Gooren, L. Hormonal and psychopharmacological interventions in the treatment of paraphilias: An update, *Journal of Sex Research, 33* (1996), 273–290; Levine, S. B., Risen, C. B., & Althof, C. B. Essay on the diagnosis and nature of paraphilia, *Journal of Sex and Marital Therapy, 16* (1990), 89–102.

In **aversion therapy** the undesirable behavior (such as masturbation for a voyeur) is paired repeatedly with a negative stimulus, such as a painful (but harmless) electric shock. The objective is that negative reactions to the paraphilic behavior will develop.

In **social training** the individual is helped to improve his or her social skills. It is hoped that if the person can better relate to people, he or she will be able to develop sexual relationships that would be considered more typical.

In **orgasmic reconditioning** the goal is to increase sexual arousal by socially appropriate stimuli. For example, if the person becomes sexually aroused by masturbating, as he or she approaches orgasm, "socially appropriate imagery" such as pictures of attractive people would be used. The hope is that orgasm will then be connected with these images and not the paraphilic ones.

aversion therapy
Pairing an undesirable sexual behavior to a painful response.

social training
Improving a person's social skills.

orgasmic reconditioning
Increasing sexual arousal to socially appropriate stimuli.

antiandrogen drugs
Chemicals that reduce the sex drive by lowering the testosterone level in the bloodstream.

nymphomania
An excessive, insatiable sexual drive in women.

satyriasis
An excessive, insatiable sexual drive in men—also called *Don Juanism.*

Drug Therapy

Although no drug can eliminate paraphilic behavior, some chemicals can sometimes be helpful in reducing the intensity of sexual drives and establishing an environment for more successful treatment using one of the other approaches. For example, Prozac, which is commonly used for treating depression, has been used to help some people reduce obsessions and compulsions. Also, **antiandrogen drugs,** chemicals that reduce the sex drive by lowering the testosterone level in the bloodstream, can reduce sexual desire and erections in males. Such a drug is Depo-Provera, which must be injected weekly to be effective. However, even Depo-Provera does not change the nature of sexual stimuli for people; it only reduces the intensity of their reactions.

Sexual Addiction

In 1998 President Clinton's sexual activity stirred up the debate over "sexual addiction." The idea that some people might have very strong, or even insatiable, sexual needs has been around a long time. The term **nymphomania** refers to an excessive, insatiable sexual drive in women. The same condition in men is referred to as **satyriasis,** or **Don Juanism.** Many professionals have argued about the appropriateness of these labels for years. They contend that the labels should not be used at all because judgments about how much sexual behavior is "normal" or "excessive" are subjective.

Some experts believe that sexual addiction is mainly a male abnormality caused by childhood trauma that usually requires intense psychotherapy. Many others say this is nonsense because there is no such thing as too much sexual behavior, unless it is with the wrong partner. They say that some people who have the symptoms do not experience conflict and are not really troubled by it. Still others are concerned that use of the label *sexual addiction* may help people inappropriately excuse their behavior.

Sexual addiction can involve a wide variety of practices. Sometimes an addict has trouble with just one unwanted behavior, sometimes with many. As in other addictions, the sexual addict experiences powerlessness over a compulsive behavior. The addict may wish to stop but repeatedly fails to do so. The consequences can be loss of relationships, difficulties with work, arrests, financial troubles, a loss of interest in matters not sexual, low self-esteem, and despair (What is sexual addiction? 2003).

Among the writings about sexual addiction have been several books by Patrick Carnes, who outlines 10 practical and useful indicators of compulsive sexual behavior.

1. A pattern of out-of-control behavior
2. Severe consequences caused by sexual behavior
3. Inability to stop despite adverse consequences
4. Persistent pursuit of self-destructive or high-risk behavior
5. Ongoing desire or effort to limit sexual behavior, usually at a partner's insistence
6. Sexual obsession and fantasy as a primary coping strategy
7. Increasing amounts of sexual experience because the current level of activity is no longer sufficient
8. Severe mood changes related to sexual activity
9. Inordinate amounts of time spent in obtaining sexual activity, being sexual, and/or recovering from sexual experience
10. Neglect of important social, occupational, and/or recreational activities caused by behavior

The main way to identify any addictive behavior is to consider whether it is causing negative or unwelcome problems and yet the person continues it anyway. Sexual addicts are often unable to make and keep commitments to themselves and others about stopping or changing particular sexual behaviors over the long term, and most have problems with real intimacy (Sex addiction frequently asked questions, 2001).

In more recent years, one form of sexual addiction is cybersex addiction. There may be many symptoms of cybersex addiction; common symptoms are (1) spending increasing amounts of online time focused on sexual or romantic intrigue or involvement, (2) failed attempts to cut back on frequency of online sexual involvement, (3) online use that interferes with work and personal life, (4) secretiveness or lying about the amount of time spent on online sexual activity, and (5) a primary focus of sexual activity related to computer activity (Cybersex addiction checklist, 2001).

Even though there is no agreement about how to deal with compulsive sexual activity—if it can be done at all—organizations have been formed to help people deal with their activities if they feel there is a problem—for example, a 12-step program modeled after Alcoholics Anonymous called Sex and Love Addicts Anonymous. Other such groups are called Sex Addicts Anonymous, Sexaholics Anonymous, and Sexual Compulsives Anonymous.

The initial process of treatment can be divided into three major stages: (1) identification of the problem, (2) behavior contracting (clearly defining specific sexual behaviors which are to be eliminated and how this will be done), and (3) relapse prevention (providing support, managing stress, improving relationships, working out financial and other problems, etc.). Recovering addicts require external sources of social reinforcement and support for changing lifelong patterns of behavior (How to approach treatment of the sexual addict, 2001).

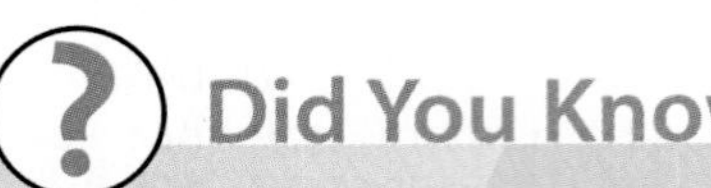

Sexual Addiction Recovery Resources

E-mail Groups
- Addict-L@listserv.kent.edu — addiction research and treatment
- Listserv@netcom.com — Internet addiction support group

Resource and Recovery Sites
- http://www.sexhelp.com
- http://addictionresearch.com

National Resources

Sexual Addicts Anonymous
(713) 869-4902
P.O. Box 70949
Houston, TX 77270

Sexaholics Anonymous
(615) 331-6230
P.O. Box 111910
Nashville, TN 37222

Recovering Couples Anonymous
(314) 830-2600
P.O. Box 11872
St. Louis, MO 63105

Source: Sex Addiction Help. [Online]. Available: http://www.sexaddicthelp.com/weblinks.html

Discussion Questions

1. Describe how sexual feelings or behaviors vary from common to atypical along a continuum.
2. What are the most common forms of paraphilia? Describe the type of person who might practice them.
3. What are the less common forms of paraphilia? Discuss why someone would practice them.
4. Describe the major types of treatment programs for paraphilias, including the ways they work and their effectiveness.
5. Is "sexual addiction" a true disorder? Explain your answer.

Application Questions

Reread the chapter-opening story and answer the following questions:

1. In spite of his well-publicized sexual behavior, Marv Albert's fiancée married him in September 1998. Would you have advised her to go through with the wedding? Explain your answer.
2. Discuss the issues of safer sex surrounding the sexual acts engaged in by Albert.
3. In addition to causing immense embarrassment, Marv Albert's sexual habits cost him his job (and probably some friends as well). What might have caused Albert to take such risks? What therapies are available to help him with his atypical behaviors?

Critical Thinking Questions

1. Look over the American Psychiatric Association's definitions for the varied paraphilias, supplied throughout the chapter. What are the common elements? On the basis of that information, how would you define "atypical sexual behavior"?
2. Given that the pornography industry takes in about $2 billion a year, are we a nation of voyeurs? What differentiates a diagnosed voyeur from someone who views porn? Explain your answers.

Critical Thinking Case

Bill and Anne, college juniors, were in a monogamous relationship for about 5 months when Bill said that he wanted to add some "variety" to their sex life. Anne's immediate reaction was to feel that she was not giving Bill enough sexual satisfaction, and so she did not respond to his suggestion. As much as she loved Bill, she felt unsure about his request for variety.

After he broached the subject several more times, she finally asked him what he wanted. He said that a former girlfriend had enjoyed having another girl join them from time to time. Anne was initially aghast at the idea of including a third person, especially a girl. But a few months later, Anne and a female friend had a brief sexual encounter after drinking heavily. Anne did not enjoy it. When she told Bill what had happened, he reacted sharply: What was she doing with another sexual partner?

Why did Bill react as he did? What did Bill really want from the encounter—another girl for his girlfriend or a threesome for himself? Why was it important for him to communicate correctly what he wanted?

You want something your partner does not want. How do you approach it? How do you make sure you are comfortable?

Exploring Personal Dimensions

Respond about only your sexual activity. If you do not participate in any sexual activity, skip this assessment. Check the following items that apply to you.

_____ 1. I tell my partner what feels good.

_____ 2. I tell my partner what hurts, if anything.

_____ 3. I avoid frequent sexual encounters because I do not like them.

_____ 4. I let myself just go with my feelings and behave the way I want to act during sexual encounters.

_____ 5. My partner and I have talked about and resolved how often to have sexual activity.

_____ 6. Sexual activity is a problem for me and my partner.

_____ 7. I have told my partner what I want during sexual activity.

_____ 8. My partner and I enjoy holding hands, kissing, and just talking as much as we do having sexual activity.

_____ 9. It is important that each time we express love or date that it culminate in sexual intercourse to be a really meaningful experience.

Scoring

Give yourself the following points for the items you check, and total your score.

1. 2	4. 2	7. 2
2. 2	5. 2	8. 2
3. −2	6. −2	9. −2

Interpretation

This exercise indicates whether you have healthy communication in your sexual relationship. Interpret your score as follows:

6–10 = Your communication is healthy.
0–5 = Your communication is moderately healthy.
−1–−6 = You need to improve your communication skills.

Source: Bruess, C. & Richardson, G. *Decisions for Health.* Madison, WI: Brown & Benchmark, 1995.

Sexuality Online

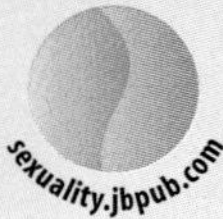

Go to the web component for *Exploring the Dimensions of Human Sexuality* at sexuality.jbpub.com for web exercises, additional resources related to this chapter, and student review tools.

Suggested Readings

Ames, A. M. & Houston, D. A. Legal, social, and biological dimensions of pedophilia, *Archives of Sexual Behavior, 19* (August 1990), 333–342.

Cole, C., O'Boyle, M., Emory, L., & Meyer, W. Comorbidity of gender dysphoria and other major psychiatric diagnoses, *Archives of Sexual Behavior, 26* (1997), 13–26.

Davison, G. & Neale, J. *Abnormal Psychology,* 6th ed. New York: Wiley, 1993.

How do I know if I am a sex addict? Sexual Recovery Institute (2001). [Online]. Available: http://www.sexualrecovery.com/sri_docs/howdoiknow.htm

Laws, Dr. R. & Marshall, W. L. A brief history of behavioral and cognitive behavioral approaches to sexual offenders, *Sexual Abuse: Journal of Research and Treatment, 15, no. 2* (April 2003), 75–92.

McCarthy, B. The wife's role in facilitating recovery from male compulsive sexual behavior, *Sexual Addiction and Compulsivity, 9, no. 4* (2002), 275–284.

Stages in a compulsive episode. *Sex Addiction Help*. [Online]. Available: http://www.sexaddicthelp.com.

CHAPTER 16

Forcible Sexual Behaviors

FEATURES

Multicultural Dimensions
Coercive Sexual Experiences

Ethical Dimensions
Should the Media Reveal the Names of Rape Survivors?

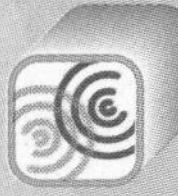

Communication Dimensions
Helping Survivors of Rape and Sexual Abuse

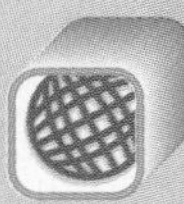

Global Dimensions
Coercive Sexual Behaviors in Japan

Ethical Dimensions
Is It Ethical to Publicly Identify Sexual Offenders?

Multicultural Dimensions
Wife Abuse in China

Gender Dimensions
Same-Sex Sexual Harassment

CHAPTER OBJECTIVES

1. Differentiate among rape, statutory rape, stranger rape, and date (acquaintance) rape. Discuss what makes someone rape. Discuss the myths surrounding rape.
2. Discuss pedophilia, including the profile of the pedophiliac, incidence and effects of pedophilia, and prevention.
3. Describe the incidence of incest and the typical effects on incest victims.
4. Summarize important information about violence in marriage, including marital rape and domestic abuse.
5. Discuss sexual harassment in the workplace, in schools, on campus, and in the military and indicate what can be done to prevent and deal with it.

sexuality.jbpub.com

Social Responses to Rape
Incidence of Pedophilia
Domestic Violence
Sexual Harassment

INTRODUCTION

After a discussion about forcible sexual behavior in my sexuality class, a female student who was in her late 20s asked to go to my office to talk for a few minutes. When we got there, she said that she had found the information and the discussion on forcible sexual behavior interesting and enlightening. She also said she was feeling personally troubled because it reminded her of something that had happened to her. She then told me about it.

She remembered when she was 15 years old. She said she was a typical middle-class high school girl. Although her parents and her teachers did not say a lot about sexuality, she had heard quite a bit about rape on TV and seen stories about it in magazines and newspapers. Her parents, as had many of her friends, warned her about being careful and about not trusting strangers. She dated Ed, a neighbor who lived just a block away. Ed's parents and her parents sometimes got together socially, and they had been friends for at least 10 years. Ed's parents had always been friendly to her, too, and she probably saw them at least two or three times each week.

Ed was 2 years older and a star basketball player. He was an excellent student and considered to be a leader and one of the most popular boys at school. She remembered that he had always seemed to be one of the best athletes as they were growing up. After a few dates, they had started to become intimate. She enjoyed the closeness with him and found him very attractive. She had some tears in her eyes when she said that on one date, after an exciting basketball game, he had intercourse with her while she was crying and asking him not to do it. Although he was a little forceful, he did not raise his voice and he did not hit her. He just paid no attention to what she was saying.

At the time she said she did not realize it was rape. She asked him why he was doing this to her, but he did not answer. Afterward she did not want to date him anymore, and her parents wondered why. Her friends thought she was crazy not to want to go out with him. She said she had not told anyone about this before, but that she just had to get it out. When we talked about forcible sexual behavior in class, all the memories rushed back to her.

Many readers of this chapter are probably survivors of forcible sexual behavior—whether it was rape, child sexual abuse, sexual harassment, or another form of forcible sexual behavior. Sometimes it can be difficult and painful to think about these topics. However, most people, such as the student in our story, find it helpful to learn more about such topics and to deal more directly with their feelings about them.

Throughout this text it has been recognized that many sexual behaviors exist and that various factors contribute to these behaviors. Most often people voluntarily choose a particular behavior, but some sexual behaviors are not voluntary. In this chapter we focus on rape and child sexual abuse because of their seriousness. By no means, however, are these the only forcible sexual behaviors. Other representative forcible sexual behaviors are also considered. A characteristic of all these behaviors is that we know very little about them because of their obvious secretive and private nature. Although knowledge about forcible sexual behavior has rapidly increased, a great need for continued study and research is evident.

Rape

Rape is a forcible act. Legal definitions of rape and law enforcement procedures for handling rape cases are changing, and they differ from state to state. However, a practical definition of **rape** is "forcible sexual intercourse." This can include forced oral sexual activity, penile–vaginal sexual activity, and anal sexual activity. If a person is forced to do any of these things when he or she does not want to, that is rape.

Within the category of rape, there are several types. For example, **statutory rape** is intercourse with a person who is younger than the age of consent (ranging from 14 to 18 years from state to state). Even with consent, statutory rape is considered to have occurred if one of the participants is not of legal age. **Stranger rape** is rape of a person by an unknown assailant. If a rape is committed by someone known to the victim, it is **acquaintance rape,** or **date rape,** both of which are discussed later in this chapter.

rape
Forcible sexual intercourse with a person who does not give consent.

statutory rape
Intercourse with a person younger than the legal age of consent.

stranger rape
Rape of a person by an unknown person.

acquaintance rape
Rape by a friend, acquaintance, or date; also known as *date rape.*

Rape Myths

In spite of the increased attention given to the topic of rape in recent years, rape myths remain prevalent (see Myth vs. Fact on pp. 622 and 623). Males seem to accept rape myths more than females, and individuals with a conservative gender-role ideology believe rape myths more than those with more liberal ideologies (Johnson, Kuck, & Schander, 1997). In addition, males who have difficulty distinguishing rape myths from fact had attitudes toward rape and its victims that are resistant to change (Gilmartin, 1994). There are many ramifications of this. For example, those who believe rape myths are more tolerant of the rapist and less tolerant of the victims (Varelas & Foley, 1998).

Men and women who are less inclined to believe rape myths assign significantly less blame to the victim and situation and more blame to the perpetrator. They are also less likely to believe the assault could have been prevented (Kopper, 1996). In general, men are more tolerant of rape, more likely to attribute blame for rape to the victim, and less negative in their views of rapists than are women (Caron & Carter, 1997).

1 IN 4 WOMEN
WILL BE RAPED IN
HER LIFETIME.
WILL IT BE
YOUR MOTHER,
YOUR SISTER,
YOUR DAUGHTER
OR YOUR WIFE?
The statistics won't improve if you pretend they aren't true.
Help stop the violence. Call 920-4642 for information.
The Violence Against Women Coalition

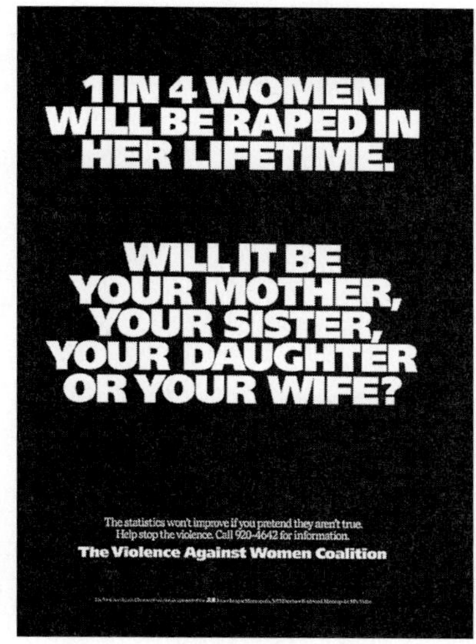

As a female, what can you do to improve your odds of preventing rape? As a male, what can you do to make sure you never are involved in forced sexual activity?

Society and Rape

Some people have wondered whether particular characteristics of a given society help promote rape. Although no definitive relationship has been established, beliefs that restrict the rights and roles of women are related to beliefs about rape, which place women at a disadvantage (Costin, 1985). In other words, myths about rape are positively related to beliefs that women's social roles and rights should be more restricted than men's. Whatever the reasons might be, statistics of the International Criminal Police Organization (Interpol) indicate that the United States has the highest number of rapes among all Western countries (Contemporary sexuality, 1996).

Many writers feel that three characteristics account for the high incidence of rape in American society: (1) Rape is a means of keeping women subordinate to men, (2) pornography provides a cultural situation that endorses and legitimizes rape, and (3) rape is a crime of violence rather than a crime motivated by a desire for sexual gratification (Baron & Straus, 1984).

Ellis (1989) has also provided possible theories of rape that relate to characteristics of society. One, the "femininist" theory, emphasizes that male domination in sociopolitical and economic arenas results in use of sexual intimidation and exploitation by males to maintain their supremacy. Another, the social learning theory, implies that sexual behavior and violence become fused through frequent exposure to their continued association (such as in movies, TV shows, rock videos, and so on). Some people feel that rape could be reasonably defined as a concrete acting out of culturally normative beliefs and images (Lisak, 1991).

It is also interesting to note a few studies that reflect attitudes about rape of some people in the United States. For example, a vignette depicting a date rape was presented to 352 male and female high school students. The vignette was accompanied by a photograph of the victim dressed provocatively, a photograph of the victim dressed conservatively, or no photograph. Subjects who viewed the photograph of the victim in provocative clothing were more likely than the other subjects to indicate that the victim was responsible for her assailant's behavior and that his behavior was justified and were less likely to judge the act of unwanted sexual intercourse as rape (Cassidy, 1995).

The responses of 531 midwestern college students to scenarios depicting nonconsensual sexual intercourse between males and females with varying degrees of prior intimacy were examined (Freetly, Hattery, & Kane, 1995). Females were more likely than males to consider the scenarios unacceptable, and the gender differences increased with the level of prior intimacy between the victim and the offender in the scenario. Respondents who reported knowing a rape victim were also more likely to consider the scenarios unacceptable.

A cross-cultural analysis comparing attitudes about women and rape victims of Asian and white college students revealed significant differences in

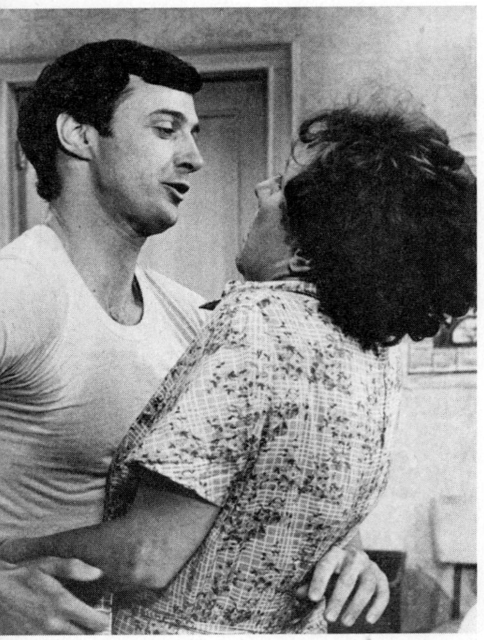

Public awareness of rape and its accompanying trauma has been raised in media depiction. An early appearance of a true-to-life rape situation appeared in the sitcom *All in the Family.* During the episode, which was written and developed by rape counselors, Edith Bunker is raped in her own home. The show, plus the publicity it created, helped many real-world victims to step forward.

attitudes as a function of ethnicity and sex. Asians and males were more likely to report negative feelings toward rape victims and greater acceptance of rape myths than whites and females, whereas Asians with greater degrees of acculturation to Western values endorsed responses similar to those of their white counterparts (Mori, et al., 1995).

Apparently, steps need to be taken to reduce the cultural acceptance of violence and to restructure male and female sex roles to specify equality, warmth, and supportiveness. In the past, male dominance, toughness, and violence have often been emphasized. A restructuring of the relationships between genders might reduce the high incidence of rape in American society. Steps to reduce your personal risk of rape are found in Table 16.1.

The Rapist

The topics of rape and rapists are hot issues in American society. Some theorists argue that rape is an act of uncontrolled passion or the result of a lack of sexual partners; others feel that it is an extreme expression of male power and violence. For others, rape is a biologically driven phenomenon whereby men forcefully try to maximize the number of women with whom they procreate (Laumann, et al., 1994).

Most rapists rape to be aggressive, to wield their power, or to degrade the victim. In most instances their motivations and satisfactions are not sex-

TABLE 16.1 How to Lessen Your Chances of Being Raped

It is impossible to act in a way that will guarantee that you will never be raped; however, you can easily develop some habits that will lessen the chances.

At Home

1. When you are returning home, have your key ready and enter immediately.
2. Be sure that doors, door frames, window frames, locks, and hinges are secure.
3. Keep valuables out of sight—outside your house (perhaps stored at a bank) if possible.
4. Have good lighting in all interior and exterior areas.

On the Street

1. Be aware of your surroundings.
2. Be alert to suspicious or unusual movements.
3. Walk in well-lighted places, avoid deserted areas, and do not take shortcuts through dark areas.
4. Walk on the left side of the street, facing traffic, so you can see oncoming cars.
5. Never hitchhike.

Personal Precautions

1. Keep doors and windows locked.
2. In the telephone directory, list only your last name and initials.
3. Be cautious how you handle telephone calls; for example, never let a stranger know you are home alone.
4. Never let an unknown person enter your residence without proper identification unless absolutely necessary.
5. Have an emergency plan in mind, just in case.

Source: Bruess, C. & Richardson, G. *Decisions for health.* Madison, WI: Brown & Benchmark, 1995.

ual. In fact, it is unlikely that they achieve any sexual satisfaction from the act of rape. Many theorists have developed typologies of rapists, some suggesting as few as two or three basic types. Others suggest five or six. Every one of these typologies is flawed by its failure to account for the fact that people who rape strangers may be very different from those who rape their wife or their date (Russell, 1984).

After extensively reviewing rape studies, Knight, Rosenberg, and Schneider (1985) found a great deal of consistency in the reasons people commit rape. They identified four well-distinguished groupings to explain why rape occurs: (1) Aggression serves to enhance the offender's sense of power, masculinity, or self-esteem or enables him to express feelings of mastery and conquest; (2) the rapist has anger toward women and wants to hurt, humiliate, or degrade the victim; (3) sadistic rapists may be sexually aroused in response to violence and the very brutal nature of the assault; and (4) for some rapists sexual offenses may be only one component of an impulsive, antisocial lifestyle and an extensive criminal history. It is common to hear patterns of rape labeled as anger, power, sadistic, gang, assaultive, explosive, psychotic, or sociopathic. Regardless of the particular label, this typology covers most rapes.

Since the mid-1970s, the motivation for rape has usually been explained in terms of hostility and power rather than sexual satisfaction. There are three major outcomes of rape: sexual intercourse, domination of the victim, and harm to the victim. Felson and Krohn (1990) have suggested that the motives might vary with the situation. For example, in rapes involving estranged couples or older offenders and victims, it appeared that rape and physical attacks during rape were more likely to be used to punish the victim. However, for rapes involving younger offenders and victims, it appeared that rape was more likely to be sexually motivated.

Although the exact reasons for rape are hard to pinpoint, there are consistent differences between rapists and nonrapists in certain psychological dimensions. Several different measures of hostility toward women and dominance motives, as well as factors that may underlie these characteristics, have successfully differentiated sexually aggressive from nonaggressive college men (Lisak, 1991).

Characteristics of rapists are viewed in other ways as well. For example, sexually aggressive behavior has been associated with the beliefs that sexual aggression is normal and that relationships contain a large element of game playing, with a conservative attitude toward female sexuality, and with an acceptance of rape myths as accurate (Koss & Leonard, 1984). The most important factor distinguishing sexually aggressive males from other males seemed to be the presence of sexually aggressive friends. This factor contributed to attitudes that legitimized sexual aggression against women (Alder, 1985). Rapists also seemed to be underassertive, to have low levels of self-esteem, to possess high levels of anxiety in social-sexual interactions, and to

Did You Know . . .

Given the current emphasis on controlling violence and respecting all people, it is interesting that an activity called "whirling" has appeared. In one instance, 13 women attending a large gathering of fraternity and sorority members reported that they were sexually assaulted by crowds of men who ripped off their clothes and molested them (Thirteen women report sexual assaults at national fraternity gathering, 1998).

express puritanical and negative attitudes toward sexuality (Baxter, et al., 1984). In addition, a majority of rapists had been sexually molested (Petrovich & Templer, 1984).

Psychological studies show, however, that rapists have varying psychological profiles. For example, some have difficulties with impulse control and tend to commit their offense during the course of another crime. Others, who typically have low self-esteem and desirability scores, tend to use restraining and control techniques during sexual encounters. Still others, who are very angry people, are more likely to want to inflict harm or degradation on others (Kalichman, 1990).

It is also common to find that rapists give excuses for their behavior. Those who denied that what they did was rape justified their actions; those who admitted it was rape attempted to excuse it or themselves. Those who admitted committing rape, although believing that rape was wrong, explained the act by appealing to forces beyond their control. Common excuses focused on alcohol/drug intoxication and emotional problems. In this way their serious mistake did not represent their "true" self. In contrast, deniers explained their behavior as appropriate in the situation. Commonly, rapists viewed men as sexually masterful and women as coy but seductive or viewed the victim as the type of woman who "got what she deserved." These explanations are related to the myths that women both enjoy and are responsible for rape (Scully & Marolla, 1984).

Some people mistakenly feel that rape is increasingly an interracial crime and even that African-American rapists seek out white victims. However, by far, in most instances of rape the rapist and the victim are of the same race. In addition, the proportion of African-American offenders who victimize whites has actually been decreasing (Koch, 1995).

High-profile cases involving athletes and sexual assault have raised questions. Some people think that athletes may be more prone to commit rape than nonathletes. In general, however, there is no significant difference between athletes and nonathletes in aggressive sexual behavior (Caron, Halteman, & Stacy, 1997).

Myth vs Fact

Myth: Rape is an impulsive act of passion—meaning that men cannot control their sex drive.
Fact: Rapists themselves do not see rape as compulsive sexual behavior. The objective for rape is not usually sexual pleasure; it is to have power and to commit violence. Sexual activity is used to carry out nonsexual needs.

Myth: Women want to be raped—meaning that women have fantasies that reflect their desire to be raped.
Fact: Rape is an act of violent aggression. No healthy individual desires to be dehumanized and violated.

Myth: Women ask to be raped—meaning they tempt the man. "She should have worn a bra," "Hitchhikers get what they deserve," and "She shouldn't have been out so late at night" are examples of this thinking.
Fact: The blame and responsibility for a criminal assault are the assailant's, not the victim's.

Myth: A woman can run faster with her skirt up than a man can with his pants down—meaning a woman cannot be raped against her will.
Fact: Rape is an aggression committed under force or the threat of force on an unconsenting person. A knife, gun, or even verbal threat is often understandably stronger than a person's will.

Myth: You cannot blame a man for trying—meaning the responsibility for stopping a man is the woman's; therefore, it is her fault if matters get out of hand.
Fact: A criminal, not a victim, is responsible for criminal acts. Rape is not an impulsive act of passion. It is done for power and control.

Date Rape

Date rape, or acquaintance rape, is much more common than most people realize, although because of its nature gathering reliable data on this topic is difficult. It is suspected that some incidents of date rape might be a result of poor communication, because many people still have a difficult time talking about sexuality. At any rate, it might help those dating to realize the following: Spending money on a date does not justify expecting sexual favors; a person who participates in other forms of sexual behavior does not necessarily find intercourse acceptable; and if a date uses sexual behavior as a means of proving masculinity or femininity, it might be better to date other people.

Unfortunately, forced sexual contact has always happened between dating partners. Women often blamed themselves for "leading a date on." It was not until the mid-1970s that the term *date rape* was coined and women had legal rights to go after assailants they had dated. Barry Burkhart has studied the topic since 1975. After conducting a number of studies, he concluded the following (Date rape is occurring too often, 1987):

1. Twenty-five percent of women say they have had coerced intercourse, but only 15% of episodes meet the legal definition of rape.
2. Only 29% of men denied any form of sexually aggressive behavior, and 15% had intercourse against the woman's will—though none described it as rape.

3. Sixty-one percent of the men admitted they had fondled a woman against her will, 42% had removed clothing, and 37% had touched a woman's genitals against her will.
4. Thirty-five percent of men had ignored a woman's protest, 11% had used physical restraint, 6% had used threats, and 3% had used physical violence to coerce sexual contact.
5. Fifty percent of the men admitted to forced sexual activity.

Burkhart reported that the men who admitted to forced sexual activity could not be characterized as "sick people." Most were ordinary, not deranged perverts, and were doing what they thought they were supposed to be doing. Most offenders were very active in heterosexual relationships but saw women as objects of sexual pleasure. The average profile of the men involved in date rape showed they were irresponsible, self-centered, lacking in social skills, and emotionally immature. The victims were likely to blame themselves for their victimization and did not view their treatment as strange or unusual. This would probably not be true today.

Date rapists were probably socialized in a way that resulted in an exaggerated sexual impulse and that placed an inordinately high value on sexual accomplishment. Female victims might have rejected coital intimacy for a variety of reasons that date rapists failed to recognize, instead focusing on whether her rejection was genuine and on whether his sexual powers were adequate. A very high aspiration level resulted in sexual frustration, which seemed to lead to date rape (Kanin, 1985).

Perhaps this social problem is compounded by the fact that, although both genders perceive sexuality as important, males report perceiving a world in which sexuality is a more pervasive and salient fact of life than it is in reports of females. Adolescents viewed sexual aggression by a man against a woman as an ever-present and sometimes acceptable possibility (Goodchilds & Zellman, 1984).

As mentioned, male and female perceptions of unwanted sexual experiences are often very different. College women report that such experiences are common; college men report they are rare (Ward, et al., 1991). Relatedly, Laumann and associates (1994) reported that 22% of all women indicated they had been forced sexually by a man. Only 2.8% of the men indicated that they had ever forced a woman sexually. Is it possible that this 2.8% of the men are doing all the forcing? Of course not. We do not know why these differences might exist.

In a study designed to assess rape and sexual force inclinations among college men, some inclination to rape or force sexual activity was reported by 34% of the respondents. Respondents who reported both inclinations indicated higher rape myth acceptance, offered more justifications for the increasing use of violence against women, were lower in rape empathy, held more gender-stereotyped attitudes toward women, and accepted interpersonal violence more than those who reported no inclinations (Osland, Fitch, & Willis, 1996).

Interestingly, females may be less sympathetic than males to victims of acquaintance rape. This is because females might feel more vulnerable if they are sympathetic, whereas they will feel more secure if they see the attack on the other female more as her fault (A crime between friends, 1990).

Although date rape has gained increased attention, no one has accurate statistics on the magnitude of the problem. Available statistics can even be misleading. For example, at one midwestern university the campus police listed 11 rapes for the entire year. However, the campus clinic had, on the average, 16 female rape victims seeking medical attention each weekend evening (Harvard establishes "date rape" prevention program, 1986).

Myth vs Fact

Myth: If a woman is going to be raped, she might as well relax and enjoy it—meaning it is just sexual activity.
Fact: Rape victims experience intense psychological and physical trauma. Rape is a violent, dehumanizing, and intimate invasion of a woman's privacy and integrity as a human being. The motive for rape is power; it is not sexual enjoyment. Rape is anything but enjoyable!

Myth: The rapist is usually of a different race from the victim—meaning rape usually reflects ethnic or racial hatred.
Fact: In most instances the rapist and the victim are of the same race (estimates indicate this is true in as many as 90–95% of the cases).

Myth: Most rapes are committed by strangers—meaning we are safe with people we know.
Fact: It is common for the rapist and the victim to know each other, to have been acquainted, or at least to have seen each other on the street, in the grocery store, in the student union, and so on.

More than 80% of the rapes on college campuses are committed by someone with whom the victim is acquainted; about 50% are committed on dates (and heavy drinking of alcohol and acquaintance rape often go together) (Abbey, 1991). Although women are fearful of walking alone on campus at night, the most common sexual assault is not the "stereotypical" rape attack but instead one that occurs as a part of the "normal" social environment on the campus (Ward, et al., 1991).

As many as one in four college women has had some experience with acquaintance rape. It can be even more traumatic than stranger rape because of circumstances that might make people very unlikely to believe the victim (A crime between friends, 1990).

Forced sexual behaviors are also a problem among high school students. Twenty-six percent of students in grades 8–12 have reported being forced into some type of sexual activity. The type of force used on dates included verbal threats, physical violence, and intimidation; persistence topped the list (Rhynard, Krebs, & Glover, 1997).

The prevalence of and risk factors associated with unwanted sexual activity by dates or boyfriends were studied over a 4-year period in a sample of young rural adolescent girls. Twenty-three percent reported such experiences with dates or boyfriends by the fourth year of the study, including forced touching, intercourse, oral sex, and/or other sexual behaviors. Fifteen percent had experienced date rape. Significant predictors of unwanted sexual activity included earlier age of menarche, earlier age of initiation of sexual activity, sexually active same-sex friends, poorer peer relationships, and poorer emotional status (Vicary, Klingaman, & Harkness, 1995).

Many women who are date raped do not report the rape to authorities because of feelings of self-blame and embarrassment. That rapes are not reported perpetuates the belief that rape is uncommon. Also, a victim of rape may feel she is the only one and may be reluctant to become the exception who reports (Finkelson & Oswalt, 1995).

In 2001 several studies related to dating violence were reported. The U.S. Department of Justice released interesting information about the prevalence and nature of sexual assault at American colleges (Fisher, et al., 2001). According to their information, about 3% of college women experience a completed and/or attempted rape during a typical college year. About 13% had been stalked during the previous college year. Of the incidents of sexual victimization, the vast majority occurred after 6 P.M. in living quarters. Nearly 60% of completed rapes that took place on campus occurred in the survivor's residence, 31% occurred in other living quarters on campus, and 10% occurred at a fraternity house. Most off-campus incidents, especially rapes, also occurred in residences. Nearly 90% of the women knew the offender, who was usually a classmate, friend, ex-boyfriend, or acquaintance. About 20% of the incidents resulted in additional injury. In about half of the incidents categorized as completed rapes, the women did not consider the incident a rape.

Halpern and colleagues (2001) reported that in heterosexual romantic relationships one-third of adolescents reported some type of sexual victimization. Twelve percent reported physical violence victimization.

Gordon (2001) reported that one in five teen girls is physically or sexually abused by someone she is dating. The incidence of violence extended across all racial groups. Girls who experienced physical dating violence had a higher risk of substance abuse, including heavy smoking, binge drinking, cocaine use, and unhealthy weight control; intercourse before age 15 years; nonuse of a condom during intercourse; and experience of three or more sexual partners within the preceding 3 months. They were also more likely to become pregnant during their teenage years and to have thoughts of suicide or attempt suicide.

According to a survey of more than 80,000 9th- and 12th-grade boys and girls in Minnesota, nearly 1 in 10 girls and 1 in 20 boys experienced violence and/or rape on a date (One out of ten female adolescents, 2001). Those who experienced violence and rape also reported higher rates of disordered eating, suicidal thoughts and attempts, and lower scores on measures of emotional well-being and self-esteem.

Ways to Help Prevent Acquaintance Rape

Because of the magnitude of date rape, many steps have been taken to help deal with and reduce the problem. Awareness is the first step, and materials have been developed to help college students understand date rape and how to prevent it. The American College Health Association (2002) has developed a pamphlet about acquaintance rape titled *Acquaintance Rape: What Everyone Should Know,* which contains suggestions for both men and women.

For example, the pamphlet indicates that alcohol and other drugs can inhibit clear thinking, make talking and listening more difficult, and make it harder to assess risk. Consenting sexual activity doesn't just happen. It requires sober, verbal communication without intimidation or threats. Many states' laws recognize that someone must be sober to give true consent. Also, being drunk or high is never an excuse for raping someone.

The pamphlet also has a section titled "What You Can Do," which indicates that you can think about how to respond to social pressures and ask yourself:

- What role does sex play in my life?
- What role do I want it to play?
- How does alcohol affect my sexual decision making?
- How do I learn someone's desires and limits?
- How do I express my own?

Another section of the pamphlet relates to challenging myths and stereotypes. It suggests that you challenge your friends who belittle rape or who accept definitions of sex and gender roles that allow forcing someone to participate in sexual activity. It suggests talking with your friends and giving one another the opportunity to be assertive, respectful, honest, and caring.

Finally, the pamphlet emphasizes the need to communicate effectively. It suggests trusting your instincts and telling your partner what you want or don't want, listening carefully to what the other person is saying, asking rather than assuming, and remembering that effective and assertive communication may not always work. Sometimes people simply don't listen. However, no one ever *deserves* to be raped!

Harvard University has developed a program to help students prevent date rape and to address issues of peer harassment. The program, initiated by the administration and strongly supported by students, enables students to communicate more clearly about sexual issues. In addition to the general informational components of the program, all incoming freshmen are exposed to information and counseling in an attempt to prevent date rape (Harvard establishes "date rape" prevention program, 1986). The Antioch College policy requiring verbal consent to sexual behavior is shown in Table 16.2.

TABLE 16.2 The Antioch College Policy Requiring Verbal Consent for Each Level of Sexual Behavior

As part of community governance, Antioch College students developed a policy requiring students to obtain verbal consent for each level of sexual behavior. It has been the subject of many articles in which varying opinions have been expressed. Here are the 10 reasons given to obtain verbal approval for sexual activities:

1. Because many partners find it sexy to be asked, as sexual behavior progresses, if it's okay.
2. Because sexual activity is better when each partner enjoys what is happening and no one is being forced to do something he or she doesn't want to do.
3. Because if your partner is having a good time and is not forced to do something against his or her will, he or she may be more likely to want to see you again. Mutual respect is the best basis for friendship and intimacy.
4. Because forcing sexual activity on another person can violate state and federal laws and your school's policy. In most instances, unwanted touching and fondling is sexual assault.
5. Because it prevents misunderstandings (silence is not a "yes").
6. Because you won't be accused of rape.
7. Because you won't go to jail or be expelled.
8. Because it's better to be safe than sorry.
9. Because if you want to impose your sexual will on someone, your behavior has more to do with dominating the person than with enjoying sexuality and an intimate relationship.
10. Why would you want to have sexual behavior with someone who doesn't like what you are doing?

Source: Antioch College. Ten reasons to obtain a verbal consent for sex, *About women on campus, 2* (winter 1994).

Situational Model of Sexual Coercion

One way to comprehend better and perhaps reduce the problem of date rape is to understand a situational model of sexual coercion (Snyder & Ickes, 1985) (Figure 16.1). The model includes individual personality characteristics, situational components, cognitive processes, and behavioral effects of participants in a social situation (Craig, 1990). In other words, people introduce certain traits or dispositions to a dating situation, but they also use manipulation to express their dispositions.

In the first step of the model, the dispositions and history of the male lead him to select situations in which he can act in a particular way. Relatedly, there seems to be a common set of characteristics that distinguish between sexually coercive and noncoercive men (Craig, 1990). Coercive males tend to be more aggressive, to believe that relationships with women are basically adversarial, and to support rape myths and sex-role stereotypes. Peer approval also seems important, and sexual behavior is emphasized as a status symbol.

In the second step of the model, coercive males use selective exposure to choose situations that are likely to match their dispositions and characteristics. They tend to select certain types of women, dating situations, and relationships. For example, although there is not total agreement among researchers, it seems that women who are selected as victims by coercive males are more sexually experienced, more sexually passive, and less likely to use methods of avoidance such as running away or screaming.

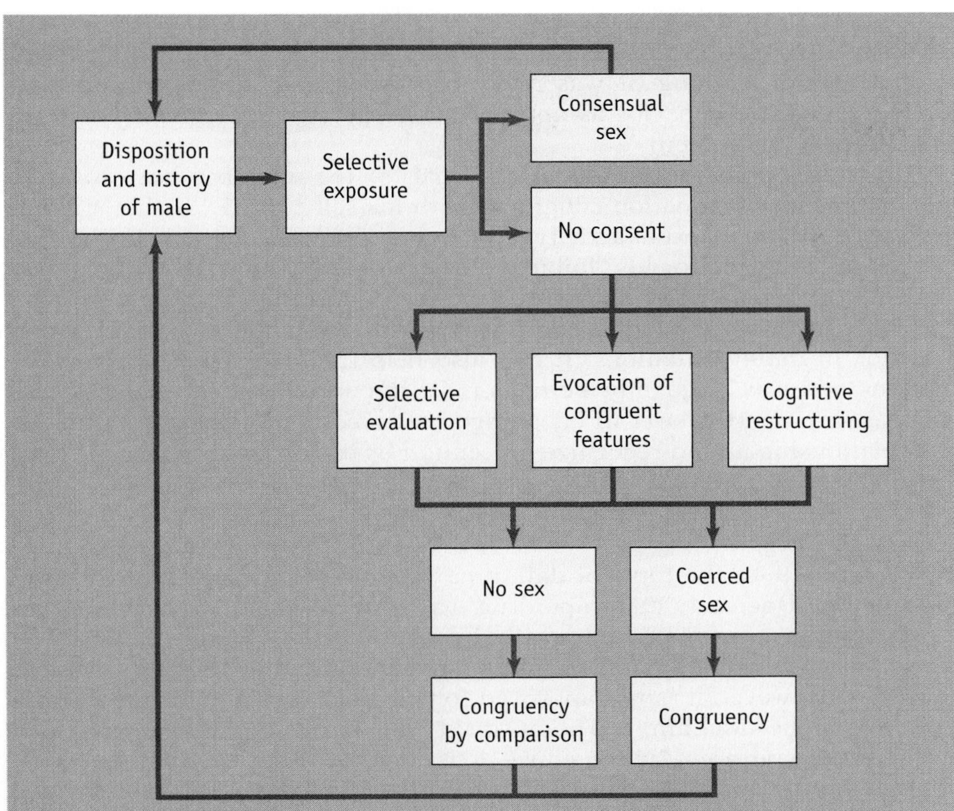

FIGURE 16.1 The situational model of coercive sexual behavior.

Regarding the dating situation, sexual coercion seems more likely to occur when the male initiated the date, paid expenses, and drove; when there was miscommunication about sexual behavior; when an isolated location was used; when there was some consensual sexual contact; and when both persons were moderately or extremely intoxicated. In terms of the dating relationship, coercion seems more likely when there is an established relationship between the partners. Also, sexual violence seems more likely when there are differences between partners in age, intelligence, and social status.

Precollege sexual victimization is also positively correlated with college victimization. In other words, women who have been sexually victimized in earlier years are the ones most likely to be sexually victimized again. However, sexual conservatism is negatively correlated with college victimization (Himelein, 1995). In addition, there is still a strong association between the amount of alcohol women drink each week and their overall experience with sexual coercion (Gross & Billingham, 1998).

If the factors suggested do not result in consensual sexual activity, there are additional components of the model. Through selective evaluation the male may place major importance on situational aspects that he believes encourage him to make sexual advances. For example, the female's friendliness, appearance, or behavior might cause a male's misperception of the situation.

Even after setting up a situation that increases his likelihood of engaging in sexual activity—and paying attention only to the cues that would seem to encourage sexual advances—the coercive male may still encounter resistance. He may then try to lower the woman's resistance by using alcohol or drugs or by making false statements or promises.

Cognitive restructuring is changing one's interpretations to better fit one's self-image. In relation to coercive sexual behavior, this could include use of alcohol, victim blaming (it was really her fault), and rationalization (perceiving aggressive behavior as appropriate or perceiving aggressive actions as acceptable to women).

Up to this point in the model, the goal for the male has been to make the features of the situation congruent with his self-concept. If that still has not happened, or if sexual activity still has not occurred, he may feel a need to externalize blame for his "failure." For example, he may indicate she was just cold or that they did not really have the opportunity.

The situational model can be helpful to understanding coercive sexual behavior in dating situations. It can also help us understand why misperceptions occur so frequently. Perhaps most importantly, it can be used in a positive way—particularly to encourage better communication at all levels of a relationship and to recognize prevention or promotion of behaviors that help prevent coercion.

date-rape drugs
Sedative hypnotic drugs used to incapacitate victims who are then sexually molested or raped.

Date-Rape Drugs

In the early 1990s the topic of date rape was further complicated by **date-rape drugs.** One early date-rape drug was flunitrazepam (Rohypnol). It is a prescription drug marketed legally in 60 countries around the world. It is used as a sedative hypnotic and as a preanesthetic medication in those countries. However, it is not approved for medical use in the United States (Lyman, Hughes-McLain, & Thompson, 1998). Because of its sedative hypnotic action and amnesialike effect, it is ideal for use in date-rape situations. It can be administered without consent to produce disinhibition and to obtain sexual activity. It has no taste or odor when mixed with alcohol. People drugged with Rohypnol may remember nothing about what happened or have only a very sketchy memory. They are often unsure that they have been raped, except that they may wake the next morning feeling genital discomfort or finding themselves undressed. Assailants typically claim the victims consented to sexual activity, and there is no way to know for sure. The time required for Rohypnol to reach its peak blood level is 1 hour, but it can be identified in the urine for 4 to 30 days after ingestion (Ledray, 1996).

Another date-rape drug is gammahydroxybutyrate (GHB). It can be used by sexual predators to render their victims almost instantly helpless and to leave them with little or no memory of the attack. It is similar to the drug Rohypnol. GHB has no approved medical use, and it can cause depression, seizures, coma, and death. Kits can be purchased to make the drug at home for less than $100. Many argue that GHB should be an illegal substance (Pryor warns of strong drug used by sex predators, 1998).

A third drug being used as a date-rape drug is ketamine hydrochloride. It is commercially referred to as Ketaject or Ketalar. It is used medically as an anesthetic for diagnostic and surgical purposes. It produces anesthesia within 40 seconds of intravenous administration and within 8 minutes of intramuscular administration. It is currently widely used by veterinarians. In the United States the popular method of use involves heating of the liquid until it turns into a white powder, which is then smoked or snorted. Full effects of ketamine occur in about 5 to 10 minutes and last up to 1 hour (Lyman, Hughes-McLain, & Thompson, 1998).

In 1996 President Clinton signed a bill outlawing Rohypnol and other date-rape drugs and adding 20 years to the sentence of a rapist who uses these drugs on a victim. The law also included increased penalties for illegal manufacturing, distribution, dispensing, or possession of the drugs. It was the first time that using a drug as a weapon was classified as a crime in the United States.

Here are some things you can do to reduce the possibility of being a victim of a date-rape drug (Lyman, Hughes-McLain, & Thompson, 1998):

1. Be extra cautious on dates until you feel convinced of your companion's integrity.
2. Buy your own drinks or be present when the drinks are delivered.
3. Never leave a drink unattended.
4. Do not trust a date more than someone else you have known for the same length of time.
5. At parties, do not drink from community punch or drink bowls.

The Incidence of Rape

Because many cases are not reported, statistics on rape leave a lot to be desired. Estimating rates of violence, especially of sexual assault and other incidents committed by intimate offenders, continues to be a difficult task. Many factors inhibit women from reporting these crimes. The private nature of the event, the perceived stigma, and the belief that no purpose would be served by reporting the crime prevent an unknown portion of the victims from talking about the attack.

The U.S. Department of Justice (Sex offenses and offenders, 1998) indicates that each year there are about 500,000 rapes or other sexual assaults. About 32% of these are reported to a law enforcement agency. About 60% of these incidents occur in the victim's home or at the home of a friend, relative, or neighbor. In addition, an estimated 91% of the victims are female, and 99% of the offenders are male. Seventy-five percent of the assaults involve offenders with whom the victim had a prior relationship—a family member, intimate, or acquaintance. There is about one rape or sexual assault victimization of a female for every 270 females in the general population; for males, the rate is substantially lower, with about one for every 5,000 males age 12 years or older.

There has been substantial variation in the number of reported forcible rapes per 100,000 females through the years. For example, in 1976 there were 52 per 100,000. The rate tended to increase until reaching its peak of 84 per 100,000 in 1992. The rate decreased to about 72 per 100,000 by 1998. The number of reported rapes continued to decline for several years (−2.2% in 1997, −5.1% in 1998, and −8.4% in 1999). Then, it increased slightly (0.7%) in 2000 (U.S. Department of Justice, 2001). The number of reported rapes increased by 4 percent when 2002 was compared with 2001. Many experts feel that the numbers may not actually be increasing, but women may just be more willing to report rapes because of the attention given to sexual assault in the news (Salant, 2003). About 80% of rape victims are younger than 30 years old, and about half of those are younger than 18 years old. Victims younger than 12 years account for 15% of those raped, and another 29% of rape victims are between 12 and 17 years.

The *Uniform Crime Reports* of the Federal Bureau of Investigation (1996) indicate that one forcible rape occurs every 6 minutes in the United States. The lowest number of rapes occurs in December, and the highest number occurs in July. Rape victims are about evenly divided among whites and African-Americans, and about 88% of the time the victim and the offender are of the same race (U.S. Department of Justice, 1998).

At least 12.1 million adult women have been victims of at least one forcible rape during their lifetime. Rape seems to be a "crime of youth" because 61% of rapes occur before the victim is 18 years old, and 29% occur before the victim is 11 years old (Schafran, 1996). Seventy-four percent of girls younger than 14 years old who have had sexual relations are the victims of rape (di Mauro, 1995).

In 2003 additional statistics about rape were provided by the Rape Abuse and Incest National Network (RAINN statistics, 2003). For example, 1 out of 6 American women are the survivors of an attempted or completed rape in their lifetime, 9 out of every 10 rape survivors are female, and 2.78 million men have experienced an attempted or completed rape. In addition, 82.5% of rape survivors are white, 13.3% are black, and 4.2% are of other races. Only about 1 in 3 rapes and sexual assaults are reported to law enforcement officials.

It is interesting to consider junior high school students' perceptions of nonconsensual sexual behavior. Three hundred and seventy-one suburban and urban students in northwest Ohio completed a survey designed to assess their attitudes and perceptions. Thirty-five percent reported they had engaged in sexual intercourse; 17% reported having been sexually coerced by a teenager; 19% reported feeling pressure from their friends to have intercourse; 7% reported having been sexually coerced by an adult; and 6% reported having sexually coerced someone else. Students also demonstrated

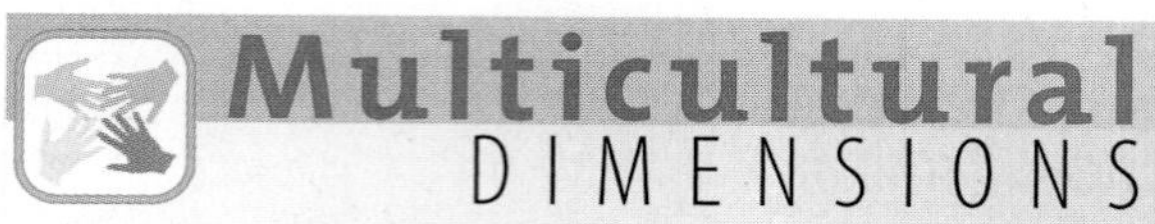

Coercive Sexual Experiences

As part of the National Health and Social Life Survey, Laumann and associates (1994) asked about coercive sexual experiences. Because of the broad nature of the question, reported incidents may not all be rape, but there are still some interesting statistics. For example, 2.8% of the men reported forcing a woman sexually, and 1.5% of the women reported forcing a man sexually. However, 1.3% of the men reported being forced by another man, and 22% of the women reported being forced by a man.

Coerced sexual activity seems to decline as people grow older. There is not a notable difference in the rate by education level. For example, 26% of women with less than a high school education reported having been coerced compared to 23% of women with a master's or advanced degree.

It is interesting to note that 31% of women with no religious affiliation reported having been coerced sexually as compared to 17% of Catholic women. This compares to an average of 23% for Protestant women.

The researchers felt that the most intriguing and unexpected pattern may be the very low rate of sexual coercion (16%) reported by women living in central cities and the relatively high rate (25%) for those living in noncity urban areas. This is not consistent with the perception of the risk of sexual assault in big cities. However, a vast majority of coerced sexual activity occurs with someone well known to the respondent, not with someone unknown, the more typical circumstance thought to predominate in large cities.

Finally, 22% of the women considered themselves to have been forced against their will to do something sexually. Asian and Hispanic women reported notably lower rates than white women, and African-American women reported rates between those extremes. By race and ethnicity, the proportions who were forced were

White = 23%
African American = 19%
Hispanic = 14%
Asian = 17%

Except for offering observations about incidents in cities versus rural areas, the researchers did not provide possible explanations for the other observed differences in coercive sexual activity. We can only speculate about the reasons for the differences related to age, educational level, religious background, and race and ethnicity.

a lack of knowledge of nonconsensual sexual behaviors (Jordan, et al., 1998).

Of all the factors that influence a victim's decision to report a rape, the relationship between the victim and the rapist is the most important. Women raped by men they know are less likely to make a report because they question their role and responsibility in the attack, whereas women in a classic rape (attacked by a stranger) have the evidence needed to convince both themselves and others that they were true rape victims (Williams, 1984). In addition, it is more likely that a rape will be reported if the offender did not have a right to be present where the assault occurred, if serious injury resulted from the assault, and if the victim is married (Lizotte, 1985). Victims of group sexual assault are also more likely than victims of individual sexual assault to seek police and crisis services (Gidycz & Koss, 1990).

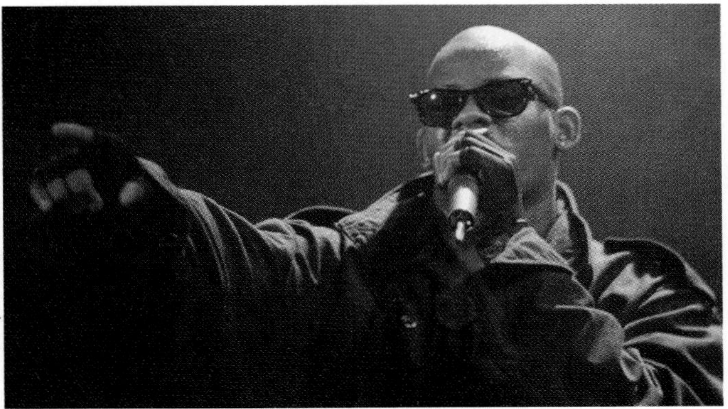

While Paul Reubens' career never quite recovered after the highly publicized charges of indecent exposure and child pornography, the same was not true for rap and R & B superstar R. Kelly, who was charged with 21 counts of child pornography stemming from a videotape that allegedly shows him having sexual activity with a 13-year-old girl. Kelly's CD in 2003 debuted at number one and the first single from the album, "Ignition," peaked at number two on the Billboard's singles chart and enjoyed consistent radio and television play, all while he faced serious charges of a sexual encounter with a minor. Does this send the message that the rap and R & B community condones such behavior?

Not only is it difficult to obtain accurate statistics about rape for reasons already mentioned, but false rape reports make it even more difficult to know for sure what is happening. For example, one study (Kanin, 1994) showed that 41% of the total reported forcible rape cases in a small midwestern community were false rape allegations. These false rape allegations seemed to serve three major functions for the complainants: providing an alibi, seeking revenge, and obtaining sympathy and attention.

Consequences of Rape

The survivor of a rape, her friends, her family, and her husband or lover usually respond to the crime's sexual aspects, instead of the violent aspects. Rape survivors and their loved ones need the same kinds of help to get through this difficult time as survivors of other violent acts. And beyond that, they need assistance with the specific problems that follow such a personally destructive attack.

Adolescent rape survivors seem to have more subsequent behavior problems than older survivors. This is probably because the adolescent experiences an attack at the time when she is developmentally trying to maintain a steady self-concept, she is establishing an independent social role, and she is undergoing many psychological and physiological changes. Immediate reactions may include not trusting herself, turning away from friends, retreating to the protection of the family, and reducing social activities. Long-term reactions include sustained unrest, sleep disturbances, fears, and avoidance of complex activities and creative skills. In addition, the experience of being forced or pressured to have sexual intercourse is associated with externalizing behavior, such as fighting, among girls, and with internalizing behavior, such as eating disorders, among boys (Shrier, et al., 1998).

Burgess (1985) described a typical **rape trauma syndrome** and stress response of rape victims. The rape trauma syndrome consists of two phases that can disrupt the survivor's life. The acute phase can last from days to weeks and is characterized by general stress response symptoms such as increased irritability, difficulty in thinking clearly, and difficulty in sleeping. The second phase, the long-term process of reorganization, consists of the survivor's restoring order to her lifestyle and reestablishing a sense of control in the world. Common symptoms experienced during the rape trauma syndrome include imagining the event is recurring and having dreams and nightmares, a numbing of responsiveness or reduced involvement with the

rape trauma syndrome
A two-phase reaction to rape. An acute phase involves intense emotional responses for several weeks. The long-term phase may last several years and involves reorganization and establishment of control.

environment, sleep disturbances, feelings of guilt, impaired concentration, and avoidance of activities that arouse recollection.

Schafran (1996) pointed out that 3.8 million women have had rape-related posttraumatic stress disorder; an estimated 1.3 million currently have it, and each year 211,000 will develop it. In addition, rape survivors have higher rates of drug and alcohol consumption and a greater likelihood of having drug- and alcohol-related problems. They are also 3 times more likely than women who have not been raped to have a major depressive episode, 4.1 times more likely to have contemplated suicide, and 13 times more likely to have attempted suicide. These are some of the devastating and potentially life-threatening effects of rape.

Rape survivors report greater fear surrounding intimacy. They report less confidence in others' dependability, less comfort with closeness, and more fear of abandonment (Thelen, Sherman, & Borst, 1998). In addition, the self-esteem of sexually assaulted women is lower in general than that of nonassaulted women (Kulkoski & Kilian, 1997).

As part of the National Health and Social Life Survey, Laumann and associates (1994) reported a number of differences between adult women who had had forced sexual activity and those who had not. All questions related to the year just before the survey. For example, 22% of the women who had not been forced were unable to experience orgasm as compared to 33% of the women who had been forced. Thirty-one percent of the women who had not been forced lacked interest in sexual activity during the last year as compared to 41% of the women who had been forced. Eighteen percent of the women who had not been forced indicated sexual activity was not pleasurable as compared to 34% of the women who had been forced.

Adult rape survivors experience a shattering effect on personal stability and adjustment. Many do not wish to confide in another person and try to hold in their feelings. Some are hesitant to participate in their usual sexual relations. Personal feelings of privacy, dignity, and trust are undermined, and feelings of vulnerability are common. Many women feel they live in a world filled with threats. Anger, rage, shame, and fear profoundly influence the recovery of rape survivors. It is not unusual for this anger to be expressed toward men in general. Although some women suffer physical trauma from rape, requiring surgical repair of the perineum, vulva, or urethra, it is emotional scars that take longest to heal.

Adjustment difficulties might not appear for a long time—even years—after the event. To help reduce these problems, as well as the feelings of self-blame and vulnerability, survivors can participate in professional counseling. In addition, family members and significant others need to be supportive and avoid victim blaming (Wyatt & Newcomb, 1990). Emotional support from friends has been found to be even better than emotional support from other sources (Ullman, 1996).

Many survivors of sexual assault do heal and do just fine in their lives. They probably do not forget, but they do move on. There is a great deal of hope today for such survivors.

Rape of Males

Almost all the information on rape presented so far has focused on females as victims. This is appropriate because the vast majority of survivors are females. However, in recent years there has been an increased recognition that males can be victims, too. Even the rape laws in many states now recognize the existence of male rape. Generally, male rape falls into one of three categories: male rape in prison, male rape by other males outside prison, and male rape by females.

More and better research is needed to determine the true prevalence of prison rape, but it appears to be an act of heterosexuals rather than homosexuals. This may sound strange at first, but in a prison situation rape is viewed as a validation of masculinity and a violent act of conquest (Scacco, 1975). The likelihood of being raped in prison is so great that some argue that a judge who sentences a young man to reform school or prison passes a sentence of male rape on him as surely as the prison sentence (Scacco, 1982).

Even outside prison, it is probable that most rapes of males are committed by heterosexual men. This is perhaps more understandable when we consider that violence and power, rather than sexual satisfaction, are the primary motivations for rape. Statistics on the frequency of male rape are almost impossible to obtain. Perhaps this is because of the lack of research on the subject combined with the hesitation of male victims to report an attack. In addition to the reasons females hesitate to report a rape, males often feel they are supposed to be strong and "macho." To report being raped would not be consistent with this image.

There has been some increased interest in the topic of the rape of males. Perhaps this is because up to 10% of survivors of rape reporting to treatment centers in the United States are men (King, 1995). In a survey of hundreds of agencies providing support for sexual assault victims, it was found that 51% of the 336 responding agencies reported encountering male victims. A total of 3,635 male victims were seen at the agencies between 1972 and 1991. Most of them were white and heterosexual. Of the rapists, 93.7% were male, and 6.3% were female. Most of the men reported experiencing the same kinds of difficulties after the rape reported by females (Isely & Gehrenbeck-Shim, 1997).

Most rapes of males are perpetrated by heterosexual men who commonly commit rape with one or more other people (Isely & Gehrenbeck-Shim, 1997; Scarce, 1997). Violence and power are usually associated with the sexual assault of men, just as they are with assault of women. One study involving 89 male rape victims found that motivations for rape were similar whether males or females were the victims. Females, however, were slightly more likely to be injured than were males. Female victims were also more likely than male victims to resist the offender (58% versus 36%) (Felson & Krohn, 1990).

A male being raped by a female is hard for many people to imagine. This is because of traditional feelings about sexuality—particularly that all males are "at the ready" for sexual activity and that males cannot be forced into submission. Although the first attitude is open to question (often based on incorrect logic), the second relates to physiological functioning. People seem to think that a male could not respond sexually while being threatened because he could not achieve a penile erection. It has been found, however, that such emotions as anger, fright, and pain can cause a sexual response, including all the usual physiological changes (Sarrel & Masters, 1982). This, of course, can be quite upsetting to the victim because it might be interpreted as indicating willingness. Guilt and other negative feelings can occur as well. Consequently, the responses of male rape survivors are very similar to those of female rape survivors.

Social Responses to Rape

In many communities, sexual assault crisis centers, workshops dealing with prevention of sexual assault, and improved methods of helping survivors have become priorities. Shelters for survivors of assault have been provided so they have a place to receive help. In general, there is a better understanding of the problems in communities and the need for more support.

On many college campuses there are laudable attempts to deal with sexual assault. An effective program (1) defines and demystifies sexual assault, (2) offers educational programs, (3) empowers women to be assertive, (4) exposes the link between alcohol abuse and unwanted sexual behavior, (5) conducts institutional surveys, and (6) identifies a specific individual on campus to coordinate efforts and clinical services (Meilman, Riggs, & Turco, 1990). There is also greater recognition on college campuses of the need for more attention to the problem of sexual assault. Lighting and security on campuses have improved; courses in sexual assault prevention and self-defense are offered, and escort services are available so women need not be alone on campus, particularly after dark.

There have also been major changes in laws related to rape in the past few decades. Many of the newer rape laws (1) establish "degrees" of rape to describe types of sexual assault more accurately; (2) are gender-neutral and do not apply only to attacks by men on women; (3) eliminate requirements that victims prove they resisted by "fighting back" and that corroborating evidence be presented; (4) shield victims from inquiries into past sexual experience; and (5) allow a husband to be charged with raping his wife. In fact, in many states the term *forced sex* or *sexual assault* has replaced the word *rape.* The convicted rapist can often be sentenced to life in prison.

Changes have also been made in relation to law enforcement personnel. Training has been designed to help them become more sensitive to the problem of sexual assault. More female officers are used, and there is improved cooperation between law enforcement personnel and medical and support personnel. Guidelines for handling survivors of sexual assault have also been established.

Overall, there is some good news. The rape rate appears to have declined since the 1970s; survivors seem to be more willing to report to the police; police and prosecutors are more likely to employ specialized sex crime units with expertise in the emotional as well as the legal aspects of the crime; and there is evidence that jurors have become more sympathetic to acquaintance rape victims (Bryden & Lengnick, 1987).

Women who have been assaulted have begun to fight back in civil court as well. For example, a Seattle woman was awarded $300,000 from three men who raped her and a fourth who prevented her escape; a Vermont woman received $450,000 even after a defendant was acquitted of rape charges; and a Minnesota woman received $21,500 from a physician (who had been her lover) for rape.

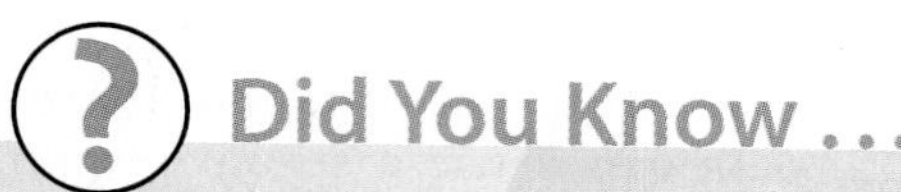

Where to Find Help

The following numbers can be helpful if you want to find out more about reporting abuse or if you want more information about abuse:

Child abuse: (800) 4-A-CHILD (422-4453)

Elder abuse: (800) 677-1116

Sexual assault: (800) 656-4673

Domestic violence: (800) 799-7233

Source: Where to find help. InteliHealth, The Harvard Medical School (2001). Available: http://intelihealth.com.

Ethical DIMENSIONS

Should the Media Reveal the Names of Rape Survivors?

The names of rape survivors traditionally have been withheld by the news media to "protect" them. Does this special treatment do rape survivors a disservice by separating them from other survivors of violent crimes? Should the privacy of rape survivors be protected more than the privacy of survivors of other violent crimes? This issue has often been debated, and it arose again in August 2002 when two California teenagers were kidnapped. Their names and pictures were widely distributed to help locate them. When, after their rescue, a sheriff said they had been raped during the abduction, "What should be done now?" asked many journalists. Some media representatives stuck to their own rule and did not refer to the teenagers by name. Others called them by name, reasoning that their names had already been released.

Some people believe that the bright lights of publicity may harm the innocent in crimes of rape. They assert that rape survivors are unwillingly thrust into the limelight, their right to choose is once again removed, and their feeling of powerlessness is perpetuated. They argue that publicly identifying rape survivors without their consent compounds the trauma of rape and may discourage future survivors from reporting crimes.

Others point out that in most states it is legal to publish the names of rape survivors, and, in fact, their names should be published just as the names of people who are victims of other violent crimes are. They point out that it is discriminatory to publish the names of alleged assailants, but not the alleged survivors. They also indicate that not naming the survivors contributes to the perception that rape is a different type of crime and helps to perpetuate the notion that there is some blame or disgrace attached. It is also argued that special treatment by the news media inhibits society from treating rape as a violent crime.

Do you think it is ethical, and the best thing to do, for the media to give the names of rape survivors?

But even with the increased emphasis on prevention, a great deal must be done. Major priorities include more changes in legislation, law enforcement policies and practices, educational intervention, and media strategies. The codification of women's equality and rights is an important part of a strategy for preventing assault. Skills training, which includes avoidance strategies, appropriate resistance, and self-defense training, is also needed.

Pedophilia

The term **pedophilia** denotes feelings of adult sexual attraction to children. Even though physical force may not be used, an adult who performs a sexual act with a child is forcing himself or herself on a helpless minor in the eyes of the law. Pedophiliacs may expose their genitals to a child or fondle and even penetrate a child. There are countless ways a child might be molested; most often the term *child molestation* refers to pedophilia. For all practical purposes the terms are used interchangeably.

pedophilia
Sexual behavior in which a child is the sexual object.

The Pedophiliac

According to the American Psychiatric Association (1998) the symptoms of pedophilia include, over a period of at least six months, intense sexually arousing fantasies, sexual urges, or behaviors involving sexual activity with a prepubescent child or children (usually age 13 years or younger). The fantasies, sexual urges, or behaviors cause significant distress or impairment in social, occupational, or other important areas of functioning.

A man or a woman can be a pedophiliac, but most commonly we hear about males' being the offenders. Unlike other men, child molesters associate sexual feelings with frustration, tension, and a sense of maladjustment and deviance. Many child molesters are narcissistic or egocentric and emotionally immature people. They tend to perceive social reality differently than do other men, and they tend to view women as big, powerful, and frightening. The child molester's apparent fear of women, his emotional immaturity, and his preoccupation with sexual activity apparently make him turn to children for sexual gratification (Johnston, 1987).

It is thought that about only 2% of child molesters are women. It is likely, however, that because of the traditional caregiving role of the female, the true incidence of female sexual contact with children is underreported. Women who molest children have a history of sexual assault as a child, tend to show severe character disorder, and are likely to be of limited intelligence (Rowan, Rowan, & Langelier, 1990).

Pedophiles report being sexually abused as children significantly more often than other people do (Freund, Watson, & Dickey, 1990). As a group, they are less prone than other sexual offenders to use drugs or alcohol. They often report being sickly as children and having chronic illnesses. They describe themselves in terms of being shy and introverted (Ames & Houston, 1990). The ratio of heterosexual to homosexual pedophiles is about 11:1 (Freund & Watson, 1992).

Incidence of Pedophilia

As with some other sexual offenses, it is difficult to know for sure how often **child sexual abuse** occurs. Even with limitations to this kind of information, it is important to consider a few studies to have a general idea about the prevalence of this problem.

child sexual abuse
Any sexual abuse involving fondling, erotic kissing, oral sexual activity, or genital penetration between an adult and a child, including pedophilia and incest.

As part of the National Health and Social Life Survey (Laumann, et al., 1994), it was found that about 12% of the men and 17% of the women had been sexually touched when they were children. The experience was reported equally by people of different ages, suggesting that there has not been an increase in rates in recent years. The females were primarily touched by men, and the males were touched more often by women but also by men. Touching genitals was by far the most common behavior for both genders. The majority of the sample reported an experience with only one adult, but about one in three reported events that occurred with more than one person.

In the survey, family friends and relatives were the primary offenders. About 34% of respondents reported they were touched one time, 38% a few times, and 27% many times. As might be expected, only 22% told someone about this sexual contact with an older person. Those who had had early childhood sexual experiences were consistently more sexually active in adulthood than those who had not had such experiences.

The most vulnerable age for sexual abuse is between 7 and 13 years. It happens to children in both rural and urban areas, in all socioeconomic and educational levels, and across all racial and cultural groups. Another study reported victimization rates of 27% of females and 16% of males (Child sexual abuse, 1998). Compare that to rates in other countries in Table 16.3.

According to the National Clearinghouse on Child Abuse and Neglect Information (1998), almost 1 million children are victims of child abuse each year. Twelve percent of these (120,000) suffer sexual abuse.

One in eight male high school students has been physically or sexually abused (The health of boys, 1998). About 5% of the males report sexual abuse, whereas 13% report physical or sexual abuse. Those in families in which the mother had less than a high school education were more than twice as likely to report abuse as those in families in which the mother was a high school graduate. Asian-American and Hispanic boys reported higher rates of abuse than did whites and African Americans. Boys who reported being abused also displayed symptoms of poor mental health at a higher rate than did boys who were not abused.

Whereas females younger than 18 years make up about 25% of the U.S. female population, they account for about 20% of the total rapes reported (U.S. Department of Justice, 1998). It is estimated that about 16% of rape survivors are younger than 12 years old. About 20% of the survivors are below 12 years, 11% of survivors are 12–17 years, and 1% of those 18 years or older were raped by their father. In 90% of the rapes of children less than 12 years old, the child knew the offender.

Over two-thirds of all incidences of sexual assault reported to law enforcement agencies involved juveniles less than 18 years old at the time of the crime. Thirty-three percent of all sexual assaults involved youth aged 12 through 17 years, and 34% involved youth younger than age 12 years. The age profile of sexual assault victims varied with the nature of the crime. Juveniles were the large majority of the victims of forcible fondling (84%), forcible sodomy (79%), and sexual assault with an object (75%). In contrast, juveniles were the victims in less than half (46%) of forcible rapes. In each sexual assault category except forcible rape, children below the age of 12 years were about half of all victims (Sexual assault of young children as reported, 2000).

TABLE 16.3 **Child Sexual Abuse Rates in Different Countries**

Although we know there can be difficulties obtaining accurate statistics about any abusive behaviors, here are reported prevalence rates of child sexual abuse in selected countries (in each case the numbers are prevalence per 100).

	Females	Males
Austria	36	19
South Africa	34	29
Netherlands	33	NA
Costa Rica	32	13
New Zealand	32	NA
Australia	28	9
UNITED STATES	27	16
Spain	23	15
Norway	19	9
Belgium	19	NA
Canada	18	8
Greece	16	6
Denmark	14	7
Great Britain	12	8
Switzerland	11	3
Germany	10	4
Sweden	9	3
France	8	5
Ireland	7	5
Finland	7	4

NA = statistics not available

Source: Adapted from Finkelhor, D. The international epidemiology of child sexual abuse, *Child Abuse and Neglect, 16* (1994), 409–417.

Effects of Pedophilia

As with rape survivors, there is a tendency to blame survivors of child molestation. Blaming survivors, in turn, may contribute to a climate conducive to child molesting. The major reason for blaming survivors is the attitude that they "should have resisted" (Waterman & Foss-Goodman, 1984).

There has been considerable debate over the harmful effects of sexual child abuse. Highly publicized accounts linking a history of sexual abuse to prostitution, drug abuse, homicide, and multiple personalities increase public and professional interest. However, professionals encounter cases in which there appears to be little or no indication of negative effects of sexual victimization (Conte, 1985). It has even been found that boys 10 to 16 years old reported that sexual contacts with an adult were predominantly positive (Sandfort, 1984). In fact, a percentage of both men and women reported the experience as positive (McConaghy, 1998).

Researchers cannot explain the relatively large numbers of sexually abused children who have no apparent adverse psychological symptoms (Finkelhor, 1990). For those children who show symptoms, initial effects of sexual abuse include fear, anxiety, depression, anger, aggression, and sexually inappropriate behavior. The most common long-term effects are depression, self-destructive behavior, anxiety, feelings of isolation, poor self-esteem, difficulty in trusting others, substance abuse, and sexual maladjustment (Adult survivors of sex-abuse in crisis, 1990; Finkelhor, 1990).

Obviously all children do not react the same way to child abuse. Some research has identified effects of child abuse that include sleeping and eating

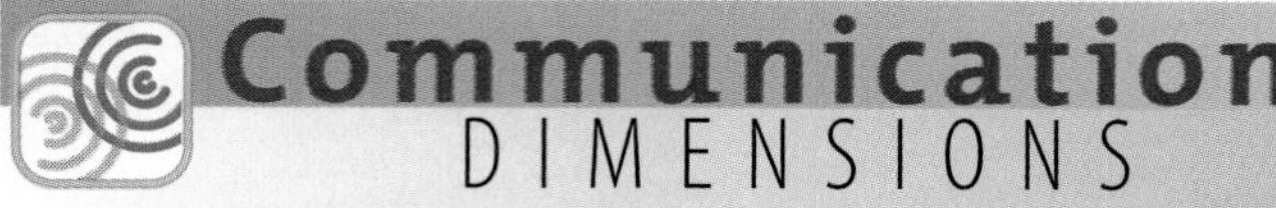

Helping Survivors of Rape and Sexual Abuse Even if you are not a trained counselor, if someone who has been raped or sexually abused talks with you about what has happened, you can be helpful by remembering the following points:

1. Listen in a supportive way, showing sympathy and concern. Ask questions and do not argue.
2. Encourage the person to express his or her feelings about the incident(s).
3. Control your own emotions. Do not react strongly and do not question the judgment of the survivor.
4. Indicate that you believe the account of what happened.
5. Let the survivor know that it was not his or her fault and that he or she is not to blame.
6. Give comfort.
7. Help the person focus on actions that might be needed, such as seeking medical treatment or reporting to police.
8. The survivor must decide what to do; you cannot force him or her or make the decision yourself.
9. Help the person find professional follow-up services—professional counseling, crisis center or domestic violence center guidance, legal assistance, medical follow-up—and accompany the person if that is appropriate and if the person desires it.
10. Survivors of rape and/or sexual abuse can respond in almost any way. They may be hysterical, amazingly calm, or anything in between. Almost any (or no) reaction is "normal."
11. Let the person know you are available to help or give support in the future.
12. Check as often as necessary to see how the person is progressing toward full recovery.

Source: Adapted from Bruess, C. & Richardson, G. *Decisions for health.* Madison, WI: Brown & Benchmark, 1995.

disturbances, anger, withdrawal, and guilt. Or there might be sexual preoccupation (excessive masturbation and an unusual interest in sexual organs and nudity) and a host of physical complaints such as rashes, vomiting, and headaches without medical explanation (Kohn, 1987).

In addition, teenage women who have been sexually abused are more likely to engage in voluntary sexual intercourse (Polit, White, & Morgan, 1990). They have more permissive attitudes about 16- to 17-year-olds' having intercourse and a younger age of first voluntary sexual intercourse for themselves. They also have higher depression scores and need more psychological help than those who do not report forced sexual intercourse (Miller, Monson, & Norton, 1995). They are also three to four times more likely to become infected with gonorrhea or syphilis and more likely to engage in unprotected intercourse with multiple partners (Vermund, 1990). Sexually abused women are the most likely to have had an STI (Kenney, Reinholtz, & Angellini, 1998). Perhaps these activities are related to the self-destructive behavior mentioned previously.

Kenney and associates (1997) explored ethnic differences in childhood and adolescent sexual abuse and the effect on teenage pregnancy rates. Almost 36% of the women reported sex abuse before age 18 years, and more than 26% were pregnant before they were 18 years old. More than one-third of pregnant teenagers in the study had been sexually abused. Coercive sexual abuse was more likely to contribute to teenage pregnancy among minority group teens, whereas rape was more likely to contribute to teenage pregnancy among whites.

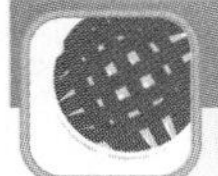

Global DIMENSIONS

Coercive Sexual Behaviors in Japan In Japan, rape is described as having sexual intercourse with a woman through force or against her will, but there is no clear legal definition. However, the victim or her parent or legal guardian must file a complaint in order for the rape to be recognized as a criminal act. Fewer than 2,000 cases are reported annually throughout the country.

Protection against sexual harassment in Japan lags far behind American and European standards. The Japanese Labor Ministry has specifically forbidden sexual harassment; however, much remains to be done.

There seems to be a tolerance of violence in Japan's male-dominated society. There is a long history of violence's being condoned as a symbol of manliness. As a result, in comic books, general sexual content has been curbed but portrayals of sexual violence are common. There are even "ladies' comic books" that seem to glorify sexual violence and rape. These are not a fringe phenomenon—the leading one claims annual sales of 400,000 copies.

Source: Hatano, Y. & Shimazaki, T. Japan, in *The international encyclopedia of sexuality,* vol. 2, R. T. Francoeur, ed. New York: Continuum Publishing, 1999.

Hillis and coworkers (2001) indicated that physical abuse and sexual abuse are related to subsequent unintended pregnancies and STI. In a study of more than 5,000 females, they found such abuse resulted in increased risk of intercourse by age 15 years and in sexual activity with multiple partners.

Exposure to childhood sexual abuse seems to be associated with increased rates of sexual risk-taking behaviors and sexual revictimization during adolescence. Young women reporting childhood sexual abuse, particularly those for whom sexual intercourse was involved, reported significantly higher rates of early-onset consensual sexual activity, teenage pregnancy, multiple sexual partners, unprotected intercourse, STIs, and sexual assault after the age of 16 years (Fergusson, Horwood, & Lynskey, 1997).

Urquiza and Goodlin-Jones (1994) studied child sexual abuse and adult revictimization. More than 65% of respondents who reported rape as an adult reported a history of childhood sexual abuse. Of those who had not been victims of childhood sexual abuse, 33% reported rape as an adult. It seems that higher rates of rape are associated with a prior history of childhood sexual abuse. This was true for white, African-American, and Latina respondents, but not for Asian-American respondents.

One of the most disturbing finds about child abuse is its strong intergenerational pattern: Boys who are abused are far more likely to turn into offenders; girls are more likely to produce children who are abused. In addition, victimization can lead to revictimization. Many who had been abused as children reported they were later victims of rape or attempted rape. Abuse victims seem to be easy targets because they do not know how to take care of themselves. This may be due to poor self-image, a lack of assertiveness, or the feeling they deserve to be punished (Kohn, 1987).

Most perpetrators of abuse are known to the majority of their female and male victims, and those reported are almost all male (McConaghy, 1998). Most child molesting is committed by family friends, relatives, or acquaintances, even though the stereotypical molester is thought of as a sex fiend who lurks in the shadows. Child molesting is directed toward other-sex children about twice as often as toward same-sex children.

Limited knowledge exists of male victims of sexual abuse. It appears that these male victims are concerned about sexual identity after the experience. When studied, most boys expressed some discomfort with their masculine identity and felt profoundly shaken by the abuse. Simple reassurance was not enough for most because they had complex feelings regarding their own sexual arousal (Male victims of sexual abuse, 1986). Because severe violence occurs in very few cases (probably only 2–3%), the danger to the child is far more likely to be psychological than physical. In fact, typical sexual activity is limited to noncoital acts such as touching or looking.

Usually such sexual experiences are less traumatic for the child than for the parents. It is important that adults understand children's feelings and reactions, because a child often suffers no lasting trauma if parents can control their reactions.

Prevention

Preventing child sexual abuse demands attention. Fortunately, in recent years programs have been designed to educate children and adults to distinguish between appropriate and inappropriate touch, to say no to unwanted or uncomfortable touch, to tell a trusted adult if inappropriate touch occurs, and to identify their family and community support systems. In addition, adolescents have been encouraged to consider the risks related to certain behaviors, the selection of a mate who will not abuse their children, and ways in which they will protect children from sexual abuse (Olson, 1985).

Educators, parents, and other adults need to learn to recognize physical and behavioral signs of sexual abuse and pay attention to indirectly related comments made by a child. Physical signs may include irritation, pain, or injury in the genital area. Behavioral signs may include nervous, aggressive, hostile, or disruptive behavior toward adults, especially parents. It is wise to remember that one sign alone may not be a positive indication, but if a number of signs are present, the possibility of sexual abuse should be considered (Child sexual abuse, 1998). One should believe the child, remain calm, avoid blaming the child, avoid leading questions such as "You did that a lot?" and know where to seek help for counseling services. Adults also need to help children learn that they do not have to agree to demands for physical closeness; that touching can be good, bad, or confusing; that some secrets should not be kept; that at times adults make mistakes and do things they should

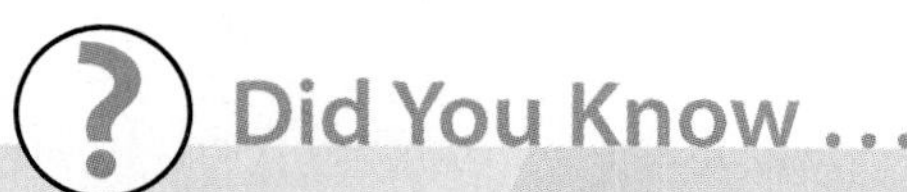

Law enforcement personnel are recognizing the need for special training to handle child sexual abuse cases. Without proper training innocent people can be falsely charged, valid cases may have to be dismissed, and children and others involved may not be treated as well as possible.

Training includes the dynamics of child sexual abuse, the science of interviewing children, and approaches to verifying and corroborating allegations. Understanding psychological needs of the victim, recognizing the sometimes vague symptoms of abuse, and knowing how to elicit sensitive information about sexual behavior from children are essential skills for law enforcement personnel (Peters, 1991).

not; and that there are times to ask for help and also to give help when asked for help by a friend (Duncan & Drolet, 1986).

Another way to help prevent sexual abuse is to screen professionals who work with children carefully. For example, in many states it is necessary for teachers and other school personnel to have a background check before they can assume their responsibilities. This is usually done by requiring fingerprinting of such professionals before they are hired.

A vivid example of the need to screen individuals working with children carefully was seen in 2002 when a Boston church scandal started a chain reaction (Kasindorf, et al., 2002). In January 2002 Boston's Cardinal Bernard Law acknowledged that he had moved a priest from parish to parish despite evidence that he had molested children. Soon afterward, church files revealed that another priest had abused children and advocated sexual activities between men and boys but still received the archdiocese's support. Before the year was over, thousands of adults filed lawsuits over abuse they said occurred when they were boys and girls—some as long as 50 years earlier. Five U.S. bishops, including Cardinal Law, resigned for reasons related to sexual abuse of children. Although not accused of abuse, Law resigned because of his failure to deal effectively with abusers who were priests.

As a result of this scandal, Roman Catholic bishops adopted a new policy for handling priests accused of sexual abuse. If a priest is found guilty by a board composed mostly of lay Catholics and at least one priest, he cannot wear a collar or give Communion, and he may be stripped of his status. In addition, most priests indicated they will tell the police about sexual abuse allegations in the future (Michaels, 2002).

In recent years, all 50 states have passed laws requiring sex offenders to alert the community to their presence. Twenty-eight states run Internet sites listing such criminals. In some states judges have ordered offenders to post signs outside their homes, mandated bumper stickers, and even required temporary placards for traveling in someone else's car. Some people argue these laws are appropriate to help protect society from sex offenders; others consider it inappropriate to brand people and even punish their families. A Washington state study found that such policies did not prevent sex offenders from committing more crimes, but they did help police find and arrest repeaters more quickly (Thomas, 2001).

In many states there is a law requiring rapists and child molesters to register each year for inclusion in a database of sex offenders. Failure to register is usually a felony and can result in more jail time. Even so, the state of California lost track of more than 33,000 sex offenders, or 44% of the total number of registered offenders. They simply vanished after registering. Nationally 52% of rapists are arrested for new crimes within 3 years of leaving prison, according to the U.S. Justice Department (Curtis, 2003).

One sex offender was chased, punched, followed by police, filmed by television helicopters, and harassed by protesters during the first 4 months after his release from prison. He was run out of Michigan, Ohio, and Kentucky and moved to several locations in New Mexico. Signs placed on the fence across the street from where he lived read "Keep Your Women/Children Away," "Molester Lives Here," and "Go Back Where You Came From—Hell." One man punched the sex offender while he was doing yard work (Stephens, 2003).

College officials have to decide how to best deal with the Campus Sex Crimes Prevention Act, a federal law that requires sex offenders, when they register with the state, to indicate whether and where they are enrolled, employed, or volunteering on a college campus. As of October 1, 2003, college officials must tell students, faculty, and administrators where informa-

Ethical DIMENSIONS

Is It Ethical to Publicly Identify Sexual Offenders?

Named after Megan Kanka, a 7-year-old New Jersey child who was raped and murdered by a convicted sex offender who lived across the street from her, "Megan's Law" requires that authorities and the community be notified when a convicted sex offender is released or moves into their neighborhood. Variations of Megan's Law are found in a number of states. For example, Alabama's Megan's Law also forbids a convicted offender to live near a school, day care center, or past victim.

Some people want a law requiring that the identity of convicted child molesters be made known to community members. This means that if a convicted child molester moved into your community, you and all your neighbors would be informed that he or she was there and that he or she had been a child molester. People support such a law because they feel they have a right to protect their children.

Other people think it is a violation of individual rights and personal privacy if a convicted child molester's identity is made public. They feel that the molester, as has any other person convicted of a crime, has paid for the crime through a prison sentence and in other possible ways, and it is not ethical to reveal his or her identity to the public. The person has a right to live privately and to start a new life if he or she desires. On the basis of these arguments, there have been legal challenges to Megan's Law in New Jersey, and similar laws have been found unconstitutional in other states.

In Virginia, state police developed a web site that lists the names of violent sex offenders. They guessed that 5,000 people would log on on the first day. But in the first 12 hours, it was visited more than 45,000 times. By the second day, the site was so jammed that many people could not get through because the site can handle only six "hits" per second. Some people expressed the point of view that we should not be concerned about former sex offenders' being harassed, because "If they don't want their names in the paper, they shouldn't commit the crime." Others question the ethics of this web site and feel it treats sex offenders unfairly.

Do you think it is ethical to require that identities of sexual offenders be made public?

tion on registered sex offenders can be obtained. Most have chosen to make the registry available for perusal in the campus police department and made its existence known either through the college's web site or by mailing of pamphlets that direct students and others to its location (Bosslett, 2003).

Incest

incest
Sexual behavior between relatives who are too closely related to be married.

Incest is sexual behavior between relatives who are too closely related to be legally married. Much of what has been said about child sexual abuse also applies to incest. However, it is helpful to consider incest separately because it is rapidly changing from a private subject to a public one.

The most commonly reported form of incest is father–daughter, but in practice, brother–sister incest probably happens more often (Canavan, Meyer, & Higgs, 1992). It has traditionally been estimated that about 10% of girls had a sexual experience with an adult relative, but the proportion is probably more like 19%. In fact, when child sexual abuse by relatives outside the basic family unit was included, a total of 38% of women reported at least one experience of sexual abuse before reaching the age of 18 years (Startling new study shows one in six women incestuously abused before age 18, 1986). Boys are less commonly molested by a parent or other older relative, although this also occurs.

Mother–child incest was often thought to be virtually nonexistent. This may be because of a cultural unwillingness to believe that women commit such acts or because female sex offenders have seldom been studied. Although many more males than females are guilty of incest, it is likely that the amount of sexual abuse of male and female children by women has been underestimated (Banning, 1989).

Children involved in incest are usually afraid to tell anyone about it. The only clues are vague symptoms such as withdrawal, fears about going to school, anxiety, nightmares, or bodily complaints (Herman, 1981). To make matters worse, victims of incest often consider it their fault. In one case a 10-year-old girl explained that it was her fault because "I never told him not to do it" (Sexually abused children believe it's their fault, 1984).

The characteristics of those involved in incest are surprising. For example, the offenders often appeared to be nice guys—conventional, independent, and often very self-assured. The mothers in homes where incest occured tended to be emotionally distant and aloof toward their children. Vulnerable family members typically viewed the father as the parent who loved them because he interacted more with them and provided significant caretaking, despite the incestual behavior (What families won't tell, 1986).

More than 95% of the offenders were male, and the family structure was strongly patriarchal. Most families involved had lived in the same place for at least 5 years, and, contrary to popular beliefs, stepfathers were not involved more often than biological fathers. When confronted, most abusive fathers appeared truly sorry for their actions, but the vast majority did not believe they had done anything particularly wrong. Incestuous fathers openly indicated they felt a right to educate their children about sex and to use their children to meet their own sexual needs. Incest was related to the father's immaturity—it was not only sex he was after but power and control. The common denominator in these men seemed to be self-indulgence. Many refused to believe that they really hurt their children. Basically, the act was so pleasurable they just did not care. It has been estimated that more than 1 million American women have been sexually abused by fathers, stepfathers, brothers, uncles, or other family members (What families won't tell, 1986).

It has generally been thought that shame and guilt made it difficult for incest survivors to tell or to seek help, and that most survivors complied passively. The pressure placed on incest survivors to maintain secrecy is substantial, but more recently it has been found that incest survivors were less resistant than survivors of other forms of family violence only in their attempts to flee. Reluctance to leave is understandable, because incest victims are characterized by relative domestic "imprisonment," often playing roles of surrogate mothers. In seeking outside help and attempting to resist sexual overtures, however, incest survivors were relatively aggressive (Gordon & O'Keefe, 1985).

Traditionally it was thought that perpetrators of incest were pathological or driven to incest by high stress levels; however, that is not true. Stress levels of incestuous adults were not found to be higher than those of people committing other crimes. The assailants were also not poorer, sicker, or more often unemployed. More than any other type of family violence, incest seems to be premeditated and not a sudden loss of control (Gordon & O'Keefe, 1985).

The incest taboo is universal in human culture. It is considered by anthropologists to be the foundation of all kinship structures and even the basis of human social

Vladimir Nabokov's book *Lolita,* the story of a middle-aged professor's sexual obsession with his 13-year-old stepdaughter, caused quite a stir when published in 1955. But by 1998, the social climate against incest had grown so intense that the European-made movie version of the book could not find a distributor in America. Although it was shown on Showtime (cable) and in very limited theatrical release, its financial failure sent a strong message throughout the movie industry.

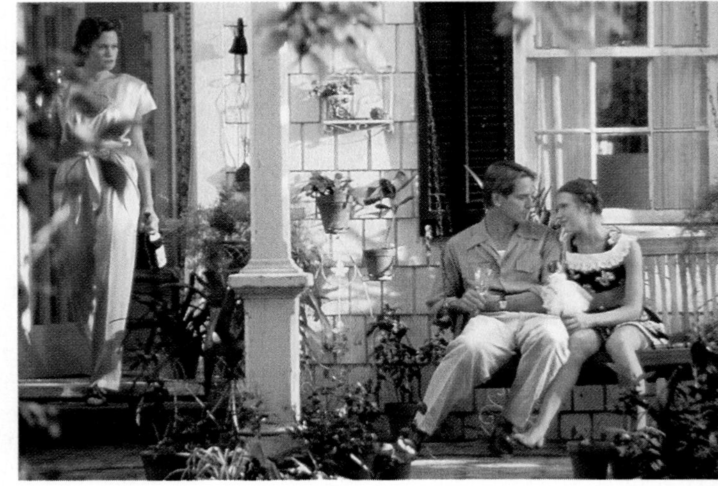

order (Herman, 1985). Nevertheless, incest occurs in all social classes, in all geographic areas, and among all ethnic and racial groups.

Incestuous families seem to have more children than the norm because the mother is unable to control her reproductive life. Incestuous fathers do not assume caretaking functions when the wife is disabled, and they expect to continue to receive female nurturance. The oldest daughter is usually "deputized" to take on a "little mother" role, and her sexual relationship with the father often evolves as an extension of her other duties. Most incestuous fathers continue to have sexual relationships with their wife as well as with their daughter. The incestuous behavior, once established, has repetitive and compulsive aspects that resemble those of addiction.

Compared to females who were not incest victims, female incest survivors report significantly higher anger level in general and more anger toward their parents; anger toward mother and father was about equal. Extent of their anger is correlated with age of victim at onset of incest, duration of incest, incest involving penetration and use of force, and perceived parental responsibility for abuse (Newman & Peterson, 1996).

It is difficult, if not impossible, to separate the long-term effects of sexual abuse of children in general from those of incest, but it is important to try to understand them. The long-term consequences that affect adults in many ways include (1) posttraumatic stress disorder (including hypervigilance, intrusive thoughts, and flashbacks of the abusive experience); (2) cognitive distortions (for example, seeing the world as a dangerous place, underestimating personal self-worth, or having chronic perceptions of helplessness); (3) emotional distress; (4) impaired sense of self (relying on the reactions of others to determine their own feelings, potential to be easily manipulated by others); (5) avoidance; (6) interpersonal difficulties; and (7) health problems (Kendall-Tackett & Marshall, 1998).

Various community organizations offer help for incest survivors and their families—for example, child-protection agencies, rape crisis centers, women's centers, and organizations that offer help for parents who are under extreme stress or are frightened about their feelings toward their children. The best strategy for preventing incest is to provide information to children, as well as to parents. This means providing sexuality education at the elementary school level and above, including specific information about incest. For example, children should be taught that Uncle Charlie or Aunt Mary does not automatically have the right to touch them all over. In addition, information about pedophilia and other sexual practices should be provided at the appropriate level of understanding.

The initial focus of crisis intervention should be on stopping the sexual abuse and establishing a safe environment in the family. Once the incest is reported, it is controversial whether or not the child should be temporarily removed from the home. This might be destructive to the child because she may feel that she has done something wrong, that she is being punished, or that both parents are against her. It is also difficult to find an appropriate place to put the child; however, removal from the home may be the only way to ensure the child's safety.

Restoration of the incestuous family centers on the mother–daughter relationship. The mother must feel strong enough to protect herself and her children, and the daughter must feel sure she can turn to her mother for protection. The father can be judged ready to return to his family when he has admitted and taken full responsibility for the incest, apologized to his daughter(s) in the presence of all family members, and promised never to abuse his children again. Given the present state of knowledge, no one can claim to "cure" incest; rather, the behavior may be controlled (Herman, 1985).

Spousal Abuse

As we have seen, the topics of childhood sexual abuse and incest overlap. The same is true of various aspects of spousal abuse. For example, the abuse may be in the form of forced sexual activity, use of violence without sexual activity, or both. Today it is recognized that husbands and wives can both be victims of spousal abuse. In fact, both males and females engage in frequent minor assaults. However, females are more often the victims of severe partner assault and injury, not necessarily because males strike more often but because males strike harder (Morse, 1995). Because the number of *reported* cases of abuse of wives far exceeds the number of *reported* cases of the abuse of husbands, because physical danger to wives is usually far greater, and because most of the studies available on this topic deal with females, most of the information here is about females as well.

Marital Rape

For hundreds of years it was not legally possible for a husband to rape his wife. It was felt that the male right to sexual activity was a fundamental part of marriage. In the 1970s the feminist movement promoted the renunciation of what was called the "marital rape exemption." Feminists argued that rape laws served to protect men's sexual right to female property rather than protect women's bodily integrity. They demanded that the laws be changed (Ryan, 1995). It is difficult to believe that as recently as 1976 no husband could be charged with raping his wife. Today it is a crime in all 50 states for a husband to rape his wife (Mahoney, 1998).

For obvious reasons, it is difficult to obtain accurate information on the frequency of spousal rape. A summary of various studies indicates that about 14% of married women reported either a completed or an attempted rape by a husband. The best estimate based on existing studies is that 1 in 10 to 1 in 7 married women will experience a rape by a husband. The incidence of sexual assault reported by battered women appears to be at least two to three times the rate of rape experienced by all ever-married women (Mahoney & Williams, 1998).

As stated earlier, there is a tendency toward repeated abuse. In this case, 53% of marital rape survivors report previous sexual abuse, 68% report previous emotional abuse, 35% report previous physical abuse, and 18% report no previous abuse (Peacock, 1998).

Why spouses are raped is a question that has not been greatly explored. The few existing studies summarize common reasons as (1) entitlement to sex (thinking that the marriage contract includes the right to sexual intercourse on demand), (2) sexual jealousy, (3) rape as punishment for some "wrong" behavior, and (4) rape as a form of control (asserting of power and control) (Bergen, 1998).

A number of factors contribute to the underreporting of spousal rape and women's reluctance to discuss such experiences. They include the following:

1. Loyalty to husband/privacy of family
2. Unwillingness to accept their own victimization
3. Reluctance to label the experience "rape"
4. Misunderstandings about a woman's role in marriage and marital responsibilities
5. Sexual inexperience and uncertainty about what constitutes "normal" and "forced" sexual relations (Mahoney & Williams, 1998)

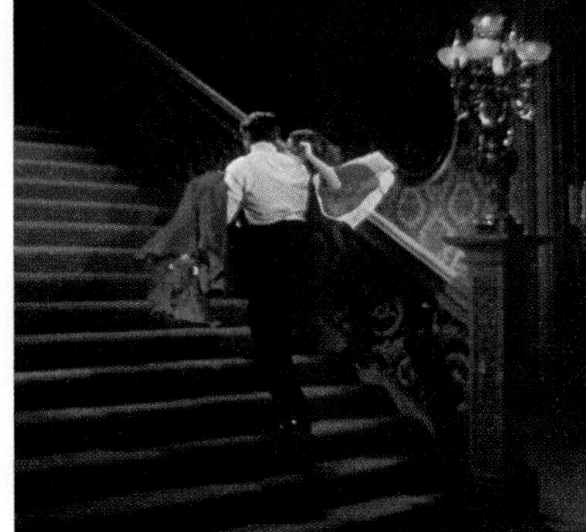

In the movie *Gone with the Wind,* the husband, Rhett Butler (played by Clark Gable), carries his wife, Scarlett O'Hara (Vivien Leigh), kicking and screaming up a staircase, implying sexual activity is to follow. Portrayed as sensual more than 60 years ago, could it be considered spousal rape by today's standards?

Victims of rape by a husband are different from other rape victims because they are violated by someone with whom they share their homes, lives, and maybe children. They are faced with a betrayal of trust and intimacy. Wife rape victims are more likely to be raped multiple times than stranger and acquaintance rape victims. Women who experience wife rape suffer long-lasting physical and psychological injuries that are as severe as or more severe than those of stranger rape victims (Mahoney, 1998).

Why would a woman stay with a man who raped her? The answers are usually very complicated but include such reasons as the following:

1. Many women believe it is part of their "duty" to have sexual intercourse with their husband, even if it is violent and against their will.
2. Many women cannot leave because they do not have the financial resources to do so.
3. Women may fear what the offender may do to her or the children.
4. Some women may not leave because of love and loyalty to the husband, which can override her own pain and suffering (Mahoney, 1998).

It seems that women raped by a spouse are more likely to experience long-term effects than are women raped by an acquaintance or a stranger. Possible long-term effects include (1) negative feelings toward men; (2) low self-esteem; (3) fear; (4) anxiety; (5) guilt; (6) embarrassment; (7) outrage; (8) changes in behaviors, including an increase in drinking and refusal to consider remarriage; (9) depression (Peacock, 1998).

Women who have been raped by a spouse reported warning signs they had seen in their husband that may be seen in other men who have the potential to rape. These warning signs include an extreme interest in and use of pornography, use of alcohol to excess, use of sex play as a payoff in the relationship, and difficulty in handling anger (Peacock, 1998).

Domestic Violence

Domestic violence is a significant health and social problem in the United States and many other industrialized societies such as Germany and Great Britain. In other industrialized societies, however, it is considered to be almost nonexistent. In a study of 86 "primitive" societies, domestic violence was present at varying levels of frequency and severity in 90%. The reasons for the variability from culture to culture have not been established. Domestic violence occurs for many reasons. It can be an indication of manhood, a means of personal control, a reflection of personal animosity, and an expression of social jealousy (Campbell, 1985).

It is a difficult task to estimate rates of domestic violence. Many factors inhibit women from reporting these crimes. The private nature of the event, the perceived stigma, and the belief that no purpose would be served by reporting the crime prevent an unknown portion of the survivors from talking about the event. Therefore, available statistics are at best estimates.

On average in recent years, 22% of all female and 3% of all male victims of violence were attacked by an intimate partner. Women were victims of intimate partner violence about five times more often than males. Half of the females were physically injured, and 37% of these sought professional medical treatment. About 11% of all murders per year are the result of intimate partner violence (Intimate partner violence, 2000). About half of all reported attacks that cause injury are committed by an intimate partner (Hoyt, 2001).

It has been estimated that in the United States, 6 million women are beaten each year by their husband or boyfriend; 4,000 of them are killed. The FBI estimates that an act of domestic violence occurs every 18 seconds (Paisner, 1991). The Feminist Majority Foundation indicates that domestic violence claims the lives of four women each day; women are 10 times more likely than men to be victimized by an intimate; and the rate at which women separated from their spouses suffer violent victimization is 128 per 1,000, or more than 12 times that of never-married women, about twice that of divorced women, and more than 6 times the rate of married women. Also, 20% of women who get treatment in emergency rooms are victims of domestic violence (Facts about domestic violence in the United States, 1999).

FOR 11,000 WOMEN EVERY DAY, THE MOON WOULD BE A SAFER PLACE TO BE.
THE NATIONAL COALITION AGAINST DOMESTIC VIOLENCE

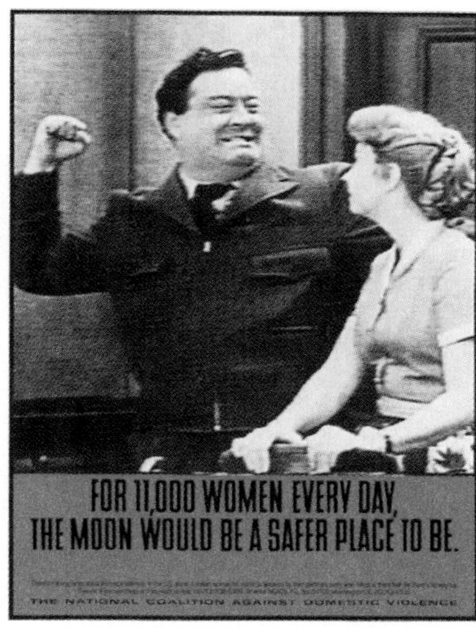

Back in the 1950s, the popular TV show *The Honeymooners* portrayed the blue-collar husband Ralph (Jackie Gleason) as getting mad at his wife and threatening, "One of these days, Alice ... Pow ... Right to the moon!" The line provoked uproarious laughter. (He never did harm her.) But there is nothing funny about domestic violence. According to the National Coalition Against Domestic Abuse, 4 million U.S. women are victims of assaults by their partners each year.

Direct physical attack is the most common abuse, but a woman is also abused when she is repeatedly placed in physical danger or controlled by the use of threats to hurt her, her children, friends, family, or pets. Physical abuse can also be sexual. A marital or live-in relationship does not give a man the right to force sexual relations or practices that are unwanted, uncomfortable, or degrading. Battered women often have low self-esteem and feel humiliated and ashamed of their body. For the battering man, daily tensions seem to lead to abusive behaviors and violent explosions. Afterward, the man most likely makes excuses, apologizes, and promises it will not happen again. He may even make a special effort to smooth things over by trying to be nice. Because his wife wants to believe him, they often make up and she tries to forget. As time passes, however, tensions again build for the man, and the battering recurs as part of this cycle of violence (Rouse, 1985).

The physical abuse associated with domestic violence is probably heard about most often; domestic violence, however, is not limited to physical abuse. The National Resource Center on Domestic Violence (*Help end domestic violence,* N.D.) defines it as a "pattern of abusive and controlling behaviors that some individuals use against their intimate partners or former partners." In addition to physical abuse such as hitting, punching, kicking, or using weapons, it can include

- *Sexual abuse:* forcing a partner to engage in unwanted sexual behaviors
- *Emotional abuse:* name calling, put-downs; stalking; treating a partner as inferior; using threatening looks, actions, or gestures; threatening children or pets
- *Property/economic abuse:* stealing or destroying property and money; refusing the partner food or medical attention; or interfering with a partner's work or education

Batterers often tend to absolve themselves of full responsibility, and, at the same time, they offer justifications for their abusiveness. The most common excuse is an appeal to loss of control—usually resulting either from drug or alcohol use or from a buildup of frustrations. Because awareness is impaired, there is a feeling that their impairment diminishes responsibility. The second major category of excuse is victim blaming. The men deny responsibility by claiming they were "provoked." Most often, batterers say their violence was a response to verbal aggressiveness; in some cases they say it was a response to physical aggressiveness (Ptacek, 1998).

Whereas excuses represent denial of responsibility, justifications are denials of wrongdoing by the offender. The first category of justification is denial of injury. Offenders deny or minimize the injuries battered women suffer. The second category involves finding fault with the woman for something—perhaps not being good at cooking, not being sexually responsive, not being deferential enough to her husband, not being faithful, and so on. The assumption of entitlement, denies the wrongness of the violence. The batterer sees himself as punishing the woman for her failure to be a good wife (Ptacek, 1998).

A number of researchers have examined the incidence of marital violence being reported to the police. So far, few consistent reasons for reporting patterns have emerged. In fact, battered women who call the police are not significantly different demographically, economically, or situationally from battered women in general (Johnson, 1990). Interestingly, complaints are rarely reported by victims of sexual abuse in marital relationships. In general, when sexual abuse is verified, it is accompanied by other forms of abuse (Grams, et al., 1997).

Jacobson and associates (1996) found that 38% of couples in a violent relationship separated or divorced over a 2-year period. This is more than had been previously thought. Many people wonder why women, or men for that matter, would remain in abusive relationships, and researchers have focused on this issue. Choice and Lemke (1997) found that the two central questions are "Will I be better off?" and "Can I do it?" Their model proposes that abused women's stay-or-leave decisions occur in a stepwise fashion. A woman may wish to leave her relationship but be inhibited because she does not feel she has control over her circumstances. Conversely, a woman may wish to remain in the relationship.

In summary, those who are battered stay with a batterer because they love their spouse, the spouse is genuinely apologetic, disclosure of the violence would cause embarrassment, the behavior is excused by circumstances (such as stress or excessive alcohol use), there are material and economic concerns, psychological dependency exists, or they fear for the safety of the children (Flynn, 1990).

Battering is rarely a one-time event, and attacks usually increase in number and severity unless intervention occurs. A battered woman may blame herself because the man tells her it is her fault or simply because women in our society are often taught to blame themselves for problems in a personal relationship. Battering men have certain characteristics in common: low self-

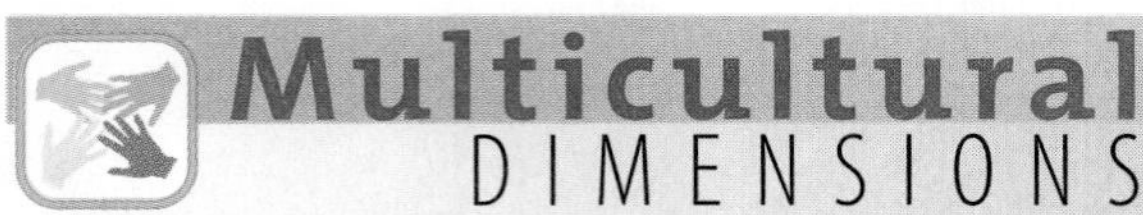

Wife Abuse in China

Don't Talk to Strangers is a 23-part TV series that ran on Chinese networks and has been marketed abroad. The series was credited with putting the uncomfortable subject of spousal abuse in the open in China. This was surprising to many because traditional Chinese culture teaches that family problems should stay within the family. Many were surprised when the show made it past Communist Party propaganda officials, who generally frown on negative portrayals of Chinese society.

Some viewers found the show too violent, too gloomy, and too hopeless. Others consider it important to get the problem out into the open. Activists say spousal abuse occurs in one in three Chinese families compared to one in four in the United States.

In China, the marriage law of 2001 gives victims the right to protection and orders abusers punished. In divorce cases, victims of abuse can also sue for damages. However, willingness to enforce the law varies widely across the country. China's first battered women's shelters were forced to close because of lack of money or authorities' unwillingness to offer protection. Some people consider it normal for couples to fight, and it is difficult to get people to see that as violence.

Source: Bodeen, C. TV show about wife abuse grips China, *The Seattle Times* (February 3, 2003), A18.

esteem, traditional sex-role expectations, jealousy, a need to control, abusive family background, a need to blame others, and denial. Programs to help battering men are based on the philosophy that violence is typically a learned reaction and that more constructive ways to deal with conflict and stress can be learned. For example, men learn to talk more openly about themselves, their feelings, and their home situations, and they learn to overcome denial and ask for help. Men must be taught to acknowledge that battering behavior is unacceptable, and they must be willing to change. Some men do change, but most do not (Rouse, 1985).

We have been slow to recognize the problem of domestic violence. In the past, laws and common practice encouraged husbands to discipline their wife by force if they saw fit. But conditions are changing. Family violence research has made it clear that the problem of battering is too widespread to ignore or to explain away by blaming the victim. Many new resources are available. Battered women's shelters are particularly helpful in providing services for battered women and their children and in continuing efforts to educate people about domestic violence.

There are ways we can combat domestic violence. Here are some possibilities (101 ways to combat domestic violence, 2003):

1. Make violence unacceptable in your life.
2. Contact your local school board and ask them to address dating violence.
3. Contact your local media representatives and remind them that October is Domestic Violence Awareness Month. Ask them what they plan to do. Tell them about the National Domestic Violence Hotline (1-800-799-SAFE), and ask them to publicize it.
4. Contact community businesses and agencies, and ask them to display the number of the National Domestic Violence Hotline in prominent places.

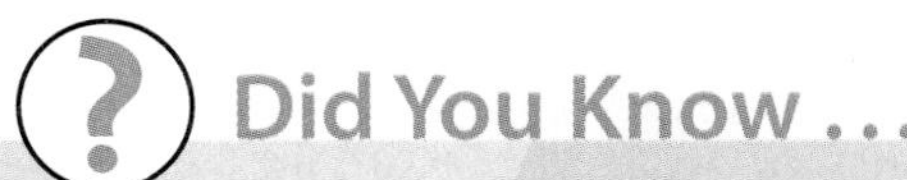

Violence by women received little attention until the mid-1970s. Now we know that women in relationships engage in violent acts as often as men. In about half of violent relationships, the violence is mutual. When there is a sole perpetrator, it is just as likely to be a female as a male. However, female use of violence, even when intended to cause harm, is mainly self-defensive.

Men tend to inflict more severe damage on women than the converse. Reasons given for this are that women tend to cease violent behaviors before causing serious injury and that men are usually physically larger and stronger than women.

The needs of battered men are somewhat different from those of battered women. Abused women have varied needs, including safety for themselves and often for their children; abused men's needs are more limited. Because they usually have the necessary resources to leave the relationship, their primary needs are legal assistance and psychological counseling.

Sources: Flynn, C. P. Relationship violence by women: Issues and implications, *Family Relations, 38, no. 2* (April 1990), 194–198; Morse, B. J. Beyond the conflict tactics scale: Assessing gender differences in partner violence, *Violence and Victims, 10, no. 4* (winter 1995), 251–272.

5. Contact local schools and colleges and let students know about resources available on the Internet concerning domestic violence.
6. Ask the local police department to be sure officers are trained in handling domestic violence.
7. Ask your priest, pastor, rabbi, or other religious leader to have a special service devoted to domestic violence.
8. Do not let jokes about violent behavior go unchallenged.
9. Work with day care centers to publish information about domestic violence to their customers.
10. Learn more about policies and facilities related to domestic violence in your community.

Sexual Harassment

sexual harassment
Unwelcome verbal, physical, or sexual conduct that has the effect of creating an intimidating, hostile, or offensive environment.

Since the mid-1970s, courts, popular and professional periodicals, newspapers, and books have focused on **sexual harassment.** Hundreds of articles have appeared in print, increasing national attention to the subject. It is not easy to define sexual harassment. Sometimes it is hard to draw the line between harassment and other behaviors, but it can include touching, verbal abuse, demanding of sexual favors, or use of threatening tones. The Canadian Association of University Teachers has defined *sexual harassment* as follows:

> *Sexual advances, requests for sexual favors, and other verbal or physical conduct of a sexual nature [when] submission to such conduct is made either explicitly or implicitly a term or condition of an individual's employment, academic status, or academic accreditation.*
>
> *Submission to or rejection of such conduct by an individual is used as the basis for employment, academic status, or academic-accreditation decisions affecting such individual, and such conduct has the purpose or effect of unreasonably interfering with an individual's work or academic performance, or creating an intimidating, hostile, or offensive working or academic environment. (The Chronicle of Higher Education, 1981)*

The U.S. Equal Employment Opportunity Commission defines *sexual harassment* as unwelcome verbal, physical, or sexual conduct that is a condition of employment, that is used as the basis for employment decisions, or that has the effect of creating an intimidating, hostile, or offensive work environment (McMillen, 1986). Sexual harassment may include verbal abuse; sexist remarks regarding a person's clothing or body; patting, pinching, or brushing up against a person's body; leering or ogling; demand for sexual favors in return for hiring, promotion, or tenure; physical assault; and rape. Two categories of sexual harassment have been described. In the first, something is to be exchanged. Perhaps a boss offers a person a job opportunity in exchange for sexual favors or threatens loss of a job opportunity if the person does not comply. In the second, there is no promise or threat; however, there are sexual remarks, touching/stroking, or lewd looks (Meyer, et al., 1981).

Legally speaking, then, there are two kinds of sexual harassment. The first is quid pro quo (Latin for "something for something"): Something is to be exchanged. The second is a hostile environment, which means that speech or conduct in itself can create a hostile environment, which in turn is sexual harassment (Cloud, 1998).

Defining sexual harassment in practice can be difficult. Although there are legal guidelines in many instances, various people may have inconsistent perceptions. For example, Blakely and associates (1995) found that more females than males viewed ambiguous sexually oriented work behavior as harassment. In addition, those who had been a target of sexual harassment tended to view the behavior as more harassing (Blakely, Blakely, & Moorman, 1995).

The topic of sexual harassment has been considered by many to be a radical-fringe by-product of feminist theory. Today it is embedded in legal decisions at all levels—including those of the Supreme Court. About 60 new sexual harassment cases are filed every day, more than 15,500 per year (Cloud, 1998).

Men who accept traditional sex roles or male sexual dominance are more likely than other men to engage in verbal sexual harassment (Muehlenhard & Falcon, 1990). Harassment tactics usually involve the inappropriate use of power. In one study it was found that 79% of the harassers had the power to fire or promote the person being harassed. The costs of sexual harassment are substantial in terms of employee turnover, creation of an unpleasant work environment, and reduced work performance. Half of all female workers have experienced sexual harassment. The most frequent types were the persistent, less severe forms (commentary and manhandling) that fall into legal limbo yet provide a continual source of irritation. Women are harassed more by superordinates but are also harassed by peers. They are more likely to receive commentary from peers and more severe forms of harassment (manhandling, negotiation, and assault) from superordinates (Loy & Stewart, 1984).

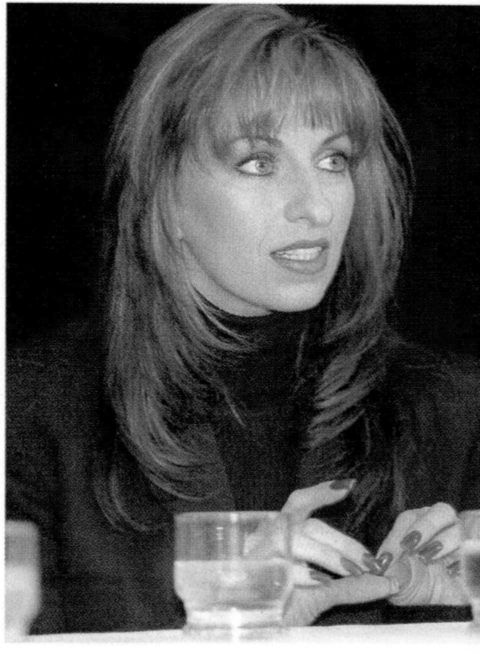

The sexual harassment suit filed by Paula Jones demonstrates how actions can have far-reaching effects. Jones's allegations resulted in President Clinton's spending millions of dollars in legal bills, paying off an $850,000 settlement, possibly committing perjury in an affidavit, and being impeached. For Jones, the case left her career and marriage in shambles.

Although men can also be victims of sexual harassment, that occurs rarely, and males seem to suffer fewer negative effects from such experiences than women do. Men with traditional sex-role attitudes and low self-esteem, and women with traditional attitudes and high self-esteem, are more tolerant of harassment behaviors and view the victim more negatively than other males and females (Malovich & Stake, 1990).

Women feel the results of harassment primarily as psychological and physical distress and with more negative symptoms from more severe harassment. They tend to deal informally with harassment and few go to their supervisor or an appropriate committee or seek legal help. Social stigmatization by peers is a common outcome for harassed individuals. Harassers ignore their victims, and coworkers tell victims not to pursue the issue. Women who ignore the harassment or complain to their boss experience the fewest negative sanctions; almost half of the women who directly confront their harassers receive some type of negative organizational sanction. Unfortunately, women who pursue active strategies in response to their harassment suffer the most personal and organizational consequences (Loy & Stewart, 1984).

Lindenberg and Reese (1996) studied sexual harassment policies and employees' attitudes about them. The employees' satisfaction with the policies was mixed, and there was a lot of uncertainly about just what the policies meant and how they would be interpreted and enforced. Reporting rates were low in relation to the actual number of harassment experiences. Recommendations for policy improvements included providing training on the nature of sexual harassment, using an ombudsperson, and increasing accountability of supervisors.

Sexual Harassment in Schools

Initial concerns about sexual harassment focused on the workplace; however, more recently additional attention has been given to schools and colleges. Di Mauro (1995) indicated that at least one in five adolescent girls in grades 8–11 are subjected to sexual harassment.

A dramatically increased number of school-related sexual harassment cases went to court in the early 1990s; they commonly involved student-to-student situations. Also, an increasing amount of research indicates that a large proportion of both male and female students are harassed; the behaviors occur frequently; most commonly the behavior is verbal, but physical actions are also common; the behavior is detrimental to all students but especially to girls; and many who have been sexually harassed also have harassed others (Moore & Rienzo, 1998).

The American Association of University Women conducted a national survey on sexual harassment in public schools in 1993 and again in 2001 (Hostile hallways: Bullying, teasing, and sexual harassment in schools, 2001). They found that students in 2001 were much more likely to say that their schools had sexual harassment policies and distribute literature on sexual harassment. As in 1993, in 2001 80% of students experienced some form of sexual harassment at some time during their school life. There was a striking increase (from 18% to 24%) in the number of boys who often experienced sexual harassment in school. In addition, 56% of boys said they experienced sexual harassment occasionally. Girls were more likely than boys to experience sexual harassment ever (83% vs. 79%). Students who experienced sexual harassment were most likely to react by avoiding the person who bothered or harassed them (40%), talking less in class (24%), wanting not to go to school (22%), changing their seat in class to get farther away from someone (21%), and finding it hard to pay attention in school (20%).

Loredo and associates (1995) found that in defining sexual harassment, high school students relied on four factors: the behavior itself, the target's reaction to the behavior, the perpetrator's intentions, and the relationship between the two participants. After viewing eight scenarios about sexual harassment, females rated the scenarios more severely than males did. Teacher perpetrators were judged more severely than student perpetrators.

As mentioned, the number of court cases related to sexual harassment in schools is increasing. Although there have been some conflicting decisions, the Supreme Court issued a major decision in 1998 in its ruling that school districts cannot be liable for damages in a private lawsuit about teacher–student sexual harassment unless an official in a position to take corrective action knew of the harassment and was "deliberately indifferent" to it. At the same time Richard W. Riley, secretary of education, indicated, "Any sexual harassment of a student—particularly sexual abuse by a teacher—is a basic breach of trust between the school and the student and the family" (Walsh, 1998).

The question of whether schools should be held liable when students sexually harass their peers is extremely sensitive (Edwards, 1999). Some people argue that schools should be responsible only for taking reasonable action rather than for ensuring that the behavior ends—although it can be hard to determine the definition of "reasonable." Others feel school personnel have a responsibility to take strong actions to prevent behaviors often associated with typical child growth and development—such as sexual comments, touching, and jeering. It is a real challenge to design appropriate policies and procedures related to students' sexually harassing their peers.

Sexual Harassment on Campus

Sexual harassment exists on all types of university campuses. In many cases it is unreported—and is often ignored altogether. In general, women are more likely to define behaviors as harassing and men are more likely to believe victims have contributed to their own problem. There are costs to individuals and to the institution. Victims tend to sacrifice self-confidence, academic and work opportunities, letters of recommendation, and grades. The student's professional development is hindered, and the university acquires a negative image (Rubin & Borgers, 1990).

Women are less tolerant of sexual harassment than are men and see it as a more serious problem. More female faculty report sexual harassment by colleagues than by students. More male faculty, however, report sexual harassment by students than by peers. Harassment is most likely to be inflicted by a colleague of higher academic rank than by one of equal or lower rank. Student harassment of male and female faculty is most often anonymous (obscene phone calls and sexual comments on course evaluations) and overall is often considered less significant in nature (body language or sexist comments) (McKinney, 1990).

The perception of sexual harassment on college campuses varies somewhat between males and females. For example, college students rated the degree to which they thought sexual harassment occurred in 20 hypothetical interactions. Men and women rated the interactions alike as long as the harasser was a man and the victim was a woman. When the perpetrator was a woman and the victim was a man, men gave significantly lower ratings than women. In contrast, women's ratings were the same regardless of the harasser's sex. Harassment ratings also varied as a function of the power differential between the harasser and the victim. The more equal the relationship, the less likely participants were to perceive the behavior as sexually harassing (Katz, et al., 1996).

There sometimes seem to be more instances of sexual harassment involving college athletes than the rest of the college population. However, a closer analysis indicates that the athletic world is similar to other social domains in the occurrence of sexual harassment (Volkwein, Schnell, & Sherwood, 1997).

Female participation in college sports has greatly increased, and about one in three women in college participates in competitive sports. Unfortunately, sexual harassment and abuse of female athletes are part of the reality of women's sports. Examples include coaches' preoccupations with athletes' bodies and weight, inappropriate comments about their bodies and

Gender DIMENSIONS

Same-Sex Sexual Harassment Sexual harassment is obviously a problem for women in the workplace—and sometimes for men. Most often, the instances we hear about involve other-sex situations. However, more and more same-sex harassment cases have been filed, and lower courts have been inconsistent in their findings. One judge allowed a case to proceed only because the supervisor, accused of harassing was admittedly gay.

The Equal Employment Opportunity Commission has for years taken the position that Title VII of the Civil Rights Act does not care which sexes are involved. In 1998 the Supreme Court allowed a case to proceed in which a man working on an oil rig charged two male coworkers with making taunting comments and threatening rape.

Men and women often deal with sexual harassment differently. Whereas a woman may be more inclined to report harassing conduct, the traditional inclination of many men is just to "deal with it." This attitude has possibly led to less frequent reporting of male same-sex harassment.

Same-sex harassment cases will probably receive heavy media coverage. Treatment in the press will likely have a strong influence on whether men (or women in same-sex harassment situations) will keep harassment complaints to themselves or report them in the future.

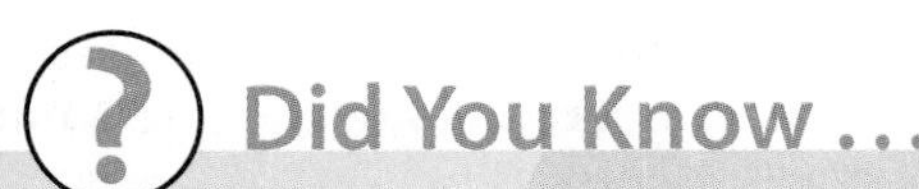

Addressing Sexual Harassment in the Military

A climate that negatively affects teamwork within a military unit impacts mission effectiveness. Consequently, the Department of Defense has specific policies and programs that support a zero-tolerance philosophy toward sexual harassment in the armed forces. Because women are essential to mission accomplishment, this is an issue that is addressed at every level of every military unit.

As gender-related incidents are investigated, they have been accompanied by a concerted effort of the Department of Defense to prevent recurrences. This has been demonstrated by the development and evaluation of programs designed to educate service members as to what constitutes sexual harassment, how to deal with it, and how to report incidents without fear of reprisal.

In an appearance before the Senate Armed Services Committee in 1997, Edwin Dorn, the undersecretary of defense for personnel and readiness, underscored the importance of military units' functioning as a team. He mentioned trust, loyalty, and self-sacrifice, issues not often relevant in large organizations. According to Mr. Dorn, a climate of discrimination and harassment will erode these elements that are essential for unit effectiveness (Dorn, 1997). Nevertheless, a policy can only be as strong as the program it supports. According to Sheila Widnall, former secretary of the air force, an Equal Opportunity program to support a zero-tolerance policy on harassment must be based on the following five principles:

1. A commander's personal commitment
2. The establishment of goals, principles, and standards of performance
3. Clear, concise written policies
4. Continual training through a military member's career
5. Complaint systems that are prompt, thorough, and fair and allow for resolution, support, reprisal prevention, and sanctions (Widnell & Dorn, 1995)

The military leadership has taken the initiative for monitoring the climate within the services. Programs have been developed to improve the climate through training, prevention, and resolution. These programs have been evaluated by using instruments such as command climate surveys, sensing sessions, and other internal review processes. They have also been examined by the media, congressional inquiry, and watchdog organizations. In 2000, an assessment of four key Department of Defense human relations programs that had been fielded or modified since 1997—the Command Climate Survey, The Army Values Program, the Consideration of Others Program, and Equal Opportunity (EO) Training Programs—was conducted. The purpose of this reassessment was to determine whether the establishment or revision of these programs had improved human relations in the Army. A total of 24,000 army leaders and soldiers were surveyed and interviewed. Among the findings were indications that although the army provides a generally effective human relations environment, many service members do not yet consider human relations an important component of combat readiness (Johnson & Harris, 2001).

Commanders are constantly working toward achieving zero tolerance for sexual harassment; they still have a way to go. The process for reporting incidents has been improved, thus increasing the prospect of investigation and resolution. This sends a clear message that members of the various armed services must be willing to report and be vigilant, and that these behaviors are not tolerated.

Susan M. Tendy, Ed.D.
Director of Assessment, Department of Physical Education
United States Military Academy
West Point, New York

Sources: Dorn, E. DoD committed to zero tolerance of sexual harassment, *Defense Issues, 12, no. 9* (1997), 1–4. Available: http://www.defenselink.mil/speeches/1997/di1209.html. Widnall, S. E. & Dorn, E. To stop harassment, leaders must lead. *Defense Issues, 10, no. 64* (May 1995), 1–5. Available: http://www.defenselink.mil/speeches/1995/di1064.html. Johnson, E. & Harris, B. Special Report 46: Human relations update 2000 executive summary (March 2001). Available: http://www.asamra.army.pentagon.mil/eo/eo_docs/human_relations.pdf.

their sexuality, forbidding of romantic relationships, and direct sexual come-ons from members of the coaching staff. It is important for college officials to establish preventive measures, such as educational training for coaches and athletes, to clarify exactly what constitutes harassment. In addition, there is a responsibility to provide resources to help deal with the problem (Heywood, 1999).

Many higher education administrators are reexamining policies on sexual harassment and finding difficult ethical and civil-liberties questions. Their goal is to write guidelines that identify and weed out harassing behavior without jeopardizing academic freedom or employees' due-process rights. Difficult questions need to be answered. The Universities of Iowa and Michigan have adopted rules declaring sexual relationships between faculty members and students unethical, but other institutions have rejected similar proposals, citing possible civil-rights violations (McMillen, 1986).

Some university officials feel there should be a general statement of the university's position on sexual harassment because it is not possible to cover specific situations adequately. Others feel that the specifics should be clearly spelled out to prevent potential confusion. Some officials feel policies should prohibit even consensual sexual relationships between students and faculty members. They argue that although such relationships may appear to be consensual, they are not because of the faculty member's position of authority. Others feel that consensual relationships are not the business of the university.

A sexual harassment policy at the University of Georgia, for example, specifically prohibits sexual relationships between faculty or staff and undergraduate students whom they are supervising or teaching. It also discourages relationships between superiors and subordinates among university employees and between faculty or staff and graduate students (Teacher–student relationships not tolerated, 1999).

Reactions to Sexual Harassment

Reactions to sexual harassment are influenced by individual characteristics and the severity of the harassing behavior. Sex, attitudes toward women, religiosity, and locus of control influence the way people say they would react to harassment (Baker, Terpstra, & Larntz, 1990).

However a person is affected by sexual harassment—as the harassee, the harasser, or as a manager—there are two common recommendations for action: responsibility and communication. Each of us has the responsibility for what we do and how we handle what others do to us. Open and honest communication is the only way to resolve a sexual harassment conflict; the manager, the harasser, and the harassee can usually work out the conflict if they remain objective and calm. A climate of responsibility and communication can prevent potential sexual harassment or resolve a problem if it occurs (Meyer, et al., 1981).

Sexual harassment responses can range from avoidance or defusion to negotiation or confrontation. Avoidance (ignoring the harassment or doing nothing) is quite common. Defusion (which includes responses such as going along, stalling, or making a joke of it) is a more active way to try to minimize the impact of conflict. Negotiation is a more assertive response and involves a direct request to the harasser to stop. This shifts the focus of the interaction to the victim's needs and priorities in the relationship. Confrontation, the most assertive response on this continuum, has two components: aggressive personal responses (such as telling the harasser to stop rather than simply asking) and use of the organizational power structure (such as making a formal complaint through channels) (Gruber, 1989).

Generally, a person being harassed has several options—personal action, company grievance, union grievance (if applicable), and legal action. Each situation influences the best way to handle the problem. There are two objectives for personal action: Attempt to stop the harassment and, if that fails, document it. If this fails and there is a grievance procedure, a complaint can be filed through prescribed channels. It is wise to be familiar with appropriate procedures and needed documentation. If this procedure also fails, and the person is a member of a union, filing a grievance with the union is another option. Again, it is important to know proper information and procedures. If none of these routes works, it may be necessary to pursue outside legal action. This involves a government agency first, such as the U.S. Equal Employment Opportunity Commission, and then, perhaps, a court system. The various legal options and procedures are confusing, but help is available. It is extremely important to document, to maintain a high performance level, and to pay attention to deadlines for filing a complaint (Meyer, et al., 1981).

Exploring the DIMENSIONS of Human Sexuality

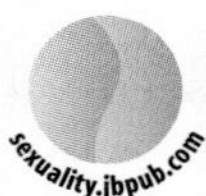

Our feelings, attitudes, and beliefs regarding sexuality are influenced by our internal and external environments. Go to sexuality.jbpub.com to learn more about the biological, psychological, and sociological factors that affect your sexuality.

Biological Factors

- Alcohol is a factor in 50% of rapes.
- Date-rape drugs produce disinhibition and an amnesialike effect, so that victims do not remember what happened.
- Younger people commit violent acts more often than older people.
- Although men and women attack each other at about the same rate (12%), as a result of the usually greater strength of men women are hurt more often and live in fear of further attacks.

Sociocultural Factors

- Socioeconomic status plays a role, as higher levels of aggression are found among lower-income populations. Pedophiles and the children they abuse are members of all socioeconomic and educational groups.
- People who believe in rape myths assign less blame to the perpetrator and more blame to the victim.
- Laws regarding sexual activity of teens vary among countries. Japanese law only prohibits sexual intercourse with someone younger than 12 years old—no other sexual activity, including child pornography, is covered.
- Deliberate interracial rape is uncommon; 88% of victims are the same race as the perpetrator.
- A cultural belief in patriarchy, whereby males have a dominant role over women, can promote abusive behavior.

Psychological Factors

- Sexual abuse in childhood contributes significantly to the risk of development of mental disorders later in life. Adolescent rape survivors have more behavioral problems than older survivors. Women with low self-esteem tend not to end an abusive relationship.

CASE STUDY

Many positive social changes have occurred over the past few decades to help the victims of forcible sexual behaviors. Although child sexual abuse has long occurred—Freud wrote about it almost 100 years ago—it was a hushed, taboo topic. Many victims thought that they were the "only one," or that they had done something wrong. Not anymore.

The media have been a positive force for change by giving coverage to forcible sexual behavior cases. The trial of O. J. Simpson—and the surrounding coverage about battered women—gave many victims the courage to step forward. Even TV shows inform children about what to do in case someone touches them in a way that makes them feel "uncomfortable."

The legal system has made huge strides in recent years, creating and enforcing laws and helping victims of forced sexual behaviors. Police have been trained to take domestic violence calls seriously, and not to let the perpetrator of violence off the hook.

Laws have been passed to help victims of sexual harassment at work or school. And, whereas in 1976 no man could be legally accused of raping his spouse, now marital rape laws have been passed in all 50 states.

Discussion Questions

1. What are the different categories of rape? Who are the rapists in these categories? What are the effects on the victims?
2. What effects does child abuse have on its survivors?
3. Describe the type of person that commits incest. What drives a seemingly "normal" individual to commit incest?
4. Explain why someone in an abusive marriage stays in the relationship. Can one be absolutely sure when a spouse should leave? Or is every situation different?
5. In what ways is sexual harassment the same and different in the workplace, in schools, in colleges, and in the military? Is the intent of harassment the same in each situation?

Application Questions

Reread the chapter-opening story and answer the following questions.

1. Is date rape a form of miscommunication or a form of sexual violence? Put another way, did Ed simply misinterpret the woman's resistance, assuming that "she wanted to be convinced to have sex"? Even if that was the case, did he have the right to continue sexual activity before she consented?
2. Assume for a moment that you are the woman who has just been date raped. What actions can and should you take? What might the consequences of those actions be for both you and the rapist?

Critical Thinking Questions

1. In 1991 a Florida federal judge ruled that pictures of naked and scantily clad women displayed in a workplace qualified as sexual harassment under Title VII of the 1964 Civil Rights Act. In his written opinion, the judge said that such a "boys' club" atmosphere is "no less destructive to workplace equality than a sign declaring 'Men Only.'" At the same time, the Florida branch of the American Civil Liberties Union denounced the decision as a possible violation of free speech. Under the federal court ruling, the company involved had to institute an antiharassment policy and take down the photos. In your opinion, what was the right decision in this situation?
2. Several women in an office complained to their human resources department that a male colleague had a photo of a woman in a bikini on his desk and that the photo created a "hostile working environment." When the man was confronted by his supervisor, he stated that the photo was of his wife, and he refused to remove it. What rights does the man have to display a photo of his wife? What rights do the women in the department have to object to the photo?

Critical Thinking Case

In the early 1990s, Paul Ingram, a deputy in the sheriff's department in Olympia, Washington, suddenly found himself accused of child abuse. His two daughters, aged 18 and 22 years, had just returned from a spiritual retreat when they suddenly recalled that their father had sexually abused them when they were children. During the retreat, a charismatic preacher had said that someone in the audience had been molested as a child—a plausible assumption in any audience given prevalence rates. The more the daughters remembered, the more their stories kept changing. The father was stunned, claiming he remembered no sexual abuse toward his daughters. But he also believed his daughters would never lie. Eventually, he confessed to abusing his daughters. In fact, the more he remembered, the clearer his memories of the events became. A psychologist tried an experiment on Paul, in which false information about abusing his children was told to him. Within days, Paul claimed to "remember" these made-up events. When told that these events had never taken place, Paul tried to retract his other statements from the legal process. Unfortunately, he was too late. Paul was convicted and sentenced to jail for his initial recalled memories (Wilson, et al., 1996).

Given this true case study of recovered memories, is it ethical to use them for treatment of a sexual abuse survivor? Is it ethical to use them to charge someone else with sexual assault or sexual abuse many years later? Explain your answer.

Exploring Personal Dimensions

Date Rape

Directions

This exercise is for those who are single and dating. Mark all that apply to you.

_____ 1. When dating, most of the excitement is to see what degree of intimacy I will be able to reach with this person (that is, how far we will go).

_____ 2. I test how far I will go (physical intimacy) with someone by progressive fondling (holding hands, putting arm around waist, rubbing back, chest, or breast and genitals) to see at what point the person will stop me.

_____ 3. When dating, I generally go with others or go somewhere public until I know someone.

_____ 4. I ask around about someone before I go out with her or him.

_____ 5. I make it very clear what my values are about physical intimacy when dating before difficult situations arise.

_____ 6. I have tried to coerce or talk someone into having sexual activity with me.

Scoring

Give yourself the following points for the items you checked, and total your score.

1.	3
2.	3
3.	−2
4.	−3
5.	−3
6.	5

Interpretation

3–11	You are potentially infringing on someone else's right to live within her or his value system and legal rights. You may be "date raping" or attempting date rape.
0–2	You have tendencies to infringe on someone else's right to live within her or his value system.
−1–−3	You are practicing moderately healthy dating precautions to avoid date rape.
−4–−8	You are practicing healthy dating precautions to avoid date rape.

Sexuality Online

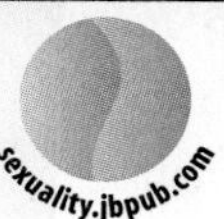

Go to the web component for *Exploring the Dimensions of Human Sexuality* at sexuality.jbpub.com for web exercises, additional resources related to this chapter, and student review tools.

Suggested Readings

Bohn, D. K. & Holz, K. A. Sequelae of abuse: Health effects of childhood sexual abuse, domestic battering, and rape, *Journal of Nurse-Midwifery, 41, no. 6* (1996), 442–456.

Brownmiller, S. *Against our will: Men, women, and rape.* New York: Simon & Schuster, 1975.

Easton, A. N., Summers, J., Tribble, J., Wallace, P. B., & Lock, R. S. College women's perceptions regarding resistance to sexual assault, *Journal of American College Health, 46, no. 3* (1997), 127–131.

Feinberg, C. Hitting home, *The American Prospect* (April 8, 2002), 30–34.

Fishbach, R. L. & Herbert, B. Domestic violence and mental health: Correlates and conundrums within and across cultures, *Social Science and Medicine, 45, no. 8* (1997), 1161–1176.

Forsyth, C. J. The structuring of vicarious sex, *Deviant-Behavior, 17, no. 3* (1996), 279–295.

King, M. & Woollett, E. Sexually assaulted males: 115 men consulting a counseling service, *Archives of Sexual Behavior, 26, no. 6* (1997), 579–588.

Kopper, B. A. Gender identity, rape myth acceptance, and time of initial resistance on the perception of acquaintance rape blame and avoidability, *Sex Roles, 34, no. 1–2* (1996), 81–93.

Lonsway, K. A. Preventing acquaintance rape through education: What do we know? *Psychology of Women Quarterly, 20* (1996), 229–265.

Lyons, P. The rape, *The Journal of Family Practice, 45, no. 6* (1997), 457–458.

Mansley, A. Caring for rape survivors, *Nursing Times, 94, no. 17* (1998), 24–26.

Schewe, P. A. & O'Donohue, W. Rape prevention with high-risk males: Short-term outcome of two interventions, *Archives of Sexual Behavior, 25, no. 5* (1996), 455–471.

Stormo, K. J., Lang, A. R., & Stritzke, W. G. K. Attributions about acquaintance rape: The role of alcohol and individual differences, *Journal of Applied Social Psychology, 27* (February 15, 1997), 279–305.

Struckman-Johnson, C. & Struckman-Johnson, D. Sexual coercion reported by women in three midwestern prisons, *Journal of Sex Research, 39, no. 3* (August 2002), 217–227.

CHAPTER 17

Sexual Consumerism

FEATURES

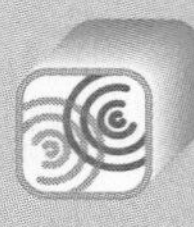

Communication Dimensions
Feelings About Sexual Themes

Ethical Dimensions
Controlling Cyberspace

Gender Dimensions
Male and Female Use of Autoerotic Materials

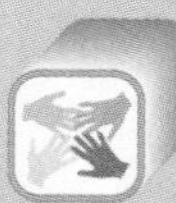

Multicultural Dimensions
"Values" of Prostitution in Other Countries?

Multicultural Dimensions
Organizations for Sex Workers

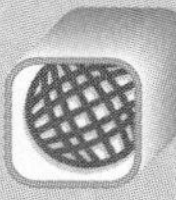

Global Dimensions
Sex Work in Other Countries

CHAPTER OBJECTIVES

1 Describe the ways in which sexuality is used in the mass media, including in advertising, TV, movies, literature, popular music and on the Internet.

2 Discuss what constitutes sexually explicit materials, the results of research on their effects, and efforts to control their distribution.

3 Describe the different types of sex workers and the economic factors associated with sex work.

sexuality.jbpub.com
Advertising
Literature
The Control of Sexually Explicit Materials

INTRODUCTION

Not long ago, in a human sexuality class, the conversation turned to the relationship between sexuality and money. Some students were surprised when others became very interested in the topic. They seemed to feel that there was nothing to be gained by continuing the conversation because they did not see a relationship between sexuality and money.

The students interested in the topic persisted. One of the communication majors pointed out that in his classes he learned that messages and products related to sexuality are big business. The saying "You've come a long way, baby" definitely applies to this topic for better or worse, he pointed out. He went on to say that we are all bombarded with sexual themes daily; that you cannot turn on TV, pick up a magazine, or see a billboard without being confronted with sexual topics and themes. This use of sexual content, he indicated, is designed to sell even products that have no relation to sexuality.

Some other students warmed up to the discussion. One student, a psychology major, mentioned that commercialism related to sexuality has taken another form as well. Products specifically related to sexuality are available in large numbers and in great variety. Whether you want to put it in, dangle it about, or place it on, there is a store where you can get whatever "it" is.

Several students started arguing about whether the use of sexual themes to influence consumers is good or bad. One health education major argued that the use of sexual themes to sell products unrelated to sexuality is sexploitation, with the potential for sexism. He said this situation could prompt people to view others as sex objects, and it could interfere with personal relationships and sexual satisfaction as well—because when one compares one's partner against the commercialized ideal seen in the media, one is likely to be disappointed. This could lead to frustration and a mean-spiritedness that might translate into poor communication, sexual and otherwise.

Another student, a business major, jumped into the fray and added that the pressure to be like people in the ads—sexy, gorgeous, hunky—may cause people to feel inferior and ashamed of their body. Feelings of inferiority and shame, as we learned earlier (Chapter 15), can progress to sexual dysfunction.

Still another student pointed out that appearance may not be the only concern. She expressed concern that as the result of observing the sexual prowess of television and movie stars on-screen, we assume that all of us should be able to affect our partners the same way. If they do not swoon at the very thought of a caress from us, if they do not get light-headed when we place an arm around them, if they do not lick their lips when they see us in a state of semiundress, we may believe that we are ineffective lovers. Thus, because of unrealistic depictions of sexual behavior in the movies and TV, ordinary people like us may fear losing our lovers because we cannot sexually satisfy them.

A nursing major argued that some people value sexual commercialization. Whether because idealized views of sexual activity are exciting, because they have potential for improving sexual relationships by indicating new ways to relate, or because they help to desensitize people to an emotionally charged topic (namely, sexuality), these views are considered a positive trend by many people, he said.

The students' discussion was useful in that it covered most of the points that the instructor wanted to raise before starting the chapter on sexuality and commercial activities. Regardless of our points of view, sexual commercialization is probably here to stay. This chapter considers how sexuality is used in a commercial sense and will help you become a better sexual consumer.

Mass Media and the Arts

Advertising

Advertisements in magazines and newspapers that use sexual themes to sell products are abundant. One need only turn at random to any page and more than likely an ad or an article that has some relationship to sex or sexual attractiveness will be evident. Most of this kind of advertising is pretty obvious if you give it a moment's thought, but in the 1970s a book called *Subliminal Seduction*—about subliminal sexual selling—created a furor (Key, 1973). The main premise of the author, Wilson Key, was that many advertisers who used sexual imagery to sell their products intended it to work on the viewer's subconscious, not conscious, awareness. To support his premise

Key cited the following kinds of imagery he had found in enlarged photographs taken from magazine ads:

1. Images of people engaged in sexual activity, hidden in the shading of ice cubes in liquor advertisements
2. The word *fuck* or *sex*, written in very small letters, hidden in the ads
3. Pictures that appeared innocent on one side of a magazine page but that made sexual suggestion when held up to the light—for example, a picture of a woman standing on the front of a blank sheet, backed by a picture of a projectile (such as an airplane or cigar) aimed at her vagina
4. Pictures composed to suggest genitals—for instance, of liquor bottles with small round objects on each side (such as oranges or apples) suggesting a penis and two testicles

Some critics have argued that Key went too far and that looking for sexual connotations in ice cubes is in itself perverse. In fact, many feel that Key had no evidence or research to support his ideas. Marketers have since produced research evidence indicating that subliminal advertising is a farce. Ads crafted to appeal to basic needs are apparently highly effective, even without the kinds of things Key described. As we shall see in this chapter, we buy many products without fully understanding why. Those selling us these products, though, know that one of the hidden motivations behind our buying habits relates to sexuality. We want to appear sexy, appeal to a potential sex mate, and feel attractive; knowing this, salespeople use these needs to persuade us to buy products, even though we think we are buying them for reasons totally divorced from sexuality.

Advertisers seem to have made a study of sexual motivation. Some research from as long ago as 1973 suggested that since oral–genital activity had become relatively acceptable and widely practiced (Hunt, 1974), it found its way into product advertising. What better way to sell cigarettes to women, for example, than to associate cigarettes with penises? For years cigarettes have been used as phallic symbols. Beginning in the 1930s, cigarette ads featured only men offering cigarettes to women, employing phallic symbolism. We remember cigarette ads with words such as *longer, firmer, rounder, more satisfying, better tasting,* and *more pleasing* (not to mention *more fully packed*).

Automobile advertisements make obvious use of sexual appeals, along with appeals to such other needs as recognition and esteem. When cars were long and well-adorned, they were presented as phallic symbols. *Real* men, the ads suggested, wanted long cars. The tips of automobiles were even ornamented. Today, although car companies sell smaller cars as a rule, their ads still associate the product with sexuality, sometimes by posing pretty, well-endowed, scantily clad, and perfectly proportioned females beside cars. At automobile shows, held in coliseums and arenas throughout the United States, companies employ young female models (again scantily clad) to adorn their displays.

A number of years ago another blatant sexual appeal to consumers was employed by the advertisers of a caffeine-containing over-the-counter "picker-upper" tablet. The ad campaign for this product was directed at the insecurity of women who did not work outside the home, presenting the pill as a remedy for that tired feeling associated with the routine of housework. The ads suggested that women owed it to their mate to greet him at the front door looking sexy and not tired. The ads exhorted female readers to pop some of the pills before their mate's arrival to be assured of eternal loyalty.

Myth vs Fact

Myth: In recent years, there has been an increased and about equal use of male and female body exposure in advertisements.
Fact: There has been an increase in breast and total female body exposure, but female body exposure is about four times more common than male body exposure.

Myth: Women appear more often than men in television beer commercials.
Fact: Men appear twice as often as women in television beer commercials.

Myth: Television is the main source of information about sexuality for teenagers.
Fact: Friends are the main source of information about sexuality for teenagers.

Myth: Fraudulent sexual aids are not among the top sources of health fraud in the United States.
Fact: According to the Food and Drug Administration, fraudulent sexual aids are among the top 10 sources of health fraud in the United States.

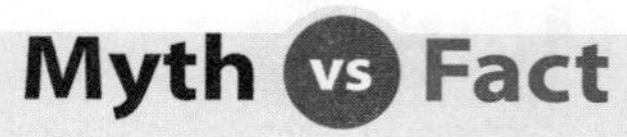

Myth: There are special exercises and/or creams that are helpful in increasing the size of a female's breasts.
Fact: Breast size and shape are the result of glandular influences and cannot be altered by exercise or by application of anything to the breast.

Myth: Prostitution is illegal in most countries around the world.
Fact: In many countries there are no laws against prostitution. In fact, the United Nations adopted a resolution in favor of decriminalization of prostitution.

Myth: It is illegal to release the names of those accused of using prostitutes or the prostitutes themselves publicly until they have been shown to be guilty in a court of law.
Fact: Although some civil liberties groups object, in some states the identities of prostitutes and their customers are made public as soon as they are arrested—before any court action occurs.

Lest male readers feel superior, remember that advertisement in which someone mistakes the man for his wife's father? His vanity wounded, the fellow dyes his hair to remove the gray, thereby keeping his wife, his pride, and his job—and lining the pockets of the dye manufacturers.

Liquor ads are particularly notable for linking sexual imagery to our aspirations for living well. The people depicted as liquor drinkers are handsome, well dressed, sophisticated, flirtatious, and the object of someone else's unconcealed attention. Readers are supposed to envy the exciting life these attractive people live and, through their choice of liquor purchases, to emulate them.

Whether intended for this purpose or not, advertisements can send sexual messages as well as messages related to gender bias. For example, over a 10-year period there was a significant increase in breast exposure and total female body exposure even though fashion trends did not account for this change. In addition, female body exposure was about four times more common than male body exposure, in part because women were displayed in underwear and bikini swimsuits more often than were men (Plous & Neptune, 1997).

The use of sexual themes to sell products has expanded in some interesting ways. For example, in 2001 Abercrombie & Fitch said its summer catalog was sexy in a wholesome sort of way. Critics called it soft porn and joined forces to boycott the trendy youth-oriented retailer. The catalog featured young unclad male and female models to woo younger customers and use sexual themes to popularize the image of the company (Crary, 2001).

In Europe, Durex, the world's number one condom maker, started a TV and print advertising campaign using humor. In one TV ad a young man walking down the street to meet his date is followed by a boisterous and excited crowd of men dressed in white sperm costumes. The sperm are suddenly trapped, squirming, in a huge condom in the middle of the street. The ad has the tagline "Durex: For a Hundred Million Reasons" (Durex condom maker using "humor" ads to sell condoms in Europe, 2001).

Television Advertising and Programming

More Americans have television sets than phones. About a third of our free time is spent watching television—TV sets in the average home are on about 7 hours per day. Content analysis shows sexuality topics are far more explicit today than they were a decade or two ago (Brown & Steele, 1996).

Kuriansky (1996) provided an interesting historical overview of sexuality and television advertising. Here are some of the highlights:

1. Beer led the way for using sexual themes to sell. One TV ad in the 1950s showed a tired husband growing perky after drinking a beer. He then chased his wife around the room while disrobing.
2. Car spots also pioneered the sexy sell by using sexy models draped over the hood or stroking the wheel suggestively.
3. In 1980 then-15-year-old Brooke Shields panted that nothing came between her and her Calvins. Though some versions of the ad were banned, jeans sales doubled.
4. In the early 1990s a group of female employees sued Stroh's brewery for sexual harassment and named the company's "Swedish Bikini Team" campaign (featuring buxom, blonde, bikini-clad women) as contributing to a "hostile work environment."
5. In 1995 the FBI investigated a Calvin Klein ad featuring an underage teen stripping for a photographer. Many pairs of jeans were sold.

6. Candies hiking boots received more free exposure than paid air time when a furor erupted over the censorship of scenes of a nude couple straddling a chair.
7. What is acceptable on U.S. TV is often tame compared to that in other parts of the world where full frontal nudity is used to sell everything from shock absorbers to sardines. In a Danish TV spot, a newspaper is draped over a man's erect penis as he spies on ladies in the steam room.
8. Cloaking sexuality in romance is one way to prevent controversy. The Taster's Choice soap-opera-like spots follow a handsome neighbor invited in for coffee and whatever else.

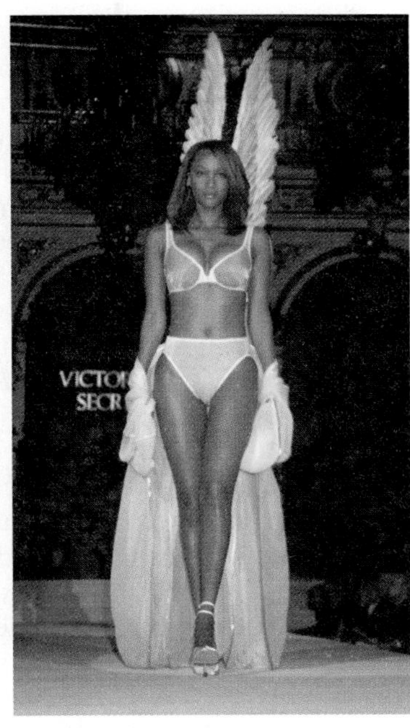

Victoria's Secret became a multibillion-dollar company by redefining the market for underwear. Here the model Tyra Banks shows off the "Angels" line of lingerie at a fashion show. After a single TV ad shown during the 1999 Super Bowl, more than 1 million people inundated the Victoria's Secret web site, hoping for a glimpse of more "fashion."

9. Humor also relieves the anxiety of sexual suggestion. In another ad, the actress Annie Potts is lifted into a hulk's arms while extolling the virtues of large popcorn kernels.
10. It seems that sexual themes will always sell. The Candies CEO said: "In 30 to 60 seconds, to keep people from going to the refrigerator, you have to astound them. And sex does."

Providing a different point of view, the consumer behaviorist Solomon (1996) pointed out that although "sex sells," using sex may actually be counterproductive to the marketer. A provocative picture can be too effective by attracting so much attention that it hinders processing and recall of the ad's contents. Sexual appeals can be ineffective if used merely as a means to grab attention. They do, however, seem to work when the product is itself sexually related, in an ad for a cologne or other product to enhance interpersonal attraction.

Interestingly, men appear twice as often as women in television beer commercials. However, women's bodies and body parts appear more often than pictures of men's bodies. Women also appear more often in swimwear than do men. Concerns have been raised about the dehumanizing influence of these images in beer commercials (Hall & Crum, 1994).

Still, before people will watch commercials, they have to be enticed to watch programs. And entertainment, as advertising, has become highly eroticized—sometimes quite explicitly in movies and now more often explicitly on television as well.

An estimated 30 million adults are regular viewers of daytime soap operas. Over a 10-year period, an analysis of several soaps showed a 35% increase in sexual activity. The frequency of sexual acts climbed from 3.7 per hour to 5 per hour. Two of the soaps averaged 7 to 11 acts per hour. At the same time that the soaps are fraught with myriad sexual relationships, stories now are dealing more frequently with younger viewers' concerns such as date rape, pregnancy, and learning to say no to sexual relations (Greenberg & Busselle, 1996).

The television sitcom has changed dramatically in the past few decades. Three of every four shows in the "family hour" contain sexually related talk or behavior. Most of this sex play does not proceed to sexual intercourse, but characters seem to talk about sexual topics all the time (Hass, 1997). Americans are exposed to more than 9,000 scenes of sexual intercourse, sexual comment, or innuendo in an average year of TV viewing. The Federal Communications Commission's indecency standard is so vague that enforcement is virtually impossible. Meanwhile, the vast majority of Americans register their approval of sexual themes in programs by tuning in more frequently (Crossen, 1991).

Relatedly, dating shows have become to the 21st century what sleazy talk and courtroom shows were to the late 1990s (Poniewozic, 2002). The popularity of shows such as *Blind Date, Temptation Island, The Bachelor, The Dating Experiment, Love Shack, Who Wants to Marry a Millionaire,* and *The Bachelorette* has shown that people want to observe others in their sexual relationships. These shows can make love and romance look phony at best, vicious at worst. But large numbers of people seem to enjoy these shows.

The Kaiser Family Foundation reported a significant increase (from 56% to 68%) in the amount of sexual content on TV from 1991 to 2001. However, they also found that awareness regarding selected topics (such as STIs) significantly increased among viewers who watched programs involving such topics (Sex on TV, 2001).

The Parents' Television Council also reported on the amount of sex and violence on TV (Elber, 2001). As compared to that in 1999, the council found that use of coarse language on TV had increased by 78% to 2.6 instances an hour. If milder curse words were included in the tally, the per-hour rate of foul language usage would reach 6.1. Although sexual material dipped 17%, to a per-hour average of 3.1 instances, it was more raw than in the past. Oral sexual behavior, pornography, masturbation, and kinky practices that a generation ago might not have been discussed even on late-evening series were mentioned on family hour shows.

Characters in MTV commercials, like those in music videos and other commercials, are stereotyped. Females appear less frequently, have more beautiful bodies, wear more sexy and skimpy clothing, and are more often the object of another's gaze than their male counterparts (Signorielli, McLeod, & Healy, 1994).

Many people have protested the television industry's portrayal of sexual themes in everyday life. Although objections to the portrayal of explicit sexual activities and the use of sexual language have been raised some time, today people are beginning to object to the nature and quality of the sexual relationships enacted—stereotypical roles, sexual violence and hostility, incessant teasing, and more physical than emotional display—and to be con-

Did You Know . . .

Personal ads in newspapers have been around for many years but are much more prevalent now. They can be found on the Internet, in newspapers, in magazines, and on the radio. A radio station that has a phone-dating service will hook you up with people of a similar demographic and music-taste level. Even legitimate regional magazines, like *Boston* magazine, carry personal ads. Your choice of whom you want may be partially influenced by where he or she advertises. For example, advertising in *Boston* magazine is much more expensive than advertising in the local newspapers, so such ads may attract a more upscale clientele.

cerned about the effects of these views of sexuality on socialization of the young.

The 1996 Telecommunications Act directed the U.S. Federal Communications Commission (FCC) to "prescribe guidelines and recommend procedures for the identification and rating of television programs that contain sexual, violent, or other indecent material about which parents should be informed before it is displayed to their children"—but only if the television industry does not itself establish voluntary labeling procedures. The American Civil Liberties Union (ACLU) objects to a government labeling scheme for three reasons:

1. Mandating labels compels private individuals and companies to say things about their creative offerings that they have no wish to say and even puts the words into their mouths. Such compelled speech is as much a violation of First Amendment rights as enforced silence.
2. The categories of expression (sexual, violent, and indecent) singled out for adverse treatment through labeling are inherently and hopelessly vague. Trying to distinguish among types of material would enmesh the government in an unconstitutional process of policing thought and censoring ideas.
3. Any FCC-prescribed ratings system would have the unconstitutional purpose and effect of restricting expression because it was unpopular or controversial (ACLU Freedom Network, 1998).

A television rating system was adopted in 1997. The ratings system includes age-based symbols like those for movies, such as TV-G, TV-PG, TV-14, and TV-MA, as well as the codes V, S, L, and D to indicate violence, sexual themes, "adult" language, and suggestive dialogue. However, in 1998 the Kaiser Family Foundation pointed out that (1) 79% of the shows with violence did not carry a V notation; (2) 92% of the shows with sexual themes did not have an S, and 91% with adult language did not include an L notation; (3) 83% of the shows with suggestive dialogue did not have the D, and 81% of the children's shows that contain violence did not carry the FV code, which warns parents of fantasy violence like that shown in cartoons. As of 1999 the ratings were used in conjunction with the v-chip blocking technology available on television sets. However, if the ratings themselves are not accurate, the v-chip will not block much of the sexual content and violence from television (The parent trap, 1998).

As mentioned earlier, TV programming affects what teenagers know about sexuality. For example, in response to the question "From what sources do teenagers today mainly learn about sex?" the proportion of adult Americans indicating TV as a main source increased from 11% in 1986 to 29% in 1998. By comparison, friends were given as the main source by 45%, followed by parents (7%) and sexuality education (3%). For better or worse, television shows filled with sexual content help shape young people's opinions (Stodghill, 1998).

As stated at the beginning of this chapter, the commercial use of sexual themes has its positive sides as well. According to a Harvard University study of 1,400 parents of children between 3 and 11 years of age, more than half the families believed that children learned more about sexuality from television than from any other source except the parents themselves. "A surprising number of parents reported that they rarely discussed sex with their children, but admitted that they noticed their children (particularly heavy viewers) picking up a great many ideas about sex—and a corresponding interest in it—from the tube." The authors who cited this study (Singer &

Singer, 1982) argue that television can be a useful means of dispensing information about sexuality and health, as, for instance, in programs on sex and pregnancy.

Furthermore, television is an excellent way to educate people about healthy sexual practices. For instance, the surgeon general of the United States warned that the spread of HIV and AIDS could be slowed only by sexual abstinence or the use of condoms during coitus. Fortunately, in recent years we have seen an increase in condom ads on television.

Some broadcasters worry that the public disapproves of condom ads, and some worry they would lose sponsors that do not want their ads run alongside condom ads. However, 71% of Americans favor allowing condom ads on TV: 37% support the ads running at any time and 34% support the ads' running at certain times, such as after 10 P.M. Even more support exists among adults less than 50 years of age, of whom 82% say that condom ads should be allowed (Pardun & Forde, 2002/2003).

Among the top 20 TV shows among teens, 83% included some sexual content, including 20% with sexual intercourse. Among shows with sexual content involving teenagers, 34% included a safer sex reference, almost twice the rate of 4 years earlier. Safer-sex messages still appear on a minority of shows that teens watch (More sex scenes, but more mention of "safer sex" on TV shows, 2003).

The topics discussed on television talk shows make the soap operas and many other television shows seem almost tame in comparison. Many talk show hosts compete for guests willing to make public confessions about intimate sexual relations and feelings. On-air confrontations and rowdy showdowns keep viewers tuned in (Brown & Steele, 1996).

On cable TV, the fastest growing segment is adult programming that portrays explicit sexual behavior. As cable availability expands to a potential 500 channels, even more such programming is expected.

Communication DIMENSIONS

Feelings About Sexual Themes In Chapter 3 we outlined a basic communication model. We also talked about common communication problems, including (1) frame of reference, (2) emotional interference, and (3) physical distractions. Talk with two or three of your classmates about difficulties two people in an intimate relationship might have in these three areas when they are discussing the following topics:

1. Which characters do you think are the sexiest in current television shows? Why?
2. Which ads on TV or in magazines do you find most offensive? Why?
3. What does it take for materials to be considered obscene?
4. What TV shows and/or movies do you think are most sexually stimulating? Why?
5. If you were a writer for a television series, how would you use sexual themes?

For example, in a discussion about sexy television shows, there could be a difference in language considered acceptable or in what might be considered sexy. This could cause emotional interference. Or perhaps one person could not relate to why something is sexually stimulating to another person. Thus, one person's frame of reference could cause a problem. Go through each of the five questions with at least two or three other people and see what other possible barriers you can identify. Why do you think these barriers exist? What might be done about them to improve communication?

Many television programs have been devoted to educating the public about HIV and AIDS, and other programs have focused on such topics as sexual orientation and extramarital sexual activities. Many of these programs follow a talk show format or are presented as documentaries; however, some sexual topics and issues are dramatized with the intent of entertaining and educating at the same time. For example, one situation comedy depicted a teenager's being instructed to use a condom with his girlfriend, and another weekly comedy show depicted an unmarried couple living together and the problems they encountered.

Addressing the media in general, a position statement of the Sexuality Information and Education Council of the United States (SIECUS, 1995) indicates that

> *the media have a powerful influence on all aspects of society. With this power goes a major responsibility to present the complexities of human sexuality at all stages of the life cycle in a manner that is accurate, sensitive to diversity, and free of exploitation, gratuitous sexual violence, and dehumanizing sexual portrayals.*

Recommendations for realistic, accurate images concerning sexuality in the media include (Edwards, 1996) the following:

1. Dialogue that shows true communication among children, their parents, and trusted adults
2. Situations that show planned mature relationships as opposed to spur-of-the-moment responses to passion
3. Situations in which unprotected sexual encounters have negative repercussions
4. Articulate responsible characters with whom teenagers can identify

In 2001 the Media Project presented SHINE (Sexual Health in Entertainment) awards to honor those in the entertainment industry who do an examplary job of incorporating accurate and honest portrayals of sexuality in their programming (Media project announces, 2001). Examples of award winners are an ABC *20/20* documentary in which children of a lesbian couple and children of a gay couple speak out about their parents and their family life, a program on Iowa Public Television in which youths discuss the risks and responsibilities of sexual activity, and a FOX drama episode related to the health risks of oral sexual activity.

Interestingly, teens 15 to 17 years old believe that sexual content on TV influences the behavior of their peers, but not their own. They also report some positive aspects of sexual content on TV. They say they had learned how to say no in an uncomfortable sexual situation, that they had learned how to communicate with a partner about safer sex, and that they had talked with their parents about a sexuality-related issue because of something they saw on TV (Notes from the research, 2002).

Sexuality and the Movies

Any cursory glance at the entertainment section of your local newspaper will show that movies are often marketed to the public by means of sexual themes—and have been for some time. In *The Blue Angel,* a 1930 film starring Marlene Dietrich (1930 was a time when women's bathing suits were much more than three small patches of flimsy cloth precariously held together by string), images of Marlene's bare thighs in a cabaret outfit made men's heads whirl. In *She Done Him Wrong,* when Mae West invited Cary

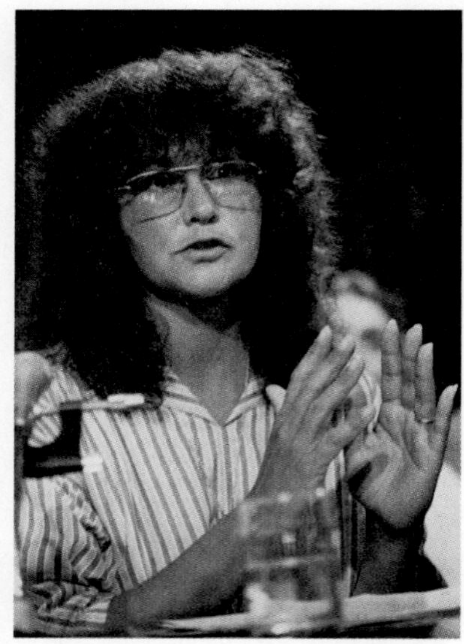

Linda Lovelace, former porn star, now openly campaigns against sexually explicit movies. Lovelace was threatened into starring in *Deep Throat* by a physically abusive husband/manager. As were countless other young actresses, Lovelace was led to believe that appearing in adult films would open the door to legitimate film work. Yet only one well-known porn star, "Traci Lords," has ever made that transition.

Grant to "come up and see me some time," men's knees knocked. When Clark Gable (Rhett Butler) carried Vivian Leigh (Scarlett O'Hara) up a flight of stairs to her bedroom in *Gone with the Wind,* women swooned; when Marlon Brando appeared in his ripped undershirt in *A Streetcar Named Desire,* they panted. People's imaginations and perceptions, rather than nudity or sexual activity on film, were integral components of cinematic sexuality during the 1930s, 1940s, and 1950s.

By the 1960s and the 1970s, sexual permissiveness and experimentation had permeated the movies, as well as other segments of society. Movies previously shown as stag films and often called blue movies were elevated to respectable status. With the showing of *I Am Curious (Yellow), Deep Throat, Beyond the Valley of the Dolls, Vixen, The Lickerish Quartet,* and *Behind the Green Door* in movie theaters (in spite of attempts by local communities to ban them), people seemed to be less shocked. Although well-known movie stars had sometimes appeared nude in films in earlier years, a new era began when Marlon Brando appeared in the X-rated *Last Tango in Paris* in the early 1970s. The films of the past 25 years leave little to the imagination and appeal more to the voyeur in us.

To help parents and others make decisions about the appropriateness of a particular movie for themselves or their children, a rating system was developed by the Motion Picture Association of America:

G—Appropriate for the general audience.

PG—Appropriate for the general audience; however, parental guidance is advised. There may be brief nudity or some brief moments of sexually explicit language.

PG-13—Parents are advised that some of the material may be inappropriate for younger children.

R—Restricted to people at least 17 years of age or those accompanied by an adult due to sexual content, sexually explicit language, or violence.

NC-17—No one under 17 years of age admitted. Extremely sexual in nature, and/or containing explicit sexual language, or extremely violent (but not necessarily pornographic).

In 1994 a Gallup Poll of 1,800 moviegoers revealed that R-rated films were the most popular, especially among 18- to 34-year-olds. Thirty-nine percent of viewers preferred them. Twenty-seven percent preferred films with PG-13 ratings, 16% preferred films with PG ratings, 7% preferred NC-17-rated films, and 6% preferred G-rated films (Smilgis & Thigpen, 1994).

Although we probably assume that there is now more sexual content in movies than there used to be, this is not necessarily the case. A content analysis of a random sample of films from a 20-year period was made by a group of trained raters, who rated sexual content in eight categories: (1) sexual acts seen or heard, (2) sexual acts implied, (3) violent sexual acts, (4) nudity, (5) anatomical slang, (6) presence in a sex-related setting (topless bar, and so on), (7) sexual jokes, and (8) sexual references (sexual gestures and descriptions of sexual encounters). The average number of sexual situations in the course of a movie was 28.9. This indicated that about every 4 minutes a sexual situation occurred. References to condom use or safer sexual activity were virtually nonexistent. Sexual relationships were, by far, most common among people who were not married to each other. However, few changes in sexual content in movies were found (Klein & Serrins, 1998).

In August 1998 a movie theater owner in South Carolina decided not to show R-rated movies in his theater even if he went bankrupt in the process. After the first month of the self-imposed ban, attendance dropped to 1,200 customers a week from 2,000. Profits were off 50% in November and 32% in December as compared to those the previous year. He estimated he lost

$20,000 at his theater in just 5 months. He had thought people supported his ban: "We had vocal support, but people were just not showing up to see the movies. If the public doesn't want it, who am I doing it for?" In January 1999 he backed off his moral stand because it was costing him too much money. He started showing R-rated movies again (Owner reinstates R-rated movies, 1999).

As with television and advertising, some people believe that the sexual explicitness of movies is detrimental to society, and others see this trend as positive. The opponents cite the weak commitments of sexual partners as partly responsible for the soaring adultery and divorce rates by setting poor examples of the meaning of intimate relationships. Those in favor of sexual explicitness in movies see this as just one sign of our increased openness about sexuality and the pleasures inherent in sexual behavior. We must make our own decisions about the appropriateness of this trend.

Videotapes

The VCR provides easy access to sexually explicit materials. Despite the R rating that supposedly restricts viewing to people 17 years or older unless accompanied by an adult, two-thirds of a sample of high school students in Michigan reported that they were allowed to rent or watch any movie they wanted, and the movies they most frequently viewed were R-rated (Brown & Steele, 1996).

The videotape rental business has grown by leaps and bounds. In almost any community, video rental shops are found. These stores stock popular movies soon after they are shown in neighborhood theaters. In addition to these popular movies, often a separate area houses the X-rated videocassette library, usually out of view so customers are not offended by the movies' enticing packages and children are not exposed to them. Shelves and shelves of the most sexually explicit films are available to rent and to view in the privacy of one's home.

The availability of sexually explicit material has alarmed some people. They consider these X-rated movies to be pure trash with the potential to instigate sexual violence and to stereotype females as sex objects. They argue that these materials are obscene and pornographic and, as such, should be prohibited. However, others view the openness toward sexual expression of various kinds to be healthy. They argue that a couple's sexual relationship can be enhanced by viewing sexually explicit films, learning about new sexual activities, or being implicitly given permission to act out sexual fantasies. The courts have ruled that people have the right to rent sexually explicit videotapes and rental shop owners have the right to make such videotapes available. However, pressure from local groups in some communities has convinced shop owners voluntarily to remove the X-rated tapes from their stock. In one view, this expression of community standards is considered healthy and the epitome of the democratic process at work. In another view, it is described as the "uptight" majority's dictating sexual mores to the more sexually comfortable minority. As we learned previously, one's view of sexual morality relates to the valuing of one's ethical principles; this is an example of that process at work.

Evidence suggests that about 70% of adult videos are rented by women. They are rented most frequently on weekend nights and used by married couples after the kids have gone to bed. Four common themes have been noted in sexually explicit videos: high levels of sexual desire, diverse sexual activity, many sexual partners readily available, and pleasure as the purpose of sexual activity (Brosius, Weaver, & Staab, 1993). In 1998 sexually explicit video rentals and sales were a $4.2 billion-a-year business (nearly 14% of all video transactions and more than a quarter of the home-video industry's revenue) (Stein, 1998).

Some videos have been produced for use by couples in their homes. Sexologists have made videos that provide explicit graphic instruction to help improve sexual relationships.

Literature

As with the content of movies, TV programs, and videos, the public has become desensitized to sexually explicit material in books. However, it was not always this way. For example, in 1928 D. H. Lawrence's *Lady Chatterly's Lover* was published. Because of its sexual explicitness, it was banned in the United States until 1959. James Joyce's *Ulysses,* published in 1934, deals with masturbation, prostitution, adultery, and voyeurism. It was not allowed into the United States for years but is now considered to be a masterpiece.

In the last few decades thousands of books of varying literary quality that openly treat sexual topics have been published. Sometimes they weave themes related to sexuality into a meaningful story, but other times their authors seem to be gratuitously writing about sexual thoughts and activity as much as possible. Many earlier works appear tame compared to what is now available. What was previously considered risque, if not actually immoral or illegal, has now come to be expected in a bestseller.

Sexually arousing material, of course, has existed for centuries. The ancient *Kamasutra* and *The Perfumed Garden,* Chaucer's *Canterbury Tales* and Boccaccio's *Decameron* (both 14th-century works), Li Yu's *Flesh Prayer Mat,* and the *Memoirs of Casanova* are examples of early erotic literature. However, more and more of our popular literature that is not primarily erotic is at least partly concerned with its characters' sexual activities. For example, romance literature relies on fantasy rather than sexual explicitness; its purpose is to tantalize and to nourish sexual fantasies, rather than to tell a good story. About 46% of all mass-market paperbacks are romance novels, read by both women and men (Bartley, 1994).

Magazines have made their mark as well. *Esquire: The Magazine for Men* appeared in 1933. Twenty years later *Playboy* appeared on the newsstands. It offered information about sexuality, an open philosophy toward sexuality, and photographs of nude women along with some stimulating stories. Its approach was followed by many other magazines. In the late 1960s other magazines, such as *Penthouse, Oui,* and *Hustler,* published pictures of nude males and females as well as people engaged in assorted sexual activities. Some even had a classified section allowing people to advertise their sexual services or request sexual partners.

As women asked for a more balanced view, magazines such as *Cosmopolitan* and *Playgirl* began printing photos of nude men and stories with appeal for women. Traditionally, women's maga-

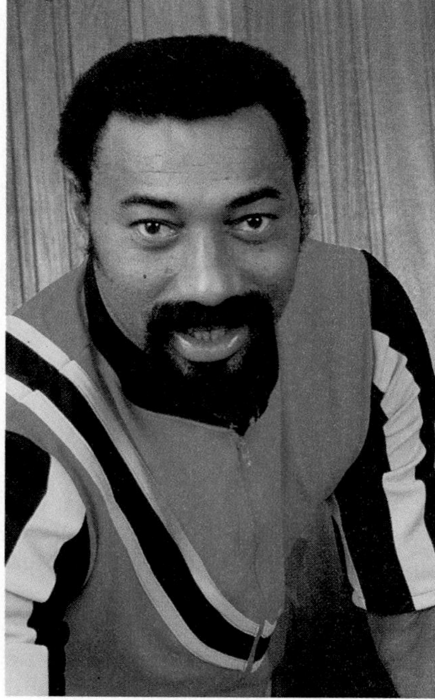

The NBA Hall of Famer Wilt Chamberlain learned the hard way that sex does not sell. After Chamberlain wrote an autobiography rich in basketball lore, published in 1991, his editor decided that it needed something extra—thus the editor came up with the idea that Chamberlain had slept with 20,000 women. Not only did the public find such a feat repulsive during the height of the AIDS epidemic, it was also inconsistent with Chamberlain's character. After the book failed, Chamberlain himself called the marketing scheme "the biggest mistake" of his life.

zines have focused on two broad topics: what a woman should do to get a man *(Cosmopolitan)* and what a woman should do once she has the man and his children *(Redbook)*. Other magazines have attempted to include other aspects of women's lives. For example, *Working Woman* and *Savvy* are aimed at women who work outside the home. *Ms.* magazine, the only women's magazine explicitly dedicated to feminism and the facts about women's sexuality, struggled for 20 years to attract enough advertising. The magazine finally gave up on advertising and now relies on a hefty subscription price for revenue. Consequently, circulation of around 500,000 dropped to 179,000 (Brown & Steele, 1996).

Magazines collectively play a role as communicators on a range of sexual health topics (Sexual health coverage in women's, men's, teen and other specialty magazines, 2000). The Kaiser Family Foundation found that 34% of articles in women's magazines, 28% of articles in men's magazines, and 42% of articles in teen magazines focused on sexual health issues. However, the emphasis is different. For example, women's magazines emphasize pregnancy, and especially planned pregnancy, contraception, and abortion. Men's magazines mainly address concerns such as STIs, including HIV and AIDS, and the few male-controlled methods of contraception; teen magazines focus on the potential adverse outcomes of sexual activity, such as STIs and unintended pregnancy. They also address the difficult decisions many teens face about whether to become sexually active.

Adult bookstores specialize in highly sexually arousing books. These stores are adult in the sense that a person must be of legal age to enter. Such establishments also sell sex-illustrated magazines, newspapers, postcards, decks of playing cards, and videotapes. Many communities have attempted to outlaw adult bookstores (through the courts and local government statute) or to limit their location to one part of the community. Nevertheless, all major cities have them, as do many smaller cities and towns. Furthermore, many conventional bookstores, recognizing a market for sexually explicit literature, maintain sections devoted to such books and magazines. As with sexuality in the movies, the cost and benefit of adult bookstores versus the risks of censorship is a topic of heated debate.

In addition to sexually explicit fiction, a how-to publishing business has developed to help people reach their sexual potential. Thus, we now have countless books about such topics as using sexual techniques, expressing gay and lesbian sexuality, helping ourselves and our partners to be sensuous women or men, improving our overall sexual relationships, and using sexual aids for pleasure.

Popular Music

The mass phenomenon that may affect more young people than any other is popular music. And in this arena, as in most others, blatant sexuality has become a style. Lyrics (words and grunts), performance (movement and costume), and provocative photos on album covers use sexual suggestion and appeal to our sexual fantasies to sell the music and the entertainer.

Perhaps the epitome of sex in music was Elvis ("The Pelvis") Presley, with his gyrating hips. Aside from his hips, however, Elvis's songs were by today's standards tame. "Heartbreak Hotel," "Love Me Tender," and "Let Me Be Your Teddy Bear," all recorded in the late 1950s, were sexually appealing mainly because of Presley's soft, sultry voice and innuendo, rather than direct sexual language—a far cry from today's popular music and music videos that contain frequent references to relationships, romance, and sexual behavior. Lyrics about sexuality are mixed with lyrics about love, violence, rejection, and loneliness.

Music videos, available on many cable networks, may be influential sources of sexual information for adolescents because they combine visuals of their favorite musicians with music. Many of the visual elements are sexual. Rap music is particularly explicit about both sexuality and violence (Brown & Steele, 1996).

Groups of citizens have attempted to ban some of this music from local radio stations and have sometimes been successful. Whether sexually explicit music is harmful (in particular, it is argued, to youths in developmental states) is debatable and depends somewhat on our values.

Online Material

Advertising, newspapers, books, magazines, television, movies, videos, and music have been around for a long time; a newer entrant on the sexual consumerism scene is online material. An increasing number of people of all ages have access to computers and the Internet and, therefore, to countless materials related to sexuality. There are at least five reasons that account for an explosion in the amount of sexual materials available via computer networks (Rimm, 1998):

1. Consumers enjoy considerable privacy on computer networks and can easily avoid the embarrassment of acquiring sexual materials elsewhere.
2. Consumers have the ability to download only those images they find most sexually arousing.

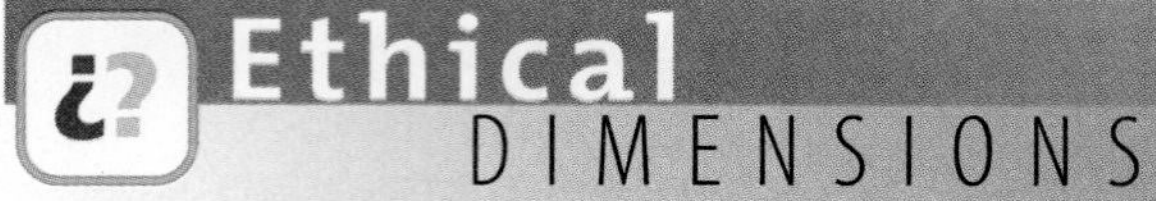

Controlling Cyberspace

In 1995 the U. S. Senate Commerce Committee proposed banning sexually explicit materials in cyberspace and considered the Communications Decency Act (CDA), which would have made the transmission of "obscene, lewd, lascivious, filthy or indecent" images, e-mail, text files, or other online communications punishable by up to $100,000 in fines and 2 years in prison. It was passed by Congress in 1996. In 1997, the Supreme Court held in a unanimous opinion that this kind of censorship could not be tolerated under the First Amendment of the U.S. Constitution.

Many people believe that attempts to ban sexually explicit materials on the Internet are, in addition to being unconstitutional, unethical. They believe that laws governing obscenity and child pornography already exist and apply to cases involving the Internet. Child pornography is not protected by free speech, so they argue that further control is not needed. In fact, they point out that such control would also deny people of all ages access to needed information about sexuality. Besides, if people want to protect children from certain information, they can do so with Internet blocking software.

Clearly, the CDA would not have been proposed if some people did not consider it ethical to ban sexually explicit materials in cyberspace. They believe such materials should not be available for viewing by anyone of any age. They also fear that even with Internet-blocking software and well-intended parents, young people will have contact with sexually explicit materials that will be harmful to them. Therefore, it is ethical to ban such materials.

Is it ethical to establish laws to ban sexually explicit materials in cyberspace? Is it ethical to transmit sexually explicit materials in cyberspace? How can the potential need for regulation be balanced with constitutional rights?

Source: Adapted from Portelli, C. J. & Meade, C. W. Censorship and the Internet: No easy answers, *SIECUS Report, 27, no. 1* (October–November 1998), 4–8.

3. Easy, discrete storage of sexually explicit images on a computer enables customers to conceal them from family members and others.
4. The prevalence and fear of HIV and AIDS and STIs have helped pornographers successfully market modem sex and autoeroticism as safe and viable alternatives to the dangers of real sex.
5. New and highly advanced computer technologies are quickly being absorbed into the mainstream, permitting an ever-expanding audience to gain access to digitized pornography available on the information superhighway.

Computer technology has influenced laws as well as behavior. For example, in 1996 federal legislation banning computer-generated depictions of children engaging in sexual conduct was passed. The act outlawed "any visual depiction" that "appears to be of a minor engaging in sexually explicit conduct." This could include scenes from a movie in which an adult portraying a minor is engaged in sexual activity (Thought police recruited in new child porn law, 1998). Although the law was challenged by sex film distributors and the ACLU, a federal judge upheld it in 1997 (New federal law upheld despite vagueness concerns, 1998).

For some people, X-rated e-mail can be a problem. Unsolicited e-mail messages that, with a click of a hot-linked Universal Resource Locator (URL), can deliver pornographic web sites to your computer screen have become relatively common intrusions online. Some have telltale IDs like "Sue2nite" or "4HotTime," but others are more deceptive. For example, in one instance an innocuous-looking message said that clicking on its hot link would provide information on how to fix a computer problem. One click of the hot link revealed a sample of sexually explicit pictures. This is probably not illegal, but it can be very annoying. The FTC encourages all consumers to forward any unsolicited, unfair, or deceptive spams to its special spam mailbox where investigators keep a database of possibly illegal e-mail solicitations.

On the Internet, people can carry on sensual conversations, play X-rated computer games with each other (for example, they can create the appearance of their characters and engage in a variety of behaviors with characters controlled by other subscribers), obtain recent information on a variety of sexual topics, leave sexual messages for other people on bulletin boards, and obtain and use software designed to help with sexual dysfunction and other problems. Computer bulletin boards and forums exist for just about all sexual interests and fetishes.

Web sites like "Persian Kitty's" provide links to free pornographic material and generate a fortune from advertisers for their operators. However, the relative ease of obtaining sexually explicit material that such a site offers raises ethical issues. Should such sites be required to provide age verification? If not, should "Persian Kitty's" be held liable if minors follow the links to sexually explicit material?

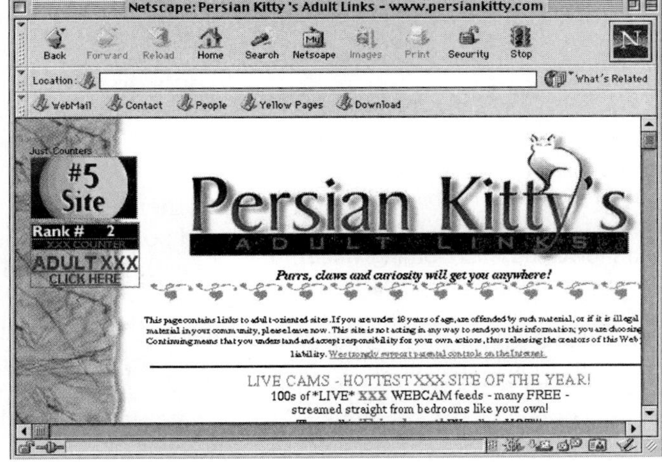

Internet chat rooms related to sexuality are also becoming more common. For example, a person can "sit" with other people or "soak" in a hot tub and discuss sexual fantasies or participate in Internet sexual activities. Flirting and discussion about sexual relationships and desires are everyday occurrences in such chat rooms.

Computers can also be used to create virtual reality (VR) sexual activity. Soon, cable TV subscribers will be able to use VR equipment, such as gloves, goggles, and body sensors, to create their own VR sexual activity.

There can be big money involved with Internet and web site activities, as Beth Mansfield discovered (Small operators can make big killings on the web, 1997). In 1995 she was a struggling accountant wondering how she and her husband would ever put their two young children through college. She decided to try her hand at creating a web site with adult content. Within 5 months people were clamoring to buy advertising on "Persian Kitty's," a directory of sexually oriented sites she named for her three cats, and now she grosses more than $900,000 a year.

One of the web's most successful adult-oriented sites is operated by Danni Ashe. It is called "Danni's Hard Drive." According to information at the web site, Danni Ashe is a former model and stripper who created and launched her own site in 1995. The site's initial 70,000 hits per day have grown to 5 million, gross revenue has grown by more than 2,000% and her original staff of 1 part-time assistant has grown to 15 full-time employees. Monthly fees of $9.95 give members access to a library of nude photos and interviews with nude models.

In 2001 the *Guinness Book of World Records* awarded Danni Ashe an award as the Most Downloaded Woman. At that time she had already been downloaded 7 million times into the computers of others. It is estimated that 1 in 5 hits on the Web is sex-related and that sexual themes are the web's top moneymaker (Pastor's column hits the growth of porn, 2001).

Danni Ashe is more popular on the Internet than many well-known stars. For example, her web site receives more hits than the web sites for Martha Stewart, Oprah Winfrey, Britney Spears, Cindy Margolis, and Cindy Crawford (How popular is Danni Ashe compared to other stars? 2003).

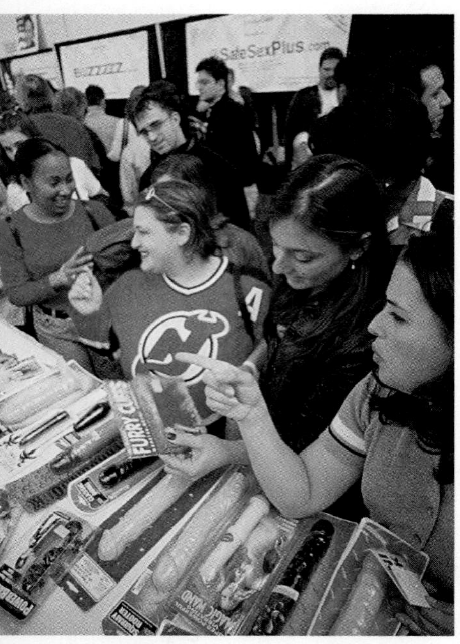

In April 1999, the Erotica USA expo was held in New York City at the Javitz Center. Billed as a 4-day sex convention for the general public, the show drew an estimated 40,000 attendees and showcased latex clothing, videos, sex toys, magazines, sex clubs, and Internet-based sex business. It is estimated that the U.S. sex industry generates $9 billion in annual sales. With so much money at stake, do you think it would be difficult to control and regulate such an industry?

Of course, the Internet also has the potential for abuse with respect to sexuality. Some people have claimed they have been sexually harassed by anonymous participants in computer bulletin boards. Others have been concerned about the transmission of sexual photos of children. There is also concern about uncontrolled access to sexual materials by underage people.

In addition, it is estimated that one in five young people aged 10–17 years who use the Internet at least once a month receives unwanted sexual solicitations. Only 10% were reported to police, school officials, or Internet service providers. Solicitations involve requests to talk on the telephone, communicate by mail, and meet strangers who have established contact online (Wong, 2001).

What seems to be a very positive use of the Internet for sexuality education occurred late in 2001 (Goodwill ambassador and former, 2001). Geri Halliwell, a former Spice Girl, launched a sexuality education web site in Britain. Titled "Like It Is," the interactive site is geared toward school-aged children and teens and offers information on reproductive health and services, including teen pregnancy, birth control, and emergency contraception. Halliwell said, "This site gives frank information, but in a way that is appropriate and safe for young people." The site can be viewed at http://www.likeitis.org.uk.

Sexual Aids

Another aspect of the commercialization of sexuality is selling the promise (and sometimes the reality) of more satisfying sexual activity through the use of sexual devices and other aids. There is a big business in the manufacture and sale of sexual aids and enhancers. Some, such as penile implants and vibrators, are used in treating sexual dysfunctions. Films on techniques for achieving orgasm and enhancing the sexual experience are often used by sex therapists as an adjunct to their treatment programs.

People use such simple aids as massage oil to heighten their sensual pleasure. They use other sexual devices to intensify sensation and to reach orgasm. It is noteworthy that according to the Food and Drug Administration, fraudulent sexual aids are among the top 10 sources of health fraud in the United States (The top ten health frauds, 1990).

Previously we discussed some of the uses of vibrators. They come in a variety of colors and shapes and can be electrically or battery operated. They can be used by either sex for solitary masturbation or as a part of heterosexual or homosexual encounters. Many are sold in ordinary retail outlets for massage purposes.

A vibratorlike device, called the Eroscillator, even has its own web page. It points out that the Eroscillator is *not* a vibrator. "It provides a totally unique, gentle 'oscillating' motion which moves naturally and softly from side to side rather than up and down like a vibrator." If you believe the ad, the Eroscillator has three different levels of intensity, is completely safe, is specifically designed to meet your needs, and has no risk of irritation.

Magazines and newspapers are full of ads claiming that women may add extra inches to their breasts with only a few minutes of specific exercise daily or by using creams, massage, or worthless gadgets—all for a price. Just as the Eroscillator does, a breast cream called Enhancia has its own web page. One woman claims she noticed a difference in about 2 weeks: an increase of almost 1 inch around her bust.

In fact, breast size and shape are the result of glandular influences that cannot be altered by applying anything to the breast. It is also impossible to increase breast size through exercise. The effect of exercise is to enlarge muscle tissue. Because there is no muscle tissue in the breast, exercise cannot enhance the breast. Only injections or implants can enlarge the breast. As discussed in In Focus: Body Image these procedures are controversial and expensive, and they can have dangerous long-term effects.

Underclothing that particularly emphasizes the genitals is manufactured to satisfy a range of tastes. It is sold by mail-order businesses, by e-mail, and by expensive boutiques. Other sexual products are more exotic. A few examples of these products will demonstrate their nature:

1. Some manufacturers have gone beyond the standard type of vibrator that therapists recommend to enhance sexual pleasure. For example, one manufacturer advertises the Sensual Encounter, a 7-inch vibrator with various attachments: natural veined penis, French tickler, fuzzy tongue, and others. This same ad describes the Anal Intruder vibrator for the novice analist.

2. A variety of aphrodisiacs and lotions are available: Motion Lotion, Joy Jelly, Korean Ginseng capsules, Man Power capsules, Spanish Fly Sugar powder, Jungle Love Sugar powder, or Wild Passion Ginseng capsules. They are unlikely to be effective.

3. A man dissatisfied with the size of his penis may be persuaded to buy a "penis enlarger vacuum," and a female dissatisfied with the size of her breasts can buy a "breast enlarger."

4. Penis extenders are used by those who want to give their partner the sensation of penetration by a larger penis. They are worn at the tip of the penis and are held in place by a condom or straps. Penis erectors vary in design, but many are like splints designed to support a nonerect penis. Another variety is a "cock ring," which fits around the base of the penis after erection and maintains the erection while it is in place. Also available is an artificial penis attached to a motor that moves the penis in a thrusting manner.

5. Artificial vaginas are available for males for masturbatory purposes; artificial penises (dildos) can be used by either males or females for insertion into the vagina or anus.
6. Another product advertises by asking men whether they have ever experienced fellatio while driving a car. If they have and enjoyed the sensation, or would like such an experience, they are invited to buy the Auto Suck Vagina. The product resembles an automobile vacuum and thus, the ad reassuringly advises, keeps its user out of trouble with the highway police should he be stopped "at the moment of climax."

Sexual aids used to be sold almost exclusively out of "porno-sleaze" shops in such places as New York's Times Square, but they have become such big business that they are now sold in women's sex-toy boutiques. Many of these boutiques run a very profitable catalogue business. An example of this type of organization is the Xandria Collection located in San Francisco. Through their catalogue one can purchase dildos, vibrators that fit over the penis for self-stimulation, prosthetic penis aids, penis extensions, clitoral stimulators, penis rings, and Ben-Wa balls (small balls to insert into the vagina that move around, thereby stimulating the woman), not to mention the various lotions and potions and underwear with holes in just the right places. In addition, the Xandria Collection sells sex manuals: *Sexual Adventures in Marriage, Yesterday's Porno, Sexual Pleasures from A to Z,* and *Sex Comic Classics.*

Another means of selling sexual aids has as its model the famous Tupperware parties (Benderly, 1986; Cool, 1998). Here is how it works: Someone volunteers the use of her house for the party and invites a group of friends, and a saleswoman shows all sorts of sexual aids, ranging from soft leather to French ticklers (penis sleeves with ribs to stimulate the vagina).

As you can see, the use of sex to sell products, combined with the manufacture and sale of sexual aids, is significant. You can hardly open a magazine or newspaper, read a book, watch television, attend the theater, or listen to popular music without encountering sexual themes; sexual explicitness (and implicitness) is part of our everyday existence. We need to be aware of its presence so that we can better control its effect on our behavior and attitudes. By way of example, knowing that the scantily clad model has no relation to our need to own a new car, we might be better able to ignore the sexual appeal of the ads and purchase a car that is suited to our needs and financial constraints.

Being aware of the uses of sexuality in the marketplace can make you a better consumer, a more enlightened citizen, and a healthier person sexually.

Sexually Explicit Materials

Terminology is critical, but somewhat confusing, in relation to sexually explicit materials. You may hear different people use the same terms to describe different things, so it is important to establish definitions. **Pornography** is visual and written material that is used for purposes of sexual arousal. It has been said that pornography, as is beauty, is in the eye of the beholder. Opinions about what it is, its possible uses, and its legal status are extremely varied.

Definitions

The legal definition of *obscenity,* established by the Supreme Court in 1973, is that for something to be obscene it must meet all three of the following conditions:

1. The average person, applying contemporary community standards, would find that the work, taken as a whole, appeals to **prurient** interest.
2. The work depicts or describes, in a patently offensive way, sexual conduct specifically defined by the applicable state (or federal) law.
3. The work, taken as a whole, lacks serious literary, artistic, political, or scientific value.

Therefore, although sexually explicit materials are legal in the United States, obscenity is not. Taking the three Supreme Court criteria just listed together, a reasonable definition of **obscenity** is a personal or societal judgment that something is offensive. Therefore, one person may consider obscene something that another does not.

Another important term is **erotica,** which usually describes sexually oriented material that can be evaluated positively, in contrast to obscenity, which is offensive. Erotica consists of "depictions of sexuality which display mutuality, respect, affection, and a balance of power" (Stock, 1985).

pornography
Visual and written materials used for the purpose of sexual arousal.

prurient
Characterized by lustful thoughts or wishes.

obscenity
Personal or societal judgment that something is offensive.

erotica
Sexually oriented material that may be artistically produced or motivated.

Effects of Sexually Explicit Materials

Traditionally many people have been opposed to sexually explicit materials. Perhaps this is because they feared that the materials had many undesirable effects, such as causing people to participate in sexual activity they might not otherwise have engaged in, increasing the number of sexual offenses, and corrupting the minds of children. It is difficult to do research in an area where there are so many personal and social variables, but a brief look at research findings about the effects of sexually explicit materials may be helpful.

The report of the Commission on Obscenity and Pornography (1970), sponsored by the federal government, and a review of this report by two researchers at Johns Hopkins University (Money & Athanasiou, 1973) give us some information about the effects of pornography. According to these sources, the following appear to be true:

1. There is little, if any, difference in males' and females' sexual responses to sexually explicit materials.
2. People are stimulated only by portrayals of sexual ideas or acts that turn them on. In other words, sexually explicit materials do not seem to plant in people's minds ideas or desires that they do not already have.
3. Exposure to sexually explicit materials does not seem to alter a person's sexual behavior patterns in the long run.
4. Continued exposure to sexually explicit materials tends to lead to indifference and boredom. John Money (1973) believes that stimuli in sexually explicit materials are effective for 2 to 4 hours. After this time a person becomes either more selective or indifferent to the stimuli.
5. Filling out questionnaires on responses to sexually explicit material may be more stimulating than the material itself. (Perhaps this is best explained by human beings' great capacity to fantasize.)
6. Convicted sex offenders have been exposed to fewer sexually explicit and sexuality education materials during their life than nonoffenders. This fact contradicts the common belief that exposure to sexually explicit materials causes people to commit sexual offenses.

Do we worry more than we should about sexually explicit material? If it causes harm, what is the nature of the harm, and whom does it affect? Money (1973, 143) summarizes the research in this area: "Pornography's influence will depend on the moral context that is set early in the sex education of children and against which erotic illustrations will be seen and read. . . . Pathology tends to incubate in secrecy as when, in a child's early development, sex and heterosexual reproduction are unmentionable, tabooed and punishable."

For many people it was surprising that evidence from the President's Commission showed that sexually explicit materials might have some educational benefit. For example, if the information is factual, it can enlighten the ignorant. It also seems to foster less inhibited attitudes toward sexuality: "Well timed in its use and supported by good moral principles, visual erotica can become a positive and constructive aid in the service of developing sexual normalcy" (Money, 1973, 143). Although there is no strong evidence, it could also be argued that sexually explicit materials can provide variety and add spice to the life of some people. Given the emphasis on safer sex alternatives today, sexually explicit materials can be helpful in providing sexual stimulation and pleasure without potential exposure to HIV.

According to the commission, approximately 85% of adult men and 70% of adult women in the United States have been exposed at some time to erotica, but only 20% to 25% of the male population have had somewhat regular experience with it. Who are the consumers of sexually explicit movies, books, and newspapers? The 1970 commission characterized them as predominantly white, middle-class, middle-aged married males, dressed in business suits or casual attire, shopping or attending a movie alone. The average patron of adult bookstores and movie houses appears to have had fewer sexually related experiences in adolescence than the average male in our society but to be more sexually oriented as an adult. Otherwise the buyers of sexually explicit materials are not very different from nonconsumers. They report frequencies of intercourse fairly similar to those of nonconsumers and report a similar degree of enjoyment from intercourse. Furthermore, activi-

Gender DIMENSIONS

Male and Female Use of Autoerotic Materials

As part of the National Health and Social Life Survey, Laumann and associates (1994) reported on the number of men and women who had used autoerotic materials in the past year. The main activities indicated by the subjects were viewing X-rated movies or videos (23% of the males and 11% of the females), going to a club that has nude or seminude dancers (22% of the males and 4% of the females), and using sexually explicit books or magazines (16% of the males and 4% of the females). Vibrators or dildos were used by 2% of the males and 2% of the females, and other sex toys were used by 1% of the males and 2% of the females. Forty-one percent of the men and 16% of the women reported using autoerotic materials during the past year.

Interestingly, thinking about sex frequently (defined as "every day" or "several times a day") was reported by 54% of the males and 19% of the females. Thinking about sex infrequently (defined as "a few times a month" to "a few times a week") was reported by 43% of the males and 67% of the females. Thinking about sex never or rarely (defined as "less than once a month") was reported by 4% of the males and 16% of the females.

Source: Laumann, E. O., Gagnon, J. H., Michael, R. T., & Michaels, S. *The social organization of sexuality.* Chicago: The University of Chicago Press, 1994.

ties most frowned on by our society, such as sadomasochism, pedophilia, bestiality, and nonconsensual sexual activity, are also outside the scope of the interests of the average patron of adult bookstores and movie houses.

In 1985, then United States attorney general, Edwin Meese III, announced the formation of a new Commission on Pornography. Surrounded by controversy from the beginning—the politically conservative administration was suspect and, therefore, the commission's conclusions would be considered preordained to meet a conservative agenda—the commission produced findings that were in direct contrast to those of the 1970 commission. In particular, the 1985 commission concluded "that the available evidence strongly supports the hypothesis that substantial exposure to sexually violent material as described here bears a causal relationship to antisocial acts of sexual violence and, for some subgroups, possibly to unlawful acts of sexual violence" (Attorney General's report on pornography, 1986, 40). Many experts disagreed with this conclusion and maintained that the 1970 commission's conclusions were more valid and relied more on scientific method and evidence than did the 1985 commission, which was accused of relying on predominantly anecdotal reports. This argument rages to this day.

Several more recent studies have considered the effects of sexually explicit materials. Stark (1997) pointed out that some researchers have advocated that sexually explicit materials be restricted on the ground that they harm women—that is, that they harm women in general, not those who consume the materials. It is argued that such materials subordinate women to men.

In exploring the relationship between men's exposure to sexually explicit materials and their beliefs about men and women, Frable and associates (1997) found that men with relatively high exposure to sexually explicit materials see a world filled with masculine men, sexy women, and, in some contexts, gender differences. Davies (1997), however, found that men who rented more sexually explicit videos did not hold significantly different attitudes about feminism and rape than men with lower exposure to sexually explicit videos. She concluded that negative attitudes toward women are not generated by sexually explicit videos and that they may be deeply ingrained in society.

Stein (1998) indicated that intellectuals have just about accepted erotica's place in pop culture. Many people are buying materials for their own use. "Of the $10 billion sex industry, it's not ten perverts [each] spending $1 billion a year." There is definitely a growing acceptance of the sex industry.

Child Pornography

So far we have considered sexually explicit materials about adults for adults. There is increasing concern about the use of children in pornographic materials and, more recently, about continued eroticization of young children in the print media and on television. One example of the eroticization of children highlighted by Women Against Pornography was a four-page spread in a national magazine. Entitled "Tiny Treasures: The Allure of the World's Best Perfumes," the ad showed a 5-year-old girl, professionally coiffed, heavily made up, and half-nude. The copy noted that the perfume was "jasmine and gardenia for seduction with just a touch of innocence." Caress soap ran an ad with a preteen girl wearing a T-shirt on which the word *Caress* invitingly covered her small bosom. The fear is that child molesters will be further enticed by images such as those presented in "Tiny Treasures" (National magazines, 1984).

The use of minors in sexually explicit media—**child pornography**—is now prohibited. In the past, many magazine publishers and film producers used their own children in sexually explicit materials they developed. Others adver-

child pornography
Use of minors in sexually explicit media.

tised in magazines catering to readers of pornography. For example, an ad in Al Goldstein's *Screw* offered $200 for young girl child models. That ad generated dozens of responses from parents eager to earn money in this way. As is pornography in general, child pornography is big business (Lederer, 1980). Still, in spite of the law, magazines and films that depict children in sexually erotic conditions are produced and sold. Given the current societal concern for child abuse (sexual and otherwise) and for missing children, law enforcement agencies have organized to crack down on the kiddie porn industry.

Child pornographers are found in large and small towns and might just be the people next door. They are not obvious criminals. In 1998 the largest child pornography operation discovered to that point was called Wonderland—and its Internet operation was called Wondernet. The group used an imposing system of codes and encryption and took full advantage of the technological capacities of the Internet (Shannon, 1998).

The Control of Sexually Explicit Materials

Should sexually explicit materials be censored and controlled? There are varying opinions. In an attempt to keep sexually explicit materials on the Internet away from the 16 million users younger than 17 years old in the United States, Congress passed the Child Online Protection Act, which forced web sites to require a credit card number or some other adult ID. The law made it a crime knowingly to communicate to a minor "for commercial purposes" any online material that is "harmful to minors." Penalties included fines up to $50,000 a day for each violation and up to 6 months in prison. At best, however, the law would make sexually explicit material a bit more difficult for minors to reach. It does not touch areas not on the web, such as e-mail or Usenet newsgroups. It also does not affect noncommercial sites or operations based outside the United States (Child online protection act of 1998, 2003). On February 1, 1999, U.S. District Judge Lowell Reed extended indefinitely a preliminary injunction against the act, ruling it violates free speech (*ACLU v. Reno II*). This law has been controversial. Some people feel that it is in society's best interest to protect children from sexually explicit materials. Free speech advocates, on the other hand, challenge the law on constitutional grounds, arguing it would affect everybody on the web.

Also in 1996 the Child Pornography and Protection Act was passed (High court to hear arguments on child porn amendment, 2001). Since then supporters have claimed that the act was an essential tool to prevent pedophiles from preying on children. Those who disagree have argued that it is so vaguely worded that there is no way to know what is over the line and what is not. Through the years court challenges related to the act have had inconsistent outcomes. For example, one federal district court judge found the law constitutional, and one U.S. court of appeals struck it down. The debate continues.

A major related event occurred in June of 2003 when the U.S. Supreme Court upheld a federal law requiring public library personnel to install pornography filters on all computers providing Internet access, as a condition of continuing to receive federal subsidies and grants (Greenhouse, 2003). The law, enacted in 2001, had been blocked by a lower court and never taken effect. Under the law, filters are required for all library users, not just children. The law authorizes, but does not require, librarians to unblock Internet sites at the request of adult users. Many opinions exist about the wisdom of this law and how it relates to First Amendment rights to free speech.

Certain segments of the public are very concerned about the increased availability of sexually explicit materials and have organized to combat this trend. As proof of the increase they point to data indicating that 40% of VCR owners report having bought or rented X-rated cassettes within a year's time (Duggan, 1985); the popularity of cable television channels, such as the Playboy Channel, that specialize in sexual broadcasts; and the success of such sexually explicit magazines as *Penthouse* and *Playboy.* These citizen groups have been encouraged by the Attorney General's Commission on Pornography (1986, 39), which reviewed numerous studies related to pornography and concluded that pornography "shows a causal relationship between exposure to material of this type and aggressive behavior toward women."

The interesting aspect of this organized opposition to sexually explicit materials is that it has united diverse groups. National conservative groups as well as some national feminist groups have joined a loose network of local groups to fight the "Porn War." Among the conservative organizations are the National Federation for Decency, the Citizens for Decency through Law, Morality in Media, the Moral Majority, and the Citizens for Legislation Against Decadence. Among the feminist groups are Women Against Pornography, Feminists Against Pornography, the Pornography Resource Center, and Women against Violence against Women.

The objections of these groups to sexually explicit materials are several. Some consider an explicit description or image of sexual acts immoral and irreligious. Others object to women's being portrayed as sex objects and believe this view of women will be generalized to "real life." Still others perceive that women in sexually explicit materials are treated violently and fear that this type of portrayal might cause more violence toward women. For example, Women Against Pornography (WAP) has demanded that sexually explicit materials be prohibited from depicting rape, whipping, or bondage. WAP believes that such depictions lead men to feel superior to women and extend that idea of superiority to nonsexual relationships (such as those in the workplace). Women Against Violence Against Women concentrates predominantly on music and advertising, asserting that commercial degradation of women fosters sexism.

Many groups of women are most vocal in their opinions. However, though not organized, men also suffer from sexploitation. When men are shown performing violent acts on women, they are being taught to be powerful and dominant over the other sex. They are learning that sexual relationships require a measure of forcefulness that in actuality interferes with sexual arousal rather than enhances it. When men learn to treat women as sexual objects, their relationships suffer. Depictions of men and women sharing equally in sexual and love relationships would teach both sexes that sexual fulfillment is a mutual responsibility; the results would be a decrease of pressure on men to know what to do and how to do it and fewer sexually frustrated women.

Some feminists have criticized the great deal of effort devoted to an antiporn position. They feel that actions, strategies, and theories promoting women's sexual opportunities and well-being as they prevent women's endangerment are still needed. They emphasize that the focus on sexually explicit materials trivializes real violence; distracts attention and drains activism from more fundamental legal, political, and economic issues; and fails to reduce violence against women. To win their battles, antipornography feminists align with the antisexual conservatives and implicitly support agendas that oppose women's sexual and reproductive rights (Tiefer, 1995). This alignment can harm women in the long run.

Leanne Katz (1994), executive director of the National Coalition Against Censorship (NCAC), makes an interesting point. NCAC believes that government agencies should not tell women or men how to think or write about their life, including their sexual life. The group's members believe that such laws

Myth vs Fact

Myth: There is no difference between obscenity and pornography.
Fact: Yes, there is. Obscenity is not protected by the Constitution. It follows the Supreme Court definition, but pornography is material designed to arouse and has no legal or consistent definition.

Myth: Sexually explicit material causes violence against women.
Fact: No reputable research in the United States, Europe, or Asia finds a causal link between pornography and violence.

Myth: Men watch pornography and imitate it or force women to do what they see.
Fact: Violence and intimidation existed for thousands of years before commercial pornography. People do not mimic what they read or view in knee-jerk fashion. Men do not learn coercion from sexual pictures.

Myth: Pornography degrades women.
Fact: Sexism, not sexual behavior, degrades women. Opponents of sexual speech do not understand that it is in everyone's interest to allow a variety of pleasurable materials that enhance well-being and sexual fulfillment.

Myth: Pornography is only for men.
Fact: Half the adult videos in the United States are bought or rented by women alone or women in couples. AIDS and other STIs have made it a public health necessity to encourage sexual fantasy material that offers women and men safe alternatives to unhealthy sexual contact.

Myth vs Fact

Myth: Women in pornography are exploited or victimized.
Fact: Women are exploited and harassed in all fields, including pornography. Exploitation will stop when it is vigorously prosecuted everywhere it occurs. Some women in pornography say their work gives them independence and a sense of accomplishment; banning it would worsen their lives.

Myth: As an aid to masturbation, pornography is action that is not protected by the First Amendment.
Fact: Pornography may lead to masturbation much as a novel or film may lead to tears or laughter. Feminists for Free Expression does not believe policing masturbation is the proper business of government or well-meaning committees.

Myth: Banning sexual material will protect or help women.
Fact: Historically, censorship has hurt women. It has prevented them from getting information about sexuality and reproduction. The best protection for women's ideas is the constitutional protection of free speech. The answer to bad pornography is good pornography, not no pornography.

are not good for anybody and are bad for women. In the name of "protecting" women from harm, family planning information has been withheld, important works of art have been removed from display, and books about women's bodies, sexuality education, HIV and AIDS, and new models of women's sexuality have been banned. They also say: "The censorship of sexually related expression may well be the greatest threat to the American system of free speech today, and attacks on sexually related expression are certainly hampering education and the open examination of sexuality."

The ACLU says that it is no accident that freedom of speech is the first freedom mentioned in the First Amendment. It is not limited to "pure speech"—books, newspapers, leaflets, and rallies. It also protects "symbolic speech"—nonverbal expression whose purpose it is to communicate ideas. It exists precisely to protect the most offensive and controversial speech from government suppression. The best means to counter obnoxious speech is speech. Persuasion, not coercion, is the solution. The ACLU also indicates that the innovation and citizen empowerment inspired by online communications will be lost if civil liberties do not also apply in cyberspace. Furthermore, there are three reasons freedom of expression is essential to a free society: (1) The right to express one's thoughts and to communicate freely with others is the foundation of self-fulfillment. (2) It is vital to the attainment and advancement of knowledge and the search for the truth. (3) It is necessary to our system of self-government and gives the American people a "checking function" against government excess and corruption.

Feminists for Free Expression (FFE) is a leading voice opposing state and national legislation that threatens free speech, defends the right of free expression in court cases, supports the rights of activists whose works have been suppressed or censored, and provides expert speakers. On the topic of sexually explicit materials, FFE published *Feminism and Free Speech: Pornography* to aid in the understanding of pornography, its uses and benefits, and its relation to violence. An overview of their scientific and cross-cultural research is provided in the Myth vs Fact box about pornography. Relatedly, there is more erotica being developed that is not sexist but feminist and gender-friendly. It is designed to portray equitable relationships.

In October 2002 the Museum of Sex opened in New York City. The purpose of the museum is to preserve and present the history, evolution, and cultural significance of human sexuality. Not everyone approves of it. William Donohue, president of the Catholic League for Religions and Civil Rights, denounced the museum for celebrating "smut as sex." He accused the museum of championing or associating with racists, pornographers, and individuals who "exhibit pathological characteristics." On the other hand, June Reinisch, a historian adviser to the museum and director emeritus of the Kinsey Institute, characterized it as a serious endeavor, in the sense that it wants to inform and educate as well as to entertain. "Sexuality is a very important part of individual life and to culture," she said. "To not understand it is to be handicapped in your understanding of human relations and culture" (James, 2002). It will be interesting to see how the Museum of Sex is regarded as time goes by.

Finally, the position of the Sexuality Information and Education Council of the United States on sexually explicit materials is as follows:

> *When sensitively used in a manner appropriate to the viewer's age and developmental level, sexually explicit visual, printed, or online materials can be valuable educational or personal aids, helping to reduce ignorance and confusion and contributing to a wholesome concept of sexuality. However, the use of violence, exploitation, or degradation, or the portrayal of children in sexually explicit materials is reprehensible. Minors should be legally protected*

from all forms of sexual exploitation.

Adults should have the right of access to sexually explicit materials for personal use. Legislative and judicial efforts to prevent the production and distribution of sexually explicit materials endanger constitutionally guaranteed freedoms of speech and press and could be employed to restrict the appropriate professional use of such materials by sexuality educators, therapists, and researchers.

Sex Workers

An important consideration in the study of sexual commercial enterprises is the topic of sex work, or prostitution. The term **prostitution** refers to any situation in which one person pays another for sexual gratification. Sex workers may be males as well as females, but primarily sex workers have been and are females. Women do sex work mainly to make money, but other factors can also motivate them. For example, the lack of education of most sex workers limits their job opportunities. In addition, some women think sex work will be exciting and glamorous, whereas others are motivated to become sex workers because they do not like the discipline and boredom of regular jobs. Some women who are drug addicts turn to sex work to support the habit. The background of many sex workers has included emotional deprivation and sexual abuse—even within the family. Some sex workers therefore feel that by providing sexual pleasure they can gain intimacy and attention.

prostitution
Participating in sexual activity for pay or profit.

call girls
Highly paid female sex workers who work by appointment only.

house (brothel) prostitutes
Sex workers who work in brothels.

streetwalkers
Sex workers who work on the streets.

Types of Sex Workers

It is difficult to estimate the number of persons who currently work or have ever worked as sex workers because there are various definitions of prostitution and because sex work is usually illegal. The National Task Force on Prostitution estimates that more than 1 million people in the United States have worked as prostitutes, or about 1% of American women (Prostitution in the United States—The statistics, 1998). There are many types of sex workers; the major types are call girls, house prostitutes, streetwalkers, massage parlor prostitutes, and bar girls and strippers.

Call Girls

Call girls are at the top of the profession. They do not solicit; rather, their "dates" are arranged by personal referral or by another person. They have regular clients who pay high fees and also pay their bills.

House Prostitutes

House (brothel) prostitutes work in more structured conditions in brothels (houses in which prostitutes work) and serve more men at cheaper rates than call girls would charge. Brothels are legal in some counties of Nevada but are illegal in all other areas of the United States.

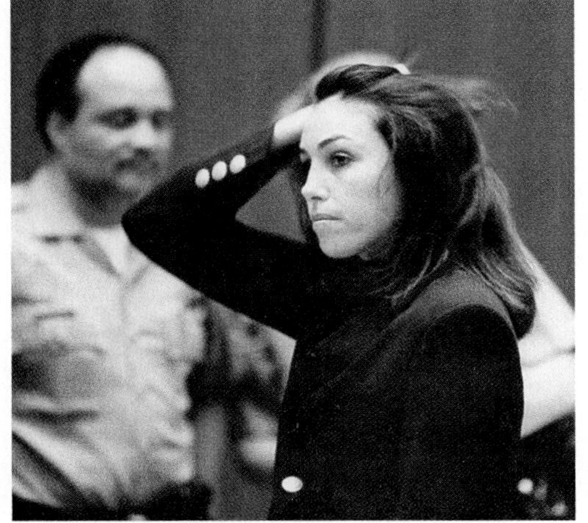

Heidi Fleiss, the so-called Hollywood Madam, ran a high-priced call girl ring in Beverly Hills. She was arrested and convicted on several charges ranging from pandering to tax evasion. However, the case raised ethical questions, because all the call girls were granted immunity and none of the clients was charged. Should prosecutors use government resources to pursue prostitutes' customers?

Streetwalkers

Streetwalkers are more independent than house prostitutes but lack the contacts or ability to become call girls. They stand or stroll on streets and approach passing males. Because of their visibility, streetwalkers are the most frequently arrested sex workers.

The ratio of on-street prostitution to off-street in cities varies with local law, police, and custom. Whereas street prostitution accounts for between 10% and 20% of the prostitution in larger cities, in some smaller cities with limited indoor venues street prostitution may constitute about 50% (Prostitution in the United States—The statistics, 1998).

Massage Parlor Sex Workers

Certainly many **massage parlors** offer only massages, but at others a client can find many "extras." The environment offers an indoor place to work that is safer than the streets, and massage parlor workers may be motivated to earn extra money by providing sexual favors. Fellatio is popular among both customers and masseuses. Many men claim they cannot get their regular partners to participate in fellatio. The masseuses appreciate it because it is efficient: They are trying to earn as much money as they can, so it is useful to be able to service a number of men in a short period.

massage parlors
Places where sex workers can be hired to perform sexual acts under the guise of giving a massage.

bar girls
Sex workers who are supposed to act available so customers will buy them drinks.

gigolo
A man who is paid to provide escort and sexual services, usually for wealthy, middle-aged women.

hustler
A male sex worker who performs homosexual acts for pay.

pimps
Individuals who set up female sex workers with clients.

Bar Girls and Strippers

Many times **bar girls** and strippers are supposed to act available so men will buy them drinks. This helps the establishment make more on the sale of liquor. Sometimes, however, paid sexual activity is also offered.

Examples of this type of activity can be found in many countries. For example, an increasing number of Cambodian "beer girls," who sell international beers, wines, and liquors at outdoor eateries and in bars, are also selling sex. If the women refuse a client's offer of sex for money, they may lose a beer sale. Because they depend heavily on commissions, they feel they have to do something to convince the client to buy. To make matters worse, beer girls are less likely than brothel workers to use condoms, and surveys show that as many as one-fifth of them are HIV-positive (Increasing number of Cambodian "beer girls" selling sex, 2003).

Japan's sex trade, estimated at $13 billion a year, is one of the nation's fastest-growing industries. Record unemployment has forced many women to work at brothels euphemistically known as fashion, health, soapland, pink salons, or telephone clubs. Only 6–25% of sex workers and the public use condoms. HIV has not been widespread in Japan, but the prevalence rate is highest among female sex workers, close to 3%. Because of the lack of HIV and AIDS education, the very small amount of condom use, and the relatively rapid increase in rates of HIV among sex workers, it is feared that HIV and AIDS could become a significant problem in Japan (Kakuchi, 2003).

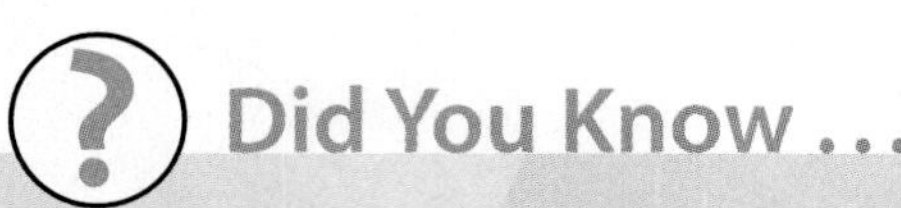

Did you know that there is a historical connection between Santa Claus and sex workers? In the third century, a rich and good hearted Turkish man named Nicholas saved poor girls from prostitution by throwing bags of gold coins through their windows or down a chimney. Over the next 700 years, with a little help from Dutch settlers in America and a poet named Clement Clarke Moore, Saint Nicholas was transposed into a merry old gent with a white beard and red suit who spends most of Christmas giving toys to good little girls and boys.

Source: Vrazo, F. Finland town, rovaniemi, *Birmingham News* (December 18, 1998), 18A.

Male Sex Workers

Whereas the majority of sex workers are women, some men also sell sexual services to women or to other men. **Gigolos** provide escort and sexual services for women, and **hustlers** are male sex workers who perform homosexual acts for pay. Male sex workers may be classified as female sex workers are, but the differences are often not obvious.

Percentages of male and female sex workers vary from city to city. Estimates in some larger cities suggest that 20% to 30% of sex workers are male. In San Francisco, it has been estimated that 25% of the female sex workers are transgendered (Prostitution in the United States—The statistics, 1998).

Pimps

The people who set up sex workers with clients are called **pimps.** Sex workers give the money they earn to their pimps in exchange for affection, concern, and love. Pimps recruit newcomers into sex work, they manage the sex workers' business and provide them counsel, bail them out of jail when necessary, and regulate the streetwalking prostitution enterprise (without a pimp, streetwalking sex workers might be in danger in certain neighborhoods).

Sexual Slavery

Various types of forced labor are increasing worldwide. One researcher concluded there were 27 million people around the world trapped in virtual prisons on farms, in sweatshops, or in brothels. Many women and girls are forced into prostitution, moved from country to country each year by criminals who sell them into virtual slavery or demand they work to pay off exorbitant "debts" (Memmott, 2001).

From the former Soviet Union alone, an estimated 50,000 women are trafficked abroad each year and forced into sexual slavery. The women are told they will be given jobs as waitresses, nannies, or dancers in foreign countries. However, once they arrive at their destination, they are told they owe hundreds of dollars in job placement fees and airfare. They are threatened with beating and rape and told their family members will be hurt if they do not comply. To ensure compliance by the women, traffickers usually confiscate passports, then beat, rape, and drug them. Profits from trafficking in women reach $7–12 billion a year (Dolgov, 2001).

Opinions About Sex Work

The subject of sex workers produces strong emotional reactions in many people. For example, Overall (1992) indicated that there is an apparent conflict among some feminists and sex workers about the value of the work (prostitution) and the right to do it. She said that it makes sense to defend sex workers' entitlement to do their work but not to defend sex work as a practice under patriarchy. That is, what is wrong with sex work is not just that it is the servicing of men's sexual needs but that it is women's servicing of men's sexual needs under capitalist and patriarchal conditions.

Satz (1995) argued that one problem with sex work is that it sustains a social world where women are subordinate, and it is wrong insofar as the sale of women's sexual labor reinforces broad patterns of sexual discrimination.

Eisler (1995) summarized the economics of prostitution and indicated that, even as a growing percentage of sex workers are infected with HIV, thousands of Asian girls and women still sell themselves as prostitutes. They do so as a way of escaping dire poverty and hunger because at least for a few years it allows them to get paid far more than they could earn doing anything else, or because they can be helpful to their family by sending large portions of their earnings home. Indeed large segments of the global economy are dependent on prostitution. This includes not only the females who work in the sex tourist industry and the places where men drink, gamble, and have sexual activity with prostitutes but also the families who sell their daughters into prostitution or are supported by them. It includes those who gain even more profit from this work than the sex workers do: the "madams" of brothels and the men who run the sex industry. It also includes the police and other government officials who collect bribes to look the other way or are paid to regulate prostitution where it is legal.

Eisler further indicates that because sex work is basically a means of survival, prostitutes have begun to organize as other workers have, trying to improve their working conditions, raise the status of their profession, and promote respect for the human rights of prostitutes. In the short run, and in the lives of the women (and men) who are sex workers, these are important efforts. In the long run, however, the problem remains that what the prostitute ultimately offers for sale is the ritualization of feminine sexual submission. The crux of the matter is that the man does the choosing, and the woman (or man taking the woman's traditional role) is available for the client's use—and all too often abuse. In short, Eisler says, prostitution is a transaction between unequals, one in which the buyers set the price deciding what kinds of women (or little girls or boys) are worth paying for and in which the sellers have little if any power to determine how their body will be used. The less powerful woman is selling her body to the more powerful man.

Of course many people would argue against sex work on moral grounds. Perhaps they feel that sexual activity should be restricted to marital relations or that it is immoral for sex workers to participate in sexual activity with many different people.

In contrast to those who organize against sex work, the National Task Force on Prostitution (NTFP) was founded in 1979 to act as an umbrella organization for prostitutes and prostitutes' rights organizations. It is a network of sex workers and their supporters that supports the rights of sex workers to organize on their own behalf, work safely and without legal repression, travel without legal restrictions, have families and raise children, and enjoy the same rights, responsibilities, and privileges as other people. The goals of the NTFP are to (1) repeal the existing prostitution laws; (2) ensure the right of prostitutes and other sex workers to bargain with their employers, when they work for third parties, to improve their working conditions; (3) inform the public about a wide range of issues related to prostitution and other forms of sex work; (4) promote the development of support services for sex workers, including HIV, AIDS, and STIs and violence-prevention projects, as well as health and social support services for sex workers (including supportive programs to deal with STIs, violence, and substance abuse), legal assistance projects, and job retraining and other programs to

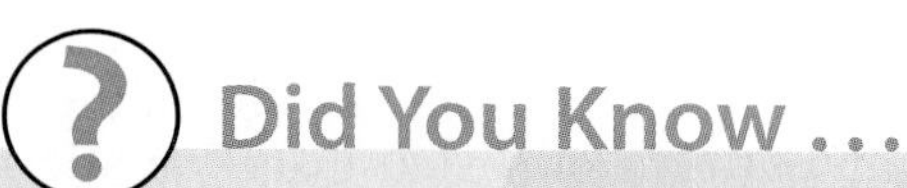

Even obtaining the services of a sex worker has changed with the advent of the Internet. For example, you can search under "prostitutes" and "[name of city]" and get a listing of the best spots to find a sex worker. Local police monitor such sites as well. Also, you can link up with an "escort" service via the Internet, ordering online.

assist prostitutes who wish to change their occupation; and (5) end the public stigma associated with sex work.

The National Organization for Women has also passed resolutions calling for union organizing and health and other protection for sex workers (NOW conference celebrates 30 years, 1998). There is also an International Committee for Prostitutes' Rights supporting all the goals of the NTFP plus elimination of laws supporting systematic zoning of prostitution, opposition to taxes on prostitutes and prostitute businesses, and support of educational programs to change social attitudes that stigmatize and discriminate against prostitutes and former prostitutes (International Committee for Prostitutes' Rights, 1998). It is interesting that in 1949 the United Nations adopted a resolution in favor of the decriminalization of prostitution, which has been ratified by 50 countries (not by the United States) (Prostitution in the United States—The statistics, 1998).

Controlling Sex Work

Some officials have tried various ways to manage sex work. For example, San Francisco took a laissez-faire approach. As a result, sex work is highly visible in tourist sections in the form of massage parlors, escort services, bar sex workers, hotel sex workers, and call girls (or boys). The major benefit of this approach has been to restrict sex work to nonresidential parts of the city. The Control Model—whereby certain neighborhoods strictly enforce laws against sex work—has been employed in North Dallas; the results have been reductions in crime and in visibility of sex workers. The Regulation Model—whereby sex work is legalized and subject to certain regulations—has been tried in rural Nevada, where it has resulted in a minimal amount of crime and where, for the most part, sex work is limited to controlled brothels. Finally, there is the Zoning Model—whereby sex work is tolerated but not legal only in certain parts of the city. With this model, sex workers are supposedly visible only in a certain part of the city, and crime associated with sex work is limited to that area. None of these approaches has been totally successful, and each has advantages and disadvantages.

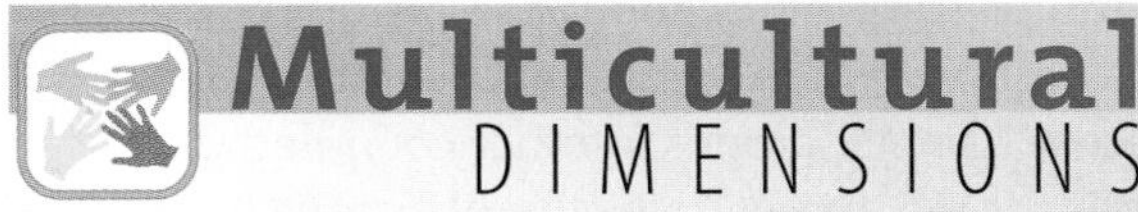

"Values" of Prostitution in Other Countries? In Russia, tens of thousands of female college students work as prostitutes or carry on exclusive relationships with so-called sponsors to pay for college. The Russian Internet is replete with web sites that offer free search engines that match potential clients with students. Most sites provide the woman's age, body measurements, types of sex she practices, corresponding costs, and even reviews by former clients. One girl used to work as an elementary teacher earning the equivalent of $60 per month. Now she works as a prostitute and earns the equivalent of $200 to $300 for a night of sexual activities. Of course, the women have expenses such as paying for a madam (agent) and use of an apartment or other appropriate facility. When asked how her parents feel about her work, one student said, "We tell them we work as waitresses. They don't ask any questions" (MacWilliams, 2002).

In some situations, prostitutes are very concerned about their rights. For example, in Paris hundreds of prostitutes wearing white masks with tears painted on them rallied in front of the French Senate to protest a high-profile government crackdown on their livelihood (French prostitutes protest crackdown, 2002).

Another method of trying to control sex work has been making public the identities of sex workers and their customers. For example, in 1997 "John TV" started in Kansas City. Every Wednesday morning viewers of the local government cable TV channel can see the names, photographs, dates of birth, and addresses of people—mostly men—who were arrested for visiting sex workers. Above each picture is this disclaimer: "This person is innocent until found guilty by a court." The ACLU has objected to this practice because it targets people before they are convicted of a crime and uses a government-controlled medium to deliver its message of humiliation (Kansas City's "John TV" tunes out rights, 1997).

Four months after the practice was started in Kansas City, officials in Stockton, California, started periodically broadcasting the names and booking photos of alleged sex workers and their customers (California TV to air information of prostitution suspects, 1997). Several months afterward, officials in St. Paul, Minnesota, started using both their cable TV show and the Internet to spread information about sex workers and their patrons (St. Paul prostitution fight may hit Internet, TV, 1997).

Another method of controlling sex workers involves organizations that provide help and support for sex workers who desire to change their life and stop being sex workers. One such organization is PROMISE:

> *PROMISE offers peer counseling, not therapy. Our model is based on addiction-recovery peer counseling and on the "strength-based" model of counseling developed at the Council for Prostitution Alternatives. Our philosophy is to reinforce the positive choices and strengths that our client demonstrates to help her achieve her goals: teaching, not preaching. (PROMISE: Our programs, 1998)*

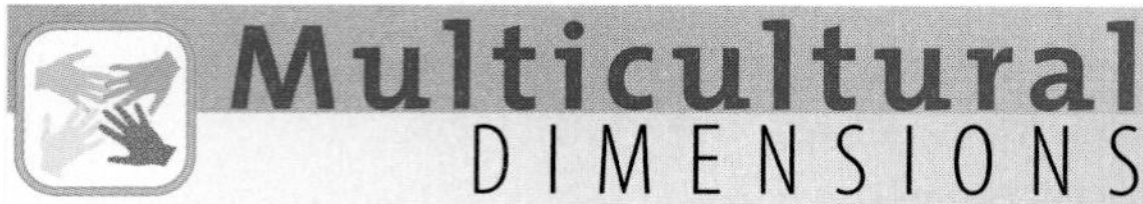

Organizations for Sex Workers One organization for sex workers is Call Off Your Tired Ethics (COYOTE), which was founded in 1973. It works for the rights of all sex workers of all genders and persuasions. COYOTE supports programs to assist sex workers if they choose to change their occupation, works to prevent the scapegoating of sex workers for AIDS and other STIs, and educates sex workers, their clients, and the general public about safer sex.

Prostitutes of New York (PONY) is a support and advocacy group for all people in the sex industry. PONY advocates the decriminalization of prostitution and calls for an end to illegal police activity in the enforcement of existing laws. It provides legal and health referrals to sex workers and encourages members to recommend doctors, therapists, and other professionals who provide high-quality service to sex workers. PONY encourages all people who sell sex or profit from sex to learn about the diversity of their industry, to promote professional standards in their sector, and to learn more about the history of the world's oldest profession (and its allied industries).

There are similar groups in other countries. One example is the Prostitutes Collective of Victoria (PCV) (Australia), which is a community-based organization developed to include and represent sex-industry workers' concerns about the issue of prostitution as a part of a worldwide prostitutes' rights movement. It works for basic human rights and occupational health and safety rights for all prostitution workers.

The Network of Sex Work Projects (NSWP) was formed in 1991. It consists of sex workers and organizations that provide services to sex workers in more than 40 countries. The NSWP focuses on issues similar to those of interest to the other groups and aims to facilitate opportunities for the voices of sex workers to be heard in relevant international forums.

The Law and Prostitution

Should prostitution be legal? This question has been argued for many years. Some people believe there are potential benefits of legalizing prostitution, such as increased human rights protection and health precautions. They argue that prostitution always has been and always will be. Legalization would increase condom use and in turn lead to a reduction of HIV and AIDS and other STIs. They feel prostitutes have the right to choose the way they earn their income; therefore, how can society stand in the way of someone's earning a good living? Opponents of prostitution argue that most prostitutes are forced into sexual slavery. They argue that legalization would give rise to a black market that would be frightening and abusive. For some opponents to prostitution, the issue is a moral one because prostitution gives rise to dehumanizing, unsafe, illegal activities. It is morally reprehensible, they say, for prostitutes to be treated as too many are treated. They conclude that the abuses and potential threat for ongoing abuse far outweigh any potential benefits of legalization. And the argument continues (Should prostitution be legal, 2003).

Child Prostitution

A particularly disturbing feature of sex work is the presence of minors selling sexual activity. Child prostitution has become more common in recent years. In some instances, children are forced by adults to perform sexual acts, and in other instances the minors may appear to be selling sexual activity by choice—though many would argue that it is not really voluntary.

Cultures exist around the world in which children, as belongings, are property to be bought and sold. Tens of millions of children are repeatedly raped, tortured, and shamed for the sexual gratification of adults. Worldwide

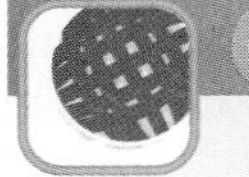

Global DIMENSIONS

Sex Work in Other Countries Sex work occurs all over the world. There has been a recent demand for Russian women (Pope, 1997). Young, pretty women have been told they have modeling jobs but are later forced into the sex industry. They are given false papers, assumed identities, and phony marriage partners so they can work abroad.

Israel is said to have a $450-million-per-year sex work ring. Young women describe hostagelike conditions, severe beatings, and rape as punishment by their captors (Pope, 1997).

Here is a sampling of sex work in other countries (Caron, 1998):

- Sex work is legal in Australia, but sex workers must be at least 18 years old. There are laws against pimping. Condoms are compulsory in sexual relationships with sex workers.
- Sex work is legal in Brazil. There are street sex workers and women working out of bars, hotels, massage parlors, saunas, and escort services. Child sex work is an expanding market in Brazil.
- Sex work is legal in Canada, but pimping and solicitation in public are not.
- In 1991 sex work was prohibited in China. Forced reeducation is punishment which includes legal and moral education and manual labor in a specified camp for 6 months to 2 years, for sex workers and johns.
- In Denmark sex work is not a criminal offense, and legal age of consent for sexual activity is 15 years old.
- In Finland prostitution is neither illegal nor regulated. Pimping and promoting sex work are forbidden.

there are perhaps as many as 100 million child prostitutes. In the United States there are about 2.4 million (Joseph, 1995).

In some Third World countries boys outnumber girls on the streets because girls are often put into brothels. These children are prostituted, or even sold, to prevent themselves and their families from starving. The customers who purchase the children and/or their services are adults who are commonly pedophiles and/or sadists.

In some instances there can be links between child prostitution and child pornography. For example, costumed children might act out a customer's fantasy in special surroundings while filming is done. The acting might be done as part of a story, such as an abduction of a virgin or a "schoolgirl tease," or the action might simply be rape and torture. There is money to be made from the prostitution activities and the selling of films or videos (Joseph, 1995).

In the United States a large number of adolescent sex workers are runaways who are looking for companionship, friendship, love, and approval, as well as a way of supporting themselves financially. Unfortunately, many of them are ideal targets for gangs, drug pushers, and pimps. To survive on the streets, runaways often sell drugs or their body, and a large number turn to other types of crime to support themselves.

It is estimated that between 300,000 and 400,000 girls and boys, aged 9–17 years, trade their body to pay for food, shelter, clothing, and other basic needs to survive on America's streets (Uhlman, 2001). Some U.S. children engage in commercial sexual activity while living at home and generally find customers among their peers. Those children at highest risk for commercial sexual exploitation are those who run away or are thrown out by their relatives. Fewer than 25% are members of impoverished families. A significant number of their customers are married men, many with children of their own. Other children at higher risk to become victims of commercial sexual activity include female gang members who get involved to raise money for the gang; foreign children; and teenagers living along the Canadian or Mexican borders who cross into those countries specifically to solicit sexual activity.

The fact that runaways make up a significant percentage of adolescent sex workers creates a particularly difficult problem for law enforcement personnel. When they arrest a child sex worker it does little good to send the child back to a poor home environment. In fact, there have been reports of children's setting up their own prostitution rings, while living at home, to earn spending money.

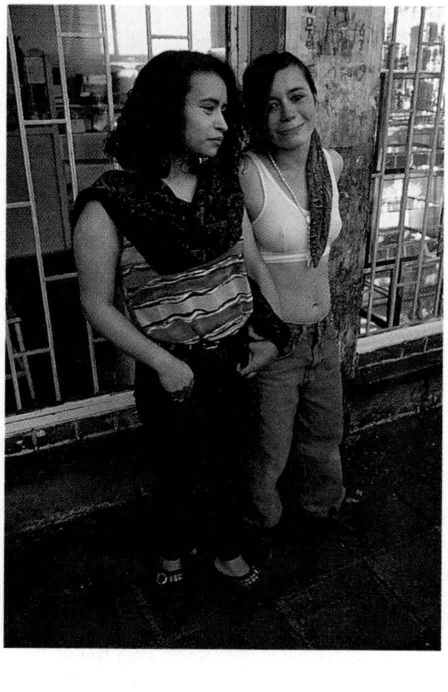

Most teenage sex workers probably are members of unstable families with many problems. Many have been victims of sexual abuse and abandoned by their families (Rio, 1991).

In response to childhood sex work, law enforcement personnel have attempted to crack down on pimps of adolescent sex workers and at the same time better coordinate with other law enforcement agencies to recognize and help runaways when possible. Service programs for runaways have incorporated a medical component to treat the physical and mental health needs of runaways who have turned to sex work

Poverty in Latin America and Asian countries has resulted in young girls' being sold into the sex trade by their parents, who are desperate for money. The children, who range in age from 6 to 15 years old, work until they have repaid their "debt"—the money given to their parents plus some profit for the pimp involved.

(and to other runaways, too). Runaway shelters provide services to help reduce the need for runaways to turn to sex work. Such services include medical services, crisis intervention services, individual and group counseling, vocational training and job placement, legal services, independent living skills training, and support and friendship. The hope is that the many shelters and service centers around the United States will help convince young people that they need not turn to pimps and sex work to meet their needs.

Thousands of British university students have turned to sex work to cover their college expenses. They work as strippers, lap dancers, escorts, and pornographic movie actors. One student said she cannot find another job that fits in with her academic obligations. Another said that taking his clothes off is easier than waiting on tables and he makes 10 times more. In Leeds, 60% of the city's sex workers are university students. One madam opened a brothel close to the University of Leeds to make it easier for students to commute to work (Birchard, 2001).

Research about all forms of sex work has changed more in recent years than at any time in the past. We now know more about the extent of sex work and its changing nature worldwide, but particularly in the West. We also have a better grasp of the reasons why some people enter the sex industry. With the growth of sex-worker organizations, there is greater access to research subjects. The existence of a pool of volunteers willing to contribute to both their own research projects and those of others has the potential of adding greatly to our knowledge about this area of human sexual behavior (Bullough & Bullough, 1996).

Exploring the DIMENSIONS of Human Sexuality

Our feelings, attitudes, and beliefs regarding sexuality are influenced by our internal and external environments. Go to sexuality.jbpub.com to learn more about the biological, psychological, and sociological factors that affect your sexuality.

Biological Factors

- Prostitutes in general have a much higher rate of HIV. About one-third of New York City streetwalkers have HIV.
- No externally used products can enlarge the penis or breasts.

Sociocultural Factors

- Fraudulent sexual aids are among the top 10 sources of health fraud in the United States.
- Prostitution is outlawed in every U.S. state except Nevada (and then only legal in a few counties).
- Many countries allow prostitution. South Korea issues identification cards to prostitutes that serve as hotel passes. South Korea and Thailand consider prostitution of young girls a tourist attraction.
- Some countries, such as Iran and China, have attempted to ban distribution of sexually explicit materials. Laws govern distribution and possession of sexually explicit photos of children.
- Media often fail to depict safer sexual practices in books, articles, TV shows, and movies.
- Sexually explicit materials helped create and expand the market for home VCRs and the Internet.

Psychological Factors

- Media images negatively impact body image and self-esteem.
- Many ads use sexual imagery to attract attention and stimulate senses.

CASE STUDY

Marketing of sexual products and use of sexual imagery to market nonsexual products are multibillion-dollar businesses. The alluring imagery may draw attention to the product but does not necessarily result in a sale unless the product is sexually related, such as a product to enhance one's appearance.

As marketers attempt to target certain groups (typically younger) with sexual imagery, they need to be aware that other people may find their ads offensive.

Marketing of sexually explicit materials to consumers in conditions of privacy (i.e., at home) has driven the markets for the VCR and the Internet.

But marketers also face legal challenges to distributing sexually explicit material. Because "community standards" are used to judge whether material is obscene, a web site operator in one state can be charged with obscenity under the community standards of a person in another state who downloads the materials.

Marketing of any sexually explicit material involving children is prosecuted harshly. Even downloading such material is a violation of the law.

Discussion Questions

1. Analyze the value of sexuality in selling products. Discuss sexually oriented ads, including the ways sex helps sell products (bikini-clad calendars, sexually explicit rap music, "dirty" classic literature, and so on).
2. Create a legal standard for distributing sexually explicit materials. Include in the standard what constitutes art, child pornography, literature, and the like.
3. Compare and contrast the varied types of sex workers. Then describe efforts to control sex work.

Application Questions

Reread the chapter-opening story and answer the following questions.

1. Of the students who had opinions about sexual consumerism, with whom do you agree? Explain your answer, citing contemporary examples.
2. In what ways do actor portrayals of sexuality—or models with "perfect" bodies—make us feel inferior? (You may want to review In Focus: Body Image when answering this question.) Could those same images be said to promote erotic feelings and thus have value?
3. Does the use of naked flesh make ads sexier? Or have ads from the past, albeit with less flesh, been just as sexually oriented?

Critical Thinking Questions

1. When planning an ad campaign, a marketer needs to think about all audiences who will view the ad. Consider the anecdotal story that has appeared in various advertising publications about the former first lady Nancy Reagan and her daughter, Patty Davis: During the early 1990s, the two women were waiting in a hotel lobby when the conversation turned to sexual consumerism. Mrs. Reagan, showing her daughter a perfume ad in a magazine, said that she did not like having to look at a nearly naked man in the ad. Her daughter replied, "Well, I sure do!" They both laughed.

   Clearly, the marketer was targeting the demographics of Reagan's daughter. But should a marketer have to be concerned about offending people in other demographics—older and more conservative people as well as minors? Describe the steps a marketer should have to take before placing ads.
2. Although it is billed as the "world's oldest profession," prostitution is not legal in the United States except in a few counties in Nevada. Should prostitution be legalized? Consider the social, legal (including tax ramifications), health, moral, and other dimensions of sexuality of both clients and prostitutes in your answer.
3. Former stars of sexually explicit films, such as Linda Lovelace and Traci Lords, have described the world of porn films as one of physical abuse (actual and threatened) and drugs. If an actress participated in explicit sexual activity under such coercion, does that constitute rape? Should distribution of such movies be illegal?
4. Distribution of photos of naked minors is illegal. But prominent "art" photographers often take photos of naked minors, and such photos are distributed in photo anthologies through major bookstore chains. How is it possible to differentiate between art and child pornography?

5. China, Iran, and other countries limit Internet access for their citizens. Two major concerns are antigovernment rhetoric and sexually explicit material. Given the ease with which minors can access sexually explicit material, should the U.S. government ban the Internet access of U.S. citizens? Should the Internet be regulated?

Critical Thinking Case

In parts of Japan, December 24 is the "hottest" night of the year. Societal pressure is strong for every unmarried person to have a date on Christmas Eve and for that date to include an overnight stay. In this respect December 24 is not dissimilar to prom night here in America. Just about every major hotel in Tokyo is sold out for that night months in advance. The Japanese describe Christmas Eve as a night to make love and refer to it as "H-Day" (for "hormone," the Japanese euphemism for sex).

This evening is quite expensive for young Japanese, as the cost typically exceeds $1,000. Men are expected to buy their date a present ($215), take her to Tokyo Disneyland ($100), provide dinner at a fancy restaurant ($385), take a room at a nice hotel (between $350 and $650), have breakfast the next morning ($35), and rent a limousine ($150)—all of this in a country less than 1% Christian and where December 25 is a normal working day.

1. Discuss H-Day in terms of the dimensions of sexuality. Include safer-sex practices, the psychological implications of engaging in sexual activity with someone because of societal pressure, religion, culture, and other factors.
2. What cultural factors would prevent H-Day from being accepted in the United States? (Assume that the date would be changed from December 24.)

Exploring Personal Dimensions

Are You a Good Sexual Consumer?

Answer the following statements with one of the following responses. When you are finished, total your points and find out how good a sexual consumer you are.

1. Rarely or never
2. Sometimes
3. Often
4. All or most of the time

_____ 1. I make sure the date on any product (such as condoms or oral contraceptives) has not expired.

_____ 2. I am not influenced by sexually alluring images to purchase products.

_____ 3. I am aware of whether any sexually explicit material I view involves minors.

_____ 4. I make sure that any sexually explicit material I view is kept away from minors.

_____ 5. I understand that sharing sexual aids (or toys) with others is a high-risk activity, capable of transmitting STIs and/or AIDS.

_____ 6. I am aware that sexual contact with sex workers or former sex workers is a high-risk activity, because of the potential for STI and/or HIV transmission.

_____ 7. I believe that aphrodisiacs offer no sexual help physiologically, and I consider their side effects before using them.

_____ 8. I evaluate "research" claims made by marketers before buying a product.

_____ 9. I consider the source of sexual health information before purchasing any product.

_____10. I have sought recommendations from friends for whom to consult in case of sexually related health care needs.

_____11. I have regular exams by a physician.

_____12. I understand that certain prescription drugs (such as antibiotics) can affect the effectiveness of oral contraceptives.

_____13. I read labels of health products and follow directions.

_____14. I do a monthly breast or testicular self-exam.

_____15. When friends state a sexual myth as though it were a fact, I use knowledge from this course to correct them tactfully.

Scoring

0–15	Your sexual consumer skills are weak.
16–30	Your sexual consumer skills are below what they should be.
31–45	Your sexual consumer skills are good but can stand improvement.

Sexuality Online

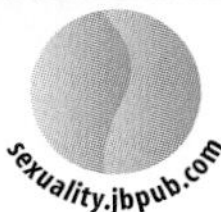

Go to the web component for *Exploring the Dimensions of Human Sexuality* at sexuality.jbpub.com for web exercises, additional resources related to this chapter, and student review tools.

Suggested Readings

Dalecki, M. G. & Price, J. Dimensions of pornography, *Sociological Spectrum, 14, no. 3* (July–September 1994), 205–219.

Eisler, R. *Sacred pleasure: Sex, myth, and the politics of the body*. San Francisco: Harper, 1995.

Feminism and sex, *Ms., 6* (November–December 1995), 48–62.

Linz, D., Donnerstein, E., Shafer, B. J., Land, K. C., McCall, P. L., & Graesser, A. C. Discrepancies between the legal code and community standards for sex and violence: An empirical challenge to traditional assumptions in obscenity law, *Law and Society Review, 29, no. 1* (1995), 127–168.

Nalezindki, A. Acceptable and unacceptable levels of risk: The case of pornography, *Social Theory and Practice, 22, no. 1* (1996), 83–104.

O'Neil, R. O. What limits should campus networks place on pornography? *The Chronicle of Higher Education, 49, no. 28* (March 21, 2003), B20.

Pardun, C. J. & Forde, K. R. Sex in the media: Do condom ads have a chance? *SIECUS Report 31, no. 2* (December 2002–January 2003), 22–23.

Rudman, W. J. & Verdi, P. Exploitation: Comparing sexual and violent imagery of females and males in advertising, *Women and Health, 20, no. 4* (1994), 1–14.

Sex on TV: Content and context, Washington, DC: The Henry J. Kaiser Family Foundation, 2001. Available: http://www.kff.org.

The San Francisco task force on prostitution: Final report, 1998. Online: Available: www.bayswan.org/2execsuon.html.

CHAPTER

18

Sexual Ethics, Morality, and the Law

FEATURES

Ethical Dimensions
Extramarital Sex

Gender Dimensions
The "Umbrelly" (A Little Humor)

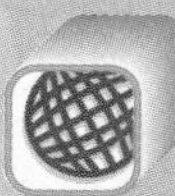

Global Dimensions
Ethical Issues Around the World

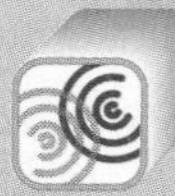

Communication Dimensions
The Morality of Requesting a Variety of Sexual Behaviors

CHAPTER OBJECTIVES

1 Define *ethics, morals, ethical principles, ethical dilemmas, values,* and the five ethical principles that serve as a basis for deciding whether a decision is moral.

2 State the ethical considerations of such sexually related topics as sexually transmitted infections, sexual activity between unmarried partners, sodomy, contraception, abortion, amniocentesis, fetal tissue implantation, prostitution, in vitro fertilization, genetic engineering, and sexual responsibility to a partner.

3 Identify the rationale for laws pertaining to homosexuality, obscenity and pornography, rape, statutory rape, adultery, and divorce.

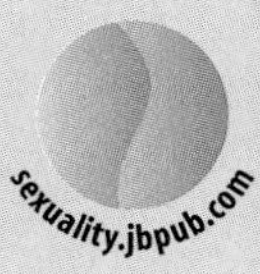

sexuality.jbpub.com
Commonly Accepted Ethical Principles
Genetic Engineering

INTRODUCTION

Wendy Weaver was a well-respected high school philosophy teacher and girls' volleyball coach in the Nebo, Utah, school district (Associated Press, 1998). Concerned about her student athletes, in the summer of 1997 she telephoned each one to ask about her summer camp schedule. That is when it happened. A student asked, "Are you gay?" Weaver answered that she was, eliciting a response from the student that she would not play on Weaver's volleyball team in the fall. When school district officials heard what Wendy Weaver disclosed to the student, they immediately fired her from her coaching responsibilities and instructed her not to speak of her sexual orientation to either students or school staff, in or outside school.

The Nebo school district officials believed they were right to protect young people in their school from what they perceived to be disclosure of immoral behavior. They believed homosexuality was wrong and that it was sinful.

Wendy Weaver, however, believed that she had a moral right to express her sexuality in any way she sought, as long as she did not impose it on her students. After all, she argued, heterosexual teachers are not forbidden to disclose their sexual orientation. Therefore, she asserted that it was wrong—immoral—to forbid her to do so.

Eventually a judge determined the legal issues involved in this case. In November, U.S. District Court Judge Bruce Jenkins ruled that Wendy Weaver's rights of free speech, equal protection under the law, and due process were violated. He ordered that the gag order be lifted and that Wendy Weaver be reinstated as coach of the girls' volleyball team. In his ruling Judge Jenkins stated, "Although the Constitution cannot control prejudices, neither this court nor any other court should, directly or indirectly, legitimize them."

This case includes issues of morality, ethics, and law. The school officials believed that they were acting morally by protecting young people from a teacher they thought might inappropriately affect their sexual orientation. Wendy believed she was acting morally when she answered the team member honestly and when she asserted her constitutional rights. And the judge believed he was acting morally when he applied a law designed to prevent prejudice from depriving a person of her rights in a democratic society. Certainly everyone could not be right; nor could everyone be wrong. Certainly, everyone was not purposefully acting immorally. We shall see in this chapter how complex issues of morality really are and how a systematic approach can manage some of this complexity when these issues relate to matters of sexuality. Furthermore, we shall see how the law is used to codify societal consensus about morality and how it is applied to express societal mores.

Many ethical dilemmas relate to sexuality. For example, whether women should use intrauterine devices (IUDs) as a means of contraception that may prevent fertilized ova from successfully implanting on the uterus's endometrial lining involves the moral question of when life begins. Whether fetal tissue or stem cells—that is, from aborted fetuses—should be made available as a treatment for such conditions as Parkinson's disease concerns the moral issue of the sanctity of the human body.

These and other questions of sexual morality are pervasive. They affect every one of us, if not directly and daily, then certainly as members of a society wrestling with their resolutions. They are also emotionally charged. This point should not be unnoticed. When issues evoke emotional reactions—as sexual issues tend to do—these emotions too often interfere with a rational investigation. Consequently, people argue their own viewpoints while ignoring other perspectives, and that method of argument is not conducive to learning.

The story of Wendy Weaver illustrates the multidimensional facets of ethics, morality, and the law.

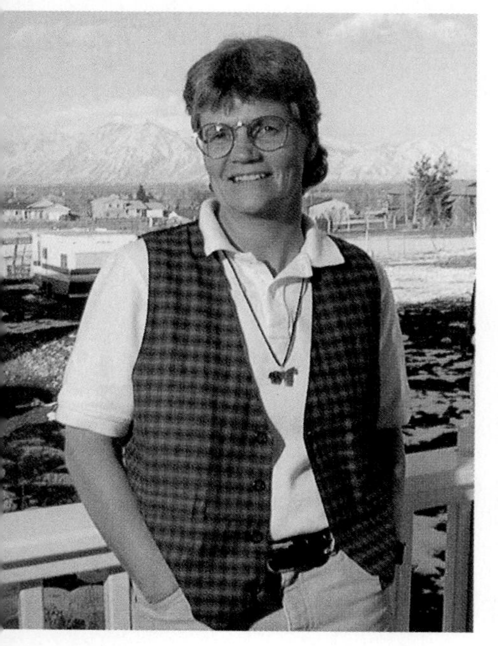

Before this discussion begins, however, we must prevent any possible confusion. The topics we consider in this chapter are all discussed elsewhere in this text in detail, and the various implications, ramifications, and idiosyncrasies associated with them are presented. The discussion of these topics here, however, serves to explore the morality and ethics of particular sexually related behaviors or decisions in a unified, systematic manner. In addition, it highlights the importance of considering the ethics and morality of all sexual matters.

Talking about sexual morality is not easy. Whose morality should we focus on? Which morals, if any, should we advocate? How can we prevent offending people whose morals differ from ours? It would be arrogant for us to insist that everyone adopt a single set of sexual morals, and it would be particularly impertinent to suggest that our own morals be the ones adopted.

Therefore, in this chapter, rather than advocating a particular set of morals or ethical principles, we describe the process of moral reasoning. We sketch our society's moral stance on sexually transmitted infections, contraception, in vitro fertilization, rape, prostitution, and so on, and describe the background and enforcement of some laws. Along the way we acknowledge some of the religious, philosophical, cultural, family-related, and experiential reasons for the differences in sexual morality among individuals and among societies.

Ethics: The Basis for Making Decisions

To begin investigating sexual morality, we need to distinguish between the terms *ethics* and *moral.* **Ethics** refers to a *system* by which we determine whether some action is moral or immoral. An action is **moral** if it is judged to be *good* or *right;* it is **immoral** if it is judged to be *bad* or *wrong.* To guide the decision of whether an action is moral or immoral, the system of ethics employs **ethical principles.** These ethical principles provide answers to abstract questions—they are general guidelines, not meant for individual cases. With regard to abortion, for example, ethicists would be more concerned with the general question of when life begins or with a woman's right to control her own reproductive capacity than with whether abortion is appropriate in a particular case. When a set of ethical principles is available and accepted by a society, the people of that society know how they are expected to behave. Professional societies attempt to develop guiding principles—or *codes of ethics*—to govern their members' behaviors. The code of ethics developed by the American Association of Sex Educators, Counselors, and Therapists, for example, sets guidelines for its members.

ethics
A system that uses ethical principles to make decisions about morality.

moral
What is judged to be right according to a system of ethics.

immoral
What is judged to be wrong according to a system of ethics.

ethical principles
Guides by which we can judge an action or decision as moral or immoral.

Ethical Principles

Table 18.1 introduces five examples of ethical principles that can be used to make moral decisions. As will be discussed, though, these kinds of principles may be in opposition to one another in any given situation.

Nonmaleficence

Is it moral to convince someone else to engage in sexual intercourse in spite of his or her reluctance? One ethical principle that speaks to this issue is

TABLE 18.1 Selected Ethical Principles

Principle	Description
1. Nonmaleficence	Whatever else, do no harm. This includes preventing harm, not inflicting harm, and removing harm when it is present.
2. Beneficence	Not only should one not do harm, but one is obligated to do good.
3. Autonomy/Liberty	People should be free to decide their own course of action as long as they do not harm others.
4. Justice/Fairness	Each person should be treated fairly.
5. Social Utility	The greatest good for the greatest number should be considered. What is best for society may outweigh what is best for the individual.

maleficence—the act of committing harm or evil. The principle of *nonmaleficence* is that whatever is moral—right or good—can be determined by asking whether it does any harm. If it does harm, it is not moral. Does coercing someone to engage in sex do physical, psychological, or spiritual harm? If so, that behavior is immoral.

Beneficence
For some ethicists, doing no harm is not enough. For an action to be moral, it has to do good. That is what is meant by the ethical principle of *beneficence.* School officials who banned Wendy Weaver from coaching volleyball thought they were doing good for the students in that school. Therefore, they thought they were acting morally. Those who opposed the ban believed they were doing good by upholding the right of people to acknowledge their sexuality in an appropriate and honest manner, regardless of their particular sexual orientation. Therefore, they thought they were acting morally. We will soon discuss how these contradictions can be resolved.

Ethical DIMENSIONS

Extramarital Sex Actually making a decision regarding sexual morality may help you comprehend the rather abstract material to come. Therefore, we quote here an argument that adultery, or extramarital relationships, can be moral and ask you to react to it. (Bear in mind that although this argument describes only men, women have extramarital affairs.)

Albert Ellis, a prominent psychologist, wrote that there is a healthy adulterer. Although Ellis's argument was presented a number of years ago, it is as applicable today as it was then. Ellis wrote (1977, 374–375):

1. The healthy adulterer is nondemanding and noncompulsive. He prefers but he does not need extramarital affairs. He believes that he can live better with than without them, and therefore he tries to have them from time to time. But he is also able to have a happy general and marital life if no such affairs are practicable.
2. The undisturbed adulterer usually manages to carry on his extramarital affairs without unduly disturbing his marriage and family relationships nor his general existence. He is sufficiently discreet about his adultery, on the one hand, and appropriately frank and honest about it with his close associates, on the other hand, so that most people he intimately knows are able to tolerate his affairs and not get too upset about them.
3. He fully accepts his own extramarital desires and acts and never condemns himself or punishes himself because of them, even though he may sometimes decide that they are unwise and may make specific attempts to bring them to a halt.
4. He faces his specific problems with his wife and family as well as his general life difficulties and does not use his adulterous relationships as a means of avoiding any of his serious problems.
5. He is usually tolerant of himself when he acts poorly or makes errors; he is minimally hostile when his wife and family members behave in a less than desirable manner; and he fully accepts the fact that the world is rough and life is often grim, but that there is no reason why it must be otherwise and that he can live happily even when conditions around him are not great. Consequently, he does not drive himself to adultery because of self-deprecation, self-pity, or hostility to others.
6. He is sexually adequate with his spouse as well as with others and therefore has extramarital affairs out of sex interest rather than for sex therapy.

Although the adulterer who lives up to these criteria may have still other emotional disturbances and may be having extramarital affairs for various neurotic reasons, Ellie argues that there is also a good chance that this is not true.

Autonomy/Liberty

The ethical principle of *autonomy* or *liberty* requires people be free to decide an issue for themselves before that decision can qualify as moral. That does not mean that every decision made freely is a moral one, only that any made under coercion is immoral. Was the decision to bar Wendy Weaver made freely by school officials, or was it coerced by a small group of vocal parents? Was Weaver allowed to decide freely whether she would discuss her sexual orientation, as could heterosexuals teaching in that school, or was she being coerced by school officials? The way you answer these questions will help you determine which actions you think were moral in this case.

Justice/Fairness

Some ethicists believe that for an action to be moral, it must treat people fairly. They term this ethical principle *justice* or *fairness*. That does not mean that people must be treated equally. For example, our culture has determined that homosexuals and heterosexuals may be treated differently by different segments of society. That is, in private clubs or homes, or in certain churches or synagogues, gays may be excluded. However, our society has determined that excluding gays from public facilities is not just or fair—it is immoral—and has codified that decision by making a law defining that behavior illegal/unconstitutional.

Social Utility

Sometimes there is a clash between individual rights and the rights of a large group of people. In these instances, some ethicists use the ethical principle of *social utility* to determine the morality of various actions being contemplated. Social utility defines the moral decision as the one that is best for society (or the large group) rather than what is best for the individual (or the small group). School officials in Nebo, Utah, determined that removing Wendy Weaver from coaching was the greater good for the greater number of people (the students). Whether they were aware of it or not, they were using social utility to justify their decision. Of course, others might argue that the greater number of people in this instance ought to have been the gay community throughout the United States whose rights have been violated for far too long.

Ethical Dilemmas

We often experience situations in which one ethical principle clashes with another. We call these clashes **ethical dilemmas.** For example, consider again the question of adultery. Suppose you held the following ethical principles: Marriage should be a sexually monogamous relationship and people have a right to a satisfying, fulfilling sexual life. Obviously if you were in a marriage in which you were sexually unfulfilled for some reason, these two ethical principles would conflict. In such a situation which principle would be operative? Which one would take precedence over the other? Sometimes religion or culture provides answers to ethical dilemmas. For instance, in Islamic countries adultery is opposed by tradition and the law; such a society has resolved our ethical dilemma—at least officially—by placing the higher value on fidelity within marriage. Where there are no such prohibitions, individuals must rank their own values in order to choose.

The existence of such dilemmas has led to the development of situation ethics, in contrast to rule ethics. **Rule ethics** are exhaustive principles intended to guide people in their moral decision making in all situations. These principles are explicit, specific, and all-encompassing. People who hold to the letter of the law and proponents of religious dogmas are rule ethicists. **Situation ethics,** in contrast, are based on the premise that all situations are unique, and

ethical dilemma
When two or more ethical principles work in opposing fashion in a particular situation, resulting in bewilderment regarding what is moral and what is immoral.

rule ethics
Guiding principles used in all situations to arrive at moral decisions, which are considered applicable to all situations.

situation ethics
A belief that no one set of rules can apply to all situations and each specific situation must be analyzed to determine which ethical principles are applicable.

therefore no one set of rules is applicable in all cases. Consequently a situation ethicist faced with a moral decision carefully reviews, analyzes, and evaluates each specific situation to determine which principles are applicable; a rule ethicist applies a given principle, regardless of the specific circumstances. As an example, a rule ethicist believes abortion is wrong in all cases. A situation ethicist may also believe abortion is wrong but may also believe it is moral in the case of a 12-year-old rape victim who becomes pregnant.

Trying to decide which viewpoint—rule ethics or situation ethics—is correct is itself an ethical dilemma. When we narrow our focus to sexual behavior, we can see that the rule/situation dichotomy has relevance. Are there general rules to guide sexual behavior, or does each situation require its own set of rules? Which rules, if any, will guide your behavior? Given your intuitive responses to the questions we raise in this chapter, see whether you consider yourself a rule or situation ethicist.

Moral Decision Making and Sexual Behavior

What influences the decisions we make about sexuality? Such factors as our knowledge or lack of knowledge; our sense of who we are; our ideals regarding fidelity and responsibility; our desire to express affection, passion, and delight; the emotional excitement we experience while facing the decision; and external cultural influences such as the double standard are all involved. The questions one asks in making moral decisions about sexuality or any other area of life are, What is *right*? What is *good*? What is *wrong*? What is *bad*? If it is right or good, it is moral! If it is wrong or bad, it is immoral! Thus morals relate to concrete decisions in particular situations.

To determine whether an action or decision is moral or immoral, we use our system of ethics. This system of ethics involves our ethical principles, which are guides by which we can judge an action or decision as moral or immoral. If the decision is inconsistent with our ethical principles, it is immoral; if it is consistent with them, it is moral.

Ethical principles specific to sexual matters include the following:

1. Sexual behavior should not be forced on anyone.
2. Sexual behavior between consenting adults is acceptable.
3. Fidelity (faithfulness) in marriage is a must.
4. Marriage partners and loved ones must be responsive to each other's needs (Bruess & Greenberg, 1988).

Unfortunately, most situations are not so cut and dried. Applying ethical principles is often a complex matter because they provide only guidance, not ready-made answers. If our principles are in conflict, we must examine our personal values to rank conflicting ethical principles in order of importance. By personal *values* we mean the worth or importance we assign to our ethical principles. If we personally value our commitment to a monogamous relationship more than we value sexual fulfillment, for example, then we resolve a conflict between the two by choosing not to have extramarital relationships. If we value sexual fulfillment more highly, then we resolve the same conflict differently.

To summarize, then, we decide the morality of an action or decision after identifying and ranking ethical principles in order of our personal values. Most people learn that the many moral decisions they make about sexual behavior are ultimately based on their personal values.

Our intention is to help you explore your own values and ethical principles so you may apply them in specific situations, and thereby act morally.

Commonly Accepted Ethical Principles

This discussion is not intended to convey that *anything goes*. Although we value and recognize the need for diversity, as a society we have reached agreement on a set of ethical principles. For example, we have societal consensus that caring, respect, honesty, responsibility, and trust ought to guide our decisions regarding morality. In fact, a whole educational movement that seeks to convey these principles to school-aged children and youth has sprouted. That movement is called *Character Education*. Its objectives are consistent with the societal consensus regarding ethical principles described: respect for the rights of all people regardless of their race, religion, gender, age, and sexual orientation; understanding, sympathy, concern, and compassion for others; and personal integrity and honesty. These are principles to which all citizens should adhere, and to emphasize their importance, society has passed laws specifying sanctions for acting contrary to them. For example, we have laws against discrimination by gender, race, and ethnicity, and in many states, sexual orientation. And we have laws punishing those who sexually abuse others. If someone lies to a sexual partner about his or her HIV status and infects that partner, we have laws to punish that behavior. If someone takes advantage of someone else by engaging in coitus with that person while he or she is incapable of deciding freely to participate (for example, if intoxicated or mentally impaired), we have laws punishing that behavior. And if someone fires someone else from a job solely because of that person's sexual orientation, we have laws to punish that behavior (as the school officials who fired Wendy Weaver found out).

In matters of sexuality and sexual morality, it is important to keep these consensually agreed-on ethical principles in the forefront. Certainly we, as the writers of this textbook, value diversity and recognize the influence of different experiences and values as they play out in various ethical dilemmas. Still, these consensually accepted ethical principles are ones to which we are committed. The problem arises when behaving consistently with one or more of these principles means violating one or more of the others. This is what we earlier described as an ethical dilemma. Ethical dilemmas apply to human sexuality, as we shall now see.

Sexually Transmitted Infections

To treat sexually transmitted infections (STIs) effectively on a large scale, health care workers often ask their patients to identify their sexual contacts. The purpose is to inform these contacts that they have been exposed to a disease and encourage them to seek treatment. Generally the carrier is inclined, at least fleetingly, to protect the anonymity of his or her sexual contacts (and perhaps his or her own identity and reputation). One of the ethical principles commonly underlying such a reaction is probably, *One should not discuss other people's private sexual behavior.* However, a competing ethical principle might be, *People should not intentionally harm the health of others.* Most individuals would probably value the second principle over the first and would therefore identify their sexual contacts. Observers who also value health over confidentiality would judge this decision to be moral. If the infected person is married and has contracted the disease through nonconsensual extramarital activity, the principle of not harming others becomes harder to apply. In this situation the patient would have to decide whether the health of the marriage partner was more valuable than potential damage to the marital relationship and the family and whether the couple had an agreement regarding fidelity that had been breached.

As we discussed in In Focus: HIV and AIDS, an important ethical issue raised by the HIV and AIDS epidemic is whether to require pregnant women to be tested for HIV. With modern medications and medical regimens, approximately two-thirds of HIV and AIDS can be prevented in babies born to infected mothers. Consequently, using the ethical principle of beneficence, some medical experts argue that all pregnant women should be required to be tested for HIV, thereby identifying mothers who ought to be treated before their babies' births and newborns who ought to be treated as soon after birth as possible. However, others argue that requiring all pregnant women to be tested would actually harm newborns (maleficence). They believe that if pregnant women are required to be tested they will refrain from identifying themselves as pregnant, thereby depriving their babies of the prenatal care that can prevent all kinds of health problems, not just HIV and AIDS. This would, in turn, increase the infant mortality rate, which is already too high, especially in low socioeconomic populations. Therefore, opponents of mandatory pregnancy testing for HIV believe testing ought to be voluntary (autonomy/liberty) with educational campaigns to communicate the advantages of being tested.

There are other ethical issues related to HIV and AIDS. For example, should research funds be used for treating AIDS patients or for finding a cure or for developing a vaccine? What is the appropriate balance in this funding? Are funds best used for education about HIV and AIDS to prevent the greatest possible number of cases?

These questions are more than issues for academic consideration: Decisions are being made on a regular basis by research institutes, the government, and insurance companies. Are these decisions being made ethically? Are they moral decisions? Your answers to these questions depend on the way you value your ethical principles. Although no one answer will meet with everyone's approval, society adopts a consensus view of morality as a matter of necessity. That is, *something* must be decided, even if the decision is to ignore the situation. Further, because we are citizens in a society that allows for our input, we are contributing to this ethical exercise by our votes, letters, and attitudes (as determined by opinion polls).

Sexual Activity Between Unmarried Partners

Whether or not to participate in sexual activity without being married is another common moral decision. Those who decide that such behavior is immoral might value the following ethical principle: *Marriage is a unique relationship blessed by God and allowing for a total expression of love.* Those who consider sexual intercourse to be moral in any circumstance, unless one participant is harmed in some way, might value another principle more, such as, *You should experience life fully.* However, decisions regarding premarital or nonmarital sexual behavior are usually more complicated than a choice between two principles. Situation ethicists pondering the morality of premarital sex in a given situation might ask the following questions:

1. How old are the people involved? Seventeen? Forty-five?
2. What do the people feel for each other?
3. Is their intention to marry or enter into a union? Soon?
4. What are their religious beliefs?
5. In which society (country, culture) do they live?

In your own situation, what special considerations are or were relevant to your decisions about the morality of your sexual behavior?

Sodomy

It is impossible to define the term **sodomy** because states lump together those sexual activities they consider immoral and codify their views by passing laws that make these sexual behaviors illegal. Usually sodomy laws refer to such sexual activities as anal intercourse, oral–genital sexual behavior, homosexual activities, and any sexual behavior with animals. In earlier years, some states defined *sodomy* as any sexual activity of anyone other than a married couple. In fact, as late as 1990, a bill was proposed by a Washington state legislator that would allow the state to prosecute anyone younger than 18 years old who was "necking" or "petting." The proposed penalty was a maximal sentence of 90 days in jail and a $5,000 fine.

sodomy
Specifically refers to anal intercourse, but is often used to refer to almost any sexual behavior someone might not consider normal.

Most sodomy laws are applied primarily against homosexuals. The penalties vary from state to state, ranging from a $200 fine to 20 years of imprisonment. Violators of sodomy laws have been imprisoned, lost their jobs and homes, lost custody of their children, and even been beaten and killed. One test of the constitutionality of sodomy laws occurred in 1986. In the *Bowers v. Hardwick* case, an Atlanta man was arrested after police officers entered his home at the request of his roommate regarding another matter and found him in bed with another man. When this case finally reached the U.S. Supreme Court, the Court upheld Georgia's sodomy law in spite of recognizing that the Constitution creates "zones of privacy." Dissenting from this decision was Justice Harry A. Blackmun, who wrote that the Court mistakenly refused to recognize "the fundamental interest all individuals have in controlling the nature of their intimate associations with others."

In 1961, every state in the United States had a sodomy law. However, in spite of the *Bowers v. Hartwick* decision, or maybe in response to it, most states have repealed their sodomy laws as they apply to consenting adults. By 2003, 38 states had either repealed their sodomy laws or declared them unconstitutional. Of the states that still have these laws, four specifically restrict their laws to homosexual activities (Figure 18.1). In fact, most

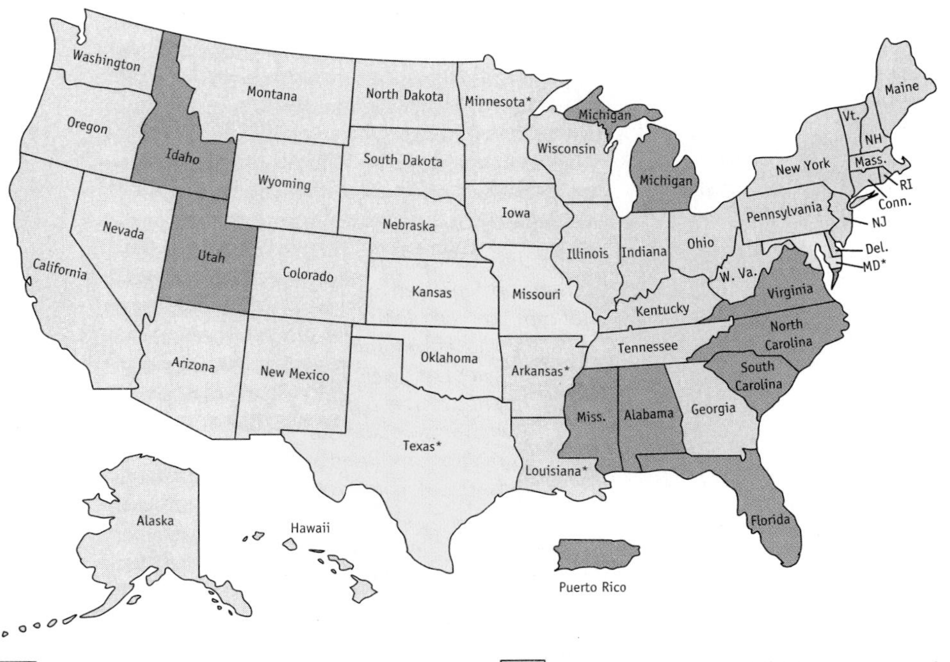

FIGURE 18.1 Four states prohibit consensual sodomy among same-sex couples only; 14 states plus Puerto Rico prohibit consensual sodomy among all couples.

Western countries have also removed sodomy laws from their statutes, considering them archaic. Supporting this view are the Universal Declaration of Human Rights, written by the United Nations Commission on Human Rights, which prohibits sodomy laws, and Amnesty International, which describes people imprisoned solely for sodomy as "prisoners of conscience" (Summersgill, 1998). In 2003, the Supreme Court ruled that laws prohibiting sexual behavior between consenting adults in private are unconstitutional. It is expected that this ruling will have significant impact for gays in particular, and others as well.

Contraception

People who oppose so-called artificial methods of contraception for religious reasons are usually guided by the ethic, *All life is sacred.* They argue that prevention of a conception that would occur without interference is interference with God's creation of life. Proponents of modern birth control, in contrast, are often guided by the ethic, *Every child deserves to be wanted and loved.* They argue that when unwanted children are born, the quality of life diminishes for the parents and the society and the children themselves often have difficult lives as well.

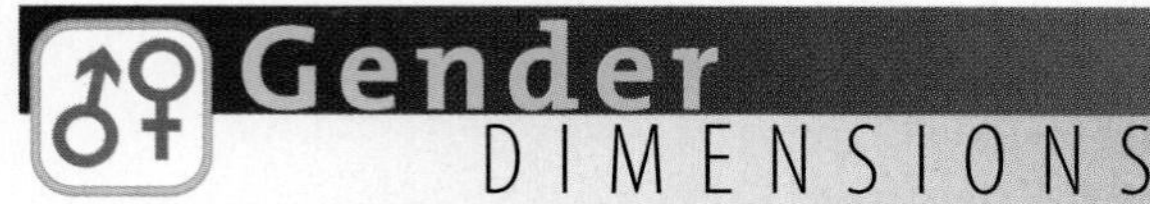

The "Umbrelly" (A Little Humor) Critics of research on contraceptive technology argue that research is immoral—that is, sexist. It focuses on female techniques, largely ignoring male methods of contraception. Others argue it is the characteristics and complexities of the male reproductive system that make the development of effective male contraception difficult. In an attempt to have males develop a greater appreciation for how the critics view the morality of contraceptive research, the following facetious description of a new male contraceptive was written:

> *The newest development in male contraception was unveiled recently at the American Women's Surgical Symposium held at the Ann Arbor Medical Center. Dr. Sophia Merkin, of the Merkin Clinic, announced the preliminary findings of a study conducted on 763 unsuspecting male grad students at a large Midwest university. In her report Dr. Merkin stated that the new contraceptive—the IPD—was a breakthrough in male contraception. It will be marketed under the trade name "Umbrelly."*
>
> *The IPD (intrapenal device) resembles a tiny folded umbrella that is inserted through the head of the penis and pushed into the scrotum with a plunger-like instrument. Occasionally there is perforation of the scrotum but this is disregarded, since it is known that the male has few nerve endings in this area of his body. The underside of the umbrella contains a spermicidal jelly, "Umbrelly."*
>
> *Experiments on a thousand white whales from the Continental Shelf (whose sexual apparatus is said to be closest to man's) proved the Umbrelly to be 100% effective in preventing production of sperm and eminently satisfactory to the female whale, since it doesn't interfere with her rutting pleasure.*
>
> *Dr. Merkin declared the Umbrelly to be statistically safe for the human male. She reported that of the 763 grad students tested with the device, only two died of scrotal infection, only 20 experienced swelling of the tissues, three developed cancer of the testicles, and 13 were too depressed to have an erection. She stated that common complaints ranged from cramping and bleeding to acute abdominal pain. She emphasized that these symptoms were merely indications that the man's body had not yet adjusted to the device. Hopefully the symptoms would disappear within a year.*
>
> *One complication caused by the IPD and briefly mentioned by Dr. Merkin was the incidence of massive scrotal infection necessitating the surgical removal of the testicles. "But this is a rare case," said Merkin, "too rare to be statistically important." She and the other distinguished members of the Women's College of Surgeons agreed that the benefits far outweighed the risk to any individual man.*

Source: Unknown.

In 1914 Margaret Sanger began publishing her newspaper *The Woman Rebel,* in which she argued that women should be free to choose whether or not to bear children. Sanger had witnessed the death of a young woman who tried to perform an abortion on herself and cited this incident as her motivation for working for a woman's right to control her fertility.

For some people, certain types of fertility-control methods are acceptable and others are not. For example, methods that prevent a fertilized egg from implanting on the endometrial lining of the uterus might be unacceptable to people who believe life begins at conception. For others, any action taken before birth is acceptable because they believe that birth is when human life begins.

Abortion

Is induced, or voluntary, abortion simply a method of fertility control and as such the right of every woman, or is it taking of life that has a right to exist? Can it be both? If so, how can the dilemma be resolved? Some people seek to solve the problem by looking for evidence—or a definition—of when life begins. Does it begin at conception or does it begin when a fetus is capable of living outside the mother (at birth, or shortly before)? Others seek to solve it by asking who controls a woman's reproductive capacity. One must decide whether preserving the life and quality of life of the living is more or less

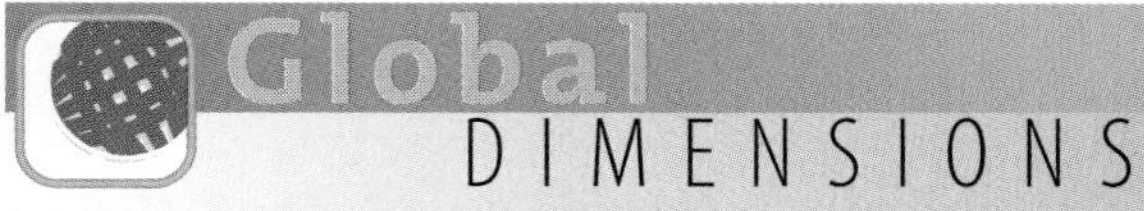

DIMENSIONS

Ethical Issues Around the World It is not surprising that different countries with different cultures have different views of ethical issues. One of these issues is age at marriage. In the United States, it is believed to be immoral for a 13-year-old girl to marry, especially an older man. We even maintain legislation defining this as a violation of law. However, in other countries, the morality of early marriage, even to an older man, is not called into question. This is especially true in Asian nations. For example, in Bangladesh, 73% of 20- to 24-year-old women report they married in their teens, in India it was 51%, and in Indonesia it was 31%. African nations also experience early marriages: Of 20- to 24-year-old women in the Ivory Coast 44% report being married when in their teens, 38% in Ghana, 31% in Zimbabwe, and 28% in Kenya. Surprisingly, these rates are lower than in the previous generation, when more young women married as teenagers. By way of comparison, 11% of U.S. women aged 20 to 24 years report being married as teens, down from 14% in the previous generation (Singh & Samara, 1996).

Another ethical dilemma relates to how much acculturation should be encouraged for populations who emigrate to the United States from other countries. We know that fitting into the new culture is important to social mobility and development. We know that future generations benefit financially, educationally, and socially by adopting many of the practices and mores of their new country. Yet, we also know that acculturation has a down side. For example, although breastfeeding is recommended for many reasons, the more acculturated Hispanic women immigrants are, the less likely they are to breastfeed. Furthermore, Hispanic women born in the United States are more likely than those born in other countries to have low birth weight babies (Fuentes-Afflick, Hessol, & Perez-Stable, 1998). This finding may be the result of foreign-born Hispanic women's having healthier diets, more and different kinds of cultural support, and other factors that can change when acculturation is encouraged.

Sources: Singh, S. & Samara, R. Early marriage among women in developing countries, *International Family Planning Perspectives, 22* (1996), 148–157, 175. Fuentes-Afflick, E., Hessol, N., & Perez-Stable, E. Maternal birthplace, ethnicity, and low birth weight in California, *Archives of Pediatric and Adolescent Medicine, 152* (1998), 1,105–1,112.

important than maintaining the existence or viability of the unborn. This ethical dilemma is one of the most divisive issues in modern society. Laws are no sooner made than they are challenged. The morality of abortion is a subject of ongoing debate in many arenas of modern life—from the purely personal to the political.

Amniocentesis

Amniocentesis involves withdrawing, via a needle inserted into the uterus through the abdominal wall, a small amount of amniotic fluid surrounding the fetus. The procedure is recommended for women whose risk of producing babies with birth defects is greater than average (for example, women older than 35 years old or women who have previously given birth to babies with birth defects). The moral question arises because if the test shows that the fetus will be deformed, mentally retarded, or seriously ill, the parents can choose to have an abortion rather than let the pregnancy run its course. Is it moral to take the risk (for example, of miscarriage) of having the test at all? Other issues are raised as well. For example, the sex of the fetus can be determined through amniocentesis. Is abortion moral when parents who have, say, four sons discover that their unborn child is a boy? Should the genes of an unborn baby be manipulated to conform with the parents'—or society's—idea of a superior human being? How much genetic manipulation is consistent with our ethical principles and values? As science becomes more sophisticated in this area, new ethical dilemmas arise.

Fetal Tissue Implantation

Parkinson's disease patients suffer tremors, muscular rigidity, and loss of balance as a result of a lack of the brain neurotransmitter dopamine. Research has discovered that fetal brain tissue, if implanted within the brain of Parkinson's patients, can produce enough dopamine to relieve many of the symptoms. However, the potential for abuse of this knowledge has prompted many groups and individuals to oppose the use of fetal tissue for implantation, or even for research purposes. One of the concerns is that a woman will become pregnant with the intention to abort the fetus and use its brain tissue for a family member suffering from Parkinson's disease. Others argue that using human tissue in this manner defiles the sanctity of the human body.

Yet there are those who strongly support the use of fetal tissue to relieve Parkinson's and other diseases. They point to the socially acceptable practice of donating and transplanting organs such as hearts, livers, kidneys, lungs, and corneas.

In 1990, Mary and Abe Ayala were told that the only chance to save their 17-year-old daughter Anissa from dying of leukemia was for her to have bone marrow transplantation. With no matching donors, the Ayalas decided to have another child (Marissa Eve) in order to use his or her bone marrow. Did the Ayalas act in a moral way? Did their physicians? What would you have done faced with such a dilemma?

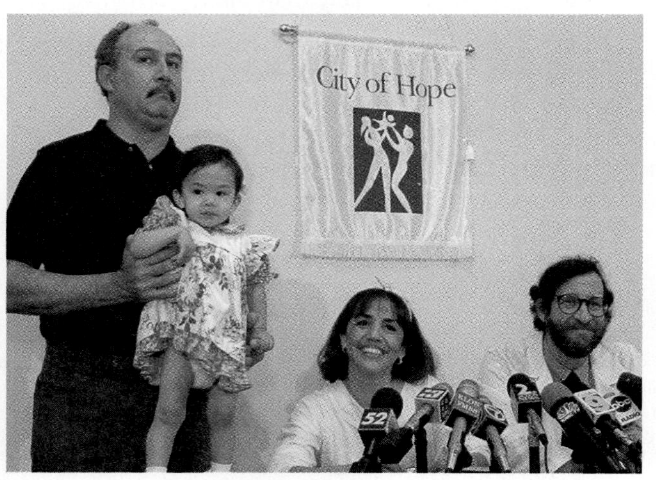

In 1988, the federal government banned the use of federal funds for research involving aborted fetal tissue implantation. Believing this policy deprives certain patients from receiving adequate care, the American College of Obstetrics and Gynecology and the American Fertility Society in February 1991 established a private advisory body to guide scientists conducting fetal tissue and fertility research. This board, the National Advisory Board on Ethics in Reproduction, sets uniform standards, reviews proposed projects, advises researchers, and serves as a clearinghouse of information.

By 1993, the federal government's ban on research with fetal tissue implantation was lifted. Since then the National Institutes of Health (NIH) has been awarded more than $23 million in grants for research involving the study, analysis, and use of human fetal tissue. Today research continues on the potential of fetal tissue in treatment of not only Parkinson's disease but also Alzheimer's disease, Huntington's disease, diabetes, multiple sclerosis, epilepsy, blindness, leukemia, hemophilia, sickle cell anemia, spinal-cord injuries, deficiencies of the immune system, birth defects, and pain (Kenney, 1997). Supporting this research are the Alzheimer's Association, the Epilepsy Foundation of America, the Cystic Fibrosis Foundation, the Parkinson's Disease Foundation, and the Society for Pediatric Research.

Part of the remaining ethical issues regarding the use of human fetal tissue pertains to the finding that tissue from miscarriages and ectopic pregnancies appears rarely to be suitable for transplantation. However, tissue from induced abortions is effective when transplanted. Researchers argue that legal barriers to harvesting tissue from induced abortions stand in the way of building up the supply of usable fetal tissue. For example, they advocate the use of fetal tissue from abortions caused by RU-486 and other drugs that induce abortion (Reuters, 1995).

Stem Cell Research

Stem cells are cells that can be found in embryos, fetuses, and adults. In adults, stem cells are specialized and can evolve into more cells of their own kind. In embryos, however, stem cells have the capacity to evolve into many different types of tissues and organs, depending on a complex of biological instructions. Embryonic stem cells are taken from embryos at the blastocyst stage of development (4 or 5 days after conception) when they are, in essence, a "blank page." At the time of this writing, scientists are working on ways of instructing stem cells to develop into specific tissue, for example, into insulin-producing pancreatic cells for implantation in diabetics.

The moral debate about stem cells involves a number of complex issues. For example, is it moral to use stem cells from aborted fetuses? Will this practice encourage more abortions? Is it moral to use stem cells from embryos created specifically for their stem cells? Is this the destruction of one human life to benefit another human life? Should scientific research, and consequently money that is devoted to scientific research, be concentrated on developing techniques for using adult stem cells rather than on embryonic stem cells? What should be the government's role in regulating and/or supporting stem cell research? Given the potential for stem cells to contribute to cures and/or treatments for Parkinson's disease, Alzheimer's disease, diabetes,

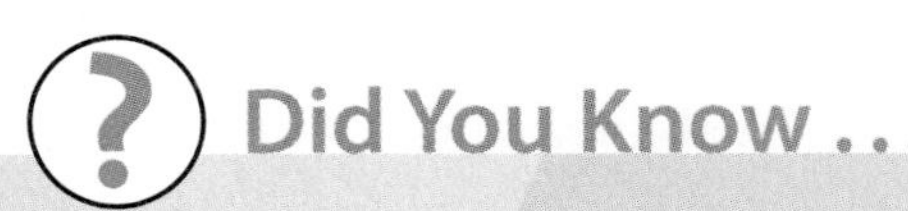

Fetal brain tissue is not the only type of fetal cell that has potential for medical use. Early in development, the fetus's blood cells are produced by stem cells in the liver. Eventually these blood cells move into the fetus's bones and become bone marrow. Therefore, injecting fetal liver cells intravenously into patients is, in effect, giving them immune system transplantation.

Fetal liver transplants hold promise for such conditions as certain leukemias, sickle cell anemia, aplastic anemia, AIDS, and severe combined immunodeficiency disease.

Diabetics have also been given fetal insulin-producing pancreas cells, and fetal brain tissue's potential to aid in the treatment of Alzheimer's disease is very real.

heart disease, and arthritis, among others, should scientific research be entailed by governmental restrictions? Is that moral?

In 2001, President George W. Bush approved a regulation that would provide government funding for limited stem cell research. Bush, a conservative politician, tried to walk the fine line between what he believed to be morally justified and the potential for the enhancement of large number of American lives—another moral consideration. He decided that, on the one hand, stem cell research had a great deal of potential to cure diseases that affect large numbers of Americans. On the other hand, he believed that developing "human life" (embryos) to harvest their stem cells was immoral. Consequently, Bush decided that the government would provide funding for scientific research that used only adult stem cells or embryonic stem cells that had already been harvested. Bush estimated that there were about 60 of those groups of embryonic stem cells around the world. Staunch conservatives viewed this decision as immoral because it did not make a statement about the sanctity of life and allowed "immorally produced" embryonic stem cells to be used for research purposes. Scientists considered this decision immoral because it limited research to a small number of embryonic stem cells that were thought to be too homogenous to produce wide-scale cures (for example, many of these existing colonies of embryonic stem cells were obtained from white populations). Furthermore, scientists argued, adult stem cells do not have the capacity to develop into a range of tissue as do embryonic stem cells but are, instead, tissue-specific. That limits their potential for a scientific breakthrough.

If you were the person deciding the role government ought to play in stem cell research, what would you decide? What moral justifications could you offer to support that decision?

Prostitution

Prostitution is the selling of sexual gratification. Examples of prostitution were recorded even in ancient times, so contemporary society can take neither credit nor blame for inventing this trade—only for the way in which it treats it.

People who consider prostitution immoral often argue that it degrades sexual intercourse, which is sanctified within marriage as an expression of love, into a mere animalistic act. Centuries ago Christianity adopted the Persian view, that the demands of the spirit and flesh were in conflict with each other, rather than the Greek view, which saw no conflict and allowed for prostitution (so long as the prostitutes were male). "Christians chose to reject the needs of the flesh in order to elevate the life of the spirit" (Nass, 1978, 47). Nevertheless making some allowances for the flesh, Christianity developed incentives for marriage and deemed sexual intercourse within marriage appropriate and outside it sinful. Our culture has largely adhered to this view of who is a legitimate and morally acceptable sexual partner. To make a judgment about prostitution, a person must decide whether the desire for sexual services and sexual outlets is more important than the principle that coitus outside marriage is immoral.

In Vitro Fertilization

In 1980 the first "test-tube" baby clinic in the United States was approved by the state of Virginia. Located at the Norfolk General Hospital in Norfolk, Virginia, this clinic offers its services to couples who wish to conceive but are infertile as a result of blocked, missing, or damaged fallopian tubes of women. (It does not treat male infertility.) The clinic, officially named the In

Vitro Clinic (for **in vitro fertilization**), had a waiting list of from 1 to 2 years just 1 week after gaining state approval.

in vitro fertilization
The creation of a pregnancy in a laboratory by uniting the sperm and egg outside the womb; sometimes termed the "test-tube" baby technique.

There are some who believe using in vitro fertilization to produce babies is immoral. For example, in March 1987 the Catholic Congregation for the Doctrine of the Faith issued "Instruction on Respect for Human Life in Its Origin and on the Dignity of Procreation," a document that defined generation of human life outside the body as "morally illicit." In addition to in vitro fertilization, other biomedical breakthroughs were condemned as immoral. Among these were genetic engineering, surrogate motherhood, cloning, and manipulations to produce human beings according to sex or other predetermined qualities. According to the document, the only approved method of human procreation is "the act of conjugal love."

Other ethical issues pertain to in vitro fertilization; for example, what will be its effect on the population of the world? Will it produce too many people for the available resources? What would that mean for the quality of life of the world's population? What should be done if the fetus develops defectively once it has been implanted in the uterus? When choosing to have a baby by artificial means, should parents be allowed to select the baby's sex, eye color, intelligence, and so on? These issues need societal attention; we as citizens need to inform our representatives of our judgments regarding what is moral and immoral relative to in vitro fertilization.

Genetic Engineering

In vitro fertilization evokes images of genetic manipulation in the minds of some people. Of course, that is not its intent. However, as science progresses and reproductive technology develops new ways to manage and enhance reproduction, fears of Huxley's *Brave New World* emerge. There are hundreds of biotechnology companies devoted to identifying genes and their functions with the hope of obtaining patents for these genes and the ways in which they can be put to use. It is envisioned that these genes will lead to designer medicines, engineered foods, and eventually custom-made kids (Achenbach, 1998), and the companies that own these patents will make a lot of money. Even the U.S. government staked out a claim to this research by funding the largest scientific project, the Human Genome Project. The $3 billion Human Genome Project, in collaboration with the private firm Celera Genomics, decoded the entire human genetic code in 2000.

All this research raises the possibility that a new generation will be genetically manipulated so that parents will be able to select the color of their babies' eyes, height, athletic and intellectual abilities, and artistic talents. However, some experts are concerned about this possibility. Jeremy Rifkin, the eminent futurist, argues that in a few generations babies will be "engineered." The biologist Lee Silver believes that the human race will be divided into two distinct species, the "Naturals" and the "GenRich" (Achenbach, 1998).

However, there are other experts who disagree. They argue that although a sheep (Dolly) has been cloned, researchers are a long way from being able to clone humans. And, even if that were possible, scientists are too ethical to do that. However, it is disconcerting that there are groups of scientists who are attempting to clone a human as of the time of this writing. Finally, experts who do not see a *Brave New World* on the horizon expect that as we approach new and more sophisticated reproductive technological advancements, ethicists, clergy, philosophers, politicians, and others, will intervene to develop gene-technology protocols that are acceptable to our societal values and mores.

Myth vs Fact

Myth: Morality is morality. What is right is right, and what is wrong is wrong.
Fact: Most people agree that what is moral in one society may not be moral in another. Furthermore, what is considered moral in one situation may not be considered moral in another situation.

Myth: There is no systematic way in which to resolve ethical and moral issues. It is mostly a matter of intuition and subjective judgment.
Fact: Ethics is a system that uses ethical principles to determine the morality of a situation or decision. Ethical principles are valued according to many factors, including experience, religious teachings, cultural background, education, and family values.

Myth: In our diverse society, there are no commonly accepted ethical principles. Different groups have different values and different views of morality.
Fact: Although it is true that in a country with many different cultural groups living together there are many different views of morality, there are some ethical principles that we can all agree on. These include caring, respect for others, honesty, responsibility, and trustworthiness.

Myth: There are some situations about which there is no disagreement regarding morality. For example, there is no disagreement about HIV and AIDS, because AIDS is such a serious and deadly disease.
Fact: HIV and AIDS provide a good example of how complex moral decisions can be. For example, there is disagreement regarding whether condom advertisements should be allowed on television and whether needle-distribution programs for intravenous drug users should be developed.

Whether we will have "designer babies" is still an open question. As citizens in a democratic society we need to keep abreast of the latest developments in this area, because the very nature of the human race may be at issue. The uses of this new technology may be as much a function of the will of the people as it is the interests of the scientists, and, if so, every person has a responsibility to become involved in some way.

The issue of bioethics is recognized throughout the world. In November, the United Nations (UN) Commission on Human Rights adopted the first international guidelines on bioethics and the human genome. The "Universal Declaration on the Human Genome and Human Rights," cosponsored by 86 countries, sets standards for people researching and using genetic information and techniques. Although it specifically recognizes the rights to freedom of research and freedom of thought, it states that "practices which are contrary to human dignity, such as reproductive cloning of human beings, shall not be permitted." The United States is one of the countries that support the UN declaration.

Sexual Responsibility to a Partner

The last sexual ethical dilemma we discuss is, What degree of responsibility do we have, sexually, with respect to others? Should our sexual behavior achieve our own ends, regardless of the desires of our sexual partners? Conversely, are we under an obligation to subjugate our own sexual needs to the needs of our sexual partners? Given that two individuals are involved, just what is moral sexual behavior?

The issue of sexual responsibility, as are all the issues discussed so far, is complex. Certainly we are all responsible for ourselves and our own behavior, but when we take care of ourselves by involving someone else, the issue becomes clouded. As an example imagine that a typical couple, Paul and Paula, love each other and are engaged to be married. Paula wants to share coitus with Paul, but Paul considers sexual intercourse outside marriage immoral. Should Paula attempt to convince Paul that they should have intercourse? Would it be reasonable for her to threaten to date someone else if he refuses? Should Paul relegate his beliefs to second place and give in to Paula? What is their responsibility to themselves? to each other? to their future? to their relationship? These questions are not easy to answer. However, when sexual behavior involves someone else, there is always potential for manipulation or coercion. The moral nature of such behavior should be explored.

During 1986 this question of sexual responsibility took on special importance. That year the U.S. surgeon general's report on AIDS was published (Koop, 1986). A major part of the government's strategy for managing the AIDS crisis was to support sexuality education. At the time, however, both the secretary of education, William Bennett, and the president, Ronald Reagan, argued that sexuality education must be taught concurrently with a particular set of morals and values. Teaching such values as responsibility, trust, and honesty, as well as the ideas that premarital sexual intercourse is to be avoided and that monogamous relationships are to be valued, was recommended. Is it morally sound to teach these specific values? Is it problematic when any set of moral imperatives are taught to young children? Or is it immoral, given the AIDS epidemic and society's interest in general, *not* to teach these values? Should parents approve of what their children are taught in the school so as to ensure these values are consistent with their cultural, ethnic, or religious beliefs? This is not as simple a matter as it might at first appear (Galli, Greenberg, & Tobin, 1987).

Communication DIMENSIONS

The Morality of Requesting a Variety of Sexual Behaviors In some sexual relationships, one partner desires more variety in sexual activities than the other. For example, one partner may prefer anal sexual intercourse, and the other may object. Or one partner may be extremely excited by oral–genital sex, and the other may be turned off by it. One person may think of certain sexual activities as immoral, another as exciting. Too often, these conflicts result in anger and resentment, thereby interfering with other aspects of the relationship, not merely the sexual part. Consequently, partners should discuss differing sexual desires and resolve these issues. Fortunately, there are ways to do just that.

To begin, each person's thoughts and feelings should be expressed. A comment like "That's sick!" short-circuits any meaningful communication. The initial part of the conversation should be devoted to understanding the viewpoint of the other person, and that requires listening. There is time to express an opposing point of view, but not until one person has had the chance to be understood. Once one person has expressed his or her viewpoint, the other should. Refrain from arguing or disagreeing at this point. Merely listen.

Once both points of view have been aired, points of agreement should be identified. For example, both partners might agree that sex is a normal and desirable part of their relationship; that variety of sexual behaviors enhances the sexual relationship and thereby positively influences other aspects of their life together; that each cares about the other's feelings and sexual satisfaction; and that they want to make each other happy.

The part of communication regarding conflicts of ethics and morality that is most difficult is finding a compromise with which both persons are satisfied. Identifying areas of agreement provides a starting point in this process. Perhaps one partner is willing to try a particular sexual activity because he or she has identified a concern for making the other person happy. Perhaps the other is willing to forgo a particular sexual activity because it will make the other unhappy. The goal is to maintain the relationship as a stimulating one, not to engage in specific behaviors. The original focus on the behaviors is what is "wanted," whereas the real issue is the "need" for excitement and stimulation. That need can be met in ways that satisfy both partners with a little ingenuity and creativity.

Remember, though, no one should be forced, coerced, or manipulated to behave in any way that he or she considers immoral. That will result only in guilt, shame, or embarrassment and will not be healthy for the person or the relationship. If your partner is trying to manipulate you, the relationship is probably not worth saving.

Even when a decision is the individual's alone, ethical dilemmas may arise. For example, should sexually active people use some means of contraception, even if their partners do not care? If not, are they behaving responsibly? What if one's religion opposes the use of contraception but one is sexually active and unwilling to risk pregnancy? As with all the issues we have explored, the means of resolving these questions is to rank the conflicting ethical principles according to our personal values.

Laws Regulating Sexual Behavior

Laws formalize moral decisions for a society. Our laws regarding sexual behavior developed from a general acceptance of specific ethical principles, values, and judgments about behaviors such as those we have explored. They have their roots in experience, in religious dogma, and in economics and politics.

Myth vs Fact

Myth: As long as two adults agree, any sexual activity in which they engage is legal, as long as it is done in private.

Fact: Not long ago, most states had sodomy laws that made certain sexual activities illegal even though they were consensual and performed by adults. Most states have repealed these laws or declared them unconstitutional. Still, some states retain their sodomy laws to this day.

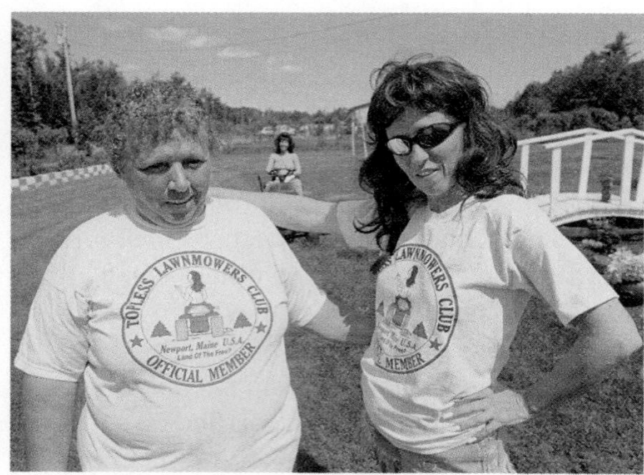

Lisa Desiree Davis of Waterville, Maine, started a topless lawnmowing service in the summer of 1998. One resident protested at the time, but no laws strictly forbade it. In November 1998, more than 70% of the town voted to allow her to continue the service. She and her mother, Shirley, also sell T-shirts and split the profits with the local fire department. Thus, what began as a moral argument to get her to stop led to legal approval by the town. *Source:* WFNX radio, November 13, 1998.

Consensus—or general agreement—about which sexual actions should be considered permissible has not always been easily achieved. Indeed, communities have sometimes had to devise ingenious compromises to keep peace among their various moral factions. Consider, for example, the "Combat Zone" in Boston, Massachusetts. To meet the needs of people who frequented bars featuring topless dancers, attended X-rated movies, and so forth, but also to protect citizens opposed to such activities from exposure to them, the municipal government restricted the bars and theaters in question to a specific part of the city, nicknamed the "Combat Zone." The Combat Zone has subsequently been abolished. For similar reasons, some European countries have established red-light districts, in an attempt to limit prostitution to a single section of town.

However, even when consensus is achieved and codified into city, state, or federal law, it is by no means stable. State laws prohibiting prostitution, which were widely acceptable when they were enacted, are periodically under attack and may well someday be modified or rejected. Supreme Court rulings on abortion and on pornography have not settled those issues. Laws prohibiting homosexuality are enforced less and less often; some are being overthrown. Such changes occur—albeit slowly—when there is a conflict between existing law and new morality. An illegal activity might begin to be seen as moral; a legal act, as immoral.

We will see in this discussion that sexual laws develop through a societal consensus of the valuing of ethical principles. The process of devising such laws involves identifying ethical principles, valuing them to define moral behavior, and then encoding laws to enforce that behavior (or prohibit it if defined as immoral). Because our values may change over time, however, we periodically reassess and change our laws governing sexual behavior.

Homosexual Activity

Some sexuality-related issues may be resolved legally, but the laws are virtually unenforceable. In these instances, accommodations on enforcement may occur. For example, although homosexuality is illegal in many states, police sometimes adopt a policy of not enforcing such laws when the sexual activity occurs in private or in the gay section of town. The gay section usually contains bars, restaurants, nightclubs and other establishments, such as bathhouses and saunas, where homosexual men and women can meet. Heterosexuals can choose to steer clear of this part of town, and homosexuals can be themselves, meeting other homosexuals and feeling relatively free to live without interference.

Laws pertaining to homosexuality provide good examples of the problems that may develop when laws thought to be specific are interpreted otherwise. We have already discussed the Supreme Court's decision regarding consensual sexual behavior conducted in private. This ruling was thought to relate specifically to homosexual behavior, but it allows states once more to vigorously apply their sodomy laws against heterosexuals as well. Furthermore, given that homosexuals are considered an "at-risk" group for AIDS—even though it is the *behavior* that places one at risk, not one's sexual orientation—such laws might be enforced to greatly curtail their liberties and, some would argue, their rights as citizens. In other words, the fear of AIDS might be used as an excuse for enforcing moral conduct as defined by the enforcers of the law. This perception is more than mere paranoia and finds support in the recent actions of local and state legislatures and law enforcement personnel who, in many areas, have closed gay bathhouses (citing health concerns as the reason) and have more closely scrutinized gay bars and their patrons.

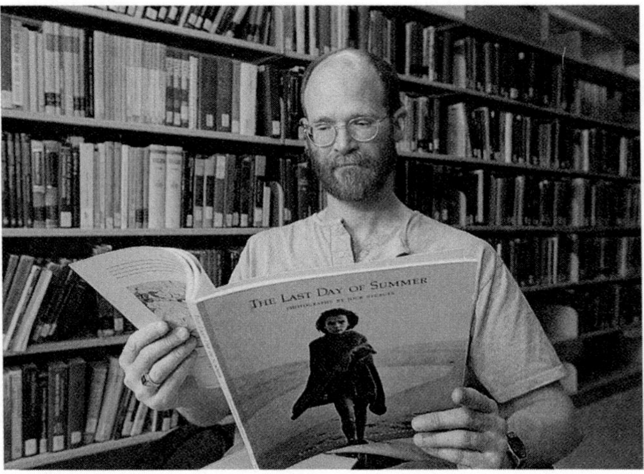

Although it is illegal for a typical person to photograph and publish nude photos of minors, many "artists" seem to have few problems getting away with it. Many bookstores sell photo albums that contain full nudity of clearly underage boys and girls, without prosecution. Is it possible to distinguish ethically or legally between nude photos of minors that are taken for the purpose of arousal from those that were taken as "art"?

Obscenity and Pornography

Some issues continue to be debated even in the face of definitive opinions from the Supreme Court. An example involves the definitions of **obscenity** and **pornography.** The Comstock Act of 1873, the first major law concerning obscenity in the United States, prohibited the mailing of obscene or lewd material. The interpretation of what was obscene or lewd was left to the Postal Service. In 1957 the Supreme Court attempted to clarify the issue by ruling that sexuality-related material and obscene material were not one and the same. Rather, sexual material was ruled obscene (and therefore outside the protection of the First Amendment) only when sexual behavior was presented in a lewd and lascivious manner. But how was it to be determined whether some particular material was lewd or lascivious? The Supreme Court stated that the standard to be applied was whether or not the average person would judge it as such.

obscenity
Something offensive to modesty or decency; often sexually related.

pornography
Sexually arousing music, art, literature, or films, a determination that may vary from individual to individual and from community to community.

Further rulings between 1957 and 1968 (55 separate legal opinions in 13 obscenity cases) attempted to define obscenity more explicitly. As a result, the phrase "utterly without redeeming social value" was added to the definition. In 1973 the Court rejected its own "utterly without redeeming social value" criterion and defined the standards of obscenity that are currently in effect:

1. Whether the average person applying contemporary community standards would find that the work, taken as a whole, appeals to the prurient (lustful) interests
2. Whether the work depicts or describes, in a patently offensive way, sexual conduct specified by state law
3. Whether the work, taken as a whole, lacks serious literary, artistic, political, or scientific value

Despite the history of legal activity, a consensus in the society as to the definition of obscenity has yet to be reached. With the advent of the Internet and the access it provides to sexually explicit material, the problem is exacerbated.

Rape

Although there is considerable debate about the psychological, sociological, and cultural causes of rape, the chief legal issue involves achieving consensus on a set of standards for enforcing the laws against rape. The legal definition of forcible rape is sexual intercourse against one's will, but because anyone might accuse another of rape, society has had to define acceptable evidence. Until recently a prosecutor had to prove that semen was present—on the woman's body or clothing—to gain a conviction of rape. However, many female victims do not have a medical exam after rape; others bathe or shower before being examined; and in many cases of true rape, the rapist fails to ejaculate. Because many rapists have been pronounced innocent because of a lack of such evidence, the presence of semen is no longer considered the sole evidence of forcible rape; bruises, the presence of a weapon, and even threats of force may now be accepted.

Defense attorneys have often focused on the victims, attempting to show that they were promiscuous and thus responsible for provoking sexual attacks. New laws reflect society's growing concern with protecting victims from unfair questioning, as well as with ensuring conviction when rape has actually occurred. These laws now prohibit questions regarding the victim's sexual experience during a rape trial. Thus the focus of the trial is on determining the guilt or innocence of the accused, not on the moral character of the victim.

Statutory Rape

Statutory rape is placed in a different legal category from forcible rape, and a situation ethicist might also put it in a different moral category. Statutory rape is sexual intercourse with a person below the legal age of consent, which varies from state to state. The statute is designed to protect children considered too immature to make sexual decisions for themselves. Even if boys or girls willingly participate in sexual intercourse, their consent is ignored for legal purposes. And even if they appear to be of age or lie about their age, the laws still apply, with few exceptions. In some states the exception is that a child proved to be sexually promiscuous or a prostitute may be considered an adult.

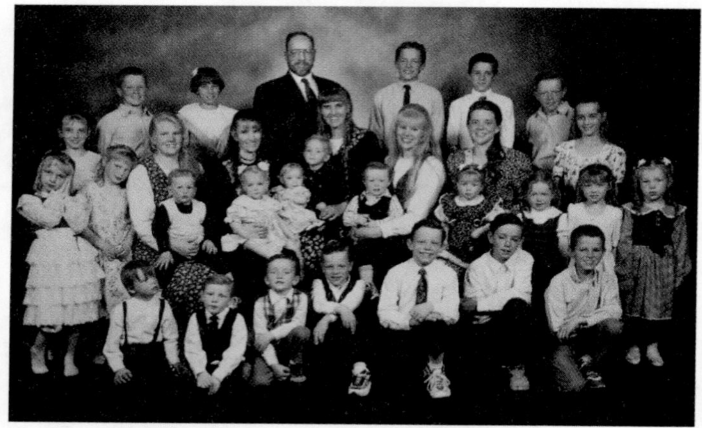

The practice of polygamy in the Mormon Church, which was a common occurrence until the mid-19th century, still continues in some small enclaves of Utah. In 2001, Tom Green, a fundamentalist Mormon, was convicted and sentenced to five years in prison in the most recent and biggest bigamy case in half a century. At the time of his trial, Green had a total of five wives and thirty children. Despite the fact that both the Mormon Church and the state of Utah are formally against the practice of polygamy as well as further charges that one of Green's wives was actually only 13 years old when he first had sexual intercourse with her, Green claims that he has been unfairly singled out. With an estimated total of 30,000 polygamists still existing in Utah and the western United States, Green maintains that he is only perpetuating a traditional religious practice.

Adultery

Adultery, or extramarital intercourse, is quite prevalent in the United States. Kinsey reported back in 1948 that more than one-third of the men in his study reported extramarital coitus; in 1953 he reported that half of the men and 26% of the women he studied had extramarital sexual intercourse by age 40 years. Many suspect that the incidence of extramarital coitus has increased since Kinsey's studies, but our concept of morality vis-à-vis marriage still leads us to sustain the laws against it. Adultery is frequently a legal ground for divorce. When adultery is the basis of divorce and custody of children is challenged in court, the adulterous partner often loses custody.

Divorce

Laws involving divorce have been reformed over the years. Originally marriage and divorce laws in the United States were based on Judeo-Christian ethical principles involving the sanctity of the family and of parenthood. These laws reinforced the idea that the family was an economic necessity, both for the individual and for the society. Consequently divorce was granted by law only if misbehavior was proved in court. In other words, one of the marriage partners had to be at fault by being adulterous, mentally or physically cruel, and so on. When the number of divorces increased, and it became a common belief that people wishing to be free of each other should not be forced to remain married, many states adopted **no-fault divorce.** No-fault divorce statutes allow courts to dissolve marriages when no fault is cited and both partners agree to end the marriage.

Some people argue that no-fault divorce laws have led to more divorces (a bad thing); others say they have led to happier people (a good thing). Another way of looking at the prevalence of divorce—regardless of fault—is to argue that we should make marriage laws stricter, rather than making divorce laws looser. People would then have to work harder to get married, and those without a strong commitment to each other would be unlikely to follow through.

Alimony is money that a judge orders the partner who earns more to pay on the granting of a divorce to the partner who earns less or no money. As are other matters related to divorce, alimony is being reevaluated. Previously alimony was handled as punishment for divorce, and the husband forced to make payments to his wife. Today judges are more likely to assess the particular circumstances in a case and award alimony to either the man or woman, on the basis of their respective resources and contributions to the marriage.

no-fault divorce
The granting of divorce without either partner's proving the other was the cause of the marriage's failure.

alimony
Money a divorced person is instructed by the courts to pay regularly to his or her ex-spouse.

Exploring the DIMENSIONS of Human Sexuality

Our feelings, attitudes, and beliefs regarding sexuality are influenced by our internal and external environments. Go to sexuality.jbpub.com to learn more about the biological, psychological, and sociological factors that affect your sexuality.

Biological Factors

- Alcohol and drugs can blur decision-making ability.

Sociocultural Factors

- Religions often establish codes of ethics, which state for members beliefs on matters including abortion, premarital sexual activity, extramarital sexual activity, same-sex sexual relations, and nonintercourse sexual activities.
- Political beliefs often suggest ethical standards. Although there are exceptions, in general, Democrats and feminists generally take a prochoice stance (not always), and Republicans and fundamentalist Christians take an antiabortion stance. Laws in the United States ban discrimination based on race, religion, gender, age, and sexual orientation for public organizations. But private organizations can still discriminate. In many Islamic countries, adultery is illegal—even punishable by death. Gender selection through female infanticide or amniocentesis coupled with abortion is tolerated in some countries.

Psychological Factors

- During the state of sexual arousal and response, it is often hard to make moral judgments that conflict with intense physiological feelings.

CASE STUDY

At the center of many ethical and moral dilemmas are cultural underpinnings—especially religious and political beliefs.

However, sometimes those cultural underpinnings clash. Consider the woman who unexpectedly finds herself pregnant. Raised as a member of the Roman Catholic religion—with its antiabortion doctrine—the woman has also been raised as a feminist, with a prochoice doctrine. Further, consider the rights of her partner, who may have a different set of sociocultural doctrines to rely on for making moral decisions.

On a more personal level, it is important to make moral decisions regarding sexual relationships before becoming sexually involved. During a state of sexual arousal and response, it is often hard to put moral feelings ahead of intense physiological feelings.

States may pass specific laws dealing with sexuality; however, such laws must not conflict with federal laws and may be challenged for their constitutionality.

Discussion Questions

1. Differentiate between ethics and morals. Apply the ethical principles of nonmaleficence, beneficence, autonomy/liberty, justice/fairness, and social utility to issues in human sexuality.
2. Discuss commonly accepted ethical principles and ways they can be applied in situations involving sexual behavior.
3. What types of sexual behavior are regulated by laws? What is the basis of those laws?

Application Questions

Reread the chapter-opening story and answer the following questions.

1. Consider the ethical principles of nonmaleficence, beneficence, autonomy/liberty, justice/fairness, and social utility as they relate to the opening story. Which of the ethical principles did Wendy Weaver and the Nebo school district follow? Then explain how the case might have been affected if Weaver and the school district had followed other principles.
2. Was it ethical for Weaver to disclose her sexual orientation to a minor student? Should Weaver have considered the student's possible religious (70% of Utah residents are Mormon) objections to homosexuality before answering?

Critical Thinking Questions

1. Is practicing safer sex an ethical or a legal issue? For example, is it unethical not to have STI and HIV tests before starting a new relationship? Can this become a legal issue?
2. An unmarried woman who has been in a steady sexual relationship for 5 months discovers she is pregnant. Is it ethical, moral, or legal for the male to decide whether the woman has the child and keeps it, gives it up for adoption, or has an abortion? What if the couple breaks up before she finds out she is pregnant? What rights, if any, does the man have in relation to the baby he helped create?
3. The ethics and morality of creating (or re-creating) life sometimes reflect technological innovations of the times. As the age of electricity dawned in the 1800s, Mary Shelley's *Frankenstein* (1818) provoked ethical and moral concerns about the use of electricity. Today, the use of electricity in the defibrillator to save a heart attack patient is accepted as ethical, moral, and legal. In fact, it would be considered unethical, immoral, and illegal not to use a defibrillator when a life could be saved. During our current age of genetic research (beginning with the 1950s discovery of DNA), Michael Crichton's *Jurassic Park* provoked similar concerns about the misuse of genetic engineering. However, even as you read this question, new technological applications are being devised that can and will save lives. Do you think people in 200 years will look back at *Jurassic Park* and wonder why we feared genetic research?

Critical Thinking Case

The ability to select the gender of a child has for years been the source of ethical debate. In some countries, cultures approve of female infanticide or amniocentesis coupled with abortion. However, the cultural morals of the United States do not favor such methods.

Would the current U.S. culture accept a scientifically based method of gender selection? The Genetics and IVF Institute (Fairfax, Virginia) announced in September 1998 that they had found a way to separate male and female sperm cells. Using specialized technology, they are able to sort out 85% of X-bearing sperm (females) and 65% of Y-bearing sperm (males). Using artificial insemination, the institute can give parents potential for gender selection, in proportion to the sperm-sorting abilities.

The technique has been used for some time on animals, which are easier to sort by gender. Testing with humans began in 1998. Human applications include preventing the birth of children with rare genetic sex-linked diseases (such as X-linked hydrocephalus) or "balancing" families with an opposite-sex sibling. The institute is not planning to market the sorting procedure to first-time parents who simply have a dream of a specific-gender child.

Do you think that sperm-sorting technology is ethically acceptable in the case of raising farm animals? How about in the name of protecting endangered species from extinction?

As far as human applications are concerned, do you find it ethical to use sperm-sorting to prevent the birth of a child who has a genetic sex-linked disease? How about to have an additional child to provide needed bone marrow for transplantion to a current child? Finally, is it ethical to use sperm sorting to have a third or fourth child of the opposite gender?

Exploring Personal Dimensions

Determining Your Ethical Compass

Several ethical dilemmas are presented to help you determine which ethical principles you use to guide your behavior and your view of morality. Choose the one option for each dilemma that best represents your views, even though you might agree with more than one.

1. Juan and Maria decide to live together and share a sexual relationship. They are thinking that they may marry in the future, but not any time soon.
   a. Juan and Maria should not move in together because we know that when men and women live together, they are not equals. Women tend to take on more of the household chores than men.
   b. Juan and Maria should be free to decide what is best for them.
   c. Juan and Maria should not live together because Maria will suffer if she does not eventually marry Juan. She will be perceived as immoral by her family and her community.
   d. No good will come of Juan and Maria's living together. In fact, it might harm society by encouraging sexual relations between people who are not married to each other.
2. Evan and Rhonda place their 2-year-old son in child care so they can both work outside the home.
   a. This is unfair because Evan and Rhonda are placing their interests above the welfare of their son.

b. Each couple should be able to decide what is best for their family unit.

c. Without the direct and extensive contact with one of his parents, Evan and Rhonda's son will not grow and develop to his potential.

d. Society will suffer if this becomes a common practice because of the emotional cost and health effects that the community will eventually have to absorb.

3. Although Juan and Maria have a sexual relationship, Juan has not disclosed to Maria that he has herpes. Juan argues that their relationship is not "serious," and, therefore, he should not have to divulge his STI to Maria. Furthermore, Juan states, he refrains from having intercourse with Maria when he has noticeable sores.

   a. Because Juan knows about his STI and Maria does not, Juan is treating Maria unfairly. He has more information than she, and that is not right.

   b. Juan has a right to decide to whom information about his health is released, as well as the nature of that information.

   c. Lacking knowledge of Juan's herpes, Maria is likely to engage in behavior that can cause her harm.

   d. If Juan continues to withhold information about his health and infects other sexual partners, society will suffer, health premiums will be raised for the rest of us, and hospital and medical staff resources may have to be redirected from other health issues.

4. Frankie and Lynn had been married for 10 years when Frankie began a sexual relationship with his coworker Flo.

   a. It is not fair that Frankie engages in sex outside his marriage whereas Lynn refrains because of her vows of fidelity. If Frankie engages in extramarital sex, why should Lynn not have affairs as well?

   b. Frankie may have many reasons for deciding to have a sexual relationship with Flo. He is an adult and should be free to decide whether the risk outweighs the benefits he derives from the relationship with Flo.

   c. If Lynn ever found out she would be devastated, and their marriage might end. If they have children, even more harm would be done.

   d. Society cannot allow extramarital affairs to be unpunished; otherwise, we would have chaos, unstable families, and dysfunctional children growing into dysfunctional adults.

5. Rose and Amber are lovers who are often seen by their neighbors holding hands as they enter their apartment building. Several of the more conservative tenants have complained about being "confronted by two lesbians flaunting their relationship to everyone else."

   a. It is not fair that heterosexual tenants can hold hands but gay couples are expected to refrain from doing so.

   b. Rose and Amber should be able to do whatever they choose. It is a free world. The other residents are free to look away.

   c. Raising this issue with Rose and Amber might make them self-conscious and lead to their questioning whether they are welcome in that apartment building. Furthermore, the strain of this confrontation might lead to stress that could harm their health.

d. It is harmful to young children, who are impressionable and in the process of developing their own sexual orientation, to see outwardly gay couples' being accepted by society. For the good of the total society, gay couples should be more discreet.

If you found yourself selecting choice (a) more often than the other choices, you are predominantly guided by the ethical principle of *justice*, believing people ought to be treated fairly. If you selected choice (b) over the others, you are guided by *autonomy*, believing people ought to be free to make their own choices without interference from others. However, if you selected choice (c) most often, you are guided by the ethical principle of nonmaleficence, believing no harm ought to be done, and, when it is, the decision is immoral. And, if you found yourself most often selecting choice (d), you are guided by *social utility*, believing a decision needs to be considered in terms of the benefit or harm to society.

Sexuality Online

Go to the web component for *Exploring the Dimensions of Human Sexuality* at sexuality.jbpub.com for web exercises, additional resources related to this chapter, and student review tools.

Suggested Readings

Falikowski, A. *Moral philosophy for modern life.* Englewood Cliffs, NJ: Prentice Hall, 1998.

Greenberg, J. S. & Gold, R. S. *The health education ethics book.* Dubuque, IA: Wm. C. Brown, 1992.

Hinman, L. M. *Applied ethics in American society.* New York: Harcourt, Brace, 1996.

Hinman, L. M. *Ethics: A pluralistic approach to moral theory.* New York: Harcourt, Brace, 1998.

May, L. *Masculinity and morality.* Ithaca, NY: Cornell University Press, 1998.

Palmer-Fernandez, G. *Moral issues: Philosophical and religious perspectives.* Englewood Cliffs, NJ: Prentice Hall, 1996.

Reich, W. T. *Bioethics: Sex, genetics, and human reproduction.* New York: Macmillan, 1997.

Roiphe, K. *Last night in paradise: Sex and morals at the century's end.* New York: Vintage, 1997.

Thiroux, J. *Ethics: Theory and practice,* 6th ed. Englewood Cliffs, NJ: Prentice Hall, 1998.

Epilogue: Taking Responsibility for Your Sexual Health

THE SEXUAL FUTURE

It was a morning of unmatched brilliance; the sun shone brightly, the robins were singing, and the spring air was morning fresh. It was a typical morning in the year 2099 for Todd and his housemates Keri, Karen, and Jerry.

Excuse me. I am being impolite. I forgot that you were from another time. I should have introduced you to our way of life before mentioning my friends. Of course we have made lots of technological advances, as you will soon see. But given what was going on in your day, you could probably see that coming, even if you could not foresee the form. Beyond that, however, we have changed our attitudes and values, our ways of doing work, and our social, sexual, and family relationships. For example, in 2099 we are altogether more respectful of individual differences than you were in your time. Questions of morality do not dominate our way of life as they did yours, and much ignorance has been dispelled. Is it a good or bad time, you ask? Let me describe our ways to you and you can answer for yourself.

Keri, Karen, Jerry, and Todd range in age from 21 to 41 years, but they are not rushing off to work today. In fact they never rush off to work, because they all work at home. Most people do. It is the computer, you see. Of course, as you did in the early part of this century, we all have computer terminals at home and we use them for work and play, as well as for banking, shopping, and communicating with one another over long and short distances. We play games on them and can program our terminals to play music for us. Our physicians even use them to diagnose illnesses and prescribe medication. (Wait until you hear about the medication we have!) Anyway, why do you think the morning air is so fresh? No cars to pollute it! In fact, there is very little transportation as you knew it. We have little need to go anywhere. Our computers meet most of our needs. Life really is easy.

Family life, as you can imagine, is also quite different from home life as you knew it. Long ago we realized that marriage was archaic—it just did not make sense in a rapidly changing society to expect two people to live together forever. People change as the society changes, but not all marriage partners change at the same pace. Once we understood this, we changed our laws to allow for a number of different marriage styles. The styles are not really new, but the legal and social ease of choosing and changing *is*. For example, we have repeating monogamous marriages (RMMs), wherein one maintains only one partner at a time but, when the marriage becomes stale, one can dissolve the marriage easily and marry another partner. Some people marry 10 or more times in this manner. Polygamy (one person married to several people at the same time) is also common, as are multiple marriage partners (MMPs). MMPs allow several males to share several female marriage partners, and vice versa.

In spite of all our attempts to adapt marriage to our society, however, most people never marry. Rather they establish informal arrangements of convenience. Some live together, some raise children together (their own or those of others), and some just share particular events together. I, for example, have an informal arrangement with Betty for sexual play, with Tina for computer game play, and with Tasha for sharing of thoughts and important feelings.

By the way, we laugh when the computer tells us stories of your struggle with sexual equality. In 2099 we cannot imagine that males would be treated differently from females. I guess our attitude evolves partly because the need for physical strength continued to decrease, just as it was in your day, and that eliminated the male's biological advantage. You see, robots do all our strenuous work, and competitive sports (other than computer games) have long since been outlawed. They were thought to contribute to warlike attitudes that, with the existence of weapons that could destroy the world, were deemed intolerable. But really that only partly explains our sexual equality. We realize that people who are discriminated against eventually revolt. It is only a matter of time—treat a group unfairly and it eventually rebels, disturbing the peace. Furthermore, our scientists have discovered treatments that allow everyone, male and female, to feel however they wish and to acquire almost any trait they want or need. Because people can change themselves nearly at will, how could we believe any one or any group to be inferior?

Scientists have made other important advances, too. Most diseases are curable now—your dreaded cancer and heart diseases among them. But perhaps the single most significant advance has been the discovery of K25W. Added to our water supply by our leaders (all of whom are scientists rather than politicians), K25W is a chemical that prepares the mind to receive and accept subliminal messages.

What are subliminal messages, you ask? Just a little trick of the media trade. The subliminal messages are verbal messages delivered so quickly and at such a low volume that those who receive them are not even aware that messages have been conveyed. Subliminal messages can be visual, too, images relayed so quickly along with other broadcast material that viewers remain unaware of them. Your society experimented with a crude form of subliminal messages when, for instance, voices were hidden beneath the pleasant music that department store customers heard while shopping reminding customers to be polite and not to shoplift. But you did not have K25W in your water! We use subliminal messages to plant many ideas, one of which is sexual equality, in the minds of our citizens.

The one problem we are still wrestling with is how to solve the discontent of our elderly. Having eradicated many of the diseases that plagued you, plus eliminating traffic accidents, we have lengthened the life span of most people, and so the size of our elderly population has grown enormously. By the way, we do not think of 70-year-olds as elderly; people live now to the ages of 120, 130, even 140 years. Mind you, our old people are quite happy (remember K25W) and able to care for themselves (remember our medications). Still, they tell stories of their past, and young people wonder whether our society is really better than the one the old folks recall. There is much ambivalence in those recollections. The old ones speak of illness, on the one hand, and the joy of life on the other; of cruelty and war, on one hand, and the Peace Corps on the other; of nursing homes, on one hand, and growing old with families to care for you on the other. No small wonder the younger ones are confused. But our scientists are working on this issue even as we speak. Before long it will be clear to all that our new society is developing in the right direction. After all, do we not live longer? Have not we eliminated sexual bias? Can not we take a pill and acquire just about any trait we want?

Well, that gives you a quick overview of some major areas of our life. Now let me tell you about my friends to show you examples of how some personal relationships work.

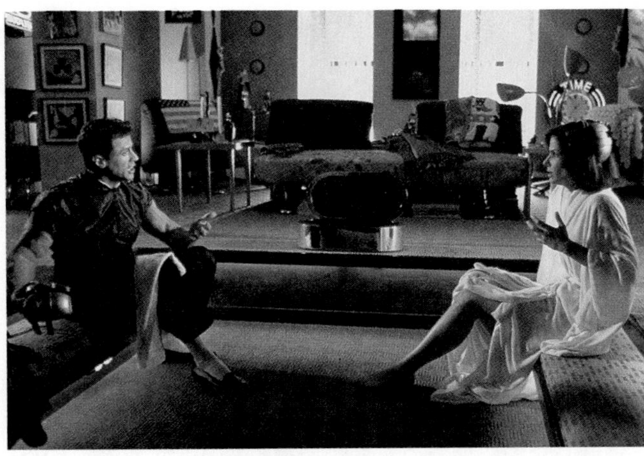

In *Demolition Man,* Sylvester Stallone plays a rogue cop put into cryogenic captivity and awakened in the year 2032. He is understandably perplexed by this strange new world, but when Sandra Bullock asks him to have sex and he realizes it involves a virtual reality helmet and no touching, he is outraged! What are the missing dimensions of sexuality in this scenario?

Todd is an Edibilist. His job relates to developing new strains of foods and nutrients. Because many of our citizens live to be 130 years old, world population has skyrocketed, and all the life-sustaining resources (food, energy, oxygen) are at a premium. Todd is married to Jerry (homosexual marriage is not uncommon among us, because people do not marry primarily to have babies). His recreational needs are met by Keri and his intellectual needs by Karen. Jerry is also Karen's sexual mate. As a matter of fact, they had a scare recently. No, not an unwanted pregnancy. That is no longer a problem. We have an enormous range of effective contraceptives (male contraceptives that prevent sperm development or immobilize sperm and female contraceptives are taken only once a year). Furthermore, someone who misuses reproductive privileges—by becoming pregnant without written approval from the Population and Parenthood Screening Bureau—is liable to be sterilized by court order. As you can imagine, population control is a major concern, and reproductive control is therefore a governmental issue. At least we have no need for abortions!

No, Jerry and Karen's problem pertained not to pregnancy but to sexual dysfunction. We have eliminated the kinds of sexual dysfunction you were familiar with. Pills are available that eliminate inhibitions to sexual response. They can also lubricate vaginas, make penises erect, and even increase sexual desire. Jerry and Karen's problem arose when she popped a "desire" pill and Jerry did not want to take his. As yet it is not a matter of policy to add these chemicals to the water supply, as we do with K25W, to make people's sexual desires compatible. The controversy is ongoing as to whether controlling sexual desire should be left to individual discretion. At present the dysfunction of the sexual union, the term for our form of sexual dysfunction, is subject to the whims of the sexual partners. Opponents of adding desire chemicals to the water supply suggest that if one person drank a glass of water, felt a rush of desire, and could not find his or her partner, hysteria, frustration, violence, or a change of partner could ensue. Well, Jerry finally took his "desire" pill and the dysfunction was eliminated. It is my guess that if this incompatibility recurs, they will be looking for new mates.

Speaking of new mates, Keri is presently looking for one. Her old mate is raising her child and Keri would like a new mate with a drastically different endowment than the last. Keri's child was a dream come true, but only after some medical intervention. The Population and Parenthood Screening Bureau tested Keri both physiologically and psychologically to determine her qualifications for parenthood and approved her application. She chose John as the father because of his blond hair, blue eyes, impressive height, and high intelligence. Several months after conception, the amniotic fluid tests revealed that the fetus was male and had brown eyes and a cleft palate—not

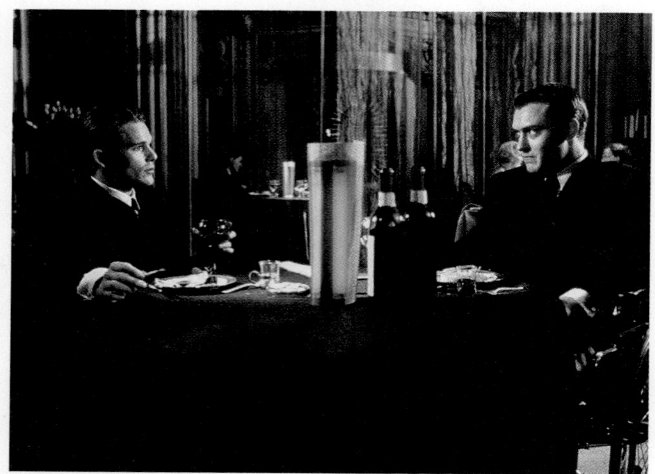

How important our genetic makeup may be in the future is explored in the film *Gattica*. Ethan Hawke plays a young man labeled an "invalid" because his parents decided not to undergo genetic engineering while he was in the womb. Barred from well-paying or respectable jobs, Ethan must take on the identity of a "valid" and risk his life to pursue his dreams. What possible effects do you think genetic engineering may have on sociocultural dimensions of sexuality?

at all like John. You can imagine how quickly Keri ordered a genetic manipulation (GM)! When her daughter was born with blue eyes and devoid of any defects, Keri was elated and decided to keep her.

Keri's friend Josie is an interesting case. In fact, her situation would make a good riddle for you: How can someone be both the biological mother and the biological father of the same child? Well, Josie was not always Josie; she was once Joseph! Joseph was born a male and as a young adult deposited sperm in one of our neighborhood sperm banks. Joseph then decided that his maleness was unsuited to his disposition (unfortunately, his mother had not ordered a GM but had let nature take its course), and he had a sex-change operation. Joseph's male genitals were surgically removed and replaced with two ovaries, two fallopian tubes, a uterus, and a vagina. Once recuperated, Joseph, now Josie, used the deposited sperm to fertilize the ovum during her ovulation period. Hence when the baby was born, its mother and father were one and the same.

But enough of unusual stories. Josie's situation is unique. Keri's case is more common. Perhaps she can soon choose another accurately genetically analyzed mate to make the kind of child she wants. If not, the GM people should be able to help, although, because they are in such demand, we encourage our citizens to do their genetic planning as much beforehand as possible (even though, as Keri's case indicates, this may result in something short of perfection).

By the way, the birthing process has changed much since your time. In 2099 women neither experience pain nor use unnatural chemicals during the delivery of babies. Instead we use endorphins. These substances were discovered more than a century ago but were not put to much use right away. Maybe you remember that endorphins are chemicals naturally produced by the human body that decrease pain and are related to relaxation. Since their discovery in the human brain, we have learned how to produce them synthetically. We administer these synthetic endorphins during childbirth (which, by the way, occurs in people's homes rather than in birthing factories—hospitals, I think you called them). Thus the birth of a baby involves nothing but joy—more joy than we have been able to develop with our medications.

For women too busy to carry the unborn for the 6 months required (we sped up the gestation process for convenience), surrogate mothers are available to do the job. A surrogate receives the fertilized ovum in her uterus and goes through the birth process as usual. The baby is then presented to the original parents and the surrogate is paid according to the birth weight and health of the baby (consequently surrogates do not smoke cigarettes, drink alcohol, or use drugs, and they monitor their nutrition carefully). Other options are available for parents of lesser financial means—animal uteruses serve as surrogate fetal development sites, as does the womb simulator (a machine in which a fetal development is maintained). These options allow the original mother to continue her usual routine unimpeded by pregnancy. However, the price she pays for this convenience is losing the joy of birthing. Moreover, a certain detachment often characterizes the mother–child relationship in such cases.

As you could probably guess, infertility does not exist today. We have so many ways of fertilizing ova and so many ways of organizing embryo and fetal development that our only problem is in restricting birth to a number that does not draw too heavily upon our society's resources.

Before you leave us, take with you the knowledge that sexual disease need not exist—it does not for us. As you can gather, I am sure, we are quite active sexually. And yet we managed to eliminate sexually transmitted diseases by the year 2047. We finally found the link among all the causative agents of STDs, including AIDS. We termed this link the *Syphgon factor,* after syphilis and gonorrhea, although a more appropriate name might be *basic biological matter–thwarting factor.* Soon after the link was found, a vaccine was developed to immunize people against STDs. Originally injected into the bloodstream, this chemical is now in pill form and is designed to dissolve under the tongue. Regarding cancer—breast, uterine, vaginal, testicular, and others—we have been able to teach people, using no medication, to control the flow of T lymphocytes to the cancerous area, thereby eliminating the cancer. Of course, to allow the technique to work, early detection is imperative; the required monthly screening (consisting only of passing through a sensitive doorway similar to that used by your generation to screen airline passengers) serves this purpose. Cancer has virtually been eliminated.

What? You want to know how we arrive at ethical and moral decisions? I am afraid you can only get into trouble asking these questions. Do you not remember the trouble they caused in your time? We leave ethical issues to our leaders. You ask why our leaders are scientists and not ethicists, philosophers, clergy, psychologists, or sociologists? Well, would you have nonscientists leading this highly technical society? We have to trust our leaders to do what is best for us.

To be honest, though, the questions you ask trouble me, too. For us, however, the opportunity to make some other choices has passed. Our society is what it is. It is, you might say, a snowball rolling downhill picking up more and more snow. But take a look at your time. Are not the seeds of our society already planted? Perhaps you still have the chance to nurture the humanizing aspects of your society and to prevent its dehumanizing aspects from developing and taking over your future.

Commentary

Interestingly, Greenberg and Bruess wrote the scenario you just read in the mid-1980s to promote discussion about the future and dimensions of sexuality (Greenberg & Bruess, 1986). As we reread this in preparation for its inclusion in this book, it struck us just how on target our predictions were. It made us think that we should be advising people on which stocks to invest in. Let us take a closer look at the future we projected two decades ago, at the characteristics of that future that already have come to pass and those that have not.

Social Dimensions

We described the year 2099 as one in which fewer people left their home and family to travel to work. Rather, they worked from home with the help of new technologies. We do not have to wait for 2099 for that to occur; it is already happening today. With the advent of the computer, paging systems, and telecommunications capabilities, more people are "telecommuting" than ever before. As in the scenario, more and more people are shopping, banking, and communicating from home. If you want a book, you need only go the web site of Amazon.com or Barnes and Noble. If you want to switch money from one bank account to another, you can hit a few keys on your home computer or a few numbers on your telephone and the transfer is completed. And, if you want to communicate with someone, you can do so by e-mail. The result should be more time for the family and for people about whom we care. However, this does not seem to be a social benefit we have as yet derived from technological advances. Too many people spend too much time at their computers, checking out Internet sites and receiving and sending e-mail messages.

Physical Dimensions

We also guessed right about the ability of physicians to use computers to treat patients better. Today, physicians can call on experts from afar, using computers and telecommunications to read X-rays, computed tomography (CT) scans, and magnetic resonance imaging (MRI) results and make a diagnosis that a local physician may be incapable of making. This technology has tremendous potential for the diagnosis and treatment of sexually transmitted diseases and other sexual illnesses.

In 2099, sexual dysfunction is not one of those matters about which citizens are concerned; they have a "desire pill." In a way, this is not much different from today's Viagra. In addition, microsurgical techniques are available to alleviate some sexual dysfunctional problems.

However, in 2099 the reason the "desire pill" is not added to the water supply is that a person who took a drink and experienced sexual desire might form a "sexual union" with a stranger who happened to be nearby and available. Today, we have a different variable serving as a barrier to "haphazard" sexual unions: HIV and AIDS. The fear of contracting HIV has led to a decrease in casual sex and an increase in condom use when sexual activity does take place. Still, research to develop an HIV and AIDS vaccine, if successful, might once again lead to a more cavalier attitude toward sex and a reemergence of the sexually free attitude of the 1960s. And yet, many Americans and others around the world are not waiting for a vaccine. Too many refuse to adopt responsible sexual behavior and engage in safer-sex practices. Furthermore, in too many places around the world, medications that are effective against HIV and postpone symptoms of AIDS are not available. The disparity between the "haves" and the "have nots" is a characteristic of today, one that has been eliminated in 2099's more egalitarian world.

Marital Dimensions

In the year 2099, there is a new form of marriage—repeating monogamous marriage (RMM). Today, with the divorce and remarriage rates as they are, we have a de facto RMM system. We have even developed a name for the convoluted family structure possible when remarriage occurs (possibly several times for the same parent): *blended families*. However, we have not institutionalized polygamy as was described in the scenario. We still believe in the fidelity of one marital partner to the other, although some might argue that the incidence of extramarital sex provides evidence of a trend in the opposite direction. And today, as in the scenario, it is common for people to live together and not be married to each other. Young couples move in together to determine whether a long-term relationship is feasible for them. Gays live together as unmarried, in the eyes of the law at least, because legislators have proscribed gay marriage. And elders cohabit because our society reinforces that arrangement through our tax codes and social welfare programs. Many Americans choose to remain unmarried, and those who do marry do so at a later age.

Gender Dimensions

We have discussed gender dimensions of sexuality throughout this book, and in 2099 attention is paid to this issue as well: Gender equality is a reality. In present-day society we have made great strides toward gender equality. It is no longer unusual for a female to be a physician or lawyer. It is no longer unusual for a male to assume such household chores as cooking, cleaning, and child rearing. And yet, women are still paid less than men even when they do the same job, and, although men do more household chores when they and their spouses work full-time outside the home, women still assume a disproportionate share. And female genital mutilation is still practiced in many parts of the world. We have yet to discover a way to remedy the disparity in the way we treat our females and males in a manner that is best for women, men, children, and the rest of society, as they did in 2099 with the magical K25W. Still, we are headed in the right direction; the trend is toward greater gender equality and fairness. We hope that we will not have to wait until 2099 to see their full development.

Pregnancy and Childbearing Dimensions

In 2099, there are no unintended pregnancies. That is certainly not where we are today. More than half of all pregnancies in the United States are unintended, and our teenage pregnancy rate is one of the highest among developed countries. As in 2099, we have a wide range of effective contraceptives. The difference is that too few Americans use them or use them irregularly or incorrectly. That leads to a greater number of unwanted births, abortions, and adoptions than would be the case otherwise.

Perhaps our descendants in 2099 have the right idea with the Population and Parenthood Screening Bureau. Today, we have too many children who are abused and neglected. We have too many children who are taken from their birth parents and placed in foster care with the intent of having them adopted, although many never do get a stable family and remain in the foster care system until they become of emancipated age. Perhaps we need to pay as much attention to enhancing parenting skills as our descendants do in 2099.

One area in which we do not have to wait for 2099 is that of genetic manipulation. With medical scientific advances, it is possible to perform surgery on fetuses in the womb to remedy structural abnormalities. Soon we will be able to apply different genes to influence eye color, intelligence, or other traits. Researchers have already isolated stem cells from embryonic tissue that can eventually be used to grow human replacement parts for transplantation. People wonder, If Dolly the sheep has been cloned, will humans eventually be cloned? The ethical implications of rapidly developing scientific advances have outstripped our society's ability to develop laws that will assure that technology will be used to enhance our culture rather than diminish it.

Want a boy baby? No need to engage in abortion or infanticide, as in some countries. Just use sperm-separation techniques to improve the odds. No, this is not part of the 2099 scenario. This is occurring today. Want a child who is likely to be an athlete or a musician? Just be selective at the sperm bank, careful to choose sperm from a male who has the characteristics you want for your child. No, this is not part of the 2099 scenario. This is occurring today. The future is here!

Tonow

As the 21st-century narrator of our story implies, being aware of present trends and considering what personal and social agreements about sexuality may be like in the future can be fun, but it can also be a responsibility.

As our society evolves we must not lose sight of our heritage and what we have learned from it. To that knowledge we must add new information—information filtered through ethical and moral awareness and values. As citizens of today and of the future, we can ill afford to shirk our responsibility to help shape our sexual society.

The physician Bernie Siegel works with cancer patients—"cancer survivors," he calls them. Knowing they probably have little time left to live, he helps them live "well" during the time left to them. This is a lesson that all of us could profit by learning. Siegel is fond of speaking of today, tomorrow, and "tonow." Using Siegel's terminology, many sexual futuristic issues are actually occurring tonow.

A woman is judged guilty of a criminal act and is considered to be a poor mother, so a judge prevents her from having other children. He offers her a choice of going to jail or having a contraceptive implant (Norplant) surgically placed on her arm. Tonow.

A society experiments on itself. Its children grow up with the majority of their mothers working full-time outside the home. In many cases, a male figure is absent from the home because of desertion, death, or divorce. What will the effects be? Tonow.

A country changes dramatically. What were once "minorities," when grouped together, become the majority. In many areas of the United States, Hispanic, Asian-American, and African-American populations have increased in numbers and in percentage of population. What will be the effects on sexuality? On attitudes toward sexual issues? On views of censorship, morality, abortion, and family life? Many believe the country will profit from this diversity. Will it? Tonow.

As people wrestle with a threat to their very lives, a threat that seems uncontrollable, AIDS stalks all segments of the population. During the sexual revolution individuals fought for the right of free sexual expression; however, in this day there can be heavy consequences for such behavior. Will behavior change? How many deaths will occur before that happens? Will relationships ever be the same? Tonow.

It is our hope that this book helps to prepare you for your sexual tonow and your sexual tomorrow. Most likely your instructor hopes your sexuality course will have the same effect. No one can predict the future, but we can anticipate trends and prepare for them. How will you prepare? When will you start?

Discussion Questions

1. Vaccines were one of the greatest wonders of the 20th century and eradicated several major diseases. However, a small percentage of people contract the disease through the vaccine and are left disabled or dead. Would you be willing to take such a risk to be vaccinated for STDs or HIV? Would you subject your infant children to such vaccines to protect their future? Explain why or why not.
2. Over the time you have taken this course, you have undoubtedly heard news stories about current research that could affect your future sexuality. Relate some of the more interesting research projects, and discuss whether they are feasible, given the biological, psychological, and sociocultural dimensions of sexuality.

Application Questions

Reread the chapter-opening story and answer the following questions.

1. Would you prefer to live in your current world or in the world of 2099 described in the story? Explain your answer.
2. Allowing government control over subliminal messages (and lacing the drinking water with K25W) would give the government complete control of the population. How could government be regulated so that only positive messages (for example, gender equality) would be conveyed? What if the government decided to convey messages like "Don't vote for the opposing political party"—or worse?

Critical Thinking Questions

1. As our society continues to accept the ideal of diversity, we seem less and less likely to unify as a nation on any issue—especially sex! Consider the use of stem cells in the United States. What sociocultural groups are likely to be in favor of their use? What groups would be against it? Is it likely the federal government would ever approve the use of fetal stem cells?
2. Aldous Huxley, in *Brave New World,* portrayed a government that kept control of its people by granting them unrestrained sexual pleasures. George Orwell, in *1984,* took the opposite position: The government keeps control by discouraging sexual contact among spouses and forbidding it among nonmarried people. Compare and contrast these methods given what you know about the many dimensions of human sexuality.

Critical Thinking Case

What Is "Quality of Life"?

The year 2099 seems to have some attractive features. Diseases are curable. Computers do a lot of the work, and the remainder can often be done at home. Cars do not pollute air. People live longer and establish numerous relationships—each designed to meet a specific need.

And yet some of the citizens in the year 2099 seem disenchanted. Their marriages often do not last very long. They cannot have children whenever they want. They cannot engage in competitive sports. Their mind is manipulated as a result of K25W in their water supply.

Given these and the other conditions we have described, would you want to live in the year 2099? Why or why not?

What in life is important to you aside from *how long you live?*

What is present and what is absent in 2099 that you need to be happy sexually?

Exploring Personal Dimensions

The form to the right might be used in our fictional story set in 2099. In our story, those individuals wishing to conceive may have to answer questions very much like those in the form. Their answers determine whether they are given permission to have a child, as well as specifying the gender and appearance of the child. As you read through this form, consider whether it is ethical to ask such questions of potential parents. What would the effects of applying such rules to parenting be on the sociocultural dimensions of sexuality?

POPULATION AND PARENTHOOD SCREENING BUREAU

Parenthood Application

Name: ____________________

Mate's Name: ____________________

Address: ____________________

Computer Access Number: ____________________

Answer all of the following questions:

1. How long have you been mating? ____________________
2. List all illnesses/diseases experienced within the last year by the female mate: ____________________
3. List all illnesses/diseases experienced within the last year by the male mate: ____________________
4. On the breakup of your relationship, what do you plan for your child? ____________________
5. What time is best for you to be interviewed by our psychological team? ____________________
6. List those traits you want ensured in your child:
   a. Sex: ____________________
   b. Eye color: ____________________
   c. Hair color: ____________________
   d. Intelligence quotient: ____________________
   e. Height: ____________________
   f. Special abilities (for example, athletic, mathematical, artistic): ____________________
7. Which method of birth control do you employ? ____________________
8. Do you have any other children? ____________________
9. What method of birthing do you plan? ____________________
10. How will your child be cared for during the workday? ____________________
11. List any parenting training you and/or your mate has received: ____________________
12. Will you agree to amniotic fluid screening during the pregnancy? ____________________

Special Note: Be aware that approval will not be granted to individuals who already have a child, who are untrained for parenthood, who do not agree to amniotic fluid screening, who have not planned for the daily care of their child-to-be, or who have not prepared for the breakup of their relationship.

An Introduction to Service–Learning

An elementary school decided to develop a schoolwide program to feed the homeless. Grades 3 and 4 organized the project. Using what they learned in their home economics and health education units, they agreed on a menu to be served in the school cafeteria. Employing the grammar, spelling, and letter writing content learned in their English unit, they wrote letters to local merchants soliciting supplies. Next, they used math skills to compute how much bread and other food they needed on the basis of the number of people they expected to feed. First and second graders also participated, using their art class skills to make placemats. Even the kitchen staff helped by mixing the tuna that was served, and the school custodian set up the lunchroom tables.

Another school adopted the school's cook's son as a pen pal. He was in the Marines and was sent to Kuwait during Desert Storm. In preparation for the letters they wrote to this young soldier, the students studied about the Middle East, including its geography, climate, customs, religions, and forms of government.

An engineering professor heard of a young quadriplegic who bemoaned the fact that he could not travel around with his friends as they scooted off on their bikes. The professor organized his engineering class around a project: Develop some way for this young quadriplegic man to participate with his friends. The result was a motorized vehicle that could be operated by the youngster's head movements.

The preceding stories are all examples of students' taking what they learned in class and applying their knowledge to help improve the lives of people in the community. This is a form of education called service–learning. In addition to being concerned with our individual needs, all of us have a responsibility to enhance the sexual health of our communities. This appendix

"Perhaps the most gratifying feeling in the world arises when you know that you played a role in making someone else's life better."

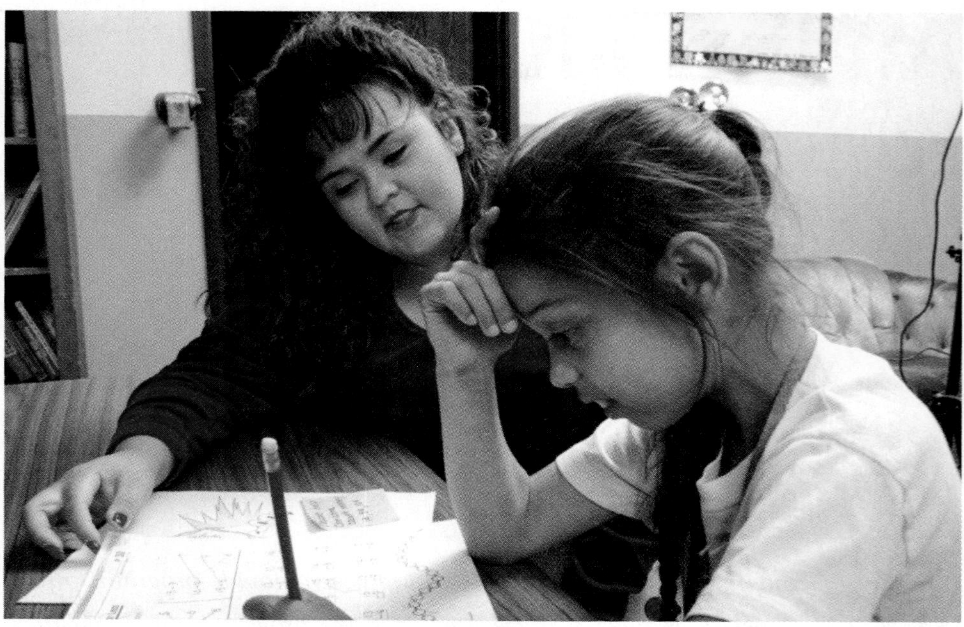

Service–learning projects can create strong bonds among the participants.

was created to provide you with a definition of service–learning, a description of its benefits to students and the community, and ideas on how to start a service–learning project.

Defining Service–Learning

Service–learning is an educational methodology through which students apply what they learn in their courses and curriculum by serving the community. The theory behind service–learning is that the students will learn more about the topic or topics they are studying by using their knowledge to help others. Service–learning is distinct from other forms of service in that it focuses equally on the service provided and on the learning that occurs. Figure SL-1 presents a way of looking at this distinction.

"Who knows what could be accomplished if more people decided to be judged not by their personal gains, but by their ability to share."

Components of Service–Learning

Service–learning consists of five phases: planning, action, reflection, evaluation, and celebration. During planning, students read books and articles, gather information, and otherwise plan to conduct the service. The action phase consists of actually performing the service. However, experience gained without processing of that experience is not very valuable. So, the reflection phase engages students in activities to draw meaning from the service they provided. There are many different methods of reflection. For example, reflection can take the form of having group discussions, maintaining a journal, writing a paper, presenting a skit, or producing a videotape. The evaluation phase is designed to determine whether the service–learning activity was successful in achieving its objectives. The evaluation should be qualitative and quantitative. For example, there may be interviews of recipients of the service and of program supervisors to obtain qualitative data, and administration of surveys, questionnaires, or observational checklists to obtain quantitative

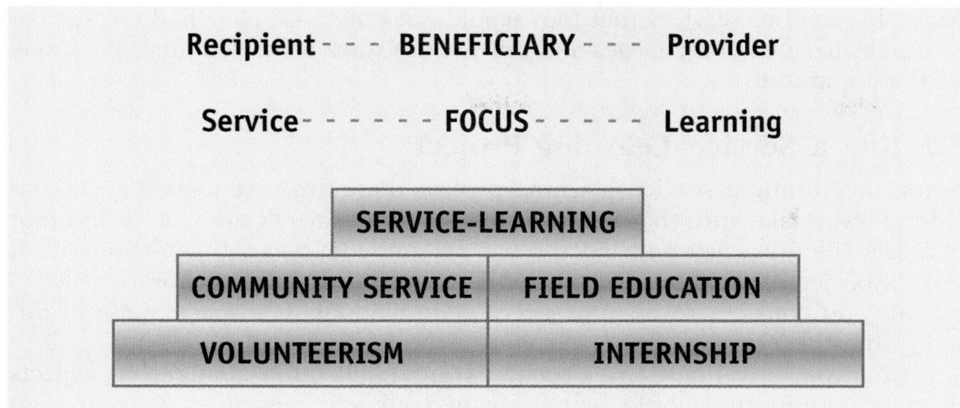

FIGURE SL-1 Distinctions among service programs.
Source: Furco, A. Service–learning: a balanced approach to experiential education, in The Corporation for National and Community Service. *Expanding Boundaries: Service and Learning.* 1996, 2–6.

data. The quantitative evaluation can be used to provide information regarding the achievement of the service–learning objectives, and the qualitative evaluation can be used to understand the quantitative data better. For example, the quantitative evaluation may tell us the objectives were not achieved, but we may have no idea why that occurred unless we also have a qualitative evaluation. Was it that the content was at too high a level for the recipients of the service, or that the instructional methods were inappropriate, or that the objectives were too ambitious given the time available? The qualitative evaluation can help us answer these questions and adjust the service accordingly the next time it is offered. Once the service–learning is complete and reflection has elicited meaning from that activity, and the evaluation has occurred, the group celebrates their accomplishment. The celebration phase also can be varied. For example, it can involve presentations to the faculty or other students, an article sent to a local newspaper or organization, or a party to which people from the organization(s) served are invited.

Benefits of Service–Learning

Because service–learning is a relatively new concept, the data on its effectiveness are just developing. However, a national study by researchers of the RAND Corporation and the University of California at Los Angeles (Astin and Sax, 1997) investigated benefits of organized service activities on college campuses. This study analyzed programs funded by the Corporation for National and Community Service through Learn and Serve America grants. The researchers identified significant benefits for students, community agencies they served, and colleges and universities when students participated in organized service activities. Students learned more and became more conscientious about their schoolwork, community agencies

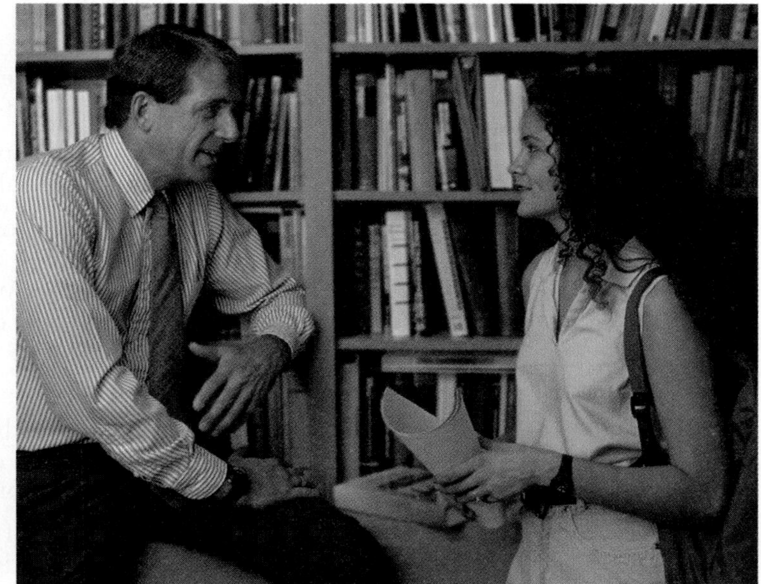

Service–learning will help you apply concepts you learn in class and in your texts to real-life situations.

"I am appreciative for this opportunity to have this experience, because it has put me more in touch with my strengths and weaknesses, and has made me feel better about myself for doing something worthwhile."

were able to offer services that they would not otherwise have had the staff or resources to offer, and colleges and universities were perceived more positively by the community.

Starting a Service–Learning Project

Before beginning a service–learning project there are several points to consider. First, make sure that you are clear on the project's guidelines and that it meets the goals your instructor has set for you. Next, think about what type of projects would interest you most. Would you prefer to work with individuals you consider to be your peers or individuals who participate in different lifestyles or are of different ages or ethnicity?

After you have made this decision you should think about what aspects of your community would benefit from your services most. Perhaps you could ask questions of your peers or instructors to get a sense of programs on your campus that could use your help. If you wish to work outside your campus, you could talk to people who know the community well.

Be sure you communicate well with your contact person at the site you have chosen for your project. Make certain that he or she understands your reasons for doing the project and exactly what you plan to learn from the project before you begin.

The following are examples of service–learning projects related to human sexuality that could apply to a variety of different interests.

- Volunteer to work with a women's studies program on your campus. They may need help with a variety of activities, and in the process of helping, you will learn more about their goals and activities and about gender roles.
- Volunteer to read to children at a local elementary school. As you review and read the books, watch for gender bias.
- Volunteer to be a Big Brother or Big Sister or Scout leader. Young people who are involved in extracurricular activities and have significant adults in their life do well in school and are less likely to become pregnant.
- Talk with your instructor or a research director to find out whether any campus researcher is working in an area of human sexuality that interests you. Offer to assist the researcher.
- Develop a slide presentation on forcible sexual behavior or any other topic of human sexuality that an instructor could use in class.
- There are a number of groups designed to protect the rights of individuals to make their own choices such as the National Organization for Women and the American Civil Liberties Union. Find out whether such groups or groups like them exist in your community and volunteer to help them send mailings, prepare for speakers, or plan programs.
- Volunteer for your school's peer education program. Many colleges and universities have programs to train students to help educate other students and sometimes community members.

There are a variety of sexual wellness and health needs in our communities. Given the knowledge and skills students learn in a sexuality course, service–learning holds tremendous potential for improving sexual health and wellness in our communities and concurrently contributing to students' learning. We hope this section helps you to realize these benefits.

References

101 Ways to Combat Domestic Violence. Feminists Against Violence Network. (2003). Available: www.geocities.com/Heartland/Meadows/7905/101.htm.

65 years and over population: 2000. Census 2000 Brief, U.S. Census Bureau, 2001.

Aamodt, A. Culture, in *Culture Child-Bearing Health Professionals,* Clark, A., ed. Philadelphia: F. A. Davis, 1978.

Abbey, A. Acquaintance rape and alcohol consumption on college campuses: How are they linked? *Journal of American College Health, 39* (1991), 165–169.

Abma, J. C., Chandra, A., Mosher, W. D., Peterson, L., & Piccinino, L. Fertility, family planning, and women's health: New data from the 1995 National Survey of Family Growth, National Center for Health Statistics, *Vital Health, 23, no. 19* (1997).

Abortion battles: More in common than we think, *USA Today* (August 13, 1996), 1.

Abortion worker shootings, *Washington Post* (October 25, 1998), A8.

Achenbach, J. Splice of life, *The Washington Post Magazine* (November 29, 1998), 12–19, 27–30.

ACLU Freedom Network. In the matter of industry for rating video programming, 1998.

Activity, *The Guttmacher Report*, 4, *no. 4* (August 2001), 2–4.

Adams, D. B., Gold, A. R., & Burt, A. D. Rise in female-initiated sexual activity at ovulation and suppression by oral contraceptives, *New England Journal of Medicine*, 299 (1978), 1145–1150.

Adamson, G. D. The new reproductive technologies—which one to choose? *Resolve Fact Sheet Series,* 1998.

Addiego, F., Belzer, E., Perry, J., & Whipple, B. Female ejaculation: A case study, *Journal of Sex Research*, 17 (1981), 13–21.

Administration for children and families, National Adoption and Foster Care Statistics (2003). Available: http://www.acf.hhs.gov/programs/cb/dis/afcars/publications/afcars.htm.

Adult survivors of sex abuse in crisis, *Behavior Today, 21* (1990), 1–3.

African awakening, *Salon Magazine.*

Age at first menstruation continues to decline, especially among African Americans, study says, *Kaiser Daily Reproductive Health Report* (October 8, 2002). Available: www.kaisernetwork.org/daily reports.

Agency for healthcare research and quality. U.S. preventive task force calls for chlamydia and lipid screening and issues two other recommendations, *Research Activities*, no. 248 (2001), 23–24.

Aids risk rising in older people, *Consumer Reports on Health*, 15, no. 1 (January 2003), 7.

AIDS virus gets new name amid feuding, *Medical World News, 27* (1986), 14–15.

Airing it out, *Time*, 160, no. 19 (November 4, 2002), 84.

Alan Guttmacher Institute. *Facts in brief: Induced abortion*, 1997.

Alan Guttmacher Institute. *Facts in brief: Induced abortion*. New York, 2000.

Alan Guttmacher Institute. *Sex and America's teenagers*, 1994.

Alder, C. An exploration of self-reported sexually aggressive behavior, *Crime and Delinquency, 31, no. 2* (1985), 306–331.

Alexander, E. & Hickner, J. First coitus for adolescents: Understanding why and when, *Journal of the American Board of Family Practice, 10, no. 2* (March-April 1997), 170–172.

Alexander, N. J. & Clarkson, T. B. Vasectomy increases the severity of diet-induced atherosclerosis in macaca fascicularis, *Science, 210* (1978), 538–541.

Allan, K. & Coltrane, S. Gender displaying television commercials: A comparative study of television commercials in the 1950s and 1980s, *Sex Roles, 35* (August 1996), 185–203.

Alter, G. New perspectives in European marriage in the nineteenth century, *Journal of Family History 16, no. 1* (1991), 1–5.

Altman, C. *You can be your own sex therapist: A systematized behavioral approach to enhancing your sensual pleasure, improving your sexual enjoyment.* Casper, WY: Casper Publishing, 1997.

Altman, C. Gay and lesbian seniors: Unique challenges of coming out in later life, *SIECUS Report, 27, no. 3* (February/March 1999), 14–17.

Alzate, H. & Hoch, Z. The G spot and female ejaculation: A current appraisal, *Journal of Sex and Marital Therapy*, 12 (1986), 211–220.

Alzate, H. & Londono, M. Vaginal erotic sensitivity, *Journal of Sex and Marital Therapy*, 10 (1984), 49–56.

America's families and living arrangements, *Current Population Reports*. U.S. Census Bureau, June 2001.

American Cancer Society. *American Cancer Society updates prostate cancer screening guidelines,* June 12, 1997.

American Cancer Society. *Cancer Facts and Figures 2001*, 2001.

American Cancer Society. *Cancer facts and figures 2003*. (2003). Atlanta, GA.

American Cancer Society. *Cancer facts and figures, 1998: Selected cancers.*

American Cancer Society. *Cancer risk report,* 1995.

American College Health Association. *Is dating dangerous?* 1997.

American College of Obstetricians and Gynecologists. *You and your baby: Prenatal care, labor and delivery, and postpartum care.* Washington, DC: American College of Obstetricians and Gynecologists Patient Education, 1994.

American College of Obstetrics and Gynecology, news release. (February 14, 2001). Washington, DC.

American Heart Association. *Sexual activity and heart disease and stroke,* 1998.

American Psychiatric Association, 1998.

American Psychiatric Association, 2000. *Diagnostic and Statistical Manual of Mental Disorders.* Washington, D.C.

American Psychiatric Association. *Diagnostic and statistical manual of mental disorders*, 4th ed, 1994.

American Public Health Association. Condoms proven effective against HIV transmission, *The Nation's Health* (September 2001), 4.

American Social Health Association. *STDs in America*, 1998.

American Society of Asethetic Plastic Surgery (2003). Available: http://surgery.org/statistics.html.

American Society of Plastic Surgeons (2003). Available: www.plasticsurgery.org.

American women waiting to begin families, InteliHealth (December 13, 2002). Available: www.intelihealth.com.

Ames, M. A. & Houston D. A., Legal, social, and biological definitions of pedophilia, *Archives of Sexual Behavior, 19* (1990), 332–342.

Ames, P. Belgian cabinet OKs gay marriages, *The Birmingham News* (June 24, 2001), 11A.

An arrangement of marriages, *Psychology Today, 26* (January/February 1993), 22.

Angell, M. *Science on trial: The clash of medical evidence and the law in the breast implant case.* New York: W. W. Norton, 1996.

Angier, J. N. Drugs, sports, body image and G. I. Joe. *New York Times* (December 22, 1998), D1.

Angier, N. *Women: An intimate geography*. Boston: Houghton Mifflin, 1999.

Annon, J. S. *The Behavioral Treatment of Sexual Problems: Brief Therapy.* New York: Harper & Row, 1976.

Anthrax threats, continued violence prompt renewed attention to clinic, client protection, The Guttmacher Report on Public Policy, 4 (2001). Available: http://www.agi-usa.org/pubs/journals/gr040613.html.

Antibiotic-resistant strains of *Neisseria Gonorrheae:* Policy guidelines for detection, management and control, *MMWR Supplement 36* (1987), 1S–18S.

Apfelbaum, B. Why we should not accept sexual fantasies, in *Expanding the boundaries of sex therapy.* Berkeley, CA: Berkeley Sex Therapy Group, 1980.

Arafat, I. & Cotton, W. L. Masturbation practices of males and females, *Journal of Sex Research, 10* (1974), 293–307.

Aries, P. & Bejin, A. *Western sexuality.* New York: Basil Blackwell, 1985.

Arndorfer, E. The gender gap in insurance coverage for women's reproductive health, *SIECUS Report, 27, no. 1* (October/November 1998), 17–20.

Artel, R. & Wiswell, R. A. Exercise prescription in pregnancy, in *Exercise in pregnancy,* Artel, R. & Wiswell, R. A., eds. Baltimore: Williams & Wilkins, 1986, 225–228.

Associated Press. Lesbian can resume coaching, judge rules, *Washington Post* (November 27, 1998), A12.

Association for voluntary sterilization. Estimate of the number of sterilizations performed in the United States, mimeo, December 1982.

Attorney General's Commission on Pornography. *Final report of the Attorney General's commission on pornography,* Washington, DC: Department of Justice, 1986.

Ault, A. U.S. Institute of Medicine panel deliberates on breast-implant safety, *The Lancet, 352, no. 9124* (August 1, 1998), 380.

Aureli, T. Day care experience and free play behavior in preschool children, *Journal of Applied Developmental Psychology, 17, no. 1* (January-March 1996), 1–17.

Azar, B. Consistent parenting helps children regulate emotions, American Psychological Association, 1998.

Badgett, M. V. L. Employment and sexual orientation: Disclosure and discrimination in the workplace, in *Sexual identity on the job: Issues and services,* Ellis, A. L. & Riggle, D. B., eds. New York: Harrington Park Press/Haworth Press, 1996, 29–52.

Baffi, C. R., Redican, K. J., Sefchick, M. K., & Impara, J. C. Gender role identity, gender role stress, and health behaviors: An exploratory study of selected college males, *Health Values, 15* (1991), 9–18.

Bailey, H. M. & Pillard, R. C., A genetic study of male sexual orientation. *Archives of General Psychiatry, 48* (1991), 1089–1086.

Bailey, J. M., Dunne, M. P., & Martin, N. G. Genetic and environmental influences on sexual orientation and its correlates in an Australian twin sample, *Journal of Personality & Social Psychology*, 78, no. 3 (2000), 524–536.

Baker, D. D., Terpstra, D. E., & Larntz, K. The influence of individual characteristics and severity of harassing behavior on reaction to sexual harassment, *Sex Roles, 22* (1990), 305–325.

Baldwin, J. D. & Baldwin, J. L. Gender differences in sexual interest, *Archives of Sexual Behavior, 16, no. 2* (1997), 181–210.

Bancroft, J. Hormones and sexual behavior, *Journal of Sex and Marital Therapy*, 10 (1984), 3–21.

Banning, A. Mother–son incest: Confronting a prejudice, *Child Abuse and Neglect, 13* (1989), 563–570.

Barbach, L. G. *For yourself: The fulfillment of female sexuality.* New York: New American Library, 1991.

Barbach, L. G. *The pause: Positive approaches to menopause.* New York: Dutton, 1993.

Barbach, L. G. *Women discover orgasm: A therapist's guide to a New Testament approach.* New York: Free Press, 1980.

Barber, J. S. & Axinn, W. G. Gender role attitudes and marriage among young women, *The Sociological Quarterly, 39* (Winter 1998), 11–31.

Barclay, A. M. Sexual fantasies in men and women. *Medical Aspects of Human Sexuality,* 7 (1973), 205–216.

Bardes, B. A., Shelley II, M. C., & Schmidt, S. W. *American government and politics today: The essentials.* Belmont, CA: West/Wadsworth, 1998.

Barker, T., ed. *The woman's book of orgasm: A guide to the ultimate sexual pleasure.* Secaucus, NJ: Citadel Press, 1998.

Barnette, M. The perfect body, *Allure* (August 1993), 197–110, 146.

Baron, L. & Straus, M. A. Sexual stratification, pornography, and rape in the United States, in *Pornography and sexual aggression,* Malamuth, N. M. & Donnerstein, E., eds. New York: Academic Press, 1984.

Baron, R. A. *Psychology,* 4th ed. Needham Heights, MA: Allyn & Bacon, 1998.

Bartell, G. Group sex among mid-Americans, *Journal of Sex Research, 6* (1970), 113–130.

Bartley, N. The return of romance: Antidote to dreary reality of the 90s, *Watertown (NY) Daily Times* (February 13, 1994), 7.

Bartoi, A. G. & Kinder, B. N. Effects of child and adult sexual abuse on adult sexuality, *Journal of Sex and Marital Therapy, 24* (1998), 75–90.

Bates, G. On the nature of the hot flash, Clinical Obstetrics and Gynecology, 24 (1981), 231–241.

Bauer, H. M., Ting, I., Greer, C. E., et al. Genital human papillomavirus infection in female university students as determined by a PCR-based method, *Journal of the American Medical Association, 265* (1991), 472–477.

Baumeister, R. F. The enigmatic appeal of sexual masochism: Why people desire pain, bondage, and humiliation in sex, *Journal of Social and Clinical Psychology, 16, no. 2* (1997), 133–150.

Baxter, D. J., Marshall, W. L., Barbaree, H. E., Davidson, P. R., & Malcolm, P. B. Deviant sexual behavior, *Criminal Justice and Behavior, 11, no. 4* (1984), 477–501.

Baxter, N. Preventive health care, 2001 update: Should women be routinely taught breast self-examination to screen for breast cancer? *Canadian Medical Association Journal,* 164, no.13 (2001), 1837–1846.

Beal, C. R. *Boys and girls: The development of gender roles.* New York: McGraw-Hill, 1994.

Bechtel, L. S., Westerfield, C., & Eddy, J. M. Autoerotic fatalities: Implications for health educators, *Health Education, 21* (1990), 38–40.

Bechtel, S. *The practical encyclopedia of sex and health: From aphrodisiacs and hormones to potency, stress, vasectomy and yeast infection.* Emmaus, PA: Rodale Press, 1993.

Bechtel, S. *Sex: A man's guide.* Emmaus, PA: Rodale Press, 1997.

Bechtel, S. & Roystains, L. *Sex: A man's guide*. Emmaus, PA: Rodale Press, 1997.

Beck, Rohter, M. L., & Friday, C. An unwanted baby boom, *Newsweek* (April 30, 1984).

Bedard, M. E. *Breaking with tradition.* Dix Hills, NY: General Hall, 1992.

Begley, S. & Brant, M. The real scandal, *Newsweek* (February 15, 1999), 48–54.

Belcastro, P. A. *The birth control book.* Boston: Jones & Bartlett, 1986.

Bell, A. P. & Weinberg, M. S. *Homosexualities: A study of diversity among men and women.* New York: Simon & Shuster, 1978.

Bell, A. P., Weinberg, M. S., & Hammersmith, S. K. *Sexual preference: Its development in men and women.* Bloomington: Indiana University Press, 1981.

Bell, R. R. & Gordon, M. *The social dimension of human sexuality.* Boston: Little, Brown, 1972.

Bell, R. R. *Premarital sex in a changing society.* Englewood Cliffs, NJ: Prentice-Hall, 1966.

Belshin, L. *The complete prostate book: Every man's guide.* Rocklin, CA: Prima Publishing, 1997.

Belzer, E. G. Orgasmic expulsions of women: A review and heuristic inquiry, *Journal of Sex Research*, 17 (1981), 1–12.

Belzer, E. G., Whipple, B., & Moger, W. On female ejaculation, *Journal of Sex Research*, 20 (1984), 403–406.

Bem, S. L. Androgyny versus the tight little lives of women and chesty men, *Psychology Today* (September 1975), 58–62.

Benderly, B. L. Modern sex, *Psychology Today* (August 1986), 68–69.

Bergen, R. K. The reality of wife rape: Women's experiences of sexual violence in marriage, in *Issues in intimate violence,* Bergen, R. K., ed. Thousand Oaks, CA: Sage Publications, 1998.

Bergfeld, J. A., Martin, M. C., Shangold, M. M., & Warren, M. P. Women in athletics: Five management problems, *Patient Care 21, no. 4* (1987), 60–82.

Bergkvist, L., Adami, H. O., Persson, J., Hoover, R., & Schairer, C. The risk of breast cancer after estrogen and estrogen-progestin replacement, *New England Journal of Medicine*, 321 (1989), 293.

Bergquist, C., Nillius, S. J., & Wide, L. Contraception in women, *Contraception, 31* (1985), 11–118.

Berkowitz, J. L., et al. Estrogen replacement therapy and fibrocystic disease in postmenopausal women. *American Journal of Epidemiology*, 121 (1985), 238–245.

Bernstein, A. C. *Flight of the stork.* Indiana: Perspectives Press, 1994.

Bestiality, Go ask alice. Columbia University (2003). [On line]. Available: www.goaskalice.columbia.edu/0707.html.

Bieber, I., Dain, H., Dince, P., Drellich, M., Grand, H., Gundlach, R., Kremer, M., Rifkin, A., Wilbur, C., & Bieber, T. *Homosexuality: A psychoanalytic perspective.* New York: Basic Books, 1962.

Bilger, B. Muscle dysmorphia syndrome, *The Sciences, 38* (January/February 1998), 10.

Bilian, X., Xueling, Z., & Dandan, F. Pharmacokimetic and pharmacodyllamic studies of vaginal rings releasing low-dosage levonorgestrel, *Contraception, 32* (1985), 455–471.

Birchard, Karen. Sex, Please, We're British: Many Students Strip to Pay Bills, BBC Reports. *The Chronicle of Higher Education*, Today's News, May 2, 2001. Available: http://chronicle.com/daily/2001/05/2001050205n.htm

Births, marriages, divorces, and deaths: 2001, *National Vital Statistics Reports*, 59, no. 14 (September 11, 2002), 1–2.

Black, J. & Underwood, J. Young, female, and gay: Lesbian students and the school environment, *Professional School Counseling, 1, no. 3* (February 1998), 15–20.

Blair, C. D. & Lanyon, R. I. Exhibitionism: Etiology and treatment, *Psychological Bulletin, 89, no. 3* (1981), 439–463.

Blair, S. L. & Lichter, D. T. Measuring the division of household labor, *Journal of Family Issues, 12* (1991), 91–113.

Blakely, G. L., Blakely, E. H., & Moorman, R. H. The relationship between gender, personal experience, and perceptions of sexual harassment in the workplace, *Employee Relationships and Rights Journal, 8, no. 4* (1995), 263–274.

Blau, M. Staying power: Bridging the gender gap in the confusing '90s, *American Health* (May 1994), 87–89.

Blood supply grows safer, *FDA Consumer, 24* (1990), 5.

Blumstein, P. & Schwartz, P. *American Couples*. New York: William Morrow, 1983.

Blumstein, P. & Schwartz, P. Bisexuality in women, *Archives of Sexual Behavior, 5* (1976), 171–181.

Bohannan, P. The binuclear family, *Science, 2* (November 1981), 28.

The boomer sandwich, *Modern Maturity*, 44w, no. 5 (September/October 2001), 94.

Boorstein, M. Test before commitment, (February 2, 1999).

Bordo, S. *The male body: A new look at men in public and private*. New York: Farrar, Straus, and Giroux, 1999.

Borysenko, J. *A woman's book of life: The biology, psychology and spirituality of the feminine life cycle*. New York: Riverhead Books, 1998.

Boslett, L. Colleges decide how to comply with new sex-offender law, *The Chronicle of Higher Education*, 49, no. 20 (January 24, 2003), A33–34.

Boston Women's Health Collective. *Our bodies, ourselves: For the new century*. New York: Simon & Schuster, 1998.

Boston Women's Health Collective. *The new our bodies, ourselves*. New York: Simon & Schuster, 1984.

Bowen, F. Is there a case for an uneven playing field? *The Birmingham News* (January 9, 2003), 7E.

Bower, S. A. & Brower, G. *Asserting yourself: A practical guide for positive change.* Reading, MA: Perseus Books, 1976.

Boyer, D. & Fine, D. Sexual abuse as a factor in adolescent pregnancy and child maltreatment, *Family Planning Perspectives, 24, 1* (1992), 4–11.

Bradford, L. J. & Beck, K. H. Development and validation of a condom self-efficacy scale for college students, *Journal of American College Health, 39* (1991), 219–225.

Brecher, E. *Love, sex, and aging.* Boston: Little, Brown, 1984.

Brennan, J. Reconciling immigrant values, in *Case studies in cultural diversity,* Ferguson, V. D., ed. Sudbury, MA: Jones & Bartlett, 1999, 185–189.

Bretschneider, J. & McCoy, N. Sexual interest and behavior in healthy 80–102 year olds, *Archives of Sexual Behavior, 17* (1988), 109–130.

Brick, P. Sexuality education in the early elementary classroom, in *The sexuality education challenge,* Drolet, J. C. & Clark, K., eds. Santa Cruz, CA: ETR Associates, 1994, 103–135.

Briton, N. J. & Hall, J. A. Beliefs about female and male nonverbal communication, *Sex Roles, 32, nos. 1 & 2* (1995), 79–90.

Broberg, A. G. Effects of day care on the development of cognitive abilities in 8-year-olds, *Developmental Psychology, 33, no. 1* (January 1997), 62–69.

Brody, J. E. Study identifies disorder afflicting body builders, *New York Times* (Late New York Edition), (January 6, 1998), F8.

Brooks, J., Ruble, D., & Clark, A. College women's attitudes and expectations concerning menstrual-related changes, *Psychosomatic Medicine*, 39 (1977), 289–298.

Brooks-Gunn, J. & Furstenberg, F. F. Coming of age in the era of AIDS: Puberty, sexuality, and contraception, *The Millbank Quarterly, 68, Suppl. 1* (1990).

Broom, S. Sex happens after 50, and so do sexually transmitted diseases, *SIECUS Report, 27, no. 3* (February/March 1999), 12–13.

Brosius, H. B., Weaver, J. B., & Staab, J. F. Exploring the social and sexual "reality" of contemporary pornography, *Journal of Sex Research, 30, no. 2* (1993), 161–170.

Brower, V. Circumcision's back, *American Health* (September 1989), 126.

Brown, J. & Hart, D. Correlates of Females' Sexual Fantasies. *Perceptual and Motor Skills* 45(1977): 819–25.

Brown, J. & Steele, J. R. Sexuality and the mass media: An overview, *SIECUS Report, 24, no. 4* (April/May 1996), 3–9.

Brown, J. E. & Story, M. Let them eat cake or a prescription for improving the outcome of pregnancy? *Nutrition Today, 25* (1990), 18–23.

Brownlee, S. The baby chase: Millions of couples have fertility problems, and many high-tech remedies. But who minds the pricey clinics they turn to? *U.S. News and World Report* (December 1995), 84–90.

Bruess, C. E. & Greenberg, J. S. *Sexuality education: Theory and practice.* Madison, WI: Brown & Benchmark, 1994.

Bruess, C. E. & Greenberg, J. S. *Sexuality education: Theory and practice,* 2nd ed. New York: Macmillan, 1988.

Bruess, C. E. & Richardson, G. *Decisions for health.* Dubuque, IA: Brown & Benchmark, 1995, 1.14–1.16.

Bryant, A. Hostile hallways: The AAUW survey on sexual harassment in American schools, *Journal of School Health, 63, no. 8* (October 1993), 355–357.

Bryden, D. P. & Lengnick, S. Rape in the criminal justice system, *The Journal of Criminal Law & Criminology, 87* (1987), 1194–1384.

Bryla, K. Y. Effects of media on female body image: myth or reality? *The Health Education Monograph Series*, 19, no. 2 (2002), 13–16.

Bullers, F. Kansas state senator says she is against women's suffrage, *The Birmingham News* (September 29, 2001), 5A.

Bullough, B. & Bullough, V. L. Are transvestites necessarily heterosexual? *Archives of Sexual Behavior, 26* (1997), 1–12.

Bullough, B. & Bullough, V. L. Female prostitution: Current research and changing interpretations, *Annual Review of Sex Research,* Society for the Scientific Study of Sexuality, 7 (1996), 158–180.

Bullough, V. L. & Bullough, B. *Human sexuality: An encyclopedia.* New York: Garland Press, 1994.

Bullough, V. L. *Sex, society & history.* New York: Science History Publications, 1976a.

Bullough, V. L. *Sexual variance in society and history,* New York: John Wiley & Sons, 1976b.

Bumpass, L. L., Sweet, J. E., & Cherlin, A. The role of cohabitation in declining rates of marriage, *Journal of Marriage and the Family, 53* (November 1991), 912–927.

Burdon, W. M. Deception in intimate relationships: A comparison of heterosexuals, homosexuals, and bisexuals, *Journal of Homosexuality, 32, no. 1* (1996), 77–93.

Bureau of Justice Statistics crime data brief, U.S. Department of Justice, 1998.

Burg, B. R. Masturbatory death and injury, *Journal of the Royal Society of Health, 107* (1987), 60–61.

Burgess, A. W., ed. *Rape and sexual assault.* New York: Garland Publishing, 1985.

Buss, D. *The evolution of desire: Strategies of human mating.* New York: Basic Books, 1994.

Buss, D., et al. International preferences in selecting mates, *Journal of Cross-Cultural Psychology, 21* (1990), 5–47.

Butler, K. L. & Byrne, T. J. Homophobia among preservice elementary teachers, *Journal of Health Education, 23* (September/October 1992), 355–359.

Butler, R. N. & Lewis, M. L. *Love and sex after 60.* Westminister, MD: Ballantine Books, 1993.

Buvat, J., Buvat-Herbaut, M., Lemaire, A., Marcolin, G., & Quittelier, E. Recent developments in the clinical assessment and diagnosis of erectile dysfunction, in *Annual review of sex research, Vol. 1,* Bancroft, J., Davis, C. M., & Weinstein, D., eds. New York: Society for the Scientific Study of Sex Research, 1990, 265–308.

Byrn, S. R., Anderson, J. G., & Anderson, M. G. New drugs for treatment for AIDS and cost implications, *The Health Education Monograph Series, 15* (1997), 14–19.

Cady, B. Breast cancer: Screening and diagnosis in a primary care practice, *Primary Care & Cancer*, 6 (1986), 23–38.

California TV to air information on prostitution suspects, American Civil Liberties Union Freedom Network, 1997.

California Vital Statistics Section. *California resident live births, 1990, by age of father, by age of mother.* Sacramento: California Vital Statistics Section, Department of Health Services, 1992.

Call, V. R. A. & Heaton, T. B. Religious influence on marital stability, *Journal for the Scientific Study of Religion, 36, no. 3* (September 1997), 382–382.

Call, V., Sprecher, S., & Schwartz, P. The incidence and frequency of marital sex in a national sample, *Journal of Marriage and the Family 57, no. 3* (August 1995), 639–652.

Cambre, S. *The sensuous heart.* Atlanta: Pritchett & Hull, 1978.

Campbell, J. C. Beating of wives: A cross-cultural perspective, *Victimology: An International Journal, 10, nos. 1–4,* (1985), 174–185.

Can we raise gender-neutral children? in *Taking sides: Issues in family and personal relationships*, Schroeder, E., ed. Guilford, CT: McGraw-Hill/Dushkin, 2003.

Canavan, M., Meyer, W., & Higgs, D. The female experience of sibling incest, *Journal of Marital and Family Therapy, 18* (1992), 129–142.

Cancer in women this year, *USA Today* (August 5, 1998), 01.A.

Cancila, C. Tissue cultures still the choice for chlamydia testing: Experts. *American Medical News, 2* (May 23, 1986), 21.

Cann, A. & Siegfried, W. D. Gender stereotypes and dimensions of effective leader behavior, *Sex Roles, 23* (1990), 413–419.

Carey, A. R. & Ward, S. Gay rights support, *USA Today* (October 26, 1998), 1.

Carnegie Corporation of New York. *A matter of time: Risk and opportunity in the out-of-school hours*, 1992a.

Carnegie Corporation of New York. *Great transitions*, 1992b.

Carnes, P. *Don't call it love.* New York: Bantam Books, 1991.

Caron, S. L. & Bertram, R. M. What college students want to know about sex, *Medical Aspects of Human Sexuality, 22* (April 1988), 18–20.

Caron, S. L. & Carter, D. B. The relationships among sex role orientation, egalitarianism, attitudes toward sexuality, and attitudes toward violence against women, *Journal of Social Psychology, 137, no. 5* (1997), 568–587.

Caron, S. L. *Cross-cultural perspectives on human sexuality.* Boston: Allyn & Bacon, 1998.

Caron, S. L., Halteman, W. A., & Stacy, C. Athletes and rape: Is there a connection? *Perceptual and Motor Skills, 83, no. 3, Pt. 2* (1997), 1379–1393.

Cassidy, L. The influence of victim's attire on adolescents: Judgment of date rape, *Adolescence, 30* (1995), 319–323.

Catania, J. A., et al. Condom use in multi-ethnic neighborhoods of San Francisco, the population-based AMEN (AIDS in multi-ethnic neighborhoods) study, *American Journal of Public Health, 82.2* (1992), 284–287.

Cates, W. Teenagers and sexual risk taking: The best of times and the worst of times, *Journal of Adolescent Health, 12, 2* (1991), 84–94.

Cates, W., Grimes, D. A., & Schulz, K. F. The public health impact of legal abortion: 30 years later, *Perspectives on Sexual and Reproductive Health*, 35, no. 1 (2003), 25.

Catholic bishops: Sterilization evil, *The Birmingham News* (June 16, 2001), 3A.

Caverject: Injections for impotence, *Consumer Reports on Health* (March 1996).

The CBS/New York Times Abortion Attitude Poll. *New York Times*, January 16, 1998.

Census shows nearly 600,000 same-sex couple homes in most comprehensive count yet of gays and lesbians, Harvard Medical School's *Consumer Health Information* (August 21, 2001). Available: http://www.intellihealth.com.

Census: More elderly live together, *InteliHealth* (July 30, 2002). Available: www.intelihealth.com.

Census: Unmarried couples increase, *InteliHealth* (May 15, 2001). Available: www.intelihealth.com.

Center for Families in Transition, Scottsdale, AZ. 2003. Online. Available: www.centerforfamilies.net/index.htm.

Center for Families in Transition. *For the sake of the children* (parental divorce-class manual). Brookline, MA: Center for Families in Transition, 1999.

Centers for Disease Control. *HIV Self-assessment quiz.* Atlanta: Centers for Disease Control.

Centers for Disease Control and Prevention, *HIV/AIDS Surveillance Report*, 13, no. 2 (2001).

Centers for Disease Control and Prevention, *Pregnancy, sexually transmitted diseases, and related risk behaviors among U.S. adolescents.* Atlanta: CDC, 1994.

Centers for Disease Control and Prevention, 1998 guidelines for treatment of sexually transmitted diseases. *MMWR, Recommendations and Reports, 47, no. RR-1* (January 23, 1998).

Centers for Disease Control and Prevention, Youth risk behavior surveillance—United States, 1995, *Morbidity and Mortality Weekly Report, 34, no. SS-4* (September 27, 1996), 1–86.

Centers for Disease Control and Prevention, Youth risk behavior surveillance—United States, 1997, *MMWR, 47, no. SS-3* (August 14, 1998), 1–92.

Centers for Disease Control and Prevention. *Fact Sheet, 2002*. Available: http://www.cdc.gov/ncidod/diseases/hepatitis/b/fact.htm.

Centers for Disease Control and Prevention. *First Marriage Dissolution, Divorce, and Remarriage in the United States.* National Center for Health Statistics. Available: http://www.cdc.gov.nchs.

Centers for Disease Control and Prevention. *Frequently Asked Questions, 2002.* Available: http://www.cdc.gov/ncidod/diseases/hepatitis/b/faqb.htm.

Centers for Disease Control and Prevention. *Hepatitis B Vaccine: Fact Sheet, 2002.* Available: http://www.cdc.gov/ncidod/diseases/hepatitis/b/factvax.htm.

Centers for Disease Control and Prevention. *HIV/AIDS surveillance report, 9, no. 1 (1997).*

Centers for Disease Control and Prevention. *Latex Fact Sheet*, 2001.

Centers for Disease Control and Prevention. *MMWR*, 49: 27 (July 14, 2000).

Centers for Disease Control and Prevention. *MMWR*, 49: SS-5 (June 9, 2000).

Centers for Disease Control and Prevention. *Tracking the Hidden Epidemics: Trends in STDs in the United States, 2000.* Washington, D.C.: Centers for Disease Control and Prevention, 2001

Centers for Disease Control and Prevention. *Youth Risk Behavior Survey*, 2003. Available: www.cdc.gov.

Centers for Disease Control and Prevention. Selected behaviors that increase risk for HIV infection among high school students, *MMWR, 41* (1992), 237.

Centers for Disease Control and Prevention. Sexual behavior among high school students, United States, 1990, *MMWR, 40* (1992), 886.

Cervical cap precautions. *Medical Selfcare* (January/February 1989), 14–15.

Chalker, R. Updating the model of female sexuality, *SIECUS Report 22, no. 5* (June/July 1994), 1–6.

Characteristics of freshmen, 2001, *The Chronicle of Higher Education*, 68, no. 1 (August 31, 2001), 22–23.

Charge upheld vs. Pee-Wee Herman actor, *FindLaw Legal News and Commentary* (March 3, 2003). Available: http://news.findlaw.com.

Charle, S. Picture imperfect, *Allure* (July 1994), 86–89.

Chen, P. & Kols, A. Population & birth planning in the People's Republic of China, *Population Reports, 25* (1982).

Cherlin, A. J., Chase-Lansdale, P. L., & McRae, C. Effects of parental divorce on mental health throughout the life course, *American Sociological Review, 63, no. 2* (1998), 239–247.

Child sexual abuse, National Committee to Prevent Child Abuse, 1998.

Child Trends. *Facts at a glance,* 1995.

Child Welfare League of America. *A survey of 17 Florence Crittenton agencies serving minor mothers,* 1994.

Chilman, C. Family life education: Promoting healthy adolescent sexuality, *Family Relations, 39, 2* (1990), 123–131.

Choi, K. H. & Catania, J. A. Changes in multiple sexual partnerships, HIV testing, and condom use among U.S. heterosexuals 18 to 49 years of age, 1990 and 1992, *American Journal of Public Health, 86* (1996), 554–556.

Choice, P. & Lemke, L. K. A conceptual approach to understanding abused women's stay/leave decisions, *Journal of Family Issues, 18, no. 3* (1997), 290–314.

Choo, P., Levine, T., & Hatfield, E. Gender, love schemas, and reactions to romantic break-ups, *Journal of Social Behavior and Personality, 11, no. 5* (1996), 143–160.

Chronicle of Higher Education. Teachers' group defines sexual harassment, *The Chronicle of Higher Education, 22, no. 3* (May 11, 1981), 14.

Chung, Y. B. Assessment of sexual orientation in lesbian/gay/bisexual studies, *Journal of Homosexuality, 30, no. 4* (1996), 49–62.

Clapp, D. Overview of assisted reproductive technologies, *Resolve Fact Sheet Series,* 1998.

Clark, T. & Epstein, R. Self-concept and expectancy for social reinforcement in noninstitutionalized male homosexuals, *Proceedings of the 77th Annual Convention of the American Psychoanalytical Association, 4* (1969), 575.

Clark, W. M. & Servivich, J. M. Twenty years and still in the dark? *Journal of Marital and Family Therapy, 23, no. 3* (July 1997), 239–253.

Clarkson, T. B. & Alexander, N. J. Long-term vasectomy: Effects on the occurrence and extent of atherosclerosis in rhesus monkeys, *Journal of Clinical Investigation, 65* (1980), 15–25.

Cleland, J. *Memoirs of a woman of pleasure.* New York: Putnam, 1963.

Clement, U. Surveys of heterosexual behavior. In *Annual Review of Sex Research, Vol. 1,* Bancroft, J., Davis, C. M., & Weinstein, D., eds. New York: Society for the Scientific Study of Sex Research, 1990, 45–74.

Clements, M. Sex in America today, *Parade* (August 7, 1994), 4–6.

Cloud, J. Sex and the law, *Times, 51, no. 11* (March 23, 1998), 48–53.

Coale, A. J. Excess female mortality and the balance of the sexes in the population: An estimate of the number of missing females, *Population and Development Review, 17* (1991), 552.

Coates, T. J. & Stall, R. D. Changes in sexual behavior among gay & bisexual men and the beginning of the AIDS epidemics, in *Psychological perspectives on AIDS,* Temoshok, L. & Baum, A., eds. Hillsdale, NJ: Erlbaum, 1990, 103–137.

Cocaine and Pregnancy *Medical Aspects of Human Sexuality, 25* (1991):16.

Cocaine: Linked to low birth weight, stillbirth, congenital defects, *Modern Medicine, 55* (1987), 165–166.

Coen, S. Sexual interviewing, evaluation, and therapy: Psychoanalytic emphasis on the use of sexual fantasy, *Archives of Sexual Behavior, 7* (1978), 229–41.

Cohen, P. Muscle mania, *New Scientist, 156* (November 22, 1997), 15.

COHIS. Anabolic steroids abuse, Community Outreach Health Information System, Boston University Medical Center. Available: gopher1.bu.edu/COHIS/subsabse/steroids/about.htm#howmany

Coker, A. L., Harlap, S., & Fortney J. A. Oral contraceptives and reproductive cancers: Weighing the risks and benefits, *Family Planning Perspectives, 25* (1993), 17–22, 36.

Colditz, G. A., et al. The use of estrogen and progestins and the risk of breast cancer in postmenopausal women, *New England Journal of Medicine, 332* (1995), 1589–1593.

Coles, R. & Stokes, F. *Sex and the American teenager.* New York: Harper & Row, 1985.

Collaborative Group on Hormonal Factors in Breast Cancer. Breast cancer and breastfeeding: Collaborative reanalysis of individual data from 47 epidemiological studies in 30 countries, including 50,302 women with breast cancer and 96,973 women without the disease, *Lancet,* 360 (2002), 187–196.

Collaborative group on hormonal factors in breast cancer: Breast cancer and hormonal contraceptives, *Lancet, 347* (1996), 405–411.

Coltrane, S. Father's role at home is under negotiation, *The Chronicle of Higher Education, 42, no. 6* (October 2, 1998), B8.

Comfort, A. *A new joy of sex: A gourmet guide to lovemaking for the nineties.* New York: Crown, 1991.

Comfort, A. *The joy of sex.* New York: Crown, 1972.

Commission on Obscenity and Pornography. *The report of the commission on obscenity and pornography.* New York: Bantam, 1970.

Communication tips for parents, Sexuality Information and Education Council of the United States, 1998.

Condoms from schools encourage safe sex, not more sex, *Health Education Reports, 20, no. 10* (May 14, 1998), 3.

Confirmation of transmission of AIDS via artificial insemination, *Infectious Diseases* (January 1986), 16, 19.

Conte, J. R. The effects of sexual abuse on children: A critique and suggestions for future research, *Victimology: An International Journal, 10, nos. 1–4* (1985), 110–130.

Contemporary Sexuality 30, no. 5. Pacific Grove, CA: Brooks/Cole, 1996.

Contraception and family planning: FDA approves use of Lunelle, the "injectable pill," *Kaiser Daily Reproductive Health Report* (2000).

Contraceptive patch, *The Contraception Report,* 12, no. 4 (2001), 12–14.

Cook, E. A., Jelen, T. G., & Wilcox, C. Measuring public attitudes on abortion: Methodological and substantive considerations, *Family Planning Perspectives, 25* (1993) 118–121, 145.

Cooksey, E. C., Rindfuss, R. R., & Guilkey, D. K. The initiation of adolescent sexual and contraceptive behavior during changing times, *Journal of Health and Social Behavior, 37, no. 1* (March 1996), 59–74.

Cool, L. C. Fantasy parties, *Penthouse* (May 1998), 112–114, 150–155.

Cooney, T. M. & Uhlenberg, P. Changes in work-family connections among highly educated men and women, *Journal of Family Issues, 12* (1991), 69–90.

Coontz, S. Marriage is fairer—and more optional, *The Chronicle of Higher Education, 45, no. 6* (October 2, 1998), B6.

Cooper, P. The art of sex: 20 ways to perfect your style, *Men's Health* (April 1990), 38–40.

Corliss, R. Objects of our affection, *Time, 152, no. 8* (1998), 73–74.

Coste, J., Job-Spira, N., & Fernandez, H. Increased risk of ectopic pregnancy with maternal cigarette smoking, *American Journal of Public Health, 81* (1991), 199–201.

Costello, C. Y. Conceiving identity: Bisexual, lesbian, and gay parents consider their children's sexual orientations, *Journal of Sociology and Social Welfare, 24, no. 3* (1997), 63–89.

Costin, F. Beliefs about rape and women's social roles, *Archives of Sexual Behavior, 14, no. 4* (1985), 319–325.

Cotton-Houston, A. & Wheeler, K. Preorgasmic group treatment: Assertiveness, marital adjustment and sexual function in women, *Journal of Sex and Marital Therapy, 9* (1983), 296–302.

Courtwright, D. T. The neglect of female children and childhood, Sex ratios in nineteenth century America: A review of the evidence, *Journal of Family History, 15* (1990), 313–323.

Coverdill, J. E., Kraft, J. M., & Manley, K. S. Employment history, the sex typing of occupations, pay and change in gender-role attitudes: A longitudinal study of young married women, *Sociological Focus, 29, no. 1* (1996), 47–60.

Craig, M. E. Coercive sexuality in dating relationships: A situational model, *Clinical Psychology Review, 10* (1990), 395–423.

Crary, D. Abercrombie & Fitch's racy catalog draws odd coalition to call for boycott, *The Birmingham News* (June 22, 2001), 7C.

Crawford, I. & Solliday, S. The attitudes of undergraduate college students toward gay parenting, *Journal of Homosexuality, 30, no. 4* (1996), 63–77.

Crawford, M. & MacLeod, M. Gender in the college classroom: An assessment of the "chilly climate" for women, *Sex Roles, 23* (1990), 101–122.

Creager, J. G. *Human Anatomy and Physiology,* 2nd ed. Dubuque, IA: Wm. C. Brown, 1992.

Crenshaw, T. Effects of psychotropic drugs in sexual functioning. Paper presented at the Annual Meeting of the Society for the Scientific Study of Sex, San Diego, CA, September 1985.

Crenshaw, T. Medical causes of sexual dysfunction. Paper presented at the Awareness AASECT 1984 Regional Conference, Las Vegas, NV, October 1984.

Crepault, C. C., et al. Erotic Imagery in Women. In Gemme, R. and C. C. Wheeler. *Progress in Sexuality*. New York: Plenum, 1977.

Crooks, R. & Baur, K. *Our sexuality,* 4th ed. Menlo Park, CA: Benjamin/Cummings, 1990.

Crossen, C. Is TV too sexy? *McCall's, 119* (October 1991), 1001.

Culross, T. Men who fake orgasm, *Cosmopolitan* (February 1990), 90–91.

Current Population Reports, Series p–20, No. 496, 1998.

Curtin, S. C. Rates of cesarean birth and vaginal birth after previous cesarean, 1991–1995, *Monthly Vital Statistics Report, 45* (July 16, 1997).

Curtis, K. California loses track of 33,000 sex offenders, *The Birmingham News* (January 8, 2003), 8A.

Cutler, W., Berg, George Preti, Abba Krieger, George R. Huggins, Celso Ramon Garcia, and Henry J. Lawley. "Human Axillary Secretions Influence Women's Menstrual Cycles: The Role of Donor Extract from Men." *Hormones and Behavior* 20(1986): 463–73.

Cybersex addiction checklist, Sexual Recovery Institute (2001). Available: http://www.sexualrecovery.com.

Dahl, D. W., Gorn, G. J., & Weinberg, C. B. Condom-carrying behavior among college students, *American Journal of Public Health, 87* (1997), 1059.

Dailard, C. Recent findings from the "add health" survey: Teens and sexual activity, *The Guttmacher Report*, 4, no.4 (August 2001), 1–3, 2–4.

Dalton, K. *Once a month*. Ramona, CA: Hunter House, 1979.

Daniel, E. L., and Levine, C. *Taking Sides: Clashing Views on Controversial Issues in Health and Society,* 5th ed. Guilford, CT: McGraw-Hill Dushkin, 2001.

Danoff, D. S. & Katz, D. *The new miracle in male genital health.* 1998.

Date rape is occurring too often, AU Professor says, *Birmingham News* (March 23, 1987), 3B.

Davenport, W. H. Sex in cross-cultural perspective, in *Human sexuality in four perspectives,* Beach, F. A., ed. Baltimore: Johns Hopkins Press, 1976.

Davies, K. A. Voluntary exposure to pornography and men's attitudes toward feminism and rape, *The Journal of Sex Research, 34, no. 2* (1997), 131–137.

Davis, D. M. Portrayals of women in prime time network television: Some demographic characteristics, *Sex Roles, 23* (1990), 325–332.

Davis, K. E. Near and dear: Friendship and love compared, *Psychology Today, 22* (February 1985).

Davis, N. J. & Robinson, R. V. Men and women's consciousness of gender inequality: Austria, West Germany, Great Britain, and the United States, *American Sociological Review, 56* (1991), 72–84.

Dawood, K., Pillard, R. C., Horvath, C., Revelle, W., & Bailey, J. M. Familial aspects of male homosexuality, *Archives of Sexual Behavior*, 29, no. 2 (2000), 155–163.

DeAngelis, B. Sexual secrets men are afraid to share, *Redbook* (February 1990), 96–97, 136.

DeBeauvoir, S. *The coming of age.* New York: Warner Books, 1973.

DeBuono, B. A., Zinner, S. H., Daamen, M., & McCormack, W. M. Sexual behavior of college women 1975, 1986, and 1989, *New England Journal of Medicine, 322* (1990), 821.

Deckers, P. & Ricci Jr., A. Pain and lumps in the female breast, *Hospital Practice* (February 28, 1992), 67–94.

DeGaston, J. F., Jensen, L., & Weed, S. Closer look at adolescent sexual activity, *Journal of Youth and Adolescence, 24, no. 4* (August 1995), 465–479.

DeGaston, J. F., Weed, S., & Jensen, L. Understanding gender differences in adolescent sexuality, *Adolescence, 31* (1996), 217–231.

Degler, C. N. *At odds: Women and the family in America from the revolution to the present.* New York: Oxford University Press, 1980.

DeJesus, I. & McCarron, B. Teens grind up dance floor—and adults freak out, *The Birmingham News* (May 20, 2002), E1, E3.

Department of Health and Human Services. Healthy People 2000 progress review: HIV infection, *Prevention Report, 12* (1997), Supplement.

DePaulo, B. M., Kirkendol, S. E., Kashy, S. E., Wyer, M. M., & Epstein, J. A. Lying in everyday life, *Journal of Personality and Social Psychology, 70, no. 5* (1996), 979–997.

DeQuine, J. Out of the closet and on to fraternity row, *Time*, 161, no. 11 (March 17, 2003), 8.

Dew, M. The effects of attitudes on inferences of homosexuality and perceived physical attractiveness in women, *Sex Roles, 12* (1985), 143–155.

DHHS. Premarital sexual experiences among adolescent women—United States, 1970–1988, *Morbidity and Mortality Weekly Report, 39* (January 4, 1991), 929–932.

Di Mauro, D. Executive summary. Sexuality research in the United States: An assessment of the social and behavioral sciences, 1995. http://www.indiana.edu/kinsey/SSRC/sexreas2.html.

Diagram Group. *Man's body.* New York: Bantam Books, 1983.

Diagram Group. *Woman's body.* New York: Bantam Books, 1978.

Diamant, L. & Simono, R. B. The relationship of homosexuality to mental disorders, in *Male and female homosexuality: Psychological approaches,* Diamant, L., ed. Washington, DC: Hemisphere, 1987, 171–186.

Dickson, A. "Men Friends." *Time, 155, no. 4* (Jan. 17, 2000), 89

Dietz, P. E., Hazelwood, R. R., & Warren, J. The sexually sadistic criminal and his offenses, *Bulletin of the Academy of Psychiatry Law, 18* (1990), 163–178.

DiIulio, J. J. Deadly divorce, *National Review, 49* (April 7, 1997), 39–401.

Division of sexually transmitted diseases. Sexually transmitted diseases treatment guidelines 2002, *Morbidity and Mortality Weekly Report*, 51 (2002). Available: http://www.cdc.gov/STD/treatment/62002TG.htm#HumanPapillomavirusInfection.

Division of STD Prevention. *Sexually transmitted disease surveillance, 1996.* U.S. Department of Health and Human Services, Public Health Service. Atlanta: Centers for Disease Control and Prevention, September 1997.

Divorce and Children. American Academy of Pediatrics, 2001. Available: http://www.aap.org/family/divorce.htm

Divorce. U.S. Centers for Disease Control. 1998.

"Do Men and Women Lead Differently?" *Leadership Strategies* 3, no. 10 (October, 2000): 8.

Do men and women speak different languages? in *Taking sides: Clashing views on controversial issues in family and personal relationships,* Vail, A. ed. Guilford, CT: Dushkin/McGraw-Hill, 1999.

Do women and men communicate differently? In *Taking Sides: Issues in Family and Personal Relationship*, Schroeder, E., ed. Guilford, CT: McGraw-Hill/Dushkin, 2003.

Doctor, R. J. & Prince, V. Transvestitism: A survey of 1,032 cross-dressers, *Archives of Sexual Behavior, 26, no. 6* (December 1997), 589–605.

Doell, R. G. Sexuality in the brain, *Journal of Homosexuality, 28, nos. 3–4* (1995), 345–354.

Does divorce create long-term negative affects for children? In *Taking Sides: Issues in Family and Personal Relationships*, Schroeder, E., ed. Guilford, CT: McGraw-Hill/Dushkin, 2003.

Dolan, B. No sex please, we're ignorant, *Time* (September 17, 1990), 71.

Dolgov, A. Russian women enslaved for sex, *The Birmingham News* (May 17, 2001), 10A.

Doll, L. S. & Beeker, C. Male bisexual behavior and HIV risk in the United States: Synthesis of research with implications for behavioral interventions, *AIDS Education & Prevention, 8, no. 3* (June 1996), 205–225.

Donatelle, R. J. & Davis, L. G. *Access to health,* 5th ed. Needham Heights, MA: Allyn & Bacon, 1998.

Donovan, P. Confronting a hidden epidemic: The Institute of Medicine's report on sexually transmitted diseases, *Family Planning Perspectives, 29* (1997), 87–89.

Dorkenoo, E. & Elworthy, S. *Female Genital Mutilation: Proposals for Change.* London: Minority Rights Group International Report, 1992.

Dorner, G. Hormonal induction and prevention of female homosexuality, *Journal of Endocrinology, 42* (1968), 162–163.

Dorner, G., Rohde, W., Stahl, F., Krell, L., & Masius, W. A neuroendocrine predisposition for homosexuality in men, *Archives of Sexual Behavior, 4* (1975), 1–8.

Dowie, M. Teratology: The loneliest science. *American Health,* June 1990, 59–67.

Downey, L. International change in sex behavior: A belated look at Kinsey's males. *Archives of Sexual Behavior, 9* (1980), 267–317.

Drummond, T. "A Win for Gays." *Time, 155, no. 12* (March 27, 2000): 38.

Duggan, L. The dubious porn war alliance: Feminists and the right agree, for once, but they're both wrong, *Washington Post* (September 1, 1985), C1, C4.

Duncan, D. F. & Drolet, J. Teach them what we ought to know, *Family Life Educator, 5, no. 2* (Winter 1986), 12–13.

Dunn, P. C., Knight, S. M., & Glascoff, M. A. Gender-specific changes in students' sexual behaviors and attitudes at a southeastern university between 1973 and 1988, *Journal of American College Health*, 41, no. 3 (1992), 99–104.

Durban, M., DiClemente, R., & Siegel, D. Factors associated with multiple sex partners among junior high school students, *Journal of Adolescent Health, 14, 3* (1993), 292–207.

Durex condom maker using "humor" ads to sell condoms in Europe, *Kaiser Network Daily HIV/AIDS Report*. The Henry J. Kaiser Family Foundation. Available: www.kaisernetwork.org.

Duxbury, L. E. & Higgins, C. A. Gender differences in work–family conflicts, *Journal of Applied Psychology, 76* (1991), 60–74.

Dying to win. *Sports Illustrated, 80* (August 8, 1994), 52–60.

Eagly, A. H. & Johnson, B. T. Gender and leadership style: A meta-analysis, *Psychological Bulletin, 108* (1990), 233–256.

Earle, J. R. & Perricone, P. J. Premarital sexuality: A ten-year study of attitudes and behavior on a small university campus, *The Journal of Sex Research, 22* (August 1986), 304–310.

The ecology of birth control. Chicago: G. D. Searle, 1971.

Ectopic pregnancy—United States, 1987, *Morbidity and Mortality Weekly Report, 39* (1990), 401–404.

Ectopic pregnancy—United States, 1990–1992, *Morbidity and Mortality Weekly Report, 44* (1995), 46–48.

Edwards, M. We have a responsibility to dialogue with the media, *SIECUS Report, 24, no. 5* (June/July 1996), 5.

Edwards, T.M. "I Surrender, Dear" *Time, 157, no. 3* (Jan. 22, 2001): 71

The effects of infant child care on infant-mother attachment security: Results of the NICHD study of early child care, *Child Development, 68, no. 5* (October 1997), 860–879.

Ehrhardt, A. A., Evers, K., & Money, J. Influence of androgen and some aspects of sexual dimorphic behavior in women with the late-treated adrenogenital syndrome, *Johns Hopkins Medical Journal, 123* (1968), 115–122.

Ehrhardt, A. A., Myer-Bahlburg, H. F. L., Rosen, L. R., Feldman, J. F., Veridiano, J. F., Zimmerman, N. P., & McEwen, B. S. Sexual orientation after exposure to exogenous estrogen, *Archives of Sexual Behavior, 14, no. 1* (1985), 57–77.

Eikson, E. H. *Identity: Youth and crisis.* New York: Norton, 1968.

Eisen, M., Zellman, G. L., & McAlister, A. L. Evaluating the impact of a theory-based sexuality and contraceptive education program, *Family Planning Perspectives, 21* (January/February 1990), 4–5.

Eisler, R. *Sacred pleasures: Sex, myth, and the politics of the body.* San Francisco: HarperCollins, 1995.

El Hadi, A. A Step forward for opponents of female genital mutilation in Egypt, *The Lancet, 349* (1997), 129–130.

Elber, L. Study: More sex and violence on TV, *The Birmingham News* (August 2, 2001), 3A.

Elchalal, U., Ben-Ami, B., Gillis, R., & Brzezinski, A. Ritualistic female genital mutilation: Current status and future outlook, *Obstetrical & Gynecological Survey 52, no. 10* (October 1997), 643–651.

Eliason, M. J. A survey of the campus climate for lesbian, gay, and bisexual university members, *Journal of Psychology and Human Sexuality, 8, no. 4* (1996), 39–58.

Elion, R. *Do you know your options: An updated guide to antiviral therapies.* Washington, DC: Georgetown University Medical Center, 1997.

Ellingson, L. Lesbian health issues: A ten year review, *The Health Education Monograph Series*, 19, no. 1 (2002), 40–45.

Elliott, J. Little consensus on prescribing estrogen for postmenopausal women, *Journal of the American Medical Association*, 243 (1979), 1951–1952.

Ellis, A. & Harper, R. *A New Guide to Rational Living.* Englewood Cliffs, NJ: Prentice-Hall, 1979.

Ellis, A. & Harper, R. *A Guide to Rational Living.* North Hollywood, CA: Melvin Powers, Wilshire Book Company, 1975.

Ellis, A. Healthy and disturbed reasons for having extramarital relations. In *Encounter with Family Realities,* Powers, E. A. & Lees, M. W., eds. St. Paul, MN: West, 1977, 374–375.

Ellis, L. *Theories of rape.* New York: Hemisphere Publishing, 1989.

Ellison, C. A critique of the clitoral model of female sexuality. Paper presented at the Annual Meeting of the American Psychological Association, Montreal, Canada, September 1980.

Elmer-Dewitt, P. Now for the truth about Americans and sex, *Time* (October 17, 1994), 64.

Emerging Issues of the Reproductive Health Technologies Project (2002). Available: http://www.rhtp.org/emerging_issues/issues_quina_statement.htm

Empower Health Corporation. Sexual dysfunction overview, 1998.

Ende, J., Rockwell, S., & Glasgow, M. The sexual history in general medical practice, *Archives of Internal Medicine, 44* (1984), 55.

Endocrinology Society. *Endocrinology and impotence (erectile dysfunction),* 1998.

Eng, T. R. & Butler, W. T., eds. *The hidden epidemic: Confronting sexually transmitted diseases.* Washington, DC: Institute of Medicine, 1996.

EngenderHealth. Sterilization most widely used contraceptive method in the world, *SIECUS Report*, 31 (2003), 19–21.

Epps, R. P., ed. *The American medical women's association guide to pregnancy and childbirth.* New York: Dell Books, 1996.

Erickson, E. H. *Childhood and society.* New York: Norton, 1950.

Erickson, E. H. *Identity: Youth and crisis.* New York: Norton, 1968.

Erlik, Y., et al. Association of waking episodes with menopausal hot flash, *Journal of the American Medical Association,* 245 (1981), 1741–1744.

Fackelmann, K. Booze and babies: How much danger? New research finds potential risk in even light drinking, *USA Today* (November 20, 2002), D9.

Facts about domestic violence in the United States. Feminist Majority Foundation (1999). [http://www.feminist.org/other/dv/dvfact:htm]

Fagot, B., Leinbach, M., & O'Boyle, C. Gender labeling, gender stereotyping, and parenting behaviors, *Developmental Psychology, 28* (1992), 225–230.

Faith, N. S. & Share, M. L. The role of body image in sexually avoidant behavior, *Archives of Sexual Behavior, 22, no. 4* (1993), 345–356.

Family Planning Perspectives, 22 (1990) 244.

Fast-tracking the first AIDS drug, *FDA Consumer* (October 1987), 13–15.

Faulkner, A. H. Correlates of same-sex sexual behavior in a random sample of Massachusetts high school students, *American Journal of Public Health, 88, no. 2* (February 1998), 262–266.

Fay, R. E., Turner, C. F., Klassen, A. D., & Gagnon, J. H. Prevalence and patterns of same-gender sexual contact among men, *Science, 243* (1989), 338–348.

FDA approved 5-year IUD, Sexhealth.com. (2002) Available: www.sexhealth.com.

FDA approves Lea's Shield, *The Contraception Report*, 13, no. 2 (2002). http://www.contraceptiononline.org/contrareport.issue.cfm.

Felson, R. B. & Krohn, M. Motives for rape, *Journal of Research in Crime and Delinquency, 27* (1990), 222–242.

Feminist Majority Foundation. *Anti-Abortion Violence Watch* (October 5, 1998).

Fergusson, D. M., Horwood, L. J., & Lynskey, M. T. Childhood sexual abuse, adolescent sexual behaviors and sexual revictimization, *Child Abuse and Neglect, 21, no. 8* (1997), 789–803.

Fernandez, E. The Latin whitewash, *Allure* (December 1993), 70–74.

Fetishism, University of Iowa Health Care (2001). Available: www.uihealthcare.com/topics/mentalemotionalhealth/ment3145.html.

Fetishism. Sinclair Intimacy Institute (2001). Available: http://www.intimacyinstitute.com.

Field, A. E., Cheung, L., Wolf, A. M., Herzog, D.B., Gortmaker, S.L., & Colditz, G. A. Exposure to the mass media and weight concerns among girls, *Pediatrics, 103, no. 3* (March 1999), 36, New York: Available: www.pediatrics.org]

Filling the gaps. Sexuality Information and Education Council of the United States, 1998.

Filomeno, A. H. Promoting parent-adolescent communication to facilitate healthy sexual socialization of youth, *The Health Education Monograph Series*, 19, no. 2 (2002),17–21.

Finkelhor, D. *A sourcebook on child sexual abuse.* Thousand Oaks, CA: Sage Publications, 1986.

Finkelhor, D. Early and long-term effects of child sexual abuse: An update, *Professional Psychology: Research and Practice, 21* (1990), 325–330.

Finkelson L. & Oswalt, R. College date rape incidence and reporting, *Psychological Reports, 77, no. 2* (1995), 526.

Fisher, B. S., Cullen, F. T., and Turner, M. G. The sexual victimization of college women. National Institute of Justice. U.S. Dept. of Justice, January 2001.

Fisher, H. E. *Anatomy of Love.* New York: W. W. Norton, 1992.

Fisher, T. D. Parent-child communication about sex and young adolescents' sexual knowledge and attitudes, *Adolescence, 21* (Fall 1986), 517–527.

Fiumara, N. J. Gonorrhea. Part I. Acute infection, *Medical Aspects of Human Sexuality, 21* (1987), 65–72.

Fiumara, N. J. Herpes simplex infection, *Medical Aspects of Human Sexuality, 20* (1986b), 72–73.

Fiumara, N. J. Nongonococcal urethritis (NGU), *Medical Aspects of Human Sexuality, 20* (1986a), 139–146.

Fletcher, J. L. Perinatal transmission of human papillomavirus, *American Family Physician, 43* (1991), 143–148.

Flewelling, R. L. & Bauman, K. E. Family structure as a predictor of initial substance abuse and sexual intercourse in early adolescence, *Journal of Marriage and the Family, 52* (1990), 171.

Flexible vaginal ring, *The Contraception Report*, 12, no. 3 (2001), 12–14.

Flynn, C. P. Relationship violence by women: Issues and implications, *Family Relations, 38* (1990), 194–198.

Folkerts, J., Lacy, S., & Davenport, L. *The media in your life.* Needham Heights, MA: Allyn & Bacon, 1998, 10–14.

Fontaine, J. H. Experiencing a need: School counselors' experiences with gay and lesbian students, *Professional School Counseling, 1, no. 3* (February 1998), 9–14.

Ford, K. Woosung, S., & Lepowski, J. Characteristics of adolescents' sexual partners and their association with use of condoms and other contraceptive methods, *Family Planning Perspectives*, 33, no.3 (May/June 2001), 100–105, 132.

Forman, R. S. & Forman, N. *Drug-induced infertility and sexual dysfunction.* Cambridge, England: Cambridge University Press, 1996.

Forrest, J. D. & Singh, S. The sexual and reproductive behavior of American women, 1982–1988, *Family Planning Perspectives, 22* (1990), 206–214.

Foster, A. Relationships between age and sexual activity in married men, *Journal of Sex Education and Therapy, 21, no. 5* (Summer 1979), 26.

Fowler, C. J. The neurology of male sexual dysfunction and its investigation by clinical neurophysiological methods, *British Journal of Urology, 81* (1998), 785–795.

Frable, D. E. S., Johnson, A. E., & Kellman, H. Seeing masculine men, sexy women, and gender differences: Exposure to pornography and cognitive constructions of gender, *Journal of Personality, 65* (June 1997), 311–355.

Frank, E. & Anderson, C. How important is sex to a happy marriage? *Reader's Digest, 115* (July 1979), 126–128.

Freeman-Longo, R. E. & Wall, R. V. Changing a lifetime of crime. *Psychology Today 20, no. 3* (March 1986), 58–64.

Freetly, A. J., Hattery, A. J., & Kane, E. W. Men's and women's perceptions of non-consensual sexual intercourse, *Sex Roles, 33* (1995), 785–802.

French prostitutes protest crackdown, *The Birmingham News* (November, 6, 2002), 9A.

Freund, K. & Watson, R. J. The proportion of heterosexual and homosexual pedophiles among sex offenders against children: An exploratory study, *Journal of Sex and Marital Therapy, 18, no. 1* (1992), 34–43.

Freund, K., Watson, R., & Dickey, R. Does sexual abuse in childhood cause pedophilia: An empirical study, *Archives of Sexual Behavior, 19* (1990), 557–568.

Friday, N. *Forbidden Flowers.* New York: Pocket Books, 1975.

Friday, N. *Men in love.* New York: Delacorte Press, 1980.

Friday, N. *My secret garden.* New York: Pocket Books, 1973.

Friday, N. *Women on top: How real life has changed women's sexual fantasies.* New York: Simon & Schuster, 1991.

Fried, P. A. Marijuana and human pregnancy. In *Drug use in pregnancy: Mother and child,* Chasnoff, I. J, ed. Boston: MTP Press, 1986, 64–74.

Friedman, R., Hurt, S., Arnoff, M., & Clarkin, J. Behavior and the menstrual cycle, *Signs*, 5 (1980), 719–738.

Friedrich, W. N., Fisher, J., Broughton, D., Houston, M., & Shafran, C. R. Normative sexual behavior in children: A contemporary sample, *Pediatrics, 101, no. r* (April 1998), e9.

Fromm, Erich. *The Art of Loving.* New York: Harper and Row, 1956.

Frye, M. Lesbian sex, in *Through the prism of difference: Readings on sex and gender,* Zinn, M. B., Hondagneu-Sotelo, P., & Messner, M. A., eds. Boston: Allyn & Bacon, 1997.

Fuentes-Afflick, E., Hessol, N. A., & Perez-Stable, E. J. Maternal birthplace, ethnicity, and low birth weight in California, *Archives of Pediatric and Adolescent Medicine, 152* (1998), 1105–1112.

Gable, C. B., Tierce, J. C., Simison, E., Ward, D., & Motte, K. Costs of HIV/AIDS at CDC counts disease stages based on treatment protocols, *Journal of Acquired Immune Deficiency Syndrome, 12* (1996), 413–420.

Gagnon, J. H. & Simon, W. *Sexual conduct: The social sources of human sexuality.* Chicago: Aldine Press, 1973.

Galinsky, E., Bond, J. T., & Friedman, E. *The changing workforce: Highlights of the national study.* New York: Families and Work Institute, 1993.

Gallardo, E., et al. Effect of age on sperm fertility potential, *Fertility and Sterility, 66* (1996), 260–264.

Gallup poll finds majority opinion of gays unchanged by AIDS, *Family Life Educator, 5* (Winter 1986), 25.

Garai, J. E. The humanistic outlook on male and female homosexuality, in *Passages beyond the gate: A Jungian approach to understanding the nature of American psychology at the dawn of the new millennium,* Jennings, G. E., ed. Needham Heights, MA: Simon & Schuster Custom Publishing, 1996, 268–274.

Gates, G. L. & Sonenstein, F. Heterosexual genital activity among adolescent males: 1988 and 1995, *Family Planning Perspectives*, 32 (2000), 295–297.

Gay and lesbian issues: A time for knowledge, understanding and acceptance, *Mental Health Update, 9* (1991), 1.

Gay, lesbian, and bisexual adolescents. SIECUS fact sheet, 1998. Online. Available: www.siecus.org/pubs/fact/fact0013.html.

Gayle, H. E. Letters to colleagues (August 2000). Available: www.cdc.gov/hiv/aids.

Gays, lesbians and bisexuals rank third in reported hate crimes. *FBI Hate Crimes Statistics* (2001). On-line. Available: http://www.hrc.org/issues/hate/stats1999.html

Gender equity in college sports: 6 views, *The Chronicle of Higher Education*, 49, no. 14, B7.

Gentili, A. & Mulligan, T. Sexual dysfunction in older adults, *Clinical Geriatric Medicine, 14* (1998), 383–393.

George, L. & Weiler, S. Sexuality in middle and late life, *Archives of General Psychiatry, 38* (1981), 919–923.

Georges, E. Abortion policy and practice in Greece, *Social Science &*

Medicine, 42, no. 4 (February 1996), 509–519.

Gerschick, T. J. & Miller, A. S. Coming to terms: Masculinity and physical disability, in *Men's lives,* 4th ed., Kimmel, M. S. & Messner, M. A., eds. Needham Heights, MA: Allyn & Bacon, 1998.

Gerstman, B. B., Gross, T. P., Kennedy, D. L., Bennett, R. C., Tomita, D. K., & Stadel, B. V. Trends in the content and use of oral contraceptives in the United States, 1964–88, *American Journal of Public Health, 81* (1991), 90–96.

Gibbs, N. & Duffy, M. We must proceed with great care, *Time*, 158, no. 7 (August 20, 2001), 15–16.

Gidycz, C. & Koss, M. P. A comparison of group and individual sexual assault victims, *Psychology of Women Quarterly, 14* (1990), 325–342.

Gill, W. B., Schumacher, G. F. B., & Bibbo, M. Pathological semen and anatomical abnormalities of the genital tract of human male subjects exposed to diethylstilbestrol in utero, *Journal of Urology*, 117 (1977), 477–480.

Gilman, L. *Before you adopt*. Adoptive Families of America, Children Youth and Family Consortium Electronic Clearinghouse.

Gilmartin, B. That swinging couple down the block, *Psychology Today, 8, no. 9* (1975), 54.

Gilmartin, P. Gender differences in college students' perceptions about rape: The results of a quasi-experimental research design, *Free Inquiry in Creative Sociology, 22, no. 1* (1994), 3–12.

Girls interested in mathematics is on the increase, *Washington Post* (April 15, 1980), C5.

Gladue, R., Green, R., & Hellman, R. Neuroendocrine response to estrogen and sexual orientation, *Science, 225* (1983), 1496–1499.

Glickauf-Hughes, C. Current conceptualizations on masochism: Genesis and object relations, *American Journal of Psychotherapy, 45* (1991), 53–68.

Gold, A. R. & Adams, D. B. Motivational factors affecting fluctuations of female sexual activity at menstruation, *Psychology of Women Quarterly*, 5 (1981), 670–680.

Goldberg, C. & Elder, J. Public still backs abortion, but wants limits, poll says, *The New York Times* (January 16, 1998), A1, A16–A17.

Goldberg, D. C., Whipple, B., Fishkin, R., Waxman, H., Fink, P., & Weisberg, M. The Grafenberg spot and female ejaculation: A review of initial hypotheses, *Journal of Sex and Marital Therapy*, 9 (1983), 27–37.

Goldstein, I., Lue, T. F., Padma-Nathan, H., Rosen, R. C., Steers, W. D., & Wicker, P. A. Oral sildenafil in the treatment of erectile dysfunction, *New England Journal of Medicine, 338* (1998), 1397–1404.

Goleman, D. Chemistry of sexual desire yields its elusive secrets, *New York Times* (October 18, 1998), C1, C15.

Goodale, K. R., Watkins, P. L., & Cardinal, B. J. Muscle dysmorphia: A new form of eating disorder? *American Journal of Health Education*, 32, no. 5 (September/October 2001), 260–266.

Goodchilds, J. D. & Zellman, G. L. Sexual signaling and sexual aggression in adolescent relationships, in *Pornography and Sexual Aggression,* Malamuth, N. M. & Donnerstein, E., eds. New York: Academic Press, 1984.

Goodwill ambassador and former "Spice Girl" Geri Halliwell to launch British sex education web site, *Kaiser Daily Reproductive Health Report* (October 25, 2001). Available: www.kaisernetwork.org.

Goosens, M., Dumey, Y., Kaplan, L., et al. Prenatal diagnosis of sickle-cell anemia in the first trimester of pregnancy, *New England Journal of Medicine, 309* (1983), 831.

Gordon, D. Dating violence among teens widespread, *InteliHealth*. Available: www.intelihealth.com.

Gordon, L. & O'Keefe, P. The normality of incest: Father-daughter incest as a form of family violence, in *Rape and Sexual Assault,* Burgess, A. W., ed. New York: Garland Publishing, 1985.

Grafenberg, E. The role of urethra in female orgasm, *International Journal of Sexology*, 3 (1950), 145–148.

Graham, J. The thinking woman's guide to liposuction, *American Health for Women, 16, no. 3* (April 1997), 70–75.

Grams, A. C., Carneiro de Sousa, M. J., Roesch, R., & Pinto de Costa, J. Sexual abuse within the marital relationship. *Medicine & Law, 16, no. 4* (1997), 743–751.

Grant, P. Face Time, *Modern Maturity,* 44, no. 2 (March/April 2001): 60–69.

Green, R. & Fleming, D. T. Transsexual surgery follow-up: Status in the 1990s, in *Annual review of sex research, 1,* Bancroft, J., Davis, C. M., & Weinstein, D., eds. New York: Society for the Scientific Study of Sex Research, 1990, 163–174.

Greenberg, B. S. & Bussele, R. What's old, what's new: Sexuality and the soaps, *SIECUS Report, 24, no. 5* (June/July 1996), 14–16.

Greenberg, J. *Comprehensive stress management* (7th ed.). Dubuque, IA: WCB/McGraw-Hill, 2002.

Greenberg, J. S. A Study of the Self-Esteem and Alienation of Male Homosexuals. *Journal of Psychology* 83(1973): 137–43.

Greenberg, J. S. *Comprehensive stress management,* 6th ed. Dubuque, IA: WCB/McGraw-Hill, 1999.

Greenberg, J. S., Bruess, C. E., & Mullen, K. D. *Sexuality: Insights and issues.* Madison, WI: WCB Brown & Benchmark Publishers, 1986.

Greenberg, J. The effects of a homophile organization on the self-esteem and alienation of its members, *Journal of Homosexuality, 1* (1976), 313–317.

Greenburg, J. S. Service-learning in health education, *Journal of Health Education, vol. 28, no. 6* (November/December 1997), 345–349.

Greenhalgh, S. & Li, J. Engendering reproductive policy and practice in peasant China: For a feminist demography of reproduction, *Signs, 20, 3* (Spring 1995), 601–640.

Greenhouse, L. "Justices Back Law to Make Libraries Use Internet Filters." *New York Times,* June 24, 2003. Online. Available: www.nytimes.com.

Greenwood, S. PMS backlash, *Medical Self-Care* (November/December 1985), 12–14.

Greenwood, S. Women's health: Menstrual Cramps, *Medical Self-Care* (November/December 1986), 20–21.

Grimsley, K. Father to get $665,000 in Maryland leave case, *The Washington Post* (August 29, 2002), EO1.

Gross, W. C. & Billingham, R. E. Alcohol consumption and sexual victimization among college women, *Psychological Reports, 82, no. 1* (1997), 743–751.

Grossman, L. SIM nation, *Time*, 160, no. 22 (November 25, 2002), 78–80.

Gruber, J. E. How women handle sexual harassment: A literature review, *Sociology and Sexual Research, 72,* (1989), 3–6.

Guerrero, L. K. Expressing emotion: Sex differences in social skills and communicative responses to anger, sadness, and jealousy, in *Sex differences and similarities in communication: Critical essays and empirical investigations of sex and gender in interaction,* Canary, D. J. & Dindia, K., eds. Mahway, NJ: Lawrence Erlbaum Associates, 1998.

Guffey, M. E. *Business communication: Process and product,* 3rd ed. Belmont, CA: Wadsworth, 1999.

Guggino, J. M. & Ponzetti, Jr., J. J., Gender differences in affective reactions to first coitus, *Journal of Adolescence, 20, no. 2* (1997), 189–200.

Guptka, G. Gender, sexuality, and HIV/AIDS: The what, the why, and the how, *SIECUS Report*, 29: 5 (June/July 2001), 6–12.

Guyot, J. F. The Defining Moment for Gender Equity, *The Chronicle of Higher Education 47, no. 32* (April 20, 2001): B15.

Haas, A. & Haas, K. *Understanding Sexuality.* St. Louis: Times Mirror/Mosby, 1990.

Haffner, D., ed. *Facing facts: Sexual health for America's adolescents.* New York: Sexuality Information and Education Council of the United States, 1995.

Haffner, D. & Casselman, M. Toy Story. *SIECUS Report* 24:4, 1996, 3–4.

Haffner, D. & Schwartz, P. *What I've learned about sex: Wisdom from leading sex educators, therapists, and researchers.* New York: Perigree Books, 1998.

Haffner, D. W. *Beyond the big talk: Every parents' guide to raising sexually healthy teens*. NY: Newmarket Press, 2001.

Haffner, D. W. & Gambrell, A. *Unfinished business.* New York: SIECUS, 1993.

Haffner, D. W. & Goldfarb, E. S. But, does it work? Improving evaluations of sexuality education. Sexuality Information and Education Council of the United States, 1988.

Haffner, D. W. & Schwartz, P. *What I've learned about sex.* New York: Perigee Books, 1998.

Haffner, D. W. & Stayton, W. R. Sexuality and reproductive health, in Hatcher, R. A., et al. *Contraceptive technology,* 7th revised ed. New York: Ardent Media, 1998.

Haignere, C. Adolescent use of condoms and abstinence, *Health Education and Behavior*, 26 (1999), 43–54.

Haines, M. R. Western fertility in mid-transition: Fertility and nuptiality in the United States and selected nations at the turn of the century, *Journal of Family History, 15* (1990) 23–48.

Hale, R. W. Diagnosis of pregnancy and associated conditions. In *Current obstetric and gynecologic diagnosis and treatment,* Benson, R. C., ed. Los Altos, CA: Lange Medical Publications, 1978.

Hales, D. R. 10 secrets of a happy marriage, *McCall's, 113* (February 1986), 26–61.

Hall, C. C. & Crum, M. J. Women and "body-isms" in television beer commercials, *Sex Roles, 31* (September 1994) 329–337.

Halpern, C. T., Oslak, S. G., Young, M. L., Martin, S. L., & Kupper, L. L. Partner violence among adolescents in opposite-sex romantic relationships: Findings from the national longitudinal study of adolescent health, *American Journal of Public Health*, 91, no. 10 (October 2001), 1679–1685.

Hamer, D. H., Hu, S., Magnuson, V. L., & Spencer, T. L. A linkage between DNA Markers on the X-chromosome and male sexual orientation, *Science, 261, no. 5119* (1993), 321–327.

Hammer, S. M., et al. A trial comparing nucleoside monotherapy and combination therapy in HIV-infected adults with CD4 cell count from 200 to 500 per cubic millimeter, *New England Journal of Medicine, 335* (1996), 1081–1099.

Hantula, R. IUDs, *Spotlight on Health, 1* (1986), 7.

Hariton, B. E. The Sexual Fantasies of Women. In *Psychology Today* (editors). *The Female Experience*. Del Mar, CA: Communications/Research/Machines, 1973.

Harrell, G. D. & Frazier, G. L. *Marketing: Connecting with customers.* Upper Saddle River, NJ: Prentice Hall, 1999, 26.

Harris, D. Physical sex differences: A matter of degree, *The Counseling Psychologist, 6, no. 2* (1976), 11.

Harris, M. B. Coming out in a school setting: Former students' experiences and opinions about disclosure, in *School experiences of gay and lesbian youth: The invisible minority,* Harris, M. B., ed. New York: Harrington Park Press/The Haworth Press, 1997, 85–100.

Harris, M., ed. *School experiences of gay and lesbian youth: The invisible minority.* New York: Harrington Park Press/The Haworth Press, Inc., 1997.

Harvard establishes date rape program, *Sexuality Today,* (October 13, 1986) 2–3.

Harvard Medical School. The premenstrual enigma, *The Harvard Medical School Health Letter*, 9 (1984), 1–2, 5.

Harvey, S. M., Beckman, L. J., & Satre, S. J. Choice of and satisfaction with methods of medical abortion among U.S. clinic patients, *Family Planning Perspectives*, 33, no. 5 (2001), 212–216.

Hass, N. Sex and today's single-minded sitcoms, *New York Times* (Late New York Edition) (January 27, 1997), 11 (sec. 2).

Hatcher, R. A., Trussell, J., Stewart, F., Cates, W., Stewart, G. K., Guestr, F., & Kowal, D. *Contraceptive technology,* 17th revised ed. New York: Ardent Media, 1998.

Hatfield, E. Passionate and compassionate love. In *The Psychology of Love,* Sternberg, R. & Barnes, M., eds. New Haven: Yale University Press, 1988.

Hausknecht, R. U. Methotrexate and misoprostol to terminate early pregnancy, *New England Journal of Medicine, 333* (1995), 537–540.

The health of boys, *Education Week, 17, no. 42* (July 8, 1998), 8.

Healthy people 2000: National health promotion and disease prevention objectives. USDHHS, PHS, Publication No. (PHS) 91-50212, 1991.

Heath, D. An investigation into the origins of a copious vaginal discharge during intercourse—enough to wet the bed—that is not urine, *Journal of Sex Research*, 20 (1984), 194–215.

Heaton, T. B. & Albrecht, S. L. The changing pattern of interracial marriage, *Social Biology, 48, no. 3–4* (Fall/Winter 1996), 203–217.

Hefner, C. Thinking outside the box, *Media Studies Journal* (Spring/Summer 1996).

Heiman, J. R., et al. Evaluating sexual dysfunction in women, *Clinical Obstetrics and Gynecology, 40* (1997), 616–629.

Hellstrom, W. J., ed. *Male infertility and sexual dysfunction.* New York: Springer-Verlag, 1997.

Help end domestic violence, National Resource Center on Domestic violence. N.D.

Henig, R. M. The sterilization option: More and more married couples choose surgical sterilization, *Washington Post, Health* (March 19, 1986), 12–16.

Henry J. Kaiser Family Foundation. *National survey of adolescents and young adults: Sexual health knowledge, attitudes and experiences*. (2003). Washington, DC.

Henry J. Kaiser Family Foundation. *Sex on TV: Content and context* (January 2001). Menlo Park, CA.

Henshaw, S. & Kost, K. Abortion patients in 1994–1995, *Family Planning Perspectives, 26* (1994), 100–106, 112.

Henshaw, S. & Van Vort, J. Abortion services in the United States, 1991 and 1992, *Family Planning Perspectives, 26* (1994), 100–106, 112.

Henshaw, S. Abortion services in the United States, 1995–1996, *Family Planning Perspectives, 28* (1996), 140–147, 158.

Henshaw, S. K. Factors hindering access to abortion services, *Family Planning Perspectives, 27* (1995), 54–59, 87.

Henshaw, S. K. Unintended pregnancy in the United States, *Family Planning Perspectives, 30* (1998), 24–29, 46.

Henslin, J. M. *Sociology,* 2nd ed. Needham Heights, MA: Allyn & Bacon, 1995.

Herbst, A. Clear cell adenocarcinoma of the genital tract of young females, *New England Journal of Medicine*, 287 (1972), 1259–1264.

Herman, J. "Father-Daughter Incest." In *Rape and Sexual Assault,* edited by A. W. Burgess. New York: Garland Publishing Co., 1985.

Herman, J. Incest, *Harvard Medical School Health Letter, 6* (March 1981), 3–4.

Herman-Giddens, M.E. Secondary sexual characteristics and menses in young girls seen in office practice. *Pediatrics* (1997) 99:4, 505–512.

Herpes without symptoms, *Family Life Education, 5* (1986), 11.

Hertica, M. A. Interviewing sex offenders, *The Police Chief, 58* (1991), 39–43.

Heston, L. & Shields, J. Homosexuality in twins, *Archives of General Psychiatry, 18* (1968), 149–160.

Heywood, L. Despite the positive rhetoric about women's sports, female athletes face a culture of sexual harassment, *The Chronicle of Higher Education, 55, no. 18* (January 8, 1999), B4.

Heywood, L. Father-daughter incest, in *Rape and Sexual Assault.* New York: Garland Publishing, 1985.

High court to hear arguments on child porn amendment, *The Birmingham News* (October 28, 2001), 20A.

Hillis, S. D., Anda, R. F., Felitti, V. J., & Marchbanks, P. A. Adverse childhood experiences and sexual risk behaviors in women: A retrospective cohort study, *Family Planning Perspectives*, 33, no. 5 (September/October 2001), 206–211.

Himelein, M. J. Risk factors for sexual victimization in dating: A longitudinal study of college women, *Psychology of Women Quarterly, 19* (1995), 31–48.

Hingson, R. W. Beliefs about AIDS, use of alcohol and drugs, and unprotected sex among Massachusetts adolescents, *American Journal of Public Health, 80* (1990), 295.

Hite, S. *The Hite report on male sexuality.* New York: Alfred Knopf, 1981.

Hite, S. *The Hite report.* New York: Macmillan, 1976.

Hite, S. *Women and love: A cultural revolution in progress.* New York: Alfred Knopf, 1987.

Hlatky, M. A., Boothroyd, D., Vittinghoff, E., Sharp, P., & Whooley, M. A. Quality-of-life and depressive symptoms in postmenopausal women after receiving hormone therapy, *Journal of the American Medical Association*, 287 (2002), 591–597.

Hochschild, A. *The second shift: Working parents and the revolution at home.* New York: Viking, 1989.

Hoff, C. C., McKusisk, L., Hilliard, B., & Coates, T. J. The impact of HIV antibody status on gay men's partner preferences: A community perspective, *AIDS Education and Prevention, 4* (1992), 197–204.

Hofferth, S. L., Kahn, J. R., & Baldwin, W. Premarital sexual activity among U.S. teenage women over the past three decades, *Family Planning Per-*

spectives, 19, no. 2 (March/April 1987), 46–53.

Hole, J. W., Jr. *Human anatomy and physiology,* 5th ed. Dubuque, IA: Wm. C. Brown, 1990.

Hollender, M. H. Women's wish to be held: Sexual and nonsexual aspects, *Medical Aspects of Human Sexuality,* (October 1970), 12–26.

Holmes, M., et al. Association of dietary intake of fat and fatty acids with risk of breast cancer, *Journal of the American Medical Association, 281* (1999), 914–920.

Hoover, E. Policing public sex, *The Chronicle of Higher Education*, 49, no. 19 (January 17, 2003), A31.

Hopkins, H. The VD that many have, few know: Chlamydiae, *FDA Consumer, 17* (1983), 4–6.

Hormone labels will warn of risks, *HealthNews* (March 2002), 10.

Hormone replacement therapy, *Time*, 161, no. 3 (January 20, 2003), 115–116.

Hort, B. E., Fagot, B. I., & Leinbach, M. D. Are people's notions of maleness more stereotypically framed than their notions of femaleness? *Sex Roles, 23* (1990), 197–212.

Hortobagyi, G. N., McLelland, R., & Reed, F. M. Your key role in breast cancer screening, *Patient Care*, 24 (1990), 82–113.

Hostile hallways: Bullying, teasing, and sexual harassment in school, *American Journal of Health Education*, 32, no. 5 (September/October 2001), 307–309.

How many F2Ms are there? International Foundation for Gender Education (2003). Available: www.ifge.org.

How Popular is Danni Ashe Compared to Other Stars? 2003. Online. Available: www.billiondownloadwoman.com/pop.html.

How the experts view androstenedione, *Washington Post* (October 20, 1998), 13, 15.

How to approach treatment of the sexual addict, Sexual Recovery Institute (2001). Available: http://www.sexualrecovery.com.

How to treat sexual addicts, *Sexuality Today, 10, no. 15* (January 26, 1987), 1–2.

Howe, H. Acting and understanding: What service-learning adds to our academic future, *Education Week, 16* (April 2, 1997), 56.

Hoyt, J. Study: Only 20% of attacks made by strangers, *The Birmingham News* (June 15, 2001), 4A. Available: http://www.intimacyinstitute.com.

Hunt, M. *Sexual Behavior in the 1970's.* Chicago: Playboy Press, 1974.

Hunter, J. Violence against lesbian and gay male youths, *Journal of Interpersonal Violence, 5* (1990), 295–300.

Hutchinson, J. B., ed. *Biological determinants of sexual behavior.* New York: John Wiley & Sons (1978).

Hyde, J. S. Gender differences in aggression, in *The Psychology of Gender,* Hyde, J. S. & Linn, M. C., eds. Baltimore: The Johns Hopkins Press, 1986.

Ibrahim, M. A. Strategies to prevent HIV infection in the United States, *American Journal of Public Health, 81.12* (1991), 155–159.

In their own right: Addressing the sexual and reproductive health needs of American men, Alan Guttmacher Institute. (2002). Available: www.agi-usa.org/pubs/exs_men.html.

Increasing number of Cambodian "beer girls" selling sex, Kaiser Daily HIV/AIDS Report (January 15, 2003). Available: www.kaisernetwork.org/daily_reports

Innala, S. M. & Ernulf, K. E. Asphyxiophilia in Scandinavia, *Archives of Sexual Behavior, 18* (1989), 181–189.

Institute of Medicine. *The best intentions.* Washington, DC: National Academy Press, 1995.

International Committee for Prostitutes' Rights, 1998.

Intimate partner violence, U.S. Dept. of Justice, Bureau of Justice Statistics (2000). Available: www.ojp.usdoj.gov.bjs.

Iovine, V. *The girlfriends' guide to pregnancy.* New York: Perigee, 1997.

Isely, P. & Gehrenbeck-Shim, D. Sexual assault of men in the community, *Journal of Community Psychology, 25* (1997), 159–166.

Ismach, J. A second look at the pill. *American Health* (July/August 1986), 47–49.

Jacobson, J. Rice U. football coach chastised for comments on gay athletes, *The Chronicle of Higher Education*, 49, no. 11 (November 18, 2002), A32.

Jacobson, J. The loneliest athletes, *The Chronicle of Higher Education*, 49, no. 10 (November 1, 2002), A36–A38.

Jacobson, N. S., Gottman, J. M., Gortner, E., Burns, S., & Shortt, J. W. Psychological factors in the longitudinal course of battering: When do the couples split up? When does the abuse decrease? *Violence and Victims, 11, no. 4* (1996), 371–392.

James, K. & MacKinnon, L. The incestuous family revisited: A critical analysis of family therapy myths, *Journal of Marriage and Family Therapy, 16* (1990), 71–88.

James, M. S. Museum of Sex to debut in New York. Available: www.ABCnews.com.

Jamison, P. L. & Gebhard, P. H. Penis size increases between flaccid and erect states: An analysis of the Kinsey data, *Journal of Sex Research*, 24 (1988), 177.

Janus, S. & Janus, C. *The Janus report on sexual behavior.* New York: John Wiley & Sons, 1993.

Jensen, S. B. Diabetic sexual dysfunction, *Archives of Sexual Behavior, 10* (1981), 493–504.

Jew, S. AIDS among California Asian and Pacific Islander sub-groups, *California HIV/AIDS Update, 4* (1991), 90–98.

Johnson, B. E., Kuck, D. L., & Schander, P. R. Rape myth acceptance and sociodemographic characteristics: A multidimensional analysis, *Sex Roles, 36* (1997), 693–707.

Johnson, I. M. A logilinear analysis of abused wives' decisions to call the police in domestic-violence disputes, *Journal of Criminal Justice, 18* (1990), 147–158.

Johnson, R. E., Nahmias, A. J., Magder, L. S., et al. A seroepidemiologic survey of the prevalence of herpes simplex virus type 2 infection in the United States, *The New England Journal of Medicine, 321* (1989), 7–12.

Johnson, R. Genital herpes and pregnancy, *American Family Physician, 33* (1986), 167–171.

Johnston, S. A. The mind of a molester, *Psychology Today 21, no. 2* (1987), 60–64.

Jones, E., et al. Teenage pregnancy in developed countries: Determinants and policy implications, *Family Planning Perspectives, 17, 2* (1985), 53–63.

Jones, E., et al. Unintended pregnancy, contraceptive practice and family planning services in developed countries, *Family Planning Perspectives, 20, 2* (1988), 53–67.

Jones, H. W. and J. P. Toner. "The Infertile Couple." *New England Journal of Medicine* 329(1993): 1710–1715.

Jones, K. L. & Smith, D. W. Recognition of the fetal alcohol syndrome in early infancy, *Lancet, 1* (1973a), 1267–1270.

Jones, K. L. & Smith, D. W. Recognition of the fetal alcohol syndrome in early infancy, *Lancet, 2* (1973b), 99.

Jones, M. M. Lessons from gay marriages, *Psychology Today, 30* (May/June 1997), 22.

Jones, W. H., Chernovetz, M. E., & Hansson, R. O. The enigma of androgeny: Differential implications for males and females, *Journal of Consulting and Clinical Psychology, 46* (1978), 293–313.

Jong, E. *Fear of Flying.* New York: Signet, 1974.

Jordan, K. M. I will never survive: Lesbian, gay, and bisexual youths' experience of high school, in *School experiences of gay and lesbian youth: The invisible minority,* Harris, M. B., ed. New York: Harrington Park Press/The Haworth Press, 1997, 17–33.

Jordan, T. R., Price, J. H., Telljohann, S. K., & Chesney, B. K. Junior high school students' perceptions regarding nonconsensual sexual behavior, *Journal of School Health, 68, no. 7* (September 1998), 289–296.

Joseph, C. Scarlet wounding: Issues of child prostitution, *Journal of Psychohistory, 23, no. 1* (1995), 2–17.

Joseph, J. Singing the push-up blues, *ABCNews.com* (September 7, 1998).

Joyce, J. *Ulysses.* New York: Random House, 1934.

Judson, F. N. Partner notification for HIV control, *Hospital Practice, 25* (1990), 63–73.

Just the facts about sexual orientation and youth. Washington, D.C., American Psychological Association, 2000.

Kahn, A. The estrogen dilemma: Osteoporosis forces hard choices on older women, *Medical Self-Care* (Winter 1984), 40–45.

Kahn, M. Parents' divorce can lead children to bad habits, Reuters/AOL, (September 9, 1998).

Kaiser Daily Health Report, fax/online bulletin (January 5, 1999). Available: http://report.kff.org/repro/contact.htm

Kaiser Family Foundation and Seventeen magazine release latest SexSmarts survey on teen sexual behavior, Kaiser Family Foundation (July 9, 2002). Available: www.kaisernetwork.org/daily_reports.

Kakuchi, S. Japan only now confronting rising HIV rate—Women in sex trade most at risk, *San Francisco Chronicle* (March 17, 2003), A8.

Kalichmen, S. C. Affective and personality characteristics of MMPI profile subgroups of incarcerated rapists, *Archives of Sexual Behavior, 19* (1990), 443–459.

Kallman, F. J. Comparative twin study on the genetic aspects of male homosexuality, *Journal of Nervous and Mental Disease, 115* (1952), 283–298.

Kandrick, M., Grant, K. R., & Segall, A. Gender differences in health related behavior: Some unanswered questions, *Social Science and Medicine, 32* (1991), 579–590.

Kanin, E. J. Date rapists: Differential sexual socialization and relative deprivation, *Archives of Sexual Behavior, 14, no. 3* (1985), 219–231.

Kanin, E. J. False rape allegations, *Archives of Sexual Behavior, 32, no. 1* (1994), 81–92.

Kann, L, Kinchen, S. A., Williams, B. I., Ross, J. G., Lowry, R., Hill, C. V., Grunbaum, J. A., Blumson, P. S., Collins, J. L., & Kolbe, L. J. Youth risk behavior surveillance—United States, 1997, *Morbidity and Mortality Weekly Report, 47, no. SS-3* (August 14, 1998), 1–92.

Kansas City's "John TV" tunes out rights, American Civil Liberties Union Freedom Network, 1997.

Kantrowitz, B. Sexism in the schoolhouse, *Newsweek* (February 24, 1992), 62–70.

Kaplan, H. S. *The sexual desire disorders: Dysfunctional regulation of sexual motivation.* New York: Brunner/Mazel, 1995.

Kaplan, S. H. *Disorders of sexual desire.* New York: Simon & Schuster, 1979.

Kaplan, S. H. *How to overcome premature ejaculation.* New York: Brunner/Mazel, 1989.

Kaplan, S. H. *Sexual aversion, sexual phobias, and panic disorder.* New York: Brunner/Mazel, 1989.

Kaplan, S. H. *The evaluation of sexual disorders.* New York: Brunner/Mazel, 1983.

Kaplan, S. H. *The new sex therapy: Active treatment of sexual dysfunction.* New York: Brunner/Mazel, 1974.

Kaplin, H. S. *The new sex therapy: Active treatment of sexual dysfunction.* New York: Brunner/Mazel, 1974.

Karofsky, P. F. Relationship between adolescent-parental communication and initiation of first intercourse by adolescents, *Journal of Adolescent Health*, 28, no. 1 (January 2001), 41–45.

Kasindorf, M., Bayles, F., & Grossman, C. L. Boston church scandal starts chain reaction, *USA Today* (December 19, 2002), 13A.

Kass, R. C., Hannon, R., & Whitten, L. Effects of gender and situation on the perception of sexual harassment, *Sex Roles, 34, nos. 1–2* (1996), 155–182.

Katz, J. E. Empirical and theoretical dimension of obscene calls to women in the United States, *Human Communication Research, 21* (1994), 155–182.

Katz, L. Censorship too close to home, *SIECUS Report, 23, no. 1* (October/November 1994), 15–18.

Katz, R. C., Hannon, R., and Whitten, L. "Effects of Gender and Situation on the Perception of Sexual Harassment." *Sex Roles* 34(Jan. 1996): 35–42.

Katzenstein, D. A., et al. The relation of virologic and immunologic markers to clinical outcomes after nucleoside therapy in HIV-infected adults with CD4 cell count from 200 to 500 per cubic millimeter, *The England Journal of Medicine, 335* (1996), 1091–1098.

Kaufman, R. H. Continued follow-up of pregnancy outcomes in diethylstilbestrol-exposed offspring, *Obstetrics and Gynecology*, 96, no. 4 (2000), 483–489.

Keenan, F. Imperfect implant, *American Health* (March 1991), 9.

Keenan, J. P., Gallup, G. G., & Goulet, N. Attributions of deception in human mating strategies, *Journal of Social Behavior and Personality, 12, no. 1* (March 1997), 45–52.

Kegel, A. Sexual functions of the pubococcygeus muscle, *Western Journal of Surgery, Obstetrics, and Gynecology*, 60 (1952), 521–524.

Kegeles, S. M., Adler, N. E., & Irvin, Jr., C. E. Adolescents and condoms: Associations of belief with intentions to use, *American Journal of Diseases of Children, 143* (1989), 911.

Kehoe, M. *Lesbians over 60 speak for themselves.* New York: Harrington Park Press, 1989.

Kellogg, A.P. Looking inward, freshman care less about politics and more about money. *The Chronicle of Higher Education 47, no. 20* (Jan. 26, 2001: A47–A50

Kendall-Tackett, K. & Marshall, R. Sexual victimization of children: Incest and child sexual abuse, in *Issues in intimate violence,* Bergen, R. K., ed. Thousand Oaks, CA: Sage Publications, 1988.

Kendler, K. S., Thornton, L. M., Gilman, S. E., & Kessler, R. C. Sexual orientation in a U.S. national sample of twin and nontwin sibling pairs, *American Journal of Psychiatry*, 157 (2000), 1843–1846.

Kenney, J. W., Reinholtz, C., & Angellini, P. J. Ethnic differences in childhood and adolescent sexual abuse and teenage pregnancy, *Journal of Adolescent Health 21, no. 1* (1997), 3–10.

Kenney, J. W., Reinholtz, C., & Angellini, P. J. Sexual abuse, sex before age 16, and high-risk behaviors of young females with sexually transmitted diseases, *Journal of Obstetric, Gynecologic, & Neonatal Nursing, 27, no. 1* (1998), 54–63.

Kerber, L. K. Moving beyond stereotypes of feminism, *The Chronicle of Higher Education, 45, no. 33* (April 23, 1999), B6–B8.

Kerr, D. L. Politics and public health: The abstinence-only debate in schools. Presentation at American School Health Association convention, 2000.

Kerssens, J. J., Bensing, J. M., & Andela, M. G. Patient preference for genders of health professionals, *Social Science and Medicine, 44, no. 10* (1997), 1531–1540.

Key, W. B. *Subliminal seduction.* Englewood Cliffs, NJ: Prentice Hall, 1973.

Keye, W. R. Update: Premenstrual syndrome, *Endocrine and Fertility Forum*, 6 (1983), 1–3.

Kiersch, T. A. Treatment of sex offenders with Depo-Provera, *Bulletin of the American Academy of Psychiatry Law, 18* (1990), 179–187.

Kilmann, P. R., Sabalis, R. F., Gearing, M. L., Bukstel, L. J., & Scovern, A. W. The sexual paraphilias: A review of the outcome research, *The Journal of Sex Research, 18, no. 3* (August 1982), 193–252.

Kilota, G. Deadliness of breast cancer in blacks defies easy answer, *The New York Times* (August 8, 1994), C10.

Kincaid, J. *Adopting for good: A guide for people considering adoption.* Grove, IL: Intervarsity Press, 1997.

Kindela, J. Dysfunctionnügen, *Flex* (January 1991), 14–15.

King, M. Sexual assaults on men: Assessment and management, *British Journal of Hospital Medicine, 53, no. 6* (1995), 245–246.

Kinsey, A. C., Pomeroy, W. B., & Martin, C. E. *Sexual behavior in the human female.* Philadelphia: Saunders, 1953.

Kinsey, A. C., Pomeroy, W. B., & Martin, C. E. *Sexual behavior in the human male*. Philadelphia: Saunders, 1948.

The Kinsey Institute. *The history and concept of sexology,* 1998.

Kirby, D. Emerging answers: Research findings on programs to reduce sexual risk-taking and teen pregnancy. Washington, DC: The National Campaign to Prevent Teen Pregnancy, 2001.

Kirby, D. & Coyle, K. Changing risk-taking behavior: Preliminary conclusions from research, in *The sexuality education challenge,* Drolet, J. C. & Clark, K., eds. Santa Cruz, CA: ETR Associates, 1994.

Klach, D. *Woman plus woman: Attitudes toward lesbianism.* New York: Simon & Schuster, 1974.

Klein, N. A. & Serrins, D. S. Sexual content of top-grossing motion pictures: A random sample from years 1973–1993, *Journal of Education, 29, no. 6* Health (1998), 354–358.

Klerman, L. V., Cliver, S. P., & Goldenberg, R. L. The impact of short interpregnancy intervals on pregnancy outcomes in a low-income population, *American Journal of Public Health, 88* (1998), 1182–1185.

Klitsch, M. Subgroups of U.S. women differ widely on exposure to sexual intercourse, *Family Planning Perspectives, 22* (1990), 94–95.

Kluger, J. What's sex got to do with it? *Time*, 161, no. 3 (January 20, 2003), 35.

Knafo, G. and Y. Jaffe. Sexual Fantasizing in Males and Females. *Journal of Research in Personality* 19(1984): 451–62.

Knight, R. A., Rosenberg, R., & Schneider, B. Classification of sexual offenders: Perspectives, methods, and validation, in *Rape and sexual assault*, Burgess, A. W., ed. New York: Garland Publishing Co., 1985.

Koch grants benefits for domestic partners, *Washington Post* (August 8, 1989), A6.

Koch, L. W. Interracial rape: Examining the increasing frequency argument, *The American Sociologist, 26, no. 1* (1995), 76–86.

Kogan, J. *Change and continuity in infancy.* New York: Wiley, 1971.

Kohn, A. Shattered innocence, *Psychology Today, 21, no. 2* (1987), 54–64.

Kolander, C. A., Ballard, D. J., & Chandler, C. K. *Contemporary women's health: Issues for today and the future.* Dubuque, IA: WCB/McGraw-Hill, 1999.

Kolata, G. Deadliness of breast cancer in blacks defies easy answer, *The New York Times* (August 3, 1994), C10.

Kolodny, R. C., Masters, W. H., & Johnson, V. E. *Textbook of sexual medicine.* Boston: Little, Brown, 1979.

Koop, C. E. *Surgeon General's Report on Acquired Immune Deficiency Syndrome.* Washington, DC: U.S. Public Health Service, October 1986.

Kopper, B. A. Gender, gender identity, rape myth acceptance, and time of initial resistance on the perception of acquaintance rape blame and avoidability, *Sex Roles, 34* (1996), 81–93.

Koss, M. P. & Leonard, K. E. Sexually aggressive men: Empirical findings and theoretical implications, in *Pornography and sexual aggression*, Kulkoski, N. & Kilian, C., eds. New York: Academic Press, 1984.

Kreiss, J. L. & Patterson, D. L. Psychosocial issues in primary care of lesbian, gay, bisexual, and transgender youth, *Journal of Pediatric Health Care, 11, no. 6* (1997) 266–274.

Krilov, L. R. What do you know about genital warts? *Medical Aspects of Human Sexuality, 25* (1991), 43–45.

Kroll, K. & Klein, E. *Enabling romance: A guide to life, sex, and relationships for the disabled (and people who love them).* Kensington, MD: Woodbine House, 1995.

Kronenberg, F. & Fugh-Berman, A. Complementary and alternative medicine for menopausal symptoms: A review of randomized, controlled trials, *Annals of Internal Medicine*, 137 (2002), 805–813.

Kulkoski, K. & Kilian, C. Sexual assault and body esteem, *Psychological Reports, 80, no. 1* (1997), 347–350.

Kuriansky, J. Sexuality and television advertising: An historical perspective, *SIECUS Report, 24, no. 5* (June/July 1996), 13.

Labi, N. A bad start? *Time, 153, 6* (February 15, 1999).

Landau, C., Cyr, M., & Morton, A. W. *The complete book of menopause.* New York: Perigee, 1994.

Latest research on marital adjustment and satisfaction, American Psychological Association.

Laumann, E. O., Gagnon, J. H., Michael, R. T., & Michaels, S. *The social organization of sexuality: Sexual practices in the United States.* Chicago: The University of Chicago Press, 1994.

Laumann, E. O., Michael, R. T., & Gagnon, J. H. A political history of the National Sex Survey of Adults, *Family Planning Perspectives, 26, no. 1* (January/February 1994), 634–638.

Lawrence, D. H. *Lady Chatterly's lover.* New York: Grove, 1959.

Lawrence, L. Partner violence among adolescents in opposite-sex romantic relationships: Findings from the National Longitudinal Study of Adolescent Health, *American Journal of Public Health*, 91 (10) (October 2001), 1679–1685.

Layng, A. What keeps women "in their place?" *USA Today Magazine* (May 1989), 89–91.

Leary, W. Older people enjoy sex, survey says, *The New York Times* (September 29, 1998), F8.

Lederer, L. *Take back the night: Women on pornography.* New York: William Morrow, 1980.

Ledray, L. E. Date rape drug alert, *Journal of Emergency Nursing, 22, no. 1* (1996), 80.

Lee, J. Love-styles, in *The psychology of love*, Sternberg, R. & Barnes, M., eds. New Haven: Yale University Press, 1988.

Legislation would provide opportunities for working moms to breastfeed. *The Nation's Health* (May/June 1998), 14.

Leiblum, S. R. & Pervin, L. A. *Principles and practice of sex therapy.* New York: Guilford Press, 1980.

Leigh, B. C., Temple, M. T., & Trocki, K. F. The sexual behavior of U.S. adults: Results from a national survey, *American Journal of Public Health, 83* (1993), 1400–1408.

Leitenberg, H. & Henning, K. Sexual fantasy, *Psychological Bulletin, 117* (1995), 469–496.

Leitenberg, H., Greenwald, E., & Tarran, M. The relation between sexual activity among children during preadolescence and/or early adolescence and sexual behavior and sexual adjustment in young adulthood, *Archives of Sexual Behavior, 18, no. 4* (1989), 299–313.

Leppard, W., Ogletree, S., & Wallen, E. Gender stereotyping in medical advertising: Much ado about something? *Sex Roles, 29* (December 1993), 829–838.

Lestger, D. The effect of alcohol consumption on marriage and divorce at the national level, *Journal of Divorce and Remarriage, 27, no. 3*–4 (1997), 159–161.

Levant, R. & Brooks, G. R. *Men and sex: New psychological perspectives.* New York: Wiley, 1997.

LeVay, S. A difference in hypothalmic structure between heterosexual and homosexual men, *Science, 253* (1991), 1034–1037.

Lever, J. & Schwartz, P. *The great sex weekend.* New York: Perigee Books, 1998.

Levin, R. & Levin, A. Sexual pleasure: The surprising preferences of 100,000 women, *Redbook* (September 1975), 38.

Lewis, J. E., Malow, R. M., & Ireland, S. J. HIV/AIDS risk in heterosexual college students: A review of a decade of literature, *Journal of American College Health*, 45, no. 4 (1997), 147–158.

Lewis, R. Genetic screening—fetal signposts on a journey of discovery, *FDA Consumer, 24* (1990), 17–23.

Lewis, R. W. Venous ligation surgery for venous leakage, *International Journal of Impotence Research, 2* (1990), 1–19.

Liebowitz, M. *The chemistry of love*. Boston: Little, Brown, 1983.

Lindenberg, K. E. & Reese, L. A. Sexual harassment policy: What do employees want? *The Policy Studies Journal, 24, no. 3* (1996), 387–403.

Lin-Fu, J. S. Asian and Pacific Islander Americans: An overview of demographic characteristics and health care issues, *Asian American and Pacific Islander Journal of Health, Inaugural Issue, 1* (1993), 20–60.

Link, A. & Copeland, P. Sexual magnetism: Pheromones—the scent of sex, *Urban Male Magazine* (Winter 2001), 38–39.

Lisak, D. Sexual aggression, masculinity, and fathers, *Journal of Women in Culture and Society, 16* (1991), 238–262.

Listening to understand, *The Pryor Report Success Workshop,* a supplement to *The Pryor Report Management Newsletter* (August 1998).

Litman, R. E. Bondage and sadomasochism, in *Sexual dynamics of anti-social behavior,* 2nd ed., Schlesinger, L. B. & Revitch, E., eds. Springfield, IL: Charles C. Thomas Publisher, 1997.

Living together before marriage may hurt—not help—chances of successful match, InteliHealth (July 25, 2002). Available: www.intelihealth.com.

Lizotte, A. J. The uniqueness of rape: Reporting assaultive violence to the police, *Crime and Delinquency, 31, no. 2* (April 1985), 169–190.

Logan, C. R. Homophobia? No, homoprejudice, *Journal of Homosexuality, 31, no. 3* (1996), 31–53.

London International Group, *1997 Durex Global Sex Survey,* 1998.

Long, G. T. & Sultan, F. E. Contributions from social psychology, in *Male and female homosexuality: Psychological approaches,* Diamant, L., ed. Washington, DC: Hemisphere, 1987, 221–236.

Long, V. E. Contraceptive choices: New options in the U.S. market, *SIECUS Report*, 31 (2002), 13–18.

LoPiccolo, J. Advances in diagnosis and treatment of sexual dysfunction. Paper presented at the annual meeting of the Society for the Study of Sex, San Diego, California, September 1985.

LoPiccolo, J. Direct treatment of sexual dysfunction in the couple, in *Hand-*

book of Sexology, Money, J. & Masaph, H., eds. Amsterdam: Elsevier/North-Holland, 1977, 1227–1244.

LoPiccolo, J. & Hieman, J. *Becoming orgasmic: A sexual and personal growth program for women.* Englewood Cliffs, NJ: Prentice Hall, 1988.

Loredo, C., Reid, A., & Deaux, K. Judgments and definitions of sexual harassment by high school students, *Sex Roles, 32, nos. 1–2* (1995), 29–45.

Lotozo, E. Pair seek to give true picture of young gay America. *Knight Ridder Newspapers* (June 4, 2003). Available: www.glsen.org.

Louis Harris and Associates, Inc. *In their own words: Adolescent girls discuss health and health care issues.* New York: The Commonwealth Fund, 1997.

Love, P. & Robinson, J. *Hot monogamy.* New York: Dutton, 1994.

Love, S. M. *Dr. Susan Love's hormone book.* New York: Random House, 1997.

Loy, P. H. & Stewart, L. P. The extent and effects of the sexual harassment of working women, *Sociological Focus, 17, no. 1* (January 1984), 31–42.

Luscombe, B. Pumping it up, *Time* 58, no. 11 (September 3, 2001), Y26.

Lyman, S. A., Hughes-McLain, C., & Thompson, G. Date-rape drugs: A growing concern, *Journal of Health Education, 29, no. 5* (1998), 271–274.

Lynberg, M. C. & Khoury, M. J. Contributions of birth defects to infant mortality among racial/ethnic minority groups, United States, 1983, *MMWR, 39* (1990), 1–11.

Lynch, A., McDuffie, R., Murphy, J., et al. Preeclampsia in multiple gestation: The role of assisted reproductive technologies, *Journal of Obstetrics and Gynecology*, 93 (2002), 445–451.

Maatman, T. & Montague, D. Diabetes mellitus and erectile dysfunction in men, *Journal of Urology, 133* (1985), 191A.

MacDonald, A., Jr. Bisexuality: Some comments on research and theory, *Journal of Homosexuality, 6* (1981), 21–35.

MacDorman, M. F. & Singh, G. K. Midwifery care, social and medical risk factors, and birth outcomes in the U.S.A., *Journal of Epidemiology and Community Health, 52* (1998), 310–317.

MacKay, H. & MacKay, T. Abortion training on obstetrics and gynecology resident programs in the United States, 1991–1992, *Family Planning Perspectives, 27* (1995), 112–115.

Macoby, E. E. & Jacklin, C. N. *The psychology of sex differences.* Stanford, CA: Stanford University Press, 1974.

MacWilliams, B. Turning tricks for tuition, *The Chronicle of Higher Education*, 49, no. 11 (November 8, 2002), A48.

Mahoney, F. R. Religiosity & sexual behavior among heterosexual college students, *Journal of Sex Research, 16, no. 1* (February 1980), 97–113.

Mahoney, P. & Williams, L. M. Sexual assault in marriage: Prevalence, consequences, and treatment of wife rape, in *U.S. Air Force Domestic Violence Literature Review,* 1998.

Malaney, G. D. Assessing campus climate for gays, lesbians, and bisexuals at two institutions, *Journal of College Student Development, 38, no. 4* (July/August 1997), 365–375.

Male contraceptive implants (July 11, 2001). Available: www.sexhealth.com

Male victims of sexual abuse: 51 case reports, *Sexuality Today, nos. 37–38* (June 30 and July 7, 1986), 2–3.

Males, females and evolution: An interview with Helen Fisher, *Family Life Matters* 43 (spring, 2001): 1, 4–5.

Mallon, R. Demonstration of vestigial prostate tissue in the human female. (October 1984). Paper presented at the Annual Regional Conference of the American Association of Sex Educators, Counselors, and Therapists, Las Vegas, NV.

Malovich, N. & Stake, J. E. Sexual harassment on campus, *Psychology of Women Quarterly, 14* (1990), 63–81.

Mancini, J. & Orthner, D. Recreational sexuality preferences among middle-class husbands and wives, *Journal of Sex Research, 14* (1978), 95–106.

Manning, W. D. Childbearing in cohabiting unions: Racial and ethnic differences, *Family Planning Perspectives*, 33, no. 5 (September/October 2001), 217–223.

Manusov, V., Floyd, K., & Kerssen-Griep, J. Yours, mine, and ours, *Communication Research, 24, no. 3* (1997), 234–260.

Many people with HIV don't tell partners and don't use condoms, study shows, *The Nation's Health* (March 1998), 2.

March of Dimes. Rubella public health education information sheet. White Plains, NY: March of Dimes Birth Defects Foundation, 1986.

Marinoble, R. M. Homosexuality: A blind spot in the school mirror, *Professional School Counseling, 1, no. 3* (February 1998), 4–7.

Marks, G., et al. Self-disclosure of HIV infection to sexual partners, *American Journal of Public Health, 81* (1991), 1321–1323.

Marshall, D. Sexual behavior on Mangaia, in *Human sexual behavior: Variations in the ethnographic spectrum,* Marshall, D. & Suggs, R., eds. Englewood Cliffs, NJ: Prentice-Hall, 1971.

Marshall, W. L., Payne, K., & Barbaree, H. E. Exhibitionists: Sexual preferences for exposing, *Behavior Research and Therapy, 29, no. 1* (1991), 37–40.

Martin, C. Attitudes and expectations about children with nontraditional and traditional gender roles, *Sex Roles, 22* (1990), 151–165.

Martin, D. & Lyon, P. *Lesbian-woman.* New York: Bantam (1972).

Martin, J. A., Hamilton, B. E, Ventura, S. J., Menacker, F., Park, M. M., & Sutton, P. D. Births: Final data for 2001, *National Vital Statistics Reports*, 51 (2002), 5, 9.

Marton, A. The Boomerangers: Adult children back in the fold, *Washington Post* (August 3, 1990), B5.

Maslow, A. H. *Toward a psychology of being,* 2nd ed. Princeton, NJ: Van Nostrand, 1968.

Masochism, University of Iowa Health Care (2001). Available: www.uihealthcare.com/topics/mentalemotionalhealth/ment3155.html.

Masters, W. H. & Johnson, V. E. *Homosexuality in perspective.* Boston: Little, Brown, 1979.

Masters, W. H. & Johnson, V. E. *Human sexual inadequacy.* Boston: Little, Brown, 1970.

Masters, W. H. & Johnson, V. E. *Human sexual response.* Boston: Little, Brown, 1966.

Masters, W. H., Johnson, V. E., & Kolodny, R. C. *Human sexuality* (2nd ed.). Boston: Little, Brown, 1985.

Matchinsky, D. J. & Iverson, T. G. Homophobia in heterosexual female undergraduates, *Journal of Homosexuality, 31, no. 4* (1996), 123–128.

Matteo, S. & Rissman, E. Increased sexual activity during the midcycle portion of the human menstrual cycle. *Hormones and Behavior,* 18 (1984), 249–255.

May, L. Many men still find strength in violence, *The Chronicle of Higher Education, 45, no. 6* (October 2, 1998), B7.

Mayo Clinic. PMS: Advances in diagnosis and treatment, Mayo Health Oasis (1998). Available: www.mayohealth.org/mayo/9609/htm/pms.htm

Mayo Health Clinic. *Dietary suggestions for premenstrual syndrome,* 1998a.

Mayo Health Clinic. *PMS: Advances in diagnosis and treatment,* 1998b.

Mays, V. M. & Cochran, S. D. Ethnic and gender differences in beliefs about sex partner questioning to reduce HIV risk, *Journal of Adolescent Research*, 8, no. 1 (1993), 77–88.

McCarthy, B. & McCarthy, E. *Male sexual awareness*. Berkeley, CA: Publishers Group West, 1998.

McCarthy, B. W., Ryan, M., & Johnson, F. A. *Sexual awareness: A practical approach.* San Francisco: Boyd & Fraser, 1975.

McCarthy, P. Ageless sex, *Psychology Today* (March 1989), 62.

McCarthy-Partoun, T. He makes a village, *Time,* 157, no. 19 (May 14, 2001), 47–48.

McCary, J. L. *Human sexuality: Second brief edition.* New York: Van Nostrand, 1979.

McConaghy, N. Pedophilia: A review of the evidence, *Australian and New Zealand Journal of Psychiatry, 32, no. 2* (1998), 252–265.

McCormack, W., ed. *Chlamydia.* Chicago: Abbott Laboratories Diagnostic Division, 1984.

McCormick, E. M. Home testing patients need pharmacist's expertise, *Pharmacy Times* (October 1994), 45–51.

McCormick, N. Come-ons and put-offs: Unmarried students' strategies for having and avoiding sexual intercourse, *Psychology of Women Quarterly, 4* (1979), 194–211.

McGuire, T. R. Is homosexuality genetic? A critical review and some suggestions, *Journal of Homosexuality, 28, nos. 1–2* (1995), 115–145.

McKinney, K. Sexual harassment of university faculty by colleagues and students, *Sex Roles, 23* (1990), 421–438.

McMillen, L. Many colleges taking a new look at policies on sexual harassment, *Chronicle of Higher Education, 33, no. 16* (December 17, 1986), 1, 16.

McQueen, A. Study: Debt, anxiety sway women from college, *AP/AOL* (June 10, 1999).

Mead, P., Miller, D., & Thomason, J. A thorough workup for vaginitis, *Patient Care, 21* (1987), 1178–1191.

Meckler, L. American family becomes more traditional, complex, *The Birmingham News* (April 13, 2001), 5A.

Media project announces winners of annual SHINE awards for sexual health in entertainment, Kaiser Daily Reproductive Health Report (October 25, 2001). Available: www.kaisernetwork.org.

Media recommendations for more realistic, accurate images concerning sexuality, SIECUS Fact Sheet, 1998. Available: www.siecus.org.

Meilman, P. W., Riggs, P., & Turco, J. H. A college health services' response to sexual assault issues, *Journal of American College Health, 39* (1990), 145–147.

Memmott, M. Slavery, related abuses growing worldwide, report says, *USA Today* (May 25, 2001), 13A.

Mendelsohn, A. You big, beautiful (and realistic) doll, *The Birmingham News* (December 23, 2002), p. D1.

Messenger, J. Sex and repression in an Irish folk community, in *Human sexual behavior: Variations in the ethnographic spectrum,* Marshall, D. & Suggs, R., eds. Englewood Cliffs, NJ: Prentice Hall, 1971.

Meyer, M. C., Berchtold, I. M., Oestreich, J. L., & Collins, F. J. *Sexual harassment at work.* New York: Petrocelli, 1981.

Michael, R. T., Gagnon, J. H., Laumann, E. O., & Kolata, G. *Sex in America: A definitive survey.* New York: Warner Books, 1995.

Michael, R., Gagnon, J., Laumann, E., & Kolata, G. *Sex in America.* Boston: Little, Brown, 1994.

Michaels, M. A church plan on sex abuse, *Time*, 160, no 22 (November 25, 2002), 25.

Miller, B. C., Monson, V. H., & Norton, M. C. The effects of forced sexual intercourse on white female adolescents, *Child Abuse and Neglect, 19, no. 10* (1995), 1289–1301.

Miller, D. W. A sociologist finds bias in sex-survey methods, *The Chronicle of Higher Education, 45, no. 33* (April 23, 1999), A25–A26.

Miller, D.W., and Sharlet, J. The Adonis complex studies men's obsession with a "male body ideal": Physicist examines "the soul-battering system" that envelops professionals, *The Chronicle of Higher Education*, Research & Publishing section, May 26, 2000. Available: http://chronicle.com/

Miller, M. More men turning to implants to enhance pecs, *The Birmingham News* (November 26, 2002), 1D, 3D.

Miller, M. & Solot, D. Organization for unmarried people condemns cohabitation report (February 8, 1999).

Milsten, R. & Slowinski, J. *The sexual male: Problems and solutions*. New York: Norton, 1999.

Minikin, M. J. & Wright, C. V. *What every woman needs to know about menopause.* New Haven, CT: Yale University Press, 1996.

Minilaparotomy and laparoscopy: Safe, effective, and widely used, *Population Reports, 13, C ser.* (May 1985).

MMWR, "Youth Risk Behavior Surveillance—United States, 1997", *47, no. SS-3* (August 14, 1998).

Moller, L., Hymel, S., & Rubin, K. Sex typing in play and popularity in middle childhood, *Sex Roles, 26* (1992), 331–335.

Money, J. *Gay, straight, and in-between.* New York: Oxford University Press, 1988.

Money, J. *Principles of developmental sexology.* New York: The Continuum Publishing Group, 1997.

Money, J. Paraphilias: Phenomenology and classification, *American Journal of Psychotherapy, 38, no. 2* (April 1984), 164–179.

Money, J. Pornography in the home, in *Contemporary sexual behavior,* Zubin, J. & Money, J., eds. Baltimore: Johns Hopkins Press, 1973.

Money, J. Sin, sickness, or status: Homosexual gender identity and psychoneuroendocrinology, *American Psychologist, 42* (1987b), 384–399.

Money, J. Status: Homosexual gender identity and psychoneuroendocrinology, *American Psychologist, 42* (1987a), 384–399.

Money, J. The concept of gender identity disorder in childhood and adolescence after 39 years, *Journal of Sex and Marital Therapy, 20, no. 3* (1994), 163–177.

Money, J. & Athanasiou, R. Pornography: Review and bibliographic annotations, *American Journal of Obstetrics and Gynecology, 115* (January 1973), 130–146.

Money, J. & Ehrhardt, A. E. *Man and woman, boy and girl.* Baltimore: Johns Hopkins Press, 1972.

Money, J. & Schwartz, M. Dating, romantic and nonromantic friendships and sexuality in 17 early-treated androgenital females, aged 16–25, in *Congenital adrenal hyperplasia,* Lee, P. A., et al., eds. Baltimore: University Park Press, 1977.

Moore, K. *Drop in teen birth rate not cause for complacency*. Washington, DC: Child Trends, 2001.

Moore, K. A., Peterson, J. L., & Furstenberg, F. F. Parental attitudes and the occurrence of early sexual activity, *Journal of Marriage and the Family, 48* (November 1986), 777–782.

Moore, M. J. & Rienzo, B. A. Sexual harassment policies in Florida school districts, *Journal of School Health, 68, no. 6* (1998), 237–242.

Moore, N. B. & Davidson, J. K., Sr. Guilt about first intercourse: An antecedent of sexual dissatisfaction among college women, *Journal of Sex and Marital Therapy, 23, no. 1* (1997), 29–46.

More sex scenes but more mention of "safer sex" on TV shows, Kaiser Daily HIV/AIDS Report (February 5, 2003). Available: www.kaisernetwork.org/daily_reports.

Morgan, P. *Who needs parents? The effects of childcare and early education on children in Britain and the USA.* London: Institute of Economic Affairs, 1996.

Morgan, R. Bisexual students face tension with gay groups, *The Chronicle of Higher Education*, 49, no. 14 (November 29, 2002), A31.

Morgan, R. The men in the mirror, *The Chronicle of Higher Education*, 49, no. 5 (September 27, 2002), A53–A54.

Morgentaler, A. *The male body: A physician's guide to what every man should know about his sexual health.* New York: Simon & Schuster, 1993.

Mori, L., Bernat, J. A., Glenn, P. A., & Selle, L. L. Attitudes toward rape: Gender and ethnic differences across Asian and Caucasian college students, *Sex Roles, 32, nos. 7–8* (1995), 457–467.

Morse, B. J. Beyond the conflict tactics scale: Assessing gender differences in partner violence, *Violence and Victims, 10, no. 4* (1995), 251–272.

Mortola, J. F. Issues in diagnosis and research of premenstrual syndrome, *Clinical Obstetrics and Gynecology, 35* (1992), 587–598.

Moseley, D., Fellingstad, D., Harley, H., & Heckel, R. Psychological factors that predict reaction to abortion, *Journal of Clinical Psychology, 37* (1981), 276–279.

Mosher, W. D. & Pratt, W. F. Contraceptive use in the United States, 1973–1988, *Advance Data, 182* (March 20, 1990).

Mosher, W. D. Contraceptive practice in the United States, 1982–1988, *Family Planning Perspectives, 22* (1990), 198–205.

Most sexually active teens first had sex at home, late at night, survey shows, The Henry J. Kaiser Family Foundation (September 26, 2002). Available: www.kaisernetwork.org/daily_reports.

Muehlenhard, C. L. & Falcon, P. L. Men's heterosocial skill and attitudes toward women as predictors of verbal sexual coercion and forceful rape, *Sex Roles, 23* (1990), 241–259.

Mulhauser, D. Dating among college students is all but dead, survey finds, *Chronicle of Higher Education*, 47, no. 48 (August 10, 2001), A51.

Mulvihill, J. J. Fetal alcohol syndrome, in *Teratogen update: Environmentally induced birth defect risks,* Sever, J. L. & Brent, R. L., eds. New York: Alan R. Liss (1986), 13–18.

Munjack, D. J. & Kanno, P. H. Retarded ejaculation: A review, *Archives of Sexual Behavior, 8* (1979), 139–150.

Munjack, D. J. & Oziel, L. *Sexual medicine and counseling in office practice.* Boston: Little, Brown, 1980.

Munroe, R. L. & Munroe, R. H. Male pregnancy symptoms and cross-sex identity in three societies, *Journal of Social Psychology, 84* (1971), 11–25.

Murphy, D. E. "Gays Celebrate, and Plan for Broader Rights." *The New York Times*, June 27, 2003. On-line. Available: www.nytimes.com.

Murray, B. More research underscores that parents' involvement shapes children's academic success, American Psychological Association.

Murray, J. B. Physiological mechanisms of sexual dysfunction side effects associated with antidepressant medication, *Journal of Psychology, 132* (1998), 407–416.

Murstein, B. L. *Love, sex, and marriage.* New York: Springer, 1974.

Myers, J. Nonmainstream body modification: Genital piercing, branding, burning, and cutting, *Journal of Contemporary Ethnography, 21* (1992), 267–306.

Nahom, D., Wells, E., Gillmore, M.R., Hoppe, M., Morrison, D. M., Archibald, M., Murowchick, E., Wilsdon, A., and Graham, L. Differences by gender and sexual experience in adolescent sexual behavior: Implications for education and HIV prevention, *Journal of School Health 71, no. 4* (April, 2001): 153–158.

Nakakuki, M. Normal and developmental aspects of masochism: Transcultural and clinical implications, *Psychiatry, 57* (1994), 244–253.

Nass, G. D. *Marriage and the family.* Reading, MA: Addison-Wesley, 1978.

Nathan, S. The epidemiology of the DSM-III psychosexual dysfunctions, *Journal of Sex and Marital Therapy, 12* (1986), 267.

The nation: Attitudes and characteristics of freshmen, *The Chronicle of Higher Education*, 49, no. 1 (August 30, 2002), 26.

National Academy of Sciences. *Nutrition during pregnancy.* Washington, DC: National Academy Press, 1990.

National Campaign to Prevent Teenage Pregnancy. No Easy Answers. Washington, D.C.: National Campaign, 1999.

National Center for Health Statistics. *Series 23, No., 19* (1996), 5–6.

National Center for Health Statistics, as reported in *The opposite of sex, Time, 152, no. 2* (July 13, 1998a), 39.

National Center for Health Statistics. *Births,* 1998b.

National Center for Health Statistics. Births, Marriages, Divorces, and Deaths: Provisional Data for 1999, *National Vital Statistics Reports, 48* (February 22, 2001).

National Center for Health Statistics. Births: Preliminary data for 2000. (July 24, 2001). Hyattsville, MD.

National Center for Health Statistics. Contraceptive use in the United States: 1982–1990, *Advance Data,* (February 14, 1995).

National Center for Health Statistics. Contraceptive utilization among widowed, divorced, and separated women in the United States, *Advance Data, 40* (September 22, 1978), 3.

National Center for Health Statistics. *Health, United States, 1998 with socioeconomic status and health chartbook.* Hyattsville, MD: National Center for Health Statistics, 1998c.

National Center for Health Statistics. Health, United States, 2002 with chartbook on trends in the health of Americans. (2002). Hyattsville, MD.

National Center for Health Statistics. Health, United States, 2000 (2000). Hyattsville, MD.

National Center for Health Statistics. Higher order multiple births drop for the first time in a decade, *News Release* (April 17, 2001).

National Center for Health Statistics. Trends in marital status of mothers at conception and birth of first child: United States, 1964–1966, 1972, and 1980, *Monthly Vital Statistics Report, 36* (May 29, 1987).

National Center for Health Statistics. Use of contraception in the United States, 1982, *Advance Data,* (December 4, 1984c).

National child abuse and neglect statistical fact sheet, National Clearinghouse on Child Abuse and Neglect Information, 1998.

National Council on the Aging. *Half of older Americans report they are sexually active: 4 in 10 want more sex, says new survey.* Press release, September 28, 1998.

National Guidelines Task Force. *Guidelines for comprehensive sexuality education,* 2nd ed. New York: Sexuality Information and Education Council of the United States, 1996.

National Institute on Aging. The menopause of life. (1986). Washington, DC: Department of Health and Human Services.

National magazines: The dangerous eroticization of children, *Sexuality Today, 7* (January 30, 1984), 1.

National Victims Center and Crime Victims Research and Treatment Center. *Rape in America.* Arlington, VA: National Victims Center, 1992.

Nearly 70 percent of elderly widows live alone, U.S. Census Bureau, 1998.

Nearly half of sexually active college women may be HPV-infected, *Medical Aspects of Human Sexuality, 25* (1991), 49.

Nederlof, K. P., Lawson, H. W., Saftias, A. F., et al. Ectopic pregnancy surveillance, United States, 1970–1987, *MMWR, 39* (1990), 9–17.

The need for comprehensive sexuality education, National Abortion and Reproductive Rights Action League Foundation, 1998. Available: http://www.naral.org

Neinstein, L. S. *Adolescent health care: A practical guide.* MD: Urban & Schwarzenberg, 1991.

Nelson, J. B. *Embodiment: An approach to sexuality and Christian theology.* Minneapolis: Augsburg, 1978.

Ness, Carol. PBS shies from show, *San Francisco Examiner (*June 6, 1999).

New federal law on computer porn upheld despite vagueness concerns, 1998.

Newcomer, S. & Udry, J. Oral sex in an adolescent population, *Archives of Sexual Behavior, 14* (1985), 41–46.

Newcomer, S. & Udry, J. Parental marital status effects on adolescent sexual behavior, *Journal of Marriage and the Family, 49* (May 1987), 235–240.

Newcomer, S. Out of wedlock childbearing in an antebellum Southern county, *Journal of Family History, 15* (1990), 357–368.

Newman, A. L. & Peterson, C. Anger of women incest survivors, *Sex Roles, 34, nos.* 7–8 (1996), 463–474.

NIAID. Chlamydial infections, *National Institutes of Health Publication No. 87–909E,* Public Health Service, Department of Health and Human Services (1987a).

NIAID. Genital herpes, *National Institutes of Health Publication No. 87–909C,* Public Health Service, Department of Health and Human Services (1987b).

NIAID. Genital warts, *National Institutes of Health Publication No. 87–909D,* Public Health Service, Department of Health and Human Services (1987c).

NIDA, Anabolic steroids, *Research Report Series,* DHHS Publication No. (ADM) 91-1810, 1999. Available: www.health.org/pubs/nidarr/index.htm

Nidus Information Services. *Ask NOAH about: Impotence (erectile dysfunction),* 1998. Available: http://noah.cuny.edu/wellconn/impotence.html

Nieschlag, E., Wickings, E., & Breuer, H. Chemical methods for male fertility control, *Contraception, 23* (1981), 1–10.

NIH panel rejects vitamin supplements, *Nutrition Week, 20* (1990), 2–3.

Nock, S. A comparison of marriages and cohabiting relationships, *Journal of Family Issues, 16* (1995), 53–73.

Noden, M. Dying to win, *Sports Illustrated* (August 8, 1994), 52–60.

Nosek, M. A. Wellness among women with physical disabilities, *Sexuality and disability, 14* (1996), 165–181.

Notes from the research, *SIECUS Development* (Summer/Fall 2002), 2.

NOW conference celebrates 30 years. Merrifield, VA: National Organization for Women, 1998.

Number of married U.S. teens increased by 50% in 1990s; Some attribute to abstinence education, *Kaiser Daily Reproductive Health Report* (November 11, 2002). Available: www.kaisernetwork.org/daily_reports.

Nutter, D. & Condron, M. Sexual fantasy and activity patterns of females with inhibited sexual desire versus normal controls, *Journal of Sex and Marital Therapy, 9* (1983), 276–282.

O'Brien, P. M. Helping women with premenstrual syndrome, *British Medical Journal, 307* (1993), 1471–1475.

O'Keefe, M. Disapproval of gay lifestyle still very strong movement, *The Birmingham News* (July 22, 2001), 4C.

O'Keefe, M. The times are trying politicians' souls, *The Oregonian* (April 20, 1995), A1.

O'Neill, A. Altered states, *People Weekly, 50, no. 16* (November 2, 1998), 110–120.

Ochs, R. Biophobia: It goes both ways, in *Bisexuality: The psychology and politics of an invisible minority,* Feinstein, B. A., ed. Thousand Oaks, CA: Sage Publications, 1996, 217–239.

Office of the Surgeon General. *The surgeon general's call to action to promote sexual health and responsible sexual behavior* (2001). Rockville, MD.

Okie, S. RU–486 joining methotrexate in reshaping abortion, *Washington Post* (October, 13, 2000), A3.

Oliver, S. T. & Toner, B. B. The influence of gender role typing on the expression of depressive symptoms, *Sex Roles, 22* (1990), 775–790.

Olson, M. A collaborative approach to the prevention of child abuse, *Victimology: An International Journal, 10, nos. 1–4* (1985), 131–139.

Oncalem, R. & King, B. Comparison of men's and women's attempts to dissuade sexual partners from the couple using condoms, *Archives of Sexual Behavior*, 30, no. 4 (August 2001), 379–391.

One out of ten female adolescents experience date violence and/or rape, says study of over 80,000 youths in Minnesota, *InteliHealth*. Available: www.intelihealth.com.

Opp, M. Habits worth breaking, *Lamaze Parents' Magazine* (1990), 30–33.

Organon. *NuvaRing, world's first vaginal birth control ring, now available in U.S.*, news release. (July 16, 2002). West Orange, NJ.

Ory, S. New options for diagnosis and treatment of ectopic pregnancy, *Journal of the American Medical Association, 267* (1992), 534–537.

Oskamp, S., Kaufman, K., & Wolterbeek, L. A. Gender role portrayals in preschool picture books, *Journal of Social Behavior and Personality, 11, no. 5* (1996), special issue, 27–39.

Osland, J. A., Fitch, M., & Willis, E. E. Likelihood to rape in college males, *Sex Roles, 35, nos. 3–4* (1996), 171–183.

Otis, C. H. Midwives still hassled by medical establishment, *Utne Reader* (November/December 1990), 32–34.

Overall, C. What's wrong with prostitution? Evaluating sex work, *Signs, 17* (Summer 1992), 705–724.

Overland, M. A. In Kashmir, militant group threatens to shoot female Muslim students who do not wear veil, *The Chronicle of Higher Education*, Today's News (September 17, 2001). Available: http://chronicle.com/daily/2001

Overview of the status of women in the states, Institute for Women's Policy Research, Washington, DC (2001). Available: www.iwpr.org/.

Owner reinstates R-rated movies, *The Birmingham News* (January 1, 1999), H1.

Packard, V. *The sexual wilderness.* New York: David McKay, 1968, 459–462.

Pageant officials advise Miss America 2003 to stop pomoting teen abstinence, *Kaiser Daily Reproductive Health Report* (October 9, 2002). Available: http://www.kaisernetwork.org/daily_reports.

Paikoff, R. & Brooks-Gunn, J. Do parent-child relationships change during puberty? *Psychological Bulletin, 110* (1991), 47–66.

Paisner, S. R. Domestic violence: Breaking the cycle, *The Police Chief, 58* (1991), 35–37.

Palmer, H. T. & Lee, J. A. Female workers' acceptance in traditionally male-dominated blue-collar jobs, *Sex Roles, 22* (1990), 607–626.

Palmer, M. *Video user's guide.* Boston: Allyn & Bacon, 1998.

Papilia, D. E. & Olds, S. W. *World: Infancy through adolescence.* New York: McGraw-Hill, 1993.

Paraphilia. Sinclair Intimacy Institute (2001). Available: http://www.intimacy.institute.com.

Pardun, C. J. & Forde, K. R. Sex in the media: Do condom ads have a chance? *SIECUS Report*, 31, no. 2 (December 2002/January 2003), 22–23.

The parent trap, *Birmingham News* (September 27, 1998), 2C.

Partner notification for preventing human immunodeficiency virus (HIV) infection: Colorado, Idaho, South Carolina, Virginia, *MMWR, 37* (1988), 393, 401.

Parts of Africa showing HIV in 1 in 4 adults, *The New York Times* (June 24, 1998).

Parulkar, B. G., Lewis, R. W., Barrett, D. M., Furlow, W. L., Castelli, G., Harris, C., & Westbrook, P. R. The role of multifunctional sleep laboratory studies in the evaluation of erectile dysfunction, Abstract 20, *Proceedings of the 3rd Biennial World Meeting on Impotence.* Boston (October 1988).

Pastor's column hits the growth of porn, *The Birmingham Post Herald* (September 1, 2001), D9.

Patterson, J. Killer cramps, *Shape* (August 1990), 20–22.

Patterson, J. The contraceptive implant, *Shape* (August 1990), 30–31.

Paul, J. P. Bisexuality: Exploring/exploding the boundaries, in *The lives of lesbians, gays, and bisexuals: Children to adults,* Savin-Williams, R. C. & Cohen, K. M., eds. Fort Worth, TX: Harcourt Brace, 1996, 436–461.

Pauly, I. Gender identity disorders: Evaluation and treatment, *Journal of Sex Education and Therapy, 16* (1990), 2–24.

Peacock, P. Marital rape, in *Issues in intimate violence,* Bergen, R. K., ed. Thousand Oaks, CA: Sage Publications, 1998.

Pearson, J. C. *Gender and Communication.* Dubuque, IA: Wm. C. Brown, 1985.

Peipert, J. F., Domangalski, L., Boardman, L., Daamen, L., Zinner, S. H., & McCormack, W. M. College women and condom use, *The New England Journal of Medicine, 335, no. 3* (July 18, 1996), 211.

Perelman, M. A. Treatment of premature ejaculation, in *Principles and Practice of Sex Therapy,* Leiblum, S. R. & Pervin, L. A., eds. New York: Guilford Press, 1980.

Perez-Stable, E. J., Otero-Sabogal, R., & Sabogal, F. Self-reported use of cancer screening tests among latinos and anglos in a prepaid health plan, *Archives of Internal Medicine, 154* (1994), 1073–1081.

Perry, J. D. Treating vaginismus with Perry brand sensors, 1992.

Perry, J. D. & Whipple, B. Pelvic muscle strength of female ejaculators: Evidence in support of a new theory of orgasm, *Journal of Sex Research*, 17 (1981), 22–39.

Person, E. S., Terestman, N., Myers, W. A., & Goldberg, E. L. Gender differences in sexual behaviors and fantasies in a college population, *Journal of Sex and Marital Therapy, 15, no. 3* (1989), 187–214.

Peters, J. M. Specialists a definite advantage in child sexual abuse cases, *The Police Chief, 58* (1991), 21–23.

Peterson, A. C. & Leffert, N. What is special about adolescence, in *Psychosocial disturbances in young people: Challenges for prevention,* Rutter, M., ed. Cambridge, England: Cambridge University Press, 1994.

Peterson, H., Xia, Z., Hughes, J., Wilcox, L. Taylor, L., & Trussell, J. The risk of ectopic pregnancy after tubal sterilization, *The New England Journal of Medicine.*

Petitti, D. B. Maternal mortality and morbidity in cesarean section, *Clinical Obstetrics and Gynecology, 28* (1985), 763.

Petrovich, M. & Templer, D. I. Heterosexual molestation of children who later become rapists, *Psychological Reports, 54* (1984), 810.

Phalen, K. F. PMS: Pretty miserable symptoms, *Washington Post Health* (August 1, 2000), 19.

Phalen, K. F. Women and yeast: A sensitive subject, *Washington Post Health* (March 6, 2000), 19.

Phalen, K. F. Your own personal heat wave, *Washington Post Health* (June 12, 2001), 19.

Phillis, D. E. & Gromko, M. H. Sex differences in sexual activity: Reality or illusion? *The Journal of Sex Research, 21, no. 4* (November 1985), 437–448.

Piccinino, L. J. & Mosher, W. D. Trends in contraceptive use in the United States: 1982–1995, *Family Planning Perspectives, 30* (1998), 4–10, 46.

Piccinino, L. J. & Mosher, W. D. Trends in contraceptive use in the United States: 1982–1995, *Family Planning Perspectives*, 30, no. 1 (1998), 4–10, 46.

Pierson, E. C. & D'Antonio, W. V. *Female and male: Dimensions of human sexuality.* Philadelphia: Lippincott, 1974.

Pietropinto, M. Sensuality scale: Test your responses, enhance your desire, *Self* (July 1990), 104–107, 152.

Planned Parenthood Federation of America. *Birth control: The condom (2003).* Available: http://www.plannedparenthood.org/bc/Condom.htm#Female.

Planned Parenthood of America, 1998.

Plaud, J. J., et al. A multivariate analysis of the sexual fantasy themes of college men, *Journal of Marital and Family Therapy, 23* (1997), 221–230.

Pleck, J., Sonnenstein, F., & Ku, L. Masculinity ideology: Its impact on adolescent males' heterosexual relationships, *Journal of Social Issues, 49, 3* (1993), 11–30.

Plotnik, R. *Introduction to psychology,* 3rd ed. Pacific Grove: CA: Brooks/Cole, 1993, 27–28.

Plous, S. & Neptune, D. Racial and gender biases in magazines and advertising, *Psychology of Women Quarterly, 21, no. 4* (December 1997), 627–644.

Polit, D. F., White, C. M., & Morgan, T. D. Child sexual abuse and premarital intercourse among high-risk adolescents, *Journal of Adolescent Health Care, 11* (1990), 231.

Polumbaum, J. China: Confucian tradition meets the market economy, *Ms.* (September/October 1992), 12–13.

Poniewozik, J. Hot tubs and cold shoulders, *Time*, 160, no. 7 (August 12, 2002), 56–58.

Pope, E. When illness takes sex out of a relationship, *SIECUS Report, 27, no. 3* (February/March 1999), 8–11.

Pope, V. Trafficking in women, *U.S. News and World Report* (April 7, 1997), 38.

Popenoe, D. Parental androgyny, *Society, 30, no. 6* (1993), 5–11.

Popenoe, D. The top ten myths of divorce, The National Marriage Project. Rutgers, The State University of New Jersey. Available: http://marriage.rutgers.edu/pubtoptenmyths.htm.

Popenoe, D. & Whitehead, B. D. The state of our unions 2000: The social health of marriage in America, The National Marriage Project. Rutgers, The State University of New Jersey (2001). Available: http://marriage.rutgers.edu/state_of_our_unions%202000%20text%20only.htm.

Popenoe, D. & Whitehead, B.D. The state of our unions 2000, *The National Marriage Project*. Available: http://marriage.rutgers.edu/state_of_our_union%202000%20text%20only.htm

Porter, J. U.S. teenage birthrate tops industrial nations, *Education Week, 17, no. 36* (May 20, 1998), 5.

Prendergast, A. Beyond the pill, *American Health* (October 1990), 37–44.

Prevalence of homosexuality, The Kinsey Institute (2003). Available: www.indiana.edu/~Kinsey/resources/FAQ.html#homosexuality.

Problems arise with the "other STDs," *The Nation's Health* (May-June 1987), 2–3.

Proctor, F., Wagner, N., & Butler, J. The differentiation of male and female orgasm: An experimental study, in *Perspectives on human sexuality*, Wagner, N., ed. New York: Behavioral Publications, 1974.

PROMISE: Our programs, 1998.

Prostitution in the United States—the statistics, 1998.

Pryor warns of strong drug used by sex predators, *Birmingham News* (August 18, 1998), 4B.

Ptacek, J. Why do men batter their wives? In *Issues in intimate violence*, Bergen, R. K., ed. Thousand Oaks, CA: Sage Publications, 1998.

Pugh, T. Mixed-race marriages on the rise, study says, *The Birmingham News* (March 23, 2001), 5A.

Quackenbush, R. L. Sex roles and social-sexual effectiveness, *Social Behavior and Personality, 18* (1990), 35–40.

Quadagno, E. D., Sly, F., Harrison, D. F., Eberstein, I. W., & Soler, H. R. Ethnic differences in sexual decisions and sexual behavior, *Archives of Sexual Behavior, 27, no. 1* (February 1998), 57–75.

Quadango, D. M., et al. The menstrual cycle: Does it affect athletic performance? *The Physician and Sports Medicine, 19* (1991), 121–124.

Quadrel, M. J., Fischoff, B., & Doris, W. Adolescent (in)vulnerability, *American Psychologist, 48, 2* (1993), 102–116.

Quinacrine Sterilization: Introduction and Overview (2002). Available: http://www.quinacrine.com/intro.html.

Quindlen, A. *Thinking out loud.* New York: Random House, 1988.

RAINN STATISTICS. The National Sexual Abuse Hotline, 2003. Online. Available: www.rainn.org/statistics.html.

Rainwater, L. *And the poor get children.* Chicago: Quadrangle Books, 1960.

Rainwater, L. *Family design: Marital sexuality, family size, and contraception.* Chicago: Aldine, 1965.

Rainwater, L. Sex in the culture of poverty, in *The individual, sex and society,* Broderick, C. B. & Bernard, J., eds. Baltimore: The Johns Hopkins Press, 1969.

Rajfer, J., Rosciszewski, A., & Mehringer, M. Prevalence of corporeal venous leakage in impotent men, *Journal of Urology, 140* (1988), 69–71.

Rankow, E. J. Sexual identity vs. sexual behavior, *American Journal of Public Health, 86, no. 12* (1996), 1822–1823.

Ransom, S. & Moldenhauer, J. Premenstrual syndrome: Systematic diagnosis and individualized therapy, *The Physician and Sportsmedicine, 26* (1998).

Recer, P. Survey: Sex rated more important than job, *The Birmingham News* (April 30, 1999), 3A.

Redfearn, S. A new ring cycle: Contraceptive woos the way, *Washington Post* (August 6, 2002), F1, F4.

Redfearn, S. Hormone questions linger: Experts address women's issues, *Washington Post* (July 7, 2002), F1, F4.

Redfield, R. R. & Burke, D. S. HIV infection: The clinical picture, in *The science of AIDS: Readings from Scientific American magazine.* New York: W. H. Freeman and Company, 1989.

Reese, S. The law and gay-bashing in schools, *The Education Digest, 62* (May 1997), 46–49.

Reid, R. L. & Yen, S. S. C. Premenstrual syndrome, *American Journal of Obstetrics and Gynecology*, 139 (1981), 85–97.

Reinisch, J. & Beasley, R. *The Kinsey Institute new report on sex.* New York: St. Martin's, 1991.

Reinisch, J. M., Hill, C. A., Sanders, S. A., & Zembia-Davis, M. High-risk sexual behavior at a midwestern university—A confirmation survey, *Family Planning Perspectives*, 27, no. 2 (March/April 1995), 79–82.

Reiss, I. L. Changing trends, attitudes & values on premarital sexual behavior in the U.S., in *Human sexuality and the mentally retarded,* de la Cruz, F. F. & La Vock, G. D., eds. New York: Brunner/Mazel, 1973, 286–289.

Remafedi, G., et al. Demography of sexual orientation in adolescents, *Pediatrics, 89, no. 4* (1992), 714–721.

Rensberger, R. Pheromones Discovered in Humans: Substances Help Regulate Female Reproductive Cycle. *Washington Post*, November 1986, A1, A7.

Renshaw, D. C. Viagra 1999, *SIECUS Report, 27, no. 3* (February/March 1999), 18–19.

Renshaw, D. Short-term therapy for sexual dysfunction: Brief counseling to manage vaginismus, *Clinical Practice in Sexuality, 6* (1990), 23–29.

Renzetti, C. M., & Curren, D. J. *Living sociology.* Needham Heights, MA: Allyn & Bacon, 1998.

Research Forecasts, Inc. *The Tampax report: A summary of survey results on a study of attitudes toward menstruation.* New York: Tampax, 1981.

Resolve conflict in four steps, *Communication Briefings, 14, no. 3* (January 1995), 2.

Responsible choices, Planned Parenthood, 1998.

Reukauf, D. & Trause, M. *Commonsense breastfeeding: A practical guide to the pleasure, problems and solutions.* New York: Atheneum, 1988.

Reuters Health Information, Sexhealth.com (July 11, 2001). Available: http://www.sexhealth.com.

Reuters. Study again clears silicone, *Washington Post* (June 22, 1999), A2.

Reuters. Viagra effective and well tolerated: Study, *Health News* (May 13, 1998).

Reynolds, K. *Pregnancy and birth: Your questions answered.* New York: DK Publishing, 1997.

Rhynard, J., Krebs, M., & Glover, J. Sexual assault in dating relationships, *Journal of School Health, 67, no. 3* (1997), 89–93.

Rice, R. The nine secrets of happy couples, *Redbook, 188* (February 1997), 92–94.

Rickert, V. I., Sanghvi, R., & Wiemann, C. M. Is lack of sexual assertiveness among adolescent and young adult women a cause for concern? *Perspectives on Sexual and Reproductive Health*, 34, no. 4 (July/August 2002), 16–28.

Rideout, V. & Hoff, T. *Sex, kids, and the family hour: A three party study of sexual content on television.* CA: Children Now and the Henry J. Kaiser Family Foundation, 1996.

Riggle, E. D., Ellis, A. L., & Crawford, A. M. The impact of "media contact" on gay men, *Journal of Homosexuality, 31, no. 3* (1996), 113–126.

Rimm, M. Marketing pornography on the information superhighway, 1998.

Rio, L. Psychological and sociological research and the decriminalization or legalization of prostitution, *Archives of Sexual Behavior, 20* (1991), 205–217.

Risch, H. A. & Howe, G. R. Menopausal hormone usage and breast cancer: A record linkage cohort study, *American Journal of Epidemiology, 139* (1994), 670–683.

Roberts, T. Gender and the influence of evaluations on self-assessments in achievement settings, *Psychological Bulletin, 109* (1991), 297–308.

Roche, J. P. Premarital sex: Attitudes and behavior by dating stage, *Adolescence, 21, no. 81* (Spring 1986), 107–121.

Rodriguez, C., Patel, A.V., Calle, E. E., Jacob, E. J., Thun, M. Estrogen replacement therapy and ovarian cancer mortality in a large prospective study of US women, *Journal of the American Medical Association*, 285, no. 11 (2001), 1460–1465.

Rome, E. S., Rybikci, L. A., & Durant, R. H. Pregnancy and other risk behaviors among adolescent girls in Ohio, *Journal of Adolescent Health, 22, no. 1* (January 1998), 50–55.

Rooney, M. Freshmen show rising political awareness and changing social views, *The Chronicle of Higher Education*, 49, no. 21 (January 31, 2003), A35–A38.

Roper Starch Worldwide. *Teens talk about sex: Adolescent sexuality in the 90s.* New York: Sexuality Information and Education Council of the United States, 1994.

Rosaria, M. The psychosexual development of urban lesbian, gay, and bisexual youth, *Journal of Sex Research, 33, no. 2* (1996), 113–126.

Rosenberg, L. Hormone replacement therapy: The need for reconsideration, *American Journal of Public Health, 83* (1993), 1670–1673.

Rosin, H. & Morin, R. As tolerance grows, acceptance remains elusive, *The Washington Post* (December 26, 1998), A1, A12, A13.

Rotherham, M. & Weiner, N. Androgeny, stress, and satisfaction, *Sex Roles, 9* (1983), 151–158.

Rouse, L. P. Battered women/battering men, *Family Life Educator, 3, no. 4* (Summer 1985), 11–15.

Rovner, S. A reversal on circumcision, *Washington Post Health* (May 15, 1990).

Rowan, E. L., Rowan, J. B., & Langelier, P. Women who molest children, *Bulletin of the American Academy of Psychiatry Law, 18* (1990), 79–83.

Rowland, D., Kallan, K., & Slob, S. Yohimbine, erectile capacity, and sexual response in men, *Archives of Sexual Behavior, 26* (1997), 49–62.

Rubenstein, C. The modern art of courtly love. *Psychology Today*, July 1983: 39–49.

Rubin, L. J. & Borgers, S. B. Sexual harassment in universities during the 1980s, *Sex Roles, 23* (1990), 397–411.

Rubinson, L. & Rubertis, L. D. Trends in sexual attitudes and behaviors of a college population over a 15-year period, *Journal of Sex Education and Therapy, 17, no. 1* (1991), 32–41.

Rubinstein, G. The decision to remove "homosexuality" from the DSM: Twenty years later, *American Journal of Psychotherapy, 49, no. 3* (Summer 1995), 416–427.

Rubinstein, S., and Caballero, B. Is Miss America an undernourished role model? *Journal of the American Medical Association*, Research Letter, *283, no. 12* (March 22/29, 2000), 1569.

Ruble, D. & Brooks-Gunn, J. Menstrual myths, *Medical Aspects of Human Sexuality*, 13 (June 1979), 110–127.

Russell, D. E. H. *Sexual exploitation.* Beverly Hills, CA: Sage Publications, 1984.

Russell, S. T. LGBTQ Youth are at risk in U.S. school environment, *SIECUS Report*, 29, no. 4 (April/May 2001), 19–22.

Russo, F. Bridal Vows Revisited, *Time 156, no. 4* (July 24, 2000), G1–G3.

Russo, F. Can the government prevent divorce? *Atlantic Monthly, 280* (October 1997), 281.

Russo, N. F. & Zierk, K. L. Abortion, childbearing, and women's well-being, *Professional Psychology: Research and Practice, 23* (1992), 269.

Rutter, V. Lessons from stepfamilies, *Psychology Today* (May/June 1994), 30–31.

Ryan, C. & Futterman, D. Social and developmental challenges for lesbian, gay, and bisexual youth, *SIECUS Report*, 29, no. 4 (April/May 2001), 5–18.

Ryan, R. M. The sex right: A legal history of the marital rape exemption, *Law and Social Inquiry, 20, no. 4* (1995), 941–1001.

Sable, M. R. & Herman, A. A. The relationship between health behavior advice and low birth weight, *Public Health Reports, 112* (1997), 332–339.

Sachs, A. Work's bad girls, *Time*, 158, no. 11 (September 3, 2001), Y7–Y8.

Sack, A. R., Billingham, R. E., & Howard, R. D. Premarital contraceptive use: A discriminant analysis approach, *Archives of Sexual Behavior, 14, no. 2* (April 1985), 165–182.

Sack, A. R., Keller, J. F., & Hinkle, D. E. Premarital sexual intercourse: A test of the effects of peer group, religiosity, and sexual guilt, *Journal of Sex Research, 20, no. 2* (May 1984), 168–185.

Sadism, University of Iowa Health Care (2001). Available: www.uihealthcare.com/topics/mentalemotionalhealth/ment3168.html.

Sadker, M. & Sadker, D. Sexism in the schoolroom of the '80s, *Psychology Today* (March 1985), 54–57.

Sadock, B. J., Kaplan, H. I., & Freedman, A. M. *The sexual experience.* Baltimore: Williams & Wilkins, 1973.

Sadomasochism, Sinclair Intimacy Institute (2001). Available: http://www.intimacyinstitute.com.

Sadowski, M. Sexuality minority students benefit from school-based support—Where it exists, Harvard Education Letter, Research Online (September/October, 2001). Available: http.//www.edletter.org/current/.

Salant, J. D. FBI: Murders, Rapes Up, Total Crime Down. *The Birmingham News*, June 17, 2003. P. 3a.

Salovey, P. & Rodin, J. The heart of jealousy, *Psychology Today* (September 1985), 22–29.

Saluter, A. F. Living status and living arrangements: March 1989, *Current Population Reports,* U.S. Bureau of the Census, P–20 series, no. 445, 1990.

Same sex weddings on campuses, *The Christian Century, 114* (August 13–21, 1997), 721–722.

Samuels, M. & Samuels, N. All about circumcision, *Medical Self-Care* (Spring 1983), 20–23.

Sanchez, R. Oregon ignites revolution in adoption, *The Washington Post* (November 26, 1998), A1.

Sanders, S. A. Midlife sexuality: The need to integrate biological, psychological, and social perspectives, *SIECUS Report, 27, no. 3* (February/March 1999), 3–7.

Sandfort, T. G. M. Relationships: An empirical investigation among a nonrepresentative group of boys, *The Journal of Sex Research, 20, no. 2* (1984), 123–142.

Sang, G. W. Gossypol—a potential contraceptive for men? *Internal Medicine for the Specialist, 6* (1985), 118–125.

Santelli, J. S., Warren, C. W., Lowry, R., Sogolow, E., Collins, J., Kaufmann, R. B., & Celentano, D. D. The use of condoms with other contraceptive methods among young men and women, *Family Planning Perspectives, 29, no. 6* (November-December 1997), 261–267.

Sarrel, P. & Masters, W. Sexual molestation of men by women, *Archives of Sexual Behavior, 11* (1982), 117–131.

Sarrel, P. & Sarrel, L. The *Redbook* report on sexual relationships, part I, *Redbook* (October 1980), 73–80.

Sato, S., et al. Transvaginal ultrasonography screening detects early-stage ovarian cancer, *Cancer* 2000, 89 (2000), 582–587.

Satran, P. R. 15 things never to say to a man: 15 things never to say to a woman, *Glamour, 94* (October 1996), 294.

Satz, D. Markets in women's sexual labor, *Ethics, 106* (October 1995), 63–85.

Saul, R. Abortion reporting in the United States: An examination of the federal-state partnership, *Family Planning Perspectives, 30* (1998), 204–211.

Saunders, E. J. Life-threatening autoerotic behavior: A challenge for sex educators and therapists, *Journal of Sex Education and Therapy, 15* (1989), 82–91.

Saxe, L. Lying: Thoughts of an applied social psychologist, *American Psychologist, 46, no. 4* (1991), 409–415.

Sayer, G. P. & Britt, H. Sex differences in prescribed medications: Another case of discrimination in general practice, *Social Science and Medicine, 45, no. 10* (1997), 1581–1587.

Scacco, A. M., Jr. (ed.). *Rape in Prison.* Springfield, IL: Chas. C. Thomas, 1975.

———. *Male Rape: A Casebook of Sexual Aggressions.* New York: AMS Press, 1982.

Scales, P. *A portrait of young adolescents in the 1990s: Implications for healthy growth and development.* Chapel Hill, NC: Center for Early Adolescence, University of North Carolina at Chapel Hill, 1991.

Scarce, M. Same-sex rape of male college students, *Journal of American College Health, 45, no. 4* (1997), 171–173.

Scarr, S. American child care today, *American Psychologist, 53, no. 2* (February 1998), 95–108.

Schafran, L. H. Topics for our times: Rape is a major public health issue, *American Journal of Public Health, 86, no. 1* (1996), 15–17.

Scheidlower, J. Sex talk, *Esquire, 127* (January 1997), 29.

Schmid, R. E. Unmarried couples top 4 million, *AP/AOL* (July 27, 1998).

———. *Male Rape: A Casebook of Sexual Aggressions*. New York: AMS Press, 1982.

Schnarch, D. *Passionate marriage: Sex, love, and intimacy in emotionally committed relationships*. New York: Norton, 1997.

Schover, L., Friedman, J., Weiler, S., Heiman, J., & LoPiccolo, J. Multiaxial problem-oriented system for sexual dysfunctions, *Archives of General Psychiatry, 39* (1982), 614–619.

Schroepfer, L. Not-so-hot seat: Impotence isn't always in the mind, *American Health* (October 1989), 40.

Schuklenk, U. & Ristow, M. The ethics of research into the cause(s) of homosexuality, *Journal of Homosexuality 31, no. 3* (1996), 5–30.

Schwartz, D. B. & Darabi, K. F. Motivations for adolescents' first visit to a family planning clinic, *Adolescence, 21, no. 83* (Fall 1986), 535–545.

Schwartz, J. Scientists find little that links breast implants to disease, *Washington Post* (December 2, 1999), A8.

Schwartz, J. L. & Gabelnick, H. L. Special report: Current contraceptive research, *Perspectives on Sexual and Reproductive Health*, 34 (2002), 310–316.

Schwartz, M. F. & Bauman, J. E. Hyperprolactinemia and sexual dysfunction in men. Paper presented at the Annual Meeting of the Society for Sex Therapy and Research, New York, March 1981.

Schwartz, P. Peer marriage, *The Family Therapy Networker* (September/October 1994), 57–61.

Schwartz, P. Sexes grow more alike, and strains emerge, *The Chronicle of Higher Education, 45, no. 6* (October 2, 1998), B7.

Schwartz, P. & Rutter, V. *The gender of sexuality.* Thousand Oaks, CA: Pine Forge Press, 1998.

Schwartz, P., Gillmore, M., & Civic, D. The social context of sexuality, in *Sexually transmitted diseases*, Cates, W., Hansfield, & Holmesk, eds. New York: McGraw-Hill, 1996.

Schwebke, J. R. Gonorrhea in the '90s, *Medical Aspects of Human Sexuality, 25* (1991a), 42–46.

Schwebke, J. R. Syphilis in the '90s, *Medical Aspects of Human Sexuality, 25* (1991b), 44–49.

Scully, D. & Morolla, J. Convicted rapists' vocabulary of motive: Excuses and justifications, *Social Problems, 31, no. 5* (1984), 530–544.

Segall, M. The American man in transition, *American Health* (January/February 1989), 59–61.

Segell, M. Homophobia doesn't lie, *Esquire, 127* (February 1997), 35.

Seigel, K. & Raveis, V. H. AIDS-related reasons for gay men's adoption of celibacy, *AIDS Education and Prevention, 5* (1993), 302–310.

Selingo, J. Students engage in behavior posing serious health risks, CDC study finds, *Chronicle of Higher Education, 44, no. 2* (September 5, 1997), 23.

Sell, R. L. Defining and measuring sexual orientation: A review, *Archives of Sexual Behavior, 26, no. 6* (December 1997), 643–658.

Selverstone, R. Adolescent sexuality: Developing self-esteem and mastering developmental tasks, *SIECUS Report, 18, 1* (1989), 1–5.

Selvin, B. W. Transsexuals are coming to terms with themselves and society, *New York Newsday* (June 1, 1993), 55, 58–59.

Semans, J. Premature ejaculation: A new approach, *Southern Medical Journal, 49* (1956), 353–358.

Serdula, M., Williamson, D. F., Kendrick, J. S., et al. Trends in alcohol consumption by pregnant women 1985 through 1988, *Journal of the American Medical Association, 265* (1991), 876–879.

Sevely, J. & Bennett, J. Concerning female ejaculation and the female prostate, *Journal of Sex Research*, 14 (1978), 1–20.

Sex addiction frequently asked questions. Sexual Recovery Institute (2001). Available: http://www.sexualrecovery.com.

Sex offenses and offenders: An analysis of data on rape and sexual assault, U.S. Department of Justice Office of Justice Programs, 1998.

Sex on TV. Menlo Park, CA: The Henry J. Kaiser Family Foundation, 2001.

Sexual and reproductive health: Women and men, 2002, The Alan Guttmacher Institute. Available: www.agi-usa.org/pubs/fb_10-02.html.

Sexual assault of young children as reported to law enforcement: Victim, incident, and offender characteristics, U.S. Dept. of Justice Bureau of Justice Statistics (July 11, 2000). Available: www.ojp.usdoj.gov/bjs/.

Sexual behavior among high school students—United States, 1990, *MMWR, 40, no. 51–52* (1992), 885–888.

Sexual health coverage in women's, men's, and teen magazines, The Henry J. Kaiser Family Foundation (2000). Available: www.kff.org.

Sexual orientation and identity, SIECUS Fact Sheet, 1998.

Sexuality and the law, *Contemporary Sexuality, 32* (1996), 7–8.

Sexuality education in the schools: Issues and answers, *SIECUS Fact Sheet,* 1998.

Sexuality Information and Education Council of the United States, Teen pregnancy. Available: www.siecus.org.

Sexuality Information and Educational Council of the United States, Teens talk about sex, *SIECUS Report, 22, no. 5* (June/July 1994), 16–17.

Sexuality update: Women with type 2 herpes at risk of cervical cancer, *Medical Aspects of Human Sexuality, 21* (1987), 17.

Sexually abused children believe it's their fault, *Sexuality Today, 7* (January 23, 1984), 1.

Sexually Transmitted Disease Summary. U.S. Department of Health and Human Services, Public Health Service, Centers for Disease Control, 1990.

Shainess, N. & Greenwald, H. Debate: Are fantasies during sexual relations a sign of difficulty? *Sexual Behavior, 1* (1971), 38–54.

Shainess, N. Masochism revisited: Reflections on masochism and its childhood antecedents, *American Journal of Psychotherapy, 51* (1997), 552–568.

Shangold, M. Causes, evaluation, and management of athletic oligomenorrhea, *Medical Clinics of North America*, 69 (1985), 83–95.

Shangold, M. The woman runner: Her body, her mind, her spirit, *Runner's World*, 16 (1981), 34.

Shannon, E. Main street monsters, *Time, 152, no. 11* (September 14, 1998), 59.

Shearer, E. L. Cesarean section: Medical benefits and costs, *Social Science and Medicine, 37* (1993), 1223–1231.

Sheehy, G. *Passages*. New York: Bantam, 1976.

Sheehy, G. *Understanding men's passages: Discovering the new map of men's lives.* New York: Random House, 1998.

Sheeran, P. *Women, society, the state and abortion: A structuralist analysis.* New York: Prager, 1987.

Sherwin, R. & Corbett, S. Campus sexual norms and dating relationships: A trend analysis, *The Journal of Sex Research, 21, no. 3* (August 1985), 258–274.

Should lesbian and gay couples be allowed to adopt? In *Taking sides: Issues in family and personal relationships*, Schroeder, E., ed. Guilford, CT: McGraw-Hill/Dushkin, 2003.

Should parents surgically alter their intersex infants? In *Taking sides: Issues in family and personal relationships*, Schroeder, E., ed. Guilford, CT: McGraw-Hill/Dushkin, 2003.

Should people not cohabit before getting married? In *Taking sides: Issues in family and personal relationships*, Schroeder, E., ed. Guilford, CT: McGraw-Hill/Dushkin, 2003.

Should prostitution be legal? In *Taking sides: Issues in family and personal relationships*, Schroeder, E., ed. Guilford, CT: McGraw-Hill/Dushkin, 2003.

Should same-sex couples be allowed to marry legally? In *Taking sides: Issues in family and personal relationships*, Schroeder, E., ed. Guilford, CT: McGraw-Hill/Dushkin, 2003.

Shrier, L. A., Emans, S. J., Woods, E. R., & DuRant, R. H. The association of sexual risk behaviors and problem drug behaviors in high school students, *Journal of Adolescent Health, 205, no. 5* (May 1997), 377–383.

Shrier, L. A., Pierce, J. D., Emans, S. J., & DuRant, F. H. Gender differences in risk behaviors associated with forced or pressured sex, *Archives of Pediatric and Adolescent Medicine, 152, no. 1* (1998), 57, 863.

SIECUS position statements on sexuality issues, 1995.

SIECUS. Policy update, November 12, 1998.

Siecus. Protecting against unwanted pregnancy: An overview of standard contraceptives, *SIECUS Report*, 31 (2003), 24–26.

SIECUS. SIECUS looks at states' sexuality laws and the sexual rights of their citizens, *SIECUS Reports, 26* (1998), 4–15.

Siegel, K. & Raveis, V. H. AIDS-related reasons for gay men's adoption of celibacy, *AIDS Education and Prevention, 5* (1993), 392–310.

Siegel, P. *Changes in you: An introduction to sexual education through an understanding of puberty.* Santa Barbara, CA: James Stanfield Company, 1991.

Sifferman, K. A. & Strohm, R. L., eds. *Adoption: A legal guide for birth and adoptive parents (layman's law guide).* Edgemont, PA: Chelsea House, 1997.

Signorielli, N., McLeod, D., & Healy, E. Gender stereotypes in MTV commercials: The beat goes on, *Journal of Broadcasting & Electronic Media, 38* (1994), 91–101.

Silberman, S. & Robinson-Kurpius, S. E. Love, marital satisfaction and duration of marriage, American Psychological Association, Washington, DC, 1998.

Silverman, J., Tores, A., & Forrest, D. Barrier to contraceptive services, *Family Planning Perspectives, 19, no. 3* (May/June 1987), 94–102.

Silverstein, J. L. Exhibitionism as countershame, *Sexual Addiction and Compulsivity, 31, no. 1* (1996), 33–42.

Singer, D. & Singer, J. Sex on TV: How to protect your child, *TV Guide, 30* (August 7, 1982), 33.

Singer, J. & Singer, I. Sex on TV: How to protect your child, *TV Guide*, 30 (1982), 33.

Singh, S. & Samara, R. Early marriage among women in developing countries, *International Family Planning Perspectives, 22* (1996), 148–157, 175.

Single parenting and today's family, American Psychological Association, 1998. http://helping.apa.org/family/single.html

Single-father homes on the rise, InteliHealth (May 29, 2001). Available: www.intelihealth.com.

Sipski, M. & Alexander, C. *Sexual functioning in people with disability and chronic disease.* Frederick, MD: Aspen Publishers, 1997.

Sivin, I., Lahteenmaki, P., Mishell, D. R., Alvarez, F., Diaz, S., Ranta, S., Grozinger, C., Lacarra, M., Brache, V., Pavez, M., Nash, H., & Stern, J. The performance of levonorgestrel rod and norplant contraceptive implants: Year randomized study, *Human Reproduction*, 13 (1998), 3371–3378.

The 65 years and over population: 2000, *Census 2000 brief*. U.S. Census Bureau, 2001.

Skene, A. Two important glands of the urethra, *American Journal of Obstetrics*, 265 (1980), 265–270.

Slade, M. Managing menopause, *American Health* (December 1994), 66–69.

Small operators can make a real killing on the web, *USA Today* (August 20, 1997), 1.

Smilgis, M. & Thigpen, E. Murder gets an R: Bad language gets NC–17, *Time, 68* (August 29, 1994).

Smith, G. L., Greenup, R., & Takafuji, E. T. Circumcision as a risk factor for urethritis in racial groups, *American Journal of Public Health*, 77 (1987), 452–454.

Smith, L., Schoonover, S., Lauver, D., & Allen, Jr., P. Sexually transmitted diseases, in *Sexual Health Promotion*, Fogel, C. I. & Lauver, D., eds. Philadelphia: Saunders, 1990.

Smith, M. & Barwin, B. Vaginal contraceptive devices, *Journal of the Canadian Medical Association, 129* (1983), 699–701.

Smith, M. D., & Morra, N. N. Obscene and threatening telephone calls to women: Data from a Canadian national survey, *Gender and Society, 8, no. 4* (1994), 584–596.

Smith, P. *National adolescent student health survey results.* Reston, VA: American School Health Association, 1988.

Snegroff, S. The stressors of non-marital sexual intercourse, *Health Education, 17* (1986), 21–23.

Snyder, M. & Ickes, W. Personality and social behavior, in *The handbook of social psychology,* Lindzey, G. & Aronsen, E., eds. New York: Random House, 1985, 883–937.

Solomon, M. *Consumer behavior,* 3rd ed. Englewood, NJ: Prentice Hall, 1996.

Sonfield, A. The states at mid-year: Major actions on reproductive health-related issues, *The Guttmacher Report on Public Policy* (August 2000), 8–9.

Sonnenstein, F., Pleck, J., & Lu, L. Levels of sexual activity among adolescent males in the United States, *Family Planning Perspectives, 23, 4* (1991), 162–167.

Sorenson, R. C. *Adolescent sexuality in contemporary America.* New York: World, 1973.

Sorenstein, F. L., Ku, L., Duberstein, L., Turner, C. F., & Pleck, J. H. Changes in sexual behavior and condom use among teenaged males: 1988 to 1995, *American Journal of Public Health, 88* (1998), 956–959.

South, S. J. & Felson, R. B. The racial patterning of rape, *Social Forces, 69* (1990), 71–93.

Spake, A. The truth about "The silent scream," *Ms.* (July 1985), 88, 91–92, 112–114.

Special report on contraception: Where will we be in the year 2010? *Sexuality Today, 9* (June 16, 1986), 1–2.

Spector, I. & Carey, M. Incidence and prevalence of sexual dysfunctions: A critical review of the empirical literature, *Archives of Sexual Behavior, 19* (1990), 389–408.

Speroff, L., et al. The comparative effect on bone density, endometrium, and lipids of continuous hormones as replacement therapy (CHART study), *Journal of the American Medical Association, 276* (1996), 1397–1403.

Spielvogel, J. J. *Western civilization,* 3rd ed. St. Paul, MN: West, 1997.

Spitz, I., et al. The safety and efficacy of early pregnancy termination with mifepristone and misoprostol: Results from the first multicenter U.S. trial, *The New England Journal of Medicine, 338* (1998), 1241–1247.

Sprecher, S. & Hatfield, E. Premarital sexual standards among U.S. college students: Comparison with Russian and Japanese students, *Archives of Sexual Behavior, 25, no. 3* (1996), 261–286.

Sprecher, S. & McKinney, K. *Sexuality.* Thousand Oaks, CA: Sage Publications, 1993.

Squires, S. Why do blacks have higher rates? *Washington Post Health* (November 21, 1995), 9, 12.

Srinivasan, K. Record low support for casual sex, *AOL/AP* (April 7, 1999).

Sroka, S. B. Common sense on custom education, *Education Week, 10* (1991).

St. Paul prostitution fight may hit Internet, TV, American Civil Liberties Union Freedom Network, 1997.

Staley, M., Hussey, W., Roe, K., Harcourt, J., & Roe, K. In the shadow of the rainbow: Identifying and addressing health disparities in the lesbian, gay, bisexual, and transgender population—A research and practice challenge, *Health Promotion Practice*, 2, no. 3 (July 2001) 207–211.

Stanton, A. Affairs part 2: Understanding what went wrong. Health and age. Novartis Foundation for Gerontology. Available: www.healthandage.com/Home/gid2=1258.

Stark, C. A. Is pornography an action? The causal vs. the conceptual view of pornography, *Social Theory and Practice, 23* (Summer 1997), 277–306.

Starr, B. & Weiner, M. *The Starr-Weiner Report on Sex and Sexuality in the Mature Years.* New York: Stein & Day, 1981.

Startling new study shows one in six women incestuously abused before age 18, *Sexuality Today, 9, nos. 37–38* (1986), 2.

Stebleton, M. J. & Rothenberger, J. H. Truth or consequence: Dishonesty in dating and HIV/AIDS-related issues in a college age population, *Journal of American College Health*, 42, no. 2 (September1993), 51.

The Status of Women in the States. Institute for Women's Policy Research. Available: www.iwpr.org

Steege, J. F. & Blumenthal, J. A. The effects of aerobic exercise on premenstrual syndrome in middle-aged women: A preliminary study, *Journal of Psychosomatic Research, 37* (1993), 127–133.

Steege, J. Female factors which contribute to premature ejaculation, *Medical Aspects of Human Sexuality, 15* (1981), 73–74.

Stein, A. P. The chlamydia epidemic: Teenagers at risk, *Medical Aspects of Human Sexuality, 25* (1991), 26–33.

Stein, J. Porn goes mainstream, *Time, 152, no. 10* (September 7, 1998), 51–52.

Stein, R. Caesarean births hit high mark, *Washington Post* (December 16, 2002), A1.

Steinberg, R. & Robinson, L. *Women's sexual health.* New York: Donald I. Fine, 1995.

Stephens, J. A. Sex offender hounded in jittery cities, *The Birmingham News* (January 17, 2003), A5.

Sternberg, R. *The triangle of love: Intimacy, passion, commitment*. New York: Basic Books, 1988.

Sternberg, R. A triangular theory of love, *Psychological Review, 93* (1986), 119–135.

Sternberg, S. U.S. AIDS threat rebounds, *USA Today* (August 14, 2001), 1A.

Stevens-Simon, C., Kelly, L., Singer, D., & Cox, A. Why pregnant adolescents say they did not use contraceptives prior to conception, *Journal of Adolescent Health, 19, no. 1* (July 1996), 48–53.

Stewart, S. D. Economic and personal factors affecting women's use of nurse-midwives in Michigan, *Family Planning Perspectives, 30* (1998), 231–235.

Stipp, D. Better prognosis: Research on impotence upsets idea that it is usually psychological, *Wall Street Journal* (April 14, 1987), 1, 25.

Stock, W. The effect of pornography on women, paper presented at a hearing of the Attorney General's Commission on Pornography. Houston, September 11–12, 1985.

Stodghill, R. Where'd you learn that? *Time, 151, no. 23* (June 15, 1998), 71–79.

Stone, A. Gay troops kept in uniform despite "Telling," report says, and report says harassment of military's gays doubles, *USA Today* (March 9, 2000): 4A–5A.

Storms, M. Theories of sexual orientation, *Journal of Personality and Social Psychology, 38* (1980), 783–792.

Strassberg, D. S., et al. Forces in women's sexual fantasies, *Archives of Sexual Behavior, 27* (1998), 403–414.

Studer, M. & Thornton, A. Adolescent religiosity and contraceptive usage, *Journal of Marriage and the Family, 49* (August 1987), 493–497.

Study eases breast cancer, estrogen fear. *USA Today,* 1998.

Substance use and risky sexual behavior: Attitudes and practices among adolescents and young adults, *American Journal of Health Education*, 33, no. 5 (September/October 2002), 278–281.

Sudden cardiac death gender gap closing in on women, *InteliHealth* (December 20, 2002). Available: www.intelihealth.com.

Sue, D. Erotic fantasies of college students during coitus, *Journal of Sex Research, 15* (1979), 299–305.

Suhr, J. Dow Corning accepts $3.2 billion settlement plan, Associated Press Press Release (July 8, 1998).

Sullivan, T. J. *Sociology,* 4th ed. Needham Heights, MA: Allyn & Bacon, 1998.

Summersgill, R. Status of state sodomy laws. http://members.aol.com/caglr/sodomlaw.htm

Survey USA public opinion poll (1998). Available: www.surveyusa.com.

Surveys show change in attitudes toward sex among high school and college students, higher incidences of "casual" and oral sex, Kaiser Daily Reproductive Health Report (January 21, 2003). Available: www.kaisernetwork.org.

Sussman, J. R. & Levitt, B. B. *Before you conceive: The complete prepregnancy guide.* New York: Bantam Books, 1989.

Swaab, D. F. & Hofman, M. A. An enlarged suprachiasmatic nucleus in homosexual men, *Brain Research, 537* (1990), 141.

Swartz, M. Buzz and Alan, *The New Yorker* (August 24 & 31, 1998), 66–78.

Swinker, M. L. Salpingitis and pelvic inflammatory disease, *American Family Physician, 31* (1985), 143–149.

Tan, C. L. Latest hot accessory for successful women: The lesser boyfriend, *The Birmingham News* (April 22, 2001), 1E, 5E.

Tanfer, K. Patterns of premarital cohabitation among never-married women in the United States, *Journal of Marriage and the Family, 49* (August 1987), 483–497.

Tanfer, K. & Horn, M. C. Contraceptive use, pregnancy, and fertility patterns among single women in their 20s, *Family Planning Perspectives, 17, no. 1* (January/February 1985), 10–19.

Tang, M-X. Effects of estrogen during menopause on risk and age at onset of Alzheimer's disease, *Lancet, 348* (1996), 429–432.

Tannen, D. *You just don't understand.* New York: Ballantine Books, 1991.

Tarnahill, R. *Sex in history.* New York: Stein & Day, 1980.

Tarvis, C. & Sadd, S. The *Redbook* report on female sexuality, *Redbook* (October 1975).

Task Force on Circumcision. Report of the task force, *Pediatrics, 84, no. 2* (August 1989) 388–391.

Tavris, C. Are girls really as mean as books say they are? *The Chronicle of Higher Education,* 48, no. 43 (July 5, 2002), B7–B9.

Teacher-student relationships not tolerated, *Academic Leader, 15, no. 1* (January 1999), 6.

Teens unsatisfied with sex ed classes, Kaiser Daily Reproductive Health Report (September 11, 2001). Available: www.kaisernetwork.org.

Telljohann, S. K., Price, J. H., Poureslami, M., & Easton, A. Teaching about sexual orientation by secondary health teachers, *Journal of School Health, 65, no. 1* (January 1995), 18–22.

Temple, M. A. Comprehensive or holistic dimensions of sexuality.

Tests confirm condoms block AIDS virus, *Medical World News, 27* (1986), 31–32.

Thabes, V. A survey analysis of women's long-term postdivorce adjustment, *Journal of Divorce and Remarriage, 27, no. 3–4* (1997), 163–175.

Thelen, M. H., Sherman, M. D., & Borst. T. S. Fear of intimacy and attachment among rape survivors, *Behavior Modification, 22, no. 1* (1998), 108–116.

Thomas, C. B. A new scarlet letter, *Time*, 157, no. 23 (June 11, 2001), 82.

Thomas, G. S. Census data show no shortage of six-figure earners, *Birmingham Business Journal*, 18, no. 33 (August 17, 2001), 10.

Thompson, B. W. A way outa no way, in *Through the prism of difference: Readings on sex and gender,* Zinn, M. B., Hondagneu-Sotelo, P., & Messner, M. A., eds. Boston: Allyn & Bacon, 1997.

Thompson, E. Reform rabbis get OK to preside at same-sex commitments. *The Birmingham News*

Thompson, S. Putting a big thing into a little hole: Teenage girls' accounts of sexual initiation, *The Journal of Sex Research, 27, 3* (1990), 341–361.

Thornton, A. Changing attitudes toward family issues in the United States, *Journal of Marriage and the Family, 51* (1989), 873.

Thought police recruited in new child porn law, 1998.

Tiefer, L. & Kring, B. Gender and the organization of sexual behavior, *The Psychiatric Clinics of North America, 18, no. 1* (March 1995), 25–36.

Tiefer, L. *Sex is not a natural act.* Boulder, CO: Westview Press, 1995.

Tiefer, L. Three crises facing sexology, *Archives of Sexual Behavior, 23, no. 4* (1994), 361–373.

Toner, J. P. & Flood, J. T. Fertility after the age of 40, *Obstetrics and Gynecology Clinics of North America, 20* (1993), 261–272.

Torgovnick, M. *Primitive passions: Men, women, and the quest for ecstasy.* New York: Random House, 1996.

The top ten health frauds, *Consumers' Research Magazine, 73* (February 1990), 34–36.

Toubia, N. Female circumcision as a public health issue, *The New England Journal of Medicine, 331* (1994), 712–716.

Toussie-Weingarten, C. & Jacobwitz, J. T. Alternatives in childbearing: Choices and challenges, in *Psychosocial Dimensions of the Pregnant Family,* Nehls Serwen, L., ed. New York: Springer, 1987, 193–218.

Tower Urology Group. *The new miracle in male genital health,* 1998.

Transvestism, University of Iowa Health Care (2001). Available: www.uihealthcare.com/topics/mentalemotionalhealth/ment3174.html.

Trends in sexual risk behaviors Among high school students—United States, 1991–2001, *Morbidity and Mortality Weekly Report*, 51, no. 38 (September 27, 2002), 856–859.

Trethowan, W. H. & Conlon, M. F. The couvade syndrome, *British Journal of Psychology, 3* (1965), 57–60.

Tripp, C. A. *The homosexual matrix.* New York: New American Library, 1976.

Trudel, G. & Proulx, S. Treatment of premature ejaculation by bibliotherapy: An experimental study, *Sexual and Marital Therapy, 2* (1987), 163–167.

Tullman, G., Gilner, F., Kolodny, R., Dornbush, R., & Tullman, G. The pre- and post-therapy measurement of communication skills of couples undergoing sex therapy at the Masters and Johnson Institute, *Archives of Sexual Behavior, 10* (1981), 95–99.

Turkey says only virgins can be nurses, *The Birmingham News* (July 20, 2001), 8A.

Twenge, J. Changes in masculine and feminine traits over time: A meta-analysis, *Sex Roles, 36, nos. 5 & 6* (1997), 305–325.

Uhlman, M. Many children trade sex to survive, study says, *The Birmingham News* (September 11, 2001), 1A.

Ullman, S. E. Do social reactions to sexual assault victims vary by support provider? *Violence and Victims, 11, no. 2* (1996), 143–157.

Uniform crime reports for the United States. Washington, DC: Federal Bureau of Investigation, U.S. Government Printing Office, 1996.

United States Code Annotated Title 47. U.S. Department of Justice (March 3, 2003). Available: www.usdoj.gov/criminal/cybercrime/47usc223NEW.htm.

University of Toronto Sexual Education and Peer Counseling Center. Premature ejaculation, 1998.

Upchurch, D. M., Levy-Storms, L., Sucoff, C. A., & Aneshensel, C. S. Gender and ethnic differences in the timing of first sexual intercourse, *Family Planning Perspectives, 30, no. 3* (May/June 1998), 121–127.

Urquiza, A. J., & Goodlin-Jones, B. L. Child sexual abuse and adult revictimization with women of color, *Violence and Victims, 9, no. 3* (1994), 223–232.

U.S. abortion rate declines overall but increases among low-income women, report says, The Henry J. Kaiser Family Foundation (October 9, 2002). Available: www.kaisernetwork.org/daily_reports.

U.S. birth rates for teens, 15–19, http://www.teenpregnancy.org.

U.S. boys may be hitting puberty sooner, *Reuters Health Service Press Release*, September 13, 2001.

U.S. Bureau of the Census. *Statistical abstract of the United States 1998.* Table 62. Washington, DC: U.S. Government Printing Office.

U.S. Bureau of the Census. Family composition begins to stabilize in the 1990s, 1998a.

U.S. Bureau of the Census. Marital status and living arrangements of adults 18 years old and over, 1998c.

U.S. Bureau of the Census. Marriage, 1998b.

U.S. Centers for Disease Control. *National Survey of Family Growth,* 1998.

U.S. Department of Health and Human Services. *Healthy People 2010: Understanding and Improving Health*. 2nd ed. Washington, DC: U.S. Government Printing Office, November 2000.

U.S. Department of Health and Human Services. Premarital sexual experience among adolescent women—United States, 1970–1988, *Morbidity and Mortality Weekly Report, 39, nos. 51 & 52* (January 4, 1991), 929–932.

U.S. Department of Health and Human Services. Teen sex down, new study shows, 1998a.

U.S. Department of Health and Human Services. Trends in adolescent pregnancy and childbearing, Office of Population Affairs (1998b).

U.S. Department of Justice, Federal Bureau of Investigation, Uniform Crime Reports, 2001. On-line. Available: http://www.fbi.gov/pressrel/pressrel00/ucrcit2000.htmU.S.

U.S. Department of Labor. *Focus on women workers.* Washington, DC: U.S. Department of Labor, 1990.

Use of AZT expanded, *FDA Consumer, 24* (1990), 17.

Utiger, R. D. A pill for impotence, *The New England Journal of Medicine, 338* (1998), 1458.

U-Va. dorm machines to sell condoms, not cigarettes, *Washington Post* (August 21, 1988), A4.

Varelas, N. & Foley, L. A. Blacks' and whites' perceptions of interracial and intraracial date rape, *Journal of Social Psychology, 138, no. 3* (1998), 392–400.

Ventura, S. J., Mathews, T. J., & Curtin, S. C. Teenage births in the United States: State trends, 1991–96, an update, *Monthly Vital Statistics Reports, 46* (1998), 1.

Vermund, S. H. History of sexual abuse in incarcerated adolescents with gonorrhea and syphilis, *Journal of Adolescent Health Care, 11* (1990), 449.

Viadero, D. Condom programs don't spur sex, study says, *Education Week, 16* (October 8, 1997), 3.

Vicary, J. R., Klingaman, L R., & Harkness, W. L. The factors associated with date rape and sexual assault of adolescent girls, *Journal of Adolescence, 18* (1995), 289–306.

Vo, K. Universities reach out to gay, lesbian students. *San Jose Mercury News* (May 25, 2003), A7.

Vobejda, B. Web site to list foster children for adoption, *Washington Post* (November 25, 1998), A5.

Volkwein, K. A. E., Schnell, F. I., & Sherwood, D. Sexual harassment in sport: Perceptions and experiences of American female student-athletes, *International Review for the Sociology of Sport, 32, no. 3* (1997), 283–295.

Voracek, M. & Fisher, M. L. Shapely centrefolds? Temporal changes in body measures: Trend analysis, *British Medical Journal*, 325 (December 21, 2002), 1447–1448.

Wagner, D. M. Divorce reform: New directions, *Current* (February 1998), 7–11.

Waldo, C. R. & Kemp, J. L. Should I come out to my students? *Journal of Homosexuality, 14, no. 2* (1997), 79–94.

Wallace, A. M. & Engstrom, J. L. The effects of aerobic exercise on the pregnant woman, fetus, and pregnancy outcome: A review, *Journal of Nurse-Midwifery, 32* (1987), 277–288.

Wallerstein, E. *Circumcision*. New York: Springer, 1980.

Wallerstein, J. S. Nine "psychological tasks" needed for a good marriage, *American Psychological Association*, 1996.

Wallick, M. M. Homophobia and heterosexism: Out of the medical school closet, *North Carolina Medical Journal, 58, no. 2* (March-April 1997), 123–125.

Walsh, A. *The science of love: Understanding love and its effects on mind and body.* Buffalo, NY: Prometheus, 1991.

Walsh, M. Riley restates rules against harassment, *Education Week, 17, no. 4* (July 8, 1998), 1, 30.

Walters, A. S. & Hayes, D. M. Homophobia within schools: Challenging the culturally sanctioned dismissal of gay students and colleagues, *Journal of Homosexuality, 35, no. 2* (1998), 1–23.

Ward, S. K., Cohn, K., White, S., & Williams, K. Acquaintance rape and the college social scene, *Family Relations, 40* (1991), 71.

Wardlow, G. *Contemporary nutrition issues and insights.* Madison, WI: Brown and Benchmark, 1997.

Wasow, M. & Loeb, M. Sexuality in nursing homes, *Journal of the American Geriatrics Society, 27* (1979), 73–79.

Waterman, C. K. & Foss-Goodman, D. Child molesting: Variables relating to attribution of fault to victims, offenders, and nonparticipating parents, *The Journal of Sex Research, 20, no. 4* (1984), 329–349.

Waters, R. Estrogen to prevent Alzheimer's, *Health, 11* (1997), 40–42.

We want to live as humans, *Human Rights Watch*, 14, no 11 (December 2002), 1–52.

Weinberg, M. S., Williams, C. J., & Moser, C. The social constituents of sadomasochism, *Social Problems, 31, no. 4* (1984), 379–389.

Weisberg, D. K. *Children of the night: A study of adolescent prostitution.* Lexington, MA: D. C. Heath, 1985.

Weisman, C. S., Nathanson, C. A., Teitelbaum, M. A., Chase, G. A., & King, T. M. Abortion attitudes and performance among male and female obstetrician-gynecologists, *Family Planning Perspectives, 18, no. 2* (March/April 1986), 67–73.

Wellington, S. Cracking the ceiling, *Time, 152, no. 23* (December 7, 1998), 187.

Werler, M., Pober, B., & Holmes, L. Smoking and Pregnancy. In Sever, John L. and Robert L. Brent. *Teratogen Update: Environmentally Induced Birth Defect Risks*. New York: Alan R. Liss, 1986, 131–139.

Wespes, E. & Schulman, C. Venous leakage: Surgical treatment of a curable cause of impotence, *Journal of Urology, 133* (1985), 796–798.

Westheimer, R. *Sex for dummies.* Indianapolis: IDG Books Worldwide, 1995.

What families won't tell, *UAB Medical Center Magazine, 2* (Fall 1986), 19–21.

What gender gap? *Kiplinger's*, 55, no. 2 (February 2001), 22, 24.

What is sexual addiction? Sex Addicts Anonymous (2003). Available: www.sexaa.org/addict.htm.

Where do babies come from? *Family Life Educator* (Winter 1987), 5–7.

Whitehurst, R. N. There are a number of equally valid forms of marriage, such as multiple marriage, swinging, adultery, and open marriage. In *Current Controversies in Marriage and the Family*, edited by H. Feldman and M. Feldman. Beverly Hills, CA, 1985.

Whitman, F. & Diamond, M. A preliminary report on the sexual orientation of homosexual twins. Paper presented at the Western Region Annual Conference of the Society for the Scientific Study of Sex, Scottsdale, AZ, January, 1986.

Why don't we hear others? *Communication Briefings, 15, no. 4* (February 1996), 1.

Why men die younger than women, *Consumer Reports on Health*, 14, no. 12 (December 2002), 1,3–4.

Wickelgren, I. Estrogen: A new weapon against Alzheimer's, *Science, 276* (1997), 676–677.

Wiest, W. Semantic differential profiles of orgasm and other experiences among men and women, *Sex roles*, 3 (1977), 399–403.

Wight, S. E. Exercise during pregnancy: Yes or no? *The Female Patient, 11* (1986), 73–84.

Wiley, D. C. Assessing the health behaviors of Texas college students, *Journal of American College Health*, 44, no. 4 (1996), 167–172.

Williams, L. S. The classic rape: When do victims report? *Social Problems, 31, no. 4* (1984), 459–467.

Williams, M. H. *Lifetime fitness and wellness.* Madison, WI: Brown and Benchmark, 1996.

Williams, M. Study: Patch could restore sex drive, *AP/AOL* (June 17, 1999).

Willis, J. Demystifying menopause, *FDA Consumer*, 22 (1988), 24–27.

Wilson, G. T., Nathan, P. E., O'Leary, K. D., & Clark, L. A. *Abnormal psychology: Integrating perspectives.* Needham, MA: Allyn & Bacon, 1996.

Wilson, M. R. & Filsinger, E. E. Religiosity and marital adjustment: Multidimensional interrelationships, *Journal of Marriage and the Family, 48* (1986), 147–151.

Wilson, R. An ill-fated sex survey, *The Chronicle of Higher Education*, 48, no. 4 (August 2, 2002), A10–A12.

Winikoff, B., et al. Acceptability and feasibility of early pregnancy termination by mifepristone-misoprostol, *Archives of Family Medicine, 7* (1998), 360–366.

Winkelstein, W. Jr., Michael, S., Padian, N. S., Wiley, J. A., Lang, W., Anderson, R. E., & Levy, J. A. The San Francisco men's health study. III. Reduction in human immunodeficiency virus transmission among homosexual/bisexual men, 1982–1986, *American Journal of Public Health, 76* (1987), 685–689.

Winn, R L. & Newton, N. Sexuality in aging: a study of 106 cultures. *Archives of Sexual Behavior* 11 (1980): 293–98.

Winship, E. *Reaching your teenager.* New York: Houghton Press, 1983.

Winters, R. A food of one's own, *Time*, 57, no. 25 (June 25, 2001), 47.

Wiswell, T. E., Smith, F. R., & Bass, J. W. Decreased incidence of urinary tract infections in circumcised male infants, *Pediatrics*, 75 (1985), 901–903.

Wolfe, S. M. & Jones, R. D. *Women's Health Alert*. Reading, MA: Addison-Wesley, 1991.

Wolpe, J. *Psychotherapy by reciprocal inhibition.* Stanford: Stanford University Press, 1958.

Women up to 10 times more likely to have poor body image than men, InteliHealth: Women's Health (May 14, 2001). Available: www.intelihealth.com.

Women usually victimized by offenders they know. U.S. Department of Justice Bureau of Justice Statistics, 1998.

Wong, N. C. Study: 1 in 5 kids pressed for sex online, *The Birmingham News* (June 21, 2001), 7A.

Woods, N. F. *Human sexuality in health and illness.* St. Louis: Mosby, 1979.

Worden, M. & Worden, B. D. *The gender dance in couples therapy.* Pacific Grove, CA: Brooks/Cole, 1998.

Working moms turn traditional when they're home. American Psychological Association, 1998.

World Health Organization. *Report on the global HIV/AIDS epidemic.* Geneva, Switzerland: World Health Organization, 1998.

World Health Organization Task Force on post-ovulatory methods of fertility regulation. Comparison of two doses of mifepristone in combination with misoprostol for early medical abortion: A randomized trial, *British Journal of Obstetrics and Gynecology*, 107, no. 4 (2000), 524–530.

The Writing Group for the PEPI Trial. Effects of hormone therapy on bone mineral density: Results from the postmenopausal estrogen/progestin interventions (PEPI) trial, *Journal of the American Medical Association, 276* (1996), 1389–1396.

Writing Group for the Women's Health Initiative randomized controlled trial. Risks and benefits of estrogen plus progestin in healthy postmenopausal women, *Journal of the American Medical Association*, 288 (2002), 321–333.

Wyatt, G. E. & Newcomb, M. Internal and external mediators of women's rape experiences, *Psychology of Women Quarterly, 14* (1990), 153–176.

Wyatt, G. E., Peters, S. D., & Guthrie, D. Kinsey revisited. Part I. Comparisons of the sexual socialization and sexual behavior of white women over 33 years, *Archives of Sexual Behavior, 71* (1988a), 210–239.

Wyatt, G. E., Peters, S. D., & Guthrie, D. Kinsey revisited. Part II. Comparisons of the sexual socialization and sexual behavior of black women over 33 years, *Archives of Sexual Behavior, 17* (1988b), 389–332.

Wyeth. Back-up contraception no longer required for women using Norplant system, news release. (July 26, 2002). Madison, WI.

Xu, F., et al. Repeat chlamydia trachomatis infection in women: Analysis through a surveillance case registry in Washington State, 1993–1998, *American Journal of Epidemiology*, 152, no. 12 (2000), 1164–1170.

Yarber, W. L. Delay in seeking prescription contraception and the health lifestyle and health locus of control of young women, *Journal of Sex Education and Therapy, 12, no. 2* (fall/winter 1986), 37–42.

Young Americans more likely than their parents' generation to oppose abortion, surveys, Kaiser Daily Reproductive Health Report (September 26, 2002). Available: www.kaisernetwork.org/daily_reports.

Young, J. R. Gay student is forced out of a campus leadership post at an Iowa college, *The Chronicle of Higher Education*, 49, no. 13 (November 22, 2002), A58.

Zaslow, J. Premarital survey may help couples choose a right mate, *The Birmingham News* (February 2, 2003), D1, D3.

Zaviacic, M., Zaviacicova, A., Holoman, I. K., & Molcan, J. Female urethral expulsions evoked by local digital stimulation of the G-spot: Differences in the response patterns, *Journal of Sex Research*, 24 (1988), 311.

Zelnik, M. & Kantener, J. F. First pregnancies to women aged 15–19: 1976 and 1971, *Family Planning Perspectives, 10* (1978), 11–20.

Zelnik, M. & Kantener, J. F. Sexual activity, contraceptive use and pregnancy among metropolitan-area teenagers: 1971–1979, *Family Planning Perspectives, 12* (1980), 230–308.

Zelnik, M. & Kantener, J. F. Sexual and contraceptive experience of young unmarried women in the U.S., 1976 and 1971, *Family Planning Perspectives, 9* (1977), 55–71.

Zidovudine for children, *FDA Consumer, 24* (1990), 5.

Zilbergard, B. *Male sexuality: A guide to sexual fulfilment.* Boston: Little, Brown, 1978.

Zilbergard, B. & Ellison, C. R. Desire discrepancies and arousal problems in sex therapy, in *Principles and practices of sex therapy*, Lieblum, S. R. & Pervin, L. A., eds. New York: Guilford, 1980.

Zilbergeld, B. *The new male sexuality: A guide to sexual fulfillment.* New York: Bantam Books, 1992.

Zilbergeld, B. & Kilmann, P. The scope and effectiveness of sex therapy, *Psychotherapy, 21* (1984), 319–326.

Zimmer, J. Body work, *Essence, 29, no. 4* (August 1998), 17–22.

Ziporyn T. LHRH: Clinical applications growing, *Journal of the American Medical Association, 253* (1985), 469–476.

Zorpette, G. You see brawny; I see scrawny, *Scientific American, 278* (March 1998), 24–25.

Zuger, B. Monozygotic twins discordant for homosexuality: Report of a pair and significance of the phenomenon, *Comprehensive Psychiatry, 17* (1976), 661–669.

Credits

Photo Credits

p. 7, © Robert Mora/Getty Images; p. 8, © The Kobal Collection; p. 9, © D. Stevens/The Kobal Collection; p. 12, © Sara Jaye/Getty Images; p. 17, © Cappella Sistina Vaticano/Art Resource; p. 19, © The Kobal Collection; p. 25, © Corbis/S.I.N.; p. 39, © CORBIS/Wolfgang Kaehler; p. 44, © (T, B) Courtesy of Behavioral Technology; p. 47, © Topham/The Image Works; p. 51, © Pat Watson/The Image Works; p. 82, © The Kobal Collection; p. 84, © (T) © IT Stock International/Index Stock Imagery, (B) © Michelle D. Bridwell/PhotoEdit; p. 95, © Bill Lai/The Image Works; p. 112, © (L, M, R) Susan Lerner/Joel Gordon Photography; p. 120, © (L) Susan Lerner/Joel Gordon Photography, (M) © Joel Gordon, (R) © Susan Lerner/Joel Gordon Photography; p. 132, © Myrleen Ferguson Cate/Photo Network/PictureQuest; p. 138, © (T, M, B) Joel Gordon; p. 142 (L), © Biophoto Associates, Science Source/Photo Researchers, (R) © Biophoto Associates, Science Source/Photo Researchers; p. 145, © Susan Lerner/Joel Gordon Photography; p. 146, © Courtesy of The Museum of Fine Arts; p. 156, © (L, M) Joel Gordon, (R) © Susan Lerner/Joel Gordon Photography; p. 167, © Joel Gordon; p. 174, © Marc Grabowski; p. 176, © The Kobal Collection; p. 179, © AP Photo/Eric Draper; p. 179 (T), © AP/Laura Rauch; p. 184 (T), © AP Photo/AP World Wide World, (B) © AP Photo/The Kansas City Star, Kelley Chin; p. 188, © Courtesy Terri DeAngelis; p. 189, © AP LaserPhoto/Ira Mark Gostin; p. 190, © Frederick M. Brown/Getty Images; p. 191, © Ben-Ari Finegold/Getty Images; p. 200, © Crandall/The Image Works; p. 210, © Kobal Collection/Tiger Aspect Pics; p. 212, © Corbis; p. 215, © The Cartoon Network/Getty Images; p. 217, © Loren Cameron/Cleis Press; p. 219, © Forty Acres and a Mule Filmworks/The Kobal Collection; p. 224, © AP Photo/Michael Caulfield; p. 236, © Wildlife Conservation Society; p. 262, © Joel Gordon; p. 265, © Reprinted with permission from Public Health - Seattle & King County.; p. 268, © C. Swartzell/Visuals Unlimited; p. 271, © Joel Gordon; p. 273, © Joel Gordon; p. 274, © Joel Gordon; p. 275, © Joel Gordon; p. 277, © Joel Gordon; p. 279, © Joel Gordon; p. 280, © Joel Gordon; p. 281, © Joel Gordon; p. 287, © Joel Gordon; p. 294, © David M. Phillips, Science Source/Photo Researchers; p. 299, © Petit Format/Nestle, Science Source/Photo Researchers; p. 306, © Larry Mulvehill, Science Source/Photo Researchers; p. 306, © B. Seitz, Science Source/Photo Researchers; p. 307, © Charles Gupton/Stock Boston; p. 322 (T), © Bob Daemmrich/Stock Boston; p. 322 (B), © Bob Daemmrich/Stock Boston; p. 323 (L), © Keith/Custom Medical Stock; p. 323 (R), © Bob Daemmrich/Stock Boston; p. 347 (T), © Joel Gordon; p. 347 (B), © Joel Gordon; p. 356, © CORBIS/Laura Dwight; p. 367, © Courtesy of AIDS Action Committee; p. 374, © Pam Ostrow/Index Stock Imagery; p. 394, © CORBIS/Bettmann; p. 403, © AP Photo/Khue Bui; p. 409, © Ralph Wilson/AP Wide World; p. 410, © AP Photo; p. 412 (T) © Paramount/Miramax/The Kobal Collection, (B) © Newsmakers/Getty Images; p. 413, © Bruce Glikas/Getty Images; p. 415, © AP Photo/Victor R. Caivano; p. 424, © AP Photo/Mike Wintroath; p. 427, © SW Production/Index Stock Imagery; p. 431, © Frank Siteman/Stock Boston; p. 433, © Family Communications; p. 438, © Barbara Haynor/Index Stock Imagery; p. 445, © Bill Aron/PhotoEdit; p. 451, © Richard Hutchings, Photo Researchers; p. 467, © Jed Share/Tony Stone Images; p. 468, © CORBIS/Courtesy of Glyndebourne Festival of Opera; Ira Nowinski; p. 488, © Steven Weinberg/Tony Stone Images; p. 489, © Kevin Winter/Getty Images; p. 494, © David Richardson/Index Stock Imagery; p. 497, © Mark Richards/PhotoEdit; p. 512 (T), © Science VU/Visuals Unlimited, (M) © Mediscan/Visuals Unlimited, (B) © Carolina Biological/Visuals Unlimited; p. 516 (T), © Science VU/Visuals Unlimited, (B) © Ken Greer/Visuals Unlimited; p. 518 (M), © Science VU/CDC/Visuals Unlimited, (B) © Ken Greer/Visuals Unlimited; p. 520, © Ken Greer/Visuals Unlimited; p. 522, © Ken Greer/Visuals Unlimited; p. 523, © Ken Greer/Visuals Unlimited; p. 524, © Carolina Biological/Visuals Unlimited; p. 526 (T), © Ken Greer/Visuals Unlimited, (B) © Ken Greer/Visuals Unlimited; p. 527, © Oliver Meckes, Science Source/Photo Researchers; p. 528, © Ken Greer/Visuals Unlimited; p. 529, © Oliver Meckes, Science Source/Photo Researchers; p. 546, © Mark Boulton, Science Source/Photo Researchers; p. 548, © Joel Gordon; p. 553, © Rob Nelson/Black Star/PNI; p. 554, © CORBIS/Neal Preston; p. 556, © Joel Gordon; p. 570, © CORBIS/Bettman; p. 587, © AP Photo/Ruth Fremson; p. 600, © AP Photo/Doug Mills; p. 601 (T), © Errol Graphics; p. 601 (B), © Fox Family Channel/The Kobal Collection; p. 605, © World of Wonder; p. 607, © Figaro Magahn, Photo Researchers; p. 619, © Courtesy of The Violence Against Women Coalition/Junior League Minneapolis; p. 620,

© The Kobal Collection; p. 631, © Tim Boyle/Getty Images; p. 643, © The Kobal Collection; p. 645, © The Kobal Collection; p. 647, © Courtesy The National Coalition against Domestic Violence; p. 651, © AP Photo/Craig Fujii; p. 667, © CORBIS/Mitchell Gerber; p. 672, © CORBIS/Bettmann; p. 674, © Gunther/MPTV; p. 677, © Courtesy of Persian Kitty; p. 678, © Joel Gordon; p. 687, © AP Photo/Chris Martinez; p. 694, © T. Ross/The Image Works; p. 702, © AP Photo/Desert News, Stuart Johnson; p. 712, © AP Photo/Julie Markes; p. 718, © David Leaming; p. 719, © Berta A. Daniels; p. 720, © Associated Press, Tom Green Defense Team/AP Wide World; p. 729, © Andrew Cooper/The Kobal Collection; p. 730, © Columbia/TriStar Motion Picture Companies/The Kobal Collection; p. 738, © Tony Freeman/PhotoEdit; p. 739, © PhotoDisc

Index

A

D

E

F

G

H

I

J

T

U

V